Mixed Models

Mixed Models

Theory and Applications with R

Second Edition

EUGENE DEMIDENKO

Dartmouth College

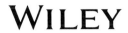

Published by John Wiley & Sons, Inc., Hoboken, New Jersey.
Published simultaneously in Canada.

For general information on our other products and services or for technical support, please contact our Customer Care Department within the United States at (800) 762-2974, outside the United States at (317) 572-3993 or fax (317) 572-4002.

Wiley also publishes its books in a variety of electronic formats. Some content that appears in print may not be available in electronic formats. For more information about Wiley products, visit our web site at www.wiley.com.

Library of Congress Cataloging-in-Publication Data:

Demidenko, Eugene, 1948–
  Mixed models : theory and applications with R / Eugene Demidenko. — Second [edition].
     p. cm. — (Wiley series in probability and statistics ; 893)
  Includes bibliographical references and index.
  ISBN 978-1-118-09157-9 (hardback)
  1. Analysis of variance. I. Title.
  QA279.D457 2013
  519.5'38—dc23   2013001306

Printed in the United States of America.

10 9 8 7 6 5 4 3 2 1

To my family

Contents

Preface

Technological advances change the world, and statistics is no exception. The cornerstone of classical statistics is the notion of *sample*. Today, data are richer: We may have repeated measurements with thousands of clusters; data may come in the form of shapes or images. This book is about statistical analysis of data that constitute a *sample of samples*. In the first ten chapters we discuss statistical models when data come in traditional form as a sequence of numbers. Chapter 11 deals with a sample (ensemble) of shapes, and in Chapter 12 we discuss how to analyze an ensemble of images.

We take the statistical model based approach to analyzing data. Then the method of analysis is a derivative. Although the method sometimes comes first, the model-based approach has obvious advantages: Assumptions are clearly formulated, and properties of several methods can be studied and compared. For example, least squares is a method of fitting, but its pros and cons can be fully understood only when a statistical model is put forward to describe how observations are obtained. Then least squares is deduced, for example, from maximum likelihood.

Statistical treatment is carried out under a unifying mixed effects approach. This approach becomes fruitful not only to analyze complex clustered data (a sample of samples) but also as a statistical model for penalization and a common ground for the Bayesian and frequentist camps.

Use of the mixed modeling technique in shape and image analysis is exciting and promising. Much work remains to reveal the full power of this statistical approach to these nontraditional statistical data.

The book is divided into three parts. The first eight chapters cover the theory of mixed models: the linear mixed effects (LME) model, the generalized linear mixed model (GLMM), and the nonlinear mixed effects (NLME) model. In Chapter 9 we discuss methods of model diagnostics and influential analysis. The final three chapters are devoted to applications: tumor regrowth, shape, and image. Major results and points of discussion in each chapter are written in lay language and are collected in *Summary Points* sections so that the reader can get a quick chapter overview.

I look forward to hearing from readers and invite them to visit the book web site at

http://www.dartmouth.edu/~eugened

where some additional information with data and images is presented.

I would like to thank the many people I worked with on various projects that have led up to this book. First, I would like to mention my long-term collaboration with Therese Stukel and Tor Tosteson and thank them for their support. I am grateful to Harold Swartz and Jack Hoopes for the exposure to biological problems, and to the team led by Keith Paulsen, including Alex Hartov, Paul Meaney, and Brian Pogue, all from Dartmouth, who introduced me to the world of image reconstruction. Many thanks to John Baron, Margaret Karagas, and Mark Israel for creating a friendly scientific atmosphere. I am grateful to Ed Vonesh for discussion and his helpful comments.

Finally, thanks to the *Scientific Workplace,* a WYSIWYG version of the LaTeX typesetting system (http://www.mackichan.com)—it is hard to imagine writing this book without this software.

Eugene Demidenko

Hanover, New Hampshire
Dartmouth College
January 2004

Preface to the Second Edition

Time proved that mixed model is an indispensable tool in studying multilevel and clustered data. Mixed model became one of the mainstreams of moderns statistics, on both the theoretical and practical fronts. Several books on the topic have been published since the first edition; see Section 1.16 for a comprehensive list. Most of these books target applications of mixed models and illustrate the examples with popular statistical software packages, such as SAS and R. This book has a distinct theoretical and research flavor. It is intended to explain what is "under the hood" of the mixed model methodology. In particular, it may be used for educational purposes by graduate and Ph.D. students in statistics.

Two major additions have been made in the second edition:

- Each section ends with a set of problems that should be important for an active understanding of the material. There are two type of problems: unmarked problems are regular problems, and problems marked with an asterisk are more difficult and are broader in scope. Usually, they involve an analytical derivation with further empirical confirmation through simulations. In many cases, I deliberately left the solution plan open so that students, together with their instructors, could use their own interpretation, and address questions to different depths. Some problems could be used for graduate or even Ph.D. research.

- Most parts of the theoretical material and methods of estimation are accompanied by respective R codes. While the first edition used S-Plus/S+, the second edition switches to the R language. The data sets and R codes can be downloaded at the author's web site,

www.dartmouth.edu/~eugened

It is suggested that they be saved on the hard drive in the directory

C:\MixedModels\

with a subdirectory that corresponds to the chapter in the book. All the codes can be distributed and modified freely.

The theory of mixed models has several important unsolved problems. I hope that the list that follows will stimulate research in this direction.

I would like to hear comments and suggestions from readers, including interesting solutions to the problems, and of course typos, which can be e-mailed to me at eugened@dartmouth.edu.

Eugene Demidenko

Hanover, New Hampshire
January 2013

R Software and Functions

R function	Description	Ch.	P.
lme	ML estimation of linear mixed model	02	44
ginverse.sym	Generalized inverse of symmetric matrix	02	51
GLSest	GLS beta-estimate for LME	02	55
lmeFS	FS ML estimation of linear mixed model	02	107
dupp	Duplication matrix $\mathcal{D}_n$	03	123
familyI	Family-specific weight-height relationship	03	149
lmeD	Simulations with lme	03	149
lmevarMINQUE	MINQUE for matrix $\mathbf{D}$	03	166
lmevarMM	Method of Moments (MM) for matrix $\mathbf{D}$	03	171
lmevarUVLS	Unbiased VLS for matrix $\mathbf{D}$	03	175
lmesim	Simulations with ML, MINQUE, MM, UVLS	03	179
calcium	Bone density in girls and boys	04	202
PRdistance	Analysis of dental growth for girls and boys	04	227
metaMLFS	MLE for meta-analysis model	05	252
ups2	Upper confidence limit for σ^2	05	262
RobustMedianML	Robust estimation of meta-analysis model	05	269
nlsMM	Simulations with Michaelis-Menten model	06	295
logG	Log-Gompertz curve with nlme and xyplot	06	301
ortree	Trunk circumference of trees fitting with nlme	06	312
phototum	Photodynamic tumor growth fitted with nlme	06	326
SSlogprob	Logistic-normal integral with integrate	07	338
gauher	Nodes and weights in GH quadrature	07	347
LNGHint	Comparison of GH with integrate	07	347
twoint	Example of double integration with gauher	07	350
threeint	Example of 3D integration with gauher	07	351
logric	Conditional logistic regression	07	361
logMLE1	ML for logistic regression using integrate	07	368
logMLEgh	ML for logistic regression using gauher	07	368
logFS	Fixed sample likelihood for logistic regression	07	370
logFSL	ML gauher fixed sample likelihood	07	370
glmmPQL	PQL for GLMM from library MASS	07	374
logVARLINK1	VARLINK for logistic regression	07	376
logsim	Simulations with logistic regression	07	374
poissfix	Poisson regression with fixed intercepts	07	400
poissGEE1	GEE Poisson regression with VLS	07	400
poissGEE	GEE Poisson regression with Newton iteration	07	400
poissHeck	Heckman method for Poisson regression	07	400
poissMLE	ML for Poisson regression using integrate	07	400
gee	GEE for GLMM using gee package	07	423

Continued

R function	Description	Ch.	P.
heightlog	nls for height of girls and boys using QLogist	08	438
heightlog2S	Two-stage method with QLogist	08	443
nlme	Example of nlme from package nlme	08	455
INT.ch08	Relative asymptotic bias using gauher	08	465
onexpML	MLE of one-parameter exponential model	08	465
onexpSIM	Simulations with one-parameter exp. model	08	476
onexpFSL	FSL method for one-parameter exp. model	08	476
nlmeFSL	FSL method for a general NLME model	08	475
callnlmeFSL	Call to nlmeFSL	08	465
heightlog.nlme	QLogist with different random effects models	08	455
wbf	*I*-influence for women's body fat	09	501
nlsnif	NLS influence for radioactive data	09	512
finney	*I*-influence for logistic regression	09	522
alckid	glm for alckid.dat	09	528
coloncancer	lme for coloncancer.dat	09	533
decE	Doubling time and SE for tumor growth	10	548
untrlme	lme for untreated tumor growth	10	553
trnlme	nlme for treated tumor regrowth	10	555
R.growth	Four groups of treated mice	10	563
rstGT	Gompertz curve with Gompertz.dat data	10	573
randtr	Plots random triangles	11	581
shapeh	Plots random polygons	11	591
maple	Opens and plots maple (x, y) shape files	11	594
potato	Opens and plots six potato images	11	604
carpet	Analyzes carpet image data	12	612
KSimage	Kolmogorov-Smirnov image comparison	12	616
lena	Plots Lena canon image	12	623
histgr	Histogram equalization	12	625
hypoxiaRAT	Hypoxia BOLD MRI rat brain	12	629
schiz	Normal and schizophrenia patients MRI	12	636
bioimage	Plots 28 cancer cell histology images	12	638
clockFIG	Clock images alignment	12	648
clockROT	Clock image rotation	12	650

Data Sets

Name	Description	Ch.	Page
Family.txt	Family height and weight data	02	44
Calcium.txt	Bone density in girls and boys	04	202
PRdistance.txt	Dental growth data for girls and boys	04	227
BerkeyMeta.txt	Efficacy of tuberculosis vaccine	05	269
TUMspher.txt	Tumor volume of spheroids	06	301
trunktree.txt	Trunk circumference of orange trees	06	310
phototumdat.csv	Photodynamic tumor therapy	06	326
psdat.r	Number of visits to doctor	07	401
height.dat	Height of girls and boys	08	437
WomenBF.dat	Women's body fat	09	500
coloncancer.dat	Colon cancer patients' treatment cost	09	509
NLSNIF.dat	Radioactivity counts in rat heart	09	512
Finney.dat	Finney data on vasoconstriction	09	522
alckid.dat	Underage alcohol consumption	09	528
DEregrowth.dat	Chemotherapy treatment comparison	10	551
tumdat.csv	Four-group mice tumor regrowth	10	563
Gompertz.dat	Gompertz transient regrowth curve	10	551
maple*.xy	Maple leaf (x, y) coordinates	11	594
pot*.pgm	Six-potato image data	11	604
carpetc.pgm	Carpet light source location	12	612
grp11.pgm	Histology images of cancer cells	12	615
EnglishLetters.txt	Frequency of English letters	12	624
Hypoxia\\Group*.pgm	Hypoxia BOLD MRI rat brain data	12	629
schiz\\case*.pgm	Normal and schizophrenia patients	12	636
\\grp*.jpg	Cancer cell histology images	12	638
clock1.pgm	Clock image alignment	12	648
\\bark\\bark*.pgm	Tree bark images	12	658

* several files exist

Open Problems in Mixed Models

- Determining how to deal with a not positive definite covariance matrix of random effects, $\mathbf{D}$, during maximum likelihood estimation algorithms. Several strategies are discussed in Section 2.15. For example, in our own R function lmeFS, we allow matrix $\mathbf{D}$ to be any (no restriction) but symmetric. As studied in Section 2.16, if matrix $\mathbf{D}$ becomes not positive definite during iterations, function lme of library nlme in R returns an error. Function lme4 of the library with the same name does not fail and returns a singular nonnegative definite matrix. The question remains how a not nonnegative definite matrix $\mathbf{D}$ can be projected on the space of nonnegative definite matrices, $\mathbb{D}_+$. In particular, shall we benefit from an expensive log-likelihood maximization on the boundary of $\mathbb{D}_+$? This question is closely related to testing what random effects variables are statistically significant.

- Testing the variance-covariance matrix of random effects, particularly testing whether a specific random effect is not statistically significant (variance=0). This question is closely related to difficulties of the numerical implementation described above. The exact F-test for a linear mixed model, as a generalization of an ANOVA test, is suggested in Section 3.5, and generalized to a nonlinear mixed model in Section 8.15.2. Tests for overdispersion in the framework of random intercepts in logistic and Poisson models are discussed in Sections 7.3.7 and 7.5.10, respectively, and the test for homogeneity in the meta-analysis model is discussed in Section 5.2.3. However, unlike its linear version most of these tests do not yield the exact/nominal significance level in a small sample, and more work is required to eliminate or reduce this discrepancy. Even the F-test by itself may not be very powerful, and a search for a better test is urgent and practically important as a tool for mixed model criticism. Several recent papers study the alternatives, including those of Giampaoli and Singer (2009), and Li and Zhu (2013).

- Testing what variables belong to fixed effects and what variables belong to random effects. Which variables affect the mean function and which variables affect the variance of the dependent variable is not a trivial matter. Existing methods of hypothesis testing work separately with fixed and random effects. We need tests that identify fixed and random parts in a mixed model simultaneously. Practically nothing has been done in this direction. Again, in asymptotic setting, when the number of clusters is large, the information matrix is block diagonal which implies that the choice of the fixed or random can be done separately. For small N, this is not true, and therefore simultaneous variable selection is required.

- Development of mixed-model-specific information criteria to address the increasing number of parameters, such as generalization of AIC/BIC, or Mallow's C_p. We have sufficient evidence that these criteria are helpful when adjusting for an increasing number of fixed effects parameters. However, random effects parameters, namely, elements of the random effects covariance matrix, have a different nature and should not be counted in the same way as fixed effects coefficients. In Section 1.6 we suggest some variants of Akaike's criterion treating the mixed model with a large number of parameters as an inverse ill-posed problem, called healthy AIC, but much work remains to be done.

- Variable selection, or more generally, model selection in the framework of mixed models. This topic is closely related to problems formulated previously. Three types of variable selection schema are available: (1) fixed effects variable selection assuming that random effects variables are known, say, random intercepts; (2) random effects variable selection assuming that fixed effects variables are known; and (3) having a set of variables, what variables go to fixed effects, what variables go to random effects, and what variables go nowhere. Only a handful of papers consider the problem, such as a recent paper by Peng and Lu (2012) in an asymptotic setting where selection is much easier. Especially important and difficult is the problem of mixed model selection when the number of potential variables is larger, sometimes much larger than the number of clusters, as in the case of genetics data. Then in addition to the difficulty of the variable selection criterion, a computational burden emerges.

- Power computation and sample size determination for mixed models. An important feature of a mixed model is that two sample sizes should be distinguished: the number of clusters, N, and the number of observations per cluster, n. Obviously, the number of clusters is more important because when the number of clusters goes to infinity and the number of observations per cluster is fixed, beta-estimates are consistent, but not otherwise. On the other hand, n plays a role in getting the power desired. From asymptotic consideration, the power function of detecting a beta-coefficient δ versus the zero null hypothesis is equal: $P = \Phi(-Z_{1-\alpha/2} + \delta/\sqrt{V(N,n)})$, where Φ is the cumulative distribution function of the standard normal distribution, α is the size of the test (typically, $\alpha = 0.05$), $Z_{1-\alpha/2} = \Phi^{-1}(1 - \alpha/2)$, and $V(N,n)$ is the variance of the beta estimate. In a particular case when $n = 1$, we arrive at the standard formula for sample size determination in the double-sided Wald test, $n = (Z_P + Z_{1-\alpha/2})^2 V/\delta^2$ (Demidenko, 2007b). For example, in the case of a linear balanced model, the variance of the beta-coefficient is a diagonal element of the matrix $N^{-1}\sigma^2 \left(\mathbf{X}'(\mathbf{I} + \mathbf{ZDZ}')^{-1}\mathbf{X} \right)^{-1}$, which is a function of N and n. A similar formula for the variance can be applied to generalized and nonlinear mixed models, but then it would require integration to obtain the Fisher information matrix. We need to extend these computations to the case of unbalanced data where the distribution of the number of observations per cluster is a part of the statistical design.

- Design of optimal experiments with mixed models. In engineering and industrial settings, fixed and random effects design matrices may be chosen as a part of experimental design. Although the theory of optimal design of experiments is well studied for linear and nonlinear regression models, not many theoretical developments exist in the mixed model framework. Similar to sample size determination, a mixed model leads to a nontrivial choice between design for fixed and random effects. Only a handful of papers exist on the topic (e.g., Dette et al., 2010) and more research is needed to address this important application of mixed models. The idea of adaptive design seems attractive (Glaholt et al., 2012).

- Statistical hypothesis testing using noniterative quadratic estimators of σ^2 and matrix $\mathbf{D}$ are discussed in Sections 3.10 to 3.12. The closed-form expression for these estimators makes it possible to study the small-sample properties and development of new statistical tests. In particular, we need extensive simulations; how these estimates behave for small number of clusters, N; and non-Gaussian, possibly skewed, distributions with long tails. The importance of noniterative estimates is explained by the possibility of using them for testing a statistical hypothesis on $\mathbf{D}$ that creates an opportunity to testing the statistical significance of the random effects.

- Studying the small-sample-size properties of the beta-estimates and the respective statistical hypothesis tests. A paramount question regarding nonlinear statistical models involves small-sample properties of estimators. The linear mixed effects model is the simplest nonlinear statistical model in which advances can be achieved. Currently, the t-test is used for the statistical significance of fixed effects coefficients assuming that the covariance matrix of random effects is fixed and known. We can adjust for the fact that an estimate of matrix $\mathbf{D}$ is used that would lead to widening the confidence intervals. More research should be done in studying how the confidence intervals and hypothesis testing can be improved using the profile likelihood; see Section 3.4 as an introduction.

- The Gauss-Markov theorem for mixed model or estimated GLS. The Gauss-Markov theorem is the cornerstone of linear models. If the scaled covariance matrix of random effects, $\mathbf{D}$, is known, the estimated generalized least squares estimator for fixed effects coefficients, $\boldsymbol{\beta}$, is BLUE (best linear unbiased estimator) and has a minimum covariance matrix (the estimator is efficient) among all (linear and nonlinear) unbiased estimators with normal observations. In Section 3.6.1 it is shown that the maximum likelihood estimator of fixed effects is unbiased in a small sample, and it remains unbiased with many other quadratic estimates of $\mathbf{D}$, such as MINQUE, MM, and VLS, discussed in Chapter 3. Thus, the set of unbiased estimator for $\boldsymbol{\beta}$ is nonempty, and therefore the question as to which is the most efficient unbiased estimator is valid. Several avenues can be taken to tackle this problem. For example, one may seek an estimate of $\mathbf{D}$ as a quadratic function of the observations that minimizes the covariance matrix of the fixed effects coefficients or its derivatives at $\mathbf{D} = \mathbf{0}$. A good start may be the simplest random effect model, the meta-analysis model, discussed in Chapter 5.

- Develop better computational algorithms for generalized linear and nonlinear mixed models, including maximum likelihood estimation based on numerical integration. Three types of quantities are computed in traditional (or approximate) log-likelihood maximization: the values of the log-likelihood function, its derivatives (the score equations), and the Hessian (or information) matrix. It should be noted that score equations are most important because the MLE is defined as the solution of these equations. The Hessian estimate is less important because any positive definite matrix provides the convergence of the maximization algorithm. While the existing methods concentrate on the log-likelihood approximation via integration, we should pay more attention to score equations. The improved Laplace approximation suggested in Section 7.1.2 can be used to approximate the integral or the Gauss-Hermite quadrature. To speed up the convergence, one can increase the number of nodes while iterations progress.

- Improve computational algorithms by recognizing that the beta-parameters, $\boldsymbol{\beta}$, and Cholesky factor elements, $\boldsymbol{\delta}$, can be combined in a linear combination $\mathbf{A}_i\boldsymbol{\beta} + \mathbf{U}_s\boldsymbol{\delta}$, as outlined in Section 8.14. The prototype of the algorithm is implemented in our function `nlmeFSL`, but more efficient C/FOTRAN code is required to see the full advantage.

- Starting values for linear and nonlinear mixed model estimation algorithms. A good choice for starting values may be crucial for a successful run, especially for generalized and nonlinear mixed models with a large number of random effects or complicated variance-covariance structure. It seems that the most important is the choice of matrix $\mathbf{D}$. Several recommendations may be explored: (1) a few iterations of the fixed-point algorithm, as discussed in Section 2.13; and (2) noniterative quadratic estimates of matrix $\mathbf{D}_*$ and σ^2, as discussed in Sections 3.10 to 3.12. Less obvious and yet more important is the choice for starting values for nonlinear mixed models. Beta-parameters may be estimated using `glm` and `nls`, and matrix $\mathbf{D}_*$ may be estimated based on the residuals. Definitely, more work is required to study theoretical properties of these starting values and to test these suggestions via extensive simulations involving 'difficult' data sets.

- Development of the criterion that the MLE of $\mathbf{D}$ is a positive definite matrix. We have developed such criterion for a linear mixed model in Section 2.6 and for a meta-analysis model in Section 5.1.2. A similar criterion is needed for generalized linear and nonlinear mixed models. This criterion can serve as a preliminary test for the adequateness of the mixed model and random effects against overspecification.

- Development of an adequate stopping criterion (criteria) for maximization of the log-likelihood function, especially with generalized linear and nonlinear models. The log-likelihood maximization may be a complex problem, especially when variables are close to collinear or when the nonlinear model has a complicated variance-covariance structure. Proximity between iterations defined as $\|\mathbf{a}_s - \mathbf{a}_{s-1}\| < \varepsilon$, where ε is a small number, does not guarantee that $\mathbf{a}_s$ is the point of the global maximum. In order to claim that iterations converged to a local maximum, the gradient of the log-likelihood function at $\mathbf{a}_s$ must be zero. A question arises: What small is small? For instance, is 10^{-1} or 10^{-8} a small gradient? The interpretable stopping criteria were developed for the nonlinear least squares, and discussed in Section 13.3.5. Similar criteria should be developed for mixed model maximization algorithms.

- Existence of the maximum likelihood estimate (MLE) for generalized linear and nonlinear mixed models. The MLE may not exist; thus, before starting a maximization algorithm one has to be sure that the maximizer exists. You may spend a lot of time on model testing and playing with the start values but eventually fail because the MLE, simply does not exist—the criteria for MLE existence are important. For a linear mixed effects model, MLE exists with probability 1, as discussed in Section 2.5. Things become more complicated for generalized and nonlinear mixed models. For example, in the case of binary dependent data, the conditions for the data separation must be fulfilled, as presented in Section 7.10. You may generalize the existence criteria developed for nonlinear regression by the author (Demidenko, 1989, 2000, 2008) to the existence of the MLE in the mixed model.

- Uniqueness of the log-likelihood maximum. The log-likelihood function is not a quadratic function even for a linear mixed model because of the presence of variances and covariances. Thus, the possibility exists of converging to a local maximum. As proven by Demidenko (2000), for many nonlinear regressions the probability that the normal equation has two or more distinct solutions is positive. We need criteria by which one can test whether the maximum log-likelihood found is global, as suggested by Demidenko (2008). As a conjecture, the log-likelihood function for a linear mixed model is unimodal (local maximum=global maximum). For a generalized linear mixed model, such as the logistic or Poisson model, this question is open A good start is to investigate the uniqueness of the maximum likelihood estimate for a Poisson model with random intercepts. The uniqueness criteria for a general nonlinear mixed model are even more difficult than those for a nonlinear regression but are not completely intractable. In general, criteria for uniqueness are model-dependent and mathematically challenging.

It should be noted that some literature exists that deals with some of the problems outlined above. We have deliberately not tried to mention all existing publications in these directions because it would require much more space. Therefore, an important part of advancing along the lines of these problems will be a careful review of work already done.

1
Introduction: Why Mixed Models?

Big ideas have many names and applications. Sometimes the mixed model is called the model for repeated measurements, sometimes a hierarchical model. Sometimes the mixed model is used to analyze clustered or panel data, sometimes longitudinal data.

Mixed model methodology brings statistics to the next level. In classical statistics a typical assumption is that observations are drawn from the same general population and are independent and identically distributed. Mixed model data have a more complex, multilevel, hierarchical structure. Observations between levels or clusters are independent, but observations within each cluster are dependent because they belong to the same subpopulation. Consequently, we speak of two sources of variation: between clusters and within clusters.

Mixed model is also well suited for the analysis of longitudinal data, where each time series constitutes an individual curve, a cluster. Mixed model is well suited for biological and medical data, which display notorious heterogeneity of responses to stimuli and treatment. An advantage of the mixed model is the ability to genuinely combine the data by introducing multilevel random effects. Mixed model is a nonlinear statistical model, due mainly to the presence of variance parameters, and thus it requires special theoretical treatment. The goal of this book is to provide systematic coverage and development of all spectra of mixed models: linear, generalized linear, and nonlinear.

The aim of this chapter is to show the variety of applications for which the mixed model methodology can be useful, or even a breakthrough. For example, application of mixed modeling methodology to shape and image analysis seems especially exciting and challenging.

Mixed models can be used for the following purposes:

- To model complex clustered or longitudinal data.

- To model data with multiple sources of variation.

- To model biological variety and heterogeneity.

- As a compromise between the frequentist and Bayesian approaches.

- As a statistical model for the penalized log-likelihood.

- To provide a theoretical basis for the Healthy Akaike Information Criterion (HAIC).

- To cope with parameter multidimensionality.

- As a statistical model to solve ill-posed problems, including image reconstruction problems.

- To model shapes and images.

An important feature of this book is that it provides numerical algorithms as a realization of statistical methods that it develops. We strongly believe that an approach is not valuable without an appropriate efficient algorithm. Each chapter ends with a summary points section that may help the reader to quickly grasp the chapter's major points.

1.1   Mixed effects for clustered data

The mixed effects approach copes with clustered data that can be viewed as a sample of samples. To illustrate, let us consider the relationship between price (x) and sales (y). Let $\{(x_k, y_k), k = 1, ..., K\}$ be the sample of observations collected on price and sales for several commodities. Plotting y versus x reveals that the relationship is close to linear with a negative slope; see the left-hand panel in Figure 1.1. In classical statistics it is assumed that pairs (x_k, y_k) are independent and identically distributed (iid) with the regression line $E(y|x) = \alpha + \beta x$. However, one may argue that we deal with clustered data, where each cluster is a commodity. In the right-hand panel, we connect observation points for each commodity and obtain a reverse picture—increase in price leads to increase in sales. A paradox?

Classical statistics assumes the model

$$y_k = \alpha + \beta x_k + \varepsilon_k, \quad k = 1, ..., K, \tag{1.1}$$

where the $\{\varepsilon_k\}$ are independent and identically distributed random variables with zero mean and constant variance σ^2. In other words, it is assumed that the data are collected from similar, homogeneous commodities. As follows from the right panel, the commodities are not homogeneous and vary substantially in terms of price and sales. An adequate model for the sales problem would be to assume that each commodity has its own commodity-specific sales (in statistical language, intercept); namely,

$$y_{ij} = \alpha_i + \beta x_{ij} + \varepsilon_{ij}, \quad i = 1, ..., N, \ j = 1, ..., n_i. \tag{1.2}$$

Note that we use a double index now because we are dealing with clustered/panel /tabular data: i corresponds to the ith commodity, j corresponds to the jth observation of the ith commodity, n_i is the number of observations for the ith commodity, and α_i is the commodity-specific intercept. The total number of observations is $K = \sum_{i=1}^{N} n_i$. Regarding the error terms $\{\varepsilon_{ij}\}$, we assume that, as previously, they are iid with the variance σ^2.

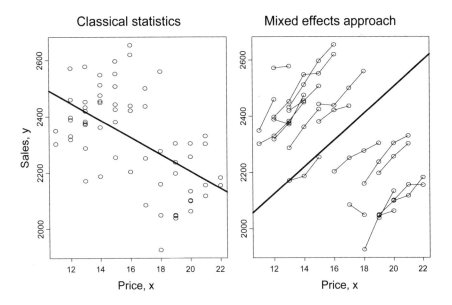

FIGURE 1.1. Classical and mixed effects approaches lead to reverse conclusions. Left: In the classical approach, it is assumed that observations are independent and identically distributed, resulting in a negative relationship. The straight line shows simple regression estimated by ordinary least squares. Right: In the mixed effects approach, it is assumed that each commodity represents a cluster and therefore that an increase in price for a specific commodity leads to an increase in sales. The straight line shows the linear mixed effects model with population-averaged slope and commodity-specific intercept.

Obviously, model (1.2) is more complex than the classical regression model (1.1), and in a special case, $\alpha_i = \alpha$, we come to (1.1). The central assumption of the mixed effects model is that intercepts $\{\alpha_i, i = 1, ..., N\}$ are random and belong to a general population that can be expressed in the second equation as

$$\alpha_i = \alpha + b_i, \tag{1.3}$$

where α is the population-averaged sale (intercept) and b_i is the random effect, or deviation of the commodity-specific sale from the population-averaged sale. Thus, on the one hand, we allow commodity-specific sales, but on the other hand, we assume that commodities represent the country market economy, and therefore one can speak of how an increase in price affects sales across all commodities. Coupled models (1.2) and (1.3) define a linear mixed effects model, parameters α and β are fixed effects (population-averaged parameters), and b_i is the random effect with zero mean and variance σ_b^2 independent of $\{\varepsilon_{ij}\}$. This is a *hierarchical* model or a model with random coefficients. The model defined by equations (1.2) and (1.3) can be combined into one as

$$y_{ij} = \alpha + \beta x_{ij} + \eta_{ij}, \quad i = 1, ..., N, \; j = 1, ..., n_i, \tag{1.4}$$

where $\eta_{ij} = \varepsilon_{ij} + b_i$ is the composite random error. As follows from (1.4), observations on the same commodity (within a cluster) correlate with the correlation coefficient:

$$\rho = \frac{\text{var}(b_i)}{\text{var}(b_i + \varepsilon_{ij})} = \frac{\sigma_b^2}{\sigma^2 + \sigma_b^2}, \tag{1.5}$$

but observations on different commodities (from different clusters) do not correlate. In a mixed effects model, there are two sources of variation: the within (or intra) -cluster variation, σ^2, and the between (or inter) -cluster variation, σ_b^2. Recall that classical regression assumes one variation. As follows from (1.5), the larger the variation between commodities, the higher the correlation within each cluster. If $\sigma_b^2 = 0$, the correlation is zero and $\alpha_i = \alpha$, ordinary linear regression. For the data in Figure 1.1, $\rho = 0.99$, so the major source of variation is the variation between commodities. That is why the slope has different signs in the two approaches.

Observations $\{y_{i1}, y_{i2}, ..., y_{i,n_i}\}$ can also be interpreted as *repeated measurements.* Therefore, model (1.4) is sometimes called the model for repeated measurements. An important example of clustered data is that of longitudinal data when subjects are observed over time. In fact, the pioneering work by Laird and Ware (1982) on the linear mixed effects model was concerned with this kind of data. Model (1.4) belongs to the family of linear mixed effects (LME) models and is studied extensively in Chapters 2 through 4. Specifically, model (1.4) is called the LME model with random intercepts, and it has many nice properties (see Section 2.4). There is more on ignoring random effects in the LME model in Section 3.9.

Summing up, ignoring clustered structure may lead to false analysis. The linear mixed effects model is an adequate model for clustered (repeated) data that involve two sources of variation, within and between clusters.

1.2 ANOVA, variance components, and the mixed model

The mixed model may be viewed as a combination of analysis of variance (ANOVA), variance component (VARCOMP), and regression models. For example, the simplest, one-way ANOVA model deals with tabular data:

$$y_{ij} = \beta_i + \varepsilon_{ij}, \quad i = 1, ..., N, \; j = 1, ..., n_i, \tag{1.6}$$

where N is the number of units (subjects or clusters), n_i is the number of observations per unit, and $\{\varepsilon_{ij}\}$ are independent and identically distributed (iid) errors with zero mean and variance σ^2. An important, sometimes not well emphasized assumption of the ANOVA model is that $\{\beta_1, ..., \beta_N\}$ are fixed parameters. Consequently, for each unit, observations $\{y_{i1}, y_{i2}, ..., y_{in_i}\}$ can be treated as replicates because they are iid with the mean β_i. A traditional hypothesis in the framework of the ANOVA model is that the units are the same, or $H_0 : \beta_1 = ... = \beta_N$.

The ANOVA model is a special case of the linear regression model,

$$\mathbf{y} = \mathbf{X}\boldsymbol{\beta} + \boldsymbol{\varepsilon}, \tag{1.7}$$

where $\mathbf{y}$ is a $K \times 1$ vector of observations, $\mathbf{X}$ is a $K \times m$ design matrix, and $\boldsymbol{\beta}$ is an $m \times 1$ vector of parameters. For example, the one-way ANOVA model (1.6) can be expressed in the regression form (1.7) if the $\{y_{ij}\}$ are arranged in the vector $\mathbf{y}$ so that $K = \sum_{i=1}^{N} n_i$, the elements of the design matrix $\mathbf{X}$ are 0 or 1, and $m = N$. A classic reference, where various ANOVA models are represented as a linear model, is Searle (1971a). All ANOVA models have two important features: (a) parameters $\{\beta_i, i = 1, ..., m\}$ are estimated by ordinary least squares, and (b) the F-test is the workhorse for linear hypothesis testing. Models (1.6) and (1.7) can also be called fixed effects models.

We come to a *different* statistical model when the $\{\beta_i\}$ are assumed random, say iid normally distributed (independent of ε_{ij}) with the common mean β and variance σ_β^2. Representing $\beta_i = \beta + b_i$, we arrive at the variance components (VARCOMP) model:

$$y_{ij} = \beta + b_i + \varepsilon_{ij}, \tag{1.8}$$

where b_i is called a *random effect*. The ANOVA is a fixed effects model and VAR-COMP is a random effects model. Although models (1.6) and (1.8) seem similar, they have different statistical properties. In ANOVA, observations do not correlate; in VARCOMP, observations correlate within each unit and the correlation coefficient is equal to $\sigma_\beta^2/(\sigma^2 + \sigma_\beta^2)$. According to the Gauss–Markov theorem, for model (1.6) the ordinary least squares coincides with the MLE and is efficient, but this does not hold for model (1.8). Moreover, if n_i are different, there is no closed-form solution for the MLE. The null hypothesis $H_0 : \beta_1 = ... = \beta_N$ for the ANOVA model transforms into $H_0 : \sigma_\beta^2 = 0$ and the F-test cannot be applied directly, as it requires substantial modification (see Section 3.5). When the number of units is relatively small (say, $N < \min n_i$), the ANOVA model is preferable. When the number of units is relatively large (say, $N > \max n_i$), the VARCOMP model may be better. The VARCOMP model has a long history (Rao, 1973; Harville, 1977; Searle et al., 1992).

The mixed model may be viewed as a combination of the ANOVA and VARCOMP models. For example, consider the problem of measuring the blood pressure for $i = 1, ..., N$ people at time points $t_{i1}, t_{i2}, ..., t_{i,n_i}$. If y_{ij} denotes the blood pressure of the ith person at time t_{ij}, the VARCOMP model (1.8) may be adequate because it reflects the fact that the blood pressure changes from person to person, but for the same time, one can speak of the population-averaged blood pressure, β. Now we realize that besides blood pressure for each person, we have information about gender, age, and so on. Also, to reflect the fact that measurements are made over a fairly long period of time, we incorporate t_{ij} into the vector of complete covariates $\mathbf{x}_{ij}$. Then the expanded VARCOMP model transforms into the mixed effects model,

$$y_{ij} = \mathbf{x}'_{ij}\boldsymbol{\beta} + b_i + \varepsilon_{ij}. \tag{1.9}$$

The similarity with the regression model (1.7) becomes evident.

In general, the linear mixed effects (LME) model is written as

$$\mathbf{y}_i = \mathbf{X}_i\boldsymbol{\beta} + \mathbf{Z}_i\mathbf{b}_i + \boldsymbol{\varepsilon}_i, \quad i = 1, ..., N, \tag{1.10}$$

where $\mathbf{b}_i$ is a vector of random effects such that $\mathrm{cov}(\mathbf{b}_i) = \sigma^2 \mathbf{D}$ and $\mathbf{Z}_i$ is the design matrix. For example, for model (1.9), the random effect is scalar and $\mathbf{Z}_i = \mathbf{1}$. The variance parameters, σ^2 and $\mathbf{D}$, are unknown and are subject to estimation along with the population-averaged parameter $\boldsymbol{\beta}$.

By combining vectors $\{\mathbf{y}_i\}$ and matrices $\{\mathbf{X}_i\}$ into $\sum n_i \times 1$ vector $\mathbf{y}$ and $\sum n_i \times m$ matrix $\mathbf{X}$, and letting $\mathbf{Z} = \mathrm{diag}(\mathbf{Z}_1, ..., \mathbf{Z}_N)$, model (1.10) can be written as one equation, $\mathbf{y} = \mathbf{X}\boldsymbol{\beta} + \mathbf{Z}\mathbf{b} + \boldsymbol{\varepsilon}$. Although some authors prefer to work with this one-equation LME model, such representation is excessive because observations across i are independent.

Although model (1.10) looks like a linear model, the fact that the variance parameters are unknown makes it a nonlinear statistical model with elaborated estimation methodology. Usually, we assume that the random effects and the error term have a normal distribution, so that model (1.10) can be written more compactly as

$$\mathbf{y}_i \sim \mathcal{N}(\mathbf{X}_i\boldsymbol{\beta}, \sigma^2(\mathbf{I} + \mathbf{Z}_i\mathbf{D}\mathbf{Z}_i')), \quad i = 1, ..., N, \tag{1.11}$$

meaning that $\mathbf{y}_i$ has a multivariate normal distribution with mean $\mathbf{X}_i\boldsymbol{\beta}$ and covariance matrix $\sigma^2(\mathbf{I} + \mathbf{Z}_i\mathbf{D}\mathbf{Z}_i')$. If $\mathbf{D}$ were known, as follows from the Gauss–Markov theorem, the generalized least squares estimator,

$$\widehat{\boldsymbol{\beta}} = \left(\sum_{i=1}^{N} \mathbf{X}'(\mathbf{I} + \mathbf{Z}_i\mathbf{D}\mathbf{Z}_i')^{-1}\mathbf{X}_i \right)^{-1} \left(\sum_{i=1}^{N} \mathbf{X}'(\mathbf{I} + \mathbf{Z}_i\mathbf{D}\mathbf{Z}_i')^{-1}\mathbf{y}_i \right),$$

would be efficient. But the variance-covariance matrix of the random effects is unknown, and its estimation becomes a central theme in the framework of the mixed effects model. Two families of estimators for the variance parameters are considered: maximum likelihood (Chapter 2) and quadratic noniterative distribution-free estimators, including MINQUE, variance least squares, and method of moments (Chapter 3).

The LME model and its generalizations are studied in the first three chapters of the book. In the first chapter we discuss computational aspects of maximum likelihood, the second chapter is about statistical properties, and in the third chapter we consider several generalizations and important special cases of the LME model. In Chapter 5, meta-analysis, a very special case of the mixed model, is studied; this model is not covered by (1.10) and therefore requires special treatment.

1.3   Other special cases of the mixed effects model

Another important special case of linear mixed effects model (1.10) is the regression model with random coefficients,

$$\mathbf{y}_i = \mathbf{X}_i\mathbf{a}_i + \boldsymbol{\varepsilon}_i, \quad \mathbf{a}_i = \boldsymbol{\beta} + \mathbf{b}_i, \quad i = 1, ..., N. \tag{1.12}$$

For example, Swamy (1971) studied this model in connection with the analysis of cross-sectional (panel) data where $\mathbf{y}_i$ is a time series of length n and i is an index economic sector. One comes to (1.12) letting $\mathbf{Z}_i = \mathbf{X}_i$ in the LME model (1.10). An interesting special case of model (1.12) is when the data are balanced, $\mathbf{X}_i = \mathbf{Z}$. For balanced data, the ordinary and generalized least squares lead to the same estimate. This model is studied in Section 2.3. In Chapter 4 we study the growth curve model, where $\mathbf{a}_i = \mathbf{A}_i\boldsymbol{\beta} + \mathbf{b}_i$ and $\mathbf{A}_i$ is the design matrix. Sometimes only a subvector $\mathbf{a}_i$ can be specified, so that other coefficients may be anything. For example, in model (1.9), only the intercept is random; this models is studied in Section 2.4, while a more general family of growth curve models is studied in Section 4.2.

Another special case of the LME model is when $n_i = 1$, which leads to a linear regression with *heteroscedastic* errors, $y_i = \boldsymbol{\beta}'\mathbf{x}_i + \eta_i$, where η_i has zero mean and variance $\text{var}(\eta_i) = \sigma^2(1 + dz_i^2)$ and d is the parameter to estimate. Many examples and treatments of the regression model with heteroscedastic errors may be found in the book by Carroll and Ruppert (1988). A nonlinear regression model with heteroscedastic errors and a nonlinear variance function defined as $\text{var}(\eta_i) = \sigma^2 w_i(\boldsymbol{\beta}, \boldsymbol{\theta})$ can be studied in the framework of the nonlinear marginal mixed model of Chapter 6.

1.4   Compromise between Bayesian and frequentist approaches

The goal of this section is to convince the reader that the mixed model may serve as a compromise between the frequentist (classical) and Bayesian approaches. Both the Bayesian and mixed model approaches are based on a hierarchical statistical model, but in the former the values for all parameters must be specified, whereas in the latter, parameters are estimated from the data.

Specifically, let $\mathbf{y}$ be the data observed. In the *Bayesian* approach, the model is specified in *hierarchical* fashion as

$$\mathbf{y}|\boldsymbol{\theta} \quad \sim \quad L(\mathbf{y}|\boldsymbol{\theta}), \tag{1.13}$$

$$\boldsymbol{\theta} \quad \sim \quad G(\boldsymbol{\theta}). \tag{1.14}$$

Equation (1.13) defines the conditional distribution of $\mathbf{y}$ given $\boldsymbol{\theta}$ through density L. The second equation, (1.14), defines *a priori* the distribution of $\boldsymbol{\theta}$ through density G. Since G is usually a member of a family of distributions, the parameter that specifies G is called the *hyperparameter*. Thus, unlike the frequentist approach, the Bayesian approach assumes that parameter $\boldsymbol{\theta}$ is random and densities L and G must be specified completely. The main computational concern in the Bayesian framework is calculation of the normalization constant

$$A = \int L(\mathbf{y}|\boldsymbol{\theta})G(\boldsymbol{\theta})d\boldsymbol{\theta} \tag{1.15}$$

in the *posterior density*

$$p(\boldsymbol{\theta}|\mathbf{y}) = \frac{1}{A}L(\mathbf{y}|\boldsymbol{\theta})G(\boldsymbol{\theta}). \tag{1.16}$$

Obviously, computation of A is required to ensure that the area under the surface defined by (1.16) is 1. Much effort has been spent on developing integration techniques for (1.15). In particular, one of the most popular approaches, based on the Markov Chain Monte Carlo (MCMC) technique, is realized in BUGS software (http://www.mrc-bsu.cam.ac.uk/bugs).

The major criticism of Bayesian theory is the requirement for complete specification of the prior distribution G. It is worthwhile to note that G directly affects the posterior density (1.16) because it acts as a factor. Consequently, sensitivity to the choice of the prior distribution in the Bayesian approach is substantial.

In the mixed model approach, the model is also specified as a hierarchical model, (1.13) and (1.14), but it is allowed to have nonrandom parameters, τ, namely,

$$\mathbf{y}|\boldsymbol{\theta} \sim L(\mathbf{y}|\boldsymbol{\theta},\boldsymbol{\tau}), \tag{1.17}$$

$$\boldsymbol{\theta} \sim G(\boldsymbol{\theta},\boldsymbol{\tau}). \tag{1.18}$$

In the Bayesian framework, τ is known and is the hyperparameter. When τ is unknown we come to the frequentist model, where τ is estimated, for example, by maximum likelihood. As in Bayesian theory, integration becomes a technical problem because ML maximizes the marginal likelihood,

$$L(\boldsymbol{\tau}) = \int L(\mathbf{y}|\boldsymbol{\theta},\boldsymbol{\tau})G(\boldsymbol{\theta},\boldsymbol{\tau})d\boldsymbol{\theta}. \tag{1.19}$$

In the framework of the mixed model, we call $\boldsymbol{\theta}$ random (or subject-specific) and $\boldsymbol{\tau}$ fixed effects (or population-averaged) parameters. Random effects are unobservable and are integrated out in (1.19), but τ is estimated. Thus, the normalizing constant, (1.15), plays the role of the likelihood in the mixed model. After $\widehat{\boldsymbol{\tau}}$ is computed, we apply standard Bayesian formulas, such as posterior density, posterior mean, and so on. In the language of the mixed model, the posterior mean is called the estimate of the random effect. We refer the reader to Sections 3.7 and 8.15, where these quantities are estimated.

In summary, a mixed model combines major features of the frequentist and Bayesian approaches. Symbolically,

mixed model = Bayesian + frequentist.

On the one hand, as in the Bayesian approach, mixed model assumes a hierarchical (conditional) model where the parameter is treated as random. On the other hand, the hyperparameter, τ, is not specified arbitrarily as in the Bayesian approach, but is *estimated* from the data. As such, a mixed model is more flexible than the Bayesian approach.

We illustrate the difference between the Bayesian and mixed model approaches by a linear model under a normal distribution,

$$\mathbf{y}|\boldsymbol{\beta} \sim \mathcal{N}(\mathbf{X}\boldsymbol{\beta},\sigma^2\mathbf{I}_n), \tag{1.20}$$

$$\boldsymbol{\beta} \sim \mathcal{N}(\mathbf{0},\sigma_\beta^2\mathbf{I}_m) \tag{1.21}$$

(Lindley and Smith, 1972; Smith, 1973). These equations are special cases of the general Bayesian model (1.13) and (1.14). In words, if the vector of regression coefficients $\boldsymbol{\beta}$ were known, $\mathbf{y}$ would have a multivariate normal distribution with mean $\mathbf{X}\boldsymbol{\beta}$ and variance σ^2. As follows from (1.21), the prior distribution for $\boldsymbol{\beta}$ is also normal with zero mean and variance σ_β^2. To complete the Bayesian specification, one needs to provide distributions for the variance parameters, σ^2 and σ_β^2. Typically, a gamma distribution with the density $\Gamma^{-1}(\alpha)\lambda^\alpha t^{\alpha-1}e^{-\lambda t}$ is used for this purpose, where α and λ are the known positive (hyper-) parameters. The idea behind the choice of α and λ is to obtain a noninformative prior. When the hyperparameter belongs to a bounded set, the noninformative prior is constant. For example, if a probability p is the hyperparameter, it is reasonable to assume that the prior density of p is 1 on $(0, 1)$. Things are complicated when the hyperparameter is not bounded, such as variance. For example, in BUGS the default values are $\lambda = 1/1000$ and $\alpha = 1/1000$. Since for the gamma distribution, $E = \alpha/\lambda$ and var$= \alpha/\lambda^2$, this choice implies that the *a priori* mean equals 1 and the variance equals 1000. In terms of the variance parameters for our linear model, such a choice would mean that $\sigma^2 = \sigma_\beta^2 = 1000$. Apparently, this choice of the hyperparameters is arbitrary.

Now we turn our attention to the mixed model approach. It uses the same hierarchical models (1.20) and (1.21) but the variance parameters are assumed unknown. We can estimate σ^2 and σ_β^2 either by maximum likelihood (ML) or by noniteratively using unbiased quadratic estimators (Chapter 3). For example, using the ML approach, the pair of models (1.20) and (1.21) imply the model

$$\mathbf{y} \sim \mathcal{N}(\mathbf{0}, \sigma^2(\mathbf{I} + d\mathbf{X}\mathbf{X}')),$$

where $d = \sigma_\beta^2/\sigma^2$ is the scaled variance parameter. In the Bayesian approach, parameters σ^2 and d have to be specified through known distributions. In the mixed model approach, we treat them as unknown parameters to be estimated from maximum likelihood. The log-likelihood, up to a constant $-n \ln \sqrt{2\pi}$, takes the form

$$l(\sigma^2, d) = -0.5n \ln \sigma^2 - 0.5 \ln \left| \mathbf{I} + d\mathbf{X}\mathbf{X}' \right| - 0.5\sigma^{-2} \mathbf{y}'(\mathbf{I} + d\mathbf{X}\mathbf{X}')^{-1}\mathbf{y}.$$

Differentiating with respect to σ^2, we obtain $\sigma^2 = n^{-1}\mathbf{y}'(\mathbf{I} + d\mathbf{X}\mathbf{X}')^{-1}\mathbf{y}$. Plugging it back into l, the variance-profile log-likelihood function simplifies to a function of one argument,

$$l(d) = -0.5n \ln \mathbf{y}'(\mathbf{I}_n + d\mathbf{X}\mathbf{X}')^{-1}\mathbf{y} - 0.5 \ln \left| \mathbf{I} + d\mathbf{X}\mathbf{X}' \right|.$$

A number of algorithms may be used to maximize this function and to obtain the MLE, $\widehat{d}$. So the hyperparameters in the Bayesian approach are estimated in the mixed model. After parameter values are determined, we compute the posterior distribution, which is also normal with mean $\widehat{\boldsymbol{\beta}} = \widehat{d}\mathbf{X}'(\mathbf{I}_n + \widehat{d}\mathbf{X}\mathbf{X}')^{-1}\mathbf{y}$. Using the dimension-reduction formula of Section 2.2.3 or Appendix 13.2, we can express $\widehat{\boldsymbol{\beta}} = (\mathbf{X}'\mathbf{X} + \widehat{d}^{-1}\mathbf{I}_m)^{-1}\mathbf{X}'\mathbf{y}$, as in Lindley and Smith (1972) but with the estimate instead of an arbitrary d.

1.5   Penalized likelihood and mixed effects

Penalized likelihood is encountered in many applications as a way to make a problem solvable by replacing an ill-posed problem with a well-posed problem. This methodology has to be proven to make a great deal of improvement in a variety of applications, from applied mathematics and computer science to engineering. However, a substantial drawback of the penalized likelihood approach is the need to know the *penalty coefficient* (sometimes called a *regularization parameter*). Strictly speaking, an ill-posed problem is merely reduced to another problem of choosing the penalty coefficient. Our aim in this section is to show how the penalized likelihood may be derived from a hierarchical statistical model so that the penalty coefficient term may be estimated along with the parameter of interest. Here we suggest the solution in general terms, and in the following sections we illustrate it by various examples.

Let $\mathbf{y}$ be an n-dimensional vector of observations with the density function L dependent on a k-dimensional parameter $\mathbf{b}$, where k may be large. Denote $l(\mathbf{b}; \mathbf{y})$ as the log-likelihood and $L(\mathbf{b}; \mathbf{y})$ as the likelihood. If n is close to k, the maximum likelihood solution

$$\max_{\mathbf{b}} l(\mathbf{b}; \mathbf{y}) \tag{1.22}$$

turns into an ill-posed problem. To improve (1.22) a penalty term is introduced, so instead one maximizes the penalized log-likelihood,

$$\max_{\mathbf{b}} \left[l(\mathbf{b}; \mathbf{y}) + \rho g(\mathbf{b}) \right], \tag{1.23}$$

where ρ is a nonnegative penalty coefficient and $g(\mathbf{b})$ is a penalty function. Typically, a quadratic term is used, $g(\mathbf{b}) = -\|\mathbf{b}\|^2$, so the penalized log-likelihood reduces to minimization of

$$-l(\mathbf{b}; \mathbf{y}) + \rho \|\mathbf{b}\|^2. \tag{1.24}$$

Sometimes, the penalized log-likelihood is used not in a statistical but in an applied mathematics framework as a regularization technique (Tikhonov and Arsenin, 1977). For example, let $\mathbf{y}$ be an $n \times 1$ normally distributed vector and $\mathbf{X}$ an $n \times k$ matrix such that $\mathbf{y} = \mathbf{Xb} + \boldsymbol{\varepsilon}$, where $\boldsymbol{\varepsilon}$ is the error term with independent identically distributed (iid) components $\varepsilon_i \sim \mathcal{N}(0, \sigma^2)$. For this linear model we have $l(\mathbf{b}; \mathbf{y}) = -(2\sigma^2)^{-1} \|\mathbf{y} - \mathbf{Xb}\|^2$, up to a constant term. If matrix $\mathbf{X}'\mathbf{X}$ is singular (e.g., when $k > n$), (1.22) is an ill-posed problem because $\mathbf{b}$ is not unique. On the other hand, if ρ is a fixed positive number, the penalized negative log-likelihood yields a unique solution, $\mathbf{b} = (\mathbf{X}'\mathbf{X} + \nu\mathbf{I})^{-1}\mathbf{X}'\mathbf{y}$, where $\nu = 2\sigma^2\rho$.

What is the value of ρ? The answer is important because if $\rho = 0$, we come to the previous ill-posed problem. If $\rho \to \infty$, we have $\mathbf{b} = \mathbf{0}$. Thus, by varying ρ, one obtains a variety of solutions, from unstable MLE to trivial $\mathbf{0}$.

To estimate ρ we assume that $\mathbf{b}$ is random, so that $L(\mathbf{b}; \mathbf{y})$ is the conditional likelihood. Let G be a density, so the density of $\mathbf{b}$ is $\omega^{-k}G(\omega^{-1}\mathbf{b})$, where ω is a positive scale parameter. Symbolically, this scheme may be expressed as a hierarchical statistical model,

$$\mathbf{y}|\mathbf{b} \sim L, \quad \mathbf{b} \sim G. \tag{1.25}$$

Since only observations on $\mathbf{y}$ are available, we need to deal with the marginal distribution

$$\int_{R^k} L(\mathbf{b}; \mathbf{y})\omega^{-k}G(\omega^{-1}\mathbf{b})d\mathbf{b},$$

where random $\mathbf{b}$ is integrated out. Letting $g = \ln G$, the marginal log-likelihood takes the form

$$l(\omega) = -k\ln\omega + \ln\int_{R^k} e^{l(\mathbf{b};\mathbf{y})+g(\omega^{-1}\mathbf{b})}d\mathbf{b}. \tag{1.26}$$

The MLE, $\widehat{\omega}$ turns l into a maximum. Now the Laplace approximation comes into play to show the link between maximum and penalized likelihood (see Section 7.7.1

for more details),

$$\int_{R^k} e^{h(\mathbf{b})}d\mathbf{b} \simeq (2\pi)^{k/2}e^{h_{\max}}\left|-\left.\frac{\partial^2 h}{\partial \mathbf{b}^2}\right|_{\mathbf{b}=\mathbf{b}_{\max}}\right|^{-1/2}, \qquad (1.27)$$

where $h_{\max} = h(\mathbf{b}_{\max})$ and $|\mathbf{H}|$ is the determinant of the negative Hessian at the maximum, $\mathbf{H} = -\partial^2 h/\partial \mathbf{b}^2$. Applying this approximation to (1.26), one obtains

$$l(\omega) \simeq -k\ln\omega + l(\mathbf{b};\mathbf{y}) + g(\omega^{-1}\mathbf{b}) - 0.5\ln|\mathbf{H}|.$$

Finally, assuming that $\ln|\mathbf{H}|$ changes little with $\mathbf{b}$, the marginal log-likelihood (1.26) can be approximated as

$$l(\omega) \simeq -k\ln\omega + l(\mathbf{b};\mathbf{y}) + g(\omega^{-1}\mathbf{b}). \qquad (1.28)$$

In the particular case when ω is known, maximization of the marginal log-likelihood is almost equivalent to maximization of

$$l(\mathbf{b};\mathbf{y}) + g(\omega^{-1}\mathbf{b}). \qquad (1.29)$$

In an important special case, when the marginal distribution of $\mathbf{b}$ is normal ($G = \mathcal{N}$) with zero mean, we have $g(\omega^{-1}\mathbf{b}) = -0.5\omega^{-2}\|\mathbf{b}\|^2$, so the maximum likelihood estimation of the hierarchical statistical model (1.25) is almost equivalent to the minimization of the penalized log-likelihood (1.24) with $\rho = 1/(2\omega^2)$. Finally, to estimate $\mathbf{b}$ and ω simultaneously, we maximize the right-hand side of (1.28), which is a well-posed problem. In the literature on mixed models, (1.28) is called *quasi-likelihood* (Breslow and Clayton, 1993). This likelihood approximation plays an important role in estimation in the generalized linear mixed models of Chapters 7 and 8, respectively. Typically, besides random effects $\mathbf{b}$, we have fixed effects (or population-averaged) parameters $\boldsymbol{\theta}$, but their presence does not alter the reasoning, described above.

Generally, any penalized log-likelihood may be derived through a mixed model. For a linear model, the penalized log-likelihood is exact; for a nonlinear model, the penalized log-likelihood is an approximation of the original log-likelihood. The Laplace approximation is the key to proving this link.

In the following sections we show some applications of this general result.

1.6   Healthy Akaike information criterion

The Akaike (1974) information criterion (AIC) became very popular as a criterion for model selection. The rationale behind this criterion is the divergence between the true distribution and a candidate measured in terms of the Kullback–Leibler information criterion, Kullback (1968). It was shown that based on this criterion, the model should be chosen such that

$$\text{AIC} = -2l_{\max} + 2k \qquad (1.30)$$

reaches a minimum, where $l_{\max}$ is the log-likelihood maximum and k is the number of unknown parameters. The smaller the AIC, the better the model. The AIC is especially useful for nonnested models; if the models are nested, standard statistical hypothesis techniques are applied. It is worthwhile to notice that (1.30) has the form of a penalized negative log-likelihood. For example, consider a linear regression model,

$$\mathbf{y} = \mathbf{X}\boldsymbol{\beta} + \varepsilon, \tag{1.31}$$

where $\boldsymbol{\beta}$ is the k-dimensional parameter vector, components ε_i are independent normally distributed random variables with zero mean and variance σ^2, and $i = 1, 2, ..., n$. Assuming that all candidate models use the same number of observations ($n =$ const), it is elementary to check that up to a constant,

$$\text{AIC} = n \ln \widehat{\sigma}^2 + 2k, \tag{1.32}$$

where $\widehat{\sigma}^2 = n^{-1} \left\| \mathbf{y} - \mathbf{X}\widehat{\boldsymbol{\beta}}_{LS} \right\|^2$ is the regression variance and $\widehat{\boldsymbol{\beta}}_{LS}$ is the least squares estimate.

Several researchers noted that there can be appreciable bias in the AIC estimate. For example, Hurvich and Tsai (1991) suggested using the term $k+(k+1)(k+2)/(n-k-2)$ instead of $2k$. Sclove (1987) and Dayton (1998) consider a generalization of the Akaike information criterion expressed as $-2l_{\max} + a(n)k$, where $a(n)$ is a function of the sample size.

Although many researchers demonstrated that the AIC is a useful quantity to characterize the information property of a statistical model, Ishiguro et al. (1997) and Mittelhammer et al. (2000), among others, pointed out a weakness of this criterion. In particular, the AIC works poorly in the case of multicollinearity. To illustrate, let us consider the problem of finding the right linear regression model using a set of independent (explanatory) variables or covariates $\{x_j, j = 1, ..., J\}$, where the number of candidate covariates, J, is quite large (perhaps even larger than the number of observations, n). Assume that an analyst has come to a satisfactory set of $k-1$ explanatory variables $x_1, ..., x_{k-1}$ and wants to try to add new variables u or v, one at a time. Consider the situation when both sets, $\{x_1, ..., x_{k-1}, u\}$ and $\{x_1, ..., x_{k-1}, v\}$, yield the same, or a very close, residual sum of squares and consequently, $\widehat{\sigma}^2$. Then, in terms of the AIC, the two models are indistinguishable because as follows from (1.32), they produce the same AIC value. For example, due to the multicollinearity between $x_1, ..., x_{k-1}$ and u, the first model yields large standard errors and low t-statistics for the least squares estimates and assume that the second model still has satisfactory t-statistics. Clearly, the second model would be better, but the AIC fails to identify it, especially when the design matrix is ill-conditioned. The model selection criterion developed below is free of this drawback.

We turn our attention to the penalized log-likelihood (1.28). Assuming that the prior distribution of parameters is normal, we obtain

$$l \simeq -\frac{k}{2} \ln \omega^2 + l(\mathbf{b}; \mathbf{y}) - \frac{1}{2\omega^2} \|\mathbf{b}\|^2.$$

The maximum of the log-likelihood function over the variance is attained at $\omega^2 = \|\mathbf{b}\|^2 / k$, so the healthy Akaike information criterion takes the form

$$\begin{aligned} HAIC \quad &- \quad H - 2l_{\max} + 2k \tag{1.33} \\ &= \quad H + AIC, \end{aligned}$$

where

$$H = k \left(\ln(\left\| \widehat{\mathbf{b}}_{ML} \right\|^2 / k) - 1 \right).$$

(1.34)

The AIC works well when two models are compared with different numbers of estimated parameters, k, but it fails to discriminate models with the same k and quality of fit when the models are ill-conditioned (ill-posed problems). To illustrate, let us come back to our linear regression example. Consider a linear regression with the number of explanatory variables equals k and the variance $\widehat{\sigma}^2$. Now add a new variable, which is highly correlated with the other variables. The result of such addition in terms of the AIC may not be well reflected because $\widehat{\sigma}^2$ will not change, due to multicollinearity. To the contrary, due to $|\mathbf{X}'\mathbf{X}| \approx 0$, the OLS estimate after addition becomes unstable, which would lead to a large value, $\left\| \widehat{\boldsymbol{\beta}}_{LS} \right\|^2$. The instability will be picked up immediately by HAIC because H becomes large. Now it is clear why the term *healthy* is used to reflect that HAIC works well for ill-posed estimation problems as well.

The healthy AIC works in both directions: when the number of parameters, k, increases and when k is constant. In the latter situation, between two models with the same log-likelihood value, the healthy AIC chooses the model with the shorter estimate length.

1.7   Penalized smoothing

Several authors have pointed out a close relationship between penalized smoothing and the mixed model (Zeger and Diggle, 1994; Wang, 1998; Zhang et al., 1998; Ruppert et al., 2003). To illustrate the connection, we start with the following simplified problem: Let $y_1, y_2, ..., y_n$ be time series data as observations at time $i = 1, 2, ..., n$ (in fact, y may be any equidistant data). We want to find $\mu_1, \mu_2, ..., \mu_n$ such that

$$y_i = \mu_i + \varepsilon_i, \quad i = 1, ..., n,$$

(1.35)

where the $\{\varepsilon_i\}$ are iid random variables with zero mean and constant variance σ^2. Clearly, without any restriction on $\{\mu_i\}$, this problem has a trivial solution, $\mu_i = y_i$. To restrict $\{\mu_i\}$, several cost functions have been suggested. The most popular is the *bending energy* cost function (for further discussion see, e.g., Chalmond, 2003). Then total criterion takes the form

$$\sum_{i=1}^{n} (y_i - \mu_i)^2 + \rho \sum_{i=2}^{n-1} (\mu_{i+1} - 2\mu_i + \mu_{i-1})^2,$$

(1.36)

where ρ is a positive parameter, the penalty coefficient. The first term in (1.36) is the usual sum of squares, and the second term is the penalty on the curvature of $\{\mu_i\}$. Indeed, if the second term is zero, then $\mu_{i+1} = 2\mu_i - \mu_{i-1}$, and by induction we express $\{\mu_i, i = 3, ..., n\}$ through μ_1 and μ_2 as $\mu_{i+1} = i\mu_2 - (i-1)\mu_1 = i(\mu_2 - \mu_1) + \mu_1$. But this is a linear function of i, so the second term puts a penalty on the non-linearity of $\{\mu_i\}$. From calculus, $\mu_{i+1} - 2\mu_i + \mu_{i-1}$ can be viewed as a discrete approximation of the second derivative, so the second term may be viewed as a discretization of the commonly used function $\int [\mu''(x)]^2 dx$ to penalize the nonlinearity.

Several different terminologies are used in the literature for the problem specified by equations (1.35) and (1.36), such as scatter plot smoothing and spline regression.

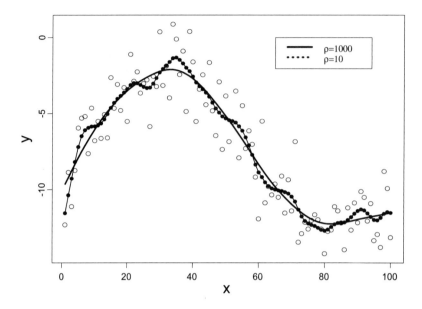

FIGURE 1.2. Penalized smoothing (1.40) with two values of the penalty coefficient, ρ. The larger the penalty coefficient, the smoother the average curve.

Since (1.36) is a quadratic function, its minimization can be expressed through matrix inverse. Indeed, introduce an $n \times (n-2)$ matrix $\mathbf{Q}$ with elements 1 and -2 parallel to the main diagonal; for example,

$$
\mathbf{Q} = \begin{bmatrix}
1 & 0 & 0 & 0 \\
-2 & 1 & 0 & 0 \\
1 & -2 & 1 & 0 \\
0 & 1 & -2 & 1 \\
0 & 0 & 1 & -2 \\
0 & 0 & 0 & 1
\end{bmatrix}
$$

for $n = 6$. Then it is elementary to see that the ith element of vector $\mathbf{Q}'\boldsymbol{\mu}$ is $\mu_i - 2\mu_{i+1} + \mu_{i+2}$, and therefore the second term in sum (1.36) can be represented as $\boldsymbol{\mu}'\mathbf{Q}\mathbf{Q}'\boldsymbol{\mu}$, so that the function to minimize takes the form

$$\|\mathbf{y} - \boldsymbol{\mu}\|^2 + \rho\boldsymbol{\mu}'\mathbf{Q}\mathbf{Q}'\boldsymbol{\mu}. \tag{1.37}$$

Let $\mathbf{X}$ be the $n \times 2$ matrix with the first column 1 and the second column $1, 2, ..., n$. It is elementary to see that $\mathbf{Q}'\mathbf{X} = \mathbf{0}$, so in (1.37) we can make a substitution $\boldsymbol{\mu} = \mathbf{X}\boldsymbol{\beta} + \mathbf{b}_n$ and come to an equivalent minimization problem,

$$\|\mathbf{y} - \mathbf{X}\boldsymbol{\beta} - \mathbf{b}_n\|^2 + \rho\mathbf{b}_n'\mathbf{Q}\mathbf{Q}'\mathbf{b}_n, \tag{1.38}$$

over $\boldsymbol{\beta}$ and $\mathbf{b}_n$, a $n \times 1$ vector. Differentiating with respect to $\boldsymbol{\beta}$, we obtain $\widehat{\boldsymbol{\beta}} = (\mathbf{X}'\mathbf{X})^{-1}\mathbf{X}'\mathbf{y}$ and

$$\widehat{\mathbf{b}}_n = (\mathbf{I} + \rho\mathbf{Q}\mathbf{Q}')^{-1}(\mathbf{y} - \mathbf{X}\widehat{\boldsymbol{\beta}}). \tag{1.39}$$

Equivalently, in terms of (1.39), one can show that the solution to penalized smoothing (1.36) is given by

$$\widehat{\boldsymbol{\mu}} = \mathbf{X}\widehat{\boldsymbol{\beta}} + \widehat{\mathbf{b}}_n = (\mathbf{I} + \rho\mathbf{Q}\mathbf{Q}')^{-1}\mathbf{y}. \tag{1.40}$$

As follows from (1.40), if $\rho = 0$, we come to the trivial solution $\widehat{\boldsymbol{\mu}} = \mathbf{y}$. When $\rho \to \infty$ we obtain the least squares prediction $\widehat{\boldsymbol{\mu}} = \mathbf{X}\widehat{\boldsymbol{\beta}}$. In Figure 1.2 we show data generated with a penalized smoothing with $\rho = 1000$ and $\rho = 10$. Clearly, the first value is more satisfactory. The choice of the penalty coefficient is crucial. Several *ad hoc* methods are available to choose ρ, such as cross-validation or Akaike information (Hurvich, 1998; Jacqmin-Gadda et al., 2002; Ruppert et al., 2003). Below we illustrate how this parameter may be chosen based on a linear mixed effects model.

Now we construct a linear mixed effects (LME) model that leads to automatic choice of the penalty coefficient. Since $\mathbf{X}$ is the fixed effects matrix, we may treat $\mathbf{b}$ as a random effect with uncorrelated components, yielding the following LME model:

$$\mathbf{y} = \mathbf{X}\boldsymbol{\beta} + \mathbf{Z}\mathbf{b} + \boldsymbol{\varepsilon},$$

where

$$\mathbf{Z} = \mathbf{Q}(\mathbf{Q}'\mathbf{Q})^{-1}, \quad \mathbf{b} \sim \mathcal{N}(\mathbf{0}, \sigma^2 d\mathbf{I}_{n-2}), \quad \boldsymbol{\varepsilon} \sim \mathcal{N}(\mathbf{0}, \sigma^2\mathbf{I}_n).$$

This model is a special case of the general LME model (1.10) where $N = 1$ and $\mathbf{D} = d\mathbf{I}_m$ (we use a subindex at the identity matrix to show its size). In brief, this model can be written as $\mathbf{y} \sim \mathcal{N}(\mathbf{X}\boldsymbol{\beta}, \sigma^2(\mathbf{I} + d\mathbf{Z}\mathbf{Z}'))$. Several methods of estimation may be suggested: ordinary or restricted maximum likelihood of Chapter 2 or distribution-free quadratic estimation such as variance least squares, MINQUE, or the method of moments of Chapter 3. As follows from Section 3.7, after d is estimated, there are two equivalent ways to estimate $\boldsymbol{\beta}$ and $\mathbf{b}$ in LME model: using the closed-form formulas

$$\widehat{\boldsymbol{\beta}} = (\mathbf{X}'(\mathbf{I} + \widehat{d}\mathbf{Z}\mathbf{Z}')^{-1}\mathbf{X})^{-1}\mathbf{X}'(\mathbf{I} + \widehat{d}\mathbf{Z}\mathbf{Z}')^{-1}\mathbf{y}, \tag{1.41}$$

$$\widehat{\mathbf{b}} = \widehat{d}(\mathbf{I}_{n-2} + \widehat{d}\mathbf{Z}'\mathbf{Z})^{-1}\mathbf{Z}'(\mathbf{y} - \mathbf{X}\widehat{\boldsymbol{\beta}}) \tag{1.42}$$

or as the minimizers of the penalized function,

$$\|\mathbf{y} - \mathbf{X}\boldsymbol{\beta} - \mathbf{Z}\mathbf{b}\|^2 + d^{-1}\|\mathbf{b}\|^2.$$

To show the equivalence among (1.41), (1.42), and (1.40), where $\rho = 1/d$, we use the dimension-reduction formula of Section 2.2.3. Then, since $\mathbf{Z}'\mathbf{X} = \mathbf{0}$ (1.41) simplifies to the OLS estimate and prediction from the LME model, $\mathbf{X}\widehat{\boldsymbol{\beta}} + \mathbf{Z}\widehat{\mathbf{b}}$ yields (1.40).

In a nonequidistant case, $x_1 < x_2 < ... < x_n$ instead of $\mu_{i+1} - 2\mu_i + \mu_{i-1} = \delta_i$, we have

$$\frac{\mu_{i+1} - \mu_i}{x_{i+1} - x_i} - \frac{\mu_i - \mu_{i-1}}{x_i - x_{i-1}} = \delta_i, \quad i = 2, ..., n-1, \tag{1.43}$$

where μ_0 and μ_{n+1} are fixed and unknown and $\delta_i \sim \mathcal{N}(0, \sigma^2 d)$. This model can be applied in a more general setting of spline (or semiparametric) regression with covariates $\mathbf{U}$: for example, $\mathbf{y} = \mathbf{U}\boldsymbol{\beta} + \mathbf{Z}\mathbf{b} + \boldsymbol{\varepsilon}$, where components of vector μ satisfy (1.43). Again, introducing an appropriate band matrix $\mathbf{Q}$, we reduce the model to LME model $\mathbf{y} = \mathbf{X}\boldsymbol{\beta} + \mathbf{Z}\mathbf{b} + \boldsymbol{\varepsilon}$, where $\mathbf{X}$ is composed of two vectors, $\mathbf{1}$ and $\mathbf{x}$, augmented by matrix $\mathbf{U}$. This method can be applied to a regression coefficient as well; for example, $y_i = \boldsymbol{\beta}'\mathbf{u}_i + \mu_i x_i + \varepsilon_i$, where the $\{\mu_i\}$ satisfy (1.43) and $\mathbf{u}_i$ is a vector of adjustment covariates.

Other more complicated LME models may be suggested: for example, to account for autocorrelation (see the literature cited at the beginning of this section).

1.8   Penalized polynomial fitting

One can apply a mixed model to any regression model where penalization is required. For example, here we use this approach for a fully parametric model with a polynomial of high degree. More specifically, without loss of generality, let $x_1 < x_2 < ... < x_n$ and

$$y_i = \boldsymbol{\beta}'\mathbf{u}_i + \sum_{k=2}^{K} b_{k-1} x_i^k + \varepsilon_i, \quad i = 1, ..., n, \tag{1.44}$$

where the $\{\mathbf{u}_i\}$ are design (explanatory) variables and the $\{b_k, k = 1, ..., K-1\}$ are unknown coefficients. For a reason to be explained later, we start from the second degree; the linear part (x) can be represented in the fixed effects $(\mathbf{u}_i)$. It is assumed that maximum polynomial degree, K, may be sufficiently large but known. To avoid multicollinearity, instead of x_i^k we can use Legendre orthogonal polynomials $P_k(x_i)$ of the kth degree, so model (1.44) can be replaced by

$$y_i = \boldsymbol{\beta}'\mathbf{u}_i + \sum_{k=2}^{K} b_{k-1} P_k(x_i) + \varepsilon_i. \tag{1.45}$$

By construction, $\sum_{i=1}^{n} P_k(x_i)P_j(x_i) = 0$ for $k \neq j$ and $\sum_{i=1}^{n} P_k^2(x_i) = 1$, which simplifies further computation. Introducing a $(K-1) \times 1$ vector $\mathbf{p}_i = (P_2(x_i), P_3(x_i), ..., P_K(x_i))'$, we come to a regression (conditional) model $y_i|\mathbf{b} = \boldsymbol{\beta}'\mathbf{u}_i + \mathbf{b}'\mathbf{p}_i + \varepsilon_i$, and in conjunction with the *a priori* distribution for the polynomial coefficients, treated as random effects, we arrive at the LME model,

$$\mathbf{y}|\mathbf{b} = \mathbf{U}\boldsymbol{\beta} + \mathbf{P}\mathbf{b} + \varepsilon, \quad \mathbf{b} \sim \mathcal{N}(0, \sigma^2 \mathbf{D}). \tag{1.46}$$

There may be several strategies to specify matrix $\mathbf{D}$. First, we can assume that $\mathbf{D}$ is proportional to the identity matrix. Second, $\mathbf{D}$ may be unstructured, but this would involve a large number of estimated parameters, $K(K-1)/2$. Third, we can penalize the high degree, in other words, nonlinearity, as we did in the penalized smoothing model (1.36). Let us take the latter approach. We note that the curvature of the elementary polynomial x^k is associated with the second derivative. Since for fixed x the second derivative of x^k is proportional to $k(k-1)$, we can assume that the diagonal elements of matrix $\mathbf{D}$ are reciprocals of the curvature. For instance, assuming that $\{b_k\}$ do not correlate for $K = 4$, we have

$$\mathbf{D} = d \begin{bmatrix} [2(2-1)]^{-2} & 0 & 0 \\ 0 & [3(3-1)]^{-2} & 0 \\ 0 & 0 & [4(4-1)]^{-2} \end{bmatrix},$$

where d is the scaled unknown variance. This choice means that the variance of $\{b_{k-1}, k = 2, ..., K\}$ is decreasing with k and proportional to $1/[k(k-1)]^2$. Combining this into (1.46), we finally arrive at the LME model,

$$\mathbf{y} \sim \mathcal{N}(\mathbf{U}\boldsymbol{\beta}, \sigma^2(\mathbf{I} + d\mathbf{PDP}')). \tag{1.47}$$

If the scaled variance d were known, we would estimate $\boldsymbol{\beta}$ and $\mathbf{b}$ from

$$\|\mathbf{y} - \mathbf{U}\boldsymbol{\beta} - \mathbf{Pb}\|^2 + d^{-2}\mathbf{b}'\mathbf{D}^{-1}\mathbf{b} \Rightarrow \min_{\boldsymbol{\beta}, \mathbf{b}},$$

so $1/d$ acts as the penalty coefficient. If the scaled variance is large, the contribution of the penalty term is negligible and we come to an unconstrained least squares estimation of model (1.45). Vice versa, if $d \to 0$, we suppress the polynomial part and simply estimate regression $\mathbf{y} = \mathbf{U}\boldsymbol{\beta} + \boldsymbol{\varepsilon}$. Thus, the d estimation becomes the first priority of the penalized polynomial fitting.

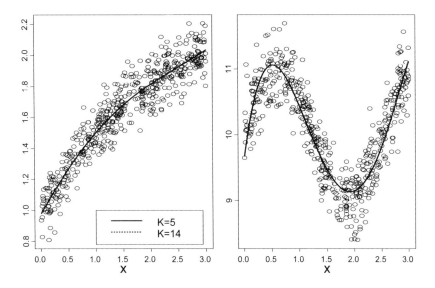

FIGURE 1.3. Two penalized polynomial fittings. The fitting is robust to the choice of the highest degree, K.

Again, several methods are available to estimate d: ordinary or restricted maximum likelihood or noniterative quadratic estimation. In Figure 1.3 we show two penalized polynomial fittings with the penalty coefficient, d, estimated from the linear mixed model (1.47). Points in the left-hand panel were generated as $y_i = x_i^{1.3}(1 + x_i)^{-1} + \varepsilon_i$ and in the right-hand panel as $y_i = \sin(2.5x_i) + 10 + \varepsilon_i$, where the $\{x_i\}$ are randomly distributed on the interval $(0, 1)$ and $\varepsilon_i \sim \mathcal{N}(0, 0.1^2)$, $i = 1, ..., 500$. For this model, the first column of matrix $\mathbf{U}$ is 1 and the second column is $\{x_i\}$. We can draw the following conclusions: (a) the penalized polynomial fitting can adequately approximate nonpolynomial functions such as sin; and (b) since the higher degree is penalized more severely, the choice of K does not make much difference. In particular, polynomials with the highest degree $K = 5$ and $K = 14$ produce almost identical approximation (polynomial curves with $K = 5$ and $K = 14$ overlap).

1.9   Restraining parameters, or what to eat

We have shown above how to restrain (penalize) coefficients in a linear model. In this section we illustrate how a mixed model may be applied to cope with multidimensionality in a nonlinear model: namely, logistic regression with a large number of parameters.

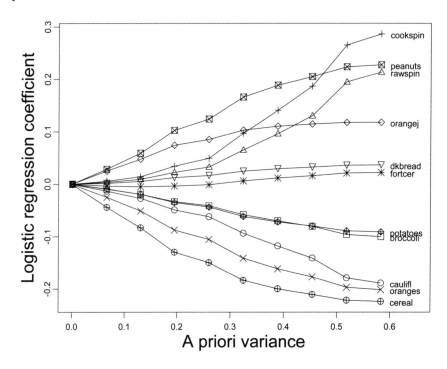

FIGURE 1.4. Coefficients in logistic regression as a function of *a priori* variance σ^2 in the penalized log-likelihood (1.51). Cauliflower, raw oranges, and cereal protect against adenoma, but eating peanuts and spinach increases risk.

A problem with a large number of parameters emerges in nutritional epidemiology (Willett, 1990). To be concrete, let us consider the effect of diet on the health status represented by a binary variable y: If the health status is satisfactory we say that $y = 0$; otherwise, $y = 1$. Let $z_{i1}, z_{i2}, ..., z_{im}$ indicate how much the jth food item was consumed monthly by the ith person, $i = 1, ..., n$. Then, to determine the diet effect, one may relate y_i to $\{z_{ij}, j = 1, ..., m\}$ through logistic regression as

$$\Pr(y_i = 1) = \frac{\exp(\beta_0 + \beta_1 z_{i1} + ... + \beta_m z_{im})}{1 + \exp(\beta_0 + \beta_1 z_{i1} + ... + \beta_m z_{im})}, \quad i = 1, ..., n. \qquad (1.48)$$

If a food item increases the probability, $\beta > 0$ ("bad" food); otherwise, $\beta < 0$ ("good" food). Typically, y codes the presence of a disease and quantities z are obtained from a questionnaire. If the number of food items is large (e.g., so large that it exceeds the number of observations), one obtains a wide range of coefficient values with high standard errors. Thus, to obtain meaningful estimates, the food coefficients should be restrained or penalized. A popular idea in epidemiology to reduce the number of food items is to consider food agglomerates, such as calories, fat, fiber, folate, and so on. This approach is realized in a special DIETSYS program developed under the National Institutes of Health, which replaces a list of original food items with a linear combination representing those agglomerates. Another approach is based on the energy adjustment method (Brown et al., 1994). A big disadvantage of those approaches is that the endpoint recommendation of what to eat is expressed in the agglomerate form, such as "eat less fat food and more vegetables" and therefore is not specific. The approach we discuss here is designed to answer the question: Exactly which food items help to improve health status? To restrain the large number of parameters, a nonlinear mixed model is used.

As an example, we consider a nutritional questionnaire study to reduce the recurrence of colorectal adenoma (Baron et al., 1998). A multicenter study was aimed to investigate the possible beneficial effects of folate intake (mostly from vegetables) based on a questionnaire of patients with at least one recent large-bowel adenoma. It was found that neither cigarette smoking nor folate intake was associated with increased risk of adenoma recurrence. The dependent variable is $y_i = 1$ if for the ith person there was adenoma recurrence and $y_i = 0$ otherwise for $i = 1, 2, ..., n = 751$ people. Thus, according to the logistic regression model (1.48), a large positive coefficient would indicate a risk-increasing food (*bad*) and a negative coefficient would indicate a risk-preventive food (*good*). We do not aim to provide a comprehensive statistical analysis but illustrate how the mixed effects methodology can help to cope with a large number of parameters. Therefore, only $m = 11$ food items were taken into consideration.

Basically, the mixed model is a Bayesian model with unknown food variance, σ^2 as in Section 1.4. More precisely, we treat (1.48) as a conditional model: If $\boldsymbol{\beta} = (\beta_1, ..., \beta_m)'$ were known, then the probability of having an adenoma recurrence is expressed by equation (1.48). *A priori*, we assume that food does not affect recurrence, so we can write

$$\boldsymbol{\beta} \sim \mathcal{N}(\mathbf{0}, \sigma^2 \mathbf{I}). \tag{1.49}$$

This means that the mean of regression coefficients is zero and that, they are independent and have variation σ^2. Equations (1.48) and (1.49) define the generalized linear mixed model (GLMM), to be studied in Chapter 7. To estimate σ^2, we obtain the marginal likelihood with $\boldsymbol{\beta}$ integrated out as

$$l(\beta_0, \sigma^2) = (2\pi\sigma^2)^{-m/2} \int_{R^m} e^{l(\beta_0, \boldsymbol{\beta}) - 0.5\sigma^{-2}\|\boldsymbol{\beta}\|^2} d\boldsymbol{\beta}, \tag{1.50}$$

where $l(\beta_0, \boldsymbol{\beta})$ is the ordinary log-likelihood for model (1.48). Direct integration is prohibitive because dimension m is large (in our case, $m = 11$). Therefore, approximate methods for integral (1.50), such as Laplace approximation or quasi-likelihood, should be used. After estimates $\widehat{\sigma}^2$ and $\widehat{\beta}_0$ are obtained, we derive the posterior means for $\boldsymbol{\beta}$ that maximize the penalized log-likelihood,

$$l(\widehat{\beta}_0, \boldsymbol{\beta}) - 0.5\widehat{\sigma}^{-2}\|\boldsymbol{\beta}\|^2. \tag{1.51}$$

Note that in the Bayesian approach we need to define values for β_0 and σ^2, but in mixed model we obtain them from the data.

In Figure 1.4 we plot posterior regression coefficients as a function of *a priori* variance, σ^2. When the variance is zero, all coefficients are zero. Indeed, the second term in the penalized log-likelihood function (1.51) then prevails, yielding $\boldsymbol{\beta} = \mathbf{0}$. Larger σ^2 implies less penalty and more variation in the regression coefficients. When $\sigma^2 \to \infty$, GLMM converges to ordinary logistic regression. Interestingly, cereal, raw oranges, and cauliflower prevent adenoma, but peanuts and spinach increase the risk.

1.10   Ill-posed problems, Tikhonov regularization, and mixed effects

Mixed models may be considered a tool for solving ill-posed problems. Let $\theta_1, \theta_2, ..., \theta_m$ be system inputs and let $f_1, f_2, ..., f_n$ be a system output. For example, consider an image reconstruction problem based on the Near-Infra Red (NIR) technique. The light goes through a semitransparent body with the absorption density θ_j at location (u_j, v_j) within the body. More details may be found in a recent book by Barrett and Myers (2004). Due to the law of optics, if $\{\theta_j, j = 1, ..., m\}$ were known, the light intensity f_i at detector i on the periphery of the body would be known exactly as a function of $\{\theta_j\}$, or in vector form, $f_i = f_i(\boldsymbol{\theta})$, where $\boldsymbol{\theta}$ is the m-dimensional unknown vector. Vector $\boldsymbol{\theta}$ is called the system vector parameter or, in statistical language, simply the parameter. Having n measurements on the periphery, $\{y_1, ..., y_n\}$, we want to reconstruct the optical properties *within* the body (absorption coefficients), $\{\theta_1, ..., \theta_m\}$, at as many points as possible—this is an inverse problem. An interested reader may read more about statistical aspects of inverse problems in a review paper by Evans and Stark (2002).

Often, inverse problems are ill-posed. In our example we would like to have as few detectors and as many points as possible, so dimensions n and m are close. Besides, the system is usually noisy, leading to a nonlinear regression problem,

$$y_i = f_i(\boldsymbol{\theta}) + \varepsilon_i, \quad i = 1, 2, ..., n. \tag{1.52}$$

To obtain estimates of $\boldsymbol{\theta}$, the least squares criterion is generally used, $\sum_{i=1}^{n} (y_i - f_i(\boldsymbol{\theta}))^2 \Rightarrow \min$. However, since $m \approx n$ and functions $f_i(\boldsymbol{\theta})$ are nonlinear, estimation (reconstruction) of $\boldsymbol{\theta}$ becomes problematic. Therefore, the problem is called *ill-posed*. A Russian mathematician, Tikhonov (Tikhonov and Arsenin, 1977), suggested augmenting the sum of squares by a quadratic term that leads to the functional

$$T(\boldsymbol{\theta}) = \sum_{i=1}^{n} (y_i - f_i(\boldsymbol{\theta}))^2 + \rho \left\| \boldsymbol{\theta} \right\|^2, \tag{1.53}$$

where ρ is called the *regularization parameter* ($\rho > 0$). The original ill-posed problem becomes a well-posed problem. Tikhonov regularization became very popular in applied mathematics and engineering, with a variety of applications: solution of an ill-conditioned linear system, integral equations, density estimation, image reconstruction, and so on. Although several heuristic techniques are available to assess the regularization parameter, such as cross-validation, there is no unified approach to the selection of ρ (Vogel, 2002). However, selection of the value of the regularization parameter is crucial: If ρ is close to 0, we come again to an ill-posed problem; if ρ is too large, the solution degenerates to $\widehat{\boldsymbol{\theta}} = \mathbf{0}$. Strictly speaking, the problem of ill-posedness is just reduced to another problem: the selection of ρ.

Tikhonov regularization may be treated from a statistical point of view, interpreting the inverse problem as a mixed model written in a hierarchical (two-stage) fashion. Indeed, following the line of the Bayesian approach, we assume that $\boldsymbol{\theta}$ is random and (1.52) is treated as a conditional equation, where the $\{\varepsilon_i\}$ are normally distributed with zero mean and constant (system) variance σ^2. Assume that our prior experience says that the component values of vector $\boldsymbol{\theta}$ are expected to be in the neighborhood of zero with certain variance σ_θ^2; or more precisely, $\theta_j \sim \mathcal{N}(0, \sigma_\theta^2)$. This is called the *prior* distribution for the parameters. Let us assume for awhile that the system variance, σ^2, and parameter variance, σ_θ^2, are known. After observations $\{y_i\}$ are collected, we may ask how our prior distribution changes to become a *posterior* distribution with the density $f(\boldsymbol{\theta}|\mathbf{y}) = C \times f(\mathbf{y}|\boldsymbol{\theta})f(\boldsymbol{\theta})$, where C is the normalizing constant, $f(\mathbf{y}|\boldsymbol{\theta})$ is the conditional density, and $f(\boldsymbol{\theta})$ is the parameter density (see Section 1.4). Since we assume normal distribution,

$$f(\mathbf{y}|\boldsymbol{\theta}) = (2\pi\sigma)^{-n/2}e^{-\frac{1}{2\sigma^2}\|\mathbf{y}-\mathbf{f}(\boldsymbol{\theta})\|^2}, \quad f(\boldsymbol{\theta}) = (2\pi\sigma_\theta)^{-m/2}e^{-\frac{1}{2\sigma_\theta^2}\|\boldsymbol{\theta}\|^2}.$$

Note that the posterior distribution, $f(\boldsymbol{\theta}|\mathbf{y})$, is not a normal distribution of $\boldsymbol{\theta}$, and the "center" of the distribution would give an idea of where the posterior values are concentrated. Let us take the *mode* of the distribution, where the density takes its maximum. In image processing and reconstruction literature the model is called MAximum a Posteriori (MAP) estimation (Geman and Geman, 1984; Besag, 1986, 1989). Since the variances are known, the MAP estimator for $\boldsymbol{\theta}$ reduces to the minimization problem,

$$\frac{1}{\sigma^2}\|\mathbf{y} - \mathbf{f}(\boldsymbol{\theta})\|^2 + \frac{1}{\sigma_\theta^2}\|\boldsymbol{\theta}\|^2 \Rightarrow \min_{\boldsymbol{\theta}}. \tag{1.54}$$

But this is the Tikhonov functional (1.53) with $\rho = \sigma^2/\sigma_\theta^2$.

Summing up:

1. The Tikhonov regularization procedure can be derived through the Bayesian approach with known variances of the system error and *a priori* parameters assuming a normal distribution.

2. The regularization (penalty) coefficient is the ratio of the system to the parameter variance.

3. The Tikhonov solution is the mode of the posterior distribution, the MAP estimator.

4. The Tikhonov solution assumes that the *a priori* value of the parameter is zero.

We make several comments. First, if the system is not too noisy but there is substantial *a priori* variation in $\boldsymbol{\theta}$, the regularization parameter should be small. Second, the assumption that the *a priori* value of the parameter is zero may be inadequate. For example, in the NIR problem this would mean that the absorption is zero, which is equivalent to assuming that the body is absolutely transparent (as a vacuum). It would be better to assume that $\theta_j \sim \mathcal{N}(\theta_0, \sigma_\theta^2)$, so that the modified Tikhonov functional takes the form

$$\sum_{i=1}^{n}(y_i - f_i(\boldsymbol{\theta}))^2 + \rho \left\| \boldsymbol{\theta} - \theta_0 \right\|^2, \tag{1.55}$$

where θ_0 is the background absorption coefficient. Although the Bayesian interpretation gives Tikhonov regularization a nice statistical interpretation, the problem of selection of the regularization parameter remains. Now we shall show that using a *mixed effects* approach, ρ can be obtained along with $\boldsymbol{\theta}$. The following reasoning follows the line of penalized likelihood of Section 1.5, the only difference being that now we apply it to reducing an ill-posed problem to a well-posed problem.

In the mixed effects approach, we change nothing in the Bayesian approach except for the assumption that σ^2 and σ_θ^2 are unknown along with $\boldsymbol{\theta}$. Thus, the mixed model is written in hierarchical fashion as

$$\mathbf{y}|\boldsymbol{\theta} \sim \mathcal{N}(\mathbf{f}(\boldsymbol{\theta}), \sigma^2 \mathbf{I}_n), \quad \boldsymbol{\theta} \sim \mathcal{N}(\boldsymbol{\theta}_0, \sigma_\theta^2 \mathbf{I}_m), \tag{1.56}$$

where $\mathbf{I}$ is an identity matrix of the appropriate size and $\boldsymbol{\theta}_0$ is known. Model (1.56) belongs to the family of nonlinear mixed effects model studied in Chapter 8. Since only the observations $\{y_i\}$ are available to estimate the parameters, we need to find the marginal distribution with the likelihood expressed via an integral as

$$L(\sigma^2, \sigma_\theta^2) = (2\pi\sigma^2)^{-n/2}(2\pi\sigma_\theta^2)^{-m/2}\int_{R^m} e^{-\frac{1}{2\sigma^2}\|\mathbf{y}-\mathbf{f}(\boldsymbol{\theta})\|^2 - \frac{1}{\sigma_\theta^2}\|\boldsymbol{\theta}-\boldsymbol{\theta}_0\|^2} \, d\boldsymbol{\theta}.$$

One could maximize L over the unknown parameters σ^2 and σ_θ^2 to obtain the maximum likelihood (ML) estimation that involves a multidimensional integration. The core of the approximation methods to the ML solution is the Laplace approximation (1.27), implemented in Section 8.8; we also refer the reader to Section 8.15. The easiest way to estimate the variance parameters is to approximate $\mathbf{f}$ by a linear function about $\boldsymbol{\theta}_0$, see Section 8.6. Then model (1.56) simplifies to a LME model $\mathbf{e} \sim \mathcal{N}(\mathbf{0}, \sigma^2(\mathbf{I}+d\mathbf{Z}\mathbf{Z}'))$, where $d = \sigma_\theta^2/\sigma^2$ and $\mathbf{Z} = \partial\mathbf{f}/\partial\boldsymbol{\theta}$ is evaluated at $\boldsymbol{\theta} = \boldsymbol{\theta}_0$. The maximum likelihood algorithm for estimation of σ^2 and d is described in the next section. When the variance parameters are known, estimation of *a posteriori* $\boldsymbol{\theta}$, as follows from the Laplace approximation (1.27), is almost equivalent to minimization of (1.55), where $\rho = 1/d$. Symbolically,

MAP estimator = mixed model ML estimator,

but unlike MAP, we do not require values for σ^2 and σ_θ^2 (specifically for their ratio), which are estimated from maximization of L. The appropriate methods are to be studied extensively in Chapter 8. In fact, the choice of ρ based on our mixed model has much in common with what other authors suggested based on the noise level, σ^2 (Kirsch, 1996; Kress, 1999; Colton et al., 2000). Notice that model (1.56) allows a combination of repeated measurements of $\mathbf{y}$, leading to a multilevel mixed model. This nonlinear mixed model technique has been applied to breast image reconstruction by microwave, with promising results (Meaney et al., 2001).

Application of the mixed model methodology to a linear image reconstruction is described in Section 1.11. We provide a constructive procedure to estimate the regularization parameter, ρ in the penalized least squares (1.54) from the data.

1.11 Computerized tomography and linear image reconstruction

Computerized (sometimes called computed) tomography (CT) reconstructs an image from projections. Thus, by measuring signals on the periphery of the body, CT reconstructs what is inside the body. This technique has many applications in radiology, and the interested reader can learn more from Andrews and Hunt (1977), Hall (1979), Herman (1980), Parker (1990), Seeram (1994), and Kak and Slaney (2001) among others. Epstein (2003) provides a comprehensive account of mathematical aspects of image reconstruction with medical applications. An up-to-date and complete discussion of image analysis is given in a book by Barrett and Myers (2004).

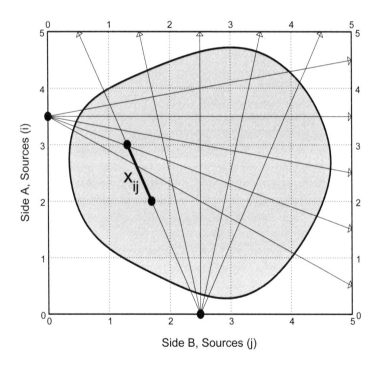

FIGURE 1.5. Principal idea of CT image reconstruction from projections. Beams penetrate the body so that the initial signal intensity is reduced. Measuring the exit intensities at several locations, CT reconstructs the attenuation coefficient in each box. Plotting these attenuation coefficients results in an image.

A CT device consists of several sources and detectors located on the periphery of a square or circle—we refer the reader to Figure 1.5, where the principal idea of a CT scan is represented schematically. Beams of x-rays or light come out of the source at a given angle, penetrate the body, and are received at detectors on an opposite side. If I_0 is the initial intensity of the beam, which comes in at one end of a homogeneous bar of length x and comes out at the other end with intensity I_1, with a certain degree of approximation we have $I_1 = I_0 e^{-\theta x}$, where θ is called the *attenuation coefficient*. If a nonhomogeneous bar is composed of m homogeneous bars of length x_i and attenuation coefficient θ_i, the intensity at the end is $I_1 = I_0 e^{-\sum_{i=1}^{m} \theta_i x_i}$, or on the log scale, $y = \sum_{i=1}^{m} \theta_i x_i$, where $y = \ln(I_0/I_1)$. This simple formula gives rise to the CT image reconstruction. Imagine that the body is divided into m small boxes (dotted lines in Figure 1.5) and within each box the attenuation coefficient θ_j is constant, $j = 1, ..., m$. If the beam comes out from the source at a given angle, we can compute the length of the ray within each box so that the following representation takes place:

$$y_i = \sum_{j=1}^{m} x_{ij} \theta_j + \varepsilon_i, \quad i = 1, ..., n, \qquad (1.57)$$

where i is the number of beams, x_{ij} is the length of the ith beam within the jth box, and ε_i is the iid random term (see Figure 1.5). Since beam angles are predefined, $\{x_{ij}, i = 1, ..., n, j = 1, ..., m\}$ are fixed numbers and can be derived from the CT hardware specification. Having n measurements $\{y_i\}$, we reconstruct (estimate in statistical terminology) m attenuation coefficients $\{\theta_j\}$. Plotting $\{\theta_j\}$ at appropriate locations yields a CT image, so the set of attenuation coefficients $\{\theta_j\}$ is called an *image*. The larger θ_j, the denser the image. This is a linear image reconstruction because it reduces to a linear problem. Special features of this problem are: (a) since we want to see as many pixels as possible, m and n are close; and (b) the number of estimated coefficients, m, is large; for example, to see a 64×64 image, we have $m = 62^2 = 3844$ unknown parameters. This makes the CT problem ill-posed. To improve the least squares solution, several approaches have been put forward, such as Tikhonov regularization and the Bayesian approach. The former requires knowledge of the regularization parameter, and the latter requires complete specification of an *a priori* image.

We apply the mixed effects approach, in which the *a priori* image is not specified completely but is up to some unknown parameters. Then the regularization parameter is estimated from the CT data along with attenuation coefficients. Introducing the $n \times m$ projection matrix $\mathbf{X}$ with elements x_{ij}, we rewrite (1.57) in vector form as

$$\mathbf{y} = \mathbf{X}\boldsymbol{\theta} + \boldsymbol{\varepsilon}, \qquad (1.58)$$

where $\boldsymbol{\varepsilon} \sim \mathcal{N}(\mathbf{0}, \sigma^2 \mathbf{I}_n)$ and $\mathbf{I}_n$ is the $n \times n$ identity matrix. Model (1.58) is an ordinary linear regression model with the efficient least squares (LS) estimator $\widehat{\boldsymbol{\theta}}_{LS} = (\mathbf{X}'\mathbf{X})^{-1}\mathbf{X}'\mathbf{y}$. This estimator is valid if $n > m$. When m approaches n, the LS estimator becomes unstable because matrix $\text{cov}(\widehat{\boldsymbol{\theta}}_{LS}) = \sigma^2 (\mathbf{X}'\mathbf{X})^{-1}$ becomes unstable as well. Consequently, a small perturbation in data leads to a large perturbation in $\widehat{\boldsymbol{\theta}}_{LS}$. To improve the solution, we use *a priori* information on the image to be reconstructed. For example, we may know how the image may look from previous experiments. Statistically, if $\boldsymbol{\theta}_0$ is the prior image, we write

$$\boldsymbol{\theta} = \boldsymbol{\theta}_0 + \mathbf{b}, \qquad (1.59)$$

where $\boldsymbol{\theta}$ is known and $\mathbf{b}$ is the deviation, a random vector. The reader will immediately recognize that $\mathbf{b}$ may be treated as the random effect, so that the couple (1.58) and (1.59) specify a linear mixed effects model, or, more precisely, a linear model with random coefficients. It is simplest to assume that $\mathbf{b} \sim \mathcal{N}(\mathbf{0}, \sigma^2 d\mathbf{I}_m)$, where d is the scaled variance.

A distinctive feature of the LME model from the Bayesian standpoint is that we do not specify variances σ^2 and d, but estimate them along with $\boldsymbol{\theta}$. In the rest of this section we provide a constructive algorithm to estimate $\boldsymbol{\theta}$ and σ^2 and d, which becomes the reciprocal of the penalty coefficient in the Tikhonov regularization (1.55).

The two equations (1.58) and (1.59) can be combined to produce a one-equation statistical model

$$\mathbf{y} \sim \mathcal{N}(\mathbf{X}\boldsymbol{\theta}_0, \sigma^2(\mathbf{I}_n + d\mathbf{X}\mathbf{X}')). \tag{1.60}$$

Our plan to estimate σ^2 and d is as follows. First we estimate σ^2 and d by maximum likelihood. Second, we apply the penalized least squares with the regularization parameter d^{-1} to derive an improved *a posteriori* image. For details, we refer the reader to Chapter 2. Another, pedagogical purpose of the following derivation is for the reader to get a flavor of the statistical and matrix algebra techniques to be used throughout the book.

Letting $\mathbf{e} = \mathbf{y} - \mathbf{X}\boldsymbol{\theta}_0$, the log-likelihood, up to a constant term, can be written as

$$l(\sigma^2, d) = -0.5 \left\{ n \ln \sigma^2 + \ln \left| \mathbf{I}_n + d\mathbf{X}\mathbf{X}' \right| + \sigma^{-2} \mathbf{e}'(\mathbf{I}_n + d\mathbf{X}\mathbf{X}')^{-1}\mathbf{e} \right\}, \tag{1.61}$$

where $\mathbf{I}_n$ is the identity matrix of the order indicated. Using the dimension-reduction formulas of Section 2.2.3, we obtain

$$\left| \mathbf{I}_n + d\mathbf{X}\mathbf{X}' \right| = \left| \mathbf{I}_m + d\mathbf{X}'\mathbf{X} \right|, \quad (\mathbf{I}_n + d\mathbf{X}\mathbf{X}')^{-1} = \mathbf{I}_n - d\mathbf{X}(\mathbf{I}_m + d\mathbf{X}'\mathbf{X})^{-1}\mathbf{X}'.$$

Let $\lambda_1, ..., \lambda_m$ be the eigenvalues and $\mathbf{p}_1, ..., \mathbf{p}_m$ the corresponding eigenvectors of matrix $\mathbf{X}'\mathbf{X}$. Then we can represent

$$\mathbf{e}'\mathbf{X}(\mathbf{I}_m + d\mathbf{X}'\mathbf{X})^{-1}\mathbf{X}'\mathbf{e} = \sum_{j=1}^{m} \frac{w_j^2}{1 + d\lambda_j}, \quad \ln \left| \mathbf{I}_m + d\mathbf{X}'\mathbf{X} \right| = \sum_{j=1}^{m} \ln(1 + d\lambda_j),$$

where $w_j = \mathbf{e}'\mathbf{X}\mathbf{p}_j$. Then (1.61) simplifies to

$$-0.5 \left\{ n \ln \sigma^2 + \sigma^{-2} \left[S - d \sum_{j=1}^{m} w_j^2(1 + d\lambda_j)^{-1} \right] + \sum_{j=1}^{m} \ln(1 + d\lambda_j) \right\},$$

where $S = \mathbf{e}'\mathbf{e}$. When d is held fixed, the maximum over σ^2 is computed exactly:

$$\sigma_s^2 = n^{-1} \left[S - d_s \sum_{j=1}^{m} \frac{w_j^2}{1 + d_s\lambda_j} \right].$$

When σ^2 is held fixed, we use the fixed-point iterations

$$d_{s+1} = d_s \frac{\sum_{j=1}^{m} w_j^2(1 + d_s\lambda_j)^{-2}}{\sigma_s^2 \sum_{j=1}^{m} \lambda_j(1 + d_s\lambda_j)^{-1}}, \quad s = 0, 1, 2, ...$$

See Appendix 13.3.4 for a general discussion of optimization algorithms, including the FP algorithm. We can start from $\sigma_0^2 = (S - \sum_{j=1}^{m} w_j^2/\lambda_j)/n$ and $d_0 = \sum_{j=1}^{m} w_j^2/\lambda_j^2/(m\sigma_0^2)$. At convergence, we obtain $\widehat{\sigma}_{ML}^2$ and $\widehat{d}_{ML}$.

To obtain the posterior image, $\widehat{\boldsymbol{\theta}}$, after σ^2 and d are determined, we can use a closed-form formula or derive $\widehat{\boldsymbol{\theta}}$ from the penalized least squares (PLS); the equivalence is proved in Section 3.7. The PLS takes the form

$$\|\mathbf{y} - \mathbf{X}\boldsymbol{\theta}_0 - \mathbf{X}\boldsymbol{\theta}\|^2 + \widehat{d}_{ML}^{-1}\|\boldsymbol{\theta} - \boldsymbol{\theta}_0\|^2 \Rightarrow \min_{\boldsymbol{\theta}}. \tag{1.62}$$

Denoting $\boldsymbol{\theta}_0 - \boldsymbol{\theta} = \mathbf{b}$, we come to the Tikhonov optimization criterion function $\|\mathbf{y} - \mathbf{X}\mathbf{b}\|^2 + \rho\|\mathbf{b}\|^2$, where $\rho = 1/\widehat{d}_{ML}$. This is a quadratic function of $\boldsymbol{\theta}$ and the closed-form solution exists. Thus, the final mixed effects (ME) CT image is given by

$$\widehat{\boldsymbol{\theta}} = \boldsymbol{\theta}_0 + \left(\mathbf{X}'\mathbf{X} + \widehat{d}_{ML}^{-1}\mathbf{I}\right)^{-1}\mathbf{X}'\mathbf{y}. \tag{1.63}$$

When the variance of the random effect is zero, we obtain $\widehat{\boldsymbol{\theta}} = \boldsymbol{\theta}_0$; when $d \to \infty$, the ME estimate converges to the LS estimate, $\widehat{\boldsymbol{\theta}}_{LS}$. The covariance matrix, $\text{cov}(\widehat{\boldsymbol{\theta}}) = \widehat{\sigma}_{ML}^2 \left(\mathbf{X}'\mathbf{X} + \widehat{d}_{ML}^{-1}\mathbf{I}\right)^{-1}$, is well-conditioned, and therefore the ME image is stable. As the reader may notice, (1.62) is the Tikhonov regularization (1.55) with the penalty coefficient equal to the reciprocal of the scaled variance estimate.

We may put other restrictions on the reconstructed image. For example, one may assume that the image is fairly smooth. Then, introducing the $(m-1) \times m$ difference matrix,

$$\mathbf{L} = \begin{bmatrix} 1 & -1 & 0 & 0 & 0 & 0 \\ 0 & 1 & -1 & 0 & 0 & 0 \\ 0 & 0 & 0 & \cdots & \cdots & 0 \\ 0 & 0 & 0 & 0 & 1 & -1 \end{bmatrix}, \tag{1.64}$$

we come to the model $\mathbf{y} \sim \mathcal{N}(\mathbf{X}\boldsymbol{\theta}_0, \sigma^2(\mathbf{I}_n + d\mathbf{W}))$, where $\mathbf{W} = \mathbf{X}\mathbf{L}'\mathbf{L}\mathbf{X}'$ is a fixed matrix. Then, nonsmoothed solutions will be penalized with PLS $\|\mathbf{y} - \mathbf{X}\boldsymbol{\theta} - \mathbf{X}\mathbf{L}'\boldsymbol{\theta}\|^2 + \widehat{d}_{ML}^{-1}(\boldsymbol{\theta} - \boldsymbol{\theta}_0)'$.

It is straightforward to generalize a mixed model (1.60) to a multilevel clustered model where, for example, repeated imaging data may be combined into one pool to detect differences between visits to the doctor, or to determine a trend, differences in gender, differences in age, and so on.

1.12 GLMM for PET

In this section we consider an image reconstruction method popular in medical applications. The statistical solution involves two components: a statistical model and an estimation algorithm. We emphasize that computational features become integral to successful implementation.

Positron emission tomography (PET) is important in nuclear medicine and has features common with x-ray computerized tomography. The difference with the linear image reconstruction considered above is that the observations are not continuous but are photon counts that imply a nonlinear statistical model. Shepp and

Vardi (1982) described PET as a probabilistic model based on the Poisson distribution. A current review of reconstruction methods for PET may be found in Lewitt and Matej (2003). The idea of PET is as follows: A subject is administered a dose of the molecules labeled with radioactive atoms. These atoms are unstable isotopes leading to the emission of gamma-ray photons, which are detected outside the body by a ring of surrounding detectors. To simplify, we consider a two-dimensional PET system. By counting the number of photons in different directions, PET attempts to reconstruct the decay rate, λ, at each point within the body. The PET image is the distribution of these rates. To make the problem solvable, instead of a continuum of points, imagine that the body is divided into m disjoint boxes. The number of decay events, n_j occurring over a fixed time in box j is random and follows the Poisson law with the rate λ_j, so that $E(n_j) = \lambda_j$, $j = 1, ..., m$. Numbers n_j are unobservable and λ_j are unknown. However, there is a ring of detectors around the body which count the total number of decay events in n cross-section tubes. Let the total number of decay events occurring in the ith tube be k_i, $i = 1, ..., n$. There exists a fixed $n \times m$ matrix $\mathbf{A}$ such that $k_i = \sum_{j=1}^{m} a_{ij} n_j$. This matrix, called the projection matrix, is derived from the geometry of the body: tube angle, size, etc. Assuming that counts n_j are independent, k_i also has a Poisson distribution with the rate $E(k_i) = \sum_{j=1}^{m} a_{ij} E(n_j) = \sum_{j=1}^{m} a_{ij} \lambda_j$. Further, assuming that $\{k_i, i = 1, ..., n\}$ are independent, we come to the likelihood function

$$L(\lambda_1, ..., \lambda_m) = \prod_{i=1}^{n} \frac{\left(\sum_{j=1}^{m} a_{ij} \lambda_j \right)^{k_i}}{k_i!} e^{-\sum_{j=1}^{m} a_{ij} \lambda_j}.$$

The log-likelihood, up to a constant term, is

$$l(\lambda_1, ..., \lambda_m) = \sum_{i=1}^{n} \left(k_i \ln \sum_{j=1}^{m} a_{ij} \lambda_j - \sum_{j=1}^{m} a_{ij} \lambda_j \right). \tag{1.65}$$

To find the maximum likelihood estimate, we need to solve m score equations,

$$\frac{\partial l}{\partial \lambda_p} = \sum_{i=1}^{n} \frac{h_{ip}}{\sum_{j=1}^{m} a_{ij} \lambda_j} - r_p = 0, \quad p = 1, ..., m, \tag{1.66}$$

where $h_{ip} = k_i a_{ip}$ and $r_p = \sum_{i=1}^{n} a_{ip}$. Usually, the EM algorithm is used to maximize (1.65):

$$\lambda_{p,s+1} = \frac{\lambda_{ps}}{r_p} \sum_{i=1}^{n} \frac{h_{ip}}{\sum_{j=1}^{m} a_{ij} \lambda_{js}}, \quad p = 1, ..., m, \tag{1.67}$$

with iterations $s = 0, 1, ...$ The iterations can be started from $\lambda_{p0} = r_p^{-1} \sum_{i=1}^{n} a_{ip}^{-1} h_{ip}$. At convergence, $\lambda_{p,s+1} = \lambda_{ps}$, satisfying the score equations (1.66) and meaning that the EM algorithms converges to the maximum likelihood estimate (MLE). Moreover, as follows from the general properties of the EM algorithm, iterations (1.67) increase the log-likelihood value, l from iteration to iteration. For a general discussion of the optimization algorithms used in statistics, including EM, see Appendix 13.3.4.

An alternative maximization algorithm for l is the Newton–Raphson (NR). We rewrite the estimating equations (1.66) in vector form, but first we need the first and second derivatives,

$$\frac{\partial l}{\partial \boldsymbol{\lambda}} = \sum_{i=1}^{n} \frac{k_i}{w_i} \mathbf{a}_i - \mathbf{r}, \qquad \frac{\partial^2 l}{\partial \boldsymbol{\lambda}^2} = -\sum_{i=1}^{n} \frac{k_i}{w_i^2} \mathbf{a}_i' \mathbf{a}_i,$$

where $\boldsymbol{\lambda} = (\lambda_1, ..., \lambda_m)'$, $\mathbf{r} = (r_1, ..., r_m)'$, $w_i = \sum_{j=1}^{m} a_{ij}\lambda_s$, and $\mathbf{a}_i$ is the ith row vector of matrix $\mathbf{A}$. Then the NR iterations are

$$\boldsymbol{\lambda}_{s+1} = \boldsymbol{\lambda}_s + \left(\sum_{i=1}^{n} \frac{k_i}{w_i^2} \mathbf{a}_i' \mathbf{a}_i \right)^{-1} \left(\sum_{i=1}^{n} \frac{k_i}{w_i} \mathbf{a}_i - \mathbf{r} \right). \tag{1.68}$$

Noticing that $E(k_i) = w_i$, we obtain the expected NR or Fisher scoring algorithm:

$$\boldsymbol{\lambda}_{s+1} = \boldsymbol{\lambda}_s + \left(\sum_{i=1}^{n} \frac{1}{w_i} \mathbf{a}_i' \mathbf{a}_i \right)^{-1} \left(\sum_{i=1}^{n} \frac{k_i}{w_i} \mathbf{a}_i - \mathbf{r} \right). \tag{1.69}$$

At the final iteration, the inverse matrix is the covariance matrix for the MLE. This matrix will be needed later for various statistical hypothesis testing. Note that the EM algorithm does not produce this matrix, which may partially explain the fact that little statistical testing has been reported in the PET literature.

Our practice shows that whereas the EM algorithm may be very slow (sometimes it requires 1000 iterations) algorithms (1.68) and (1.69) are very fast and require only four or five iterations to obtain the MLE with the same precision. However, an advantage of the EM algorithm is that it does not require a matrix inverse. Since the number of reconstructed nodes/pixels is typically large, a matrix inverse at each iteration may become a limitation. We can modify the NR or FS to avoid the matrix inverse by employing the idea of the Unit Step (US) algorithm (see also Section 7.1.5). The idea of this algorithm is to obtain an approximation of the matrix inverse from above. For example, for the FS algorithm, we have

$$\sum_{i=1}^{n} w_i^{-1} \mathbf{a}_i' \mathbf{a}_i \le \nu^{-1} \sum_{i=1}^{n} w_i^{-1} \mathbf{a}_i' \mathbf{a}_i = \nu^{-1} \mathbf{A}' \mathbf{A},$$

where $\nu = \min w_i$. Then the US algorithm, as an economical version of the FS algorithm, takes the form

$$\boldsymbol{\lambda}_{s+1} = \boldsymbol{\lambda}_s + \nu_s \left(\mathbf{A}' \mathbf{A} \right)^{-1} \left(\sum_{i=1}^{n} k_i w_i^{-1} \mathbf{a}_i - \mathbf{r} \right), \tag{1.70}$$

where $(\mathbf{A}'\mathbf{A})^{-1}$ is computed once beforehand. Although the US algorithm is usually slower than NR or FS, it is faster than EM and requires a dozen iterations rather than hundreds or even thousands.

PET is, as are many image reconstruction problems, an ill-posed problem because we want to have the number of pixels as large as possible and the number of measurements as small as possible, so that m is close to n. If no *a priori* information is available, the ML estimate is unstable. The Bayesian approach gained much popularity for PET image reconstruction (Hebert and Leahy, 1989; Kaufman, 1993; Fessler, 1994; Qi and Huesman, 2001; De Pierro and Yamagishi, 2001; Nuyts and Fessler, 2003). As mentioned above, under the Bayesian approach *a priori* image does not allow unknown parameters, whereas the mixed model does.

In the following parameterization, we assume that the rate, λ, is expressed through an exponential function as $\lambda = e^\gamma$, which is convenient because (a) one does not have to care about the positiveness of the rate, and (b) it is easy to penalize γ using a normal distribution. Following the line of the generalized linear mixed model (GLMM) technique of Chapter 7, we write the conditional log-likelihood in the form

$$l(\gamma_1, ..., \gamma_m) = \sum_{i=1}^{n} \left(k_i \ln \sum_{j=1}^{m} a_{ij} e^{\gamma_j} - \sum_{j=1}^{m} a_{ij} e^{\gamma_j} \right),$$

where $\gamma_1, ..., \gamma_m$ are iid random rates specified in the second equation as

$$\gamma_j \sim \mathcal{N}(\gamma_0, \sigma^2), \quad j = 1, ..., m,$$

where γ_0 is known and σ^2 is unknown. To obtain a marginal likelihood, we need to use integration,

$$L(\gamma_1, ..., \gamma_m) = \frac{1}{\sigma\sqrt{2\pi}} \int_{R^m} e^{l(\gamma_1, ...\gamma_m) - \frac{1}{2\sigma^2} \sum_{j=1}^{m} (\gamma_j - \gamma_0)^2} d\gamma_1 ... d\gamma_m.$$

This mixed model belongs to the family of Poisson models with random intercepts (see Section 7.5). Since m is large, exact integration is prohibitive. Several methods were developed to avoid integration using approximate estimation. Importantly, to obtain *a posteriori* rates, as follows from Laplace approximation (1.27), we maximize the penalized log-likelihood

$$P = \sum_{i=1}^{n} \left(k_i \ln \sum_{j=1}^{m} a_{ij} e^{\gamma_j} - \sum_{j=1}^{m} a_{ij} e^{\gamma_j} \right) - \sigma^{-2} \sum_{i=1}^{n} (\gamma_i - \gamma_0)^2$$

after σ^2 and γ_0 are estimated. If the image is close to the prior image, σ^2 is small and the second term in P overshadows the first. If the image is far from the prior image, the penalizing term is small. After σ^2 is estimated, one can maximize P by the NR or FS algorithm. The inverse matrix at the final iteration gives the covariance matrix of the mixed model MLE. Many *a priori* assumptions may be realized in the mixed model. For example, if one wants to penalize nonsmoothness $\gamma \sim \mathcal{N}(\gamma_0 \mathbf{1}, \sigma^2 \mathbf{L'L})$, where L is the difference matrix defined in (1.64).

1.13   Maple leaf shape analysis

The mixed model is an adequate statistical model to describe individual variety within a biological category. Indeed, the milestone concepts of the mixed model, the within- and between-subject variation, exactly match the principles of biological variety. Look at Figure 1.6: Nine maple leaves from the same tree have significant individual variation, but at the same time look similar. In the language of the mixed model, population-averaged parameters specify the common biological type (such as average maple leaf), and subject-specific parameters specify subject individuality. In classical statistics, observations are assumed to be independent and identically distributed; in the mixed effects approach, observations from the same individual constitute a cluster and therefore are correlated.

Shape is perhaps the simplest characteristic of a biological subject. We apply mixed model techniques to shape analysis in Chapter 11. Importantly, ordinary shape analysis deals with one shape, whereas a mixed model processes a sample (ensemble) of shapes simultaneously.

An important step in shape analysis is shape quantification, or in other terms, representation of a two-dimensional geometrical object numerically as a sequence of numbers. Typically, different quantification methods lead to different statistical models.

For example, for this maple leaf analysis, we use the Random Fourier Descriptor (RFD) model (see Section 11.7.2 for details). This model deals with pair coordinates, $\{(x_{ij}, y_{ij}), j = 1, 2, ..., n_i\}$ for each shape $i = 1, 2, ..., N$: for example, the outlines of maple leaf images in Figure 1.6. To obtain these coordinates, a characteristic (original) point on each shape should be identified manually, this point is shown by the circle at the top of each maple leaf. Then a traverse technique is implemented. Moving counterclockwise along the image outline, we record (x, y) coordinates, so that eventually we come to the same point/circle (Gonzalez and Woods, 2002). In Figure 1.7 we plot x and y versus the point for each leaf—these are the data with which the mixed model works.

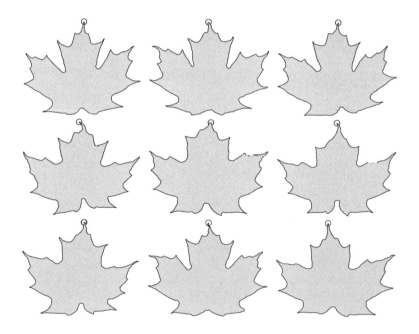

FIGURE 1.6. Nine maple leaf shapes. The circle on the top of each leaf is the starting point where the traverse starts.

An important feature of this shape quantification is that x and y are periodic functions because moving along the shape, one comes to the original point. Therefore, Fourier analysis is an adequate mathematical tool to describe x and y through a linear combination of a finite number of harmonics (see Section 11.7). Ordinarily, such analysis assumes that the Fourier coefficients $\{a_k, k = 1, 2, ..., K\}$ are fixed, where K is the number of harmonics. According to the mixed model methodology, the coefficients vary from shape to shape but stay constant within the population: namely, $a_{ik} = \alpha_k + b_{ik}$, where a_{ik} is the kth Fourier coefficient for the ith shape and α_k is the population-averaged coefficient. The RFD model for shape reduces to a LME model with appropriate formulas and algorithms.

Shape analysis is complicated by the fact that shapes may have different sizes and may be rotated arbitrarily. Fortunately, the traverse method is not affected by rotation, but the size and the specific location of the original point should be taken into account. Thus, before analyzing data in Figure 1.7, normalization and rescaling are required.

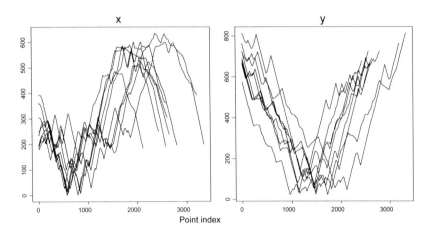

FIGURE 1.7. Quantified maple leaf shapes; x and y coordinates as a function of the traverse point for each shape. Before doing the analysis, these curves must be properly normalized and rescaled.

1.14   DNA Western blot analysis

Western blot analysis (or immunoblotting) is a popular DNA imaging analysis used for the detection of specific proteins. In this technique DNA is electrophoresed through a gel matrix to separate the individual fragments by size. The result of this procedure is a bandlike image. Two typical Western blot images, for a normal patient and a cancer patient, are shown in Figure 1.8.

Special interpretation skills are required to identify blocks and to detect the difference between two sample tissues. Besides general difficulties of interpretation and identification, the variation between samples, laboratories, and patients becomes overwhelming. Needless to say, often the DNA analysis becomes imprecise

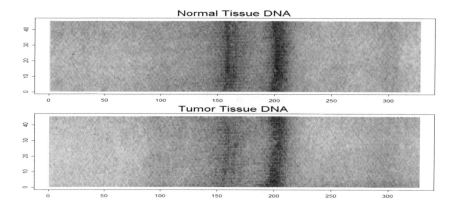

FIGURE 1.8. Typical Western blot 45×327 image for normal- and cancer-patient DNA.

and subjective. Moreover, since the human eye cannot compare hundreds of images, the analysis is reduced to just a few comparisons—biased and false results are unavoidable.

To address sample, laboratory, and patient heterogeneity, a multilevel mixed model should be applied. We quantify the two images and show the result in Figure 1.9. The result of quantification is two matrices with integer values in the range from 0 (absolute black) to 255 (absolute white). The reader may learn more about image quantification in Chapter 12. The columns are interpreted as repeated measurements, and therefore averaging is allowed. Assuming that values are normally distributed (not integers), perhaps the simplest statistical model takes the form

$$\text{Control:} \qquad y_{ij1} = \mu_{j1} + \varepsilon_{ij1},$$
$$\text{Patient:} \qquad y_{ij2} = \mu_{j2} + \varepsilon_{ij2}, \qquad (1.71)$$

where μ_{j1} and μ_{j2} are the mean values at the jth vertical readings and $\varepsilon_{ijk} \sim \mathcal{N}(0, \sigma^2)$ are iid random variables ($k = 1, 2$) and $i = 1, ..., m = 45$ and $j = 1, ..., n = 327$. The null hypothesis is $H_0 : \mu_{1,1} = \mu_{1,2}, \mu_{2,1} = \mu_{2,2}, ..., \mu_{327,1} = \mu_{327,2}$. In this setting, this hypothesis may be tested by the paired t-test applied to average data, $y_{j1} = \sum_{i=1}^{m} y_{ij1}/m$ and $y_{j2} = \sum_{i=1}^{m} y_{ij2}/m$. Several improvements may be made to model (1.71). First, one may assume that observations along the x-axis are dependent. A parsimonious correlation structure can be described by a Toeplitz (band) matrix assuming that observations follow a stationary random process, see Section 4.3.4. Second, one can address the curvature along the y-axis using the model $y_{ijk} = \mu_{j1} + \nu_k(i - m/2) + \alpha_k(i - m/2)^2 + \varepsilon_{ijk}$. Then ν_k and α_k are nuisance curvature coefficients. Again, we are concerned with the same null hypothesis, H_0.

More important, model (1.71) can be used as a building block to test H_0 when repeated measurements are available, such as from different laboratories, tissue samples, etc. For example, if DNA analysis is available for M_1 controls and M_2 cancer patients, we introduce an additional index p so that $y_{ijpk} = \mu_{jk} + b_{pk} + \varepsilon_{ijk}$, where b_{pk} is the subject-specific random effect. Moreover, one may be interested in the dependence of DNA analysis on age, gender, or other covariates $\mathbf{x}_{pk}$, leading to a linear mixed effects model

$$y_{ijpk} = \mu_{jk} + \boldsymbol{\beta}'\mathbf{x}_{pk} + b_{pk} + \varepsilon_{ijpk}.$$

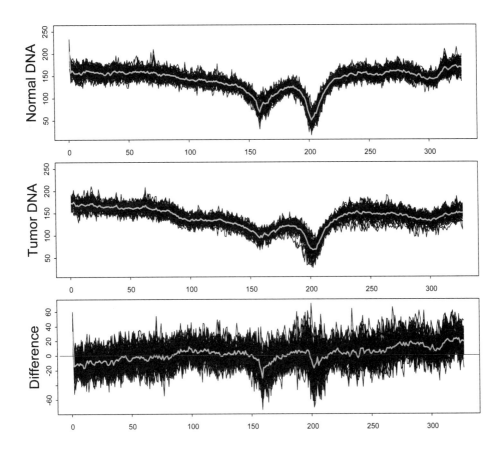

FIGURE 1.9. Quantified Western blot images with the difference. The average across vertical readings is shown by the bold line. The paired t-test produced a p-value of 0.0001.

Obviously, it takes the form (1.10) after combining observations in vectors and matrices. If the covariance matrix ε_{ijpk} is modeled via a Toeplitz matrix, we come to the LME model with linear covariance structure (see Section 4.3).

1.15 Where does the wind blow?

In this section we illustrate how a mixed model may be applied to analyze moving objects. In Figure 1.10 four images of the same sky are taken at 15-second intervals (the camera position was held fixed). From an analysis of these images, we want to determine where the wind blows, or in other words, in what direction/angle the clouds move and with what speed. First, we solve this problem assuming that the shape of the clouds does not change with time. Second, we show how to describe this problem via a nonlinear mixed model under the more realistic assumption that the moving clouds change.

A grayscale image is a $P \times Q$ matrix with integer entries from 0 (absolute black) to 255 (absolute white). Let $M_t(p,q)$ be the intensity of the image at time t at pixel (p,q), where $p = 1, 2, ..., P$ and $q = 1, 2, ..., Q$. In our example, $P = 576$ and $Q = 432$, $t = 1, 2, 3, 4 = T$. See Chapter 12 for more discussion.

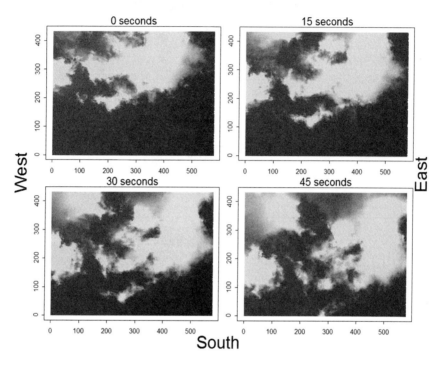

FIGURE 1.10. Pictures of the sky taken at 15-second intervals. Where does the wind blow? We apply the mixed modeling technique to answer this question.

To fix the idea, we consider the case when only two sky images, M_1 and M_2, are available. If pixel (p,q) moved to a new position $(p+\alpha, q+\beta)$, we could identify α and β from nonlinear least squares by minimizing the mean squared error

$$S(\alpha, \beta) = \frac{1}{PQ} \sum_{p=1}^{P} \sum_{q=1}^{Q} [M_1(p,q) - M_2(p+\alpha, q+\beta)]^2.$$

Although $M_1(p,q)$ and $M_2(p,q)$ are discrete functions, actually matrices, we can find the minimum of S; we refer the reader to Section 12.7.7, where a derivative-free algorithm is discussed. In image analysis, we treat elements as functions of p and q, and therefore we use the notation $M(p,q)$ rather than M_{pq}.

Next we assume that there are $t = 1, 2, ..., T$ images moving with a constant speed. Let $M(p,q)$ be the image of the moving object, which is unknown. Since after time t, pixel (p,q) on image M moved to pixel $(p+\alpha t, q+\beta t)$ on image M_t, we find α and β which minimize the MSE,

$$S(\alpha, \beta) = \sum_{t=1}^{T} \left[\frac{1}{|\mathcal{M}|} \sum_{(p,q)\in\mathcal{M}} [M_t(p+\alpha t, q+\beta t) - M(p,q)]^2 \right], \qquad (1.72)$$

where $\mathcal{M}$ is the index set (p, q), so that $1 \leq p + \alpha t \leq P$ and $1 \leq q + \alpha t \leq Q$; $|\mathcal{M}|$ is the number of pair elements in $\mathcal{M}$, or in other words, the number of summation terms. We use MSE rather than a simple sum of squares to account for the number of summation terms; this technique is called affine image registration, see Section 12.7.1 for more details. From (1.72), we immediately obtain the fact that the optimal M is the average,

$$M(p, q) = \overline{M}(p, q) = \frac{1}{T |\mathcal{M}|} \sum_{(p,q) \in \mathcal{M}} M_t(p + \alpha t, q + \beta t), \qquad (1.73)$$

so M is replaced in (1.72) with (1.73) after each iteration for α and β.

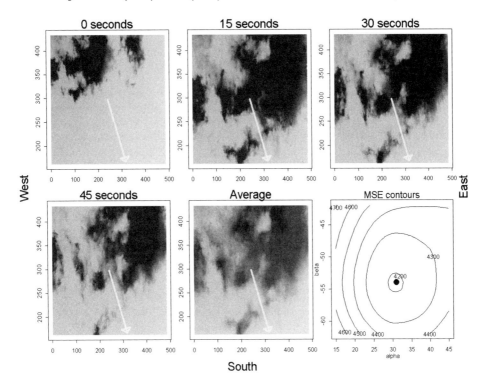

FIGURE 1.11. Reconstructed sky and wind direction indicated by an arrow. The wind blows at -60^0 with speed of 62 pixels per 15 seconds.

After a few iterations we get $\widehat{\alpha} = 31$ and $\widehat{\beta} = -54$, so the angle at which the wind blows is -60^0, indicated by an arrow on the images in Figure 1.11. After α and β are estimated, we estimate the speed as $(\widehat{\alpha}^2 + \widehat{\beta}^2)^{1/2} = 62$ pixels per 15 seconds. In Figure 1.11 we show four images $M_t(p + \widehat{\alpha}t, q + \widehat{\beta}t)$ at $t = 0, 15, 30, 45$, the average image (1.73), and the contours for the mean squared error (1.72) in coordinate system (α, β).

Now we set up a nonlinear mixed effects model (studied in Chapter 8 in a general form). In the least squares criterion (1.72), it was assumed that the moving clouds do not change, which clearly is not true. To account for change, we allow coefficients

α and β to be random, leading us to a statistical model,

$$M_t(p + \alpha(p,q)t, q + \beta(p,q)t) = M(p,q) + \varepsilon(p,q), \qquad (1.74)$$

where $\alpha(p,q)$ and $\beta(p,q)$ are random variables with means α and β, or more specifically,

$$\alpha(p,q) = \alpha + b_\alpha(p,q), \quad \beta(p,q) = \beta + b_\beta(p,q). \qquad (1.75)$$

In this model, $\varepsilon(p,q)$ is the iid error term with zero mean and variance σ^2, and $b_a(p,q)$ and $b_\beta(p,q)$ are treated as random effects with zero mean and the 2×2 covariance matrix $\sigma^2\mathbf{D}$. The stochastic equations (1.74) and (1.75) define a nonlinear mixed effects model. When $\mathbf{D} = \mathbf{0}$, we come to an ordinary nonlinear regression model and criterion (1.72): otherwise, the population-averaged parameters α and β should be estimated using approximate methods from Chapter 8, such as those based on the Laplace approximation.

1.16   Software and books

There are several statistical packages for linear and nonlinear mixed effects model estimation. The most advanced are `proc mixed` for SAS (SAS Institute, Inc.) and library `nlme` (or `lme4`) for R (R Development Core Team, 2011). Other relevant R packages/libraries are `gee` and `MASS` (function `glmmPQL`); all these can be downloaded from `http://www.R-project.org`. The documentation for R functions is usually too succinct for immediate programming. For example, there is no explanation of how to extract the variance-covariance matrix of random effects, $\mathbf{D}_* = \sigma^2\mathbf{D}$, from `lme` or `lme4`, or how to keep these functions running in the case of a failure during simulations—we illustrate these features. However, providing details on the use of this software is beyond the scope of this book. The relevant coverage of linear and nonlinear mixed models within S-Plus is given in the book by Pinheiro and Bates (2000). For SAS users we recommend books by Verbeke and Molenberghs (2009) and Vonesh (2012), which have numerous examples.

A number of books on mixed models have been published. Below is a list arranged in order of similarity to this book:

- McCulloch, C.E. and Searle, S.R. (2001). *Generalized, Linear and Mixed Models*. New York: Wiley.

- Vonesh, E.F. and Chinchilli, V.M. (1997). *Linear and Nonlinear Models for the Analysis of Repeated Measurements*. New York: Marcel Dekker.

- Vonesh, E.F. (2012). *Generalized Linear and Nonlinear Models for Correlated Data. Theory and Applications Using SAS*. Cary, NC: SAS Institute.

- Davidian, M. and Giltinan, D.M. (1995). *Nonlinear Models for Repeated Measurement Data*. London: Chapman & Hall.

- Pan, J.X. and Fang, K.T. (2002). *Growth Curve Models and Statistical Diagnostics*. New York: Springer-Verlag.

- Davis, C.S. (2002). *Statistical Methods for the Analysis of Repeated Measurements*. New York: Springer-Verlag.

- Diggle, P., Heagerty, P., Liang, K.-Y., and Zeger, S. (2002). *Analysis of Longitudinal Data*. Oxford, UK: Oxford University Press.

- Fahrmeir, L. and Tutz, G. (2001). *Multivariate Statistical Modelling Based on Generalized Linear Models*. New York: Springer-Verlag.

- Agresti, A. (2002). *Categorical Data Analysis*. New York: Wiley.

- Pinheiro, J.C. and Bates, D.M. (2000). *Mixed Effects Models in S-Plus*. New York: Springer-Verlag.

- Fitzmaurice, G.M., Laird, N.M., and Ware, J.H. (2011). *Applied Longitudinal Analysis*. Hoboken, NJ: Wiley.

- Hedeker, D. and Gibbons, R.D. (2006). *Longitudinal Data Analysis*. Hoboken: Wiley.

- Verbeke, G. and Molenberghs, G. (2009). *Linear Mixed Models for Longitudinal Data*. New York: Springer-Verlag.

- Fitzmaurice, G., Davidian, M., Verbeke, G., and Molenberghs, G. (Eds.) (2009). *Longitudinal Data Analysis*. Boca Raton, FL: CRC Press.

- Hsiao, C. (2003). *Analysis of Panel Data*. Cambridge, UK: Cambridge University Press.

- Searle, S.R., Casella G., and McCulloch, C.M. (1992). *Variance Components*. New York: Wiley.

1.17   Summary points

- Often, data have a clustered (panel or tabular) structure. Classical statistics assumes that observations are independent and identically distributed (iid). Applied to clustered data, this assumption may lead to false results. In contrast, the mixed effects model treats clustered data adequately and assumes two sources of variation, within cluster and between clusters. Two types of coefficients are distinguished in the mixed model: population-averaged and cluster (or subject)-specific. The former have the same meaning as in classical statistics, but the latter are random and are estimated as posteriori means.

- The linear mixed effects (LME) model may be viewed as a generalization of the variance component (VARCOMP) and regression analysis models. When the number of clusters is small and the number of observations per cluster is large, we treat the cluster-specific coefficients as fixed, and ordinary regression analysis with dummy variables applies, as in the ANOVA model. Such a model is called a fixed effects model. Vice versa, when the number of clusters is large but the number of observations per cluster is relatively small, a random effects model would be more adequate—then the cluster-specific coefficients are random.

- The mixed model technique is a child of the marriage of the frequentist and Bayesian approaches. Similar to the Bayesian approach, a mixed model specifies the model in a hierarchical fashion, assuming that parameters are random. However, unlike the Bayesian approach, hyperparameters are estimated from the data as in the frequentist approach. As in the Bayesian approach, one has to make a decision as to the prior distribution, but that distribution may contain unknown parameters that are estimated from the data, as in the frequentist approach.

- Penalized likelihood is frequently used to cope with parameter multidimensionality. We show that the penalized likelihood may be derived from a mixed model as an approximation of the marginal likelihood after applying the Laplace approximation. Moreover, the penalty coefficient, often derived from a heuristic procedure, is estimated by maximum likelihood as an ordinary parameter.

- The Akaike information criterion (AIC) is used to compare statistical models and to choose the most informative. The AIC has the form of a penalized log-likelihood with the penalty equal to the dimension of the parameter vector. A drawback of the AIC is that it does not penalize ill-posed statistical problems, as in the case of multicollinearity among explanatory variables in linear regression. We develop a healthy AIC that copes with ill-posedness as well because the penalty term involves the average length of the parameter vector. Consequently, among models with the same log-likelihood value and number of parameters, HAIC will choose the model with the shortest parameter vector length.

- Since the mixed model naturally leads to penalized likelihood, it can be applied to penalized smoothing and polynomial fitting. Importantly, the difficult problem of penalty coefficient selection is solved using the mixed model technique by estimating this coefficient from the data. In penalized smoothing, we restrain the parameters through the bending energy, in polynomial fitting through the second derivative.

- The mixed model copes with parameter multidimensionality. For example, if a statistical model contains a large number of parameters, one may assume that *a priori* parameters have zero mean and unknown variance. Estimating this variance from the data, after Laplace approximation we come to the penalized log-likelihood. We illustrate this approach with a dietary problem in conjunction with logistic regression where the number of food items consumed may be large.

- Tikhonov regularization aims to replace an ill-posed problem with a well-posed problem by adding a quadratic penalty term. However, selection of the penalty coefficient is a problem. Although Tikhonov regularization receives a nice statistical interpretation in the Bayesian framework, the problem of the penalty coefficient remains. A nonlinear mixed model estimates the penalty coefficient from the data along with the parameter of interest, $\boldsymbol{\theta}$.

- Computerized tomography (CT) reconstructs an image from projections and belongs to the family of linear image reconstruction. Since the number of image pixels is close to the number of observations, CT leads to an ill-posed problem. To obtain a well-posed problem, *a priori* assumptions on the reconstructed image should be taken into account. We show that a mixed model may accommodate various prior assumptions without complete specification of the prior distribution.

- Positron emission tomography (PET) uses the Poisson regression model for image reconstruction and the EM algorithm for likelihood maximization. Little statistical hypothesis testing has been reported, perhaps due to the fact that the EM algorithm does not produce the covariance image matrix. The Fisher scoring or Unit step algorithms are much faster and allow computation of the covariance matrix needed for various hypothesis testing as if two images in the area of interest are the same. To cope with ill-posedness, Bayesian methods and methods of penalized likelihood have been widely applied. The generalized linear mixed model (GLMM), studied extensively in Chapter 7, also follows the line of the Bayesian approach, but enables estimation of the regularization parameter from PET data. A multilevel GLMM model can combine repeated PET measurements and process them simultaneously, increasing statistical power substantially.

- The mixed model is well suited for the analysis of biological data when, on the one hand, observations are of the same biological category (maple leaf), but on the other hand, individuals differ. Consequently, there are two sources of variation: variation between individuals (intersubject variance) and variation within an individual (intrasubject variance). The common biological type corresponds to population-averaged parameters and individuality corresponds to subject-specific parameters. Shape is the simplest biological characteristic. Its analysis is complicated by the fact that shapes may be rotated and translated arbitrarily. Several mixed models for shape analysis are discussed in Chapter 11.

- Image science enables us to derive a large data set of repeated structure; thus, application of the repeated-measurements model, such as a mixed model, seems natural. Until now, image comparison in medicine has been subjective and based on "eyeball" evaluation of a few images (often, just a couple). Statistical thinking in image analysis is generally poor. For example, a proper DNA Western blot image evaluation should be based on several tissue samples analyzed by a multilevel mixed model.

- Mixed models can be applied for statistical image analysis, particularly to analyze an ensemble of images (see Chapter 12). As with shape analysis, two sources of variation are considered, the within-image and between-images variation. Since an image may be described as a large matrix, we may treat the element as a nonlinear function of the index and apply the nonlinear mixed effects model of Chapter 6. The mixed model can also be applied to study the motion of fuzzy objects such as clouds.

2
MLE for the LME Model

In this chapter the Linear Mixed Effects (LME) model, as it was originally introduced by Laird and Ware (1982), is estimated by the method of maximum likelihood (ML), assuming that distribution of the random terms is normal. It is worthwhile to mention that the variance-covariance matrix of the random effects $\mathbf{D}$ is the key parameter because if this matrix is known, an estimate of the beta coefficients (fixed effects) is found by generalized least squares. This chapter concerns numerical issues in the log-likelihood maximization; statistical issues are considered in Chapter 3.

The reader can consult other books published on the topic (see Section 1.16); in no way we can claim that this chapter covers all computational aspects of the maximum likelihood estimation of the LME model. Section 2.16 compares our own code with a widely known `lme` function in R.

There are several equivalent parameterizations of the log-likelihood function. In particular, the log-likelihood can be simplified by eliminating the within-subject variance σ^2 that leads to the variance-profile log-likelihood function. The dimension-reduction formulas apply to reduce the dimension of the inverse matrices, leading to economical computations. One should remember that the linear mixed effects model is an example of nonlinear statistical estimation on restricted parameter space for matrix $\mathbf{D}$, and therefore special care should be taken to ensure that this matrix stays nonnegative definite during computations. In this chapter several algorithms for the likelihood maximization are considered, with a detailed discussion of their numerical properties. Our choice is the Fisher scoring algorithm because the inverse matrix is always positive definite and its inverse provides the covariance matrix for the entire vector of estimated parameters, including variance parameters.

Matrix algebra, common to all linear models, is the major apparatus in our developments (Searle, 1971a). The reader is referred to several books on matrix algebra with statistical emphasis: Searle (1982), Graybill (1983), Lancaster and Tismenetsky (1985), Magnus (1988), Harville (1997), and Schott (1997).

2.1   Example: weight versus height

To illustrate application of the LME model, let us consider a simple statistical relationship between weight and height using family data in the format (F_k, H_k, W_k), where F_k is the family code/id for the kth person, H_k is his/her height in inches, and W_k is his/her weight in pounds. Typical tabular data on 18 family members (a total of 71 people) are given below, where members of the same family are represented by the family id, from 1 to 18:

F	H (inches)	W (pounds)
1	67	215
1	64	155
1	63	145
1	71	227
1	61	120
1	68	220
...	...	...
18	65	144
18	59	120

Obviously, one can expect that family members have somewhat similar weight and height. Can we use linear regression $W_k = \alpha + \beta H_k + \varepsilon_k$, estimating coefficients α and β by Ordinary Least Squares (OLS), and minimizing the sum of squares of residuals,

$$\sum_{k=1}^{71}(W_k - \alpha - \beta H_k)^2 \ ? \tag{2.1}$$

Apparently, minimization (2.1) ignores the within-family correlation and treats each person/observation independently. Even though ordinary least squares produces unbiased estimates, even when observations are correlated, we may obtain more efficient estimates of α and β accounting for familial correlation. However, to provide a better estimation, we have to specify the correlation structure and construct an estimation procedure that takes that familial correlation into account. The objective of the chapter is to formulate a relevant statistical model that handles data like these and estimate the model by maximum likelihood under the normal distribution assumption. The consequences of ignoring familial correlation are studied in Section 3.9, where we show that the OLS estimator remains unbiased but has larger standard errors (is less efficient).

Now we specify how to address familial correlation using the mixed effects approach. A proper model for the familial relationship between weight and height makes use of double indexing (i, j), where i denotes the ith family and j denotes the jth member of the ith family (cluster). Then, if a family consists of n_i members, the vectors $\mathbf{W}_i = (W_{i1}, W_{i2}, ..., W_{in_i})'$ and $\mathbf{H}_i = (H_{i1}, H_{i2}, ..., H_{in_i})'$ would represent the weight and height data of individuals, with a total number of observations $\sum_{i=1}^{18} n_i = 71$. We can model clustered correlation assuming that there is a positive constant correlation coefficient ρ between members of the same family, $\text{cor}(W_{ij}, W_{ik}) = \rho$ for $j \neq k$ for all $i = 1, 2, ..., N$, where N denotes the number of families (in our case, $N = 18$). However, in the spirit of mixed effects modeling, we come to the same statistical model, introducing a random intercept. (The model with random intercepts is considered in detail in Section 2.4.) Indeed, it is more realistic to assume that each family has its own intercept, $a_i = \alpha + b_i$, where b_i is a random variable (random effect) with zero mean and unknown variance σ_d^2, and α is the common intercept. In the language of the mixed effects approach, we call a_i a subject (or family)-specific and parameter α the population-averaged parameter (Davidian and Giltinan, 1995; Vonesh and Chinchilli, 1997). Thus, if the linear model with random intercepts is written in the form $\mathbf{W}_i = a_i + \beta \mathbf{H}_i + \boldsymbol{\varepsilon}_i$, where $\boldsymbol{\varepsilon}_i$ is the random vector with zero mean and uncorrelated components with variance σ^2, replacing a_i with $\alpha + b_i$ one arrives at the linear mixed effects model,

$$\mathbf{W}_i = \alpha + \beta \mathbf{H}_i + b_i \mathbf{Z}_i + \boldsymbol{\varepsilon}_i, \quad i = 1, ..., N, \tag{2.2}$$

where $\mathbf{Z}_i = \mathbf{1}_i = (1, 1, ..., 1)'$ is a vector column of dimension n_i. It is easy to see that the covariance matrix of $\mathbf{W}_i$ has the form $\sigma^2 \mathbf{V}_i$, where the $n_i \times n_i$ matrix $\mathbf{V}_i$ is defined as

$$\mathbf{V}_i = \begin{bmatrix} 1 + \sigma_d^2/\sigma^2 & \cdots & \sigma_d^2/\sigma^2 \\ \vdots & \ddots & \vdots \\ \sigma_d^2/\sigma^2 & \cdots & 1 + \sigma_d^2/\sigma^2 \end{bmatrix}. \tag{2.3}$$

Clearly, this covariance structure implies an equivi-correlation (compound symmetry) structure because $\mathrm{cor}(W_{ij}, W_{ik}) = \rho = \sigma_d^2/(\sigma^2 + \sigma_d^2)$. The key point of the mixed effects model is that we obtain more efficient estimates for α and β, minimizing the weighted sum of squares

$$\sum_{i=1}^{N=18} (\mathbf{W}_i - \alpha - \beta \mathbf{H}_i)' \mathbf{V}_i^{-1} (\mathbf{W}_i - \alpha - \beta \mathbf{H}_i), \tag{2.4}$$

which produces the generalized least squares estimate. Obviously, one needs the ratio σ_d^2/σ^2 to realize the weighted least squares; this ratio may be estimated by maximum likelihood assuming normal distribution—this method is discussed in this chapter. Also, the variance parameters may be estimated by a quadratic function of $\mathbf{W}_i$, without assuming the normal distribution (see Chapter 3).

In Section 2.4.2 we investigate how the generalized least squares estimate for β is affected by σ_d^2/σ^2.

2.1.1 The first R script

In this section we show how to estimate the simplest linear mixed model, or more specifically, the linear model with random intercepts, using the function `lme` in R with the family data discussed previously. You have to install the library `nlme` in your R before running the scripts shown below. The library `nlme` contains all necessary software components to estimate linear and nonlinear mixed models. Go to R page `http://www.r-project.org/` and type 'nlme' in the search box (located at left) using a Google search (you can also search other libraries and packages this way). Put the zipped version of the package in some directory on your computer (the default subdirectory is \\Downloads) and unzipp to the `library` subdirectory of R (you may see other libraries as well). Then issue `library(nlme)` in the command line.

The data on 18 families are contained in the text file `Family.txt` with variable names (headers) in the first row. Assuming that this file is located in the directory `c:\\MixedModels\\R\\`, we use the `read.table` function to open the file

```
famdat=read.table("c:\\MixedModels\\Chapter02\\Family.txt",header=T,
                                                       stringsAsFactors=F)
```

The dataframe `famdat` has six columns: `Height`, `Weight`, `Sex`, `ParentChild`, `Age`, and `FamilyID`. In this particular example, we shall use only three variables, `Height`, `Weight`, and `FamilyID`. The option `stringsAsFactors=F` means that the input data are treated as purely numeric (the default value is T). Other variables will be used in future examples to estimate more complicated mixed models. To estimate the relationship between weight and height with a family-specific intercept, we issue the following command:

```
out.lme=lme(fixed=Weight~Height,random=~1|FamilyID,data=famdat)
```

Two parts should be specified in `lme`: the fixed effects part (`fixed`) and the random effects part (`random`). The syntax for both parts is the same as the specification of a standard linear regression model in R (function `lm`). In the fixed effects part ~ separates the dependent variable at the left from the list of independent variables at the right (in our case one independent variable, `Height`); `random=~1` means that the only intercept is random. Clusters are specified via the vertical bar |. In our example, |`FamilyID` means that observations with the same `FamilyID` value constitute a cluster. The `lme` function is dicussed further in Section 2.16.

The call to `lme` described above produces the following output after issuing the `summary(out.lme)`:

```
Linear mixed-effects model fit by REML
 Data: famdat
 Log-restricted-likelihood: -331.6369
 Fixed: Weight ~Height
(Intercept) Height
-206.832149 5.345309
Random effects:
 Formula: ~1 | FamilyID
 (Intercept) Residual
StdDev: 14.07057 24.70590
Number of Observations: 71
Number of Groups: 18
```

As follows from this output, the common intercept is $\widehat{\alpha} = -206.83$ and the slope is $\widehat{\beta} = 5.35$, so that weight and height are related as $W = -206.83 + 5.35H$. The estimates of the standard deviations are $\widehat{\sigma}_d = 14.07$ and $\widehat{\sigma} = 24.71$. We estimate the correlation coefficient of weights among individuals of the same family as $\widehat{\rho} =$

$14.07^2/(14.07^2 + 24.71^2) = 0.244$. Other parts of the output, such as `REML` and `Log-restricted-likelihood`, are explained in Section 2.2.7.

Problems for Section 2.1

1. Estimate slope β using the data `Family.txt`, assuming that the family-specific intercepts are fixed, using the dummy variable technique. [Hint: Estimate the linear regression model with 1+18=19 parameters using `lm(y~X-1)`, where `y=famdat$Weight` and `X` is the 71×19 matrix with the first column `famdat$Height` and the other 18 columns as dummy variables.]

2. Denote $d = \sigma_d^2/\sigma^2$ as the scaled (or relative) variance of the random intercept. Express the covariance matrix (2.3) in the form $\mathbf{I}+d\mathbf{1}\mathbf{1}'$, where $\mathbf{1}$ is the column-vector of 1s.

3. Write an R code to plot the slope estimate, $\widehat{\beta} = \left(\sum_{i=1}^{18} \mathbf{X}_i' \mathbf{V}_i^{-1} \mathbf{X}_i\right)^{-1} \times \left(\sum_{i=1}^{18} \mathbf{X}_i' \mathbf{V}_i^{-1} \mathbf{y}_i\right)$, the weighted sum of squares minimizer of (2.4), where $\mathbf{X}_i = [\mathbf{1}_i, \mathbf{H}_i]$ and $\mathbf{V}_i$ is defined in (2.3), as a function of d in the range $0 \leq d \leq 20$. Show three estimates on this plot using lines of different color (use `legend`): (1) OLS, (2) REML, and (3) the family-specific intercept approach from Problem 1.

4. Incorporate `Sex` (and possibly `Age`) into the model using `fixed=Weight~Height +Age`. Is `Age` statistically significant? Provide an interpretation for the model.

2.2   The model and log-likelihood functions

In this section we formulate the linear mixed effects model under the normal assumption and provide several equivalent parameterizations of the log-likelihood function.

2.2.1   The model

In this chapter we study the Linear Mixed Effects (LME) model in the form developed by Laird and Ware (1982),

$$\mathbf{y}_i = \mathbf{X}_i\boldsymbol{\beta} + \mathbf{Z}_i\mathbf{b}_i + \boldsymbol{\varepsilon}_i, \qquad i = 1, ..., N, \tag{2.5}$$

where:

- $\mathbf{y}_i$ is an $n_i \times 1$ vector of responses of the ith subject; also called an individual or cluster.

- $\mathbf{X}_i$ is an $n_i \times m$ design matrix of explanatory variables; also called covariates or fixed effects.

- $\boldsymbol{\beta}$ is an $m \times 1$ vector of population parameters; also called population-averaged or fixed effects coefficients.

- $\mathbf{Z}_i$ is an $n_i \times k$ design matrix of random effects.

- $\boldsymbol{\varepsilon}_i$ is an $n_i \times 1$ error term with independent components, each of them having zero mean and the within-subject variance σ^2.

- $\mathbf{b}_i$ is an $k \times 1$ vector of random effects with zero mean and covariance matrix $\mathbf{D}_* = \sigma^2 \mathbf{D}$.

It is assumed that all random vectors $\{\mathbf{b}_i, \boldsymbol{\varepsilon}_i, i = 1, ..., N\}$ are mutually independent.

Throughout the book we use boldface type to denote vectors and matrices. Usually, we use lowercase for vectors and uppercase for matrices. The inequality sign for matrices, as in $\mathbf{A} \le \mathbf{B}$ $(\mathbf{A} < \mathbf{B})$, means that matrix $\mathbf{B} - \mathbf{A}$ is nonnegative (positive) definite. Recall that a symmetric matrix $\mathbf{C}$ is called nonnegative definite if $\mathbf{a}'\mathbf{Ca} \ge 0$ for all nonzero $\mathbf{a}$ (matrix $\mathbf{C}$ is said to be positive definite if $\mathbf{a}'\mathbf{Ca} > 0$). We often use Greek letters to denote random unobservable variables such as error terms.

To make the LME model identifiable for $\boldsymbol{\beta}$, we assume that matrix $\sum \mathbf{X}_i'\mathbf{X}_i$ is nonsingular and that $\sum n_i > m$. To make the LME model identifiable for σ^2 and $\mathbf{D}$, we assume that at least one matrix $\mathbf{Z}_i'\mathbf{Z}_i$ is positive definite and

$$\sum_{i=1}^{N}(n_i - k) > 0 \tag{2.6}$$

(see the details in Section 3.2). We call a LME model *balanced* if $n_i = $const and the design matrices of random effects $\mathbf{Z}_i$ are the same for all subjects/clusters, $\mathbf{Z}_i = \mathbf{Z}$. We call a random-coefficient model (1.12) *balanced* if, in addition, the design matrix of fixed effects is the same for all individuals, $\mathbf{X}_i = \mathbf{X}$ (see Section 2.3). Balanced models are important special cases of (2.5) because they admit closed-form solutions for the maximum likelihood estimate (MLE). We call a LME model a balanced growth curve model if $\mathbf{X}_i = \mathbf{X}$ and $\mathbf{Z}_i = \mathbf{I} \otimes \mathbf{q}_i$, where $\mathbf{q}_i$ is a vector column (see Section 4.1.5 for details).

The log-likelihood function for the LME model is simpler if the *scaled* covariance matrix of the random effects is used,

$$\mathbf{D} = \frac{1}{\sigma^2}\mathbf{D}_* = \frac{1}{\sigma^2}\text{cov}(\mathbf{b}_i). \tag{2.7}$$

With this parameterization, σ^2 can be factored out, that is expressed in the closed form holding other parameters fixed (that is why we prefer to work with matrix $\mathbf{D}$). We use the asterisk $_*$ for the usual (non-scaled) covariance matrix of the random effects; we use this notation particularly in Chapter 3 when considering a distribution-free quadratic estimation.

Getting back to the family data example, the model for the relationship between weight and height (2.2) is a special case of (2.5) with one random effect $(k = 1)$, where $\mathbf{y}_i = \mathbf{W}_i$,

$$\boldsymbol{\beta} = \left[\begin{array}{c} \alpha \\ \beta \end{array} \right], \quad \mathbf{X}_i = [\mathbf{1}_i; \mathbf{H}_i], \quad \mathbf{Z}_i = \mathbf{1}_i,$$

where $\mathbf{1}_i$ is the $n_i \times 1$ vector-column of 1s.

N equations of (2.5) can be compressed into one as

$$\mathbf{y} = \mathbf{X}\boldsymbol{\beta} + \mathbf{Z}\mathbf{b} + \boldsymbol{\varepsilon} \tag{2.8}$$

after stacking the data in a single vector and matrix form as follows:

$$
\mathbf{y} = \begin{bmatrix} \mathbf{y}_1 \\ \mathbf{y}_2 \\ \vdots \\ \mathbf{y}_N \end{bmatrix}, \ \mathbf{X} = \begin{bmatrix} \mathbf{X}_1 \\ \mathbf{X}_2 \\ \vdots \\ \mathbf{X}_N \end{bmatrix}, \ \mathbf{Z} = \begin{bmatrix} \mathbf{Z}_1 & 0 & 0 \\ 0 & \ddots & 0 \\ 0 & 0 & \mathbf{Z}_N \end{bmatrix},
$$

$$
\mathbf{b} = \begin{bmatrix} \mathbf{b}_1 \\ \mathbf{b}_2 \\ \vdots \\ \mathbf{b}_N \end{bmatrix}, \ \boldsymbol{\varepsilon} = \begin{bmatrix} \boldsymbol{\varepsilon}_1 \\ \boldsymbol{\varepsilon}_2 \\ \vdots \\ \boldsymbol{\varepsilon}_N \end{bmatrix} \tag{2.9}
$$

are of order $N_T \times 1$, $N_T \times m$, $N_T \times Nk$, $Nk \times 1$ and $N_T \times 1$ respectively, where

$$
N_T = \Sigma_{i=1}^{N} n_i \tag{2.10}
$$

is the total number of observations, and $\mathrm{cov}(\mathbf{b}) = \sigma^2 (\mathbf{I} \otimes \mathbf{D})$. Model (2.8) can be rewritten with one error term as

$$
\mathbf{y} = \mathbf{X}\boldsymbol{\beta} + \boldsymbol{\eta}, \tag{2.11}
$$

where

$$
\boldsymbol{\eta} = \begin{bmatrix} \boldsymbol{\eta}_1 \\ \boldsymbol{\eta}_2 \\ \vdots \\ \boldsymbol{\eta}_N \end{bmatrix} = \begin{bmatrix} \boldsymbol{\varepsilon}_1 + \mathbf{Z}_1 \mathbf{b}_1 \\ \boldsymbol{\varepsilon}_2 + \mathbf{Z}_2 \mathbf{b}_2 \\ \vdots \\ \boldsymbol{\varepsilon}_N + \mathbf{Z}_N \mathbf{b}_N \end{bmatrix}. \tag{2.12}
$$

$E(\boldsymbol{\eta}) = \mathbf{0}$, and the $N_T \times N_T$ covariance matrix of $\boldsymbol{\eta}$ has block diagonal form:

$$
\mathbf{V} = \sigma^2 \begin{bmatrix} \mathbf{I}_{n_1} + \mathbf{Z}_1 \mathbf{D} \mathbf{Z}_1' & 0 & 0 & 0 \\ 0 & \mathbf{I}_{n_2} + \mathbf{Z}_2 \mathbf{D} \mathbf{Z}_2' & 0 & 0 \\ \vdots & \vdots & \ddots & \vdots \\ 0 & 0 & \ldots & \mathbf{I}_{n_N} + \mathbf{Z}_N \mathbf{D} \mathbf{Z}_N' \end{bmatrix}. \tag{2.13}
$$

Hereafter, the LME model written in one matrix equation (2.8) or (2.11) will be referred to as "long" notation.

In this chapter it is assumed that $\mathbf{b}_i$ and $\boldsymbol{\varepsilon}_i$ are normally distributed as

$$
\boldsymbol{\varepsilon}_i \sim \mathcal{N}(\mathbf{0}, \sigma^2 \mathbf{I}), \qquad \mathbf{b}_i \sim \mathcal{N}(\mathbf{0}, \sigma^2 \mathbf{D}),
$$

where $\mathbf{I} = \mathbf{I}_{n_i}$ is an $n_i \times n_i$ identity matrix. Therefore, the LME model (2.5) with normally distributed random variables can be written in marginal form as

$$
\mathbf{y}_i \sim \mathcal{N}\left(\mathbf{X}_i \boldsymbol{\beta}, \sigma^2 (\mathbf{I} + \mathbf{Z}_i \mathbf{D} \mathbf{Z}_i') \right), \quad i = 1, ..., N. \tag{2.14}
$$

In the first two chapters we study the LME model specified by (2.5), which assumes that the components of the error vector are uncorrelated [$\mathrm{cov}(\boldsymbol{\varepsilon}_i)$ is proportional to the identity matrix]. In Chapter 4, particularly in Section 4.3, we extend the model to the case when this covariance matrix has a more complex structure, such as autocorrelation, when the dependent variable is the time series. The reader is referred to Section 4.4, where the normal distribution is viewed as a second-order approximation to the original distribution.

2.2.2 Log-likelihood functions

Dropping the constant term $C = -(N_T/2)\ln(2\pi)$, the log-likelihood function for the LME model is given by

$$
l(\boldsymbol{\theta}) = -\frac{1}{2}\Big\{ N_T \ln\sigma^2 + \sum_{i=1}^{N}\Big[\ln|\mathbf{I} + \mathbf{Z}_i\mathbf{D}\mathbf{Z}_i'|
$$

$$
+\sigma^{-2}(\mathbf{y}_i - \mathbf{X}_i\boldsymbol{\beta})'(\mathbf{I} + \mathbf{Z}_i\mathbf{D}\mathbf{Z}_i')^{-1}(\mathbf{y}_i - \mathbf{X}_i\boldsymbol{\beta})\Big]\Big\}, \tag{2.15}
$$

where

$$
\boldsymbol{\theta} = (\boldsymbol{\beta}', \sigma^2, \text{vech}'(\mathbf{D}))
$$

is a combined vector of unknown parameters. Hereafter vech($\mathbf{D}$) denotes the $k(k+1)/2$ vector of unique elements of symmetric matrix $\mathbf{D}$ (Magnus, 1988). Hence, the total dimension of the parameter vector $\boldsymbol{\theta}$ is $m + 1 + k(k+1)/2$. The Maximum Likelihood Estimate (MLE) maximizes the function l over the parameter space

$$
\boldsymbol{\Theta} = \{\boldsymbol{\theta} : \boldsymbol{\beta} \in R^m, \sigma^2 > 0, \mathbf{D} \text{ is nonnegative definite}\}. \tag{2.16}
$$

Note that we seek an estimate of matrix $\mathbf{D}$ on the set of all nonnegative definite matrices, which will be denoted $\mathbb{D}_+$ with a finite boundary, where matrix $\mathbf{D}$ is singular. The parameter space (2.16) will be referred to as Nonnegative Definite (ND). It is used traditionally in the literature on mixed models for maximization of the likelihood function. Sometimes, a more restrictive parameter space is used, assuming that matrix $\mathbf{D}$ is positive definite. For example, this assumption is used in the library nlme in R. The disadvantage of parameter space with a positive definite matrix $\mathbf{D}$ is that the MLE may not exist when the maximum of the likelihood function occurs on the boundary (see more detail in Section 2.5). For example, the chance to hit the boundary of $\boldsymbol{\Theta}$ is very high, especially for relatively small N, and special attention should be given to recognize this situation during the maximization algorithm because the value of the log-likelihood function is finite when $|\mathbf{D}| = 0$. Some remedies are discussed in Section 2.15. It is easy to show that the ND parameter space is convex. Moreover, we show that $\boldsymbol{\Theta}$ is a convex cone: If $\boldsymbol{\theta}_1, \boldsymbol{\theta}_2 \in \boldsymbol{\Theta}$ then $\lambda_1\boldsymbol{\theta}_1 + \lambda_2\boldsymbol{\theta}_2 \in \boldsymbol{\Theta}$ for any nonnegative scalars λ_1, λ_2. This follows from the fact that a nonnegative linear combination of two nonnegative (positive) definite matrices is a nonnegative (positive) definite matrix.

There exists an alternative approach taken by Rao and Kleffé (1988), who assumed that matrix $\mathbf{D}$ may not necessarily be nonnegative (or positive) definite provided that matrix (2.13) is positive definite. The latter holds if and only if all matrices $\mathbf{I} + \mathbf{Z}_i\mathbf{D}\mathbf{Z}_i'$ are positive definite. Thus, Rao-Kleffe (RK) parameter space is defined as

$$
\boldsymbol{\Theta} = \{\boldsymbol{\theta} : \boldsymbol{\beta} \in R^m, \sigma^2 > 0, \mathbf{I} + \mathbf{Z}_i\mathbf{D}\mathbf{Z}_i' \text{ is positive definite for every } i = 1, ..., N\}. \tag{2.17}
$$

Maximization of the log-likelihood function over this parameter space is somewhat easier because $l \to -\infty$ with probability 1 when $\mathbf{D}$ approaches the boundary of this parameter space (see more detail in Section 2.15.2).

Omission of the term C in (2.15) does not affect l maximization and ML estimates. However, when the likelihood values are compared with a different number of observations or when the exact likelihood function is compared to its approximate value via statistical simulations, this constant should be taken into account. We omit C for simplification.

The scaled covariance matrix of the vector of the dependent variable $\mathbf{y}_i$ is given by

$$\mathbf{V}_i = \mathbf{V}_i(\mathbf{D}) = \mathbf{I} + \mathbf{Z}_i \mathbf{D} \mathbf{Z}_i'; \tag{2.18}$$

this notation is used throughout the chapter. Random effects induce within-cluster correlation between components of vector $\mathbf{y}$, because the matrix $\mathbf{V}_i$ is not diagonal.

Using the notation $\mathbf{V}_i$, the log-likelihood function (2.15) can be rewritten as

$$l(\boldsymbol{\theta}) = -\frac{1}{2} \left\{ N_T \ln \sigma^2 + \sum_{i=1}^{N} \left[\ln |\mathbf{V}_i| + \sigma^{-2} \mathbf{e}_i' \mathbf{V}_i^{-1} \mathbf{e}_i \right] \right\}, \tag{2.19}$$

where

$$\mathbf{e}_i = \mathbf{e}_i(\boldsymbol{\beta}) = \mathbf{y}_i - \mathbf{X}_i \boldsymbol{\beta} \tag{2.20}$$

is an $n_i \times 1$ residual vector for the ith cluster, $i = 1, ..., N$.

Three equivalent types of parameterization for the log-likelihood function (2.15) exist:

1. *Dimension-reduction parameterization.* Standard log-likelihood function (2.15) involves $n_i \times n_i$ matrix inverse and determinant calculation. One can reduce the dimension to k using the dimension-reduction formulas provided below.

2. *Profile-likelihood.* One can take advantage of the fact that the optimum vector of fixed effects $\boldsymbol{\beta}$ and the within-subject variance σ^2 may be expressed via matrix $\mathbf{D}$, so that they can be eliminated from the log-likelihood function. Two profile-functions will be considered: variance-profile and full-profile.

3. *Inverse $\mathbf{D}$ (or precision matrix) parameterization.* In the dimension-reduction parameterization, one notices that the log-likelihood function can be expressed via $\mathbf{D}^{-1}$, which excludes the matrix inverse. From computational point of view, the most economical form of the log-likelihood is full-profile inverse $\mathbf{D}$ parameterization.

2.2.3   Dimension-reduction formulas

We will use the following *dimension-reduction* formulas:

$$\begin{aligned} \mathbf{V}_i^{-1} &= (\mathbf{I}_{n_i} + \mathbf{Z}_i \mathbf{D} \mathbf{Z}_i')^{-1} = \mathbf{I}_{n_i} - \mathbf{Z}_i (\mathbf{I}_k + \mathbf{D} \mathbf{Z}_i' \mathbf{Z}_i)^{-1} \mathbf{D} \mathbf{Z}_i' \\ &= \mathbf{I}_{n_i} - \mathbf{Z}_i \mathbf{D} (\mathbf{I}_k + \mathbf{Z}_i' \mathbf{Z}_i \mathbf{D})^{-1} \mathbf{Z}_i' = \mathbf{I}_{n_i} - \mathbf{Z}_i (\mathbf{D}^{-1} + \mathbf{Z}_i' \mathbf{Z}_i)^{-1} \mathbf{Z}_i', \end{aligned} \tag{2.21}$$

where matrix $\mathbf{V}_i$ is given by (2.18). These formulas may be verified by direct multiplication (the last identity holds when matrix $\mathbf{D}$ is nonsingular). A similar dimension-reduction formula holds for the determinant:

$$| \mathbf{V}_i | = | \mathbf{I}_{n_i} + \mathbf{Z}_i \mathbf{D} \mathbf{Z}_i' | = | \mathbf{I}_k + \mathbf{D} \mathbf{Z}_i' \mathbf{Z}_i | . \tag{2.22}$$

As we see, the left-hand sides in formulas (2.21) and (2.22) involve a $n_i \times n_i$ matrix, but the right-hand sides involve $k \times k$ matrices. Further, to shorten the notation, the subscript at $\mathbf{I}$ will be suppressed. If matrix $\mathbf{D}$ is nonsingular, we can express the log of the determinant as a function of $\mathbf{D}^{-1}$, namely,

$$\ln|\mathbf{V}_i| = \ln\left(|\mathbf{D}|\left|\mathbf{D}^{-1}+\mathbf{Z}_i'\mathbf{Z}_i\right|\right) = \ln\left|\mathbf{D}^{-1}+\mathbf{Z}_i'\mathbf{Z}_i\right| - \ln\left|\mathbf{D}^{-1}\right|, \tag{2.23}$$

which will constitute the basis for the inverse $\mathbf{D}$ parameterization.

Another matrix formula, which may be derived from (2.21), will be used:

$$\mathbf{Z}_i'\mathbf{V}_i^{-1}\mathbf{Z}_i = (\mathbf{I} + \mathbf{Z}_i'\mathbf{Z}_i\mathbf{D})^{-1}\mathbf{Z}_i'\mathbf{Z}_i = \mathbf{Z}_i'\mathbf{Z}_i(\mathbf{I} + \mathbf{D}\mathbf{Z}_i'\mathbf{Z}_i)^{-1}, \tag{2.24}$$

which can also be verified by direct multiplication. If matrix $(\mathbf{Z}_i'\mathbf{Z}_i)^{-1}$ exists, formula (2.24) takes a simpler form,

$$\mathbf{Z}_i'\mathbf{V}_i^{-1}\mathbf{Z}_i = \mathbf{Z}_i'(\mathbf{I} + \mathbf{Z}_i\mathbf{D}\mathbf{Z}_i')^{-1}\mathbf{Z}_i = \left((\mathbf{Z}_i'\mathbf{Z}_i)^{-1} + \mathbf{D}\right)^{-1}. \tag{2.25}$$

Using these formulas, the log-likelihood function (2.15) can be rewritten in an equivalent and economical form as

$$\begin{aligned}
l(\boldsymbol{\theta}) = & -\frac{1}{2}\left\{ N_T\ln\sigma^2 + \sum_{i=1}^{N}\ln|\mathbf{I} + \mathbf{D}\mathbf{Z}_i'\mathbf{Z}_i| \right. \\
& \left. +\sigma^{-2}\sum_{i=1}^{N}\left[S_i - (\mathbf{Z}_i'\mathbf{e}_i)'(\mathbf{I} + \mathbf{D}\mathbf{Z}_i'\mathbf{Z}_i)^{-1}\mathbf{D}(\mathbf{Z}_i'\mathbf{e}_i)\right]\right\},
\end{aligned} \tag{2.26}$$

where

$$S_i = S_i(\boldsymbol{\beta}) = \mathbf{e}_i'\mathbf{e}_i = \|\mathbf{y}_i - \mathbf{X}_i\boldsymbol{\beta}\|^2 \tag{2.27}$$

is the residual sum of squares of the ith cluster and $\mathbf{I}$ is the $k \times k$ identity matrix.

A characteristic feature of model (2.14) is that holding matrix $\mathbf{D}$ constant, l is maximized by the Generalized Least Squares (GLS) estimator,

$$\widehat{\boldsymbol{\beta}}_{GLS} = \left[\sum_{i=1}^{N}\mathbf{X}_i'(\mathbf{I} + \mathbf{Z}_i\mathbf{D}\mathbf{Z}_i')^{-1}\mathbf{X}_i\right]^{-1}\left[\sum_{i=1}^{N}\mathbf{X}_i'(\mathbf{I} + \mathbf{Z}_i\mathbf{D}\mathbf{Z}_i')^{-1}\mathbf{y}_i\right]. \tag{2.28}$$

An economical formula for computation of the GLS estimate is given in Section 2.2.5.

One can show that the matrix $\sum_i \mathbf{X}_i'(\mathbf{I} + \mathbf{Z}_i\mathbf{D}\mathbf{Z}_i')^{-1}\mathbf{X}_i$ is positive definite if matrix $\sum_i \mathbf{X}_i'\mathbf{X}_i$ is not singular, as assumed at the beginning of the section. In a special case when $\mathbf{D} = \mathbf{0}$, the GLS estimator collapses to the Ordinary Least Squares (OLS) estimator,

$$\widehat{\boldsymbol{\beta}}_{OLS} = \left(\sum \mathbf{X}_i'\mathbf{X}_i\right)^{-1}\left(\sum \mathbf{X}_i'\mathbf{y}_i\right). \tag{2.29}$$

Another extreme case is when matrix $\mathbf{D}$ becomes infinite, or more precisely, $\mathbf{D} = d\mathbf{I}$, $d \to \infty$. Then, using the dimension-reduction formula (2.21) and denoting $\delta = 1/d \to 0$, we obtain

$$\lim_{d\to\infty}\mathbf{V}_i^{-1} = \lim_{d\to\infty}[\mathbf{I} - \mathbf{Z}_i(d^{-1}\mathbf{I} + \mathbf{Z}_i'\mathbf{Z}_i)^{-1}\mathbf{Z}_i'] = \mathbf{I} - \mathbf{Z}_i\lim_{\delta\to0}(\delta\mathbf{I} + \mathbf{Z}_i'\mathbf{Z}_i)^{-1}\mathbf{Z}_i'.$$

But the last limit is the Moore–Penrose generalized matrix inverse (Albert 1972), so that

$$\mathbf{Z}_i^+ = \lim_{\delta \to 0} (\delta \mathbf{I} + \mathbf{Z}_i' \mathbf{Z}_i)^{-1} \mathbf{Z}_i'. \qquad (2.30)$$

Note that if matrix $\mathbf{Z}_i$ has full rank, then matrix $\mathbf{Z}_i' \mathbf{Z}_i$ is nonsingular and $\mathbf{Z}_i^+ = (\mathbf{Z}_i' \mathbf{Z}_i)^{-1} \mathbf{Z}_i'$. Thus, the GLS (OLS) estimator for infinite matrix $\mathbf{D}$ becomes

$$\widehat{\boldsymbol{\beta}}_\infty = \left[\sum \mathbf{X}_i'(\mathbf{I} - \mathbf{Z}_i \mathbf{Z}_i^+)\mathbf{X}_i \right]^+ \left[\sum \mathbf{X}_i'(\mathbf{I} - \mathbf{Z}_i \mathbf{Z}_i^+)\mathbf{y}_i \right]. \qquad (2.31)$$

Note that this formula works even when the inverse matrix $\sum \mathbf{X}_i'(\mathbf{I} - \mathbf{Z}_i \mathbf{Z}_i^+)\mathbf{X}_i$ is zero (e.g., it happens when $\mathbf{X}_i = \mathbf{Z}_i \mathbf{A}_i$ in the growth curve model, Chapter 4). Since the generalized inverse of the null matrix is the null matrix $\widehat{\boldsymbol{\beta}}_\infty = \mathbf{0}$ for this case. More on the generalized matrix inverse is given in Appendix 13.2.

Below we suggest an R function that computes the generalized inverse of a symmetric matrix:

```
ginverse.sym=function(A,eps=10^(-8))
{
    #Generalized inverse of a symmetric matrix A
    PV=eigen(A,symmetric=T)
    V0=IV=PV$values
    IV[abs(V0)>eps]=1/V0[abs(V0)>eps]
    IV[abs(V0)<=eps]=0
    Ainv=PV$vectors%*%(IV*(t(PV$vectors)))
    return(Ainv)
}
```

This method uses the spectral decomposition of matrix $\mathbf{A} = \mathbf{P}\boldsymbol{\Lambda}\mathbf{P}'$, where $\mathbf{P}$ is the orthogonal matrix and $\boldsymbol{\Lambda}$ is the diagonal matrix with eigenvalues on the diagonal. The eigenvalue is zero if its absolute value is less than ε, the numerical precision for computation of the eigenvalue (the user-defined *small* value). Using this decomposition, the Moore-Penrose generalized inverse is $\mathbf{A}^+ = \mathbf{P}\boldsymbol{\Lambda}^+\mathbf{P}'$, where $\boldsymbol{\Lambda}^+$ is the diagonal matrix with reciprocal nonzero eigenvalues and zero values otherwise.

In combination with (2.30), we can write

$$\mathbf{M}^+ = (\mathbf{M}'\mathbf{M})^+\mathbf{M}'$$

for any rectangular matrix $\mathbf{M}$. Therefore, by computing the generalized inverse of a symmetric matrix we can compute the generalized inverse of any matrix.

Estimator (2.31) has a nice interpretation as the *fixed effects* estimator. Indeed, let us consider the fixed effects model as an alternative to the LME model with random effects, namely,

$$\mathbf{y}_i = \mathbf{X}_i\boldsymbol{\beta} + \mathbf{Z}_i\mathbf{b}_i + \boldsymbol{\varepsilon}_i, \qquad \mathbf{b}_i \text{ is fixed}, \qquad (2.32)$$

and as earlier, the $\{\boldsymbol{\varepsilon}_i\}$ are independent random vectors with zero mean and variance σ^2. In the fixed effects approach, $\{\mathbf{b}_i, i = 1, ..., N\}$ are unknown nuisance parameters. Since the $\{\mathbf{b}_i\}$ are fixed and $\text{cov}(\mathbf{y}_i) = \sigma^2\mathbf{I}$, the OLS estimator is the Best

Linear Unbiased Estimator (BLUE), which minimizes the total sum of squares,

$$\min_{\boldsymbol{\beta},\mathbf{b}_1,\ldots,\mathbf{b}_N} \sum_{i=1}^{N} \parallel \mathbf{y}_i - \mathbf{X}_i\boldsymbol{\beta} - \mathbf{Z}_i\mathbf{b}_i \parallel^2 = S_{\min}. \tag{2.33}$$

We can rewrite this optimization problem as a standard least squares problem introducing a composite $N_T \times (m + Nk)$ matrix,

$$\mathbf{W} = [\mathbf{X},\mathbf{Z}] = \begin{bmatrix} \mathbf{X}_1 & \mathbf{Z}_1 & \mathbf{0} & \mathbf{0} \\ \vdots & \mathbf{0} & \ddots & \mathbf{0} \\ \mathbf{X}_N & \mathbf{0} & \mathbf{0} & \mathbf{Z}_N \end{bmatrix}, \tag{2.34}$$

with $\boldsymbol{\nu} = (\boldsymbol{\beta},\mathbf{b}')'$. Then (2.33) is equivalent to $\parallel \mathbf{y} - \mathbf{W}\boldsymbol{\nu} \parallel^2$, where $\mathbf{y}$ and $\mathbf{X}$ are as defined in (2.9). The OLS solution to the latter sum of squares has the minimum

$$S_{\min} = \mathbf{y}'(\mathbf{I} - \mathbf{W}\mathbf{W}^+)\mathbf{y}. \tag{2.35}$$

Alternatively, we can derive an economical formula for (2.35) holding $\boldsymbol{\beta}$ constant and minimizing the sum of squares over $\{\mathbf{b}_i\}$. Indeed, if $\boldsymbol{\beta}$ is fixed, the quadratic forms in (2.33) can be minimized for $\mathbf{b}_i$ separately. As follows from the theory of least squares with the design matrix not necessarily of full rank (Rao, 1973; Graybill, 1983), the estimates are $\widehat{\mathbf{b}}_i = \mathbf{Z}_i^+(\mathbf{y} - \mathbf{X}\boldsymbol{\beta})$, with the minimum

$$\min_{\mathbf{b}_i} \parallel \mathbf{y}_i - \mathbf{X}_i\boldsymbol{\beta} - \mathbf{Z}_i\mathbf{b}_i \parallel^2 = (\mathbf{y}_i - \mathbf{X}_i\boldsymbol{\beta})'(\mathbf{I} - \mathbf{Z}_i\mathbf{Z}_i^+)(\mathbf{y}_i - \mathbf{X}_i\boldsymbol{\beta}). \tag{2.36}$$

Next, minimizing $\sum(\mathbf{y}_i - \mathbf{X}_i\boldsymbol{\beta})'(\mathbf{I} - \mathbf{Z}_i\mathbf{Z}_i^+)(\mathbf{y}_i - \mathbf{X}_i\boldsymbol{\beta})$ for $\boldsymbol{\beta}$ leads finally to (2.31). We can interpret this result by saying that the fixed effects model corresponds to the random effects model with infinite covariance matrix, $\mathbf{D} = \infty$.

Which model, (2.5) or (2.32), is better: random or fixed effects? One cannot answer this question because this choice is, in fact, an assumption; some discussion on this topic may be found in the variance components literature (Searle, 1971b, Lindman, 1992). Clearly, a fixed effects model is less restrictive and is easy to handle because it reduces to a standard linear model, but the price is that the number of nuisance parameters increases with the number of subjects (clusters). In particular, the fixed effects approach would be preferable if the number of clusters (N) is small and the number of observations per cluster is large. A general linear growth curve model (considered in Chapter 4), is a reasonable compromise between fixed and random effects models. As follows from (2.31), the fixed-effect OLS estimator, $\widehat{\boldsymbol{\beta}}_\infty$, is consistent for $\boldsymbol{\beta}$ when $N \to \infty$, despite an increasing number of nuisance parameters, if the inverse matrix is nonsingular. A special case of a linear model with a cluster-specific intercept term is considered in Section 2.4. In Section 3.2.1 we explain why the combination of random and fixed effects leads to an invalid model.

As we shall learn later, the quantity $S_{\min}$ plays an important role in the LME model; particularly, as we shall learn later, the inequality

$$S_{\min} = \sum_{i=1}^{N}(\mathbf{y}_i - \mathbf{X}_i\widehat{\boldsymbol{\beta}}_\infty)'(\mathbf{I} - \mathbf{Z}_i\mathbf{Z}_i^+)(\mathbf{y}_i - \mathbf{X}_i\widehat{\boldsymbol{\beta}}_\infty) > 0 \tag{2.37}$$

provides a necessary and sufficient condition for the existence of the maximum likelihood estimate (Section 2.5). Also, $S_{\min}$ is the key characteristic of statistical testing for the presence of random effects (Section 3.5) and MINQUE for parameter σ^2 (Section 3.10.2).

We shall prove that $S_{\min}$ is the lower bound for the weighted sum of squares, or more precisely,

$$\sum_{i=1}^{N}(\mathbf{y}_i - \mathbf{X}_i\boldsymbol{\beta})'(\mathbf{I} + \mathbf{Z}_i\mathbf{D}\mathbf{Z}_i')^{-1}(\mathbf{y}_i - \mathbf{X}_i\boldsymbol{\beta}) \geq S_{\min} \tag{2.38}$$

for any $\boldsymbol{\beta}$ and $\mathbf{D}$.

Proof. First we show that $(\mathbf{I} + \mathbf{Z}_i\mathbf{D}\mathbf{Z}_i)^{-1} \geq \mathbf{I} - \mathbf{Z}_i\mathbf{Z}_i^+$. It follows from multiplying both sides of this inequality by $\mathbf{I} + \mathbf{Z}_i\mathbf{D}\mathbf{Z}_i'$ and the following straightforward matrix algebra:

$$\begin{aligned}(\mathbf{I} - \mathbf{Z}_i\mathbf{Z}_i^+)(\mathbf{I} + \mathbf{Z}_i\mathbf{D}\mathbf{Z}_i') &= \mathbf{I} + \mathbf{Z}_i\mathbf{D}\mathbf{Z}_i' - \mathbf{Z}_i\mathbf{Z}_i^+ - \mathbf{Z}_i\mathbf{Z}_i^+\mathbf{Z}_i\mathbf{D}\mathbf{Z}_i' \\ &= \mathbf{I} + \mathbf{Z}_i\mathbf{D}\mathbf{Z}_i' - \mathbf{Z}_i\mathbf{Z}_i^+ - \mathbf{Z}_i\mathbf{D}\mathbf{Z}_i' = \mathbf{I} - \mathbf{Z}_i\mathbf{Z}_i^+ \leq \mathbf{I}.\end{aligned}$$

Hence, the left-hand side of (2.38) is greater than or equal to

$$\sum_{i=1}^{N}(\mathbf{y}_i - \mathbf{X}_i\boldsymbol{\beta})'(\mathbf{I} - \mathbf{Z}_i\mathbf{Z}_i^+)(\mathbf{y}_i - \mathbf{X}_i\boldsymbol{\beta})$$

$$\geq \min_{\boldsymbol{\beta}}\sum_{i=1}^{N}(\mathbf{y}_i - \mathbf{X}_i\boldsymbol{\beta})'(\mathbf{I} - \mathbf{Z}_i\mathbf{Z}_i^+)(\mathbf{y}_i - \mathbf{X}_i\boldsymbol{\beta}) = S_{\min}$$

2.2.4 Profile log-likelihood functions

Taking the derivative of (2.15) with respect to σ^2, it is easy to see that function l is maximized at

$$\widehat{\sigma}^2 = \frac{1}{N_T}\sum_{i=1}^{N}(\mathbf{y}_i - \mathbf{X}_i\boldsymbol{\beta})'(\mathbf{I} + \mathbf{Z}_i\mathbf{D}\mathbf{Z}_i')^{-1}(\mathbf{y}_i - \mathbf{X}_i\boldsymbol{\beta}). \tag{2.39}$$

Lindstrom and Bates (1988) and Wolfinger et al. (1994), among others, take advantage of formula (2.39) and suggest the *variance-profile* log-likelihood function substituting (2.39) back into (2.15). This leads to an equivalent maximization problem with σ^2 eliminated,

$$l_p(\boldsymbol{\beta}, \mathbf{D}) = -\frac{1}{2}\left\{N_T\ln\sum_{i}(\mathbf{y}_i - \mathbf{X}_i\boldsymbol{\beta})'\mathbf{V}_i^{-1}(\mathbf{y}_i - \mathbf{X}_i\boldsymbol{\beta}) + \sum_{i}\ln|\mathbf{V}_i|\right\}, \tag{2.40}$$

where constant $c = \frac{1}{2}N_T(\ln N_T - 1)$ is ignored (the subscript p indicates that the function is profiled). Applying formulas (2.21) and (2.23) and assuming that $\mathbf{D}$ is nonsingular, we obtain an economical dimension-reduction parameterization of the profile function,

$$l_p(\boldsymbol{\beta}, \mathbf{D}) = -\frac{1}{2}\left\{N_T\ln\left(\sum_{i}[S_i - \mathbf{r}_i'(\mathbf{D}^{-1} + \mathbf{M}_i)^{-1}\mathbf{r}_i]\right) + \sum_{i}\ln|\mathbf{I} + \mathbf{D}\mathbf{M}_i|\right\}, \tag{2.41}$$

where $S_i = S_i(\boldsymbol{\beta})$ is as defined in (2.27),

$$\mathbf{r}_i = \mathbf{Z}'_i \mathbf{e}_i, \quad \mathbf{M}_i = \mathbf{Z}'_i \mathbf{Z}_i. \tag{2.42}$$

Further, in the last parameterization we can consider $\mathbf{D}_- = \mathbf{D}^{-1}$ as the argument; sometimes $\mathbf{D}^{-1}$ is called a precision matrix. This leads to the *precision matrix* parameterization

$$
\begin{aligned}
l_p(\boldsymbol{\beta}, \mathbf{D}_-) = &-\frac{1}{2} \left\{ N_T \ln \left(\sum_i [S_i - \mathbf{r}'_i (\mathbf{D}_- + \mathbf{M}_i)^{-1} \mathbf{r}_i] \right) \right. \\
&\left. + \sum_i \ln |\mathbf{D}_- + \mathbf{M}_i| - N \ln |\mathbf{D}_-| \right\}.
\end{aligned} \tag{2.43}
$$

A further possibility is to exclude $\boldsymbol{\beta}$ using the GLS formula (2.28). We need the following general result to derive the ultimate $(\sigma^2, \boldsymbol{\beta})$-profile log-likelihood function.

Proposition 1 *Let* $\mathbf{y}$ *and* $\mathbf{X}$ *be an* $N \times 1$ *vector and an* $N \times m$ *matrix of full rank* $(m < N)$, *respectively, and* $\mathbf{V}$ *be a* $N \times N$ *positive definite matrix. Then*

$$\min_{\boldsymbol{\beta} \in R^m} (\mathbf{y} - \mathbf{X}\boldsymbol{\beta})' \mathbf{V}^{-1} (\mathbf{y} - \mathbf{X}\boldsymbol{\beta})$$

$$= \mathbf{y}' \mathbf{V}^{-1} \mathbf{y} - (\mathbf{X}' \mathbf{V}^{-1} \mathbf{y})' (\mathbf{X}' \mathbf{V}^{-1} \mathbf{X})^{-1} (\mathbf{X}' \mathbf{V}^{-1} \mathbf{y}).$$

Proof. The minimum of the quadratic form at the left is attained at $\widehat{\boldsymbol{\beta}} = (\mathbf{X}' \mathbf{V}^{-1} \mathbf{X})^{-1} \mathbf{X}' \mathbf{V}^{-1} \mathbf{y}$, so that the minimum value is

$$(\mathbf{y} - \mathbf{X}\widehat{\boldsymbol{\beta}})' \mathbf{V}^{-1} (\mathbf{y} - \mathbf{X}\widehat{\boldsymbol{\beta}})$$

$$= \mathbf{y}' \left[(\mathbf{I} - \mathbf{X}(\mathbf{X}' \mathbf{V}^{-1} \mathbf{X})^{-1} \mathbf{X}' \mathbf{V}^{-1})' \mathbf{V}^{-1} (\mathbf{I} - \mathbf{X}(\mathbf{X}' \mathbf{V}^{-1} \mathbf{X})^{-1} \mathbf{X}' \mathbf{V}^{-1}) \right] \mathbf{y}.$$

But the matrix in brackets can be rewritten as

$$
\begin{aligned}
& \mathbf{V}^{-1} - 2\mathbf{V}^{-1} \mathbf{X} (\mathbf{X}' \mathbf{V}^{-1} \mathbf{X})^{-1} \mathbf{X}' \mathbf{V}^{-1} \\
& + \mathbf{V}^{-1} \mathbf{X} (\mathbf{X}' \mathbf{V}^{-1} \mathbf{X})^{-1} \mathbf{X}' \mathbf{V}^{-1} \mathbf{X} (\mathbf{X}' \mathbf{V}^{-1} \mathbf{X})^{-1} \mathbf{X}' \mathbf{V}^{-1} \\
= \ & \mathbf{V}^{-1} - \mathbf{V}^{-1} \mathbf{X} (\mathbf{X}' \mathbf{V}^{-1} \mathbf{X})^{-1} \mathbf{X}' \mathbf{V}^{-1},
\end{aligned}
$$

which proves the proposition. ∎

Using "long" notation (2.9), the total sum of squares can be rewritten as

$$\sum_{i=1}^{N} (\mathbf{y}_i - \mathbf{X}_i \boldsymbol{\beta})' \mathbf{V}_i^{-1} (\mathbf{y}_i - \mathbf{X}_i \boldsymbol{\beta}) = (\mathbf{y} - \mathbf{X}\boldsymbol{\beta})' \mathbf{V}^{-1} (\mathbf{y} - \mathbf{X}\boldsymbol{\beta}).$$

Then, applying Proposition 1, we obtain

$$q = \min_{\boldsymbol{\beta}} \sum (\mathbf{y}_i - \mathbf{X}_i \boldsymbol{\beta})' \mathbf{V}_i^{-1} (\mathbf{y}_i - \mathbf{X}_i \boldsymbol{\beta}) \tag{2.44}$$

$$= \sum \mathbf{y}'_i \mathbf{V}_i^{-1} \mathbf{y}_i - \left(\sum \mathbf{X}'_i \mathbf{V}_i^{-1} \mathbf{y}_i \right)' \left(\sum \mathbf{X}'_i \mathbf{V}_i^{-1} \mathbf{X}_i \right)^{-1} \left(\sum \mathbf{X}'_i \mathbf{V}_i^{-1} \mathbf{y}_i \right).$$

Consequently, if $\mathbf{V}_i$ is known, the GLS estimator (2.28) leads to the following formula for (2.39):

$$\hat{\sigma}^2_{GLS} = \min_{\boldsymbol{\beta}} \frac{1}{N_T} \sum (\mathbf{y}_i - \mathbf{X}_i\boldsymbol{\beta})' \mathbf{V}_i^{-1} (\mathbf{y}_i - \mathbf{X}_i\boldsymbol{\beta}) = \frac{q}{N_T}.$$

The *full-profile* log-likelihood function, as a function of $\mathbf{D}_-$, is given by

$$l_P(\mathbf{D}_-) = -\frac{1}{2}\left[N_T \ln q(\mathbf{D}_-) + \sum_i \ln |\mathbf{D}_- + \mathbf{M}_i| - N \ln |\mathbf{D}_-| \right], \qquad (2.45)$$

where q is defined in (2.44). Using the dimension-reduction formula (2.21), the quantities in (2.44) can be found as

$$\begin{aligned}
\sum \mathbf{y}_i' \mathbf{V}_i^{-1} \mathbf{y}_i &= \sum \mathbf{y}_i' \mathbf{y}_i - \sum (\mathbf{Z}_i' \mathbf{y}_i)' (\mathbf{D}_- + \mathbf{Z}_i' \mathbf{Z}_i)^{-1} (\mathbf{Z}_i' \mathbf{y}_i), \\
\sum \mathbf{X}_i' \mathbf{V}_i^{-1} \mathbf{y}_i &= \sum \mathbf{X}_i' \mathbf{y}_i - \sum (\mathbf{X}_i' \mathbf{Z}_i) (\mathbf{D}_- + \mathbf{Z}_i' \mathbf{Z}_i)^{-1} (\mathbf{Z}_i' \mathbf{y}_i), \\
\sum \mathbf{X}_i' \mathbf{V}_i^{-1} \mathbf{X}_i &= \sum \mathbf{X}_i' \mathbf{X}_i - \sum (\mathbf{X}_i' \mathbf{Z}_i) (\mathbf{D}_- + \mathbf{Z}_i' \mathbf{Z}_i)^{-1} (\mathbf{X}_i' \mathbf{Z}_i)'.
\end{aligned}$$
$$(2.46)$$

This form of the log-likelihood function is perhaps the most economical because quantities such as $\sum \mathbf{y}_i' \mathbf{y}_i$, $\mathbf{Z}_i' \mathbf{y}_i$, $\mathbf{X}_i' \mathbf{y}_i$, and $\mathbf{X}_i' \mathbf{X}_i$ can be computed beforehand. The profile-likelihood parameterization is well suited for profile-likelihood confidence interval construction (see Section 3.4).

2.2.5   Dimension-reduction GLS estimate

In this section we use the dimension-reduction formulas (2.46) to compute the GLS estimate,

$$\begin{aligned}
\hat{\boldsymbol{\beta}}_{GLS} &= \left[\sum \mathbf{X}_i' \mathbf{X}_i - \sum (\mathbf{X}_i' \mathbf{Z}_i)(\mathbf{I}_k + \mathbf{D}\mathbf{Z}_i' \mathbf{Z}_i)^{-1} \mathbf{D}(\mathbf{X}_i' \mathbf{Z}_i)' \right]^{-1} \\
&\quad \times \left[\sum \mathbf{X}_i' \mathbf{y}_i - \sum (\mathbf{X}_i' \mathbf{Z}_i)(\mathbf{I}_k + \mathbf{D}\mathbf{Z}_i' \mathbf{Z}_i)^{-1} \mathbf{D}(\mathbf{Z}_i' \mathbf{y}_i) \right]. \qquad (2.47)
\end{aligned}$$

Note that the direct use of formula (2.28) requires N inverses of a $n_i \times n_i$ matrix. Using the dimension-reduction formulas, we reduce the computation to N inverses of a $k \times k$ matrix. This method is used in our economical R code for maximization of the log-likelihood function based on Fisher scoring algorithm in Section 2.16.

The R code based on the economical formula (2.47) is given below. In this code the data are supplied in the matrix argument d: The first column is the cluster id, the second column contains observations of $\mathbf{y}$, columns from 3 to $(2 + m)$ contain observations of $\mathbf{X}$, and the rest is matrix $\mathbf{Z}$. This data format and R syntax are used in the following codes.

```
GLSest=function(d,m,k,D)
#computes beta_GLS
{
 id <- d[, 1]
 undi <- unique(id)
 y <- d[, 2]
 X <- as.matrix(d[, 3:(2 + m)], ncol = m)
 Z <- as.matrix(d[, (3 + m):(2 + m + k)], ncol = k)
 Xty=t(X)%*%y #matrix ∑ X'_i y_i
 XtX=t(X)%*%X #matrix ∑ X'_i X_i
 Ik=diag(rep(1,k),k,k)
 for(i in undi)
 {
    yi <- y[id == i]
    Xi <- X[id == i, ]
    Zi <- Z[id == i, ]
    ZtZ <- t(Zi)%*%Zi
    XtZ <- t(Xi)%*%Zi
    Zty <- t(Zi)%*%yi
    iM=solve(Ik+D%*%ZtZ)%*%D #matrix (I + DZ'_i Z_i)^{-1}D
    Xty=Xty-XtZ%*%iM%*%Zty
    XtX=XtX-XtZ%*%iM%*%t(XtZ)
 }
 beta.GLS=solve(XtX)%*%Xty
 return(beta.GLS)
}
```

2.2.6 Restricted maximum likelihood

It is known that maximum likelihood estimation of variances is biased for finite samples. For example, in a standard linear regression model $\mathbf{y} \sim \mathcal{N}(\mathbf{X}\boldsymbol{\beta}, \sigma^2 \mathbf{I})$, the MLE of the variance, $\hat{\sigma}^2_{ML} = SS/n$, underestimates σ^2, where SS is the residual sum of squares, n is the number of observations, and m is the number of regression coefficients. The unbiased estimator of σ^2 is $SS/(n-m)$, which takes the degrees of freedom into account. To reduce the bias in the variance components model, Patterson and Thompson (1971), and later Harville (1974), suggested modifying the standard log-likelihood function using generalized least squares residuals. The resulting method is referred to as Restricted (or perhaps more precisely, Residual) Maximum Likelihood Estimation (RMLE). Laird and Ware (1982) applied this method to LME model (2.14).

First we derive the RML for the general linear model and then apply it to the LME model.

Let the general linear model be defined as $\mathbf{y} \sim \mathcal{N}(\mathbf{X}\boldsymbol{\beta}, \mathbf{V})$ where $\mathbf{X}$ is an $n \times m$ matrix of full rank and $\mathbf{V}$ is the $n \times n$ covariance matrix, dependent on some parameter $\boldsymbol{\theta}$. In RML estimation we maximize the log-likelihood function for the residual vector $\widehat{\mathbf{e}} = \mathbf{y} - \mathbf{X}\widehat{\boldsymbol{\beta}}$, where $\widehat{\boldsymbol{\beta}}$ is the GLS estimator, $\widehat{\boldsymbol{\beta}} = (\mathbf{X}'\mathbf{V}^{-1}\mathbf{X})^{-1}\mathbf{X}'\mathbf{V}^{-1}\mathbf{y}$. Notice that since $\mathbf{y}$ has normal distribution, $\widehat{\boldsymbol{\beta}}$ and $\widehat{\mathbf{e}}$ are linear functions of $\mathbf{y}$ and have normal distribution as well. Moreover, $\widehat{\boldsymbol{\beta}}$ and $\widehat{\mathbf{e}}$ are independent because

$$
\begin{aligned}
\text{cov}(\mathbf{X}'\mathbf{V}^{-1}\mathbf{y}, \widehat{\mathbf{e}}) &= \mathbf{X}'\mathbf{V}^{-1}\mathbf{V}[\mathbf{I} - \mathbf{V}^{-1}\mathbf{X}(\mathbf{X}'\mathbf{V}^{-1}\mathbf{X})^{-1}\mathbf{X}'] \\
&= \mathbf{X}' - \mathbf{X}'\mathbf{V}^{-1}\mathbf{X}(\mathbf{X}'\mathbf{V}^{-1}\mathbf{X})^{-1}\mathbf{X}' = \mathbf{0}.
\end{aligned}
$$

This implies that the likelihood function for $\mathbf{y}$ is the product of the likelihood functions for $\widehat{\mathbf{e}}$ and for $\widehat{\boldsymbol{\beta}}$. But $\widehat{\boldsymbol{\beta}} \sim \mathcal{N}(\boldsymbol{\beta}, (\mathbf{X}'\mathbf{V}^{-1}\mathbf{X})^{-1})$, and therefore the log-likelihood function for the residual vector $\widehat{\mathbf{e}}$, up to a constant, is

$$
\begin{aligned}
l(\widehat{\mathbf{e}}, \boldsymbol{\theta}) &= l(\mathbf{y}, \boldsymbol{\theta}) - l(\widehat{\boldsymbol{\beta}}, \boldsymbol{\theta}) = -\frac{1}{2}\{\ln|\mathbf{X}'\mathbf{V}^{-1}\mathbf{X}| + \ln|\mathbf{V}| \\
&\quad + (\mathbf{y} - \mathbf{X}\boldsymbol{\beta})'\mathbf{V}^{-1}(\mathbf{y} - \mathbf{X}\boldsymbol{\beta}) - (\widehat{\boldsymbol{\beta}} - \boldsymbol{\beta})'\mathbf{X}'\mathbf{V}^{-1}\mathbf{X}(\widehat{\boldsymbol{\beta}} - \boldsymbol{\beta})\}.
\end{aligned}
$$

But since

$$
\begin{aligned}
&(\mathbf{y} - \mathbf{X}\boldsymbol{\beta})'\mathbf{V}^{-1}(\mathbf{y} - \mathbf{X}\boldsymbol{\beta}) \\
&= (\mathbf{y} - \mathbf{X}\widehat{\boldsymbol{\beta}})'\mathbf{V}^{-1}(\mathbf{y} - \mathbf{X}\widehat{\boldsymbol{\beta}}) + (\widehat{\boldsymbol{\beta}} - \boldsymbol{\beta})'\mathbf{X}'\mathbf{V}^{-1}\mathbf{X}(\widehat{\boldsymbol{\beta}} - \boldsymbol{\beta}),
\end{aligned} \tag{2.48}
$$

we can rewrite the log-likelihood function for $\widehat{\mathbf{e}}$ as

$$
l(\widehat{\mathbf{e}}, \boldsymbol{\theta}) = -\frac{1}{2}\left[\ln|\mathbf{X}'\mathbf{V}^{-1}\mathbf{X}| + \ln|\mathbf{V}| + \widehat{\mathbf{e}}'\mathbf{V}^{-1}\widehat{\mathbf{e}}\right].
$$

Clearly, the maximization of this function is equivalent to

$$
l_R(\boldsymbol{\beta}, \boldsymbol{\theta}) = -\frac{1}{2}\left[\ln|\mathbf{X}'\mathbf{V}^{-1}\mathbf{X}| + \ln|\mathbf{V}| + (\mathbf{y} - \mathbf{X}\boldsymbol{\beta})'\mathbf{V}^{-1}(\mathbf{y} - \mathbf{X}\boldsymbol{\beta})\right], \tag{2.49}
$$

because maximization of l_R for $\boldsymbol{\beta}$ gives $\widehat{\mathbf{e}} = \mathbf{y} - \mathbf{X}\widehat{\boldsymbol{\beta}}$. Function l_R is called the residual log-likelihood function. Notice that l_R differs from the standard log-likelihood function by the term $-\frac{1}{2}\ln|\mathbf{X}'\mathbf{V}\mathbf{X}|$. As a word of caution, l_R is not a *real* log-likelihood function and consequently the covariance matrix for $\boldsymbol{\theta}$ cannot be derived as the inverse of the expected second derivative. Although asymptotically, ML and RML and the respective covariance matrices coincide (see Section 3.6.3).

An alternative way to come to the restricted likelihood function (2.49) is to use a Bayesian approach with a non-informative/uniform prior distribution for $\boldsymbol{\beta}$ (Laird and Ware, 1982). More precisely, let $\boldsymbol{\beta}$ be treated as random with uniform distribution on R^m. Then, to obtain the marginal distribution for σ^2 and $\mathbf{D}$, we need to integrate out $\boldsymbol{\beta}$,

$$
L_R(\sigma^2, \mathbf{D}) = \int_{\boldsymbol{\beta} \in R^m} L(\boldsymbol{\beta}, \sigma^2, \mathbf{D}) d\boldsymbol{\beta},
$$

where L is the standard likelihood function,

$$
L(\boldsymbol{\beta}, \sigma^2, \mathbf{D}) = (2\pi)^{-n/2} |\mathbf{V}|^{-1/2} e^{-\frac{1}{2}(\mathbf{y} - \mathbf{X}\boldsymbol{\beta})'\mathbf{V}^{-1}(\mathbf{y} - \mathbf{X}\boldsymbol{\beta})}.
$$

Again using identity (2.48) we rewrite the integral above as

$$(2\pi)^{-n/2} \left|\mathbf{V}\right|^{-1/2} e^{-\frac{1}{2}(\mathbf{y}-\mathbf{X}\widehat{\beta})'\mathbf{V}^{-1}(\mathbf{y}-\mathbf{X}\widehat{\beta})} \int_{\beta \in R^m} e^{-\frac{1}{2}(\widehat{\beta}-\beta)'\mathbf{X}'\mathbf{V}^{-1}\mathbf{X}(\widehat{\beta}-\beta)} d\beta.$$

Now we use a well known result on the integration of an exponential function of quadratic form, $\int e^{-\frac{1}{2}(\mathbf{z}-\mathbf{m})'\mathbf{A}(\mathbf{z}-\mathbf{m})} d\mathbf{z} = (2\pi)^{m/2} \left|\mathbf{A}\right|^{-1/2}$ for any $m \times 1$ vector $\mathbf{m}$ and any positive definite $m \times m$ matrix $\mathbf{A}$ (Graybill, 1983, p. 332). Applying this result, we obtain

$$L_R(\sigma^2, \mathbf{D}) = (2\pi)^{-(n-m)/2} \left|\mathbf{V}\right|^{-1/2} \left|\mathbf{X}'\mathbf{V}^{-1}\mathbf{X}\right|^{-1/2} e^{-\frac{1}{2}(\mathbf{y}-\mathbf{X}\widehat{\beta})'\mathbf{V}^{-1}(\mathbf{y}-\mathbf{X}\widehat{\beta})},$$

which is equivalent to the previously derived restricted log-likelihood function (2.49). Due to this derivation RML is sometimes called marginal ML.

Since the regular and restricted versions of the log-likelihood differ by the term $-0.5 \ln \left|\mathbf{X}'\mathbf{V}^{-1}\mathbf{X}\right|$, which translates into $\ln \left|\sum \mathbf{X}_i'\mathbf{V}_i^{-1}\mathbf{X}_i\right|$ for the LME model, we come to the RML function

$$l_R(\boldsymbol{\theta}) = -\frac{1}{2} \left\{ (N_T - m) \ln \sigma^2 + \ln \left|\sum_{i=1}^{N} \mathbf{X}_i'\mathbf{V}_i^{-1}\mathbf{X}_i\right| \right. \tag{2.50}$$

$$\left. + \sum_{i=1}^{N} \left[\ln \left|\mathbf{V}_i\right| + \sigma^{-2}(\mathbf{y}_i - \mathbf{X}_i\beta)'\mathbf{V}_i^{-1}(\mathbf{y}_i - \mathbf{X}_i\beta)\right] \right\}.$$

Notice that this is the standard log-likelihood function (2.15) augmented by the term

$$-\frac{1}{2} \left(-m \ln \sigma^2 + \ln \left|\sum_{i=1}^{N} \mathbf{X}_i'\mathbf{V}_i^{-1}\mathbf{X}_i\right|\right), \tag{2.51}$$

and the constant term is augmented by $0.5 m \ln(2\pi)$.

The log-likelihood function for RML may be reparameterized following the line of previous reparameterization. For example, we come to the σ^2-profile RML function by substituting

$$\widehat{\sigma}_R^2 = \frac{1}{N_T - m} \sum_{i=1}^{N} (\mathbf{y}_i - \mathbf{X}_i\beta)'(\mathbf{I} + \mathbf{Z}_i\mathbf{D}\mathbf{Z}_i')^{-1}(\mathbf{y}_i - \mathbf{X}_i\beta) \tag{2.52}$$

into (2.50), which leads to the variance-profile log-likelihood function (up to a constant term)

$$l_{Rp}(\beta, \mathbf{D}) = -\frac{1}{2} \left\{ (N_T - m) \ln \left[\sum_{i=1}^{N} (\mathbf{y}_i - \mathbf{X}_i\beta)'\mathbf{V}_i^{-1}(\mathbf{y}_i - \mathbf{X}_i\beta)\right] \right.$$

$$\left. + \ln \left|\sum_{i=1}^{N} \mathbf{X}_i'\mathbf{V}_i^{-1}\mathbf{X}_i\right| + \sum_{i=1}^{N} \ln \left|\mathbf{V}_i\right| \right\}. \tag{2.53}$$

Notice that the degrees of freedom in the restricted version of the σ^2 estimator (2.52) are adjusted by the number of fixed effects, m. However, if the total number of observations is much greater than m, the adjustment will be negligible.

We can further reduce the computational burden using the dimension-reduction formulas (2.21) to (2.25). In fact, we can use all previously derived log-likelihood parameterizations augmented by the term (2.51). Clearly, one can use formula (2.21) to reduce the dimension of the inverse matrix in (2.51).

2.2.7 Weight versus height (continued)

We continue working on the begun started in Section 2.1 and modify the R code to account for possible excessive variation due to the age and sex of individuals. But before that we note that lme has two method options to estimate a linear mixed model. The default method is REML, which means that if the user does not specify the method of estimation, the model will be estimated by the restricted maximum likelihood described in Section 2.2.6. Thus, the log-restricted-likelihood $= -331.6369$ in the output of the lme call in Section 2.1.1 equals (2.49) $-(N-m)/2\ln(2\pi)$, where for our example, $N = 71$, the total number of observations, and $m = 2$, the number of fixed effects parameters. Below we show the output with the option method="ML".

```
Linear mixed-effects model fit by maximum likelihood
 Data: famdat
 Log-likelihood: -334.7041
 Fixed: Weight ~Height
(Intercept) Height
-205.015367 5.319309
Random effects:
 Formula: ~1 | FamilyID
 (Intercept) Residual
StdDev: 13.34261 24.50155
Number of Observations: 71
Number of Groups: 18
```

The difference in the log-likelihoods is $-\frac{1}{2}\ln|\mathbf{X}'\mathbf{V}\mathbf{X}|$, where $\mathbf{X}$ is the 71×2 matrix with the first column of 1 and the second column of Height, and $\mathbf{V}$ is the 72×72 block diagonal covariance matrix with $1+d$ on the diagonal and d off diagonal, where $d = \sigma_d^2/\sigma^2$, the relative variance intercept. The difference between ML and REML is visible but not considerable. In general, this difference vanishes quickly with the growing sample size —the consequence that maximum and restricted maximum likelihoods are asymptotically equivalent.

Problems for Section 2.2

1. Prove that if $\mathbf{S}$ is a convex cone then $\mathbf{S}$ is a convex set. More precisely, if for every pair $\mathbf{s}_1, \mathbf{s}_2 \in \mathbf{S}$ and every pair of positive scalars λ_1 and λ_2 we have $\lambda_1\mathbf{s}_1 + \lambda_2\mathbf{s}_2 \in \mathbf{S}$ then $\lambda\mathbf{s}_1 + (1-\lambda)\mathbf{s}_2 \in \mathbf{S}$ for all $0 < \lambda < 1$. This means that the parameter space (2.16) is convex.

2. Find the GLS estimator that minimizes the weighted sum of squares in Proposition 1, where $\mathbf{V} = \mathbf{I} + \rho\mathbf{X}\mathbf{X}'$, using formula (2.21).

3*. Experiment with the generalized inverse function `ginverse.sym` to find the optimal parameter ε: Generate random rectangular matrices $\mathbf{X}$ and use this function to compute the generalized inverse of matrix $\mathbf{I} - \mathbf{X}(\mathbf{X}'\mathbf{X})^{-1}\mathbf{X}'$. Find the true theoretical generalized inverse of this matrix. Find ε such that the difference between the computed and the true generalized inverse matrices is minimum. You can generate random matrices using `runif` or `rnorm` or generate determininstic matrices with columns $\mathbf{x}_1 = \mathbf{1}, \mathbf{x}_2 = (1, 2, ..., n)', \mathbf{x}_3 = (1^2, 2^2, ..., n^2)'$, and so on.

4. Derive the full-profile likelihood (2.45) in the case of one random effect (matrix $\mathbf{D}$ is scalar). Write an R program which generates data according to $y_{ij} = \alpha + \beta t_{ij} + b_i + \varepsilon_{ij}$, where $i = 1, 2, ..., N = 10$ and $t_{ij} = j$ for $j = 1, 2, ..., n_i$, and n_i are random integers in the range specified.

5. Prove that the ordinary least squares remains unbiased for the beta-coefficients in mixed model (2.5). Explain why one should bother with sophisticated estimation if OLS is unbiased.

6. Use the dummy variable approach to estimate mixed model (1.4) assuming that $\{b_i\}$ are fixed and unknown (these estimates are reffered to as *fixed effects*). Represent the model as $\mathbf{y} = \mathbf{X}\boldsymbol{\gamma} + \boldsymbol{\varepsilon}$, where $\mathbf{y}$ and $\mathbf{X}$ are the $(\sum n_i) \times 1$ vector and the $(\sum n_i) \times (N + 1)$ matrix, respectively. Write an R code to compute the fixed effects and compare them with the random effects model. Use the command `outLME$coefficients$random` to extract the random effects, where `outLME` is the variable that contains the output of `lme`.

7. Prove that $S_{\min} = \left\| \mathbf{y} - \mathbf{W}\widehat{\boldsymbol{\beta}}_\infty \right\|^2$.

8. Express the GLS estimator (2.47) in terms of $\mathbf{D}_-$.

9. Show that the restricted log-likelihood function term (2.51) is on the order of $\ln(N)$ when N goes to infinity. To simplify the derivation, assume balanced data: $n_i = n$ and $\mathbf{X}_i = \mathbf{X}, \mathbf{Z}_i = \mathbf{Z}$. This exercise implies that the restricted and regular likelihood approaches converge when the number of clusters increases.

2.3 Balanced random-coefficient model

In this section we consider a very special case of the LME model (2.5), the balanced random-coefficient model. In this model all clusters have the same size ($n_i = n$) and

$$\mathbf{Z} = \mathbf{X}_i = \mathbf{Z}_i, \quad i = 1, ..., N, \tag{2.54}$$

where matrix $\mathbf{Z}$ has full rank. In view of (1.12), it can be called the balanced random-coefficient model. This model is attractive because it allows us to obtain maximum likelihood estimates in closed forms. A more general situation when MLEs admit closed forms is considered in Section 4.1.5.

First, we notice that for model (2.5) with data (2.54), the fixed effects estimate (2.31) is zero because the matrix to invert, $\mathbf{Z}'(\mathbf{I} - \mathbf{Z}(\mathbf{Z}'\mathbf{Z})^{-1}\mathbf{Z}')\mathbf{Z}$, is null, and therefore the generalized inverse is null as well. Second, the model with balanced data may be represented in rectangular format as $\mathbf{Y} = \mathbf{Z}\boldsymbol{\beta}\mathbf{1}' + \mathbf{E}$, where $\mathbf{Y}$ is an $n \times N$ matrix and $\mathbf{1}$ is an $N \times 1$ vector of 1s; $\mathbf{E}$ is the $N \times n$ matrix of error terms with zero mean, mutually independent rows, with the covariance matrix $\sigma^2\mathbf{V} = \sigma^2(\mathbf{I} + \mathbf{Z}\mathbf{D}\mathbf{Z}')$. This model is a special case of the classical growth curve model $\mathbf{Y} = \mathbf{Z}\boldsymbol{\beta}\mathbf{X} + \mathbf{E}$, where the vector columns of $\mathbf{E}$ are iid with unstructured $n \times n$ covariance matrix $\mathbf{\Omega}$, studied by many authors. The early authors were: Potthoff and Roy (1964), Rao (1965), Khatri (1966), and Grizzle and Allen (1969). See Vonesh and Chinchilli (1997) for an overview, where it was termed the generalized multivariate analysis of variance model, and a book by Pan and Fang (2002), where it was termed simply the growth curve model. In particular, the latter authors derive closed-form expressions for variance parameters, as we do below in Theorem 2.

We start by proving that for model (2.5) with data (2.54), the GLS estimator (2.28) collapses to the OLS estimator and therefore does not depend on the matrix $\mathbf{D}$. More precisely,

$$\widehat{\boldsymbol{\beta}}_{GLS} = \widehat{\boldsymbol{\beta}}_{OLS} = (\mathbf{Z}'\mathbf{Z})^{-1}\mathbf{Z}'\overline{\mathbf{y}}, \tag{2.55}$$

where $\overline{\mathbf{y}} = \sum_{i=1}^{N} \mathbf{y}_i / N$.

Proof. By definition, the GLS estimate minimizes the weighted sum of squares,

$$\sum_{i=1}^{N}(\mathbf{y}_i - \mathbf{Z}\boldsymbol{\beta})'\mathbf{V}^{-1}(\mathbf{y}_i - \mathbf{Z}\boldsymbol{\beta}) = \sum(\mathbf{y}_i - \overline{\mathbf{y}})'\mathbf{V}^{-1}(\mathbf{y}_i - \overline{\mathbf{y}})$$

$$+2\sum(\mathbf{y}_i - \overline{\mathbf{y}})'\mathbf{V}^{-1}(\overline{\mathbf{y}} - \mathbf{Z}\boldsymbol{\beta}) + N(\overline{\mathbf{y}} - \mathbf{Z}\boldsymbol{\beta})'\mathbf{V}^{-1}(\overline{\mathbf{y}} - \mathbf{Z}\boldsymbol{\beta}). \tag{2.56}$$

But the middle term vanishes because

$$\sum(\mathbf{y}_i - \overline{\mathbf{y}})'\mathbf{V}^{-1}(\overline{\mathbf{y}} - \mathbf{Z}\boldsymbol{\beta}) = \left[\sum(\mathbf{y}_i - \overline{\mathbf{y}})'\right]\mathbf{V}^{-1}(\overline{\mathbf{y}} - \mathbf{Z}\boldsymbol{\beta}) = 0,$$

and therefore minimization of the weighted sum is equivalent to minimization of $(\overline{\mathbf{y}} - \mathbf{Z}\boldsymbol{\beta})'\mathbf{V}^{-1}(\overline{\mathbf{y}} - \mathbf{Z}\boldsymbol{\beta})$, because the first term in (2.56) is constant. Further, denoting $\widehat{\boldsymbol{\beta}} = (\mathbf{Z}'\mathbf{Z})^{-1}\mathbf{Z}'\overline{\mathbf{y}}$ and applying the dimension-reduction formula (2.21) for the last term of (2.56), we obtain

$$(\overline{\mathbf{y}} - \mathbf{Z}\boldsymbol{\beta})'\mathbf{V}^{-1}(\overline{\mathbf{y}} - \mathbf{Z}\boldsymbol{\beta}) \tag{2.57}$$

$$= [\widehat{\mathbf{e}} - \mathbf{Z}(\boldsymbol{\beta} - \widehat{\boldsymbol{\beta}})]'[\mathbf{I} - \mathbf{Z}(\mathbf{D}^{-1} + \mathbf{Z}'\mathbf{Z})^{-1}\mathbf{Z}'][\widehat{\mathbf{e}} - \mathbf{Z}(\boldsymbol{\beta} - \widehat{\boldsymbol{\beta}})],$$

where $\widehat{\mathbf{e}} = \overline{\mathbf{y}} - \mathbf{Z}\widehat{\boldsymbol{\beta}}$ is a residual vector. But as in the standard linear model, regressors and residuals are orthogonal, $\mathbf{Z}'\widehat{\mathbf{e}} = \mathbf{0}$, because

$$\mathbf{Z}'\widehat{\mathbf{e}} = \mathbf{Z}'[\mathbf{I} - \mathbf{Z}(\mathbf{Z}'\mathbf{Z})^{-1}\mathbf{Z}']\overline{\mathbf{y}} = \mathbf{0}.$$

Hence, the sum (2.57) simplifies to

$$\widehat{\mathbf{e}}'\widehat{\mathbf{e}} + (\boldsymbol{\beta} - \widehat{\boldsymbol{\beta}})'\mathbf{Z}'\mathbf{V}^{-1}\mathbf{Z}(\boldsymbol{\beta} - \widehat{\boldsymbol{\beta}}).$$

Finally, since the matrix $\mathbf{Z}'\mathbf{V}^{-1}\mathbf{Z}$ is positive definite, the minimum of (2.57) occurs at $\boldsymbol{\beta} = \widehat{\boldsymbol{\beta}}$; thus, (2.55) is proved.
∎

Thus, from (2.55) we see that for a balanced random-coefficient regression model, OLS = GLS = MLE. For example, for a balanced linear trend model with random parameters

$$y_{ij} = a_i + b_i t_j + \varepsilon_{ij}, \tag{2.58}$$

$$a_i = \alpha + \eta_i, \ b_i = \beta + \xi_i \quad i = 1, 2, ..., N, \ j = 1, 2, ..., n,$$

one obtains efficient estimates for α and β by applying the OLS to the mean data, $\bar{y}_j = \alpha + \beta t_j + \varsigma_j, \ j = 1, 2, ..., n$, namely,

$$\widehat{\beta} = \frac{\sum (\bar{y}_j - \bar{\bar{y}})(t_j - \bar{t})}{\sum (t_j - \bar{t})^2}, \quad \widehat{\alpha} = \bar{\bar{y}} - \widehat{\beta}\bar{t}.$$

Now we find the MLEs and RMLEs for σ^2 and $\mathbf{D}$ (Laird et al., 1987). As we learn in Chapter 4, $\widehat{\sigma}^2_{ML}$ and $\widehat{\sigma}^2_{ML}\widehat{\mathbf{D}}_{RML}$ are unbiased, but $\widehat{\sigma}^2_{ML}\widehat{\mathbf{D}}_{ML}$ is not. As a word of caution, the unbiasedness of the restricted MLE for variance parameters is not a general property—that is true only for balanced models.

Theorem 2 *The MLEs and RMLEs for the balanced random-coefficient model* $(\mathbf{Z} = \mathbf{X}_i = \mathbf{Z}_i)$ *are given by*

$$\widehat{\sigma}^2_{ML} = \widehat{\sigma}^2_{RML} = \frac{1}{N(n-m)} \sum_{i=1}^{N} \mathbf{y}'_i (\mathbf{I} - \mathbf{Z}(\mathbf{Z}'\mathbf{Z})^{-1}\mathbf{Z}')\mathbf{y}_i, \qquad (2.59)$$

$$\widehat{\mathbf{D}}_{ML} = \frac{1}{N\widehat{\sigma}^2_{ML}}(\mathbf{Z}'\mathbf{Z})^{-1}\mathbf{Z}'\widehat{\mathbf{E}}\widehat{\mathbf{E}}'\mathbf{Z}(\mathbf{Z}'\mathbf{Z})^{-1} - (\mathbf{Z}'\mathbf{Z})^{-1}, \qquad (2.60)$$

$$\widehat{\mathbf{D}}_{RML} = \frac{1}{(N-1)\widehat{\sigma}^2_{ML}}(\mathbf{Z}'\mathbf{Z})^{-1}\mathbf{Z}'\widehat{\mathbf{E}}\widehat{\mathbf{E}}'\mathbf{Z}(\mathbf{Z}'\mathbf{Z})^{-1} - (\mathbf{Z}'\mathbf{Z})^{-1}, \qquad (2.61)$$

where

$$\widehat{\mathbf{E}}\widehat{\mathbf{E}}' = \sum_{i=1}^{N} (\mathbf{y}_i - \mathbf{Z}\widehat{\beta}_{GLS})(\mathbf{y}_i - \mathbf{Z}\widehat{\beta}_{GLS})'$$

is the $n \times n$ matrix of the sum of residuals cross-product, and $\widehat{\beta}_{GLS} = \widehat{\beta}_{OLS}$ is as defined in (2.55).

Proof. Denote $\mathbf{e}_i = \mathbf{y}_i - \mathbf{Z}\widehat{\beta}_{GLS}$, the $n \times 1$ residual vector of the ith cluster, and $\widehat{\mathbf{E}} = [\mathbf{e}_1, ..., \mathbf{e}_N]$, the matrix $n \times N$, so that $\widehat{\mathbf{E}}\widehat{\mathbf{E}}' = \sum_{i=1}^{N} \mathbf{e}_i\mathbf{e}'_i$. Note that $\mathbf{e}_i$ does not depend on $\mathbf{D}$. First, we express σ^2, given by (2.39), through matrix $\mathbf{D}$ using dimension-reduction formula (2.21). We obtain

$$\begin{aligned}
\sigma^2 &= \frac{1}{Nn} \sum_{i=1}^{N} \mathbf{e}'_i \mathbf{V}^{-1} \mathbf{e}_i = \frac{1}{Nn} \text{tr}\left(\sum_{i=1}^{N} \mathbf{e}_i \mathbf{e}'_i \mathbf{V}^{-1} \right) = \frac{1}{Nn} \text{tr}(\widehat{\mathbf{E}}\widehat{\mathbf{E}}'\mathbf{V}^{-1}) \\
&= \frac{1}{Nn} \text{tr}\left[\widehat{\mathbf{E}}\widehat{\mathbf{E}}'(\mathbf{I} - \mathbf{Z}(\mathbf{D}^{-1} + \mathbf{Z}'\mathbf{Z})^{-1}\mathbf{Z}') \right] \\
&= \frac{1}{Nn} \text{tr}\widehat{\mathbf{E}}\widehat{\mathbf{E}}' - \frac{1}{Nn} \text{tr}\left[\widehat{\mathbf{E}}\widehat{\mathbf{E}}'\mathbf{Z}(\mathbf{D}^{-1} + \mathbf{Z}'\mathbf{Z})^{-1}\mathbf{Z}' \right] \\
&= \frac{1}{Nn} \text{tr}\widehat{\mathbf{E}}\widehat{\mathbf{E}}' - \frac{1}{Nn} \text{tr}\left[\widehat{\mathbf{E}}\widehat{\mathbf{E}}'\mathbf{Z}\mathbf{D}(\mathbf{D} + (\mathbf{Z}'\mathbf{Z})^{-1})^{-1}\mathbf{T} \right], \qquad (2.62)
\end{aligned}$$

where it is denoted $\mathbf{T} = (\mathbf{Z}'\mathbf{Z})^{-1}\mathbf{Z}'$. Second, we work on matrix $\mathbf{D}$. The MLE for $\mathbf{D}$ satisfies the score equation, the partial derivative of the log-likelihood function with respect to matrix $\mathbf{D}$. In a general case the derivative is provided by formula (2.105). In the balanced case the score equation for $\mathbf{D}$ simplifies to

$$N\mathbf{Z}'\mathbf{V}^{-1}\mathbf{Z} - \sigma^{-2}\mathbf{Z}'\mathbf{V}^{-1}\widehat{\mathbf{E}}\widehat{\mathbf{E}}'\mathbf{V}^{-1}\mathbf{Z} = \mathbf{0}. \qquad (2.63)$$

We have

$$\mathbf{Z}'\mathbf{V}^{-1} = \mathbf{Z}'(\mathbf{I} - \mathbf{Z}(\mathbf{D}^{-1} + \mathbf{Z}'\mathbf{Z})^{-1}\mathbf{Z}')$$
$$= [\mathbf{I} - \mathbf{Z}'\mathbf{Z}(\mathbf{D}^{-1} + \mathbf{Z}'\mathbf{Z})^{-1}]\mathbf{Z}' = \mathbf{D}^{-1}(\mathbf{D}^{-1} + \mathbf{Z}'\mathbf{Z})^{-1}\mathbf{T} = \mathbf{M}^{-1}\mathbf{T},$$

where it is denoted $\mathbf{M} = (\mathbf{Z}'\mathbf{Z})^{-1} + \mathbf{D}$. Next, using formula (2.25) we rewrite (2.63) as $N\mathbf{M}^{-1} - \sigma^{-2}\mathbf{M}^{-1}\mathbf{T}\mathbf{R}\mathbf{T}'\mathbf{M}^{-1} = \mathbf{0}$, which gives the equation for $\mathbf{D}$,

$$\mathbf{D} = \frac{1}{N\sigma^2}\mathbf{T}\widehat{\mathbf{E}}\widehat{\mathbf{E}}'\mathbf{T}' - (\mathbf{Z}'\mathbf{Z})^{-1}. \qquad (2.64)$$

Substituting this formula into (2.62), one obtains

$$\sigma^2 = \frac{1}{Nn}\mathrm{tr}\widehat{\mathbf{E}}\widehat{\mathbf{E}}' - \frac{\sigma^2}{n}\mathrm{tr}\widehat{\mathbf{E}}\widehat{\mathbf{E}}'\mathbf{Z}\left(\frac{1}{N\sigma^2}\mathbf{T}\widehat{\mathbf{E}}\mathbf{T}' - (\mathbf{Z}'\mathbf{Z})^{-1}\right)(\mathbf{T}\widehat{\mathbf{E}}\widehat{\mathbf{E}}'\mathbf{T}')^{-1}\mathbf{T}$$

$$= \frac{1}{Nn}\mathrm{tr}(\widehat{\mathbf{E}}\widehat{\mathbf{E}}'(\mathbf{I} - \mathbf{P_Z})) + \frac{\sigma^2}{n}\mathrm{tr}(\widehat{\mathbf{E}}\widehat{\mathbf{E}}'\mathbf{T}'(\mathbf{T}\widehat{\mathbf{E}}\mathbf{T}')^{-1}\mathbf{T}),$$

where $\mathbf{P_Z} = \mathbf{Z}(\mathbf{Z}'\mathbf{Z})^{-1}\mathbf{Z}$ is a projection matrix. But for the third term we have $\mathrm{tr}(\widehat{\mathbf{E}}\widehat{\mathbf{E}}'\mathbf{T}'(\mathbf{T}\widehat{\mathbf{E}}\mathbf{T}')^{-1}\mathbf{T}) = \mathrm{tr}((\mathbf{T}\widehat{\mathbf{E}}\widehat{\mathbf{E}}'\mathbf{T}')^{-1}\mathbf{T}\widehat{\mathbf{E}}\widehat{\mathbf{E}}'\mathbf{T}') = m$, and hence, solving for σ^2, we finally obtain the MLE:

$$\widehat{\sigma}^2_{ML} = \frac{1}{N(n-m)}\mathrm{tr}(\widehat{\mathbf{E}}(\mathbf{I} - \mathbf{P_Z}))$$

$$= \frac{1}{N(n-m)}\sum_{i=1}^{N}(\mathbf{y}_i - \mathbf{Z}\widehat{\boldsymbol{\beta}}_{GLS})'(\mathbf{I} - \mathbf{P_Z})(\mathbf{y}_i - \mathbf{Z}\widehat{\boldsymbol{\beta}}_{GLS}).$$

Since $(\mathbf{I} - \mathbf{P_Z})\mathbf{Z} = \mathbf{0}$, the preceding formula may be rewritten as (2.59). Replacing σ^2 with $\widehat{\sigma}^2_{ML}$ in (2.64), we arrive at the MLE

$$\widehat{\mathbf{D}}_{ML} = \frac{1}{N\widehat{\sigma}^2_{ML}}(\mathbf{Z}'\mathbf{Z})^{-1}\mathbf{Z}'\widehat{\mathbf{E}}\widehat{\mathbf{E}}'\mathbf{Z}(\mathbf{Z}'\mathbf{Z})^{-1} - (\mathbf{Z}'\mathbf{Z})^{-1}.$$

Again, using the fact that $(\mathbf{I} - \mathbf{P_Z})\mathbf{Z} = \mathbf{0}$, the preceding formula is equivalent to (2.60).

For the restricted maximum likelihood the expressions for σ^2 and the score equation for $\mathbf{D}$ become (2.52) and (2.129), respectively. Hence, equation (2.63) transforms to $(N-1)\mathbf{Z}'\mathbf{V}^{-1}\mathbf{Z} - \sigma^{-2}\mathbf{Z}'\mathbf{V}^{-1}\widehat{\mathbf{E}}\widehat{\mathbf{E}}'\mathbf{V}^{-1}\mathbf{Z} = \mathbf{0}$, and consequently (2.64) changes to

$$\mathbf{D} = \frac{1}{(N-1)\sigma^2}\mathbf{T}\widehat{\mathbf{E}}\widehat{\mathbf{E}}'\mathbf{T}' - (\mathbf{Z}'\mathbf{Z})^{-1}. \qquad (2.65)$$

Then, analogous to (2.62), for the RML estimator,

$$\sigma^2$$
$$= \frac{\mathrm{tr}\widehat{\mathbf{E}}\widehat{\mathbf{E}}'}{Nn-m} - \frac{1}{Nn-m}\mathrm{tr}\left[\widehat{\mathbf{E}}\widehat{\mathbf{E}}'\mathbf{Z}\mathbf{T} + (N-1)\sigma^2\widehat{\mathbf{E}}\widehat{\mathbf{E}}'\mathbf{T}'(\mathbf{T}\widehat{\mathbf{E}}\widehat{\mathbf{E}}'\mathbf{T}')^{-1}\mathbf{T}\right]$$
$$= \frac{\mathrm{tr}(\widehat{\mathbf{E}}\widehat{\mathbf{E}}'(\mathbf{I} - \mathbf{P_Z}))}{Nn-m} + \frac{(N-1)\sigma^2}{Nn-m}\mathrm{tr}\left[\widehat{\mathbf{E}}\widehat{\mathbf{E}}'\mathbf{T}'(\mathbf{T}\widehat{\mathbf{E}}\widehat{\mathbf{E}}'\mathbf{T}')^{-1}\mathbf{T}\right]$$
$$= \frac{\mathrm{tr}(\widehat{\mathbf{E}}\widehat{\mathbf{E}}'(\mathbf{I} - \mathbf{P_Z}))}{Nn-m} + \frac{(N-1)m}{Nn-m}\sigma^2.$$

Solving for σ^2, we come to the same MLE, (2.59). The estimator (2.61) follows from (2.65).   ∎

Since, according to our convention, $\mathbf{D}$ denotes the scaled covariance matrix, the estimator for the covariance matrix of random effects is $\widehat{\sigma}^2_{ML}\widehat{\mathbf{D}}$, where $\widehat{\mathbf{D}}$ is either an ML or RML estimator (we prefer RML because it is unbiased).

$\widehat{\sigma}^2_{ML}$ is positive if at least one $\mathbf{y}_i$ is not a linear combination of vector columns of matrix $\mathbf{Z}$ (we learn in Section 2.5 that this is a necessary and sufficient condition for the existence of MLE). However, there is no guarantee that $\widehat{\mathbf{D}}_{ML}$ or $\widehat{\mathbf{D}}_{RML}$ is a positive definite matrix (there is a slightly better chance for $\widehat{\mathbf{D}}_{RML}$ to be positive definite). If either of the matrices is not nonnegative definite, one could project the matrix on the space of all nonnegative definite matrices, as defined in Section 2.15. Notice that for balanced data, $\widehat{\mathbf{D}}_{ML} < \widehat{\mathbf{D}}_{RML}$. This makes perfect sense because $\widehat{\mathbf{D}}_{ML}$ is negatively biased and $\widehat{\mathbf{D}}_{RML}$ is unbiased.

In Section 3.3.1 we show that the RML estimators are efficient, i.e., their variance/covariance matrix attains the lower bound. We use the results of this section for identification of the star shape in Chapter 11 (see Section 11.7). We will encounter the balanced random-coefficient model in the analysis of shape in Chapter 11.

Problems for Section 2.3

1. Why are balanced data favorable in practice? Justify your answer by referring to mathematical results from this section.

2. Use model (2.58) to illustrate numerically that the parameters and their variances from lme give the same results as those given by formulas for $\widehat{\beta}$, $\widehat{\alpha}$ and Theorem 2. Pick n, N, and t_j, values for α and β and variances, generate random intercept and random slope data, and compute estimates using formulas; then run lme.

3*. Can we claim that the RML estimates for σ^2 and $\sigma^2\mathbf{D}$ are unbiased? Either prove or carry out a simulation study (use the model specification from Problem 2).

4*. Do the results of this section hold if only some coefficients are random, say, the slope is fixed but the intercept is random? Adjust Theorem 2 to cover this more general case.

2.4   LME model with random intercepts

In this section a very special LME model with one random effect is considered in detail, the LME model with random intercepts. This model will serve as a benchmark to compare estimators and numerical procedures for log-likelihood maximization.

The LME model with random intercepts is written

$$y_{ij} = a_i + \boldsymbol{\gamma}'\mathbf{u}_{ij} + \varepsilon_{ij}, \quad j = 1, ..., n_i, \ i = 1, ..., N, \quad (2.66)$$

where y_{ij} is interpreted as the jth observation of the ith subject. The individual intercept is the sum of a population-averaged parameter α and a random effect, $a_i = \alpha + b_i$. It is assumed that $\varepsilon_{ij} \sim \mathcal{N}(0, \sigma^2)$ and $b_i \sim \mathcal{N}(0, \sigma^2 d)$ are independent, where σ^2 is the within-subject variance and d is the scaled variance of the random effect. The simplest case of model (2.66), when there are no covariates, reduces to a one-variance component model (1.8).

The LME model with individual (random) intercepts can emerge in the following longitudinal setting. Consider a group of N patients. Each patient has his/her own covariates, such as age, gender, weight, diet, and physical performance. Let the treatment outcome be represented by a longitudinal variable, such as the blood pressure y_{ij} of the ith patient measured at time t_{ij}. Then the vector of covariates is $\mathbf{u}_{ij} = (\text{Age}_{ij}, \text{Gender}_i, \text{Weight}_{ij}, \text{Diet}_{ij})$. If longitudinal observations cover a fairly long period of time, Age, Weight, and Diet are time-varying covariates, so they are supplied with subindex j. We are interested in how the blood pressure is affected by these covariates. The key assumption is that the relationship does not vary from patient to patient, meaning that $\boldsymbol{\gamma}$ is a fixed vector. However, we admit that at the time the study begins, each patient may have a different baseline blood pressure, even for patients of the same age, gender, weight, and diet. Certainly, one could design the experiment to involve patients with the same initial conditions: the same age, gender, weight, and diet. However, the reader will agree how difficult it would be to obtain such data. A model with individual intercepts would be more realistic because it allows the analysis of patients with different baseline blood pressures.

The LME model with random intercepts also emerges in econometrics as the model for panel data in the cross-sectional analysis (see Maddala, 1987 for a review). In the variance components literature this model is called a *linear model with nested error structure* (Christensen, 1996; Wang and Ma, 2002).

In matrix notation, the LME model with random intercepts can be written as

$$\mathbf{y}_i \sim \mathcal{N}(\mathbf{X}_i\boldsymbol{\beta}, \sigma^2(\mathbf{I}_i + d\mathbf{1}_i\mathbf{1}_i')), \qquad i = 1, ..., N, \tag{2.67}$$

where $\mathbf{X}_i$ is an $n_i \times m$ design matrix of full rank with the jth row $\mathbf{x}_{ij}' = (1, \mathbf{u}_{ij}')$; $\boldsymbol{\beta} = (\alpha, \boldsymbol{\gamma}')'$ is an $m \times 1$ vector of fixed effects; $\mathbf{1}_i$ is an $n_i \times 1$ unit vector; σ^2 is the within-subject variance; and $\sigma^2 d$ is the variance of the random effect. In the notation of (2.14), $k = 1$, $\mathbf{1}_i = \mathbf{Z}_i$, $d = \mathbf{D}$. Model (2.66) has an exchangeable (compound symmetry) correlation structure because the correlation coefficient between y_{ij} and y_{ik} is constant, $d/(1 + d)$ for $j \neq k$. In fact, our LME model of Section 2.1 with family data on weight and height has the form (2.66).

The variance-profile log-likelihood function, written in the form (2.40), is

$$l_p(\boldsymbol{\beta}, d) = -\frac{1}{2}\left\{\sum_{i=1}^N \ln|\mathbf{I} + d\mathbf{1}_i\mathbf{1}_i'| + N_T \ln[\sum_{i=1}^N \mathbf{e}_i'(\mathbf{I} + d\mathbf{1}_i\mathbf{1}_i')^{-1}\mathbf{e}_i]\right\}, \tag{2.68}$$

where $\mathbf{e}_i = \mathbf{y}_i - \mathbf{X}_i\boldsymbol{\beta}$ is an $n_i \times 1$ residual vector. The dimension-reduction formulas (2.21) and (2.22) simplify to

$$|\mathbf{I} + d\mathbf{1}_i\mathbf{1}_i'| = 1 + n_i d, \quad (\mathbf{I} + d\mathbf{1}_i\mathbf{1}_i')^{-1} = \mathbf{I} - \frac{d}{1 + n_i d}\mathbf{1}_i\mathbf{1}_i'. \tag{2.69}$$

Thus, the GLS estimator (2.28) for this model is

$$\widehat{\boldsymbol{\beta}}_{GLS} = \left[\sum_i\left(\mathbf{X}_i'\mathbf{X}_i - \frac{n_i^2 d}{1 + n_i d}\overline{\mathbf{x}}_i\overline{\mathbf{x}}_i'\right)\right]^{-1} \times \left[\sum_i\left(\mathbf{X}_i'\mathbf{y}_i - \frac{n_i^2 d}{1 + n_i d}\overline{\mathbf{x}}_i\overline{y}_i\right)\right], \tag{2.70}$$

where

$$\overline{\mathbf{x}}_i = \frac{1}{n_i}\mathbf{X}_i'\mathbf{1}_i = \frac{1}{n_i}\sum_{j=1}^{n_i}\mathbf{x}_{ij}, \quad \overline{y}_i = \frac{1}{n_i}\mathbf{y}_i'\mathbf{1}_i = \frac{1}{n_i}\sum_{j=1}^{n_i}y_{ij}.$$

The fixed-effects estimator (2.31) is the limit of (2.70) when $d \to \infty$. We notice that the inverse matrix in (2.70) becomes singular when $d \to \infty$ because the first row and column are zero. We could use the generalized inverse as in (2.31), but it is easier to minimize the quadratic form (2.33) as a function of $N + m$ parameters $a_1, ..., a_N, \boldsymbol{\gamma}$ directly,

$$\sum_{i=1}^{N} \sum_{j=1}^{n_i} (y_{ij} - a_i - \mathbf{u}_{ij}'\boldsymbol{\gamma})^2 \Rightarrow \min.$$

The minimum is attained at $\widehat{a}_i = \overline{y}_i - \widehat{\boldsymbol{\gamma}}_\infty' \overline{\mathbf{u}}_i$, which leads to the Fixed Effects (FE) estimator,

$$\widehat{\boldsymbol{\gamma}}_\infty = \left[\sum_{i=1}^{N} \left(\sum_{j=1}^{n_i} \mathbf{u}_{ij}\mathbf{u}_{ij}' - n_i \overline{\mathbf{u}}_i \overline{\mathbf{u}}_i' \right) \right]^{-1} \left[\sum_{i=1}^{N} \left(\sum_{j=1}^{n_i} \mathbf{u}_{ij} y_{ij} - n_i \overline{\mathbf{u}}_i \overline{y}_i \right) \right]. \quad (2.71)$$

This estimator could also be obtained by centering observations around the individual means for each i (differencing out) and applying OLS. Interestingly, the estimator $\widehat{\boldsymbol{\gamma}}_\infty$ is consistent despite the fact that the number of nuisance parameters (subject-specific intercepts) increases with the number of clusters $N \to \infty$. In fact, this is true only for linear models, and we shall establish similar asymptotic properties for the general linear growth curve model, as a compromise between the fixed and random effect models. Contrary to the linear model, as we shall learn in Section 7.2.2, the MLE for the logistic regression model with fixed subject-specific intercept is not consistent, but the conditional maximum likelihood is—although, as shown in Section 3.2.1, the simultaneous presence of fixed and mixed effects leads to an invalid statistical model.

In a special case of the VARCOMP model (1.8), we obtain

$$\widehat{\alpha}_{GLS} = \frac{\sum_{i=1}^{N} \frac{n_i}{1+dn_i}\overline{y}_i}{\sum_{i=1}^{N} \frac{n_i}{1+dn_i}}, \quad \widehat{\alpha}_\infty = \frac{1}{N} \sum_{i=1}^{N} \overline{y}_i. \quad (2.72)$$

Note that these estimates coincide when $n_i =$ const (i.e., when the design is balanced).

Recall that the fixed effects approach assumes that intercepts are fixed and different for each person. On the contrary, the mixed effects model assumes that a_i are independent identically distributed (iid) random variables with the same mean, α. An economical version of the variance-profile log-likelihood function, based on the dimension-reduction formulas (2.69), has the form

$$l_p(\boldsymbol{\beta}, d) = -\frac{1}{2} \left\{ \sum_{i=1}^{N} \ln(1 + n_i d) + N_T \ln \left(S - d \sum_{i=1}^{N} \frac{n_i^2 h_i^2}{1+n_i d} \right) \right\}, \quad (2.73)$$

and as a special case of (2.53) for the restricted ML

$$l_{Rp}(\boldsymbol{\beta}, d) = -\frac{1}{2} \left\{ \sum \ln(1 + n_i d) + \ln \left| \sum \left(\mathbf{X}_i'\mathbf{X}_i - \frac{n_i^2 d}{1+n_i d}\overline{\mathbf{x}}_i\overline{\mathbf{x}}_i' \right) \right| \right.$$
$$\left. + (N_T - m) \ln \left(S - d \sum \frac{n_i^2 h_i^2}{1+n_i d} \right) \right\}, \quad (2.74)$$

where the scalars S and h_i are defined as

$$
\begin{aligned}
S &= S(\boldsymbol{\beta}) = \sum_{i=1}^{N} \|\mathbf{y}_i - \mathbf{X}_i\boldsymbol{\beta}\|^2, \\
h_i &= h_i(\boldsymbol{\beta}) = \frac{1}{n_i}\sum_{j=1}^{n_i}(y_{ij} - \mathbf{x}'_{ij}\boldsymbol{\beta}) = \bar{y}_i - \boldsymbol{\beta}'\bar{\mathbf{x}}_i.
\end{aligned} \tag{2.75}
$$

The log-likelihood function l_p may be simplified for balanced data ($n_i = n$). In this case the function admits a closed-form solution for the maximum over d. Indeed, if $n_i = n$, then (2.73) takes the form

$$
-\frac{1}{2}\left\{ N\ln(1+nd) + Nn\ln\left(S - \frac{n^2 dA}{1+nd} \right) \right\},
$$

where $A = \sum_{i=1}^{N} h_i^2$. The MLE for d turns the partial derivative to zero, which yields

$$
d = \frac{n^2 A - S}{n(S - nA)} = \frac{n^2\sum(\bar{y}_i - \boldsymbol{\beta}'\bar{\mathbf{x}}_i)^2 - \sum\|\mathbf{y}_i - \mathbf{X}_i\boldsymbol{\beta}\|^2}{n\left(\sum\|\mathbf{y}_i - \mathbf{X}_i\boldsymbol{\beta}\|^2 - n\sum(\bar{y}_i - \boldsymbol{\beta}'\bar{\mathbf{x}}_i)^2\right)}. \tag{2.76}
$$

Below we consider the case when a linear model with random intercepts admits a closed-form solution. Comprehensive coverage of the random-intercept model with an equal number of observations per cluster ($n_i =$const) with econometric applications may be found in a book by Hsiao (2003).

2.4.1 Balanced random-intercept model

In this section we consider the case when $n_i = n$ and $\mathbf{X}_i = \mathbf{X}$, the balanced data. Our aim is to derive closed-form expressions for ML estimates as we did in Section 2.3. First we show that the GLS estimate (2.70) does not depend on d and coincides with the OLS estimate. As we shall see later, a similar result holds for the Poisson regression model with random intercepts if the data are balanced (see Section 7.5.7 for details).

If $\mathbf{X}_i = \mathbf{X}$, it takes the form

$$
\widehat{\boldsymbol{\beta}}_{GLS} = \left(\mathbf{XX} - \frac{n^2 d}{1+nd}\overline{\mathbf{x}}\overline{\mathbf{x}}' \right)^{-1} \left(\mathbf{X}'\overline{\mathbf{y}} - \frac{n^2 d}{1+nd}\overline{\mathbf{x}}\overline{\bar{y}} \right), \tag{2.77}
$$

where $\bar{\bar{y}} = \bar{\mathbf{y}}'\mathbf{1}/n$. We use the formula

$$
(\mathbf{A} - c\mathbf{b}\mathbf{b}')^{-1} = \mathbf{A}^{-1} + c\frac{\mathbf{A}^{-1}\mathbf{b}\mathbf{b}'\mathbf{A}^{-1}}{1 - c\mathbf{b}'\mathbf{A}^{-1}\mathbf{b}}
$$

to invert the matrix in (2.77). Using this formula, we obtain

$$
\left(\mathbf{XX} - \frac{n^2 d}{1+nd}\overline{\mathbf{x}}\overline{\mathbf{x}}' \right)^{-1} = (\mathbf{X}'\mathbf{X})^{-1} + \frac{(\mathbf{X}'\mathbf{X})^{-1}\overline{\mathbf{x}}\overline{\mathbf{x}}'(\mathbf{X}'\mathbf{X})^{-1}}{1/c - \overline{\mathbf{x}}'(\mathbf{X}'\mathbf{X})^{-1}\overline{\mathbf{x}}}, \tag{2.78}
$$

where $c = n^2 d/(1+nd)$. The following simple fact is very useful in studying the random-intercept model.

Lemma 3 *Let* $\mathbf{X} = [\mathbf{1}, \mathbf{U}]$ *be an* $n \times m$ *matrix of full rank, where* $\mathbf{1} = (1, ..., 1)'$ *is an* $n \times 1$ *vector of 1s,* $\mathbf{U}$ *be an* $n \times (m-1)$ *matrix of full rank, and* $\overline{\mathbf{x}} = \mathbf{X}'\mathbf{1}/n$ *be a vector of averages. Then: (a)* $(\mathbf{X}'\mathbf{X})^{-1}\mathbf{X}'\mathbf{1} = (1, \mathbf{0})'$*; (b)* $\mathbf{X}(\mathbf{X}'\mathbf{X})^{-1}\mathbf{X}'\mathbf{1} = \mathbf{1}$*; (c)* $\mathbf{1}'\mathbf{X}(\mathbf{X}'\mathbf{X})^{-1}\mathbf{X}'\mathbf{1} = n$*; (d)* $\overline{\mathbf{x}}'(\mathbf{X}'\mathbf{X})^{-1}\overline{\mathbf{x}} = 1/n$*.*

Proof. It is easy to see that

$$(\mathbf{X}'\mathbf{X})^{-1}\mathbf{X}'\mathbf{1} = \begin{bmatrix} n & \mathbf{1}'\mathbf{U} \\ \mathbf{U}'\mathbf{1} & \mathbf{U}'\mathbf{U} \end{bmatrix}^{-1} \begin{bmatrix} n \\ \mathbf{U}'\mathbf{1} \end{bmatrix}.$$

Now we use the matrix block-inverse formula

$$\begin{bmatrix} a & \mathbf{b}' \\ \mathbf{b} & \mathbf{H} \end{bmatrix}^{-1}$$

$$= \frac{1}{a - \mathbf{b}'\mathbf{H}^{-1}\mathbf{b}} \begin{bmatrix} 1 & -\mathbf{b}'\mathbf{H}^{-1} \\ -\mathbf{H}^{-1}\mathbf{b} & (a - \mathbf{b}'\mathbf{H}^{-1}\mathbf{b})\mathbf{H}^{-1} + \mathbf{H}^{-1}\mathbf{b}\mathbf{b}'\mathbf{H}^{-1} \end{bmatrix},$$

$$\tag{2.79}$$

where a is a positive scalar, $\mathbf{H}$ is a positive definite matrix, and $\mathbf{b}$ is a vector of appropriate size. Denoting $\mathbf{q} = (\mathbf{U}'\mathbf{U})^{-1}\mathbf{U}'\mathbf{1}$ and $\kappa = \mathbf{1}'\mathbf{U}\mathbf{q}$, we obtain (a),

$$(\mathbf{X}'\mathbf{X})^{-1}\mathbf{X}'\mathbf{1} = \frac{1}{n-\kappa} \begin{bmatrix} 1 & -\mathbf{q}' \\ -\mathbf{q} & (n-\kappa)(\mathbf{U}'\mathbf{U})^{-1} + \mathbf{q}\mathbf{q}' \end{bmatrix} \begin{bmatrix} n \\ \mathbf{U}'\mathbf{1} \end{bmatrix}$$

$$= \frac{1}{n-\kappa} \begin{bmatrix} n-\kappa \\ \mathbf{0} \end{bmatrix} = \begin{bmatrix} 1 \\ \mathbf{0} \end{bmatrix}.$$

Statement (b) follows directly from (a) because

$$\mathbf{X}(\mathbf{X}'\mathbf{X})^{-1}\mathbf{X}'\mathbf{1} = [\mathbf{1}, \mathbf{U}] \begin{bmatrix} 1 \\ \mathbf{0} \end{bmatrix} = \mathbf{1}.$$

Statements (c) and (d) are apparent consequences of (b). ∎

Due to statement (b) of Lemma 3, the denominator in (2.78) simplifies to $(1 + nd)(n^2d) - 1/n = 1/(n^2d)$. Thus, letting $\mathbf{M} = (\mathbf{X}'\mathbf{X})^{-1}$ to shorten the notation, we obtain

$$\begin{aligned}
\widehat{\boldsymbol{\beta}}_{GLS} &= (\mathbf{M} + n^2d\mathbf{M}\overline{\mathbf{x}}\overline{\mathbf{x}}'\mathbf{M}) \left(\mathbf{X}'\overline{\mathbf{y}} - \frac{n^2d}{1+nd}\overline{\mathbf{x}\overline{y}} \right) \\
&= \mathbf{M}\mathbf{X}'\overline{\mathbf{y}} - \frac{n^2d}{1+nd}\mathbf{M}\overline{\mathbf{x}\overline{y}} + n^2d\mathbf{M}\overline{\mathbf{x}}\overline{\mathbf{x}}'\mathbf{M}\mathbf{X}'\overline{\mathbf{y}} - \frac{n^4d^2}{1+nd}\mathbf{M}\overline{\mathbf{x}}\overline{\mathbf{x}}'\mathbf{M}\overline{\mathbf{x}\overline{\overline{y}}} \\
&= \mathbf{M}\mathbf{X}'\overline{\mathbf{y}} - \frac{n^2d}{1+nd}\mathbf{M}\overline{\mathbf{x}\overline{y}} + n^2d\mathbf{M}\overline{\mathbf{x}}\overline{\mathbf{x}}'\mathbf{M}\mathbf{X}'\overline{\mathbf{y}} - \frac{n^3d^2}{1+nd}\mathbf{M}\overline{\mathbf{x}\overline{\overline{y}}} \\
&= \mathbf{M}\mathbf{X}'\overline{\mathbf{y}} - \left(\frac{n^2d}{1+nd} + \frac{n^3d^2}{1+nd} \right) \mathbf{M}\overline{\mathbf{x}\overline{\overline{y}}} + n^2d\mathbf{M}\overline{\mathbf{x}}\overline{\mathbf{x}}'\mathbf{M}\mathbf{X}'\overline{\mathbf{y}} \\
&= \mathbf{M}\mathbf{X}'\overline{\mathbf{y}} - n^2d(\overline{\overline{y}} - \overline{\mathbf{x}}'\mathbf{M}\mathbf{X}'\overline{\mathbf{y}})\mathbf{M}\overline{\mathbf{x}}, \tag{2.80}
\end{aligned}$$

where $\overline{\mathbf{y}} = \sum_{i=1}^{N} \mathbf{y}_i/N$. We observe that $\overline{\overline{y}} - \overline{\mathbf{x}}'\mathbf{M}\mathbf{X}'\overline{\mathbf{y}} = 0$ follows directly from (b) of Lemma 3. Indeed,

$$\overline{\overline{y}} - \overline{\mathbf{x}}'\mathbf{M}\mathbf{X}'\overline{\mathbf{y}} = (1/n - \overline{\mathbf{x}}'\mathbf{M}\mathbf{X}')\overline{\mathbf{y}} = n^{-1}(\mathbf{1}' - \mathbf{1}'\mathbf{X}(\mathbf{X}'\mathbf{X})^{-1}\mathbf{X}')\overline{\mathbf{y}} = 0.$$

Thus, the second term in the last expression of (2.80) vanishes, and for balanced data we obtain

$$\widehat{\boldsymbol{\beta}}_{GLS} = \widehat{\boldsymbol{\beta}}_{OLS} = (\mathbf{X}'\mathbf{X})^{-1}\mathbf{X}'\overline{\mathbf{y}}. \tag{2.81}$$

From standard regression theory with an intercept term, it follows that the OLS estimates for slopes and intercept may be expressed further as

$$\widehat{\boldsymbol{\gamma}}_{OLS} = (\widetilde{\mathbf{U}}'\widetilde{\mathbf{U}})^{-1}\widetilde{\mathbf{U}}'\overline{\mathbf{y}}, \quad \widehat{\alpha}_{OLS} = \overline{\overline{y}} - \overline{\mathbf{u}}'\widehat{\boldsymbol{\gamma}}_{OLS}$$

where $\widetilde{\mathbf{U}}$ is the centerized matrix, and $\widetilde{\mathbf{U}} = \mathbf{U} - \mathbf{1}\overline{\mathbf{u}}'$, where $\overline{\mathbf{u}} = \mathbf{U}'\mathbf{1}/n$.

Now we work on σ^2 and d. Since $\widehat{\boldsymbol{\beta}}_{ML} = \widehat{\boldsymbol{\beta}}_{OLS}$ does not depend on d, from (2.39) we obtain

$$
\begin{aligned}
\widehat{\sigma}^2_{ML} &= \frac{1}{Nn} \sum_{i=1}^N (\mathbf{y}_i - \mathbf{X}\widehat{\boldsymbol{\beta}}_{OLS})' \left(\mathbf{I} - \frac{\widehat{d}_{ML}}{1 + n\widehat{d}_{ML}} \right) (\mathbf{y}_i - \mathbf{X}\widehat{\boldsymbol{\beta}}_{OLS}) \\
&= \frac{1}{Nn} \left[\sum \left\| \mathbf{y}_i - \mathbf{X}\widehat{\boldsymbol{\beta}}_{OLS} \right\|^2 - \frac{\widehat{d}_{ML}}{1 + n\widehat{d}_{ML}} \sum \left((\mathbf{y}_i - \mathbf{X}\widehat{\boldsymbol{\beta}}_{OLS})'\mathbf{1} \right)^2 \right] \\
&= \frac{1}{Nn} \left(S - \frac{\widehat{d}_{ML} n^2 A}{1 + n\widehat{d}_{ML}} \right), \tag{2.82}
\end{aligned}
$$

where $S = \sum \|\widehat{\mathbf{e}}_i\|^2$, $\widehat{\mathbf{e}}_i = \mathbf{y}_i - \mathbf{X}\widehat{\boldsymbol{\beta}}_{OLS}$ is an $n \times 1$ vector of the OLS residuals, and $A = \sum (\overline{y}_i - \overline{\overline{y}})^2$ as above. From (2.76) we have

$$\widehat{d}_{ML} = \frac{n^2 A - S}{n(S - nA)} = \frac{1}{N\widehat{\sigma}^2_{ML}} \sum (\overline{y}_i - \overline{\overline{y}})^2 - \frac{1}{n}, \tag{2.83}$$

where

$$\widehat{\sigma}^2_{ML} = \frac{S - nA}{N(n-1)} = \frac{1}{N(n-1)} \sum_{i=1}^N \left(\|\mathbf{e}_i\|^2 - n(\overline{y}_i - \overline{\overline{y}})^2 \right). \tag{2.84}$$

Next we find the RML estimates for a balanced random-intercept model. Using the formula for the determinant

$$\left| \mathbf{A} - a\mathbf{b}\mathbf{b}' \right| = |\mathbf{A}| \left(1 - a\mathbf{b}'\mathbf{A}^{-1}\mathbf{b} \right)$$

and the fact that $\overline{\mathbf{x}}'\mathbf{X}(\mathbf{X}'\mathbf{X})^{-1}\overline{\mathbf{x}} = 1/n$, we can simplify the log-likelihood function (2.74) to an equivalent function,

$$-\frac{1}{2} \left\{ N\ln(1 + nd) + (Nn - m)\ln\left(S - \frac{n^2 dA}{1 + nd} \right) - \ln(1 + nd) \right\}.$$

Letting $v = 1 + nd$ and taking the derivative with respect to v, we come to the closed-form solution

$$\widehat{d}_{RML} = \frac{[N(n-1) - m + 1]An - (N-1)(S - An)}{n(N-1)(S - An)}. \tag{2.85}$$

Analogous to (2.82), we obtain the relationship between RML estimates of σ^2 and d,

$$\widehat{\sigma}^2_{RML} = \frac{1}{Nn - m} \left(S - \frac{\widehat{d}_{RML} n^2 A}{1 + n\widehat{d}_{RML}} \right). \tag{2.86}$$

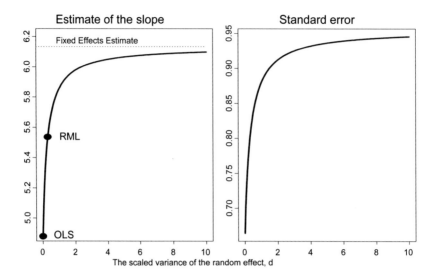

FIGURE 2.1. Generalized least squares estimate of the slope in the random intercept model (compound symmetry correlation structure) as a function of the scaled variance of the random effect d, family data (weight versus height). When $d = 0$, GLS = OLS. When $d \to \infty$, the GLS estimate approaches the fixed effects estimate $\widehat{\gamma}_\infty$. The standard error (SE) of the slope estimate is an increasing function of d. The estimate and SE are not constants because the family data are not balanced. For balanced data the estimate and SE do not depend on d.

Substituting (2.85) into (2.86), we finally obtain the closed-form RML estimate for σ^2, d, and $d_* = \sigma^2 d$:

$$\widehat{\sigma}^2_{RML} = \frac{1}{N(n-1) - m + 1} \sum_{i=1}^{N} \left(\|\widehat{\mathbf{e}}_i\|^2 - n(\overline{y}_i - \overline{\overline{y}})^2 \right), \qquad (2.87)$$

$$\widehat{d}_{RML} = \frac{1}{(N-1)\widehat{\sigma}^2_{ML}} \sum_{i=1}^{N}(\overline{y}_i - \overline{\overline{y}})^2 - \frac{1}{n}, \qquad (2.88)$$

$$\widehat{d}_{*RML} = \frac{1}{N-1} \sum_{i=1}^{N}(\overline{y}_i - \overline{\overline{y}})^2 - \frac{\widehat{\sigma}^2_{RML}}{n}. \qquad (2.89)$$

We make a few comments on the restricted ML estimates for the variance parameters. Generally, RML estimates are close to standard ML estimates. The difference is in degrees of freedom/denominator. For σ^2, the denominator is adjusted by the number of fixed effects slopes $(m - 1)$ and for d by 1. As we shall learn in Section 3.14, the RMLEs for the random-intercept model with balanced data are unbiased and coincide with other quadratic unbiased estimators: minimum norm, method of moments, and variance least squares. Interestingly, for the balanced random-coefficient model of the preceding section, ML = RML for σ^2, but it is different for the balanced random-intercept model.

2.4.2   How random effect affects the variance of MLE

Before advancing to mixed effects business, it is important to know how the presence of the random effect would affect the variance of the maximum likelihood estimate. Does the introduction of the random effect reduce or increase the variance of the ordinary least squares estimate? Is the variance of the MLE an increasing or decreasing function of the variance of the random effect? We answer this question for a balanced model with a random intercept where a closed-form solution exists. We shall find out how the scaled variance of the random effect d affects the covariance matrix of the generalized least squares estimate (2.77) in the balanced random-intercept model.

The covariance matrix for the GLS estimator is given by

$$\text{cov}(\widehat{\boldsymbol{\beta}}_{GLS}) = \sigma^2 \left(\sum_{i=1}^{N} \mathbf{X}_i' \mathbf{V}_i^{-1} \mathbf{X}_i \right)^{-1}.$$

For the balanced random-intercept model, the covariance matrix of (2.77) reduces to

$$
\begin{aligned}
\text{cov}(\widehat{\boldsymbol{\beta}}_{GLS}) &= \frac{\sigma^2}{N} (\mathbf{X}'\mathbf{V}^{-1}\mathbf{X})^{-1} = \frac{\sigma^2}{N} \left(\mathbf{X}'\mathbf{X} - \frac{n^2 d}{1+nd} \overline{\mathbf{x}}\,\overline{\mathbf{x}}' \right)^{-1} \\
&= \frac{\sigma^2}{N} \left((\mathbf{X}'\mathbf{X})^{-1} + n^2 d (\mathbf{X}'\mathbf{X})^{-1} \overline{\mathbf{x}}\,\overline{\mathbf{x}}' (\mathbf{X}'\mathbf{X})^{-1} \right) \\
&= \frac{\sigma^2}{N} (\mathbf{X}'\mathbf{X})^{-1} + \frac{d_*}{N} \begin{bmatrix} 1 & \mathbf{0} \\ \mathbf{0} & \mathbf{0} \end{bmatrix}
\end{aligned}
$$

because of statement (a) of Lemma 3.

Thus, one infers the following:

- The variance of the random intercept in the random-intercept model with balanced data affects only the variance of the intercept term.

- The variances of the slopes do not change with d_*.

One can interpret this result by saying that an equal correlation for balanced data does not affect the estimates of slopes: (a) the GLS/ML estimates do not change; (b) the variance of the estimates do not change either (the same result holds for Poisson regression; see Section 7.5.7). We emphasize that this is true only for balanced data. To illustrate, we consider our previous example with family unbalanced data.

Example (continued). We consider the family data from Section 2.1, where the LME model (2.2) with equal correlation within the family has the form of the random-intercept model (2.66). The data are not balanced and we want to know whether the GLS estimate (2.70) or its variance depends on d. In Figure 2.1 we plot the slope at height and its SE as a function of d. Since the data are not balanced, $\widehat{\boldsymbol{\beta}}_{GLS}$ and $SE(\widehat{\boldsymbol{\beta}}_{GLS})$ change with d. Two extremes are the OLS ($d = 0$) and the FE estimator ($d = \infty$). Note that the difference between two extremes values of the slope is fairly small. ∎

An attractive feature of the random-intercept model is that exact tests are available for a linear hypothesis on coefficients $\boldsymbol{\beta}$ (see Section 3.8 for details).

Problems for Section 2.4

1. Is it true to say that the fixed effects model with cluster (or subject) -specific intercepts is the limiting case of the random intercept model when its variance goes to infinity? Use theory to justify your answer.

2. Is it true that GLS slope estimates given by formula (2.70) are monotonic functions of the scaled variance of the random intercept, d? If this is true provide a proof; if this is not true, provide a counterexample.

3*. Confirm by statistical simulations that the MLE or RMLE of the slope with random intercept is unbiased in a small sample. For balanced data it follows from the fact that OLS=GLS [see equation (2.81)], so unbalanced data should be used for simulations (you can use `famdat` for this purpose).

4. Reproduce Figure 2.1 in R. Prove that SE is an increasing function of d.

2.5 Criterion for MLE existence

The aim of this section is to provide a criterion for the existence of the MLE in the LME model. There is an opinion that such a criterion would be of purely theoretical interest: Let an algorithm for the log-likelihood function maximization start. If it finds the solution, the MLE exists; if it fails, the MLE does not exist. Such a pragmatic and naive approach relies completely on the effectiveness of the maximization algorithm. However, the failure of the algorithm does not mean that the MLE does not exist! It may fail because (a) matrix $\mathbf{D}$ becomes nonnegative definite; (b) the sequence of points generated by an iterative algorithm may not converge due to a poor starting point; or (c) a computer program may terminate due to overflow, memory shortage, etc. Then, what is the reason: a poorly specified model, a wrong starting value, a poor algorithm, an error in the computer program, or perhaps the maximum of the log-likelihood function cannot be attained because the MLE does not exist? Therefore, before starting a maximization process, one has to be sure that the MLE exists. We need criteria for MLE existence!

Below, we formulate and prove a necessary and sufficient condition for the existence of the MLE in the LME model. A similar condition for a variance components model has been derived by Rao and Kleffé (1988) and modified by Demidenko and Massam (1999).

A practical implication of the following theorem is that the MLE in the LME model exists with probability 1 if the total number of observations is sufficiently large, particularly if $\sum(n_i - k) - m > 0$. However, the MLE existence does not guarantee that matrix $\widehat{\mathbf{D}}_{ML}$ is positive definite, and we discuss this issue in the next section.

Theorem 4 *Under the assumptions of Section 2.2, the ML and RML estimates for the mixed effects model (2.14) on the parameter space (2.16) exist if and only if there does not exist such a $\boldsymbol{\beta} \in R^m, \boldsymbol{\gamma}_1, ..., \boldsymbol{\gamma}_N \in R^k$, that*

$$\mathbf{y}_i = \mathbf{X}_i\boldsymbol{\beta} + \mathbf{Z}_i\boldsymbol{\gamma}_i, \quad i = 1, ..., N, \tag{2.90}$$

or, equivalently, that inequality (2.37) holds.

Proof is given in Section 2.17 (for RML we assume that at least $m+1$ matrices $\mathbf{Z}_i'\mathbf{Z}_i$ are nonsingular).

Remarks

1. Let the $N_T \times (m + Nk)$ matrix $\mathbf{W} = [\mathbf{X}; \mathbf{Z}]$ be defined as in (2.34). If

$$\mathrm{rank}(\mathbf{W}) < N_T, \tag{2.91}$$

the MLE exists with probability 1. Indeed, $\mathbf{y} \in R^{N_T}$ has normal distribution with a positive definite covariance matrix $\mathbf{V}$. Condition (2.90) means that the MLE does not exist if $\mathbf{y}$ belongs to the linear space generated by the vector columns of matrix $\mathbf{W}$. But this probability is zero if (2.91) holds. Clearly, condition (2.91) holds if $\sum(n_i - k) > m$.

2. One can verify inequality (2.37) in two ways. First, we can construct a stacked vector and matrix

$$\mathbf{y_Z} = \begin{bmatrix} \mathbf{y}_{1\mathbf{Z}} \\ \vdots \\ \mathbf{y}_{N\mathbf{Z}} \end{bmatrix}, \quad \mathbf{X_Z} = \begin{bmatrix} \mathbf{X}_{1\mathbf{Z}} \\ \vdots \\ \mathbf{X}_{N\mathbf{Z}} \end{bmatrix}, \tag{2.92}$$

where $\mathbf{y}_{i\mathbf{Z}} = (\mathbf{I} - \mathbf{Z}_i\mathbf{Z}_i^+)\mathbf{y}_i$ and $\mathbf{X}_{i\mathbf{Z}} = (\mathbf{I} - \mathbf{Z}_i\mathbf{Z}_i^+)\mathbf{X}_i$. Then the MLE exists if and only if the sum of squares of the OLS residuals in the regression of $\mathbf{y_Z}$ on $\mathbf{X_Z}$ is positive. Second, one can compute the OLS regression $\mathbf{y}$ on $\mathbf{W}$. Again, the MLE exists if and only if the sum of squares is positive; if matrix $\mathbf{W}'\mathbf{W}$ is singular, one needs to take the generalized inverse.

3. If the MLE exists, then $\boldsymbol{\beta}'\boldsymbol{\beta} \to \infty$ or $\sigma^2 \to 0$ or $\mathbf{D} \to \infty$ implies that $l \to -\infty$. Therefore, under (2.37), the level set $S_0 = \{\boldsymbol{\theta} : l(\boldsymbol{\theta}) \geq l(\boldsymbol{\theta}_0)\}$ is compact. Moreover, for any starting point $\boldsymbol{\theta}_0$ the sequence of parameters generated by any iterative maximization algorithm, which increases the value of the log-likelihood function from iteration to iteration, converges (Demidenko, 1989). In particular, this implies convergence of the EM algorithm.

4. If the MLE exists, the estimate of σ^2 must be strictly positive.

5. Assumption of the nonnegative definiteness of matrix $\mathbf{D}$ is important for proof of MLE existence. If one looks for the maximum of the log-likelihood over the set of positive definite matrices $\mathbf{D}$, this maximum may be outside the parameter space if the maximum point in (2.16) belongs to the boundary (i.e., where $|\mathbf{D}| = 0$).

Interestingly, the MLE may exist but make no sense for matrix $\mathbf{D}$ (see the example in the next section).

Problems for Section 2.5

1. Formulate Theorem 4 for the classical linear regression model ($N = 1$, $k = 0$). What happens with the log-likelihood when $\sigma^2 \to 0$ if (2.90) holds?

2. Does Theorem 4 hold for the Rao and Kleffé (1988) parameter space: that is when matrices $\mathbf{I} + \mathbf{Z}_i \mathbf{D} \mathbf{Z}_i'$ are positive definite for all $i = 1, 2, ..., N$?

3. Regarding Remark 3, construct an example of a function $f(x)$ bounded from below, where $x \in (-\infty, \infty)$, so that a sequence of values x_k minimizes the value from iteration to iteration, $f(x_{k+1}) < f(x_k)$, yet the sequence does not converge when $k = 1, 2, ...$

4. Reduce the criterion for the existence of the MLE to a least squares solution with the block diagonal matrix $\mathbf{Z}$.

5. Write an R function that tests whether the MLE exists (it should return 1 if MLE exists and 0 otherwise). Use the `ginverse` function listed in Section 2.2.3.

6. Prove that the MLE exists for the data `famdat` by means of inequality (2.37).

2.6 Criterion for the positive definiteness of matrix $\mathbf{D}$

Sometimes the maximum likelihood procedure fails during likelihood function maximization. Certainly, this might be the case when (2.90) holds, so that there is no solution to the maximum likelihood estimation. In cases where (2.90) does not hold, perhaps the only reason for failure is that during iterations the covariance matrix of random effects does not become nonnegative definite. In particular, the diagonal elements of matrix $\mathbf{D}$ might become negative. A primary question is posed: are random effects relevant? That is, perhaps, the covariance matrix of random effects is zero. Obviously, if random effects are irrelevant, one might expect different kinds of problems from divergence to computer program overflow. Before getting into trouble, is it possible to find out if a positive solution exists ? The aim of this section is to provide a relevant criterion for the LME model (2.5). A statistical criterion regarding the presence of random effects is considered in Section 3.5.

Theorem 5 *Let $\widehat{\mathbf{e}}_i = \mathbf{y}_i - \mathbf{X}_i \widehat{\boldsymbol{\beta}}_{OLS}$ denote the $n_i \times 1$ OLS residual vector and $\widehat{\sigma}_{OLS}^2 = \sum \| \widehat{\mathbf{e}}_i \|^2 / N_T$ denote the OLS variance. If the $k \times k$ matrix*

$$\sum \mathbf{Z}_i' \widehat{\mathbf{e}}_i \widehat{\mathbf{e}}_i' \mathbf{Z}_i - \widehat{\sigma}_{OLS}^2 \sum \mathbf{Z}_i' \mathbf{Z}_i \qquad (2.93)$$

is nonzero nonnegative definite, the MLE of $\mathbf{D}$ is a nonzero matrix.

Proof. It suffices to show that there exists a nonzero nonnegative definite matrix $\mathbf{D}_*$ such that $\max_{\boldsymbol{\beta}, \sigma^2} l(\boldsymbol{\beta}, \sigma^2, \mathbf{D}_*) > l(\widehat{\boldsymbol{\beta}}_{OLS}, \widehat{\sigma}_{OLS}^2, \mathbf{0})$. First we find the derivatives of l with respect to $\mathbf{D}$ using the formulas

$$\frac{\partial \ln | \mathbf{V}_i |}{\partial \mathbf{D}} = \mathbf{Z}_i' \mathbf{V}_i^{-1} \mathbf{Z}_i, \quad \frac{\partial \mathbf{e}_i' \mathbf{V}_i^{-1} \mathbf{e}_i}{\partial \mathbf{D}} = -\mathbf{Z}_i' \mathbf{V}_i^{-1} \mathbf{e}_i \mathbf{e}_i' \mathbf{V}_i^{-1} \mathbf{Z}_i. \qquad (2.94)$$

Hence, the derivative of the log-likelihood function (2.19) with respect to $\mathbf{D}$ is given by

$$\frac{\partial l}{\partial \mathbf{D}} = -\frac{1}{2} \sum_{i=1}^{N} [\mathbf{Z}_i' \mathbf{V}_i^{-1} \mathbf{Z}_i - \sigma^{-2} \mathbf{Z}_i' \mathbf{V}_i^{-1} \mathbf{e}_i \mathbf{e}_i' \mathbf{V}_i^{-1} \mathbf{Z}_i], \qquad (2.95)$$

see Section 2.9. Now we use the following fact of multivariate calculus: if $F(\mathbf{x})$ is a function of a vector argument and $\mathbf{g} = \partial F(\mathbf{x} = \mathbf{0})/\partial \mathbf{x} \neq \mathbf{0}$, there exists such a positive scalar λ that for $\mathbf{x}_* = \lambda \mathbf{g}$, we have $F(\mathbf{x}_*) > F(\mathbf{0})$. If matrix (2.93) is nonnegative definite, then

$$\frac{\partial l}{\partial \mathbf{D}}\bigg|_{\boldsymbol{\beta}=\widehat{\boldsymbol{\beta}}_{OLS}, \sigma^2=\widehat{\sigma}^2_{OLS}, \mathbf{D}=\mathbf{0}} \qquad \text{is not zero and is a nonnegative defined matrix.}$$

Therefore, there exists a nonzero nonnegative definite matrix $\mathbf{D}_*$ such that

$$\max_{\boldsymbol{\beta},\sigma^2} l(\boldsymbol{\beta},\sigma^2,\mathbf{D}_*) \geq l(\widehat{\boldsymbol{\beta}}_{OLS}, \widehat{\sigma}^2_{OLS}, \mathbf{D}_*) > l(\widehat{\boldsymbol{\beta}}_{OLS}, \widehat{\sigma}^2_{OLS}, \mathbf{0}) = \max_{\boldsymbol{\beta},\sigma^2} l(\boldsymbol{\beta},\sigma^2,\mathbf{0}),$$

which proves the theorem.

∎

For one random effect ($k = 1$) we obtain the following simple criterion: if

$$\widehat{\sigma}^2_{OLS} < \frac{\sum(\mathbf{z}'_i(\mathbf{y}_i - \mathbf{X}_i\widehat{\boldsymbol{\beta}}_{OLS}))^2}{\sum \mathbf{z}'_i \mathbf{z}_i}, \tag{2.96}$$

then $\widehat{D}_{ML}$ is positive, where $\mathbf{Z}_i = \mathbf{z}_i$ is an $n_i \times 1$ design vector of the random effect. The proof follows from the fact that under condition (2.96), the derivative of the log-likelihood function at $\boldsymbol{\beta} = \widehat{\boldsymbol{\beta}}_{OLS}$ and $\sigma^2 = \widehat{\sigma}^2_{OLS}$ is positive, and therefore there exists a positive D that gives a greater value of the log-likelihood function than that at $D = 0$.

In the preceding section it was shown that the MLE exists with probability 1 if $\sum(n_i - k) > m$. As follows from this section, there is always a positive probability that $\widehat{\mathbf{D}}_{ML} = \mathbf{0}$.

2.6.1 Example of an invalid LME model

In this section a peculiar LME model is considered for which the MLE exists but $\widehat{\mathbf{D}}_{ML} = \mathbf{0}$. For that model the condition of Theorem 4 holds with probability 1, but the condition of Theorem 5 does not. A more general LME model for which the MLE of **D** is zero, linear regression with random coefficients, is considered in Section 3.2.1.

Consider a simple example of a LME model, in fact, a VARCOMP model. Let y_{ij} denote a characteristic of subject j in experimental group i. For example, y_{ij} could measure the response to treatment of individual j under treatment plan i. It is assumed that all subjects in the same group behave similarly; that is all $\{y_{ij}, j = 1, ..., n_i\}$ have common mean β_i and the same variance, where n_i is the number of subjects in the ith group and there are N groups. We believe that subjects from different groups behave independently but within one group react to experimental conditions somewhat similarly (i.e., y_{ij} and y_{il} correlate). Taking all of the above into account, it seems that an adequate model to describe data $\{y_{ij}\}$ is

$$y_{ij} = \beta_i + b_i + \varepsilon_{ij}, \quad i = 1, ..., N, \ j = 1, ..., n_i, \tag{2.97}$$

where ε_{ij} is the error term with zero mean and variance σ^2, b_i is the random effect with zero mean and variance $d_* = d\sigma^2$, and β_i is the fixed effect. Also, it is assumed that $\{\varepsilon_{ij}, b_i\}$ are mutually independent and normally distributed. The reader can recognize that model (2.97) looks like the VARCOMP model (1.8) but the $\{\beta_i\}$ are different. As follows from model (2.97), the subjects from different groups are independent, but within the group they have compound symmetry correlation, $\text{cor}(y_{ij}, y_{ik}) = d_* / (d_* + \sigma^2) = d/(1+d)$. This, a seemingly valid statistical model, is inadequate because the maximum likelihood estimator does not exist. We will show this using Theorem 4. For this model $\mathbf{X}_i$ is an $n_i \times N$ matrix, with $\mathbf{1}_{n_i}$ as the ith column and zero elsewhere, and $\boldsymbol{\beta} = (\beta_1, ..., \beta_N)'$, $\mathbf{Z}_i = \mathbf{z}_i = \mathbf{1}_{n_i}$ is an $n_i \times 1$ vector. The rank of matrix $\mathbf{W}$ is N and, as follows from Theorem 4, if at least for one i we have $n_i > 1$, the MLE exists with probability 1. For model (2.97), $\mathbf{X}_i\boldsymbol{\beta} = \beta_i \mathbf{z}_i$ and the log-likelihood function (2.26) takes the form

$$-\frac{1}{2}\left\{ N_T \ln \sigma^2 + \sum_{i=1}^{N} \ln(1 + dn_i) + \sigma^{-2} \sum_{i=1}^{N} \frac{\|\mathbf{y}_i - \beta_i \mathbf{1}_i\|^2}{1 + dn_i} \right\}. \tag{2.98}$$

This function reaches its maximum at $\widehat{\beta}_i = \overline{y}_i$ regardless of d, so that $\widehat{d}_{ML} = 0$. In fact, we could obtain this result from Theorem 5 because $\mathbf{Z}_i \widehat{\mathbf{e}}_i = 0$, and therefore (2.93) is a nonzero negative definite matrix.

In the literature on the variance components model, it is usually assumed that fixed effects are not confounded with random effects. This excludes pathological models such as (2.97) (Hartley and Rao, 1967). A valid model is to assume that all β_i are the same, which leads us to (1.8).

Problems for Section 2.6

1. Derive a sufficient criterion for the positiveness of the variance MLE in the random intercept model using (2.96).

2. Does Theorem 5 hold for RML?

3. Give a nonformal explanation as to why model (2.97) is a *greedy* (overspecified) model.

4. Provide a formal proof that the maximum of function (2.98) is attained at $\beta_i = d = 0$.

5*. Test the performance of criterion (2.93) via simulations. More specifically, test criterion (2.96) for a linear model with a random intercept using the family data (you may use the results of Problem 1). Set the true parameter values as $\alpha = -204$ and $\beta = 5.3$. Generate $N_{\exp} = 100$ dataframes using the same cluster id as `FamilyID` and `x=famdat$Height`; generate `y=alpha+beta*x+rnorm(N,mean=0,sd=sigma)`, where `sigma=24` as in the family example. Note that the y-generation assumes zero variance of the random intercept, or in other words, all intercepts are the same. Estimate the model using `lme` under an assumption of random intercepts. Count the number of times the estimate of the variance of the random effect is greater than 10^{-4} and count the number of times inequality (2.96) holds at the same time. How many times the estimate of the random effect variance less than 10^{-4}? Does (2.96) hold if and only if the MLE of the random intercept variance is greater than 10^{-4}? Summarize your findings.

2.7   Pre-estimation bounds for variance parameters

In this section pre-estimation bounds for the MLE of variance parameters σ^2 and $\mathbf{D}$ are derived under model (2.5). These bounds provide some insight into the interpretation of the variance components and its relationship to the fixed effects approach when the $\mathbf{b}_i$ are treated as fixed.

Let $\widehat{\sigma}^2_{ML}$ be the MLE of σ^2 in the LME model. We shall prove that

$$\widehat{\sigma}^2_{XZ} \leq \widehat{\sigma}^2_{ML} \leq \widehat{\sigma}^2_{OLS}, \tag{2.99}$$

where

$$\widehat{\sigma}^2_{XZ} = \frac{S_{\min}}{N_T} = \frac{1}{N_T} \min_{\boldsymbol{\beta}} \parallel \mathbf{y_Z} - \mathbf{X_Z}\boldsymbol{\beta} \parallel^2 = \frac{1}{N_T} \mathbf{y}'_\mathbf{Z}(\mathbf{I} - \mathbf{X_Z}\mathbf{X}^+_\mathbf{Z})\mathbf{y_Z}, \tag{2.100}$$

and $S_{\min}$ is as defined in (2.37) with $\mathbf{y_Z}$ and $\mathbf{X_Z}$ as defined in (2.92), and $\widehat{\sigma}^2_{OLS}$ as defined in Theorem 5 in Section 2.6.

Proof. To prove the left inequality (2.99), we note that as follows from (2.21), $\mathbf{V}^{-1}_i \geq \mathbf{I} - \mathbf{Z}_i\mathbf{Z}^+_i$, meaning that the difference between the left and right sides is a nonnegative definite matrix. Applying this inequality to (2.39), we obtain

$$
\begin{aligned}
\widehat{\sigma}^2_{ML} &\geq \frac{1}{N_T} \min_{\boldsymbol{\beta}} \sum (\mathbf{y}_i - \mathbf{X}_i\boldsymbol{\beta})'\mathbf{V}^{-1}_i(\mathbf{y}_i - \mathbf{X}_i\boldsymbol{\beta}) \\
&\geq \frac{1}{N_T} \min_{\boldsymbol{\beta}} \sum (\mathbf{y}_i - \mathbf{X}_i\boldsymbol{\beta})'(\mathbf{I} - \mathbf{Z}_i\mathbf{Z}^+_i)(\mathbf{y}_i - \mathbf{X}_i\boldsymbol{\beta}) \\
&= \frac{1}{N_T} \mathbf{y}'_\mathbf{Z}[\mathbf{I} - \mathbf{X_Z}(\mathbf{X}'_\mathbf{Z}\mathbf{X_Z})^{-1}\mathbf{X}'_\mathbf{Z}]\mathbf{y_Z} = \widehat{\sigma}^2_{XZ},
\end{aligned}
$$

which proves the left side of (2.99). To prove the right inequality in (2.99), we let $\mathbf{D} = \mathbf{0}$, $\sigma^2 = \widehat{\sigma}^2_{OLS}$, and $\boldsymbol{\beta} = \widehat{\boldsymbol{\beta}}_{OLS}$, which gives the value of the log-likelihood function at OLS,

$$l = l_{OLS} = -\frac{1}{2}(N_T \ln \widehat{\sigma}^2_{OLS} + N_T).$$

Since $\widehat{\sigma}^2_{ML}$ satisfies (2.39), we obtain

$$
\begin{aligned}
l_{OLS} &\leq \max l = l_{ML} \\
&= -\frac{1}{2}\left\{N_T \ln \widehat{\sigma}^2_{ML} + N_T + \sum \ln \mid \mathbf{I} + \widehat{\mathbf{D}}_{ML}\mathbf{Z}'_i\mathbf{Z}_i \mid\right\} \\
&-\frac{1}{2}\left\{N_T \ln \widehat{\sigma}^2_{ML} + N_T\right\},
\end{aligned}
$$

which implies that $\widehat{\sigma}^2_{OLS} \leq \widehat{\sigma}^2_{ML}$. ∎

There is a nice interpretation of inequality (2.99): The least squares variance $\widehat{\sigma}^2_{OLS}$, in a sense, estimates the total variation, which is the sum of the variance of the random term $\boldsymbol{\varepsilon}_i$ and the variance of the random effect $\mathbf{Z}_i\mathbf{b}_i$. The variance $\widehat{\sigma}^2_{XZ}$ estimates the variance of $\mathbf{y}_i$ in the fixed effects model approach, and therefore is the minimal variance. Inequality (2.99) means that the MLE variance of σ^2 lies between them.

Now we find a similar inequality for the MLE of the covariance matrix $\mathbf{D}$. Using the left side of (2.99), we obtain

$$
\begin{aligned}
l_{OLS} &= -\tfrac{1}{2}\{N_T \ln \widehat{\sigma}^2_{OLS} + N_T\} \le l_{ML} \\
&= -\tfrac{1}{2}\{N_T \ln \widehat{\sigma}^2_{ML} + N_T + \sum \ln \mid \mathbf{I} + \widehat{\mathbf{D}}_{ML}\mathbf{Z}'_i\mathbf{Z}_i \mid\} \\
&\le -\tfrac{1}{2}\{N_T \ln \widehat{\sigma}^2_{XZ} + N_T + \sum \ln \mid \mathbf{I} + \widehat{\mathbf{D}}_{ML}\mathbf{Z}'_i\mathbf{Z}_i \mid\},
\end{aligned}
$$

which implies that

$$
\sum_{i=1}^{N} \ln \mid \mathbf{I} + \widehat{\mathbf{D}}_{ML}\mathbf{Z}'_i\mathbf{Z}_i \mid \; \le N_T \ln \frac{\widehat{\sigma}^2_{OLS}}{\widehat{\sigma}^2_{XZ}}. \tag{2.101}
$$

As seen from this inequality, the magnitude of matrix $\widehat{\mathbf{D}}_{ML}$ depends on how close the variance $\widehat{\sigma}^2_{XZ}$ is to the variance $\widehat{\sigma}^2_{OLS}$. If these two variances are the same, $\widehat{\mathbf{D}}_{ML} = \mathbf{0}$. Actually, this fact is the basis for our F-test in Section 3.5 in the presence of random effects.

Inequality (2.101) yields an upper bound for the MLE matrix $\mathbf{D}$. It is possible to find the exact upper bound for one random effect when $\mathbf{D} = d$ is a scalar ($k = 1$). Then, inequality (2.101) can be rewritten as

$$
\sum_{i=1}^{N} \ln(1 + dp_i) \le A, \tag{2.102}
$$

where $p_i = \mathbf{Z}'_i\mathbf{Z}_i$ is scalar and $A = N_T \ln(\widehat{\sigma}^2_{OLS}/\widehat{\sigma}^2_{XZ})$. Since the left side of (2.102) is an increasing and concave function of d, the upper bound is the solution to the equation $\sum \ln(1 + dp_i) = A$. The Newton algorithm with a starting value $d_0 = 0$ leads to an increasing iterative sequence of d_s that converges to the upper bound of the variance of the random effect. The reader can derive an explicit bound for $\widehat{d}_{ML}$ in the balanced random-intercept model of Section 2.4.

Generally, inequality (2.101) defines a compact set in $\mathbf{D}$-space. If the matrices $\{\mathbf{Z}_i\}$ are of full rank, applying the matrix inequality $\mathbf{I} + \widehat{\mathbf{D}}_{ML}\mathbf{Z}'_i\mathbf{Z}_i \ge \widehat{\mathbf{D}}_{ML}\mathbf{Z}'_i\mathbf{Z}_i$, we obtain a rough approximation to the upper bound for the general variance as

$$
\mid \widehat{\mathbf{D}}_{ML} \mid \le \exp\left(\frac{N_T \widehat{\sigma}^2_{OLS}}{\widehat{\sigma}^2_{XZ} \sum \ln \mid \mathbf{Z}'_i\mathbf{Z}_i \mid} \right).
$$

Applying the further matrix inequality $\ln(|\mathbf{M}|) \le k \ln(k^{-1}\mathrm{tr}(\mathbf{M}))$ for any positive definite $k \times k$ matrix $\mathbf{M}$, we obtain the inequality $\sum_i \ln(t_i + \tau) \le B$, where it is denoted $\tau = \mathrm{tr}(\mathbf{D})$, and

$$
B = \frac{1}{k}\left[A - \sum_i \ln \mid \mathbf{Z}'_i\mathbf{Z}_i \mid \right] + N \ln k, \quad t_i = \mathrm{tr}(\mathbf{Z}'_i\mathbf{Z}_i)^{-1}.
$$

Again, this inequality may be solved for τ successfully using the Newton algorithm starting from $\tau = 0$.

Problems for Section 2.7

1. Show that $\widehat{\sigma}^2_{XZ} > 0$ is a necessary and sufficient criterion for the existence of the MLE (see Section 2.5).

2. Prove the inequality $\ln(|\mathbf{M}|) \leq k \ln(k^{-1} \mathrm{tr}(\mathbf{M}))$ for any positive definite $k \times k$ matrix $\mathbf{M}$ using the fact that the geometric mean is equal or less than the arithmetic mean, namely, $\left(\prod_{i=1}^{m} \lambda_i \right)^{1/m} \leq \frac{1}{m} \sum_{i=1}^{m} \lambda_i$, where $\lambda_i \geq 0$.

3. Derive pre-estimation bounds for the model with random intercepts.

4*. Using the results from Problem 2, compute the upper bound for the MLE of the scaled variance of the random intercept in the weight versus height example of Section 2.1.1 by solving the equation $\sum_{i=1}^{18} \ln(t_i + d) = B$. You can use either the R built-in function `uniroot` or write your own function using Newton iterations, $d_{s+1} = d_s - \left(\sum_{i=1}^{18} \ln(t_i + d_s) - B \right) / \sum_{i=1}^{18} 1/(t_i + d_s)$, where s is the iteration index. Is the upper bound sharp? Find conditions when the inequality turns into an equality.

5*. Generalize the pre-estimation bounds for the restricted MLE.

2.8   Maximization algorithms

Three general types of algorithms are used in statistics to maximize the log-likelihood function: Expectation-Maximization (EM), Fisher scoring (FS), and Newton–Raphson (NR). All these algorithms can be applied in the framework of the linear mixed effects model (Jennrich and Schluchter, 1986; Laird et al., 1987; Lindstrom and Bates, 1988; Jamshidian and Jennrich, 1993; Wolfinger et al., 1994). These algorithms have the generic form

$$\mathbf{t}_{s+1} = \mathbf{t}_s + \lambda_s \boldsymbol{\delta}_s, \quad s = 0, 1, ..., \qquad (2.103)$$

where $\mathbf{t}_s$ is the ML estimate at the sth iteration, $\mathbf{t}_{s+1}$ is the updated vector, $0 < \lambda_s \leq 1$ is the step length, and $\boldsymbol{\delta}_s$ is the direction vector or adjustment vector, calculated as

$$\boldsymbol{\delta}_s = \mathbf{H}_s^{-1} \mathbf{g}_s, \qquad (2.104)$$

where

$$\mathbf{g}_s = \left. \frac{\partial l}{\partial \mathbf{t}} \right|_{\mathbf{t}=\mathbf{t}_s}$$

is the gradient of the log-likelihood function l, and $\mathbf{H}_s$ is a positive definite matrix. The step length λ_s is required to ensure the increase in function l from iteration to iteration. In fact, the three algorithms mentioned above differ by matrix $\mathbf{H}$. For the NR algorithm, $\mathbf{H}$ is the negative Hessian matrix (negative matrix of the second derivatives, $-\partial^2 l / \partial \boldsymbol{\theta}^2$), and for the FS algorithm $\mathbf{H}$ is the information matrix (the expected matrix $-\partial^2 l / \partial \boldsymbol{\theta}^2$). For convergence, the matrix $\mathbf{H}$ must be positive definite. For the NR algorithm, one may expect that $\mathbf{H}$ is positive definite in a neighborhood of the maximum. For the FS algorithm, this matrix is always positive definite if the statistical model is specified correctly. For the EM algorithm, the matrix $\mathbf{H}$ is also positive definite, and $\lambda_s = 1$ is fixed. Characteristically, for this algorithm, the log-likelihood function increases from iteration to iteration, $l(\mathbf{t}_{s+1}) > l(\mathbf{t}_s)$, if the gradient at $\mathbf{t}_s$ is not zero, so λ_s is redundant. Unfortunately, this is not true for the other two algorithms, and λ_s should be found empirically (e.g., by halving starting from $\lambda = 1$). As follows from multivariate calculus, at each iteration there exists a positive λ_s that provides an increase in the log-likelihood if $\mathbf{g}_s \neq \mathbf{0}$. Also theoretically, the Newton–Raphson algorithm has a quadratic speed of convergence in a neighborhood of the maximum. However, if iterations are far from the maximum, the NR algorithm may fail. In particular, it happens when the negative matrix of the second derivatives does not become positive definite. Conversely, the EM algorithm seems more robust at the starting point, although it may exhibit slower convergence. Often, in the framework of mixed effects modeling, the failure to converge is associated with the fact that some diagonal elements of matrix $\mathbf{D}$ become close to zero or, more generally, $\mathbf{D}$ does not become positive definite (Jennrich and Schluchter, 1986). Theoretically, the Fisher scoring algorithm provides positive definiteness of $\mathbf{H}$ and potentially inherits positive properties of the other two algorithms, at least for large N. A big advantage of the NR and FS algorithms over the EM algorithm is that they produce the asymptotic covariance matrix of the estimated parameters, $\mathbf{H}_s^{-1}$, as a by-product of the maximization process. We prefer using the expected negative Hessian to estimate the covariance matrix rather than empirical Hessian (second derivatives) because the latter may lead to an undesirable statistical paradox (Demidenko and Spiegelman, 1998).

The EM algorithm was suggested initially by Laird and Ware (1982) in their pioneering work on linear mixed effects models. The Newton–Raphson algorithm for the LME model was developed by Lindstrom and Bates (1988), and Wolfinger et al. (1994). They give formulas for the first and second derivatives of the log-likelihood function in coordinate form that make the algorithm presentation quite cumbersome. The NR algorithm is used in statistical packages SAS (the procedure mixed) and the R package nlme (function lme) and the recent lme4 (the function lme4). In subsequent sections we consider matrix versions of the NR, EM, and FS algorithms and their modifications based on a perturbation formula for the inverse matrix. Matrix formulation makes these algorithms compact and facilitates study of their properties. The important part is to obtain updates for matrix $\mathbf{D}$ because beta coefficients are derived from GLS.

The choice of starting point in any nonlinear optimization problem is important. A good idea is to start the maximization algorithm from an unbiased quadratic estimate of $\mathbf{D}$, such as MINQUE, method of moments, or variance least squares, developed in Chapter 4. They produce the exact MLE for balanced data so that the iterative maximization converges at the first iteration.

In this chapter we use $(\sigma^2, \mathbf{D})$ parameterization; in Section 6.4.4 we consider log-likelihood maximization, under parameterization $(\sigma^2, \mathbf{D}_*)$, as an illustration of the total generalized estimating equations approach. The reader can find more discussion on optimization issues in Appendix 13.3.

Problems for Section 2.8

1. Let function $f(\mathbf{x})$ be continuous on R^m and bounded from above, $f(\mathbf{x}) < K$. Let a sequence $\{\mathbf{x}_k\}$ gradually increase the value of f, i.e. $f(\mathbf{x}_{k+1}) > f(\mathbf{x}_k)$. Does the sequence $\{\mathbf{x}_k, k = 1, 2, ...\}$ converge? Does the sequence $\{\mathbf{x}_k\}$ have at least one limiting point (is there a subsequence that converges)? Prove the statements

or provide counterexamples. Does converence imply that $\{\mathbf{x}_k\}$ converge to a local maximum? Refer to Section 13.3 in the Appendix for a general discussion.

2. Does MLE always exist? Is it unique? Does the solution of the score equation (the derivative of the log-likelihood function with respect to parameter is zero) yield maximum likelihood? Give conditions and examples when it does. Does MLE (with the maximum likelihood value) satisfy the score equation?

3. How often can one find a solution of the score equation that is neither minimum nor maximum (sometimes this solution is called the saddle point)? What is the probability of this event?

2.9 Derivatives of the log-likelihood function

All maximization algorithms require derivatives of function (2.15) with respect to the parameters. Using standard formulas we obtain

$$
\begin{aligned}
\frac{\partial l}{\partial \boldsymbol{\beta}} &= \sigma^{-2} \sum \mathbf{X}_i' \mathbf{V}_i^{-1} (\mathbf{y}_i - \mathbf{X}_i \boldsymbol{\beta}), \\
\frac{\partial l}{\partial \sigma^2} &= -\frac{1}{2} N_T \sigma^{-2} + \frac{1}{2} \sigma^{-4} \sum (\mathbf{y}_i - \mathbf{X}_i \boldsymbol{\beta})' \mathbf{V}_i^{-1} (\mathbf{y}_i - \mathbf{X}_i \boldsymbol{\beta}), \\
\frac{\partial l}{\partial \mathbf{D}} &= -\frac{1}{2} \sum [\mathbf{Z}_i' \mathbf{V}_i^{-1} \mathbf{Z}_i - \sigma^{-2} \mathbf{Z}_i' \mathbf{V}_i^{-1} (\mathbf{y}_i - \mathbf{X}_i \boldsymbol{\beta})(\mathbf{y}_i - \mathbf{X}_i \boldsymbol{\beta})' \mathbf{V}_i^{-1} \mathbf{Z}_i].
\end{aligned}
\tag{2.105}
$$

We use formulas (2.94) to obtain $\partial l / \partial \mathbf{D}$; the first two derivatives are straightforward. The maximum likelihood estimate maximizes function l or, equivalently, solves the system of nonlinear equations

$$
\frac{\partial l}{\partial \boldsymbol{\beta}} = \mathbf{0}, \quad \frac{\partial l}{\partial \sigma^2} = 0, \quad \frac{\partial l}{\partial \mathbf{D}} = \mathbf{0},
$$

for $\boldsymbol{\beta}$, σ^2 and $\mathbf{D}$, where the last equation is the $k \times k$ matrix equation. For the Newton–Raphson algorithm, we also need the second derivatives. We could obtain them by differentiating (2.105) again, but then we would have to differentiate a matrix with respect to a matrix to find $\partial^2 l / \partial \mathbf{D}^2$. Fortunately, we can avoid this cumbersome procedure by applying the following *perturbation formula* for the inverse matrix (Schott 1997).

Proposition 6 *Let $\mathbf{M}$ be a positive definite matrix and $\mathbf{C}$ a nonnegative definite matrix of the same order. Then for sufficiently small $\mathbf{C}$,*

$$
(\mathbf{M} + \mathbf{C})^{-1} = \mathbf{M}^{-1} - \mathbf{M}^{-1} \mathbf{C} \mathbf{M}^{-1} + \boldsymbol{\Delta},
\tag{2.106}
$$

where (i) $\boldsymbol{\Delta} = \boldsymbol{\Delta}(\mathbf{C})$ is a positive definite matrix, and (ii) $\| \boldsymbol{\Delta} \| = o(\| \mathbf{C} \|)$.

Proof. First we prove that $\boldsymbol{\Delta}$ is a positive definite matrix. We use the following matrix inequality: $(\mathbf{I} + \mathbf{C})^{-1} \geq \mathbf{I} - \mathbf{C}$ for all nonnegative definite matrices $\mathbf{C}$. This inequality follows from

$$
\begin{aligned}
\mathbf{I} - (\mathbf{I} + \mathbf{C})^{-1} &= (\mathbf{I} + \mathbf{C})^{-1/2} (\mathbf{I} + \mathbf{C} - \mathbf{I})(\mathbf{I} + \mathbf{C})^{-1/2} \\
&= (\mathbf{I} + \mathbf{C})^{-1/2} \mathbf{C} (\mathbf{I} + \mathbf{C})^{-1/2} \leq \mathbf{C},
\end{aligned}
$$

because $(\mathbf{I} + \mathbf{C})^{-1} \leq \mathbf{I}$. As follows from this inequality,

$$
\begin{aligned}
(\mathbf{M} + \mathbf{C})^{-1} &= \mathbf{M}^{-1/2}(\mathbf{I} + \mathbf{M}^{-1/2}\mathbf{C}\mathbf{M}^{-1/2})^{-1}\mathbf{M}^{-1/2} \\
&\geq \mathbf{M}^{-1/2}(\mathbf{I} - \mathbf{M}^{-1/2}\mathbf{C}\mathbf{M}^{-1/2})\mathbf{M}^{-1/2} \\
&= \mathbf{M}^{-1} - \mathbf{M}^{-1}\mathbf{C}\mathbf{M}^{-1},
\end{aligned}
$$

which proves the first statement of the proposition. To prove the second statement, we apply the following well known matrix result (Graybill, 1983):

$$
(\mathbf{I} - \mathbf{A})^{-1} = \mathbf{I} + \mathbf{A} + \mathbf{A}^2 + ...,
$$

if all eigenvalues of matrix $\mathbf{A}$ are less than 1 in absolute value. Applying this result to the left-hand side of (2.106) with sufficiently small $\mathbf{C}$ (more precisely for $\mathbf{C}$ with eigenvalues in absolute value less than 1), we obtain

$$
\begin{aligned}
(\mathbf{M} + \mathbf{C})^{-1} &= \mathbf{M}^{-1/2}[\mathbf{I} - (-\mathbf{M}^{-1/2}\mathbf{C}\mathbf{M}^{-1/2})]^{-1}\mathbf{M}^{-1/2} \\
&= \mathbf{M}^{-1/2} \sum_{k=0}^{\infty} (-1)^k (\mathbf{M}^{-1/2}\mathbf{C}\mathbf{M}^{-1/2})^k \mathbf{M}^{-1/2} \\
&= \mathbf{M}^{-1} - \mathbf{M}^{-1}\mathbf{C}\mathbf{M}^{-1} + \mathbf{\Delta},
\end{aligned}
$$

where

$$
\mathbf{\Delta} = \mathbf{M}^{-1/2} \sum_{k=2}^{\infty} (-1)^k (\mathbf{M}^{-1/2}\mathbf{C}\mathbf{M}^{-1/2})^k \mathbf{M}^{-1/2}.
$$

Clearly, $\| \mathbf{\Delta} \| = o(\| \mathbf{C} \|)$, meaning that matrix $\mathbf{\Delta}$ is of smaller order than matrix $\mathbf{C}$.   ∎

In the next section we use perturbation formula (2.106) to derive the matrix version of the NR algorithm and its modifications.

Problems for Section 2.9

1. Derive approximation (2.106) for numbers.

2. Derive approximation (2.106) for a special case when $\mathbf{C} = c\mathbf{1}\mathbf{1}'$ and compare it with the exact formula inverse. (Hint: Use the matrix inverse formula from Section 2.4.1.)

3. Derive approximation (2.106) in a special case when $\mathbf{M} = \mathbf{I}$ (the identity matrix) and $\mathbf{C} = \lambda\mathbf{1}\mathbf{1}'$, where $\lambda > 0$ and $\mathbf{1}$ is a vector of 1s. Check Proposition, using the exact matrix inverse (2.69) by showing that $\lim_{\lambda \to 0} \mathbf{\Delta} = \mathbf{0}$. Also prove that $\mathbf{\Delta}$ is a positive definite matrix for $\lambda > 0$.

4*. Is matrix $\mathbf{\Delta}$ in the proof positive definite if $\mathbf{C}$ is positive definite? Start with the case when matrices are scalars. Compute $\mathbf{\Delta}$ and test its positive definiteness for several $\mathbf{M}$ and $\mathbf{C}$ before proving the general case.

2.10   Newton–Raphson algorithm

As mentioned above, all iterative maximization algorithms have generic forms (2.103) and (2.104). For the NR algorithm, $\mathbf{H}$ is the Hessian (second derivatives) matrix.

One could obtain second derivatives by differentiating (2.15) directly as Lindstrom and Bates (1988) and Wolfinger et al. (1994) did, but we suggest another, less cumbersome matrix approach based on the perturbation formula derived in the preceding section.

Let $\boldsymbol{\beta}_s, \sigma_s^2$, and $\mathbf{D}_s$ be approximations to the ML estimate at the sth iteration. We update these approximations as

$$\boldsymbol{\beta} = \boldsymbol{\beta}_s + \boldsymbol{\delta}_\beta, \ \sigma^2 = \sigma_s^2 + \delta_{\sigma^2}, \ \mathbf{D} = \mathbf{D}_s + \boldsymbol{\Delta}_\mathbf{D}, \tag{2.107}$$

where $\boldsymbol{\delta}_\beta$, δ_{σ^2}, and $\boldsymbol{\Delta}_\mathbf{D}$ are parameter adjustments (presumably small). We use the following first-order approximations to the nonlinear terms of (2.105):

$$\sigma^{-2} \simeq \sigma_s^{-2} - \sigma_s^{-4}\delta_{\sigma^2}, \quad \sigma^{-4} \simeq \sigma_s^{-4} - 2\sigma_s^{-6}\delta_{\sigma^2}.$$

We apply perturbation formula (2.106) to update the inverse matrix $\mathbf{V}$. Letting $\mathbf{M} = \mathbf{V}_{is}$, $\mathbf{C} = \mathbf{Z}_i\boldsymbol{\Delta}_\mathbf{D}\mathbf{Z}_i'$, we obtain a first-order approximation to the updated inverse,

$$\mathbf{V}_i^{-1} = [\mathbf{I} + \mathbf{Z}_i(\mathbf{D}_s + \boldsymbol{\Delta}_\mathbf{D})\mathbf{Z}_i']^{-1} = (\mathbf{V}_{is}+\mathbf{Z}_i\boldsymbol{\Delta}_\mathbf{D}\mathbf{Z}_i')^{-1} \simeq \mathbf{V}_{is}^{-1} - \mathbf{V}_{is}^{-1}\mathbf{Z}_i\boldsymbol{\Delta}_\mathbf{D}\mathbf{Z}_i'\mathbf{V}_{is}^{-1}. \tag{2.108}$$

Now we substitute the updated values into system (2.105) leaving only the first-order terms, i.e., quadratic and product terms are omitted. As is easy to see, this substitution produces two parts: the first part contains no adjustments and corresponds to the derivative of l at iteration s; the second (adjusted) part contains three adjustment components. We do not write the first part because it corresponds to derivatives (2.105) at iteration s; also, the subindex i is omitted to shorten the notation. The adjusted part for equation (2.105) has the form

$$[\sigma_s^{-2} \sum \mathbf{X}'\mathbf{V}^{-1}\mathbf{X}]\boldsymbol{\delta}_\beta + [\sigma_s^{-4} \sum \mathbf{X}'\mathbf{V}^{-1}\mathbf{e}]\delta_{\sigma^2} + [\sigma_s^{-2} \sum \mathbf{X}'\mathbf{V}^{-1}\mathbf{Z}\boldsymbol{\Delta}_\mathbf{D}\mathbf{Z}'\mathbf{V}^{-1}\mathbf{e}].$$

The adjusted part for the second equation has the form

$$[\sigma_s^{-4} \sum \mathbf{e}'\mathbf{V}^{-1}\mathbf{X}]\boldsymbol{\delta}_\beta + [\sigma_s^{-6} \sum \mathbf{e}'\mathbf{V}^{-1}\mathbf{e} - 0.5N_T\sigma_s^{-4}]\delta_{\sigma^2}$$
$$+[0.5\sigma^{-4} \sum \mathbf{e}'\mathbf{V}^{-1}\mathbf{Z}\boldsymbol{\Delta}_\mathbf{D}\mathbf{Z}'\mathbf{V}^{-1}\mathbf{e}],$$

and for the third equation

$$[\sigma_s^{-2} \sum \mathbf{e}'\mathbf{V}^{-1}\mathbf{Z}\boldsymbol{\Delta}_\mathbf{D}\mathbf{Z}'\mathbf{V}^{-1}\mathbf{X}]\boldsymbol{\delta}_\beta + [0.5\sigma^{-4} \sum \mathbf{e}'\mathbf{V}^{-1}\mathbf{Z}\boldsymbol{\Delta}_\mathbf{D}\mathbf{Z}'\mathbf{V}^{-1}\mathbf{e}]\delta_{\sigma^2}$$
$$+0.5[\sum \{\sigma_s^{-2}(\mathbf{R}\boldsymbol{\Delta}_\mathbf{D}\mathbf{Z}'\mathbf{V}^{-1}\mathbf{e}\mathbf{e}'\mathbf{V}^{-1}\mathbf{Z} + \mathbf{Z}'\mathbf{V}^{-1}\mathbf{e}\mathbf{e}'\mathbf{V}^{-1}\mathbf{Z}\boldsymbol{\Delta}_\mathbf{D}\mathbf{R}) - \mathbf{R}\boldsymbol{\Delta}_\mathbf{D}\mathbf{R}\}],$$

where $\mathbf{R} = \mathbf{Z}'\mathbf{V}^{-1}\mathbf{Z}$ is the $k \times k$ matrix. Importantly, this method produces terms at the adjustments corresponding to the second derivative of l or the Jacobian of system (2.105). To use the NR algorithm we need to represent matrix $\boldsymbol{\Delta}_\mathbf{D}$ in vector form using formulas from Appendix 13.2.3, so we let $\boldsymbol{\delta}_\mathbf{D} =\text{vec}(\boldsymbol{\Delta}_\mathbf{D})$. For example, taking the vec operation of the last term in the equation above, we obtain

$$\sigma_s^{-2} \sum \mathbf{X}'\mathbf{V}^{-1}\mathbf{Z}\boldsymbol{\Delta}_\mathbf{D}\mathbf{Z}'\mathbf{V}^{-1}\mathbf{e}$$
$$= \text{vec}[\sigma_s^{-2} \sum \mathbf{X}'\mathbf{V}^{-1}\mathbf{Z}\boldsymbol{\Delta}_\mathbf{D}\mathbf{Z}'\mathbf{V}^{-1}\mathbf{e}] = [\sigma_s^{-2} \sum \mathbf{e}'\mathbf{V}^{-1}\mathbf{Z} \otimes \mathbf{X}'\mathbf{V}^{-1}\mathbf{Z}]\boldsymbol{\delta}_\mathbf{D}.$$

After rewriting the estimating equations above in the vector form, we come to the following negative Hessian matrix of the log-likelihood function (2.15) in terms of the $(m + 1 + k^2) \times 1$ vector $(\boldsymbol{\beta}', \sigma^2, \text{vec}'(\mathbf{D}))'$:

$$\mathbf{H} = \begin{bmatrix} \mathbf{H}_{11}^{m \times m} & \mathbf{H}_{12}^{m \times 1} & \mathbf{H}_{13}^{m \times k^2} \\ \mathbf{H}_{12}' & H_{22}^{1 \times 1} & \mathbf{H}_{23}^{1 \times k^2} \\ \mathbf{H}_{13}' & \mathbf{H}_{23}' & \mathbf{H}_{33}^{k^2 \times k^2} \end{bmatrix},$$

where

$$\mathbf{H}_{11} = \sigma^{-2} \sum \mathbf{X}_i' \mathbf{V}_i^{-1} \mathbf{X}_i, \quad \mathbf{H}_{12} = \sigma^{-4} \sum \mathbf{X}_i' \mathbf{V}_i^{-1} \mathbf{e}_i,$$

$$\mathbf{H}_{13} = \sigma^{-2} \sum \mathbf{e}_i' \mathbf{V}_i^{-1} \mathbf{Z}_i \otimes \mathbf{X}_i' \mathbf{V}_i^{-1} \mathbf{Z}_i, \quad H_{22} = \sigma^{-6} \sum \mathbf{e}_i' \mathbf{V}_i^{-1} \mathbf{e}_i - 0.5 N_T \sigma^{-4},$$

$$\mathbf{H}_{23} = 0.5 \sigma^{-4} \sum \mathbf{e}_i' \mathbf{V}_i^{-1} \mathbf{Z}_i \otimes \mathbf{e}_i' \mathbf{V}_i^{-1} \mathbf{Z}_i,$$

$$\mathbf{H}_{33} = 0.5 \sum \{ \sigma^{-2} (\mathbf{Z}_i' \mathbf{V}_i^{-1} \mathbf{e}_i \mathbf{e}_i' \mathbf{V}_i^{-1} \mathbf{Z}_i \otimes \mathbf{R}_i + \mathbf{R}_i \otimes \mathbf{Z}_i' \mathbf{V}_i^{-1} \mathbf{e}_i \mathbf{e}_i' \mathbf{V}_i^{-1} \mathbf{Z}_i) - \mathbf{R}_i \otimes \mathbf{R}_i \}.$$

Thus, the Newton–Raphson algorithm is written as

$$\begin{bmatrix} \boldsymbol{\beta}_{s+1} \\ \sigma_{s+1}^2 \\ \text{vec}(\mathbf{D}_{s+1}) \end{bmatrix} = \begin{bmatrix} \boldsymbol{\beta}_s \\ \sigma_s^2 \\ \text{vec}(\mathbf{D}_s) \end{bmatrix} \quad (2.109)$$

$$+ \lambda_s \begin{bmatrix} \mathbf{H}_{11} & \mathbf{H}_{12} & \mathbf{H}_{13} \\ \mathbf{H}_{12}' & H_{22} & \mathbf{H}_{23} \\ \mathbf{H}_{13}' & \mathbf{H}_{23}' & \mathbf{H}_{33} \end{bmatrix}_s^{-1} \begin{bmatrix} \frac{\partial l}{\partial \boldsymbol{\beta}} \\ \frac{\partial l}{\partial \sigma^2} \\ \text{vec}(\frac{\partial l}{\partial \mathbf{D}}) \end{bmatrix}_s,$$

where the first derivatives of the log-likelihood are calculated by formulas (2.105). The step length λ_s is chosen by the following rule: Start with $\lambda_s = 1$; if $l_{s+1} > l_s$, accept $\lambda_s = 1$ and go to the next iteration. If $l_{s+1} \le l_s$, take $\lambda_s = 1/2, 1/2^2,\dots$ until $l_{s+1} > l_s$. We cannot find positive λ_s in two cases: in the first case the gradient of the log-likelihood is zero or very small—the maximum (at least local) is found. In the second case, which occurs more often, the gradient is not zero; the NR algorithm fails because the Hessian matrix is not positive definite. Unfortunately, the Hessian may not be positive definite, especially when iterations are far from the maximum point, and this is the main drawback of the NR algorithm. As we shall see later, Fisher scoring is as fast as the NR algorithm but more reliable in the sense that the inverse matrix (the information matrix) is always positive definite for a well-defined LME model (see the next section for more detail). In fact, one can interpret the FS algorithm as the "expected version" of the NR algorithm, meaning that the information matrix is the expected (average) negative Hessian matrix.

Problems for Section 2.10

1. Derive NR iterations (2.109) for a linear mixed model with a univariate random effect (vec is not necessary in this case).

2. Prove that the NR algorithm leads to a symmetric matrix $\mathbf{D}$ at each iteration.

3*. Implement NR iterations in R for a linear mixed model with a univariate random effect. Test your code with lme using simulated data.

4*. Implement NR iterations in R for a general linear mixed model (2.5). Use kronecker for $\otimes$ and as.vector for vec. Test your code with lme.

2.11   Fisher scoring algorithm

The Fisher Scoring (FS) algorithm is a general algorithm for log-likelihood maximization with matrix $\mathbf{H}$ as the expected negative Hessian, the information matrix, $\mathcal{I}$. The formula for the information matrix for parameters $\boldsymbol{\beta}, \sigma^2, \text{vec}(\mathbf{D})$, which are derived in Chapter 4, is given by

$$\mathcal{I} = \left[\begin{array}{ccc} \sigma^{-2} \sum \mathbf{X}_i' \mathbf{V}_i^{-1} \mathbf{X}_i & \mathbf{0} & \mathbf{0} \\ \mathbf{0} & 0.5 N_T \sigma^{-4} & 0.5\sigma^{-2} \sum \text{vec}'(\mathbf{R}_i) \\ \mathbf{0} & 0.5\sigma^{-2} \sum \text{vec}(\mathbf{R}_i) & 0.5 \sum \mathbf{R}_i \otimes \mathbf{R}_i \end{array} \right],$$

(2.110)

where $\mathbf{R}_i = \mathbf{Z}_i' \mathbf{V}_i^{-1} \mathbf{Z}_i$, so that iterations take the form (2.103) with $\mathbf{H} = \mathcal{I}$, adjustments (2.104), and the gradient calculated by formulas (2.105). Since this information matrix has a block diagonal structure (the MLEs for $\boldsymbol{\beta}$ and variance parameters $(\sigma^2, \mathbf{D})$ are asymptotically independent), we adjust fixed effects and variance parameters separately. The new $\boldsymbol{\beta}_{s+1}$ is estimated by GLS (2.28), replacing $\mathbf{D}$ with $\hat{\mathbf{D}}_s$, and σ^2 and $\mathbf{D}$ are recalculated using the bottom-right block of matrix $\mathcal{I}$.

There are three reasons to prefer Fisher scoring to the Newton–Raphson algorithm:

1. The negative Hessian matrix $, -\partial^2 l / \partial \boldsymbol{\theta}^2$, or *empirical* information matrix, may not be positive definite (more precisely, not nonnegative definite), especially when the current approximation is far from the MLE. When this happens, the NR algorithm slows down or even fails. On the contrary, the *expected* information matrix (2.110), used in the FS algorithm, is always positive definite if the LME model is well defined (see Proposition 13 in Chapter 4).

2. The expected information matrix at the final iteration leads to a better estimate of the asymptotic covariance than does the empirical information matrix (Demidenko and Spiegelman, 1997). Additionally, the expected information matrix is robust to possible outliers, unlike the empirical information matrix. To illustrate this point, let us consider the nonlinear regression model $y_i = f_i(\theta) + \varepsilon_i$, with normally distributed errors and a scalar parameter θ. Then the empirical Fisher information is proportional to $\sum (df_i/d\theta)^2 - \sum (d^2 f_i/d\theta^2) e_i$, where e_i is the ith residual and the expected information is proportional to $\sum (df_i/d\theta)^2$. Clearly, in the presence of an outlier (e_i is large in absolute value), the empirical information will be influenced by that outlier. On the contrary, the expected information is not affected by the outlier. In fact, in nonlinear regression use of the expected information to calculate the variance of the least squares estimate is the rule (Bates and Watts, 1988; Seber and Wild, 1989).

3. Use of the expected information matrix simplifies construction of different versions of maximization algorithms based on profile log-likelihood functions and the restricted MLE (see Section 3.6.3). For instance, if we want to apply the FS algorithm to the variance profile log-likelihood function, we use matrix (3.20). If we want to use the RMLE, we use the same information matrix because the asymptotic properties of MLE and RMLE are the same, see Section 3.6.3.

Therefore, we prefer the Fisher scoring algorithm over the Newton–Raphson or EM algorithms; in practical maximization the FS algorithm is almost as fast as the NR algorithm but is more robust to the starting point. As will follow from Section 3.12, the FS algorithm may be interpreted as the least squares solution.

We apply the FS algorithm to the nonlinear marginal model of Chapter 7 in the framework of the total generalized estimating equations approach (see Section 6.4).

2.11.1 Simplified FS algorithm

Since maximization over σ^2 admits a closed-form solution (2.39), if $\boldsymbol{\beta}$ and $\mathbf{D}$ hold, we can use the $(3,3)$ block of matrix (2.110) to find the adjustment for $\mathbf{D}$; that is,

$$
\begin{aligned}
\operatorname{vec}(\mathbf{D}_{s+1}) \;=\;& \operatorname{vec}(\mathbf{D}_s) + \lambda_s \left(\sum \mathbf{R}_{is} \otimes \mathbf{R}_{is} \right)^{-1} \\
& \times \operatorname{vec} \left(\sum [\sigma_s^{-2} \mathbf{Z}_i' \mathbf{V}_{is}^{-1} \mathbf{e}_{is} \mathbf{e}_{is}' \mathbf{V}_{is}^{-1} \mathbf{Z}_i - \mathbf{R}_{is}] \right),
\end{aligned}
\tag{2.111}
$$

where the subscript s indicates that quantities are computed at the sth iteration. Then σ^2 and $\boldsymbol{\beta}$ are recalculated by (2.39) and (2.28) using $\mathbf{D}_{s+1}$, and iterations continue. Iterations (2.111) may be derived directly from the score equation $\partial l / \partial \mathbf{D} = \mathbf{0}$, rewriting

$$
\begin{aligned}
\mathbf{Z}_i' \mathbf{V}_i^{-1} \mathbf{Z}_i \;=\;& \mathbf{Z}_i' \mathbf{V}_i^{-1} \mathbf{V}_i \mathbf{V}_i^{-1} \mathbf{Z}_i = \mathbf{Z}_i' \mathbf{V}_i^{-1} (\mathbf{I} + \mathbf{Z}_i \mathbf{D} \mathbf{Z}_i') \mathbf{V}_i^{-1} \mathbf{Z}_i \\
\;=\;& \mathbf{Z}_i' \mathbf{V}_i^{-2} \mathbf{Z}_i + \mathbf{R}_i \mathbf{D} \mathbf{R}_i'.
\end{aligned}
$$

Then the score equation for $\mathbf{D}$ is equivalent to

$$
\sum \mathbf{R}_i \mathbf{D} \mathbf{R}_i' = \sum [\sigma^{-2} \mathbf{Z}_i' \mathbf{V}_i^{-1} \mathbf{e}_i \mathbf{e}_i' \mathbf{V}_i^{-1} \mathbf{Z}_i - \mathbf{Z}_i' \mathbf{V}_i^{-2} \mathbf{Z}_i].
\tag{2.112}
$$

Applying the vec operator to both sides, we obtain

$$
\operatorname{vec}(\mathbf{D}_{s+1}) = \left(\sum \mathbf{R}_{is} \otimes \mathbf{R}_{is} \right)^{-1} \operatorname{vec} \left(\sum [\sigma_s^{-2} \mathbf{Z}_i' \mathbf{V}_{is}^{-1} \mathbf{e}_{is} \mathbf{e}_{is}' \mathbf{V}_{is}^{-1} \mathbf{Z}_i - \mathbf{Z}_i' \mathbf{V}_{is}^{-2} \mathbf{Z}_i] \right).
$$

It is straightforward to show that the last equation is equivalent to (2.111) with $\lambda_s = 1$. One can use the dimension-reduction formulas; for example, if the $\mathbf{Z}_i$ have full rank, then $\mathbf{R}_i = ((\mathbf{Z}_i' \mathbf{Z}_i)^{-1} + \mathbf{D})^{-1}$ and the matrices $(\mathbf{Z}_i' \mathbf{Z}_i)^{-1}$ can be computed beforehand. In the next subsection we use the dimension-reduction formulas for variance-profile parameterization.

2.11.2 Empirical FS algorithm

One can use first derivatives to approximate the information matrix. This idea comes from the fact that, generally, for the information matrix,

$$
\mathcal{I} = -E \left(\frac{\partial^2 l}{\partial \boldsymbol{\theta}^2} \right) = E \left(\frac{\partial l}{\partial \boldsymbol{\theta}} \right) \left(\frac{\partial l}{\partial \boldsymbol{\theta}} \right)'.
$$

Thus, approximately,

$$
\mathbf{H} \sim \sum_{i=1}^{N} \left(\frac{\partial l_i}{\partial \boldsymbol{\theta}} \right) \left(\frac{\partial l_i}{\partial \boldsymbol{\theta}} \right)'
$$

for a sufficiently large N. An attractive feature of the Empirical FS (EFS) algorithm is that it does not require second derivatives at all and it may work well when N is fairly large, due to asymptotic theory. We use this algorithm in Chapter 5 for ML estimation of the robust/median meta-analysis model and in Chapters 7 and 8 for nonlinear mixed models, where computation of second derivatives becomes cumbersome.

2.11.3 Variance-profile FS algorithm

The FS algorithm can be applied to the variance-profile log-likelihood function (2.41) derived in Section 2.2.4. As follows from formula (3.20), the information matrix for $\text{vec}(\mathbf{D})$ in the variance-profile log-likelihood function is given by

$$\mathbf{H} = 0.5 \left[\sum_{i=1}^{N} \mathbf{R}_i \otimes \mathbf{R}_i - \frac{1}{N_T} \text{vec}(\sum_{i=1}^{N} \mathbf{R}_i) \text{vec}'(\sum_{i=1}^{N} \mathbf{R}_i) \right], \qquad (2.113)$$

where

$$\mathbf{R}_i = \mathbf{Z}_i'\mathbf{Z}_i(\mathbf{I}_k + \mathbf{D}\mathbf{Z}_i'\mathbf{Z}_i)^{-1} = (\mathbf{I}_k + \mathbf{Z}_i'\mathbf{Z}_i\mathbf{D})^{-1}\mathbf{Z}_i'\mathbf{Z}_i$$

is a symmetric matrix. Hence, to apply the FS algorithm, we need only the first derivatives of (2.41) with respect to $\mathbf{D}$, where the beta coefficients are recalculated by formula (2.28). Applying the dimension-reduction formulas, we come to an economical expression for the beta-vector:

$$\boldsymbol{\beta} = [\mathbf{N} - \sum \mathbf{T}_i(\mathbf{D}^{-1} + \mathbf{M}_i)^{-1}\mathbf{T}_i']^{-1}[\mathbf{t} - \sum \mathbf{T}_i(\mathbf{D}^{-1} + \mathbf{M}_i)^{-1}\mathbf{p}_i], \qquad (2.114)$$

where in addition to notation (2.42) we denote

$$\mathbf{T}_i = \mathbf{X}_i'\mathbf{Z}_i, \quad \mathbf{p}_i = \mathbf{Z}_i'\mathbf{y}_i, \quad \mathbf{t} = \sum \mathbf{X}_i'\mathbf{y}_i, \quad \mathbf{N} = \sum \mathbf{X}_i'\mathbf{X}_i. \qquad (2.115)$$

Notice that these quantities are fixed and may be computed beforehand.

To obtain the derivative of (2.41) with respect to matrix $\mathbf{D}$ we use the general formula (Appendix 13.2.4)

$$\frac{\partial \mathbf{r}'(\mathbf{D}^{-1} + \mathbf{M})^{-1}\mathbf{r}}{\partial \mathbf{D}} = (\mathbf{I} + \mathbf{M}\mathbf{D})^{-1}\mathbf{r}\mathbf{r}'(\mathbf{I} + \mathbf{D}\mathbf{M})^{-1}, \qquad (2.116)$$

which yields

$$\frac{\partial l_p}{\partial \mathbf{D}} = \frac{1}{2} \sum_{i=1}^{N} \left[\frac{N_T}{S}(\mathbf{I} + \mathbf{M}_i\mathbf{D})^{-1}\mathbf{r}_i\mathbf{r}_i'(\mathbf{I} + \mathbf{D}\mathbf{M}_i)^{-1} - \mathbf{M}_i(\mathbf{I} + \mathbf{D}\mathbf{M}_i)^{-1} \right],$$

where

$$S = \sum_i [S_i - \mathbf{r}_i'(\mathbf{D}^{-1} + \mathbf{M}_i)^{-1}\mathbf{r}_i].$$

Finally, matrix $\mathbf{D}$ updates as

$$\text{vec}(\mathbf{D}_{s+1}) = \text{vec}(\mathbf{D}_s) + \lambda_s\mathbf{H}_s^{-1}\text{vec}\left(\frac{\partial l_p}{\partial \mathbf{D}}\bigg|_{\mathbf{D}=\mathbf{D}_s}\right), \qquad (2.117)$$

where matrix (2.113) and the derivative are computed at the sth iteration. In practice, often $\lambda_s = 1$; however, we cannot guarantee that the unit step always increases the value of the log-likelihood function.

Problems for Section 2.11

1. State conditions under which the Fisher information matrix given by (2.110) is positive definite.

2. Prove that matrix $\mathbf{R}_i$ is symmetric.

3. Prove that (3.20) implies (2.113).

4. Check the matrix derivative (2.116) for scalars (all matrices and vectors are scalars).

2.12   EM algorithm

The Expectation-Maximization (EM) algorithm was one of the first to maximize the log-likelihood function for the LME model. See Laird and Ware (1982), Jennrich and Schluchter (1986), Laird et al. (1987), Lindstrom and Bates (1988). The derivation of this algorithm may be found in Laird and Ware (1982), and for a multilevel nested random effect model in Longford (1987). Jamshidian and Jennrich (1993) discuss several improvements to speed up the algorithm. A comprehensive account of the EM algorithm may be found in a book by McLachan and Krishnan (1996). A general discussion of the EM algorithm, along with other optimization algorithms, is given in Appendix 13.3.4.

In a version of the EM algorithm applied to the LME model, variance parameters are updated by the formulas

$$\Delta\sigma^2 = \frac{2\sigma^2}{N_T}\frac{\partial l}{\partial\sigma^2}, \qquad \Delta\mathbf{D} = \frac{2}{N}\mathbf{D}\frac{\partial l}{\partial\mathbf{D}}\mathbf{D}, \tag{2.118}$$

and $\boldsymbol{\beta}$ is recalculated by formula (2.28). Since the updates are linear combinations of the derivatives, the EM algorithm can be viewed as a special form of the generic algorithm (2.103) with $\lambda_s = 1$. Using formulas for derivatives (2.105), we can represent the EM algorithm (2.118) explicitly in a form suitable for computation as

$$\sigma_{s+1}^2 = \sigma_s^2 - 1 + \frac{1}{\sigma_s^2 N_T}\sum_{i=1}^{N}(\mathbf{y}_i - \mathbf{X}_i\boldsymbol{\beta}_s)'\mathbf{V}_{is}^{-1}(\mathbf{y}_i - \mathbf{X}_i\boldsymbol{\beta}_s), \tag{2.119}$$

$$\mathbf{D}_{s+1} = \mathbf{D}_s - \frac{1}{N}\sum_{i=1}^{N}[\mathbf{D}_s\mathbf{Z}_i'\mathbf{V}_{is}^{-1}\mathbf{Z}_i\mathbf{D}_s - \sigma_s^{-2}\mathbf{D}_s\mathbf{Z}_i'\mathbf{V}_{is}^{-1}\mathbf{e}_{is}\mathbf{e}_{is}'\mathbf{V}_{is}^{-1}\mathbf{Z}_i\mathbf{D}_s], \tag{2.120}$$

where the beta coefficients are recalculated by the GLS formula,

$$\boldsymbol{\beta}_{s+1} = \left[\sum_{i=1}^{N}\mathbf{X}_i'(\mathbf{I} + \mathbf{Z}_i\mathbf{D}_s\mathbf{Z}_i')^{-1}\mathbf{X}_i\right]^{-1}\sum_{i=1}^{N}\mathbf{X}_i'(\mathbf{I} + \mathbf{Z}_i\mathbf{D}_s\mathbf{Z}_i')^{-1}\mathbf{y}_i.$$

At convergence, the limit point turns the derivatives (2.105) to zero, so that the EM iterations converge to the MLE. Precisely, let the EM iterations converge, $\lim_{s\to\infty}\boldsymbol{\beta}_s = \lim_{s\to\infty}\boldsymbol{\beta}_{s+1} = \widehat{\boldsymbol{\beta}}_*$, $\lim_{s\to\infty}\sigma_s^2 = \lim_{s\to\infty}\sigma_{s+1}^2 = \widehat{\sigma}_*^2$ and $\lim_{s\to\infty}\mathbf{D}_s = \lim_{s\to\infty}\mathbf{D}_{s+1} = \widehat{\mathbf{D}}_*$, a positive definite matrix. Then, taking limits in (2.119) and (2.120) as $s \to \infty$, we come to the pair of equations

$$\widehat{\sigma}_*^2 = \widehat{\sigma}_*^2 - 1 + \frac{1}{\widehat{\sigma}_*^2 N_T}\sum_{i=1}^{N}(\mathbf{y}_i - \mathbf{X}_i\widehat{\boldsymbol{\beta}}_*)'\widehat{\mathbf{V}}_i^{-1}(\mathbf{y}_i - \mathbf{X}_i\widehat{\boldsymbol{\beta}}_*),$$

$$\widehat{\mathbf{D}}_* = \widehat{\mathbf{D}}_* - \frac{1}{N}\sum_{i=1}^{N}[\widehat{\mathbf{D}}_*\mathbf{Z}_i'\widehat{\mathbf{V}}_i^{-1}\mathbf{Z}_i\widehat{\mathbf{D}}_* - \widehat{\sigma}_*^{-2}\widehat{\mathbf{D}}_*\mathbf{Z}_i'\widehat{\mathbf{V}}_i^{-1}\mathbf{e}_{is}\mathbf{e}_{is}'\widehat{\mathbf{V}}_i^{-1}\mathbf{Z}_i\widehat{\mathbf{D}}_*],$$

which are equivalent to $\partial l/\partial\sigma^2 = 0$ and $\partial l/\partial\mathbf{D} = \mathbf{0}$. The second equation is equivalent to $\partial l/\partial\mathbf{D} = \mathbf{0}$ if matrix $\mathbf{D}_*$ is nonsingular. We use the dimension-reduction formula (2.25) to facilitate matrix inverse, especially when the n_i are much larger than k.

The EM algorithm has two *merits*:

1. It maximizes the log-likelihood function from iteration to iteration, $l_{s+1} > l_s$, if the gradient is not zero (Laird and Ware, 1982).

2. Formula (2.120) generates positive definite matrices $\{\mathbf{D}_s\}$ if the starting matrix $\mathbf{D}_0$ is positive definite. To see this, we rewrite the right-hand side of (2.120) times N as follows:

$$\sum\mathbf{D}_s(\mathbf{D}_s^{-1} - \mathbf{Z}_i'\mathbf{V}_{is}^{-1}\mathbf{Z}_i)\mathbf{D}_s + \sigma_s^{-2}\mathbf{D}_s\sum(\mathbf{Z}_i'\mathbf{V}_{is}^{-1}\mathbf{e}_{is}\mathbf{e}_{is}'\mathbf{V}_{is}^{-1}\mathbf{Z}_i)\mathbf{D}_s. \quad (2.121)$$

We prove that (2.121) is a positive definite matrix for all s by induction. Let $\mathbf{D}_s$ be positive definite. Then the second matrix term in (2.121) is a nonnegative definite matrix. For the first term, at least for one i matrix $\mathbf{Z}_i$ has full rank and therefore the first term is a positive definite matrix due to the matrix identity (2.25). Since the sum of a positive and a nonnegative matrix is a positive definite matrix, (2.121) is positive definite. It is worthwhile to note that the NR and FS algorithms do not produce the nonnegative matrix even if at the previous iteration the matrix was nonnegative definite; thus special care should be taken to ensure nonnegative definiteness, See details in Section 2.15, where several methods to control $\mathbf{D}$ are discussed.

A major drawback of the EM algorithm is that it may exhibit a slow convergence when matrix $\mathbf{D}$ is close to zero (recall that when we showed convergence of the EM algorithm, we assumed that matrix $\widehat{\mathbf{D}}_*$ is positive definite). It can be seen from formula (2.118) that the EM algorithm stops at zero since $\mathbf{D}_0 = \mathbf{0}$ generates all $\mathbf{D}_s = \mathbf{0}$. Note that although each matrix $\mathbf{D}_s$ is positive definite, the limit matrix may not be positive definite. A slow convergence of the algorithm in the neighborhood of zero is illustrated at length below.

The EM algorithm belongs to the class of fixed-point iterative algorithms,

$$\mathbf{w}_{s+1} = \mathbf{R}(\mathbf{w}_s), \quad s = 0, 1, ..., \quad (2.122)$$

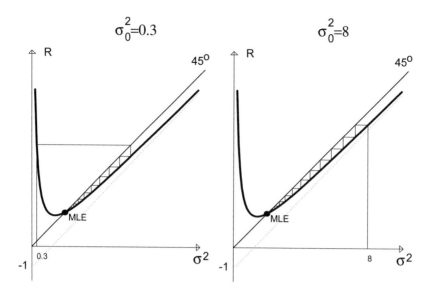

FIGURE 2.2. EM algorithm $\sigma_{s+1}^2 = \sigma_s^2 - 1 + 2/\sigma_s^2$. In the left-hand graph the starting point is to the left and in the right-hand graph the starting point is to the right of the solution $\sigma_*^2 = 2$. For large σ^2 the function $R(\sigma^2)$ may be well approximated by $\sigma^2 - 1$, the dotted line. The dot 'MLE' with coordinates (2,2), is the intersection of $R(\sigma^2)$ with the 45° line.

where $\mathbf{w}$ is a vector and $\mathbf{R}$ is a vector function. When (2.122) converges, the limit (fixed) point $\mathbf{w}_* = \lim_{s \to \infty} \mathbf{w}_s$ satisfies the equation $\mathbf{w}_* = \mathbf{R}(\mathbf{w}_*)$. However, iterations may diverge, and in particular, their behavior may depend crucially on the starting point, $\mathbf{w}_0$.

To illustrate the fixed-point nature of the EM algorithm, we consider a simplified version of the algorithm where $\boldsymbol{\beta}$ and $\mathbf{D}$ are held fixed. Then, as follows from formula (2.119), the EM algorithm for σ^2 takes the form $\sigma_{s+1}^2 = R(\sigma_s^2)$ where $R(\sigma^2) = \sigma^2 - 1 + A/\sigma^2$ and $A = \sum (\mathbf{y} - \mathbf{X}\boldsymbol{\beta})' \mathbf{V}^{-1} (\mathbf{y} - \mathbf{X}\boldsymbol{\beta})/N_T > 0$ is fixed. It is easy to see that $\lim_{\sigma^2 \to \infty} R(\sigma^2) = \lim_{\sigma^2 \to 0} R(\sigma^2) = \infty$ with the minimum attained at $\sigma_{min}^2 = \sqrt{A}$ and the unique fixed-point $\sigma_*^2 = A$. Two possible iteration patterns are shown in Figure 2.2. At the left, the starting point $\sigma_0^2 = 0.3$ is to the left of the solution; at the right, the starting point is to the right of the solution.

Now we illustrate iterations (2.120) in fixed-point form for $k = 1$ (one random effect) holding parameters $\boldsymbol{\beta}$ and σ^2 constant. Then, denoting $a_i = \|\mathbf{z}_i\|^2$ and $r_i = \mathbf{z}_i' \mathbf{e}_i$, after using formulas (2.21) and (2.25), we come to the following fixed-point function:

$$R(D) = \frac{D}{\sigma^2 N} \sum_{i=1}^{N} \frac{\sigma^2 + (\sigma^2 a_i + r_i^2)D}{(1 + a_i D)^2}. \tag{2.123}$$

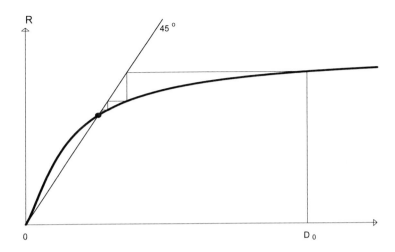

FIGURE 2.3. EM (fixed-point) algorithm $D_{s+1} = R(D_s)$ for one random effect when other parameters are held constant. The first derivative of R at zero is 1, and for this case the second derivative is positive. These imply that the MLE is positive (dot).

As is easy to see, the value of function R at $D = 0$ is zero and has an asymptote when $D \to \infty$,

$$R(0) = 0, \quad R(\infty) = \frac{1}{\sigma^2 N} \sum_{i=1}^{N} \frac{\sigma^2 a_i + r_i^2}{a_i^2} = \text{const},$$

see Figures 2.3 and 2.4. Also, we find that the slope of function R at zero is 1 and

$$R''(0) = \frac{2}{\sigma^2 N} \sum_{i=1}^{N} (r_i^2 - \sigma^2 a_i).$$

Since $R(D)$ is a continuous function and $R'(0) = 1$, we conclude that the equation $D = R(D)$ has a positive solution if $R''(0) > 0$, which is equivalent to $\sigma^2 < \sum r_i^2 / \sum a_i^2$. This inequality corresponds exactly to the condition on the positiveness of the MLE derived in Section 2.6. On the contrary, if $R''(0) < 0$, the MLE is zero as shown in Figure 2.4.

In case of balanced data (BRC model), we have $a_i = a$ and $r_i^2 = r^2$, so that EM iterations become

$$D_{s+1} = \frac{D_s}{\sigma^2} \frac{\sigma^2 + (\sigma^2 a + r^2)D_s}{(1 + aD_s)^2}.$$

As we see, even for balanced data the EM algorithm may be very slow if D is close to zero. Recall that for balanced data the NR and FS algorithms produce the MLE after the first iteration.

Summarizing, (a) when the MLE for $\mathbf{D}$ is on the boundary of the parameter space, the EM algorithm converges very slow; (b) even for balanced data the EM algorithm requires many iterations; and (c) a good starting point for the EM algorithm is $\mathbf{D} = \infty$.

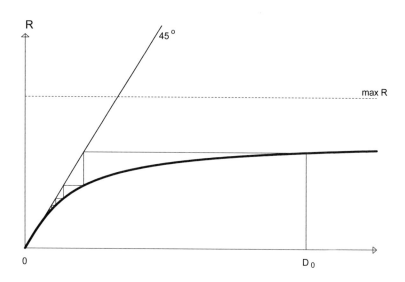

FIGURE 2.4. EM (fixed-point) algorithm $D_{s+1} = R(D_s)$ when $R''(0) < 0$. The MLE is zero and iterations converge to zero very slowly.

2.12.1 Fixed-point algorithm

In this section we derive a Fixed-Point (FP) algorithm using the dimension-reduction formulas, which may be viewed as a version of the EM algorithm. An attractive feature of this algorithm is that instead of inverting an $n_i \times n_i$ matrix, one needs to inverse a $k \times k$ matrix, see also Appendix 13.3.4.

First, applying these formulas to the GLS estimator, we recompute $\boldsymbol{\beta}$ using formula (2.114), which gives

$$\boldsymbol{\beta}_{s+1} = [\mathbf{N} - \sum \mathbf{T}_i \mathbf{F}_i^{-1} \mathbf{T}_i']^{-1} [\mathbf{t} - \sum \mathbf{T}_i \mathbf{F}_i^{-1} \mathbf{p}_i], \qquad (2.124)$$

where $\mathbf{F}_i = \mathbf{D}_s^{-1} + \mathbf{M}_i$. Second, applying the dimension-reduction formulas to $\partial l_p / \partial \mathbf{D} = \mathbf{0}$, we come to an equivalent matrix equation,

$$\sum [\frac{N_T}{S} \mathbf{F}_i^{-1} \mathbf{p}_i \mathbf{p}_i' \mathbf{F}_i^{-1} + \mathbf{F}_i^{-1}] - N\mathbf{D} = \mathbf{0},$$

which we rewrite in fixed-point form as

$$\mathbf{D}_{s+1} = \frac{1}{N} \left[\frac{N_T}{\sum [\|\mathbf{e}_i\|^2 - \mathbf{p}_i' \mathbf{F}_{is}^{-1} \mathbf{p}_i]} \sum_{i=1}^{N} \mathbf{F}_{is}^{-1} \mathbf{p}_i \mathbf{p}_i' \mathbf{F}_{is}^{-1} + \sum_{i=1}^{N} \mathbf{F}_{is}^{-1} \right]. \qquad (2.125)$$

This algorithm has the same merits and demerits as those of the EM algorithm. Note that the denominator $\sum [\|\mathbf{e}_i\|^2 - \mathbf{p}_i' \mathbf{F}_{is}^{-1} \mathbf{p}_i]$ is positive at each iteration if the condition on the MLE existence (2.37) holds. Again, a good start for (2.125) is to take $\mathbf{D}_0 = \kappa \mathbf{I}$, where κ is a big positive number. However, the FP algorithm has all the drawbacks outlined above as for the EM algorithm.

Problems for Section 2.12

1. What are the advantages of using large σ_0^2 and $\mathbf{D}_0$ in recursive formulas (2.119) and (2.120)? Illustrate your answer using Figures 2.2 and 2.3.

2. Estimate the weight versus height LME model from Section 2.1 using the EM algorithm. Plot iterations for σ^2 and d as in Figures 2.2 and 2.3.

3*. Write your own R function which estimates the LME model using the EM algorithm. Test the performance of the EM algorithm using simulations. Generate the LME model with random intercept and estimate it with lme and your own function. Compare the results. In how many cases are the results identical?

2.13   Starting point

Every iterative procedure requires a starting point (value), and maximization of the log-likelihood function is not an exception. Since the maximum of the log-likelihood function admits a closed-form solution for $\boldsymbol{\beta}$ and σ^2, it suffices to provide a starting point for matrix $\mathbf{D}$. Here we suggest two starting points for matrix $\mathbf{D}$ based on the FS and FP algorithms. Another strategy to find a satisfactory starting point is to use a distribution-free estimate such as the MINQUE or MM estimate (see the next chapter). The advantage of this starting point is that if data are close to balanced, the starting point is close to the MLE/RMLE.

It is especially useful to have several starting points when an algorithm converges to a matrix $\mathbf{D}_*$ on the boundary of the parameter space, i.e., when $|\mathbf{D}_*| = 0$ (see Section 2.15).

2.13.1   FS starting point

We derive the starting point for $\mathbf{D}$ as the first iteration of the FS algorithm based on the OLS solution ($\mathbf{D} = \mathbf{0}$). Let $\widehat{\boldsymbol{\beta}}_{OLS}$ be the OLS estimate derived from (2.28) letting $\mathbf{D} = \mathbf{0}$, and $\widehat{\mathbf{e}}_i$ be the OLS residual vector for the ith individual (object, cluster). The OLS estimate of σ^2 is $\widehat{\sigma}_{OLS}^2 = N_T^{-1} \sum \widehat{\mathbf{e}}_i' \widehat{\mathbf{e}}_i$. When $\mathbf{D} = \mathbf{0}$ we have simply $\mathbf{V}_i = \mathbf{I}$, and in the previous notation, $\mathbf{R}_i = \mathbf{Z}_i' \mathbf{Z}_i$. Then the derivative of the log-likelihood function with respect to $\mathbf{D}$ at zero, as follows from (2.105), is written as

$$\left. \frac{\partial l}{\partial \mathbf{D}} \right|_{\mathbf{D}=\mathbf{0}} = \frac{1}{2} \sum_{i=1}^{N} [\widehat{\sigma}_{OLS}^{-2} \mathbf{Z}_i' \widehat{\mathbf{e}}_i \widehat{\mathbf{e}}_i' \mathbf{Z}_i - \mathbf{Z}_i' \mathbf{Z}_i]. \tag{2.126}$$

Since we are interested in the solution for $\mathbf{D}$, we take the (3,3)-block of the information matrix (2.110). Hence, repeating arguments of the matrix version of the NR algorithm we come to the starting point $\widehat{\mathbf{D}}_0$ as the solution to the following matrix equation:

$$\sum_{i=1}^{N} (\mathbf{Z}_i' \mathbf{Z}_i) \mathbf{D} (\mathbf{Z}_i' \mathbf{Z}_i) = \sum_{i=1}^{N} [\widehat{\sigma}_{OLS}^{-2} \mathbf{Z}_i' \widehat{\mathbf{e}}_i \widehat{\mathbf{e}}_i' \mathbf{Z}_i - \mathbf{Z}_i' \mathbf{Z}_i].$$

We notice that matrix $\mathbf{D}$ cannot simply be derived from this equation unless all $\mathbf{Z}_i' \mathbf{Z}_i$ are the same. Therefore, we take the vec operator of both sides, which leads us to an explicit form,

$$
\mathrm{vec}(\widehat{\mathbf{D}}_0) = \left[\sum_{i=1}^{N}(\mathbf{Z}_i'\mathbf{Z}_i) \otimes (\mathbf{Z}_i'\mathbf{Z}_i)\right]^{-1}
$$

$$
\times \mathrm{vec}\left[\sum_{i=1}^{N}[\widehat{\sigma}_{OLS}^{-2}\mathbf{Z}_i'\widehat{\mathbf{e}}_i\widehat{\mathbf{e}}_i'\mathbf{Z}_i - \mathbf{Z}_i'\mathbf{Z}_i]\right]. \tag{2.127}
$$

As follows, this starting point, $\widehat{\mathbf{D}}_0$, is a positive definite matrix if the derivative (2.126) is positive definite, in accordance with the criterion of the positive definiteness of the MLE, Section 2.6. We need the following matrix result to prove this statement (we refer the reader to Appendix 13.2.3 for matrix algebra formulas to be used in the proof).

Proposition 7 *Let $\{\mathbf{R}_i, i = 1, ..., N\}$ be $k \times k$ symmetric nonnegative definite matrices such that at least one of them is positive definite, and let $\mathbf{B}$ be a positive definite matrix of the same order. Then (a) matrix $\sum_i \mathbf{R}_i \otimes \mathbf{R}_i$ is positive definite, and (b) matrix $\mathbf{D}$, as the solution to the matrix equation $\sum_i \mathbf{R}_i\mathbf{D}\mathbf{R}_i = \mathbf{B}$, is symmetric and positive definite.*

Proof. (a) Let $\mathbf{u}$ be any nonzero $k^2 \times 1$ vector; we want to prove that $\mathbf{u}'\sum_i \mathbf{R}_i \otimes \mathbf{R}_i\mathbf{u} > 0$. Let $\mathbf{U}$ be the $k \times k$ matrix such that $\mathrm{vec}(\mathbf{U}) = \mathbf{u}$. Then

$$
\mathbf{u}'\sum_i \mathbf{R}_i \otimes \mathbf{R}_i\mathbf{u} = \mathrm{vec}'(\mathbf{U})\sum_i \mathbf{R}_i \otimes \mathbf{R}_i\mathrm{vec}(\mathbf{U})
$$

$$
= \sum_i \mathrm{vec}'(\mathbf{U})\mathrm{vec}(\mathbf{R}_i\mathbf{U}\mathbf{R}_i) = \sum_i \mathrm{tr}(\mathbf{R}_i\mathbf{U})^2.
$$

Thus, $\mathbf{u}'\sum_i \mathbf{R}_i \otimes \mathbf{R}_i\mathbf{u} = 0$ if and only if $\mathbf{R}_i\mathbf{U} = \mathbf{0}$ for all i. (b) Note that matrix $\mathbf{D}$ is positive definite if and only if $\mathrm{tr}(\mathbf{D}\mathbf{U})$ is positive for any $k \times k$ positive definite matrix $\mathbf{U}$. Since $\mathrm{vec}(\mathbf{D}) = (\sum \mathbf{R}_i \otimes \mathbf{R}_i)^{-1}\mathrm{vec}(\mathbf{B})$ we have

$$
\mathrm{tr}(\mathbf{D}\mathbf{U}) = \mathrm{vec}'(\mathbf{U})(\sum \mathbf{R}_i \otimes \mathbf{R}_i)^{-1}\mathrm{vec}(\mathbf{B}) = \mathrm{tr}(\mathbf{U}\mathbf{R}_i^2\mathbf{B}) > 0.
$$

To prove (b), we find a large enough ω that $\mathbf{R}_i \leq \omega\mathbf{I}$. This inequality implies that $\mathbf{B} \leq \omega^2\mathbf{D}$, and therefore, matrix $\mathbf{D}$ is positive definite. ∎

As follows from this proposition the starting point is a positive definite matrix if the derivative (2.126) is a positive definite matrix.

2.13.2   FP starting point

This starting point is derived from equation (2.125), letting $\mathbf{D} = \infty$. Recall that infinite matrix $\mathbf{D}$ corresponds to the fixed effects approach, see the discussion around formula (2.37). Then we set $\mathbf{F}_i^{-1} = (\mathbf{Z}_i'\mathbf{Z}_i)^{-}$ and, as follows from Section 2.5, $S_{\min} > 0$ implies the existence of the MLE. We use notation $\widehat{\sigma}_{XZ} = N_T^{-1}S_{\min}$ and interpret it as the lower bound for the variance estimate, (2.100). Then, as follows from

(2.125), we obtain

$$\widehat{\mathbf{D}}_0 = \frac{1}{N} \left[\widehat{\sigma}_{XZ}^{-2} \sum_{i=1}^{N} (\mathbf{Z}_i'\mathbf{Z}_i)^- \mathbf{r}_i \mathbf{r}_i' (\mathbf{Z}_i'\mathbf{Z}_i)^- + \sum_{i=1}^{N} (\mathbf{Z}_i'\mathbf{Z}_i)^- \right], \tag{2.128}$$

where $\widehat{\sigma}_{XZ}^2$ is defined in (2.100) and $\mathbf{r}_i = \mathbf{Z}_i'(\mathbf{y}_i - \mathbf{X}_i\widehat{\boldsymbol{\beta}}_\infty - \mathbf{Z}_i\mathbf{Z}_i^+\mathbf{y}_i)$.

Problems for Section 2.13

1. Express the starting point (2.127) explicitly in matrix form when $\mathbf{Z}_i = \mathbf{Z}$, where $\mathbf{Z}$ is a full-rank matrix.

2*. Compare starting point matrices (2.127) and (2.128) when $\mathbf{Z}_i = \mathbf{Z}$, where $\mathbf{Z}$ is a full-rank matrix and variances σ^2 are known replacing the empirical values with their expectation. Under what additional conditions will the two matrices coincide? Use simulations to support and verify your analytical derivation.

3*. Compare starting point matrices (2.127) and (2.128) with a single random effect assuming that variances σ^2 and σ_d^2 are known. Can one prove that one point is always smaller than another? Under what additional conditions do the two points coincide? Under what conditions do the starting points coincide with the MLE of d? Use simulations to support and verify your analytical derivation. Use the random intercept model for simulations (consult the next chapter).

4*. Use simulations in R to determine which starting point yields the higher value of the log-likelihood function. Use the random intercept and slope model for simulations (consult the next chapter).

2.14 Algorithms for restricted MLE

In this section we discuss briefly how to maximize the restricted maximum likelihood in the form (2.50) or (2.53).

2.14.1 Fisher scoring algorithm

As a result of the asymptotic equivalence of RML and ML, they have the same asymptotic covariance matrices. Consequently, the Fisher scoring algorithm applied to the restricted log-likelihood function may use the same matrix $\mathbf{H}_s$ but different gradient $\mathbf{g}_s$, in view of the generic maximization algorithm (2.104). The gradient $\mathbf{g}$ of function (2.50) has three components. The first component, the derivative with respect to $\boldsymbol{\beta}$, is the same as for the ML method, $\partial l_R / \partial \boldsymbol{\beta} = \sigma^{-2} \sum \mathbf{X}_i' \mathbf{V}_i^{-1} \mathbf{e}_i$. The second component, the derivative with respect to σ^2 for the RML log-likelihood function, is

$$\frac{\partial l_R}{\partial \sigma^2} = -0.5\sigma^{-2}(N_T - m) + 0.5\sigma^{-4} \sum \mathbf{e}_i' \mathbf{V}_i^{-1} \mathbf{e}_i.$$

The third component, the derivative with respect to $\mathbf{D}$, is

$$\frac{\partial l_R}{\partial \mathbf{D}} = -0.5 \sum [\mathbf{Z}_i' \mathbf{V}_i^{-1} \mathbf{Z}_i - \sigma^{-2} \mathbf{Z}_i' \mathbf{V}_i^{-1} \mathbf{e}_i \mathbf{e}_i' \mathbf{V}_i^{-1} \mathbf{Z}_i$$

$$- \mathbf{Z}_i' \mathbf{V}_i^{-1} \mathbf{X}_i (\sum_{j=1}^{N} \mathbf{X}_j' \mathbf{V}_j^{-1} \mathbf{X}_j)^{-1} \mathbf{X}_i' \mathbf{V}_i^{-1} \mathbf{Z}_i]. \tag{2.129}$$

Thus, the FS algorithm for the RML estimation, which maximizes the log-likelihood function (2.50), has the form (2.104), where $\mathbf{g}_s$ is the $(m + 1 + k^2) \times 1$ vector

$$\mathbf{g}_s = \left(\left(\tfrac{\partial l_R}{\partial \boldsymbol{\beta}} \right)', \left(\tfrac{\partial l_R}{\partial \sigma^2} \right)', \operatorname{vec}' \left(\tfrac{\partial l_R}{\partial \mathbf{D}} \right) \right)' \text{ evaluated at } \boldsymbol{\beta} = \boldsymbol{\beta}_s, \sigma^2 = \sigma_s^2, \mathbf{D} = \mathbf{D}_s, \text{ with}$$

matrix $\mathbf{H}_s$ defined by (2.110).

2.14.2   EM algorithm

We use the fixed-point approach to create an EM/FP version for RMLE as we did in Section 2.12.1. Indeed, the estimating equation for $\mathbf{D}$ is $\mathbf{0} = \partial l_R / \partial \mathbf{D}$, where $\partial l_R / \partial \mathbf{D}$ is given by (2.129), which can be rewritten equivalently as

$$\mathbf{0} = \mathbf{D} - \sum_{i=1}^{N} \mathbf{D}[\mathbf{D}^{-1} - \mathbf{Z}_i' \mathbf{V}_i^{-1} \mathbf{Z}_i] \mathbf{D}$$

$$-\sigma^{-2} \sum_{i=1}^{N} \mathbf{D} \mathbf{Z}_i' \mathbf{V}_i^{-1} [\mathbf{e}_i \mathbf{e}_i' - \mathbf{X}_i (\sum_{j=1}^{N} \mathbf{X}_j' \mathbf{V}_j^{-1} \mathbf{X}_j)^{-1} \mathbf{X}_i'] \mathbf{V}_i^{-1} \mathbf{Z}_i \mathbf{D}.$$

Moving $\mathbf{D}$ to the left-hand side leads to the fixed-point iterations

$$\mathbf{D}_{s+1} = \sum_{i=1}^{N} \mathbf{D}_s [\mathbf{D}_s^{-1} - \mathbf{Z}_i' \mathbf{V}_{is}^{-1} \mathbf{Z}_i] \mathbf{D}_s \qquad (2.130)$$

$$+\sigma_s^{-2} \sum_{i=1}^{N} \mathbf{D}_s \mathbf{Z}_i' \mathbf{V}_{is}^{-1} [\mathbf{e}_{is} \mathbf{e}_{is}' - \mathbf{X}_i (\sum_{j=1}^{N} \mathbf{X}_j' \mathbf{V}_{js}^{-1} \mathbf{X}_j)^{-1} \mathbf{X}_i'] \mathbf{V}_{is}^{-1} \mathbf{Z}_{is} \mathbf{D},$$

where $\mathbf{e}_{is}$ is the ith residual vector, as in standard ML. Parameter σ_s^2 may be updated as in the ML algorithm: $\widehat{\sigma}_s^2 = \sum_{i=1}^{N} \mathbf{e}_{is}' \mathbf{V}_{is}^{-1} \mathbf{e}_{is} / (N_T - m)$. The restricted EM algorithm has the same properties as the standard EM algorithm; namely, it increases the log-likelihood value at each iteration but may be slow, especially when the determinant of matrix $\mathbf{D}$ is close to zero.

Problems for Section 2.14

1. Prove that the expected values for the derivatives (2.129) are zero.

2. Plot several functions of d to illustrate the fixed-point iterations (2.130), similar to Figure 2.3. Use the random intercept model to generate the data.

3*. Construct starting points FS and FP for RMLE following the derivation from Section 2.13.

2.15   Optimization on nonnegative definite matrices

As mentioned earlier, during likelihood maximization one may encounter a matrix $\mathbf{D}$ that is not nonnegative definite (some eigenvalues are negative) or even negative definite (all eigenvalues are negative). Thus, strictly speaking, we need to deal with *constrained* maximization over the space of nonnegative definite matrices. This problem is common to maximum likelihood estimation of random effects models, so that the following discussion is applicable to variance components or nonlinear mixed effects models as well. A routine practice in variance components model is to set the MLE to zero if the log-likelihood maximum is attained at a negative value (Searle et al., 1992). In fact, the chance of getting a negative definite matrix $\mathbf{D}$ in the course of the maximization procedure is a typical reason for failure of commercial statistical packages. Usually, the problem with matrix $\mathbf{D}$ arises when the number of clusters, N, is too small (see the simulations below). Note that when an iterative algorithm converges to a nonnegative definite singular matrix, the gradient of the log-likelihood function is not zero, which may be interpreted as the failure to converge. However, the gradient cannot be zero if one deals with constrained maximization with the solution on the boundary of the parameter set (Ortega and Rheinboldt, 1970; Polak, 1971; Dennis and Schnabel, 1983). The problem of a nonnegative definite matrix does not apply to EM or FP algorithms because they produce nonnegative definite matrices if the starting matrix is nonnegative definite. Thus, the following discussion concerns the NR and FS algorithms. For a general discussion of optimization algorithms, we refer the reader to Appendix 13.3.

There are three strategies to cope with matrix $\mathbf{D}$ over the course of likelihood maximization:

1. Allow the matrix $\mathbf{D}$ to be negative definite, but replace it with a nonnegative definite matrix *after* iterations converged (in SAS this corresponds to the option NONBOUND).

2. Force the matrix $\mathbf{D}$ to stay nonnegative definite (constrained maximization).

3. Use matrix reparameterization such that $\mathbf{D}$ is always nonnegative definite, e.g., use Cholesky decomposition $\mathbf{D} = \mathbf{L}'\mathbf{L}$ and accomplish maximization for matrix $\mathbf{L}$.

These methods are discussed in detail below. But before moving to the remedies we shall investigate how often $\widehat{\mathbf{D}}_{ML}$ belongs to the boundary of the parameter space.

2.15.1 How often can one hit the boundary?

To assess the chance during maximization of hitting the boundary of the parameter space (2.16), where matrix $\mathbf{D}$ becomes singular, we conducted the following statistical experiment. We use the fact that a closed-form solution exists for the balanced random-coefficient model; see Section 2.3. Hence, we take a random-coefficient linear trend model (2.58) with $n = 4$ and true $\sigma^2 = 1$, $\alpha = 1$, $\beta = 0.1$, $t_j = j$, and true scaled covariance matrix for the intercept and the slope,

$$\mathbf{D} = \begin{bmatrix} 1 & 0.3 \\ 0.3 & 0.5 \end{bmatrix}.$$

Five hundred data sets for each N have been generated, and for each data set we computed the exact MLE and RMLE using formulas (2.60) and (2.61). Then we computed eigenvalues of each 2×2 matrix and percent simulations in which the minimal eigenvalue is negative. This assesses the chance that during maximization of the log-likelihood we "hit the wall" (e.g., the solution will be on the boundary

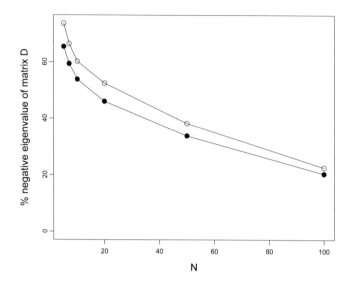

FIGURE 2.5. Percent of simulations when matrix $\widehat{\mathbf{D}}_{ML}$ (empty circles) and matrix $\widehat{\mathbf{D}}_{RML}$ (filled circles) are singular. The chance of hitting the boundary of the parameter space during likelihood maximization is high: 50% for $N = 20$ and 20% for $N = 100$.

of the parameter space). As one can see from Figure 2.5, the chance to obtain a deficient estimate of $\mathbf{D}$ is substantial, although it is a little less for RML because $\widehat{\mathbf{D}}_{ML} < \widehat{\mathbf{D}}_{RML}$ always. For instance, for $N = 20$ there is 50% chance that one confronts a constrained optimization problems. This phenomenon was also mentioned by Jennrich and Schluchter (1986). Even for large N, the chance to get a deficient $\mathbf{D}$ is quite high, 1 out of 5.

2.15.2 Allow matrix $\mathbf{D}$ to be not nonnegative definite

This is the case when the parameter space is defined by (2.17). From a numerical point of view, this means that matrix $\mathbf{D}$ does not necessarily have to stay nonnegative definite during a maximization process. However, matrix $\mathbf{V}_i = \mathbf{I} + \mathbf{Z}_i\mathbf{D}\mathbf{Z}_i'$ must be positive definite for each $i = 1, ..., N$ to be able to compute the log-likelihood function. Thus, we can expand the parameter space to $\mathbb{D}_- = \{\mathbf{D} : \mathbf{I} + \mathbf{Z}_i\mathbf{D}\mathbf{Z}_i'$ is positive definite for each $i = 1, ..., N\}$, which is less restrictive than $\mathbb{D}_+ = \{\mathbf{D}$ is nonnegative definite$\}$; namely, $\mathbb{D}_+ \subset \mathbb{D}_-$. As mentioned in Section 2.2.2, $\mathbb{D}_-$ was used by Rao and Kleffé (1988) in their general variance components model. The RK parameter space (2.17) is convex as an intersection of N convex sets (see the problems at the end of the section). After the point of maximum is found, we transform a possible not nonnegative definite matrix $\mathbf{D}$ into a nonnegative definite matrix (see the end of this section).

To illustrate the difference between the two parameter sets, we consider the following example with two uncorrelated random effects.

Example. *The LME model with two uncorrelated random effects, $k = 2$:*

$$\mathbf{D} = \begin{bmatrix} D_{11} & 0 \\ 0 & D_{22} \end{bmatrix}, \quad \mathbf{Z}_i = [\mathbf{z}_{1i}, \mathbf{z}_{2i}], \quad \mathbf{V}_i = \mathbf{I} + D_{11}\mathbf{z}_{1i}\mathbf{z}_{1i}' + D_{22}\mathbf{z}_{2i}\mathbf{z}_{2i}'.$$

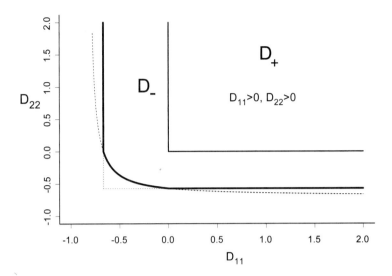

FIGURE 2.6. Two parameter spaces for the 2×2 diagonal matrix $\mathbf{D}$. The parameter space $\mathbb{D}_+$ consists of all nonnegative numbers. The boundary of $\mathbb{D}_-$ is shown in bold.

It is assumed that neither vector $\mathbf{z}$ is zero. Since the matrix $\mathbf{D}$ has only two free elements, we can depict $\mathbb{D}_+$ and $\mathbb{D}_-$ graphically on the plane in the coordinate system (D_{11}, D_{22}), see Figure 2.6. $\mathbb{D}_+$ is the first quadrant on the plane $(D_{11} \geq 0, D_{22} \geq 0)$. Now we determine $\mathbb{D}_-$ where some diagonal elements may be negative. As follows from linear algebra, matrix $\mathbf{V}_i$ has $n_i - 2$ eigenvalues 1 and two non-1 eigenvalues coinciding with the eigenvalues of the matrix

$$\begin{bmatrix} 1 + D_{11} \left\| \mathbf{z}_{1i} \right\|^2 & D_{11} \mathbf{z}'_{1i} \mathbf{z}_{2i} \\ D_{22} \mathbf{z}'_{1i} \mathbf{z}_{2i} & 1 + D_{22} \left\| \mathbf{z}_{2i} \right\|^2 \end{bmatrix}.$$

Thus, the matrix $\mathbf{V}_i$ is positive definite if and only if the diagonal elements are positive,

$$1 + D_{11} \left\| \mathbf{z}_{1i} \right\|^2 > 0, \; 1 + D_{22} \left\| \mathbf{z}_{2i} \right\|^2 > 0, \tag{2.131}$$

and the determinant is positive,

$$(1 + D_{11} \left\| \mathbf{z}_{1i} \right\|)(1 + D_{22} \left\| \mathbf{z}_{2i} \right\|^2) - D_{11} D_{22} (\mathbf{z}'_{1i} \mathbf{z}_{2i})^2 > 0. \tag{2.132}$$

Inequalities (2.131) yield the lower bounds for D_{11} and D_{22} :

$$D_{11} > -\min_i \left\| \mathbf{z}_{1i} \right\|^{-2}, \; D_{22} > -\min_i \left\| \mathbf{z}_{2i} \right\|^{-2}. \tag{2.133}$$

Inequality (2.132) yields a hyperbolic region that superimposes the rectangular region specified by (2.133). A typical parameter space $\mathbb{D}_-$ is depicted in Figure 2.6. The dotted rectangular region is determined by inequalities (2.131); the curve is determined by inequalities (2.132), $i = 1, 2, ..., N$. ∎

There is the jeopardy that maximization over $\mathbb{D}_-$ leads to an indefinite solution; more precisely, $l \to +\infty$ when $|\mathbf{V}_i| \to 0$ for some i. Indeed, let us examine what happens when for certain i the matrix $\mathbf{V}_i = \mathbf{I} + \mathbf{Z}_i \mathbf{D} \mathbf{Z}_i'$ becomes singular. Dropping i and the σ^2-term, to shorten the notation, the ith log-likelihood contribution is $-0.5 \left\{ \ln |\mathbf{V}| + \mathbf{e}' \mathbf{V}^{-1} \mathbf{e} \right\}$. Let $\lambda_1 \leq \lambda_2 \leq \ldots \leq \lambda_n$ denote eigenvalues of matrix $\mathbf{V}$ and $\mathbf{p}_1, \mathbf{p}_2, \ldots, \mathbf{p}_n$ denote its eigenvectors. Then from eigenvalue decomposition, $\mathbf{V}^{-1} = \sum_{j=1}^{n} \lambda_j^{-1} \mathbf{p}_j \mathbf{p}_j'$ and $\ln |\mathbf{V}| = \sum_{j=1}^{n} \ln \lambda_j$. Hence, the ith log-likelihood contribution is rewritten as

$$-\frac{1}{2} \left\{ \sum_{j=1}^{n} \left[\ln \lambda_j + \lambda_j^{-1} (\mathbf{p}_j' \mathbf{e})^2 \right] \right\}. \tag{2.134}$$

If, during iterations, $\mathbf{D}$ comes close to a boundary point of $\mathbb{D}_-$, the matrix $\mathbf{V}$ becomes close to singular, i.e., $\min \lambda_i = \lambda_1 \to 0$. However, taking $\boldsymbol{\beta}$ such that $\mathbf{p}_1' \mathbf{e} = \mathbf{p}_1' (\mathbf{y} - \mathbf{X} \boldsymbol{\beta}) = 0$ the log-likelihood function approaches $+\infty$ since the first term in (2.134) approaches $+\infty$ and the second term is zero.

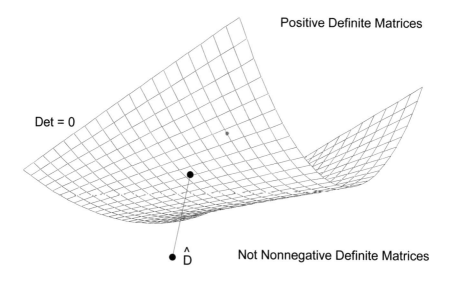

FIGURE 2.7. The space of 2×2 nonnegative definite matrices $\mathbb{D}_+$ defined by the inequalities Det $= |\mathbf{D}| = D_{11} D_{22} - D_{12}^2 \geq 0$ and $D_{11} \geq 0, D_{22} \geq 0$. Positive definite matrices lie *within* the surface, nonnegative singular matrices lie *on* the surface, and nonnegative definite matrices lie *under* the surface. $\widehat{\mathbf{D}}$ is not a nonnegative definite matrix; however, we can find the projection of $\widehat{\mathbf{D}}$ onto $\mathbb{D}_+$.

The good news is that $\mathbf{p}_1' (\mathbf{y} - \mathbf{X} \boldsymbol{\beta}) = 0$ happens with probability 0 because $\mathbf{y}$ has a continuous (actually normal) distribution. Numerically, this means that if the direction of the log-likelihood increase is determined, the log-likelihood goes to $-\infty$

almost surely on the ray approaching the boundary of the RK parameter space, i.e. where for some j we have $|\mathbf{V}_j| = 0$. This property serves as a justification for our unconstrained log-likelihood maximization algorithm realized in R; see Section 2.16 for details.

We can easily satisfy the condition $\mathbf{D}_s \in \mathbb{D}_-$ during the maximization process. Indeed, at each iteration (2.103), we check whether matrix $\mathbf{V}_i$ is positive definite for each i by computing eigenvalues of matrix $\mathbf{Z}_i'\mathbf{Z}_i\mathbf{D}$. If for at least one i the minimum eigenvalue is zero or negative, we reduce λ_s by 2 (the step length should be reduced further to satisfy the monotonicity, $l_{s+1} > l_s$).

Now let the log-likelihood maximum on $\mathbb{D}_-$ be found and $\widehat{\mathbf{D}}$ correspond to the final iteration. If $\widehat{\mathbf{D}}$ is a nonnegative definite matrix, we call it the MLE. If $\widehat{\mathbf{D}}$ is not nonnegative definite, we project it onto the space of all nonnegative definite matrices $\mathbb{D}_+$. In the previous example, $k = 2$ and $D_{12} = 0$, so that $\mathbb{D}_+$ is the first quadrant R^+. In the general case, $D_{12} \neq 0$, and the set of all nonnegative matrices is defined by the square-root envelope $D_{12} = \pm\sqrt{D_{11}D_{22}}$ in the coordinate system $(D_{11}, D_{12}, D_{22}) =$vech$(\mathbf{D})$ with nonnegative D_{11} and D_{22}, see Figure 2.7. If $\widehat{\mathbf{D}}$ is outside the envelope, we must find the closest point (projection) on $\mathbb{D}_+$. In the next theorem we determine how to find this projection.

Theorem 8 *Let a symmetric $k \times k$ matrix $\widehat{\mathbf{D}}$ be represented via eigenvalue decomposition as $\widehat{\mathbf{D}} = \mathbf{P}\mathbf{\Lambda}\mathbf{P}'$, where $\mathbf{P}$ is the $k \times k$ matrix of eigenvectors and $\mathbf{\Lambda} =$diag$(\lambda_1, \lambda_2, ..., \lambda_k)$ is the diagonal matrix of eigenvalues. Then the projection of $\widehat{\mathbf{D}}$ onto $\mathbb{D}_+$ is defined as $\mathbf{P}\mathbf{\Lambda}_+\mathbf{P}'$, where*

$$\mathbf{\Lambda}_+ =\text{diag}(\max(0, \lambda_1), \max(0, \lambda_2), .., \max(0, \lambda_k)).$$

Proof. We want to find a $k \times k$ nonnegative definite (symmetric) matrix $\mathbf{D}$ such that

$$\text{tr}(\widehat{\mathbf{D}} - \mathbf{D})^2 = \sum_{i,j=1}^{k} (\widehat{D}_{ij} - D_{ij})^2 = \min. \tag{2.135}$$

From the properties of the trace, since $\mathbf{P}'\mathbf{P} = \mathbf{P}\mathbf{P}' = \mathbf{I}$, it follows that

$$
\begin{aligned}
\text{tr}(\widehat{\mathbf{D}} - \mathbf{D})^2 &= \text{tr}(\mathbf{P}\mathbf{\Lambda}\mathbf{P}' - \mathbf{D})^2 = \text{tr}\left[\mathbf{P}(\mathbf{\Lambda} - \mathbf{P}'\mathbf{D}\mathbf{P})\mathbf{P}'\right]^2 \\
&= \text{tr}\left[\mathbf{P}(\mathbf{\Lambda} - \mathbf{P}'\mathbf{D}\mathbf{P})\mathbf{P}'\right]\left[\mathbf{P}(\mathbf{\Lambda} - \mathbf{P}'\mathbf{D}\mathbf{P})\mathbf{P}'\right] \\
&= \text{tr}\left[\mathbf{P}(\mathbf{\Lambda} - \mathbf{P}'\mathbf{D}\mathbf{P})(\mathbf{\Lambda} - \mathbf{P}'\mathbf{D}\mathbf{P})\mathbf{P}'\right] \\
&= \text{tr}\left[(\mathbf{\Lambda} - \mathbf{P}'\mathbf{D}\mathbf{P})(\mathbf{\Lambda} - \mathbf{P}'\mathbf{D}\mathbf{P})\mathbf{P}'\mathbf{P}\right] \\
&= \text{tr}(\mathbf{\Lambda} - \mathbf{P}'\mathbf{D}\mathbf{P})^2 = \sum_{i=1}^{k}(\lambda_i - M_{ii})^2 + \sum_{i \neq j} M_{ij}^2, \tag{2.136}
\end{aligned}
$$

where $\mathbf{M} = \mathbf{P}'\mathbf{D}\mathbf{P}$ is a nonnegative definite matrix. But minimum (2.136) is attained at

$$M_{ii} = \Lambda_{+ii} = \begin{cases} \lambda_i \text{ if } \lambda_i > 0 \\ 0 \text{ if } \lambda_i \leq 0 \end{cases}$$

and $M_{ij} = 0$ for $i \neq j$. Doing the back transformation, we come to the solution to (2.135) as $\mathbf{P}\mathbf{\Lambda}_+\mathbf{P}'$, where $\mathbf{\Lambda}_+$ is the diagonal matrix with the ith diagonal element $\Lambda_{+ii} = \max(0, \lambda_i)$, $i = 1, 2, ..., k$. ∎

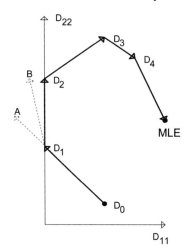
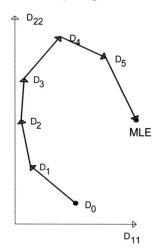

FIGURE 2.8. Two strategies to stay within the space of nonnegative definite matrices. Maximization on the boundary: stay on the boundary by projecting the direction vector on the maximization space (here $D_{11} \geq 0, D_{22} \geq 0$). Reduced step length: reduce the length of the direction vector to stay within the maximization space (easy to implement). However, the latter approach may lead to a slower convergence.

Thus, if $\widehat{\mathbf{D}}$ is not nonnegative definite, we define the MLE as a nonnegative definite matrix closest to $\widehat{\mathbf{D}}$, namely,

$$\widehat{\mathbf{D}}_{ML} = \mathbf{P}\boldsymbol{\Lambda}_+\mathbf{P}', \tag{2.137}$$

where $\mathbf{P}$ and $\boldsymbol{\Lambda}_+$ are eigenvectors and nonnegative eigenvalues of $\widehat{\mathbf{D}}$ as defined in Theorem 8.

However, we may not be satisfied with (2.137) and seek further simplification. Indeed, if $\widehat{\mathbf{D}}_{ML}$ is singular, it may indicate that we have too many random effects in the LME model (overspecification). What random effects should be eliminated? This leads to the following question: what rows and columns of matrix $\widehat{\mathbf{D}}_{ML}$ should be set to zero to make the matrix as close as possible to the original matrix and positive definite? Clearly, the number of zero rows and columns must be equal to the number of zero eigenvalues. This problem can be solved by simple enumeration since k is usually not big.

Example. For $k = 2$ a nonnegative definite singular matrix has the form

$$\widehat{\mathbf{D}}_{ML} = \begin{bmatrix} a^2 & ab \\ ab & b^2 \end{bmatrix}.$$

What row and row/column should be set to zero with the least distortion while minimizing the trace of the squared difference, as in (2.135)? When $k = 2$, we have two possibilities: to zero the first row and column, or to set the second row and column. For the first case, the trace of the squared difference is $a^4 + 2a^2b^2$, and for the second case the trace is $b^4 + 2a^2b^2$. Thus, for $k = 2$ we zero the row and column with the larger diagonal element. This rule makes perfect statistical sense: we leave the random effect with lesser variance.

■

The method to cope with a matrix that is not nonnegative definite may be viewed as a multivariate generalization of routine MLE adjustment in the variance components model when the MLE is set to zero if the log-likelihood maximization produces a negative variance (Searle et al., 1992).

2.15.3   Force matrix $\mathbf{D}$ to stay nonnegative definite

We may force matrix $\mathbf{D}$ to stay nonnegative in the course of the log-likelihood maximization. We assume that the starting point for matrix $\mathbf{D}$ in the NR or FS algorithm, $\mathbf{D}_0$, is nonnegative definite. Let $\mathbf{D}_s$ be nonnegative definite at the sth iteration. Then, the $(s+1)$th approximation to the MLE is computed as

$$\mathbf{D}_{s+1} = \mathbf{D}_s + \lambda_s \mathbf{\Delta}_s, \tag{2.138}$$

where $0 < \lambda_s \leq 1$ is the step length and $\mathbf{\Delta}_s$ is the adjustment matrix. Two situations may occur, Figure 2.8:

1. Matrix $\mathbf{D}_s$ is positive definite. Then, for any $\mathbf{\Delta}_s$ there exists a positive λ_s such that $\mathbf{D}_{s+1} = \mathbf{D}_s + \lambda_s \mathbf{\Delta}_s$ is positive definite and $\mathbf{D}_{s+1}$ increases the log-likelihood. An appropriate λ_s may be found by a simple halving procedure, or more precisely we can set $\lambda_s = \min |\lambda_-(\mathbf{D}_s\mathbf{\Delta}_s^-)|$, where $\mathbf{\Delta}_s^-$ is the generalized inverse of matrix $\mathbf{\Delta}_s$ and λ_- is the negative eigenvalue (if matrix $\mathbf{\Delta}_s$ is nonnegative definite we set $\lambda_s = 1$). It is easy to prove that $\mathbf{D}_s + \lambda\mathbf{\Delta}_s$ is positive definite for any $0 < \lambda < \lambda_s$ but that matrix $\mathbf{D}_s + \lambda_s\mathbf{\Delta}_s$ is singular if matrix $\mathbf{\Delta}_s$ has at least one negative eigenvalue.

2. Matrix $\mathbf{D}_s$ is singular but nonnegative definite, i.e., belongs to the boundary of the set of all nonnegative definite matrices $\mathbb{D}_+$ defined in the previous section; refer to Figure 2.7 for a geometrical illustration for $k = 2$. This case is more complex and requires more attention. If matrix $\mathbf{\Delta}_s$ is nonnegative definite then any positive λ_s leaves us within $\mathbb{D}_+$, so we can proceed without complications and find the step length to satisfy the increase of the log-likelihood, the right-hand graph in Figure 2.8. Now let us consider the case when $\mathbf{\Delta}_s$ is not nonnegative definite. Then positive λ_s may lead to a not nonnegative definite matrix; that is we cannot use $\mathbf{\Delta}_s$ to stay in the parameter space $\mathbb{D}_+$. However, instead of $\mathbf{\Delta}_s$ we may take the projection of $\mathbf{\Delta}_s$ onto $\mathbb{D}_+$ as in Section 2.15.2. Thus, when $\mathbf{D}_s$ is singular and $\mathbf{\Delta}_s$ is not nonnegative definite, we take $\mathbf{D}_{s+1} = \mathbf{D}_s + \lambda_s\mathbf{\Delta}_{+s}$, where $\mathbf{\Delta}_{+s}$ is the projection of $\mathbf{\Delta}_s$ onto $\mathbb{D}_+$ derived similarly to (2.137). Namely, $\mathbf{\Delta}_{+s} = \mathbf{P}\mathbf{\Lambda}_+\mathbf{P}'$, where $\mathbf{P}$ is the eigenvector matrix and $\mathbf{\Lambda}_+$ is the diagonal matrix with $\max(0, \nu_i)$ as the ith diagonal element and ν_i is the eigenvalue of $\mathbf{\Delta}_s$. Such a modification makes the matrix $\mathbf{D}_{s+1}$ nonnegative definite for any positive λ_s.

Two ways to control matrix $\mathbf{D}$ are depicted in Figure 2.8, with $k = 2$ and $D_{12} = 0$ as in the preceeding example. Matrix $\mathbf{D}_0$ is positive definite ($D_{11} > 0, D_{22} > 0$).

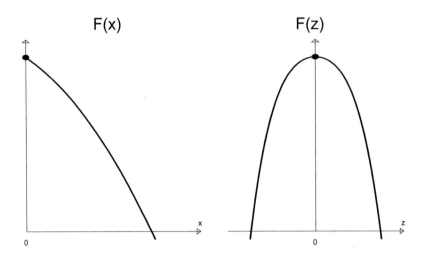

FIGURE 2.9. Original constrained optimization function $F(x)$, $x \geq 0$, and the equivalent unconstrained optimization function $F(z)$, $-\infty < z < \infty$, after reparameterization $x = z^2$.

Vector $\boldsymbol{\Delta}_0 = \overrightarrow{\mathbf{D}_0 \mathbf{A}}$ is the adjustment to $\mathbf{D}_0$, which leads to a not nonnegative matrix since the $(1,1)$ element is negative (left-hand graph). However, $\lambda_0 = 1/2$ leads to a positive definite matrix $\mathbf{D}_1$ (left graph), which corresponds to case 1. Taking $\lambda_s = \min |\lambda_-(\mathbf{D}_s \boldsymbol{\Delta}_s^-)|$ leads to the approximation $\mathbf{D}_1$, which is the boundary point of $\mathbb{D}_+$. Then the next adjustment, $\boldsymbol{\Delta}_1 = \overrightarrow{\mathbf{D}_1 \mathbf{B}}$, is not a nonnegative definite matrix, and therefore we need to take the projection of $\boldsymbol{\Delta}_1$ on the D_{22}-axis that gives $\mathbf{D}_2$; further adjustments provide positive definite matrices $\{\mathbf{D}_s, s > 2\}$, and eventually the maximization leads to the MLE. On the right-hand graph we come to the same MLE using a halving procedure, but it would require more steps.

2.15.4   Matrix $\mathbf{D}$ reparameterization

The idea of replacing matrix $\mathbf{D}$ with a nonnegative definite matrix has been suggested by Pinheiro and Bates (1996). The simplest and intuitively appealing reparameterization, proposed by Lindstrom and Bates (1988) in the framework of linear mixed effects models, is based on Cholesky decomposition, $\mathbf{D} = \mathbf{L}'\mathbf{L}$, where $\mathbf{L}$ is an upper triangular matrix (some authors define $\mathbf{D} = \mathbf{L}\mathbf{L}'$, where $\mathbf{L}$ is a lower triangular matrix). Then, substituting $\mathbf{L}'\mathbf{L}$ for $\mathbf{D}$ in the log-likelihood function, one comes to an unconstrained maximization problem with $\mathbf{L}$ as the argument. However, despite the fact that this reparameterization reduces a constrained problem to an unconstrained problem, there is a price—slower convergence. To illustrate this point, let us take a simple function,

$$F(x) = 1 - (1+x)^2, \quad x \geq 0 \qquad (2.139)$$

to be maximized over nonnegative values x (see the left-hand plot in Figure 2.9). This function attains its absolute maximum on $(-\infty, \infty)$ at $x_{\max} = -1$; however, the constrained maximum point is $x_{\max} = 0$, with the maximum value F zero. We can reduce optimization problem (2.139) to an equivalent unconstrained maximization

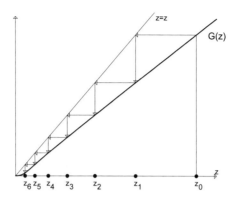

FIGURE 2.10. Newton–Raphson algorithm for $F(z)$ maximization with fixed-point iterations $z_{s+1} = G(z_s)$.

problem, taking the reparameterization $x = z^2$, which leads to a function $F(z) = 1 - (1 + z^2)^2$ to be maximized over $-\infty < z < \infty$. Below we compare constrained and unconstrained optimization problems assuming that the Newton–Raphson (NR) algorithm is used.

First, we consider the NR maximization algorithm when x is allowed to be negative. Since $F(x)$ is a quadratic function, the NR algorithm gives $x_1 = -1$ at the first iteration starting from any initial value x_0. Taking the closest nonnegative point to $x_1 = -1$, which may be viewed as the projection of $x = -1$ on the set of nonnegative numbers in the line of Section 2.15.2, leads to the constrained maximum, zero. Second, we apply the NR algorithm to the unconstrained function $F(z) = 1 - (1 + z^2)^2$, where $-\infty < z < \infty$. It is easy to verify that the NR algorithm leads to iterations $z_{s+1} = z_s - F'(z_s)/F''(z_s) = 2z_s^3/(3z_s^2 + 1)$, which can be written symbolically as $z_{s+1} = G(z_s)$, where the function $G(z)$ is $2z^3/(3z^2 + 1)$; see Figure 2.10. Slow convergence to zero is obvious.

Summing up, for function (2.139) the NR algorithm applied to the constrained optimization problem converges at the first iteration, but the same algorithm applied to an equivalent unconstrained optimization problem requires many iterations to converge.

2.15.5 Criteria for convergence

Some optimization algorithms stop when two consecutive iterations give close results in terms of either the value of the optimization function or the argument value (*parameters* in statistical terminology). Then, when either or both absolute differences are less than some small number (ε), it is claimed that iterations converged to an optimum (maximum). Unfortunately, being close neighboring iterations does not guarantee that the iterations converged to an optimum–strictly speaking, it says only that further iterations do not increase the log-likelihood. To be sure that iterations in fact converged to a maximum, we need to check whether the gradient is zero, assuming that at the final iteration the matrix $\mathbf{D}$ is positive definite. Therefore, a necessary output parameter of the log-likelihood function maximization is its gradient, $\|\partial l/\partial\boldsymbol{\theta}\|$. In optimization theory, $\|\partial l/\partial\boldsymbol{\theta}\| = 0$ is called the first-order condition. It provides a necessary condition for the unconstrained local maximum (or minimum), e.g. Ortega and Rheinboldt (1970), Polak (1971), Dennis and Schnabel (1983). In the Newton–Raphson algorithm it is better to use a relative gradient, which leads to a criterion for convergence (stopping criterion),

$$\left(\frac{\partial l}{\partial\boldsymbol{\theta}}\right)' \mathbf{H}^{-1} \left(\frac{\partial l}{\partial\boldsymbol{\theta}}\right) \leq \varepsilon^2, \tag{2.140}$$

where the inverse matrix is the Hessian. Similarly, in the Fisher scoring algorithm, we use an information matrix instead of the Hessian. The value $\varepsilon \approx 10^{-5}$ seems to be appropriate. Since there are closed-form formulas for the maximum over $\boldsymbol{\beta}$ and σ^2 which turn the respective derivatives to zero, we may take only the derivative with respect to $\mathbf{D}$ in expression (2.140). Good practical advice is to start the algorithm from another starting point, especially when, at the final iteration, it hit the boundary of the parameter set ($\mathbf{D}$ is singular)—it should converge to the same value. If the algorithm arrives at different points with zero gradient, two local maxima of the log-likelihood function are encountered (this seldom happens). However, often, two limiting points emerge due to the algorithm's failure to compute the gradient. Then it would be premature to claim that the maximum of the log-likelihood is achieved. In fact, we do not know if the log-likelihood function of the LME model is generally unimodal. In particular, it would be desirable to obtain constructive criteria to test whether a specific local minimum is a global minimum. Some approaches to sum of squares in nonlinear regression are discussed by Demidenko (2000).

It is important to understand that the first-order criterion works only when at the final iteration, the matrix $\mathbf{D}$ is positive definite. If iterations lead to matrix $\mathbf{D}$, which is nonnegative definite but singular, the derivative cannot be zero and another convergence criterion should be used, because a constrained optimization takes place and the maximum lies on the boundary of the parameter space (2.16). To derive a first-order condition for the constrained log-likelihood maximum, we adopt Kuhn–Tucker conditions for the optimization problem

$$F(\mathbf{x}) \Rightarrow \max \text{ under restriction } g(\mathbf{x}) = 0, \tag{2.141}$$

where $\mathbf{x} \in R^K$ and F and g are differentiable functions (Hestenes, 1975; Walsh, 1975). The Kuhn–Tucker condition says that for $\widehat{\mathbf{x}}$ to be a solution to (2.141), derivatives of F and g evaluated at $\widehat{\mathbf{x}}$ should be negative proportional, or more precisely there exists $\lambda < 0$ that $\partial F(\widehat{\mathbf{x}})/\partial\mathbf{x} = \lambda\partial g(\widehat{\mathbf{x}})/\partial\mathbf{x}$. In our case, F is the log-likelihood function, $\mathbf{x}$ is the matrix $\mathbf{D}$, and g is the determinant function. Since $\partial|\mathbf{D}|/\partial\mathbf{D} = adj(\mathbf{D})$, where adj means adjoint matrix, we find that the necessary condition to reach the maximum of the log-likelihood is that elements of $\partial l/\partial\mathbf{D}$, defined in (2.105), and $adj(\mathbf{D})$ are negative proportional (for $k = 1$ we formally take $adj = 1$ because then $\partial|\mathbf{D}|/\partial\mathbf{D} = 1$).

Summing up, the Kuhn–Tucker condition for a local maximum of the log-likelihood function at $\widehat{\mathbf{D}}$ is as follows:

1. All eigenvalues of $\widehat{\mathbf{D}}$ are zero or positive. (This implies that all diagonal elements are nonnegative.)

2. There is a nonpositive λ such that $\partial l/\partial\mathbf{D} = \lambda \times adj(\mathbf{D})$.

Clearly, if $\partial l/\partial \mathbf{D} = \mathbf{0}$, one can take $\lambda = 0$, showing that the Kuhn–Tucker condition works in regular situations as well.

It is easy to confirm that $\lambda \leq 0$ exists. Indeed, let $\mathbf{A} = \partial l/\partial \mathbf{D}$ and $\mathbf{B} = adj(\mathbf{D})$. Condition 2 holds if and only if $B_{ij} = 0$ implies that $A_{ij} = 0$ and that for all $B_{ij} \neq 0$, the ratio A_{ij}/B_{ij} is constant and negative.

We illustrate this stopping criterion by a one- and a two-random effects LME model ($k = 1, 2$).

For $k = 1$, if an algorithm converged to $\widehat{D} = 0$, the Kuhn–Tucker condition becomes $\partial l/\partial D \leq 0$, where the derivative is evaluated at $D = \widehat{D}$.

For $k = 2$, we assume that $\mathbf{D} = \mathrm{diag}(D_{11}, D_{22})$, as in the example of Section 2.15.2. Thus, let the final $\widehat{\mathbf{D}}$ lie on the boundary $\mathbb{D}_+$, or, more precisely, $\widehat{D}_{11} = 0$ and $\widehat{D}_{22} > 0$. Hence, to satisfy the Kuhn–Tucker condition, we need to have $\partial l/D_{22} = 0$ and $\partial l/D_{11} \leq 0$.

According to the manuals, in current commercial software such as `nlme` and `proc mixed`, the Kuhn–Tucker condition is not checked.

Problems for Section 2.15

1. Is it true that for any linear model with random intercept, the probability that the derivative (2.126) is negative is positive?

2. Prove that $\mathbb{D}_-$ and $\mathbb{D}_+$ defined in Section 2.15.2 are convex sets (the set is convex if for every pair of elements from this set the segment that connects these elements belongs to this set as well). Are $\mathbb{D}_-$ and $\mathbb{D}_+$ convex sets (a set is a cone if for every pair of elements from this set a linear combination with positive coefficients belongs to this set)? Find $\mathbf{Z}_1$, $\mathbf{Z}_2$, and $\mathbf{D}$ such that $\mathbf{D} \in \mathbb{D}_-$ but $\mathbf{D} \notin \mathbb{D}_+$.

3. Explain why maximization on the boundary requires a solution to a generally nonlinear equation. What is that equation when the boundary of the maximization domain is defined by equation $|\mathbf{D}| = 0$?

4. Generalize function (2.139) from Section 2.15.4 to maximization on the matrix space, $F(\mathbf{D}) = 1 - \mathrm{tr}(\mathbf{I}_k + \mathbf{D})^2$, where $\mathbf{D}_k$ is the $k \times k$ symmetric matrix, using the parameterization $\mathbf{D} = \mathbf{L}'\mathbf{L}$. Write down the iterative NR algorithm and demonstrate a slow convergence. To simplify, you may assume that $k = 2$.

5. Give a geometric illustration for the Kuhn–Tucker condition when (a) $k = 1$, and (b) $k = 2$ as discussed at the end of Section 2.15.5.

2.16 lmeFS and lme in R

In this section we discuss our own R code for the estimation of a linear mixed effects model, `lmeFS`, and compare it with a widely popular `lme` function in package `nlme`. When it comes to the implementation of any algorithm for the log-likelihood maximization, the major question is how to deal with cases when the matrix $\mathbf{D}$ during iterations becomes not positive definite. To illustrate complications with `lme`, we suggest a short simulation study for a simple linear mixed model with random intercept and slope,

$$y_{ij} = (\alpha + a_i) + (\beta + b_i)j + \varepsilon_{ij}, \quad j = 1, 2, ..., n_i, \quad i = 1, 2, .., N, \qquad (2.142)$$

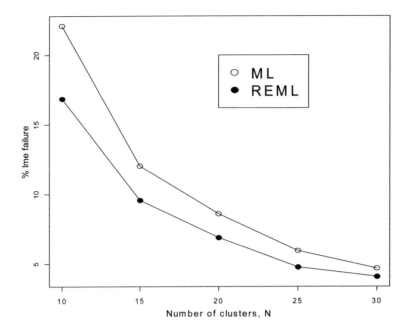

FIGURE 2.11. Simulation results with model (2.142); number of simulations = 5,000.

where a_i and b_i are random effects with zero mean, variance σ_a^2 and σ_b^2, and correlation coefficient ρ. In these simulations, we use $\alpha = -1, \beta = 0.2, \sigma^2 = \sigma_a^2 = \sigma_b^2 = 0.1, \rho = 0.5$ with the number of observations per cluster, n_i, varying from 3 to 7. To keep simulations running even in case of failure to converge we use the command `try`. Below is a fragment of the R code using `method=ML` with the default values for the number of iterations and tolerance convergence (`dL` is the dataframe with the simulated data):

```
out<-try(lme(fixed=y~X2,random=~Z2|id,data=dL,method="ML"))
if(attr(out,"class")=="try-error") lmeF=lmeF+1/Nexp
```

The variable `lmeF` is the proportion of `Nexp=5000` experiments when `lme` fails to converge. The result of this simulation study for N ranging from 10 to 30 is displayed in Figure 2.11 (we have tried increasing the maximum number of iterations using command `lmeControl`, but the percent `lme` failure did not change). As follows from this simulation study, even when the model is specified correctly, `lme` may fail, especially for a small number of clusters. Not surprisingly, the percent failure increases when the model becomes more complicated, i.e. when the number of random effects is large. We assert that these failures are due to the fact that in the `lme` software matrix, $\mathbf{D}$ is forced to be positive definite. Indeed, matrix $\mathbf{D}$ is factorized via Cholesky decomposition in the `nlme` library. Of course, the `lme` failure does not always mean that the matrix $\mathbf{D}$ tends to be not positive definite, but in most cases it is the reason (our code below confirms this assertion).

Several sophisticated strategies to cope with the nonnegative definiteness of matrix $\mathbf{D}$ have been discussed in this chapter. After rigorous testing and simulations we came to the conclusion that the best way to cope with the nonnegative definiteness is not to cope at all, that is to maximize l on the Rao-Kleffé parameter space (2.17), that is, allow $\mathbf{D}$ to be *not* positive definite and even not nonnegative definite during iterations. There are three reasons for this strategy: (1) the algorithms simplify, (2) the maximum of the log-likelihood function does not belong to the boundary of the parameter set (the function goes to $-\infty$ when the point approaches the boundary that keeps iterations away from it, see Section 2.15.2), and (3) the post-maximization analysis of matrix $\mathbf{D}$ may shed light on what random effects lead to negative variance estimate and therefore can be omitted. Thus we follow the principle that it is better to get any solution than no solution at all, as in the case of lme failure.

The call to our own linear mixed model estimation function lmeFS is as follows:

```
lmeFS(d,m,k,D=matrix(0,k,k),MLRML="ML",MaxIter=25,epspar=0.0001,pr=F)
```

The parameters have the following meaning:

- d is the data matrix (or a dataframe); the first column is id, which specifies what cluster the observation belongs to, the second column is the y-variable ($\mathbf{y}_i$); the next m columns are fixed effects ($\mathbf{X}_i$); and the next k columns are random effects ($\mathbf{Z}_i$).

- m is the number of fixed effects, the number of columns in matrix $\mathbf{X}_i$, including vector of ones for the intercept.

- k is the number of random effects, the number of columns in matrix $\mathbf{Z}_i$.

- D is the starting values for the $k \times k$ matrix $\mathbf{D} = \sigma^{-2}\mathrm{cov}(\mathbf{b}_i)$, the scaled matrix of the random effects; the default starting matrix is zero.

- MLRML specifies ML or RML; the default method is maximum likelihood.

- MaxIter is the maximum number of iterations; the default value is 25.

- epspar is the ε for parameter change from iteration to iteration; iterations stop if $\max|\mathrm{change}| < \varepsilon$.

- pr controls the output at each iteration; by default there is no printout.

If the file lmeFS.r is saved in the directory c:\\MixedModels\\Chapter02, it can be downloaded into R by issuing the

```
source("c:\\MixedModels\\Chapter02\\lmeFS.r")
```

This function implements the Fisher scoring algorithm with an information matrix given by formula (2.110). The inverse of this matrix gives the covariance matrix for all estimated parameters. Our practice showed that the unit length strategy, $\lambda_s = 1$, works well; and it saves time. We suggest starting the log-likelihood maximization from $\mathbf{D} = \mathbf{0}$ which corresponds to the Variance Least Squares (VLS) estimate, see Section 3.12.4 for detail. Choice of the unction lmeFS converged in all simulations, unlike lme, including those presented in Figure 2.11. In those simulations where lme did not converge, our function returned matrix $\mathbf{D}$, which was not positive definite (in most cases one of the diagonal elements was negative). Thus, we conclude that the reason for the lme failure was that matrix **D** was not positive definite.

An example of the output/return of this function is shown below.

```
$solcode
[1] 0
$iterdone
[1] 7
$loglik
[1] -201.2231
$b
 [,1]
X1 -1.0473094
X2 0.2205644
$s2
[1] 0.1071485
$covbeta
 [,1] [,2]
[1,]  0.0017939030 -0.0006319487
[2,] -0.0006319487  0.0003536507
$cov.s2vecD
 [,1] [,2] [,3] [,4] [,5]
[1,]  0.000106666 -0.00157912 0.000538691 0.000538691 -0.000301641
[2,] -0.001579123 0.07751204 -0.026673063 -0.026673063 0.010846980
[3,]  0.000538691 -0.02667306  0.013193838  0.009101669 -0.005098106
[4,] 0.000538691 -0.02667306  0.009101669  0.013193838 -0.005098106
[5,] -0.000301641 0.01084698 -0.005098106 -0.005098106  0.002854657
$grad
[1] 0.0002057721
$D
 [,1] [,2]
[1,] 0.2388303 -0.1136758
[2,] -0.1136758 0.1368344
```

The output of this function is a list with the following components:

1. `solcode`: 0 means normal solution (the iterations converged); 1 means that the iterations reached maximum, `MaxIter`; 2 means that the returned matrix **D** is not positive definite (there are negative eigenvalues).

2. `iterdone`: the number of iterations made until convergence.

3. `loglik`: the maximum log-likelihood function (including the constant).

4. `b`: the ML beta estimate at the final iteration.

5. s2: the estimate of σ^2.

6. covbeta: the $m \times m$ covariance matrix of the beta-parameter.

7. cov.s2vecD: the $(1+k^2) \times (1+k^2)$ matrix of the variance-covariance matrix, $(\sigma^2, \text{vec}(\mathbf{D}))$.

8. grad: the gradient; it must return a small value.

9. D: matrix ML estimate of $\mathbf{D}$. If the matrix returned is not positive definite, say, some diagonal elements are negative that may be interpreted as an advice to remove the respective random effect from the model.

In a recent package by D. Bates, lme4, another version of lme is offered, lmer (this package contains functions for estimation of generalized linear and nonlinear mixed models as well; we consider them later). Unlike lme, a new version does not break down when the matrix $\mathbf{D}$ tends to be not positive definite. Instead, this function returns matrix $\mathbf{D}_* = \text{cov}(\mathbf{b}_i)$ with one of the variances (diagonal elements of matrix $\mathbf{D}_*$) almost equal zero. Our function lmeFS returns a matrix $\mathbf{D}$ estimate, which may have negative diagonal elements. It may be further projected on the space of nonnegative definite matrices, as discussed in Section 2.15.2.

Problems for Section 2.16

1. Use lmeFS for the weight example from Section 2.1.1.
2. Reproduce Figure 2.11.

2.17   Appendix: proof of the existence of MLE

We start with the MLE; proof of the existence of RMLE is considered later.
A. Existence of the MLE
Sufficient condition. Assume that for any $\boldsymbol{\beta} \in R^m, \boldsymbol{\gamma}_1, ..., \boldsymbol{\gamma}_N \in R^k$, there exists at least one i such that $\mathbf{y}_i \neq \mathbf{X}_i\boldsymbol{\beta} + \mathbf{Z}_i\boldsymbol{\gamma}_i$. We then prove that the MLE exists. The latter inequality implies that

$$S_{\min} \equiv \min_{\boldsymbol{\beta}, \boldsymbol{\gamma}_1, ..., \boldsymbol{\gamma}_N} \sum_{i=1}^{N} \| \mathbf{y}_i - \mathbf{X}_i\boldsymbol{\beta} - \mathbf{Z}_i\boldsymbol{\gamma}_i \|^2 > 0, \qquad (2.143)$$

and as follows from (2.36), $S_{\min} = \min_{\boldsymbol{\beta}} \sum_i (\mathbf{y}_i - \mathbf{X}_i\boldsymbol{\beta})'(\mathbf{I} - \mathbf{Z}_i\mathbf{Z}_i^+)(\mathbf{y}_i - \mathbf{X}_i\boldsymbol{\beta}) > 0$. For further proof, we need the following log-likelihood function representation:

$$l(\boldsymbol{\beta}, \sigma^2, \mathbf{D}) = -\frac{1}{2}N_T \ln \sigma^2 - \frac{1}{2}\sum_{i=1}^{N}\{\ln |\mathbf{I} + \mathbf{DZ}_i\mathbf{Z}_i'|$$
$$+ \sigma^{-2}[\mathbf{e}_i'(\mathbf{I} - \mathbf{Z}_i\mathbf{Z}_i^+)\mathbf{e}_i + \mathbf{e}_i'\mathbf{Q}_i\mathbf{e}_i]\}, \qquad (2.144)$$

where $\mathbf{Q}_i$ is an $n_i \times n_i$ symmetric matrix defined as $\mathbf{Q}_i = \mathbf{Z}_i\mathbf{Z}_i^+ - \mathbf{Z}_i(\mathbf{I}+\mathbf{DZ}_i'\mathbf{Z}_i)^{-1}\mathbf{DZ}_i'$, and the residual vector $\mathbf{e}_i$ is defined as (2.20). We show that $\mathbf{Q}_i$ is a nonnegative definite matrix. Indeed, using the formula for the generalized inverse (2.30), we obtain

$$\mathbf{Q}_i = \lim_{\delta \to 0}[\mathbf{Z}_i(\mathbf{Z}_i'\mathbf{Z}_i + \delta\mathbf{I})^{-1}\mathbf{Z}_i' - \mathbf{Z}_i(\mathbf{I} + \mathbf{D}\mathbf{Z}_i'\mathbf{Z}_i)^{-1}\mathbf{D}\mathbf{Z}_i']$$
$$= \lim_{\delta \to 0}\mathbf{Z}_i(\mathbf{I} + \mathbf{D}\mathbf{Z}_i'\mathbf{Z}_i)^{-1}[\mathbf{I} + \mathbf{D}\mathbf{Z}_i'\mathbf{Z}_i - \mathbf{D}(\mathbf{Z}_i'\mathbf{Z}_i + \delta\mathbf{I})](\mathbf{Z}_i'\mathbf{Z}_i + \delta\mathbf{I})^{-1}\mathbf{Z}_i'$$
$$= \lim_{\delta \to 0}[\mathbf{Z}_i(\mathbf{I} + \mathbf{D}\mathbf{Z}_i'\mathbf{Z}_i)^{-1}(\mathbf{I} - \delta\mathbf{D})(\mathbf{Z}_i'\mathbf{Z}_i + \delta\mathbf{I})^{-1}\mathbf{Z}_i'].$$

Since for small δ the matrix in the last set of brackets is nonnegative definite, $\mathbf{Q}_i$ is also a symmetric nonnegative definite matrix, as a limit of nonnegative definite matrices. Moreover, using (2.30) for the last limit, we obtain $\mathbf{Q}_i = \mathbf{Z}_i(\mathbf{I} + \mathbf{D}\mathbf{Z}_i'\mathbf{Z}_i)^{-1}\mathbf{Z}_i^+$. In particular, this implies that $\mathbf{e}_i'\mathbf{Q}_i\mathbf{e}_i \geq 0$ for all $i = 1, ..., N$.

To prove the existence of the MLE, it suffices to show that when the parameter vector $\boldsymbol{\theta}$ approaches a boundary point of the parameter set $\boldsymbol{\Theta}$ that does not belong to this set, then $l(\boldsymbol{\theta}) \to -\infty$, Demidenko (1997). There are four such possibilities:

$$\begin{array}{ll} (1)\ \mathbf{D} \to \infty & (2)\ \sigma^2 \to 0 \\ (3)\ \sigma^2 \to +\infty & (4)\ \|\boldsymbol{\beta}\| \to \infty. \end{array} \qquad (2.145)$$

We aim to prove that each case implies that $l \to -\infty$.

Case 1: $\mathbf{D} \to \infty$, which means that at least for one element (r, s) we have $D_{rs} \to \infty$. The following elementary inequality will be used:

$$A \ln \lambda + \lambda^{-1}B \geq 1 + A \ln B, \quad \lambda > 0, \qquad (2.146)$$

where $A > 0, B > 0$. We seek an upper bound for l as a function of $\mathbf{D}$ only. Since $\mathbf{Q}_i$ is a nonnegative definite matrix, we can drop the term $\mathbf{e}_i'\mathbf{Q}_i\mathbf{e}_i$. Further, applying (2.146) to (2.144) with $A_i = n_i$, $B = \sum \mathbf{e}_i'(\mathbf{I} - \mathbf{Z}_i\mathbf{Z}_i^+)\mathbf{e}_i \geq S_{\min} > 0$, $\lambda = \sigma^2$, we obtain

$$l \leq -\frac{N}{2} - \frac{N_T}{2}\ln S_{\min} - \frac{1}{2}\sum_i \ln |\mathbf{I} + \mathbf{D}\mathbf{Z}_i'\mathbf{Z}_i|. \qquad (2.147)$$

By assumption, there exists at least one matrix $\mathbf{Z}_j$ of full rank, i.e., at least for one j there exists a positive scalar ν such that $\mathbf{Z}_j'\mathbf{Z}_j \geq \nu\mathbf{I}$. This implies that $|\mathbf{I} + \mathbf{Z}_i'\mathbf{Z}_i\mathbf{D}| \geq |\mathbf{I} + \nu\mathbf{D}|$ for $i = j$ and $|\mathbf{I} + \mathbf{Z}_i'\mathbf{Z}_i\mathbf{D}| \geq 1$ for $i \neq j$. Now we prove that

$$D_{rs} \to \infty \ \text{implies} \ \ln |\mathbf{I} + \nu\mathbf{D}| \to +\infty. \qquad (2.148)$$

Indeed, since matrix $\mathbf{D}$ is nonnegative definite $D_{rs}^2 \leq D_{rs}D_{ss}$ which implies that at least one diagonal element goes to infinity and consequently $\text{tr}(\mathbf{D}) \to \infty$. Therefore, the maximum eigenvalue, $\lambda_{\max}(\mathbf{D}) \to \infty$ because $\lambda_{\max} \geq k^{-1}\sum_{q=1}^{k}\lambda_q = k^{-1}\text{tr}(\mathbf{D}) \to \infty$, where λ_q is the qth eigenvalue of matrix $\mathbf{D}$. Hence,

$$\ln |\mathbf{I} + \nu\mathbf{D}| = \sum_{q=1}^{k}\ln(1 + \nu\lambda_q) \geq (k-1)\ln(1 + \nu\lambda_{\min}) + \ln(1 + \nu\lambda_{\max}) \to \infty,$$

when $\lambda_{\max} \to \infty$, which proves (2.148). Now taking the limit on the right side of (2.147) when $\mathbf{D} \to \infty$, we obtain $l \to -\infty$.

Case 2 or 3: $\sigma^2 \to 0$ or $\sigma^2 \to \infty$. Since $|\mathbf{I} + \mathbf{D}\mathbf{Z}_i'\mathbf{Z}_i| \geq 1$, we obtain

$$l \leq -\frac{N_T}{2}\ln\sigma^2 - \frac{1}{2\sigma^2}\sum \mathbf{e}_i'(\mathbf{I} - \mathbf{Z}_i\mathbf{Z}_i^+)\mathbf{e}_i \leq -\frac{N_T}{2}\ln\sigma^2 - \frac{S_{\min}}{2\sigma^2}.$$

Obviously, this implies that $l \to -\infty$ if either $\sigma^2 \to 0$ or $\sigma^2 \to \infty$.

Case 4: $\| \boldsymbol{\beta} \| \to \infty$. Without loss of generality, we can assume that for some $\mu > 0$ we have $\mathbf{D} \le \mu \mathbf{I}$ because otherwise we have case 1. Then there exists a constant $\rho > 1$ such that $\mathbf{I} + \mathbf{Z}_i \mathbf{D} \mathbf{Z}_i' \le \rho \mathbf{I}$ for all $i = 1, ..., N$. Applying inequality (2.146) to the log-likelihood function (2.15), we obtain $l \le -N/2 - (N_T/2) \ln \rho^{-1} \sum_{i=1}^N \| \mathbf{y}_i - \mathbf{X}_i \boldsymbol{\beta} \|^2$. But by assumption $\sum \mathbf{X}_i' \mathbf{X}_i$ has full rank, which implies that $\sum \| \mathbf{y}_i - \mathbf{X}_i \boldsymbol{\beta} \|^2 \to \infty$ if $\| \boldsymbol{\beta} \| \to \infty$. Then, from the inequality above, $l \to -\infty$.

Necessary condition. Let us assume that (2.90) holds for some $\boldsymbol{\beta} \in R^m, \boldsymbol{\gamma}_1, ..., \boldsymbol{\gamma}_N$. We aim to find a sequence of parameters that leads to $l \to +\infty$. Indeed, if (2.90) holds, then $S_{\min} = 0$ and maximization over σ^2 gives

$$\max_{\boldsymbol{\theta}} l \ge -\frac{N}{2} - \frac{1}{2} N_T \ln[\sum_i \mathbf{e}_i' \mathbf{Z}_i (\mathbf{I} + \mathbf{D} \mathbf{Z}_i' \mathbf{Z}_i)^{-1} \mathbf{Z}_i^+ \mathbf{e}_i] - \frac{1}{2} \sum_i \ln |\mathbf{I} + \mathbf{D} \mathbf{Z}_i' \mathbf{Z}_i|.$$

We let $\mathbf{D} = d\mathbf{I}$, $d > 0$. Let λ_{ij} denote the jth eigenvalue of matrix $\mathbf{Z}_i' \mathbf{Z}_i$; then the right-hand side of the last inequality can be rewritten as

$$
\begin{aligned}
&-\frac{N}{2} - \frac{N_T}{2} \ln d \\
= &-\frac{N_T}{2} \ln[\sum_i \mathbf{e}_i' \mathbf{Z}_i (\mathbf{I} d^{-1} + \mathbf{Z}_i' \mathbf{Z}_i)^{-1} \mathbf{Z}_i^+ \mathbf{e}_i] - \frac{1}{2} \sum_i \ln |\mathbf{I} + d\mathbf{Z}_i' \mathbf{Z}_i| \\
= &-\frac{N}{2} - \frac{N_T}{2} \ln[\sum_i \mathbf{e}_i' \mathbf{Z}_i (\mathbf{I} d^{-1} + \mathbf{Z}_i' \mathbf{Z}_i)^{-1} \mathbf{Z}_i^+ \mathbf{e}_i] + \frac{1}{2} (N_T - Nk) \ln d \\
&-\frac{1}{2} \sum_{i=1}^N \sum_{j=1}^k \ln[(1 + d\lambda_{ij})/d].
\end{aligned}
\tag{2.149}
$$

Consider the limit of each term in (2.149) when $d \to \infty$. For the second term we have

$$-\frac{N_T}{2} \ln \lim_{d \to \infty} \sum_i \mathbf{e}_i' \mathbf{Z}_i (\mathbf{I} d^{-1} + \mathbf{Z}_i' \mathbf{Z}_i)^{-1} \mathbf{Z}_i^+ \mathbf{e}_i = -\frac{N_T}{2} \ln \sum_i \| \mathbf{Z}_i^+ \mathbf{e}_i \|^2,$$

which is either $+\infty$ or a finite number. The third term in (2.149) tends to $+\infty$ because by assumption, $N_T > Nk$. For the fourth term we have

$$-\frac{1}{2} \lim_{d \to \infty} \sum_{i=1}^N \sum_{j=1}^k \ln[(1 + d\lambda_{ij})/d] = \left\{ \begin{array}{l} -\frac{1}{2} \sum_{ij} \ln \lambda_{ij} \text{ if } \forall \lambda_{ij} > 0 \\ \infty \text{ otherwise} \end{array} \right. .$$

Combining all the limits, we find that l goes to $+\infty$ when $d \to \infty$, so the MLE does not exist.

B. Existence of the RMLE with the log-likelihood function defined by (2.50)

Sufficient condition. We need to show that in four cases shown in (2.145), the log-likelihood function approaches $-\infty$. Since $N_T - m > 0$, it suffices to consider only case 1. Let $\delta_1, ..., \delta_k$ denote eigenvalues of matrix $\mathbf{D}$ in ascending order, i.e., δ_k is the maximum eigenvalue. We shall prove that function

$$\Psi(\mathbf{D}) = \ln | \sum_{i=1}^N \mathbf{X}_i' (\mathbf{I} + \mathbf{Z}_i \mathbf{D} \mathbf{Z}_i')^{-1} \mathbf{X}_i| + \sum_{i=1}^N \ln |\mathbf{I} + \mathbf{Z}_i \mathbf{D} \mathbf{Z}_i'|$$

approaches $+\infty$ when $\mathbf{D} \to \infty$. By assumption, there are $m + 1$ matrices $\mathbf{Z}_i$ that have full rank. This implies the existence of a positive scalar ϕ such that $\mathbf{Z}_i' \mathbf{Z}_i \ge \phi \mathbf{I}$ for at least $m + 1$ indices i. Then for the second term of $\Psi(\mathbf{D})$, we have

$\sum \ln |\mathbf{I}_{n_i} + \mathbf{Z}_i \mathbf{D} \mathbf{Z}_i'| = \sum \ln |\mathbf{I}_k + \mathbf{D} \mathbf{Z}_i' \mathbf{Z}_i|$, and thus this term is bounded from below by $(m+1)\ln |\mathbf{I} + \phi \mathbf{D}| = (m+1)\sum_{j=1}^{k} \ln(1 + \phi \delta_j)$. To find the lower bound for the first term, we denote $\varsigma = \max_{i=1,...,N} \lambda_{\max}(\mathbf{Z}_i' \mathbf{Z}_i)$ so that $\mathbf{Z}_i \mathbf{Z}_i' \le \varsigma \mathbf{I}$. Then the first term of $\Psi(\mathbf{D})$ can be bounded from below as follows: $\ln |\sum \mathbf{X}_i'(\mathbf{I} + \mathbf{Z}_i \mathbf{D} \mathbf{Z}_i')^{-1} \mathbf{X}_i| \ge \ln |\sum \mathbf{X}_i'(\mathbf{I} + \delta_k \mathbf{Z}_i \mathbf{Z}_i')^{-1} \mathbf{X}_i| \ge \ln |\sum_{i=1}^{N} \mathbf{X}_i'(\mathbf{I} + \varsigma \delta_k \mathbf{I})^{-1} \mathbf{X}_i| = \ln |\sum_{i=1}^{N} \mathbf{X}_i' \mathbf{X}_i| - m \ln(1 + \varsigma \delta_k)$. By assumption, the matrix $\sum_{i=1}^{N} \mathbf{X}_i' \mathbf{X}_i$ is not singular and thus $\ln |\sum \mathbf{X}_i' \mathbf{X}_i|$ exists. Combining the two bounds, we obtain $\Psi(\mathbf{D}) \ge \ln |\sum \mathbf{X}_i' \mathbf{X}_i| - m \ln(1 + \varsigma \delta_k) + (m+1)\sum_{j=1}^{k} \ln(1 + \phi \delta_j)$ so that $\Psi(\mathbf{D}) \ge \ln |\sum \mathbf{X}_i' \mathbf{X}_i| - m \ln \frac{1 + \phi \delta_k}{1 + \varsigma \delta_k} + \sum_{j=1}^{k} \ln(1 + \phi \delta_j) \to \infty$, when $\delta_k \to \infty$. This implies that $l \to -\infty$ when $\mathbf{D} \to \infty$.

Necessary condition. The proof is similar to the MLE. Since $\mathbf{I} + \mathbf{Z}_i \mathbf{D} \mathbf{Z}_i' \ge \mathbf{I}$, we have $\mathbf{V}_i^{-1} \le \mathbf{I}$ and therefore $\ln |\sum \mathbf{X}_i'(\mathbf{I} + \mathbf{Z}_i \mathbf{D} \mathbf{Z}_i')^{-1} \mathbf{X}_i| \le \ln |\sum \mathbf{X}_i' \mathbf{X}_i|$. Hence, for the RML log-likelihood function we come to a slightly different inequality, $\max_{\boldsymbol{\theta}} l \ge -0.5N - 0.5(N_T - m)\ln[\sum \mathbf{e}_i' \mathbf{Z}_i(\mathbf{I} + \mathbf{D} \mathbf{Z}_i' \mathbf{Z}_i)^{-1} \mathbf{Z}_i^+ \mathbf{e}_i] - 0.5\sum \ln |\mathbf{I} + \mathbf{D} \mathbf{Z}_i' \mathbf{Z}_i| - 0.5 \ln |\sum \mathbf{X}_i' \mathbf{X}_i|$. Again, letting $\mathbf{D} = d\mathbf{I}$ and $d \to \infty$, we find that the right side approaches $+\infty$ meaning that the RMLE does not exist.

2.18   Summary points

- The Linear Mixed Effects (LME) model developed by Laird and Ware (1982) is a generalization and combination of the VARCOMP and linear regression models. This model is adequate to describe clustered/panel/tabular data for the dependent variable where the rows are independent but observations within each row constitute a cluster and therefore are dependent. This dependence is modeled via random effects in the manner of the VARCOMP model.

- There are many equivalent parameterizations of the log-likelihood function for the linear mixed effects model under normal assumption. In particular, one can eliminate variance σ^2 and/or fixed effects $\boldsymbol{\beta}$ to yield the profile parameterization. Dimension-reduction formulas apply which reduce the $n_i \times n_i$ to the $k \times k$ matrix inverse, where n_i is the number of observations per individual (subject or cluster) and k is the number of random effects. If the covariance matrix of random effects $\mathbf{D}$ is known, the Generalized Least Squares (GLS) estimator is the best unbiased estimator because it has minimum variance among all unbiased estimators under normal distribution. However, matrix $\mathbf{D}$ in most cases is unknown, so that we need to estimate it along with the fixed effects coefficients. This makes the estimation problem nonlinear.

- Random effects in the LME model may be treated as fixed unknown nuisance parameters. The fixed effects approach leads to a large number of nuisance parameters, and the least squares estimator for $\boldsymbol{\beta}$ in this approach may be formally derived from the GLS estimator, letting $\mathbf{D}$ go to infinity. The fixed effects approach is theoretically easier to handle because it can be reduced to standard linear regression. It is preferable when the number of subjects is small and the number of observations per cluster is large.

- Balanced data (equal cluster size and no missing values, rectangular format) are preferred in the mixed effects model because then the ML, GLS, and OLS estimates coincide and there exists a closed-form solution for the variance parameters. Two important balanced LME models are the random-intercept and random-coefficient models. In a balanced random-intercept model, the variance of the random effect affects neither the MLE of the slopes nor their variances. The ML estimator is unbiased and efficient among all unbiased estimators of the fixed effects coefficients under normal distribution for balanced data.

- The MLE exists with probability 1 if the rank of the combined design matrices of fixed and random effects is less than the total number of observations. More precisely, the MLE exists if the vector of the response variable does not belong to the linear space spanned by the vector columns of the matrices of fixed and random effects. Equivalently, the MLE exists if the residual sum of squares in the fixed effects approach is positive. However, this existence does not guarantee that $\widehat{\mathbf{D}}_{ML}$ is positive definite.

- Condition (2.93) provides a numerical criterion that the MLE of $\mathbf{D}$ is not zero, i.e., random effects are present. This condition should be checked before the log-likelihood maximization algorithm begins.

- The MLE of σ^2 lies within bounds specified by inequality (2.99): the OLS estimate of σ^2 is the upper bound and the OLS estimate of σ^2 in the fixed effects approach is the lower bound for $\widehat{\sigma}^2_{ML}$.

- Generally, there are three types of algorithms for the log-likelihood maximization: the Newton–Raphson (NR), Fisher scoring (FS), and EM (Expectation-Maximization) algorithms; they all have generic form (2.103) and differ by matrix $\mathbf{H}$. The log-likelihood function for the linear mixed effects model is not convex, and therefore the Hessian matrix may not be positive definite. However, one can expect positive definiteness of the Hessian in a neighborhood of the maximum. Hence, if the starting point in the NR algorithm is far from the maximum, the algorithm may fail, but if the starting point is relatively close to the maximum, the NR algorithm is fast. The FS algorithm is more robust to the choice of starting point because its (information) matrix is always positive definite (under mild assumptions). The EM algorithm may be slow when the matrix $\mathbf{D}$ is close to zero. We recommend use of the FS algorithm with the starting point for $\mathbf{D}$ derived from a few iterations of the EM algorithm, starting from $\mathbf{D} = \infty$. Quadratic estimation of the variance parameters developed in Chapter 3 suggests another way to obtain starting points.

- The most economical and reliable algorithm for likelihood maximization is the FS for variance-profile or full-profile parameterization with the precision matrix as the argument and the starting point as a quadratic estimate of matrix $\mathbf{D}$ from Chapter 4. The inverse to the negative Hessian matrix gives an asymptotic covariance matrix for variance parameters.

- There exists a risk that during iterations the matrix $\mathbf{D}$ does not become nonnegative definite. For example, for a balanced growth curve model with random coefficients and number of individuals $N = 20$, the chance that $\widehat{\mathbf{D}}_{ML}$ or $\widehat{\mathbf{D}}_{RML}$ lie on the boundary of the parameter space (i.e., are singular) is about 50%. However, when N grows, the chances become less.

- The matrix $\mathbf{D}$ needs special attention in the course of the log-likelihood maximization procedure because it must be nonnegative definite. Three approaches may be suggested to cope with the nonnegative definiteness of $\mathbf{D}$. In the first approach, we allow matrix $\mathbf{D}$ to be negative definite during the iteration process, but all matrices $\mathbf{V}_i$ must stay positive definite to be able to compute the log-likelihood function. This approach makes the parameter space less restrictive, and under certain conditions the log-likelihood function approaches infinity when $\mathbf{V}_i$ becomes singular. After maximization is finished, we project the solution $\widehat{\mathbf{D}}$ onto the space of all nonnegative definite matrices $\mathbb{D}_+$. In the second approach, one may force matrix $\mathbf{D}$ to stay nonnegative definite in the course of maximization. There are two ways to do this. The easiest way is to take a shorter step to ensure that the next approximation is a positive definite matrix. A more sophisticated way is to project the adjustment matrix on $\mathbb{D}_+$. In the third approach the matrix $\mathbf{D}$ is reparameterized in such a way that it remains nonnegative definite. For example, using Cholesky decomposition, we can write $\mathbf{D} = \mathbf{L}'\mathbf{L}$, where $\mathbf{L}$ is an upper triangular matrix, and maximize the log-likelihood over $\mathbf{L}$.

- Stopping criteria must include evaluation of the gradient or the relative gradient of the log-likelihood function, which must be zero at the final iteration if the matrix $\widehat{\mathbf{D}}$ is positive definite. If the final $\widehat{\mathbf{D}}$ is not positive definite (singular), the gradient is not zero and another first-order condition should be employed that makes use of the Kuhn–Tucker condition for constrained optimization. It should be remembered that maximization of the log-likelihood function is a nonlinear constrained optimization problem, and, in particular, it may have several local maxima. A good practice is to start from a different initial point to confirm that iterations converge to the same estimate. This check is especially important when at the final iteration, the matrix $\widehat{\mathbf{D}}$ is found to be singular.

- The R function `lme` of the package `nlme` may fail when matrix $\mathbf{D}$ tends to be not positive definite during iterations. We recommend using the R function `lme4` of the package `lme4` which protects the code from the abnormal ending. Unfortunately, the syntax in `lme4` is different from that in `lme`, so programs written for `lme` will not run with `lme4`. The output matrix $\widehat{\mathbf{D}}_*$ may be nonnegative definite and singular. Our own R function `lmeFS` converges in most cases but may return a not nonnegative definite matrix $\mathbf{D}$, so that the user needs to decide what random effects are excessive and should therefore be eliminated to make the LME model well specified.

3

Statistical Properties of the LME Model

3.1 Introduction

In this chapter we continue studying the Linear Mixed Effects (LME) model defined in (2.5). In Chapter 2, we were concerned primarily with numerical algorithms for the likelihood maximization. In this chapter our attention is on the statistical properties of the LME model, particularly the distribution-free estimation of the variance parameters. Once the covariance matrix of the random effects is estimated, we use a generalized least squares estimator to estimate the fixed effects (beta) coefficients. In this chapter we shall learn that this *estimated* GLS leads to unbiased estimates of the fixed effects coefficients, even in a small sample.

3.2 Identifiability of the LME model

In Section 2.2 we formulated conditions under which the LME model is identifiable. The identifiability of a statistical model is essential. In this section we provide more detail on identifiability and prove that under the conditions formulated, the LME model is identifiable. We start with a general definition.

Definition 9 *Let a statistical model be defined by a family of distributions for* $\mathbf{y}$ *parameterized by the vector* $\boldsymbol{\theta}$, $\{P_{\boldsymbol{\theta}}, \boldsymbol{\theta} \in \boldsymbol{\Theta}\}$, *where* $\boldsymbol{\Theta}$ *is the parameter space and* $P_{\boldsymbol{\theta}}$ *denotes the distribution associated with* $\boldsymbol{\theta}$. *We say that the model is identifiable on* $\boldsymbol{\Theta}$ *if* $P_{\boldsymbol{\theta}_1} = P_{\boldsymbol{\theta}_2}$ *implies that* $\boldsymbol{\theta}_1 = \boldsymbol{\theta}_2$.

Identifiability may be viewed as a necessary property for the adequacy of a statistical model. Briefly, it provides the uniqueness of the distribution as a function of the parameter. Clearly, if $\boldsymbol{\theta}_1 \neq \boldsymbol{\theta}_2$ but $P_{\boldsymbol{\theta}_1} = P_{\boldsymbol{\theta}_2}$, one cannot distinguish two parameters, regardless of the number of observations. Consequently, if the model is not identifiable, there are no consistent estimators for $\boldsymbol{\theta}$. For example, in the standard linear regression model $\mathbf{y} \sim \mathcal{N}(\mathbf{X}\boldsymbol{\beta}, \sigma^2\mathbf{I})$, the necessary and sufficient condition for the identifiability of $\boldsymbol{\beta}$ is that the matrix $\mathbf{X}$ have full rank (sometimes this condition is called the *estimability* of $\boldsymbol{\beta}$). Interestingly, the condition of full rank is not necessary for σ^2. A well known example of a nonidentifiable statistical model is the measurement error (errors-in-variables) model, where the dependent and independent variables are iid (called the *structural case*): It has been proven by Kendall and Stuart (1961) that the model with normally distributed variables is not identifiable unless the ratio of the measurement error variances is known.

Apparently, a necessary condition for identifiability is the uniqueness of the first two moments as functions of the model parameters:

$$E_{\boldsymbol{\theta}_1}(\mathbf{y}) = E_{\boldsymbol{\theta}_2}(\mathbf{y}) \text{ and } \text{cov}_{\boldsymbol{\theta}_1}(\mathbf{y}) = \text{cov}_{\boldsymbol{\theta}_2}(\mathbf{y}) \text{ imply } \boldsymbol{\theta}_1 = \boldsymbol{\theta}_2. \tag{3.1}$$

It is worthwhile to note that, generally, (3.1) is just a necessary, not a sufficient, condition for identifiability. However, for regression models with normal distribution, condition (3.1) is sufficient because the normal distribution is uniquely specified by the first two moments. More precisely, this statement is formulated as follows.

Proposition 10 *Let a regression model be defined as*

$$\mathbf{y} \sim \mathcal{N}(\mathbf{f}(\boldsymbol{\beta}), \mathbf{V}(\boldsymbol{\beta}, \boldsymbol{\theta})),$$

where $\mathbf{y}$ is an $n \times 1$ vector of data, $\mathbf{f}(\boldsymbol{\beta})$ is a linear or nonlinear $n \times 1$ vector function of an $m \times 1$ vector parameter $\boldsymbol{\beta}$, and $\mathbf{V}(\boldsymbol{\beta}, \boldsymbol{\theta})$ is the $n \times n$ covariance matrix dependent on $\boldsymbol{\beta}$ and the $k \times 1$ vector parameter $\boldsymbol{\theta}$. Then the regression model is identifiable if and only if $\mathbf{f}(\boldsymbol{\beta}_1) = \mathbf{f}(\boldsymbol{\beta}_2)$ and $\mathbf{V}(\boldsymbol{\beta}_1, \boldsymbol{\theta}_1) = \mathbf{V}(\boldsymbol{\beta}_2, \boldsymbol{\theta}_2)$ imply that $\boldsymbol{\beta}_1 = \boldsymbol{\beta}_2$, $\boldsymbol{\theta}_1 = \boldsymbol{\theta}_2$.

Now we apply this result to the linear mixed effects model with normally distributed random variables (2.14). The following conditions imply the nonsingularity of the information matrix (see Proposition 13 in Section 3.3).

Theorem 11 *If matrix $\mathbf{X}$ has full rank, at least one matrix $\mathbf{Z}_i$ has full rank, and $\sum(n_i - k) > 0$, the LME model (2.14) is identifiable.*

Proof. Since the expectation and covariance matrix do not have common parameters, the conditions of Proposition 10 may be separated for $\boldsymbol{\beta}$ and $\boldsymbol{\theta} = (\sigma^2, \text{vech}(\mathbf{D}))$. The condition $\mathbf{f}(\boldsymbol{\beta}_1) = \mathbf{f}(\boldsymbol{\beta}_2)$ for the LME model is written as $\mathbf{X}\boldsymbol{\beta}_1 = \mathbf{X}\boldsymbol{\beta}_2$, which implies that $\boldsymbol{\beta}_1 = \boldsymbol{\beta}_2$ if and only if matrix $\mathbf{X}$ has full rank. Now we prove that the covariance matrix $\mathbf{V}$ is uniquely specified by $(\sigma^2, \text{vech}(\mathbf{D}))$ if at least one matrix $\mathbf{Z}_i$ has full rank and $\sum(n_i - k) > 0$. Indeed, it suffices to prove that N equations $(\sigma_1^2 - \sigma_2^2)\mathbf{I}_{n_i} + \mathbf{Z}_i(\mathbf{D}_{*1} - \mathbf{D}_{*2})\mathbf{Z}_i' = \mathbf{0}$ imply that $\sigma_1^2 = \sigma_2^2$ and $\mathbf{D}_{*1} = \mathbf{D}_{*2}$. Taking the vec transformation, we obtain

$$\text{vec}\left((\sigma_1^2 - \sigma_2^2)\mathbf{I}_{n_i} + \mathbf{Z}_i(\mathbf{D}_{*1} - \mathbf{D}_{*2})\mathbf{Z}_i'\right)$$
$$= (\sigma_1^2 - \sigma_2^2)\text{vec}(\mathbf{I}_{n_i}) + (\mathbf{Z}_i \otimes \mathbf{Z}_i)\,\text{vec}(\mathbf{D}_{*1} - \mathbf{D}_{*2}).$$

Hence, introducing a $\left(\sum n_i^2\right) \times \left(1 + k^2\right)$ matrix $\mathbf{E}$ with the ith $n_i \times (1 + k^2)$ matrix block $(\text{vec}(\mathbf{I}_{n_i}), \mathbf{Z}_i \otimes \mathbf{Z}_i)$, the identifiability for the second moments is equivalent to the condition that matrix $\mathbf{E}$ have rank k^2. Obviously, matrix $\mathbf{E}$ has full rank if and only if the matrix

$$
\begin{aligned}
\mathbf{E}'\mathbf{E} &= \begin{bmatrix} \sum \mathrm{vec}'(\mathbf{I}_{n_i})\mathrm{vec}(\mathbf{I}_{n_i}) & \sum \mathrm{vec}'(\mathbf{I}_{n_i})(\mathbf{Z}_i \otimes \mathbf{Z}_i) \\ \sum(\mathbf{Z}_i' \otimes \mathbf{Z}_i')\mathrm{vec}(\mathbf{I}_{n_i}) & \sum \mathbf{Z}_i'\mathbf{Z}_i \otimes \mathbf{Z}_i'\mathbf{Z}_i \end{bmatrix} \\
&= \begin{bmatrix} N_T & \sum \mathrm{vec}'(\mathbf{Z}_i'\mathbf{Z}_i) \\ \sum \mathrm{vec}(\mathbf{Z}_i'\mathbf{Z}_i) & \sum(\mathbf{Z}_i'\mathbf{Z}_i \otimes \mathbf{Z}_i'\mathbf{Z}_i) \end{bmatrix}
\end{aligned}
$$

is nonsingular. The proof that matrix $\mathbf{E}'\mathbf{E}$ has full rank if at least one matrix $\mathbf{Z}_i$ has full rank and $\sum(n_i - k) > 0$ is provided in Proposition 13 of Section 3.3. ∎

As a word of caution, the identifiability of a statistical model does not imply that the maximum likelihood estimation will not fail. For instance, in linear model (2.66) with fixed intercepts $\{a_i\}$ and bounded $\{n_i\}$, the MLE of a_i is not consistent when $N \to \infty$. This is a classical example of a statistical model with a large number of (nuisance) parameters, introduced by Neyman and Scott (1948). In the next subsection we provide a peculiar example of an identifiable statistical model, where the MLE does not make much sense, although it does exist.

3.2.1 Linear regression with random coefficients

Identifiability is not a sufficient condition for the validity of a statistical model. Here we consider a linear regression model with random coefficients, $\mathbf{y} = \mathbf{X}\mathbf{b} + \boldsymbol{\varepsilon}$, where $\boldsymbol{\varepsilon}$ is an $n \times 1$ normally distributed error term with zero mean and variance σ^2. This model may be viewed as a generalization of (2.97). The vector of regression coefficients, $\mathbf{b}$, is random: $\mathbf{b} = \boldsymbol{\beta} + \boldsymbol{\delta}$, where $\boldsymbol{\delta} \sim \mathcal{N}(\mathbf{0}, \sigma^2\mathbf{D})$ and $\boldsymbol{\beta} = E(\mathbf{b})$ is the parameter of interest. Variance parameters σ^2 and $\mathbf{D}$ are assumed unknown. Also, we shall assume that the $n \times m$ design matrix, $\mathbf{X}$, has full rank and $m < n$. Compactly, this model can be written as

$$
\mathbf{y} \sim \mathcal{N}(\mathbf{X}\boldsymbol{\beta}, \sigma^2(\mathbf{I} + \mathbf{X}\mathbf{D}\mathbf{X}')). \tag{3.2}
$$

Applying Proposition 10, it is possible to show that model (3.2) is identifiable. We estimate this model maximizing the log-likelihood function, which, up to a constant term, is

$$
l(\boldsymbol{\beta}, \sigma^2, \mathbf{D}) = -\frac{1}{2}\{n \ln \sigma^2 + \ln|\mathbf{I} + \mathbf{X}\mathbf{D}\mathbf{X}'| + \sigma^{-2}(\mathbf{y} - \mathbf{X}\boldsymbol{\beta})'(\mathbf{I} + \mathbf{X}\mathbf{D}\mathbf{X}')^{-1}(\mathbf{y} - \mathbf{X}\boldsymbol{\beta})\}.
$$

Let $\widehat{\boldsymbol{\beta}}_{OLS} = (\mathbf{X}'\mathbf{X})^{-1}\mathbf{X}'\mathbf{y}$ be the OLS estimator and $\widehat{\mathbf{e}} = \mathbf{y} - \mathbf{X}\widehat{\boldsymbol{\beta}}_{OLS}$ be an $n \times 1$ OLS residual vector. We simplify the weighted sum of squares using the matrix inverse formulas (2.21) and (2.25) and the fact that for the least squares, $\mathbf{X}'\widehat{\mathbf{e}} = \mathbf{0}$ as follows:

$$
\begin{aligned}
&(\mathbf{y} - \mathbf{X}\boldsymbol{\beta})'(\mathbf{I} + \mathbf{X}\mathbf{D}\mathbf{X}')^{-1}(\mathbf{y} - \mathbf{X}\boldsymbol{\beta}) \\
&= (\widehat{\mathbf{e}} - \mathbf{X}(\boldsymbol{\beta} - \widehat{\boldsymbol{\beta}}_{OLS}))'(\mathbf{I} + \mathbf{X}\mathbf{D}\mathbf{X}')^{-1}(\widehat{\mathbf{e}} - \mathbf{X}(\boldsymbol{\beta} - \widehat{\boldsymbol{\beta}}_{OLS})) \\
&= \widehat{\mathbf{e}}'\left[\mathbf{I} - \mathbf{X}(\mathbf{D}^{-1} + \mathbf{X}'\mathbf{X})^{-1}\mathbf{X}'\right]\widehat{\mathbf{e}} - 2\widehat{\mathbf{e}}'\left[\mathbf{I} - \mathbf{X}(\mathbf{D}^{-1} + \mathbf{X}'\mathbf{X})^{-1}\mathbf{X}'\right]\mathbf{X}(\boldsymbol{\beta} - \widehat{\boldsymbol{\beta}}_{OLS}) \\
&\qquad + (\boldsymbol{\beta} - \widehat{\boldsymbol{\beta}}_{OLS})'((\mathbf{X}'\mathbf{X})^{-1} + \mathbf{D})^{-1}(\boldsymbol{\beta} - \widehat{\boldsymbol{\beta}}_{OLS}) \\
&= \|\widehat{\mathbf{e}}\|^2 + (\boldsymbol{\beta} - \widehat{\boldsymbol{\beta}}_{OLS})'((\mathbf{X}'\mathbf{X})^{-1} + \mathbf{D})^{-1}(\boldsymbol{\beta} - \widehat{\boldsymbol{\beta}}_{OLS}).
\end{aligned}
$$

Furthermore, the maximum of l over σ^2 admits a closed-form solution so that we come to the minus twice variance-profile log-likelihood function,

$$\ln|\mathbf{I} + \mathbf{X}\mathbf{D}\mathbf{X}'| + n\ln[\|\widehat{\mathbf{e}}\|^2 + (\boldsymbol{\beta} - \widehat{\boldsymbol{\beta}}_{OLS})'((\mathbf{X}'\mathbf{X})^{-1} + \mathbf{D})^{-1}(\boldsymbol{\beta} - \widehat{\boldsymbol{\beta}}_{OLS})], \qquad (3.3)$$

after omitting a constant term. But this function reaches its maximum when the second term under the logarithm vanishes, $\boldsymbol{\beta} - \widehat{\boldsymbol{\beta}}_{OLS} = \mathbf{0}$. Therefore, the GLS/ML estimator for model (3.2) coincides with the OLS estimator, $\widehat{\boldsymbol{\beta}}_{ML} = \widehat{\boldsymbol{\beta}}_{OLS}$. Consequently, the log-likelihood function l collapses to $-0.5\{\ln|\mathbf{I} + \mathbf{X}\mathbf{D}\mathbf{X}'| + n\ln\|\widehat{\mathbf{e}}\|^2\}$. Since $\|\widehat{\mathbf{e}}\|^2$ does not depend on $\mathbf{D}$, the latter maximum corresponds to the minimum of $|\mathbf{I} + \mathbf{X}\mathbf{D}\mathbf{X}'|$, which leads to the trivial solution, $\widehat{\mathbf{D}}_{ML} = \mathbf{0}$. Thus, the MLE for model (3.2) coincides with the OLS estimator, and the variance-covariance matrix is zero—thus matrix $\mathbf{D}$ fails to estimate. We can interpret this result by saying that model (3.2) is not specific enough to identify the "randomness" of $\mathbf{b}$.

Model (3.2) would make more sense if observations are collected over several individuals, namely,

$$\mathbf{y}_i \sim \mathcal{N}(\mathbf{X}_i\boldsymbol{\beta}, \sigma^2(\mathbf{I} + \mathbf{X}_i\mathbf{D}\mathbf{X}_i')), \quad i = 1, ..., N. \qquad (3.4)$$

But this model is a special case of the LME model (2.5) with $\mathbf{Z}_i = \mathbf{X}_i$, and is studied in the next chapter. This example explains why we need observations on individuals (repeated measurements) to estimate a random-coefficient model.

Another illustration of an invalid model is when fixed and mixed effects are present in the model at the same time. To be specific, let us consider the random-intercept model of Section 2.4 but where intercepts have different means,

$$y_{ij} = \alpha_i + \boldsymbol{\gamma}'\mathbf{u}_{ij} + b_i + \varepsilon_{ij}. \qquad (3.5)$$

Here $b_i \sim \mathcal{N}(0, \sigma^2 d)$, $\varepsilon_{ij} \sim \mathcal{N}(0, \sigma^2)$, and α_i are fixed and unknown. This model is similar to (3.2), with the difference that in (3.5) only the intercept is random. It is easy to see that for model (3.5) the log-likelihood is given by (2.73) with $h_i = 0$ because $\widehat{\alpha}_i = \overline{y}_i - \boldsymbol{\gamma}'\overline{\mathbf{u}}_{ij}$. Therefore, similarly to model (3.2), we obtain $\widehat{d}_{ML} = 0$ and $\widehat{\boldsymbol{\gamma}}_{ML} = \widehat{\boldsymbol{\gamma}}_\infty$ given by (2.71). In Section 11.6 we confront the problem with simultaneous estimation of fixed and random effects in the statistical analysis of shape.

Problems for Section 3.2

1. Is it true that if a statistical model is not identifiable, the ML estimator is inconsistent? Provide an example.

2. Is it possible that a LME model is not identifiable but the variance parameters MLE are unique and consistent?

3. Prove that for model (3.5) we have $\widehat{d}_{ML} = 0$ and $\widehat{\boldsymbol{\gamma}}_{ML} = \widehat{\boldsymbol{\gamma}}_\infty$ given by (2.71). Provide a layperson explanation that $\widehat{d}_{ML} = 0$. Why is (2.71) an overspecified model?

3.3   Information matrix for variance parameters

Besides estimates of fixed effects coefficients, we may be interested in the covariance matrix of variance parameters *per se*. The aim of this section is to provide formulas for the asymptotic covariance matrix of $\boldsymbol{\theta} = (\sigma^2, \text{vech}'(\mathbf{D}))'$, derived as the inverse of the information matrix. The information matrix for the variance components model is usually expressed element-wise in terms of matrix trace (Searle et al., 1992). Here we derive a more compact formula using the duplication matrix and its properties, see Appendix 13.2.3.

Because observations are independent for different subjects, we can drop subindex i for simplicity of notation. Then the log-likelihood function for the ith individual is written as

$$l = -\frac{1}{2}\left\{n\ln\sigma^2 + \sigma^{-2}(\mathbf{y} - \mathbf{X}\boldsymbol{\beta})'(\mathbf{I} + \mathbf{Z}\mathbf{D}\mathbf{Z}')^{-1}(\mathbf{y} - \mathbf{X}\boldsymbol{\beta}) \right.$$
$$\left. + \ln|\mathbf{I} + \mathbf{Z}\mathbf{D}\mathbf{Z}'|\right\}. \tag{3.6}$$

The $(1 + k(k+1)/2) \times (1 + k(k+1)/2)$ information matrix for $\boldsymbol{\theta}$ is calculated as the covariance matrix of the first derivatives of (3.6) with respect to σ^2 and vech($\mathbf{D}$), where vech denotes the vector collection of unique elements of matrix $\mathbf{D}$ (we refer the reader to formula (2.105) and Appendix 13.2). Differentiating (3.6) with respect to σ^2, we obtain

$$\frac{\partial l}{\partial \sigma^2} = -\frac{n}{2\sigma^2} + \frac{1}{2\sigma^2}\mathbf{u}'\mathbf{u}, \tag{3.7}$$

where $\mathbf{u} = \sigma^{-1}(\mathbf{I} + \mathbf{Z}\mathbf{D}\mathbf{Z})^{-1/2}\boldsymbol{\eta} \sim \mathcal{N}(\mathbf{0}, \mathbf{I})$. Further, using the formula for the variance of a quadratic form with a normally distributed vector (Graybill, 1983; Schott, 1997), one obtains

$$\text{var}\left(\frac{\partial l}{\partial \sigma^2}\right) = \frac{1}{4\sigma^4}\text{var}(\mathbf{u}'\mathbf{u}) = \frac{n}{2\sigma^4}.$$

The derivative of l with respect to $\mathbf{D}$ in terms of $\mathbf{u}$ can be expressed as

$$\frac{\partial l}{\partial \mathbf{D}} = \frac{1}{2\sigma^2}\mathbf{Z}'(\mathbf{I} + \mathbf{Z}\mathbf{D}\mathbf{Z}')^{-1}\mathbf{e}\mathbf{e}'(\mathbf{I} + \mathbf{Z}\mathbf{D}\mathbf{Z}')^{-1}\mathbf{Z} - \frac{1}{2}\mathbf{Z}'(\mathbf{I} + \mathbf{Z}\mathbf{D}\mathbf{Z}')^{-1}\mathbf{Z}$$
$$= \frac{1}{2}(\mathbf{T}\mathbf{u})(\mathbf{T}\mathbf{u})' - \frac{1}{2}\mathbf{Z}'\mathbf{V}^{-1}\mathbf{Z}, \tag{3.8}$$

where $\mathbf{T} = \mathbf{Z}'(\mathbf{I} + \mathbf{Z}\mathbf{D}\mathbf{Z}')^{-1/2}$, see Section 2.9.

For the LME model, the information about beta and variance parameters is orthogonal (corresponding derivatives are uncorrelated, or more precisely, independent), which can be expressed mathematically as

$$\text{cov}\left(\frac{\partial l}{\partial \boldsymbol{\beta}}, \frac{\partial l}{\partial \sigma^2}\right) = \mathbf{0}, \quad \text{cov}\left(\frac{\partial l}{\partial \boldsymbol{\beta}}, \frac{\partial l}{\partial \mathbf{D}}\right) = \mathbf{0}. \tag{3.9}$$

To show the first orthogonality, we rewrite the derivative with respect to beta parameters as

$$\frac{\partial l}{\partial \boldsymbol{\beta}} = \sigma^{-2}\mathbf{X}'(\mathbf{I} + \mathbf{Z}\mathbf{D}\mathbf{Z}')^{-1}(\mathbf{y} - \mathbf{X}\boldsymbol{\beta}) = \mathbf{X}'\mathbf{V}^{-1/2}\mathbf{u}.$$

Then the independence of $\partial l/\partial\boldsymbol{\beta}$ and $\partial l/\partial\sigma^2$ follows from the fact that the third moment of the normal distribution is zero,

$$\text{cov}\left(\frac{\partial l}{\partial \boldsymbol{\beta}}, \frac{\partial l}{\partial \sigma^2}\right) = E\left(\frac{1}{2\sigma^2}\mathbf{u}'\mathbf{u}\mathbf{X}'\mathbf{V}^{-1/2}\mathbf{u}\right) = \mathbf{0}.$$

A similar proof works for the independence of $\partial l/\partial \boldsymbol{\beta}$ and $\partial l/\partial \mathbf{D}$. Indeed, considering the covariance between $\partial l/\partial \boldsymbol{\beta}$ and $\mathbf{c}'(\partial l/\partial \mathbf{D})\mathbf{c}$ for any fixed vector $\mathbf{c}$, we obtain

$$\text{cov}\left(\frac{\partial l}{\partial \boldsymbol{\beta}}, \mathbf{c}'\frac{\partial l}{\partial \mathbf{D}}\mathbf{c}\right) = E\left(\frac{1}{4\sigma^2}\mathbf{X}'\mathbf{V}^{-1/2}\mathbf{u}(\mathbf{c}'\mathbf{T}\mathbf{u})^2\right) = \mathbf{0},$$

which again follows from the fact that the third moment of the normal distribution is zero. Since the information matrix is block diagonal, without loss of generality, we can assume that $\boldsymbol{\beta}$ is the true vector when calculating the asymptotic covariance matrix for the variance parameter $\boldsymbol{\theta}$. The fact that the information matrix in the LME model for $(\boldsymbol{\beta}, \boldsymbol{\theta})$ is block diagonal has been known for a long time (Jennrich and Schluchter, 1986). We refer the reader to Appendix 13.1.3 for a general discussion. Consequently, the asymptotic covariance matrix for $\widehat{\boldsymbol{\beta}}_{ML}$ is approximated as

$$\text{cov}(\widehat{\boldsymbol{\beta}}_{ML}) = \widehat{\sigma}^2\left(\sum_{i=1}^{N}\mathbf{X}_i'(\mathbf{I} + \mathbf{Z}_i\widehat{\mathbf{D}}\mathbf{Z}_i')^{-1}\mathbf{X}_i\right)^{-1}. \tag{3.10}$$

In the rest of this section we consider variance parameters; our objective is to calculate the information matrix for $\boldsymbol{\theta}$. For this, we need more advanced use of vector functions vec and vech to represent symmetric matrices. These matrix-to-vector operators are described at length by Lancaster and Tismenetsky (1985), Fuller (1987), Magnus (1988), Schott (1997), and Harville (1997), among others. Many facts of matrix algebra and calculus used in this book are collected in Appendix 13.2. The vec function applies to a matrix and represents the matrix as a vector by stacking the columns into a column-vector. By vech we denote a similar function, but applied to a symmetric matrix, with columns starting from the main diagonal. The *duplication* matrix, described by Magnus (1988), relates the two functions in a simple way: let $\mathbf{M}$ be any $k \times k$ symmetric matrix; then the $k^2 \times k(k+1)/2$ duplication matrix $\mathcal{D}_k$ of full rank is such that $\text{vec}(\mathbf{M}) = \mathcal{D}_k\text{vech}(\mathbf{M})$. Based on $\mathcal{D}_k$ it is possible to construct a generalized inverse matrix $\mathcal{D}_k^+ = (\mathcal{D}_k'\mathcal{D}_k)^{-1}\mathcal{D}_k'$ for the back representation, $\text{vech}(\mathbf{M}) = \mathcal{D}_k^+\text{vec}(\mathbf{M})$. Magnus provides explicit expressions for $\mathcal{D}_k$ and $\mathcal{D}_k^+$; following are examples for $k = 3$:

$$\mathcal{D}_3^{9\times 6} = \begin{bmatrix} 1 & 0 & 0 & 0 & 0 & 0 \\ 0 & 1 & 0 & 0 & 0 & 0 \\ 0 & 0 & 1 & 0 & 0 & 0 \\ 0 & 1 & 0 & 0 & 0 & 0 \\ 0 & 0 & 0 & 1 & 0 & 0 \\ 0 & 0 & 0 & 0 & 1 & 0 \\ 0 & 0 & 1 & 0 & 0 & 0 \\ 0 & 0 & 0 & 0 & 1 & 0 \\ 0 & 0 & 0 & 0 & 0 & 1 \end{bmatrix}, \quad (\mathcal{D}_3^+)' = \begin{bmatrix} 1 & 0 & 0 & 0 & 0 & 0 \\ 0 & \frac{1}{2} & 0 & 0 & 0 & 0 \\ 0 & 0 & \frac{1}{2} & 0 & 0 & 0 \\ 0 & \frac{1}{2} & 0 & 0 & 0 & 0 \\ 0 & 0 & 0 & 1 & 0 & 0 \\ 0 & 0 & 0 & 0 & \frac{1}{2} & 0 \\ 0 & 0 & \frac{1}{2} & 0 & 0 & 0 \\ 0 & 0 & 0 & 0 & \frac{1}{2} & 0 \\ 0 & 0 & 0 & 0 & 0 & 1 \end{bmatrix}.$$

We will use duplication matrices to calculate the information and covariance matrices for $\mathbf{D}$. Note that the covariance matrix for $\text{vec}(\mathbf{D})$ is deficient (singular) because matrix $\mathbf{D}$ is symmetric. To shorten the notation, we introduce the function *covh* which denotes the covariance matrix of $\text{vech}(\mathbf{M})$, where $\mathbf{M}$ is a symmetric matrix, i.e., $covh(\mathbf{M}) = \text{cov}(\text{vech}(\mathbf{M}))$.

Below is the R code for computation of the duplication matrix $\mathcal{D}_n$ based on the Magnus representation:

```
dupp<-function(n)
{
    d1 <- n^2
    d2 <- (n * (n + 1))/2
    D <- matrix(rep(0, d1 * d2), nrow = d1)
    for(i in 1:n)
        for(j in 1:i) {
            u <- matrix(rep(0, d2), ncol = 1)
            u[(j - 1) * n + i - (j * (j - 1))/2, 1] <- 1
            Tm <- matrix(rep(0, d1), ncol = n)
            if(i == j)
                Tm[i, i] <- 1
            else Tm[i, j] <- Tm[j, i] <- 1
            D <- D + matrix(as.vector(Tm), ncol = 1) %*% t(u)
        }
    return(D)
}
```

We can use Dplus <- solve(t(D) %*% D) %*% t(D) to compute $\mathcal{D}^+$, where D=dupp(n).

Since we are interested in covariance, the nonrandom term, $0.5\mathbf{Z}'\mathbf{V}^{-1}\mathbf{Z}$ in (3.8) can be omitted, so that

$$covh\left(\frac{\partial l}{\partial \mathbf{D}}\right) = covh\left(\frac{1}{2}(\mathbf{Tu})(\mathbf{Tu})'\right). \tag{3.11}$$

To express (3.11) in terms of $\mathbf{Z}$ and $\mathbf{D}$, the following result will be used (the commutation matrix $\mathbf{K}_n$ is defined in Appendix 13.2.3).

Lemma 12 *Let* $\mathbf{u}$ *be an* $n \times 1$ *vector,* $\mathbf{u} \sim N(\mathbf{0}, \mathbf{I}_n)$. *Then* $cov(\mathbf{u} \otimes \mathbf{u}) = 2\mathbf{N}_n$, *where* $\mathbf{N}_n = (\mathbf{I}_{n^2} + \mathbf{K}_n)/2$, $\mathbf{I}_{n^2}$ *is an* $n^2 \times n^2$ *identity matrix, and* $\mathbf{K}_n$ *is a commutation matrix.*

The proof is given in Magnus (1988). Then, using this lemma, we obtain

$$covh\left(\frac{1}{2}(\mathbf{Tu})(\mathbf{Tu})'\right)$$

$$= \mathcal{D}^+ cov\left(\frac{1}{2}(\mathbf{Tu})(\mathbf{Tu})'\right)\mathcal{D}^{+'} = \frac{1}{4}\mathcal{D}^+ cov\left(\mathbf{Tu} \otimes \mathbf{Tu}\right)\mathcal{D}^{+'}$$

$$= \frac{1}{4}\mathcal{D}^+ cov\left((\mathbf{T} \otimes \mathbf{T})(\mathbf{u} \otimes \mathbf{u})\right)\mathcal{D}^{+'} = \frac{1}{2}\mathcal{D}^+(\mathbf{T} \otimes \mathbf{T})\mathbf{N}_n(\mathbf{T}' \otimes \mathbf{T}')\mathcal{D}^{+'}.$$

Now we find the expectation of the cross-product. As it is easy to see, we can write $\mathbf{u}'\mathbf{u} = (\mathbf{u} \otimes \mathbf{u})'\text{vec}(\mathbf{I}_n)$, so that

$$\text{cov}\left(\frac{\partial l}{\partial \sigma^2}, \frac{\partial l}{\partial \text{vech}(\mathbf{D})}\right) = \frac{1}{4\sigma^2}\mathcal{D}^+ (\mathbf{T} \otimes \mathbf{T})\,\text{cov}(\mathbf{u} \otimes \mathbf{u})\text{vec}(\mathbf{I}_n)$$

$$= \frac{1}{2\sigma^2}\mathcal{D}^+ (\mathbf{T} \otimes \mathbf{T})\,\mathbf{N}_n\text{vec}(\mathbf{I}_n).$$

Thus, the information matrix for $(\sigma^2, \text{vech}(\mathbf{D}))$ is given by

$$\mathcal{I} = \frac{1}{2}\left[\begin{array}{cc} n\sigma^{-4} & \sigma^{-2}\text{vec}'(\mathbf{I}_n)\mathbf{N}_n (\mathbf{T}' \otimes \mathbf{T}')\mathcal{D}^{+\prime} \\ \sigma^{-2}\mathcal{D}^+ (\mathbf{T} \otimes \mathbf{T})\,\mathbf{N}_n\text{vec}(\mathbf{I}_n) & \mathcal{D}^+ (\mathbf{T} \otimes \mathbf{T})\,\mathbf{N}_n (\mathbf{T}' \otimes \mathbf{T}')\mathcal{D}^{+\prime} \end{array}\right]. \tag{3.12}$$

In fact, this matrix can be simplified further as follows. The following property of matrix $\mathbf{N}_n$ will be used:

$$(\mathbf{A} \otimes \mathbf{A})\mathbf{N}_n = \mathbf{N}_n(\mathbf{A} \otimes \mathbf{A}), \quad \mathcal{D}^+\mathbf{N}_n = \mathcal{D}^+, \tag{3.13}$$

where $\mathbf{A}$ is a matrix of appropriate size. Then, for the (1,2)th block of $\mathcal{I}$, we obtain

$$\mathbf{N}_n (\mathbf{T}' \otimes \mathbf{T}')\mathcal{D}^{+\prime} = (\mathbf{T}' \otimes \mathbf{T}')\mathbf{N}_n\mathcal{D}^{+\prime} = (\mathbf{T}' \otimes \mathbf{T}')\mathcal{D}^{+\prime}.$$

The analogous transformation is valid for the (2,1)th block. For the last term of (3.12), we have

$$\mathcal{D}^+ (\mathbf{T} \otimes \mathbf{T})\,\mathbf{N}_n (\mathbf{T}' \otimes \mathbf{T}')\mathcal{D}^{+\prime}$$
$$= \mathcal{D}^+ (\mathbf{T} \otimes \mathbf{T})(\mathbf{T}' \otimes \mathbf{T}')\mathcal{D}^{+\prime} = \mathcal{D}^+ (\mathbf{TT}' \otimes \mathbf{TT}')\mathcal{D}^{+\prime}.$$

But $\mathbf{TT}' = \mathbf{R}$, where

$$\mathbf{R} = \mathbf{Z}'(\mathbf{I} + \mathbf{ZDZ}')^{-1}\mathbf{Z}, \tag{3.14}$$

and using the identity

$$\text{vec}(\mathbf{ABF}) = (\mathbf{F}' \otimes \mathbf{A})\text{vec}(\mathbf{B}) \tag{3.15}$$

for any matrices of appropriate size, we obtain

$$(\mathbf{T} \otimes \mathbf{T})\,\text{vec}(\mathbf{I}_n) = \text{vec}(\mathbf{TT}') = \text{vec}(\mathbf{Z}'(\mathbf{I} + \mathbf{ZDZ}')^{-1}\mathbf{Z}).$$

Combining all derivations, we finally arrive at the information matrix for $\boldsymbol{\theta}$ from cluster i,

$$\mathcal{I} = \frac{1}{2}\left[\begin{array}{cc} n_i\sigma^{-4} & \sigma^{-2}\text{vec}'(\mathbf{R}_i)\mathcal{D}^{+\prime} \\ \sigma^{-2}\mathcal{D}^+\text{vec}(\mathbf{R}_i) & \mathcal{D}^+ (\mathbf{R}_i \otimes \mathbf{R}_i)\mathcal{D}^{+\prime} \end{array}\right]. \tag{3.16}$$

In a special case of uncorrelated random effects, this matrix is found in Harville (1997). The asymptotic covariance matrix of the variance parameters, based on the entire sample $i = 1, ..., N$, is the inverse to the total information matrix,

$$\text{cov}(\widehat{\boldsymbol{\theta}}_{ML}) = 2\left[\begin{array}{cc} N_T\sigma^{-4} & \sigma^{-2}\text{vec}'(\sum \mathbf{R}_i)\mathcal{D}^{+\prime} \\ \sigma^{-2}\mathcal{D}^+\text{vec}(\sum \mathbf{R}_i) & \mathcal{D}^+ (\sum \mathbf{R}_i \otimes \mathbf{R}_i)\mathcal{D}^{+\prime} \end{array}\right]^{-1}, \tag{3.17}$$

where the $k \times k$ matrix $\mathbf{R}_i$ is defined as

$$\mathbf{R}_i = \mathbf{Z}_i'(\mathbf{I} + \mathbf{Z}_i\mathbf{D}\mathbf{Z}_i')^{-1}\mathbf{Z}_i = \left((\mathbf{Z}_i'\mathbf{Z}_i)^{-1} + \mathbf{D}\right)^{-1}.$$

Note that this identity holds if matrix $\mathbf{Z}_i$ has full rank. Using matrix block-inverse, we can find the asymptotic variance for $\widehat{\sigma}_{ML}^2$ and the covariance matrix of the random effects ($N_T = \sum n_i$),

$$\mathrm{var}(\widehat{\sigma}_{ML}^2) = \frac{2\sigma^4}{N_T - \omega}, \tag{3.18}$$

where

$$\omega = \mathrm{vec}'\left(\sum \mathbf{R}_i\right)\mathcal{D}^{+\prime}\left(\mathcal{D}^+\left(\sum \mathbf{R}_i \otimes \mathbf{R}_i\right)\mathcal{D}^{+\prime}\right)^{-1}\mathcal{D}^+\mathrm{vec}\left(\sum \mathbf{R}_i\right), \tag{3.19}$$

and

$$\begin{aligned}
covh(\widehat{\mathbf{D}}_{ML}) \\
= \; 2\left[\mathcal{D}^+\left(\sum \mathbf{R}_i \otimes \mathbf{R}_i - \frac{1}{N_T}\mathrm{vec}\left(\sum \mathbf{R}_i\right)\mathrm{vec}'\left(\sum \mathbf{R}_i\right)\right)\mathcal{D}^{+\prime}\right]^{-1}.
\end{aligned} \tag{3.20}$$

Notice that this covariance matrix does not depend on σ^2.

The covariance matrix for restricted ML may be found from the sandwich formula, see Appendix 13.1.4. For the variance components model this matrix is found in Searle et al. (1992) and McGilchrist (1994).

Using matrix identities (3.13), it is possible to show that in expression (3.19) one can get rid of the duplication matrix, or more precisely,

$$\omega = \mathrm{vec}'(\sum \mathbf{R}_i)\left(\sum \mathbf{R}_i \otimes \mathbf{R}_i\right)^{-1}\mathrm{vec}(\sum \mathbf{R}_i). \tag{3.21}$$

Proof. Indeed, using the definition of $\mathcal{D}^+$, we have

$$\begin{aligned}
\omega &= \mathrm{vec}'(\sum \mathbf{R}_i)\mathcal{D}^{+\prime}(\mathcal{D}'\mathcal{D})\left(\mathcal{D}^+\left(\sum \mathbf{R}_i \otimes \mathbf{R}_i\right)\mathcal{D}\right)^{-1}\mathcal{D}^+\mathrm{vec}(\sum \mathbf{R}_i) \\
&= \mathrm{vec}'(\sum \mathbf{R}_i)\mathcal{D}\left(\mathcal{D}^+\left(\sum \mathbf{R}_i \otimes \mathbf{R}_i\right)\mathcal{D}\right)^{-1}\mathcal{D}^+\mathrm{vec}(\sum \mathbf{R}_i).
\end{aligned}$$

But

$$\left(\mathcal{D}^+\left(\sum \mathbf{R}_i \otimes \mathbf{R}_i\right)\mathcal{D}\right)^{-1} = \mathcal{D}^+\left(\sum \mathbf{R}_i \otimes \mathbf{R}_i\right)^{-1}\mathcal{D} \tag{3.22}$$

because

$$\begin{aligned}
&\mathcal{D}^+\left(\sum \mathbf{R}_i \otimes \mathbf{R}_i\right)^{-1}\mathcal{D}\mathcal{D}^+\left(\sum \mathbf{R}_i \otimes \mathbf{R}_i\right)\mathcal{D} \\
&= \mathcal{D}^+\left(\sum \mathbf{R}_i \otimes \mathbf{R}_i\right)^{-1}\sum \mathbf{N}(\mathbf{R}_i \otimes \mathbf{R}_i)\mathcal{D} \\
&= \mathcal{D}^+\left(\sum \mathbf{R}_i \otimes \mathbf{R}_i\right)^{-1}\left(\sum \mathbf{R}_i \otimes \mathbf{R}_i\right)\mathbf{N}\mathcal{D} = \mathcal{D}^+\mathbf{N}\mathcal{D} = \mathbf{I}.
\end{aligned}$$

Thus, continuing, we have

$$\omega = \text{vec}'(\sum \mathbf{R}_i)\mathcal{D}\mathcal{D}^+ \left(\sum \mathbf{R}_i \otimes \mathbf{R}_i\right)^{-1} \mathcal{D}\mathcal{D}^+ \text{vec}(\sum \mathbf{R}_i).$$

But for a symmetric matrix, $\mathcal{D}\mathcal{D}^+\text{vec}(\mathbf{A}) =\text{vec}(\mathbf{A})$; therefore, we finally come to (3.21).   ∎

Analogously, using the identity (3.22) and the fact that $\mathbf{N}\text{vec}(\mathbf{A}) =\text{vec}(\mathbf{A})$ for symmetric matrix $\mathbf{A}$, one can show that (3.20) is equivalent to

$$2\mathcal{D}' \left[\sum \mathbf{R}_i \otimes \mathbf{R}_i - \frac{1}{N_T}\text{vec}(\sum \mathbf{R}_i)\text{vec}'(\sum \mathbf{R}_i)\right]^{-1} \mathcal{D}. \qquad (3.23)$$

As follows from classical mathematical statistics, (3.18) and (3.20) define the lower bound for the variance and covariance of unbiased estimators for σ^2 and $\mathbf{D}$, the Cramér–Rao inequality. See, for example, Rao (1973) or Casella and Berger (1990). In the next subsection we prove that this bound is attained for σ^2 when the data are balanced, i.e., $n_i =$const and $\mathbf{Z}_i =$const.

In practice, we estimate $\text{cov}(\widehat{\boldsymbol{\theta}}_{ML})$ by replacing σ^2 and $\mathbf{D}$ with their MLEs.

Sometimes we need the covariance matrix for the MLE of $\mathbf{D}_* = \sigma^2\mathbf{D}$. Since $\text{vech}(\widehat{\mathbf{D}}_{*ML}) = \widehat{\sigma}^2_{ML}\text{vech}(\widehat{\mathbf{D}}_{ML})$, by the delta-method (Rice 1995) we yield

$$\begin{aligned}
covh(\widehat{\mathbf{D}}_{*ML}) &= \text{var}(\widehat{\sigma}^2_{ML})\text{vech}(\widehat{\mathbf{D}}_{ML})\text{vech}'(\widehat{\mathbf{D}}_{ML}) + \sigma^4 covh(\widehat{\mathbf{D}}_{ML}) \\
&\quad +\sigma^2[\text{cov}(\widehat{\sigma}^2_{ML}, \text{vech}(\widehat{\mathbf{D}}_{ML}))\text{vech}'(\widehat{\mathbf{D}}_{ML}) \\
&\quad +\text{vech}(\widehat{\mathbf{D}}_{ML})\text{cov}'(\widehat{\sigma}^2_{ML}, \text{vech}(\widehat{\mathbf{D}}_{ML}))], \qquad (3.24)
\end{aligned}$$

where $\text{var}(\widehat{\sigma}^2_{ML})$ and $covh(\widehat{\mathbf{D}}_{ML})$ are defined by (3.18) and (3.20), respectively, and $\text{cov}(\widehat{\sigma}^2_{ML}, \text{vech}(\widehat{\mathbf{D}}_{ML}))$ is the $(2,1)$th block of matrix (3.17).

It is well known that the information matrix is always nonnegative definite because essentially it is a covariance matrix. However, to make the statistical model correct, we have to be sure that the information matrix is positive definite (nonnegative definite and nonsingular). Conditions on positive definiteness of the information matrix provide minimal requirements for the validity of the model. In particular, these conditions imply that in a large sample, the variance-covariance matrix of $\widehat{\mathbf{D}}$ approaches zero with the order N^{-1}.

Proposition 13 *The information matrix for the LME model is positive definite if (2.6) holds and at least for one i matrix, $\mathbf{Z}_i$ is not zero.*

Proof. We use the following simple matrix fact: If matrix $\mathbf{M}$ is partitioned as

$$\mathbf{M} = \begin{bmatrix} c & \mathbf{b}' \\ \mathbf{b} & \mathbf{H} \end{bmatrix}, \qquad (3.25)$$

where $c > 0$, then matrix $\mathbf{M}$ is positive definite if and only if matrix $\mathbf{H} - c^{-1}\mathbf{b}\mathbf{b}'$ is positive definite. Since matrix $\mathcal{D}^+$ has full rank, the inverse matrix in (3.17) is positive definite if and only if the matrix

$$\sum \mathbf{R}_i \otimes \mathbf{R}_i - N_T^{-1}\text{vec}(\sum \mathbf{R}_i)\text{vec}'(\sum \mathbf{R}_i) \qquad (3.26)$$

is positive definite. Let $\mathbf{U}$ be any nonzero $k \times k$ matrix. Without loss of generality, we can assume that this matrix is normalized, $\text{tr}(\mathbf{U}'\mathbf{U}) = 1$. To show that matrix (3.26) is positive definite, it suffices to prove that

$$\text{vec}'(\mathbf{U}) \left(\sum \mathbf{R}_i \otimes \mathbf{R}_i - \frac{1}{N_T} \text{vec}(\sum \mathbf{R}_i) \text{vec}'(\sum \mathbf{R}_i) \right) \text{vec}(\mathbf{U})$$

$$= \text{vec}'(\mathbf{U})[\sum \mathbf{R}_i \otimes \mathbf{R}_i] \text{vec}(\mathbf{U}) - \frac{1}{N_T} [\text{vec}'(\mathbf{U}) \text{vec}(\sum \mathbf{R}_i)]^2 > 0. \quad (3.27)$$

For the first term in (3.27), we apply the formula

$$\text{vec}'(\mathbf{U})(\mathbf{A} \otimes \mathbf{B}) \text{vec}(\mathbf{U}) = \text{tr}(\mathbf{U}\mathbf{A}\mathbf{U}'\mathbf{B}'), \quad (3.28)$$

which yields $\text{vec}'(\mathbf{U})[\sum \mathbf{R}_i \otimes \mathbf{R}_i] \text{vec}(\mathbf{U}) = \sum \text{tr}(\mathbf{U}\mathbf{R}_i\mathbf{U}'\mathbf{R}_i)$. For the second term of (3.27), we apply the formula $\text{vec}'(\mathbf{A}) \text{vec}(\mathbf{B}) = \text{tr}(\mathbf{A}'\mathbf{B})$, which yields

$$\frac{1}{N_T} [\text{vec}'(\mathbf{U}) \text{vec}(\sum \mathbf{R}_i)]^2 = \frac{1}{N_T} [\sum \text{tr}(\mathbf{U}\mathbf{R}_i)]^2.$$

Then, denoting $\mathbf{A}_i = \mathbf{U}\mathbf{R}_i$, it suffices to show that the quantity

$$Q = \sum_{i=1}^{N} \text{tr}(\mathbf{A}_i\mathbf{A}_i') - \frac{1}{N_T} [\sum_{i=1}^{N} \text{tr}(\mathbf{A}_i)]^2 \quad (3.29)$$

is positive. We have

$$\begin{aligned}
Q &= \sum_{i=1}^{N} \text{tr}(\mathbf{A}_i - \overline{\mathbf{A}})(\mathbf{A}_i - \overline{\mathbf{A}})' + N \left[\text{tr}(\overline{\mathbf{A}\mathbf{A}}') - \frac{N}{N_T} \text{tr}^2(\overline{\mathbf{A}}) \right] \\
&= \sum_{i=1}^{N} \text{tr}(\mathbf{A}_i - \overline{\mathbf{A}})(\mathbf{A}_i - \overline{\mathbf{A}})' + N \left[\text{tr}(\overline{\mathbf{A}\mathbf{A}}') - \frac{1}{k} \text{tr}^2(\overline{\mathbf{A}}) \right] \\
&\quad + \frac{N(N_T - Nk)}{N_T k} \text{tr}^2(\overline{\mathbf{A}}),
\end{aligned}$$

where $\overline{\mathbf{A}} = \sum \mathbf{A}_i / N$. The middle term is nonnegative because $\text{tr}(\mathbf{M}\mathbf{M}') \geq k^{-1} \text{tr}^2(\mathbf{M})$ for any $k \times k$ matrix $\mathbf{M}$. Let, on the contrary, $Q = 0$; then $\mathbf{A}_i = \overline{\mathbf{A}}$, so $\mathbf{R}_i$ does not depend on i. Since $N_T - Nk \geq 0$ and $\sum_{i=1}^{N} \text{tr}(\mathbf{A}_i) = 0$ it follows from (3.29) that $\text{tr}(\mathbf{U}'\mathbf{R}^2\mathbf{U}) = \text{vec}'(\mathbf{U})(\mathbf{R} \otimes \mathbf{R}) \text{vec}(\mathbf{U}) = 0$, which implies that $\mathbf{Z}_i'(\mathbf{I} + \mathbf{Z}_i\mathbf{D}\mathbf{Z}_i')^{-1}\mathbf{Z}_i = \mathbf{0}$ for all i, a contradiction. ∎

Remarks

1. In the absence of random effects ($\mathbf{D} = \mathbf{0}$), from formula (3.17) we obtain a familiar asymptotic variance of $\widehat{\sigma}^2_{ML}$, namely, $\text{var}(\widehat{\sigma}^2) = 2\sigma^4/N_T$, where N_T is the total number of observations.

2. The covariance matrix of variance parameters does not depend on the fixed effects, $\boldsymbol{\beta}$.

3. For one random effect ($k = 1$) we have $R_i = \|\mathbf{z}_i\|^2 / (1 + \|\mathbf{z}_i\|^2)$, and the Kronecker product is replaced by the standard product. Then matrix $\mathcal{D}^+$ vanishes and the covariance simplifies to

$$\operatorname{cov}\left[\begin{array}{c} \widehat{\sigma}^2_{ML} \\ \widehat{d}_{ML} \end{array}\right] = 2 \left[\begin{array}{cc} N_T \sigma^{-4} & \sigma^{-2} \sum \frac{\|\mathbf{z}_i\|^2}{1+d\|\mathbf{z}_i\|^2} \\ \sigma^{-2} \sum \frac{\|\mathbf{z}_i\|^2}{1+d\|\mathbf{z}_i\|^2} & \sum \frac{\|\mathbf{z}_i\|^4}{(1+d\|\mathbf{z}_i\|^2)^2} \end{array}\right]^{-1},$$

where $\sigma^2 d$ is the variance of the random effect. Using the standard formula for the 2×2 matrix inverse, we obtain

$$\operatorname{var}(\widehat{d}_{ML}) = \frac{2}{\sum \frac{\|\mathbf{z}_i\|^4}{(1+d\|\mathbf{z}_i\|^2)^2} - \frac{1}{N_T}\left(\sum \frac{\|\mathbf{z}_i\|^2}{1+d\|\mathbf{z}_i\|^2}\right)^2}.$$

We illustrate the calculation of the asymptotic covariance matrix of variance parameters with the LME model with random intercepts (2.67), where $\mathbf{Z}_i = \mathbf{1}_i$. Then $R_i = n_i/(1 + n_i d)$ and

$$\operatorname{cov}\left[\begin{array}{c} \widehat{\sigma}^2_{ML} \\ \widehat{d}_{ML} \end{array}\right] = 2 \left[\begin{array}{cc} N_T \sigma^{-4} & \sigma^{-2} \sum \frac{n_i}{1+n_i d} \\ \sigma^{-2} \sum \frac{n_i}{1+n_i d} & \sum \left(\frac{n_i}{1+n_i d}\right)^2 \end{array}\right]^{-1}. \tag{3.30}$$

As follows from formula (3.24),

$$\operatorname{var}(\widehat{d}_{*ML}) = 2\sigma^4 \frac{N_T + \sum \left(\frac{n_i}{1+n_i d}\right)^2 d^2 - 2d \sum \frac{n_i}{1+n_i d}}{N_T \sum \left(\frac{n_i}{1+n_i d}\right)^2 - \left(\sum \frac{n_i}{1+n_i d}\right)^2}. \tag{3.31}$$

For balanced data ($n_i = n$), we obtain

$$\operatorname{cov}\left[\begin{array}{c} \widehat{\sigma}^2_{ML} \\ \widehat{d}_{ML} \end{array}\right] = \frac{2}{Nn} \left[\begin{array}{cc} \sigma^{-4} & \frac{\sigma^{-2}}{1+nd} \\ \frac{\sigma^{-2}}{1+nd} & \frac{n}{(1+nd)^2} \end{array}\right]^{-1},$$

with diagonal elements

$$\operatorname{var}(\widehat{\sigma}^2_{ML}) = \frac{2\sigma^4}{N(n-1)}, \quad \operatorname{var}(\widehat{d}_{ML}) = \frac{2(1+nd)^2}{Nn(n-1)} \tag{3.32}$$

and

$$\operatorname{var}(\widehat{d}_{*ML}) = \frac{2\sigma^4}{Nn(n-1)}[(1+(n-1)d)^2 + (n-1)d^2]. \tag{3.33}$$

As follows from these formulas, the variance of $\widehat{\sigma}^2_{ML}$ has the order $(Nn)^{-1}$ and the order of the variance of $\widehat{d}_{ML}$ is N^{-1}. This means that we can consistently estimate σ^2, even having a finite number of subjects/clusters when the cluster size increases. However, we cannot consistently estimate the variance of the random effect without having a large number of clusters.

A comparison of the MLE for the variance parameters with quadratic unbiased estimators such as MINQUE and the method of moments for unbalanced data is deferred to Section 3.14.

3.3.1 Efficiency of variance parameters for balanced data

The aim of this section is to investigate whether the MLEs of the variance parameters with balanced data for the random-coefficient and random-intercept model of Sections 2.3 and 2.4.1 are efficient, i.e., if they reach the Cramér–Rao bound. We prove that the estimator of σ^2 is efficient in the random-coefficient model; however, other estimators are not.

Theorem 14 *For the random-coefficient model with balanced data, $\widehat{\sigma}^2_{ML} = \widehat{\sigma}^2_{RML}$, given by formula (2.59), is efficient, i.e., it reaches the Cramér–Rao bound.*

Proof. Using the fact that $\mathrm{var}(\boldsymbol{\eta}'\mathbf{A}\boldsymbol{\eta}) = 2tr(\mathbf{VA})^2$ for $\boldsymbol{\eta} \sim \mathcal{N}(\mathbf{0}, \mathbf{V})$, we find that

$$
\begin{aligned}
\mathrm{var}(\widehat{\sigma}^2_{ML}) &= \frac{1}{(N(n-m))^2} \sum \mathrm{var}(\boldsymbol{\eta}'_i(\mathbf{I} - \mathbf{Z}(\mathbf{Z}'\mathbf{Z})^{-1}\mathbf{Z})\boldsymbol{\eta}_i) \\
&= \frac{2N\sigma^4}{(N(n-m))^2} tr((\mathbf{I} + \mathbf{ZDZ}')(\mathbf{I} - \mathbf{Z}(\mathbf{Z}'\mathbf{Z})^{-1}\mathbf{Z}))^2 \\
&= \frac{2N\sigma^4}{(N(n-m))^2} tr(\mathbf{I} - \mathbf{Z}(\mathbf{Z}'\mathbf{Z})^{-1}\mathbf{Z})) = \frac{2\sigma^4}{N(n-m)}.
\end{aligned}
$$

In view of (3.18) and (3.21), the efficiency of $\widehat{\sigma}^2_{ML}$ would follow from $\omega = Nm$. However,

$$
\mathrm{vec}'(\mathbf{R})(\mathbf{R} \otimes \mathbf{R})^{-1}\mathrm{vec}(\mathbf{R}) = tr(\mathbf{RR}^{-1}\mathbf{RR}^{-1}) = m,
$$

which proves its efficiency. ∎

However, the RMLE for σ^2 in the random-intercept model is not efficient, i.e., its variance does not reach the lower bound. To simplify, we consider the balanced random-intercept model of Section 2.4.1 in the form $\mathbf{y}_i = a_i + \boldsymbol{\gamma}'\mathbf{u} + \boldsymbol{\varepsilon}_i$, where $a_i \sim \mathcal{N}(\alpha, d_*)$, $\boldsymbol{\varepsilon}_i \sim \mathcal{N}(0, \sigma^2)$, and $\mathbf{u}$ is an $(m-1) \times 1$ vector. The RML unbiased estimate for σ^2 is given by (2.87), and it may be shown that

$$
\mathrm{var}(\widehat{\sigma}^2_{RML}) = \frac{2\sigma^4}{N(n-1) - m + 1};
$$

see Section 3.10.2. But from (3.32) it follows that the efficiency of the RMLE, as the ratio of the lower bound to the variance of the estimate, is

$$
\frac{N(n-1) - m + 1}{N(n-1)} = 1 - \frac{m-1}{N(n-1)}.
$$

This means that if $m = 1$, then $\widehat{\sigma}^2_{RML}$ is efficient, but this is the case when the random-intercept model collapses to the random-coefficient model. Otherwise, $\mathrm{var}(\widehat{\sigma}^2_{RML})$ does not reach its lower bound, but the efficiency does approach 1 with the order $1/N$.

Now we look at the efficiency of $\widehat{d}_{*RML}$ given by formula (2.89). The lower bound for $\mathrm{var}(\widehat{d}_{*RML})$ is given by (3.33). Since $\widehat{d}_{*RML}$ is unbiased and is a quadratic function of observations, its variance may be computed based on the formula $\mathrm{var}(\boldsymbol{\eta}'\mathbf{A}\boldsymbol{\eta})$

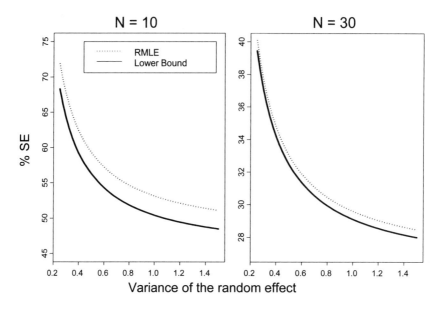

FIGURE 3.1. Cramér–Rao lower bound for the MLE and the percent standard error (SE) of $\widehat{d}_{*RML}$ for different true values of d_* and $N = 10, 30$ in the random-intercept model. For small N, the RML estimator does not reach the lower bound; for relatively large N, the difference becomes negligible.

$= 2tr(\mathbf{AV})^2$, where $\boldsymbol{\eta} \sim \mathcal{N}(\mathbf{0}, \mathbf{V})$. In Figure 3.1 we compare $\mathrm{var}(\widehat{d}_{*RML})$ with the lower bound as a function of the true d_* for $N = 10$ and $N = 30$ in terms of

$$\%SE = \frac{\sqrt{\mathrm{var}(\widehat{d}_{*RML})}}{d_*} \times 100\%,$$

the relative SE. As the reader can see, $\%$SE decreases with increasing d_* and reaches a plateau. For the small sample ($N = 10$), we lose a few percent of efficiency; for $N = 30$, the efficiency is pretty high. The efficiency of the variance parameter estimation for unbalanced data in the random-intercept model is considered in Section 3.14.

Problems for Section 3.3

1. Prove representation (3.7).

2. Write an R code for computation of the commutation matrix $\mathbf{K}_n$ using the representation in Appendix 13.2.3.

3. Check Lemma 12 using simulations.

4. Express (3.24) in closed form using (3.18), (3.20), and (3.17).

5. Is it true that $\%$ SE decreases with N for the fixed value of the random effect, as shown in Figure 3.1?

6*. Does Theorem 14 hold for random effects? If not, why? Support your statement with simulations.

3.4   Profile-likelihood confidence intervals

Confidence interval (CI) construction and statistical testing on beta parameters in the LME model are usually based on the asymptotic covariance matrix (3.10). For example, the statistical significance of the jth component of vector $\boldsymbol{\beta}$ uses the ratio $\widehat{\beta}_j/s_j$, where s_j is the MLE standard error calculated as the square root of the (j, j)th diagonal element of matrix (3.10). Approximately, or more precisely, asymptotically (when the number of clusters is large), $\widehat{\beta}_j/s_j \sim \mathcal{N}(0, 1)$ under the null hypothesis, which will be referred to as the Wald CI because of its association with Wald hypothesis testing. If the number of estimated parameters is relatively large (say, $N_T - m < 30$), one can use the t-ratio:

$$\frac{\widehat{\beta}_j}{s_j} \sim t(N_T - m), \tag{3.34}$$

where $N_T = \sum n_i$ is the total number of observations and $N_T - m$ is the degrees of freedom (d.f.). It is worthwhile to note that the ratio in (3.34) does not have a t-distribution, as in a standard linear regression model, because we use an estimate of matrix $\mathbf{D}$, not the true value.

Many authors have indicated that profile-likelihood (PL) intervals perform better than usual Wald CIs in a nonlinear statistical model (Bates and Watts, 1988; Ritter and Bates, 1996). The idea of a PL confidence interval is as follows. Let j be fixed and we want to construct a confidence interval of the jth component of the vector $\boldsymbol{\gamma} = (\gamma_1, \gamma_2, ..., \gamma_k)'$ based on the log-likelihood $l(\boldsymbol{\gamma})$. Let $\widehat{\boldsymbol{\gamma}}$ be the MLE with the log-likelihood maximum, $l_{\max} = l(\widehat{\boldsymbol{\gamma}})$. We fix γ_j and denote the $(k - 1) \times 1$ vector $\widetilde{\boldsymbol{\gamma}} = (\gamma_1, ..., \gamma_{j-1}, \gamma_{j+1}, ..., \gamma_k)'$, with the jth component removed and find the maximum of the log-likelihood function over $\widetilde{\boldsymbol{\gamma}}$, which we denote $\widetilde{l}(\gamma_j)$, the constrained maximum. Then the $(1 - \alpha)100\%$ profile-likelihood CI for γ_j are the roots, x, of the equation

$$\widetilde{l}(x) = l_{\max} - \frac{1}{2}Z_{1-\alpha/2}^2, \tag{3.35}$$

where $Z_{1-\alpha/2}$ is the $(1 - \alpha/2)$th quantile of the normal distribution. Supposedly equation (3.35) has two roots, $x_1 < x_2$ (it may happen that either of the roots is infinity). Then the PL $(1-\alpha)100\%$ CI for γ_j is (x_1, x_2). To account for d.f. following the line of (3.34), we use the t-distribution to take another critical value that leads to the PL CI

$$\widetilde{l}(x) = l_{\max} - \frac{1}{2}q_{1-\alpha/2, t(n-m)}^2, \tag{3.36}$$

where $q_{1-\alpha/2, t(n-m)}$ is the $(1 - \alpha/2)$-quantile of the t-distribution with $n - m$ d.f. and n is the sample size. The advantage of (3.36) over (3.35) is that the former gives the exact CI for the linear model, e.g., when matrix $\mathbf{D}$ is known in the LME model. The reader is also referred to Section 4.3.4, where the profile-likelihood region is constructed for the growth curve model with random intercepts and autocorrelated residuals. Also, it is worthwhile to mention that, since confidence intervals and hypothesis testing are equivalent (Rao, 1973), the PL CI leads to a better test of $H_0 : \beta_j = 0$. We accept H_0 if the CI covers 0.

Now we come back to the LME model. The key point of the PL CI for the beta coefficient in the LME model is that computation of the constrained $\widetilde{l}$ reduces to another LME model. Indeed, assume that we want to find the PL CI for β_j. Denoting the $(m-1) \times 1$ vector $\widetilde{\boldsymbol{\beta}} = (\beta_1, ..., \beta_{j-1}, \beta_{j+1}, ... , \beta_m)'$ and a key dependent variable $\widetilde{\mathbf{y}}_i = \mathbf{y}_i - \beta_j \mathbf{x}_j$, under fixed β_j, the LME model can be written as

$$\widetilde{\mathbf{y}}_i = \widetilde{\mathbf{X}}_i \widetilde{\boldsymbol{\beta}} + \mathbf{Z}_i \mathbf{b}_i + \boldsymbol{\varepsilon}_i, \tag{3.37}$$

where $\widetilde{\mathbf{X}}_i$ is an $n_i \times (n-1)$ matrix with the jth column removed from $\mathbf{X}_i$. Since (3.37) is the LME model, we apply the same software as for the initial LME model to find maximum $\widetilde{l}$. The profile likelihood parameterizations of Section 2.2.4 are well suited for PL confidence interval construction.

Several numerical algorithms can be used to find the two roots of equation (3.36). Since computation of the constrained maximum $\widetilde{l}$ does not require new software, we can easily plot the graph of $\widetilde{l}$ against β_j in the interval where the roots of (3.36) are expected. For instance, if $\alpha = 0.05$, we may plot $\widetilde{l}$ in the interval $(\widehat{\beta}_j \pm 3 \times s_j)$ to obtain rough confidence limits by bracketing. More accurate limits can be computed using the derivative-free bisection or secant algorithms (Press et al. , 1992). Venzon and Moolgavkar (1988) suggest a Newton–Raphson procedure to find exact roots, but its realization requires special software.

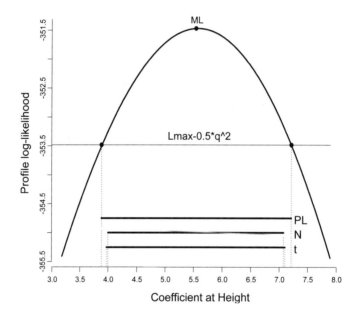

FIGURE 3.2. Profile-likelihood (PL)-based confidence interval for the coefficient at height, β in the LME model with family data. The PL confidence limits are the roots of the equation $l(\beta) = l_{\max} - 0.5q_t^2$, where q_t is the $(1 - \alpha/2)$th quantile of the t-distribution with $\sum n_i - m$ d.f. (in our example, $\alpha = 0.05$, $\sum n_i = 75$, $m = 2$). The PL interval is the widest; the narrowest is the Wald CI (N), $\widehat{\beta} \pm 1.96 \times SE$. The t-Wald CI (t) is a little wider because the t-quantile with 73 d.f. is $1.99 > 1.96$.

Example. We illustrate the profile-likelihood CI by the weight-height LME model with family data of Section 2.1; $\mathbf{W}_i = \alpha + \beta \mathbf{H}_i + b_i + \varepsilon_i$. If we are concerned with the CI for the slope β, we fix its value and come to the single random-intercept model $\mathbf{y}_i = \alpha + b_i + \varepsilon_i$ where

$$\mathbf{y}_i = \mathbf{W}_i - \beta\mathbf{H}_i. \tag{3.38}$$

Using the `lme` function in R, we issue

```
lme(y~., random=~1|Family, data=FamilyData)$logLik
```

which returns the value $\tilde{l}$, where `y` computed by formula (3.38) belongs to the dataframe `FamilyData`. By default, the method of estimation is RML, and we could use the ML-based CI using `method="ML"`. Three confidence intervals for β are depicted in Figure 3.2; 95% confidence intervals N and t are classical Wald CI based on $\hat{\beta}/s_\beta$. The former is (3.97, 7.10) and takes the coefficient 1.96 at s_β. The latter is (3.99, 7.07) and takes 1.99, the 0.975 quantile of the t-distribution with 73 d.f. The PL CI is wider, (3.88, 7.21).

Problems for Section 3.4

1. Prove that the profile-likelihood CI defined by (3.36) coincides with the standard CI for linear regression.

2. Write an R function that finds two roots of (3.36) using the `uniroot` function. This function requires specification of a segment such that the left-hand side of (3.36) has values with opposite signs at the ends. The ML estimate may serve one point and the four fold estimate SE may serve as another point.

3*. Compare the profile likelihood CI with the standard CI for the slope coefficient in a small sample using simulations. Use a linear model with a random intercept (2.66) for this purpose. Compute the coverage probability and the average width for a sequence of N and a variance of the random intercept. Can you defend the statement that the profile CI is better for small N and that the difference is negligible for large N?

3.5   Statistical testing of the presence of random effects

A question of essential importance in the LME model is whether random effects are relevant. In statistical language, this translates into hypothesis testing,

$$H_0 : \mathbf{D} = \mathbf{0}. \tag{3.39}$$

A "computational" answer is suggested in Section 2.6: if (2.93) is a positive definite matrix, then $\widehat{\mathbf{D}}_{ML}$ is not zero. But what if $\widehat{\mathbf{D}}_{ML}$ is very small; can we still claim that the true $\mathbf{D}$ is zero? What is small? Recall that the idea of statistical hypothesis testing is to find what is small in the language of the type I error.

Hypothesis (3.39) belongs to the *nonstandard* testing situation described by Self and Liang (1987) because $\mathbf{D} = \mathbf{0}$ is the boundary point of the parameter space. This is a well-recognized problem in statistics and several authors have addressed this problem in general terms (Chernoff, 1954; Moran, 1971). In particular, the consequences of the fact that $\mathbf{D} = \mathbf{0}$ lies on the boundary of the parameter set in the LME model have been described in detail by Stram and Lee (1994) and more recently by Stern and Welsh (2000). The point of complication comes from the fact that if $\boldsymbol{\theta}_0$ is a boundary point, the likelihood ratio-test does not have a limiting χ^2-distribution. Indeed, the optimal properties of the MLE and likelihood ratio test are developed for the case when the true parameter is an inner point to be able to apply the Taylor series expansion. Consequently, the likelihood ratio test for (3.39) would lead to a lower power even in large samples. A large-sample adjustment of the likelihood ratio test in variance components model has been suggested by Stern and Welsh (2000). The score test for the LME model has been discussed by Verbeke and Molenberghs (2003).

One can expect that the actual significance level of the likelihood ratio test will be less than nominal—this is the conclusion of Morrell (1998) after extensive simulation study. We shall illustrate this statement by a simple example in which the power function admits a closed-form solution.

Example: *Statistical testing on the boundary of the parameter space.* We consider a simple example that illustrates the difficulty of hypothesis testing, particularly the failure of the likelihood ratio test when the null hypothesis is on the boundary of the parameter space. Let $y_i \sim \mathcal{N}(\mu, \sigma^2)$ be iid $(i = 1, ..., N)$, where μ is nonnegative and σ^2 is known. The null hypothesis is $H_0 : \mu = 0$, with the alternative $H_A : \mu > 0$. The standard test, which is equivalent to the likelihood ratio test with the alternative $H_A : \mu \neq 0$, is based on the MLE $\overline{y} = \sum_{i=1}^{N} y_i/N$ and uses the fact that under $\mu = 0$,

$$N\sigma^{-2}\overline{y}^2 \sim \chi^2(1), \tag{3.40}$$

meaning that under the null hypothesis, the left-hand side is distributed as χ^2 with 1 degree of freedom. The standard test statistic (3.40) assumes implicitly that the parameter μ is unrestricted, $\mu \in (-\infty, \infty)$. What is wrong when it applies to the parameter space $\mu \geq 0$? When the parameter μ is restricted, the likelihood should be maximized on the interval $[0, \infty)$, which leads to the MLE different from the average, namely,

$$\widehat{\mu} = \max(0, \overline{y}) = \begin{cases} 0 \text{ if } \overline{y} < 0 \\ \overline{y} \text{ if } \overline{y} \geq 0. \end{cases} \tag{3.41}$$

Now the likelihood ratio test breaks down for (3.41) because $N\sigma^{-2}\widehat{\mu}^2$ is no longer distributed as $\chi^2(1)$! Let us examine the consequences of the use of the standard likelihood ratio test for the restricted parameter space. Let the significance level be fixed, α. Then, as follows from (3.40), the critical value of the likelihood ratio test, c, is the $(1 - \alpha)$th quantile of the χ^2-distribution with 1 degree of freedom. We compute the real power of the test, where instead of $\overline{y}$, one uses the restricted MLE, $\widehat{\mu}$:

$$\begin{aligned} \text{Power}(\mu) &= \Pr(\text{Reject } H_0|\mu) = \Pr(N\sigma^{-2}\widehat{\mu}^2 > c|\mu) \\ &= 1 - \Pr(N\sigma^{-2}\widehat{\mu}^2 \leq c|\mu) = 1 - \Pr(y < \sqrt{c}|\mu)], \end{aligned}$$

where μ is the true parameter and $y \sim \mathcal{N}(0, 1)$. Thus, the true power function for the standard likelihood ratio test, which ignores the fact that $\mu = 0$ is the boundary point, is

$$\text{Power}(\mu) = 1 - \frac{1}{\sqrt{2\pi}} \int_{-\infty}^{\sqrt{c}} e^{-\frac{1}{2}(t-\mu)^2} dt = 1 - \Phi(\sqrt{c} - \mu).$$

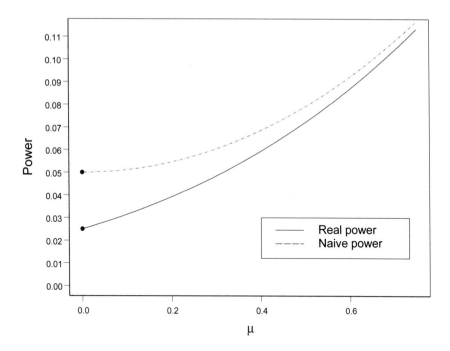

FIGURE 3.3. Two power functions for the likelihood ratio test: for example, $H_0 : \mu = 0$ with parameter space $\{\mu : \mu \geq 0\}$. The real power is less, especially in the neighborhood of small μ. This leads to a double increase in type II error when μ is close to zero.

Recall that if $\mu = 0$ would not be a boundary point then the naive power would be

$$
\begin{aligned}
1 - \Pr(N\sigma^{-2}\overline{y}^2 \;\; &\leq \;\; c|\mu) = 1 - \Pr(y < \sqrt{c}|\mu) + \Pr(y < -\sqrt{c}|\mu) \\
&= \;\; 1 - \Phi(\sqrt{c} - \mu) - \Phi(-\sqrt{c} - \mu).
\end{aligned}
$$

The two power functions are shown in Figure 3.3. When applying the likelihood ratio test to $H_0 : \mu = 0$, it is wrongly believed that the power function is dashed. The real power is less; the difference is particularly striking at small positive values of μ. Specifically, the significance level of the test is half as large as believed. Practically, it means that using the restricted MLE and standard likelihood ratio test, we will increase type II error, i.e., we will accept $\mu = 0$ when in fact $\mu > 0$.

∎

Next we develop an *exact* F-test for hypothesis (3.39) for the LME model (2.14). That test may be viewed as a generalization of the F-test for the variance components model. The attractive feature of the test is that it has an exact significance level and it should work in small samples as well.

The idea of the test is that when $\mathbf{D} = \mathbf{0}$, the difference between the minimum sum of squares with random effects, $S_{\min}$, and the minimum sum of squares without random effects (OLS) should be close. Thus, we compute the residual SS:

$$
S_{OLS} = \sum_{i=1}^{N} \left\| \mathbf{y}_i - \mathbf{X}_i \widehat{\boldsymbol{\beta}}_{OLS} \right\|^2
$$

assuming no random effects. Next we compare it to the minimum sum of squares in the presence of random effects, i.e., the minimum (2.33), $S_{\min} = \min_\gamma \|\mathbf{y} - \mathbf{W}\gamma\|^2$, where matrix the $\mathbf{W}$ is defined by (2.34) and $\gamma = (\beta', \mathbf{b}_1', ..., \mathbf{b}_N')'$. The next result is crucial to our test.

Theorem 15 *Let $r = rank(\mathbf{W})$. Then under (3.39), the ratio of the two quadratic forms has F-distribution, or more precisely,*

$$\frac{(S_{OLS} - S_{\min})/(r - m)}{S_{\min}/(N_T - r)} \sim F(r - m, N_T - r). \tag{3.42}$$

Proof. We shall prove that if $\mathbf{D} = \mathbf{0}$, the two quadratic forms $\sigma^{-2}S_{\min}$ and $\sigma^{-2}(S_{OLS} - S_{\min})$ follow a χ^2-distribution, with $N_T - r$ and $r - m$ degrees of freedom respectively, and are independent. We start with the denominator. Since $\mathbf{P_W} = \mathbf{W}(\mathbf{W}'\mathbf{W})^+\mathbf{W}'$ is the projection matrix and $\mathbf{X}$ is a submatrix of $\mathbf{W}$, we have $(\mathbf{I} - \mathbf{P_W})\mathbf{X} = \mathbf{0}$ and therefore

$$S_{\min} = \mathbf{y}'(\mathbf{I} - \mathbf{P_W})\mathbf{y} = (\mathbf{X}\beta + \varepsilon)'(\mathbf{I} - \mathbf{P_W})(\mathbf{X}\beta + \varepsilon) = \varepsilon'(\mathbf{I} - \mathbf{P_W})\varepsilon.$$

But $\mathbf{I} - \mathbf{P_W}$ is an idempotent matrix with the rank and trace equal to $N_T - r$ and therefore $\sigma^{-2}S_{\min} \sim \chi^2(N_T - r)$. Further, we have $S_{OLS} = \mathbf{y}'(\mathbf{I} - \mathbf{P_X})\mathbf{y} = \varepsilon'(\mathbf{I} - \mathbf{P_X})\varepsilon$ and $S_{OLS} - S_{\min} = \varepsilon'(\mathbf{P_W} - \mathbf{P_X})\varepsilon = \varepsilon'\mathbf{T}\varepsilon$ where $\mathbf{T} = \mathbf{P_W} - \mathbf{P_X}$, the matrix of quadratic form in the numerator. It is easy to see that $(\mathbf{I} - \mathbf{P_W})\mathbf{T} = \mathbf{0}$ because $(\mathbf{I} - \mathbf{P_W})\mathbf{X} = \mathbf{0}$ and $(\mathbf{I} - \mathbf{P_W})\mathbf{W} = \mathbf{0}$.

Now we shall prove that matrix $\mathbf{T}$ is idempotent. First, we see that

$$(\mathbf{I} - \mathbf{P_X})(\mathbf{I} - \mathbf{P_W}) = (\mathbf{I} - \mathbf{P_W})(\mathbf{I} - \mathbf{P_X}) = \mathbf{I} - \mathbf{P_W}.$$

Then

$$\begin{aligned}
\mathbf{T}^2 &= (\mathbf{P_W} - \mathbf{P_X})(\mathbf{P_W} - \mathbf{P_X}) \\
&= [(\mathbf{I} - \mathbf{P_X}) - (\mathbf{I} - \mathbf{P_W})][(\mathbf{I} - \mathbf{P_X}) - (\mathbf{I} - \mathbf{P_W})] \\
&= \mathbf{I} - \mathbf{P_X} - \mathbf{I} + \mathbf{P_W} - \mathbf{I} + \mathbf{P_W} + \mathbf{I} - \mathbf{P_W} = \mathbf{P_W} - \mathbf{P_X} = \mathbf{T},
\end{aligned}$$

so the matrix $\mathbf{T}$ is idempotent. Now we find the trace (rank) $\text{tr}(\mathbf{T}) = \text{tr}(\mathbf{P_W}) - \text{tr}(\mathbf{P_X}) = r - m$, and therefore $\sigma^{-2}(S_{OLS} - S_{\min}) \sim \chi^2(r - m)$. The F-distribution (3.42) follows from the fact that the ratio of two independent quadratic forms divided by their degrees of freedom has F-distribution. ∎

When random effects are present in the LME model (2.14) ($\mathbf{D} \neq \mathbf{0}$), $S_{\min}$ should be relatively small, and therefore the ratio (3.42) becomes large. Recall that the relationship between $S_{OLS}/S_{\min}$ and the magnitude of matrix $\widehat{\mathbf{D}}_{ML}$ was noticed in Section 2.7. Thus, we reject $H_0 : \mathbf{D} = \mathbf{0}$ if the left-hand side of (3.42) is large. More precisely, the F-test for hypothesis $H_0 : \mathbf{D} = \mathbf{0}$ works as follows. Let $1 - \alpha$ be a chosen significance level (e.g., $\alpha = 0.05$) and $f_{0.95}$ be the quantile of F-distribution with $r - m$ and $N_T - r$ degrees of freedom. Then H_0 is rejected when

$$\frac{(S_{OLS} - S_{\min})/(r - m)}{S_{\min}/(N_T - r)} > f_{0.95}. \tag{3.43}$$

In another interpretation, the null is rejected when the ratio $S_{OLS}/S_{\min}$ exceeds $1 + (r - m)/(N_T - r)f_{0.95}$.

This test may be viewed as a generalization of the F-test developed for the VARCOMP models; see Searle et al. (1992), and Mathew and Sinha (1992), and for a mixed effects model with one random effect, Khuri et al. (1998). Indeed, for the VARCOMP model of Section 1.2 we have

$$y_{ij} = \beta + b_i + \varepsilon_{ij}, \quad j = 1, ..., n_i, i = 1, ..., N, \tag{3.44}$$

where $\varepsilon_{ij} \sim \mathcal{N}(0, \sigma^2)$ and $b_i \sim \mathcal{N}(0, \sigma^2 d)$. Then (3.42) for hypothesis $H_0 : d = 0$ collapses to a well known F-test

$$\frac{\sum n_i(\overline{y}_i - \sum_{j=1}^{N} n_j \overline{y}_j / N_T)^2 / (N - 1)}{\left(\sum_{i,j} y_{ij}^2 - \sum_{i=1}^{N} n_i \overline{y}_i^2\right) / (N_T - N)} \sim F(N - 1, N_T - N); \tag{3.45}$$

see Searle et al. (1992, p. 77). We prove that for model (3.44) our F-test (3.42) collapses to (3.45). Indeed, for (3.44) we have $r = N$, and for the denominator of (3.42),

$$S_{\min} = \sum_i \sum_j (y_{ij} - \overline{y}_i)^2 = \sum_{i,j} y_{ij}^2 - \sum_{i=1}^{N} n_i \overline{y}_i^2.$$

For the numerator, after some algebra,

$$
\begin{aligned}
&S_{OLS} - S_{\min} \\
&= \sum_i \sum_j (y_{ij} - \overline{\overline{y}})^2 - \sum_{i,j} y_{ij}^2 + \sum_i n_i \overline{y}_i^2 = \sum_i n_i(\overline{y}_i - \sum_j n_j \overline{y}_j / N_T)^2.
\end{aligned}
$$

Thus, (3.42) for the VARCOMP model collapses to (3.45). It is possible to show that our F-test collapses to existing tests in other special cases described by Khuri et al. (1998). Since the statistic in (3.42) is expressed in terms of the minimum sum of squares, one can easily generalize it to nonlinear models, e.g., see Section 7.7.5.

Problems for Section 3.5

1. Confirm by simulations the two power functions displayed in Figure 3.3.

2. Under what assumption $r > m$?

3*. Estimate the power of the F-test for VARCOMP model (3.44) using simulations. Derive the power analytically using the noncentral F-distribution.

4*. Compare the F-test (3.42) with the likelihood ratio test. Take note of the fact that the size of the latter test is not equal to α (the nominal size of the test).

3.6   Statistical properties of MLE

3.6.1   Small-sample properties

Little is known about small-sample properties of estimators in linear mixed effects models. Here we recover and prove the often-forgotten important fact that the ML estimator for $\boldsymbol{\beta}$ is unbiased in small samples. Also we prove that the variance parameters in a balanced random growth curve model are unbiased as well.

Fixed effects coefficients

It is well known that the OLS estimator is unbiased in linear regression model. Also, the GLS estimator is unbiased if the variance-covariance matrix is known. Generally, if an estimator depends on an unknown parameter and we replace that parameter with its estimate, the resulting estimator is biased. Perhaps because of this fact, many believe that the estimated GLS (EGLS); i.e., the GLS estimator with estimated variance-covariance matrix is biased. Indeed, the fact that the estimated GLS is unbiased in small samples is known, but not widely; see Kackar and Harville (1984) or Kenward and Roger (1997). The unbiasedness simply follows from the facts that in most cases (a) the estimate of the covariance matrix is an even function of residuals and (b) the EGLS estimator can be expressed as an odd function of residuals. Therefore, the resulting expected value is the true beta because the distribution is symmetric about $\boldsymbol{\beta}$.

Below, we provide conditions on the unbiasedness of the GLS estimator with an estimated variance-covariance matrix and prove that the MLE for $\boldsymbol{\beta}$ in the LME model is unbiased in small samples.

Lemma 16 *Let the general linear model be defined as* $\mathbf{y} = \mathbf{X}\boldsymbol{\beta} + \boldsymbol{\eta}$, *where* $\mathbf{y}$ *is an* $n \times 1$ *vector of the dependent variable,* $E(\boldsymbol{\eta}) = \mathbf{0}$, *and* $cov(\boldsymbol{\eta}) = \sigma^2 \mathbf{V}$. *The estimated GLS estimator is*

$$\widehat{\boldsymbol{\beta}}_{GLS} = (\mathbf{X}'\widehat{\mathbf{V}}^{-1}\mathbf{X})^{-1}(\mathbf{X}'\widehat{\mathbf{V}}^{-1}\mathbf{y}),$$

where $\widehat{\mathbf{V}} = \widehat{\mathbf{V}}(\boldsymbol{\eta})$ *is an estimator of* $\mathbf{V}$. *If (a)* $\boldsymbol{\eta}$ *has a symmetric distribution, i.e.,* $f(\boldsymbol{\eta}) = f(-\boldsymbol{\eta})$, *where* f *is the density of* $\boldsymbol{\eta}$, *and (b)* $\widehat{\mathbf{V}}$ *is an even function of* $\boldsymbol{\eta}$, *i.e.,* $\widehat{\mathbf{V}}(\boldsymbol{\eta}) = \widehat{\mathbf{V}}(-\boldsymbol{\eta})$, *the EGLS estimator is unbiased.*

Proof. Since $\widehat{\boldsymbol{\beta}}_{GLS} - \boldsymbol{\beta} = (\mathbf{X}'\widehat{\mathbf{V}}^{-1}\mathbf{X})^{-1}(\mathbf{X}'\widehat{\mathbf{V}}^{-1}\boldsymbol{\eta})$, it suffices to show that $E\mathbf{p}(\boldsymbol{\eta}) = \mathbf{0}$ where $\mathbf{p}(\boldsymbol{\eta}) = \widehat{\boldsymbol{\beta}}_{GLS} - \boldsymbol{\beta}$. But $\mathbf{p}$ is an odd function of $\boldsymbol{\eta}$ because $\widehat{\mathbf{V}}(-\boldsymbol{\eta}) = \widehat{\mathbf{V}}(\boldsymbol{\eta}) = \widehat{\mathbf{V}}$ and

$$\mathbf{p}(-\boldsymbol{\eta}) = (\mathbf{X}'\widehat{\mathbf{V}}^{-1}\mathbf{X})^{-1}(\mathbf{X}'\widehat{\mathbf{V}}^{-1}(-\boldsymbol{\eta})) = -\mathbf{p}(\boldsymbol{\eta}).$$

It follows from multivariate calculus that an odd function has a zero integral:

$$E\mathbf{p}(\boldsymbol{\eta}) = \int \mathbf{p}(\boldsymbol{\eta})f(\boldsymbol{\eta})d\boldsymbol{\eta} = \mathbf{0},$$

because $\mathbf{p}(\boldsymbol{\eta})f(\boldsymbol{\eta})$ is an odd function. Thus, $\widehat{\boldsymbol{\beta}}_{GLS}$ is unbiased for any n.   ∎

Now we apply this lemma to the maximum/restricted maximum likelihood estimator $\widehat{\boldsymbol{\beta}}_{ML}$, which is (2.28) with $\mathbf{D}$ replaced by $\widehat{\mathbf{D}}_{ML}$ or $\widehat{\mathbf{D}}_{RML}$.

Theorem 17 *The maximum likelihood estimator* $\widehat{\boldsymbol{\beta}}_{ML}$ *in the linear mixed effects model with normal errors is unbiased.*

Proof. We write the LME model (2.14) in one equation as (2.8), with $\mathbf{y}, \mathbf{X}$, and $\boldsymbol{\eta}$ defined by (2.9). We notice that since $\boldsymbol{\varepsilon}_i$ and $\mathbf{b}_i$ are normally distributed, $\boldsymbol{\eta}$ has a symmetric distribution so that condition (a) of Lemma 16 holds. Since $\widehat{\boldsymbol{\beta}}_{ML}$ has the form of the GLS estimator (2.28) with $\mathbf{D}$ replaced by $\widehat{\mathbf{D}}_{ML}$, it suffices to show that $\widehat{\mathbf{D}}_{ML}$ is an even function of $\{\boldsymbol{\eta}_i\}$. The log-likelihood function (2.15) in terms of $\boldsymbol{\eta}_i$, up to a constant term, can be rewritten as

$$-\frac{1}{2}\{N_T \ln \sigma^2 + \sum_{i=1}^{N}[\ln |\mathbf{I} + \mathbf{Z}_i \mathbf{D} \mathbf{Z}_i'| + \sigma^{-2}\boldsymbol{\eta}_i'(\mathbf{I} + \mathbf{Z}_i \mathbf{D} \mathbf{Z}_i')^{-1}\boldsymbol{\eta}_i]\},$$

which is an even function of $\{\boldsymbol{\eta}_i\}$. Therefore, $\widehat{\mathbf{D}}_{ML}$ is also an even function as its maximizer. All conditions of Lemma 16 are fulfilled and the MLE for $\boldsymbol{\beta}$ is unbiased. ∎

The unbiasedness of $\widehat{\boldsymbol{\beta}}$ in small samples holds when $\mathbf{D}$ is estimated by any of the methods considered below, such as MINQUE and method of moments, because $\widehat{\mathbf{D}}$ can be expressed as an even function of $\{\boldsymbol{\eta}_i\}$.

Variance parameters

Generally, maximum likelihood estimators of variance parameters σ^2 and $\mathbf{D}$ are biased. Some have the mistaken impression that the RML estimators of the variance parameters are unbiased in a small sample (Brown and Prescott, 1999). In fact, the RML estimators are unbiased in *balanced* models. Here, we prove that these estimators are unbiased for the balanced random-coefficient (BRC) model of Section 2.3. This unbiasedness follows from the fact that for the BRC model the unbiased quadratic estimators MINQUE, MM, and VLS (considered later) collapse to the MLE. Nevertheless, the following theorem is instructive.

Theorem 18 *The variance parameters $\widehat{\sigma}^2_{ML}$ and $\widehat{\sigma}^2_{ML}\widehat{\mathbf{D}}_{RML}$ given by formulas (2.59) and (2.61) are unbiased for the balanced random-coefficient model.*

Proof. First, we prove the unbiasedness of $\widehat{\sigma}^2_{ML}$. If $\mathbf{P}_\mathbf{Z}$ denotes the projection matrix, then taking the expectation, we obtain

$$\begin{aligned} E\left[\mathbf{y}_i'(\mathbf{I} - \mathbf{P}_\mathbf{Z})\mathbf{y}_i\right] &= E\left[(\mathbf{Z}\boldsymbol{\beta} + \boldsymbol{\eta}_i)'(\mathbf{I} - \mathbf{P}_\mathbf{Z})(\mathbf{Z}\boldsymbol{\beta} + \boldsymbol{\eta}_i)'\right] \\ &= E\left[\boldsymbol{\eta}_i'(\mathbf{I} - \mathbf{P}_\mathbf{Z})\boldsymbol{\eta}_i'\right], \end{aligned}$$

where $E(\boldsymbol{\eta}_i) = \mathbf{0}$ and $\text{cov}(\boldsymbol{\eta}_i) = \sigma^2(\mathbf{I} + \mathbf{Z}\mathbf{D}\mathbf{Z}')$. Next, using the formula for the expected value of the quadratic form, the expectation above simplifies to

$$\sigma^2 \text{tr}\left[(\mathbf{I} + \mathbf{Z}\mathbf{D}\mathbf{Z}')(\mathbf{I} - \mathbf{P}_\mathbf{Z})\right] = \sigma^2 \text{tr}(\mathbf{I} - \mathbf{P}_\mathbf{Z}) = \sigma^2(n - m),$$

which yields $E\sigma^2_{ML} = \sigma^2$.

Second, we prove the unbiasedness of $\widehat{\sigma}^2_{ML}\widehat{\mathbf{D}}_{RML}$. Since $\mathbf{e}_i = \boldsymbol{\eta}_i - N^{-1}\mathbf{P}_\mathbf{Z}\sum_{j=1}^{N}\boldsymbol{\eta}_j$, we have

$$\begin{aligned} \sum_{i=1}^{N}\mathbf{e}_i\mathbf{e}_i' &= \sum_{i=1}^{N}\boldsymbol{\eta}_i\boldsymbol{\eta}_i' - N^{-1}(\sum_{i=1}^{N}\boldsymbol{\eta}_i)(\sum_{j=1}^{N}\boldsymbol{\eta}_j)'\mathbf{P}_\mathbf{Z} \\ &\quad - N^{-1}\mathbf{P}_\mathbf{Z}(\sum_{j=1}^{N}\boldsymbol{\eta}_j)(\sum_{i=1}^{N}\boldsymbol{\eta}_i)' + N^{-1}\mathbf{P}_\mathbf{Z}(\sum_{j=1}^{N}\boldsymbol{\eta}_j)(\sum_{j=1}^{N}\boldsymbol{\eta}_j)'\mathbf{P}_\mathbf{Z}. \end{aligned}$$

The expected value of the first term is $N\sigma^2(\mathbf{I} + \mathbf{Z}\mathbf{D}\mathbf{Z}')$. The expected value of the second and third terms is $\sigma^2(\mathbf{P}_\mathbf{Z} + \mathbf{Z}\mathbf{D}\mathbf{Z}')$. The expected value of the fourth term is also $\sigma^2(\mathbf{P_Z}+\mathbf{ZDZ'})$. Combining all four expectations yields $E(\widehat{\mathbf{E}}\widehat{\mathbf{E}}') = \sigma^2\left[N\mathbf{I} - \mathbf{P_Z} + (N-1)\mathbf{ZDZ'}\right]$, and finally, since $\widehat{\sigma}^2_{ML}$ is unbiased,

$$
\begin{aligned}
E(\widehat{\sigma}^2_{ML}\widehat{\mathbf{D}}_{RML}) &= \frac{\sigma^2}{N-1}\left[(N-1)(\mathbf{Z'Z})^{-1} + (N-1)\mathbf{D}\right] - \sigma^2(\mathbf{Z'Z}) \\
&= \sigma^2\mathbf{D},
\end{aligned}
$$

which proves the unbiasedness.

3.6.2 Large-sample properties

A characteristic property of the linear mixed effects model with normally distributed errors is that the information matrix for beta coefficients and variance parameters is block diagonal, which means that the MLEs for $\boldsymbol{\beta}$ and $(\sigma^2, \mathbf{D})$ are asymptotically independent (Section 3.3). There are two consequences of this fact. The numerical consequence is that maximization of the log-likelihood function may be accomplished separately for $\boldsymbol{\beta}$ and the variance parameters $(\sigma^2, \mathbf{D})$ because the expected Hessian matrix has a block diagonal form (one may expect that the off-diagonal elements of the actual Hessian are close to zero, especially in a large sample). The statistical consequence, in the line of the pseudo-likelihood theory (Gong and Saminiego, 1981; Parke, 1986), is that the use of *any* consistent estimate of $\mathbf{D}$ in the GLS formula (2.28) would lead to an efficient estimator of $\boldsymbol{\beta}$. See Section 3.15, where the LME model with not necessarily random variables is considered. As we shall learn from the following chapters, this fact remains true for nonlinear marginal mixed models. See Appendix 13.1.3 for a general theory on pseudo-likelihood.

To make mathematically correct asymptotic statements about $\widehat{\boldsymbol{\beta}}$ and $\widehat{\mathbf{D}}$, we need to specify the behavior of matrices $\mathbf{X}_i$ and $\mathbf{Z}_i$ on infinity when $N \to \infty$. There are two ways to do it: to assume that these matrices are fixed (deterministic scheme or fixed design) or random (stochastic scheme or random design). In the *deterministic* scheme, we need to assume the boundedness of matrix elements and the existence of certain matrix limits. In the *stochastic* scheme, we assume that $\mathbf{X}_i$ and $\mathbf{Z}_i$ are random, or more precisely, independent and identically distributed (iid), meaning that there exists a multivariate distribution from which $\mathbf{X}_i$ and $\mathbf{Z}_i$ are drawn. Notice that if matrices $\mathbf{X}_i$ and $\mathbf{Z}_i$ are fixed, the $\{\mathbf{y}_i\}$ are not iid even when $n_i =$const. To the contrary, if $\mathbf{X}_i$ and $\mathbf{Z}_i$ are random independent and identically distributed then the $\{\mathbf{y}_i\}$ are iid as well. The major advantage of the stochastic scheme is that we can apply maximum likelihood or estimating equation theory because the observations are iid. However, in the deterministic approach, one needs to provide individual asymptotic study because $\{\mathbf{y}_i\}$ are not iid.

To illustrate the difference between the deterministic and stochastic schemes, we consider the linear regression model.

Asymptotic properties of the OLS estimator in linear regression

We consider the standard linear regression model in the form

$$
y_i = \boldsymbol{\beta}'\mathbf{x}_i + \varepsilon_i, \tag{3.46}
$$

where the $\{\varepsilon_i\}$ are iid, $E(\varepsilon_i) = 0$, $\text{var}(\varepsilon_i) = \sigma^2$, $i = 1, ..., N$. Note that the distribution of the ε_i may or may not be normal. The Ordinary Least Squares (OLS) estimator is

$$\widehat{\boldsymbol{\beta}}_N = (\mathbf{X}'\mathbf{X})^{-1}\mathbf{X}'\mathbf{y} = \left(\sum_{i=1}^{N}\mathbf{x}_i\mathbf{x}_i'\right)^{-1}\left(\sum_{i=1}^{N}\mathbf{x}_i'y_i\right).$$

We use the index N to emphasize the dependence on the sample size. We want to provide conditions on consistency and asymptotic normality of the OLS estimator when $N \rightarrow \infty$. Surprisingly, in the literature there is not much clarity on the issue of whether the independent variables $\{\mathbf{x}_i\}$ are deterministic or random (stochastic). A deterministic scheme is convenient and broadly accepted when the statistical properties of the OLS estimator are studied in a small sample; then (3.46) is referred to as a *linear model*. In fact, the celebrated Gauss–Markov theorem about the optimality of $\widehat{\boldsymbol{\beta}}_N$ works for fixed $\mathbf{x}_i$. However, it is less well known that the Gauss–Markov theorem is not true for random $\mathbf{x}_i$, i.e., in the stochastic approach, as shown by Demidenko (1981) and Shaffer (1991).

Deterministic scheme: $\mathbf{x}_i$ are fixed vectors. It is important to note that if the $\{\mathbf{x}_i\}$ are fixed, the $\{y_i\}$ are not identically distributed because they have different means, $E(y_i) = \boldsymbol{\beta}'\mathbf{x}_i \neq$const. To prove the asymptotic properties of the OLS estimator we use a multivariate version of the Central Limit Theorem (CLT) of Appendix 13.1.1. In view of that theorem, and to provide the penalized and asymptotic normality of the OLS estimator, we need to assume that

$$\|\mathbf{x}_i\| \leq B, \quad \lim_{N\rightarrow\infty}\frac{1}{N}\sum_{i=1}^{N}\mathbf{x}_i\mathbf{x}_i' = \mathbf{A}, \tag{3.47}$$

where B is a constant and $\mathbf{A}$ is a nonsingular matrix. Then it is easy to show that under conditions (3.47), the OLS estimator is consistent,

$$p\lim_{N\rightarrow\infty}\widehat{\boldsymbol{\beta}}_N = \boldsymbol{\beta},$$

and asymptotically normal: namely,

$$\sqrt{N}(\widehat{\boldsymbol{\beta}}_N - \boldsymbol{\beta}) \simeq \mathcal{N}(\mathbf{0}, \sigma^2\mathbf{A}^{-1}).$$

To prove that the OLS estimator is asymptotically efficient requires more work because observations $\{y_i\}$ are not iid. To the contrary, we do not have such a problem in the stochastic scheme because then the $\{y_i\}$ are iid and we simply refer to the estimating equation or M-theory; see Appendix 13.1.4.

Stochastic scheme: $\mathbf{x}_i$ are random vectors. Following Gallant (1987), we assume that there is a general multivariate distribution F_x from which the $\mathbf{x}_i$ is drawn; thus the $\{\mathbf{x}_i\}$ are iid. More precisely, we assume that the marginal mean and covariance matrix exist,

$$E(\mathbf{x}) = \int \mathbf{z}\,dF(\mathbf{z}), \quad E(\mathbf{x}\mathbf{x}') = \int \mathbf{z}\mathbf{z}'\,dF_x(\mathbf{z}), \tag{3.48}$$

and moreover, the matrix $E(\mathbf{x}\mathbf{x}')$ is not singular. Also, as part of the standard regression analysis, it is assumed that ε_i and $\mathbf{x}_i$ are independent. The marginal distribution F may have unknown parameters $\boldsymbol{\xi}$, so that the complete linear regression model with random $\mathbf{x}_i$ is written as

$$y_i|\mathbf{x}_i = \boldsymbol{\beta}'\mathbf{x}_i + \varepsilon_i, \quad \mathbf{x}_i \sim F(\cdot; \boldsymbol{\xi}).$$

Importantly, $\boldsymbol{\xi}$ must be unrelated to $\boldsymbol{\beta}$. In the special case when $\varepsilon_i \sim \mathcal{N}(0, \sigma^2)$, the complete log-likelihood function is

$$l(\boldsymbol{\beta}, \sigma^2; \boldsymbol{\xi}) = -\frac{1}{2} \left\{ n \ln \sigma^2 + \frac{1}{\sigma^2} \sum_{i=1}^{N} (y_i - \boldsymbol{\beta}' \mathbf{x}_i)^2 \right\} + \sum_{i=1}^{N} \ln f(\mathbf{x}_i; \boldsymbol{\xi}),$$

where $f = F'$. Since the information matrix for $(\boldsymbol{\beta}, \sigma^2, \boldsymbol{\xi})$ is block diagonal, estimation of $(\boldsymbol{\beta}, \sigma^2)$ and $\boldsymbol{\xi}$ may be accomplished separately without efficiency loss. Consequently, $\boldsymbol{\xi}$ does not affect the efficiency of the estimation of the regression parameters $\boldsymbol{\beta}$ and σ^2. A characteristic feature of this scheme is that it leads to iid $\{y_i, \mathbf{x}_i, \varepsilon_i\}$. Conditions (3.48) suffice to prove consistency and asymptotic normality of the OLS estimator. For example, to see that equation (3.48) implies consistency, we write

$$\widehat{\boldsymbol{\beta}}_N - \boldsymbol{\beta} = \left(\frac{1}{N} \sum_{i=1}^{N} \mathbf{x}_i \mathbf{x}_i' \right)^{-1} \left(\frac{1}{N} \sum_{i=1}^{N} \mathbf{x}_i' \varepsilon_i \right).$$

Then, by the Law of Large Numbers (LLN), $p \lim_{N \to \infty} N^{-1} \sum_{i=1}^{N} \mathbf{x}_i \mathbf{x}_i' = E(\mathbf{x}\mathbf{x}')$. Further, since the $\{\mathbf{x}_i' \varepsilon_i\}$ are iid, $p \lim_{N \to \infty} N^{-1} \sum_{i=1}^{N} \mathbf{x}_i' \varepsilon_i = E(\mathbf{x}'\varepsilon) = E(\mathbf{x}')E(\varepsilon) = 0$, due to the independence of ε and $\mathbf{x}$. Similarly, one proves the asymptotic normality of the OLS estimator because the $\{\mathbf{x}_i' \varepsilon_i\}$ are iid with zero mean and finite covariance matrix. Finally, by CLT we have

$$\sqrt{N}(\widehat{\boldsymbol{\beta}}_N - \boldsymbol{\beta}) \simeq \mathcal{N}\left(\mathbf{0}, \sigma^2 \left(\int \mathbf{z}\mathbf{z}' dF_x(\mathbf{z}) \right)^{-1} \right) \tag{3.49}$$

when $N \to \infty$.

Deterministic or stochastic scheme? When asymptotic properties are studied, the stochastic scheme is more convenient because the observations $\{(y_i, \mathbf{x}_i), i = 1, ..., N\}$ are then iid, which allows one to refer to standard maximum likelihood or estimating equation theory (see Appendix 13.1.4).

Asymptotic properties of the LME model

In view of the preceding discussion, we prefer to take the stochastic scheme when studying large-sample properties of the linear mixed effects model, i.e., to assume that matrices $\mathbf{X}_i$ and $\mathbf{Z}_i$ are random and independent of $\boldsymbol{\varepsilon}_i$ and $\mathbf{b}_i$. The assumption that matrices $\mathbf{X}_i$ and $\mathbf{Z}_i$ are random and iid greatly simplifies the asymptotic study and has been utilized in several papers (Hooper, 1993). A little trickier is specification of the number of observations per individual/cluster, n_i. In the stochastic scheme we assume that $\{n_i\}$ are random with a distribution defined on positive integers. Thus, observations $(\mathbf{X}_i, \mathbf{Z}_i, n_i)$ may be carried out first by sampling n_i and then sampling $(\mathbf{X}_i, \mathbf{Z}_i)$ conditional on n_i. The distribution of $\mathbf{X}_i$, $\mathbf{Z}_i$, or n_i may depend on unknown parameters, but importantly, those parameters do not contain $\boldsymbol{\beta}, \sigma^2$, or $\mathbf{D}$. We assume that in addition to the $\{\varepsilon_i\}$, the triples $\{(\mathbf{X}_i, \mathbf{Z}_i, n_i)\}$ are iid. Let the density of $(\mathbf{X}_i, \mathbf{Z}_i, n_i)$ be denoted f dependent on an unknown parameter $\boldsymbol{\xi}$. Then the complete LME model in the stochastic scheme can be written as

$$\mathbf{y}_i | (\mathbf{X}_i, \mathbf{Z}_i, n_i) \sim \mathcal{N}(\mathbf{X}_i \boldsymbol{\beta}, \sigma^2(\mathbf{I} + \mathbf{Z}_i \mathbf{D} \mathbf{Z}_i')), \quad (\mathbf{X}_i, \mathbf{Z}_i, n_i) \sim f(\cdot; \boldsymbol{\xi}),$$

with the complete log-likelihood function

$$l(\boldsymbol{\beta}, \sigma^2, \mathbf{D}) + \sum_{i=1}^{N} \ln f(\mathbf{X}_i, \mathbf{Z}_i, n_i; \boldsymbol{\xi}),$$

where l is the log-likelihood function for the LME model. It is important to observe that $\boldsymbol{\xi}$ does not affect estimation of $(\boldsymbol{\beta}, \sigma^2, \mathbf{D})$; in particular, the estimating equations are the same and the information matrix for $(\boldsymbol{\beta}, \sigma^2, \mathbf{D})$ and $\boldsymbol{\xi}$ is block diagonal. Since $\{(\mathbf{X}_i, \mathbf{Z}_i, n_i)\}$ are iid, so are $\{\mathbf{y}_i\}$ and $\{(\mathbf{y}_i, \mathbf{X}_i, \mathbf{Z}_i, n_i)\}$. This property is crucial: Since the observations are iid, we can legitimately refer to the maximum likelihood theory, and therefore the ML estimator is consistent, asymptotically normally distributed, and efficient, without additional proof. In particular, the information matrix for the variance parameters is $E_\mathbf{Z}\mathcal{I}$, where $\mathcal{I}$ is given by (3.16) and (3.17) is a consistent estimator of the covariance matrix. For example, for a random-coefficient model (1.12), as follows from formula (2.25), the asymptotic normality of the ML estimator can be written as

$$\sqrt{N}(\widehat{\boldsymbol{\beta}}_N - \boldsymbol{\beta}) \simeq \mathcal{N}\left(\mathbf{0}, \sigma^2 \left(\sum_{j=1}^{\infty} p_j \int \mathbf{z}\mathbf{z}' dF_j(\mathbf{z})\right)^{-1} + \mathbf{D}_*\right),$$

where F_j is the distribution function of $\mathbf{z}_j$ and $p_j = \Pr(n = n_j)$. Here we interpret the integral as the conditional expectation of $\mathbf{Z}'\mathbf{Z}$ at $n = n_j$ and p_j as the marginal probability that n takes value n_j.

What happens when n_i goes to infinity?

In some situations it is difficult to expect that the number of individuals/clusters N goes to infinity, as in the previous asymptotic. Can one still yield consistent estimates by infinitely increasing the number of observations per individual, n_i, while keeping N bounded? The answer is negative. To illustrate, let us take the random-coefficient model, $\mathbf{X}_i = \mathbf{Z}_i$. Using formula (2.25), we obtain

$$\text{cov}(\widehat{\boldsymbol{\beta}}) = \sigma^2 \left(\sum_{i=1}^{N} \mathbf{X}_i'(\mathbf{I} + \mathbf{X}_i\mathbf{D}\mathbf{X}_i')^{-1}\mathbf{X}_i\right)^{-1} = \sigma^2 \left(\sum_{i=1}^{N} \left((\mathbf{X}_i'\mathbf{X}_i)^{-1} + \mathbf{D}\right)^{-1}\right)^{-1}.$$
$$(3.50)$$

When $n_i \to \infty$ and N is fixed, we have $(\mathbf{X}_i'\mathbf{X}_i)^{-1} = O(n_i^{-1}) \to \mathbf{0}$, so that $\text{cov}(\widehat{\boldsymbol{\beta}}) \to \sigma^2\mathbf{D}/N$. Thus, for the LME model, an increasing number of individuals is a requirement for consistency, and $N \to \infty$ cannot be compensated by increasing the number of observations per individual.

Certainly, if both N and n_i go to infinity, the MLE regains its consistency: Then N times the covariance matrix is approximately $\sigma^2\mathbf{D}$. For a special balanced random-coefficient model, $\mathbf{X}_i = \mathbf{X}$ and $n_i = n =$ const, and as follows from (3.50), the N times covariance matrix is

$$\sigma^2 \left((\mathbf{X}'\mathbf{X})^{-1} + \mathbf{D}\right) \geq \sigma^2\mathbf{D}.$$

Thus, although large $\{n_i\}$ improve estimates, one needs to have as many subjects as possible. Loosely speaking, N is more important than n_i. Interestingly, a similar result holds for the nonlinear mixed effects model (see Section 8.4 for details).

3.6.3 ML and RML are asymptotically equivalent

In many instances, ML and RML estimates are close. For example, as follows from Section 4.1.5, for balanced data the difference between $\widehat{\sigma}^2_{ML}$ and $\widehat{\sigma}^2_{RML}$ is on the order m/N_T^2. The fact that the two methods give close estimates comes from their asymptotic equivalence: if N is relatively large, one may expect that the two methods are close.

The aim of this section is to prove that ML and RML have identical statistical properties in large samples. Since $\widehat{\boldsymbol{\beta}}$ and $\widehat{\sigma}^2$ are functions of $\widehat{\mathbf{D}}$, it suffices to prove the asymptotic equivalence of $\widehat{\mathbf{D}}$. This equivalence implies that the expected negative Hessian of the RML will be close to the standard ML for sufficiently large N. Thus, we can use the information matrix derived for ML when applying the Fisher scoring algorithm to RML, see Section 2.14.

As follows from Section 2.2.6, the log-likelihood functions for RML and ML differ by the term $\ln \left| \sum_{i=1}^N \mathbf{X}_i'(\mathbf{I} + \mathbf{Z}_i\mathbf{D}\mathbf{Z}_i')^{-1}\mathbf{X}_i \right|$. We show that the contribution of this term vanishes when $N \to \infty$. Indeed, normalizing the log-likelihood function by dividing by N, we obtain

$$\frac{1}{N} \ln \left| \sum_{i=1}^N \mathbf{X}_i'(\mathbf{I} + \mathbf{Z}_i\mathbf{D}\mathbf{Z}_i')^{-1}\mathbf{X}_i \right| = \frac{1}{N} \ln \left| \frac{1}{N} \sum_{i=1}^N \mathbf{X}_i'(\mathbf{I} + \mathbf{Z}_i\mathbf{D}\mathbf{Z}_i')^{-1}\mathbf{X}_i \right|$$

$$+ \frac{1}{N} \ln N = O\left(\frac{1}{N} \ln |\mathbf{M}| + \frac{1}{N} \ln N\right) = 0,$$

assuming that $\mathbf{M} = \lim_{N\to\infty} N^{-1} \sum_{i=1}^N \mathbf{X}_i'(\mathbf{I} + \mathbf{Z}_i\mathbf{D}\mathbf{Z}_i')^{-1}\mathbf{X}_i$ is a constant matrix. The fact that the augmented term vanishes serves as a heuristic proof. To prove that the two estimators are equivalent, we shall show that the estimating equations for ML and RML coincide for large N.

Proposition 19 *The statistical properties of the standard and restricted MLE are equivalent in large samples, or, more precisely, the augmented term in the estimating equation for* $\mathbf{D}$ *vanishes when* $N \to \infty$:

$$\lim_{N\to\infty} \frac{1}{N} \frac{\partial}{\partial \mathbf{D}} \ln \left| \sum_{i=1}^N \mathbf{X}_i'(\mathbf{I} + \mathbf{Z}_i\mathbf{D}\mathbf{Z}_i')^{-1}\mathbf{X}_i \right| = \mathbf{0}.$$

Proof. The estimating equations for ML and RML differ by the term

$$\frac{\partial}{\partial \mathbf{D}} \ln \left| \sum_{i=1}^N \mathbf{X}_i'(\mathbf{I} + \mathbf{Z}_i\mathbf{D}\mathbf{Z}_i')^{-1}\mathbf{X}_i \right|$$

$$= \sum_{i=1}^N \mathbf{Z}_i'\mathbf{V}_i^{-1}\mathbf{X}_i \left(\sum_{j=1}^N \mathbf{X}_j'\mathbf{V}_j^{-1}\mathbf{X}_j \right)^{-1} \mathbf{X}_i'\mathbf{V}_i^{-1}\mathbf{Z}_i,$$

where $\mathbf{V}_i = \mathbf{I} + \mathbf{Z}_i\mathbf{D}\mathbf{Z}_i'$. We shall show that this term vanishes when $N \to \infty$; that is, $\lim_{N\to\infty} N^{-1}\mathbf{G}_N = \mathbf{0}$, where

$$\mathbf{G}_N = \sum_{i=1}^N \mathbf{Z}_i'\mathbf{V}_i^{-1}\mathbf{X}_i \left(\sum_{j=1}^N \mathbf{X}_j'\mathbf{V}_j^{-1}\mathbf{X}_j \right)^{-1} \mathbf{X}_i'\mathbf{V}_i^{-1}\mathbf{Z}_i$$

is an $m \times m$ nonnegative definite matrix. Since $\mathbf{G} \leq \mathbf{I}\text{tr}(\mathbf{G})$, it suffices to prove that $\lim_{N \to \infty} N^{-1}\text{tr}(\mathbf{G}_N) = 0$. But

$$
\begin{aligned}
\text{tr}(\mathbf{G}_N) &= \left(\sum_{j=1}^{N} \mathbf{X}_j' \mathbf{V}_j^{-1} \mathbf{X}_j \right)^{-1} \text{tr} \left(\sum_{i=1}^{N} \mathbf{Z}_i' \mathbf{V}_i^{-1} \mathbf{X}_i \mathbf{X}_i' \mathbf{V}_i^{-1} \mathbf{Z}_i \right) \\
&= \left(\sum_{j=1}^{N} \mathbf{X}_j' \mathbf{V}_j^{-1} \mathbf{X}_j \right)^{-1} \sum_{i=1}^{N} \text{tr} \left(\mathbf{Z}_i' \mathbf{V}_i^{-1} \mathbf{X}_i \mathbf{X}_i' \mathbf{V}_i^{-1} \mathbf{Z}_i \right) \\
&= \left(\sum_{j=1}^{N} \mathbf{X}_j' \mathbf{V}_j^{-1} \mathbf{X}_j \right)^{-1} \sum_{i=1}^{N} \text{tr} \left(\mathbf{X}_i' \mathbf{V}_i^{-1} \mathbf{Z}_i \mathbf{Z}_i' \mathbf{V}_i^{-1} \mathbf{X}_i \right).
\end{aligned}
$$

Finally, we note that $\mathbf{V}_i^{-1} \mathbf{Z}_i \mathbf{Z}_i' \mathbf{V}_i^{-1} \leq \mathbf{V}_i^{-1}$ which gives $\text{tr}(\mathbf{G}_N) \leq \text{tr}(\mathbf{I}) = m$. This implies that $\lim_{N \to \infty} N^{-1}\text{tr}(\mathbf{G}_N) = 0$.

∎

More detail on the asymptotic properties of ML and RML may be found in Cressie and Lahiri (1993) and Richardson and Welsh (1994).

Problems for Section 3.6

1. Prove that the statistic $X = \boldsymbol{\beta}' \boldsymbol{\varepsilon} / g(\boldsymbol{\varepsilon}' \mathbf{A} \boldsymbol{\varepsilon})$ has zero mean, where $\boldsymbol{\varepsilon} \sim \mathcal{N}(0, \boldsymbol{\Omega})$, $\boldsymbol{\beta}$ is a fixed vector, $\mathbf{A}$ is a positive definite fixed matrix, and g is a positive function.

2. Prove that a limiting point of the sequence $X_n = \boldsymbol{\beta}_n' \boldsymbol{\varepsilon} / g_n(\boldsymbol{\varepsilon}' \mathbf{A}_n \boldsymbol{\varepsilon})$, $n \to \infty$ with the entries defined as in the previous problem has zero mean (this sequence may be thought of as the iteration sequence of an algorithm, such as Newton's algorithm).

3. Describe in a few words the difference between stochastic and deterministic approaches to studying the asymptotic properties of estimators.

4. Derive the asymptotic normality of the LS estimator of β in the form (3.49) for the simple regression model $y = \alpha + \beta x + \varepsilon$, where x is a binary variable.

5*. Prove the asymptotic equivalence between ML and RML by demonstrating that the information matrices converge to the same limit as $N \to \infty$ under a stochastic scheme. Use information matrices from Section 3.3.

3.7   Estimation of random effects

A peculiar property of the mixed effects model is that one is able to make individual predictions even if the number of observation points for a specific individual is less than the number of estimated parameters (fixed effects). This property of the mixed effects model comes from the principal assumption that each individual (cluster) has its own subject-specific parameter with the common (population-averaged) mean. Obviously, individual predictions may be accomplished in standard linear regression model as well, but then the beta parameters are not subject-specific as in the mixed model.

Let us first assume that $\boldsymbol{\beta}$ and variance parameters σ^2 and $\mathbf{D}$ are known. We want to find an estimate for the random effect $\mathbf{b}_i$ as the conditional expectation of $\mathbf{b}_i$ given $\mathbf{y}_i$. Assuming normal distribution, from model (2.14) it follows that $\text{cov}(\mathbf{b}_i, \mathbf{y}_i) = \sigma^2 \mathbf{D} \mathbf{Z}_i'$. Therefore, using the formula for the conditional mean (Rao 1973) we yield the posterior mean of the random effect,

$$E(\mathbf{b}_i|\mathbf{y}_i) = \text{cov}(\mathbf{b}_i, \mathbf{y}_i)\text{cov}^{-1}(\mathbf{y}_i)\,(\mathbf{y}_i - E(\mathbf{y}_i)) = \mathbf{D}\mathbf{Z}_i'(\mathbf{I} + \mathbf{Z}_i\mathbf{D}\mathbf{Z}_i')^{-1}(\mathbf{y}_i - \mathbf{X}_i\boldsymbol{\beta}).$$

This estimator has a strong Bayesian flavor, as noted by many authors: Laird and Ware (1982), Pinheiro and Bates (2000), to name a few. Hence, an estimator for random effect (if $\boldsymbol{\beta}$ and $\mathbf{D}$ are given) is

$$\widehat{\mathbf{b}}_i = \mathbf{D}\mathbf{Z}_i'(\mathbf{I} + \mathbf{Z}_i\mathbf{D}\mathbf{Z}_i')^{-1}(\mathbf{y}_i - \mathbf{X}_i\widehat{\boldsymbol{\beta}}), \tag{3.51}$$

where $\widehat{\boldsymbol{\beta}}$ is the generalized least squares estimator (2.28). This formula may be simplified using the dimension-reduction formula (2.21) and noting that

$$\begin{aligned}
\mathbf{Z}_i'(\mathbf{I} + \mathbf{Z}_i\mathbf{D}\mathbf{Z}_i')^{-1} &= \mathbf{Z}_i' - \mathbf{Z}_i'\mathbf{Z}_i\mathbf{D}(\mathbf{I} + \mathbf{Z}_i'\mathbf{Z}_i\mathbf{D})^{-1}\mathbf{Z}_i' \\
&= (\mathbf{I} + \mathbf{Z}_i'\mathbf{Z}_i\mathbf{D} - \mathbf{Z}_i'\mathbf{Z}_i\mathbf{D})\,(\mathbf{I} + \mathbf{Z}_i'\mathbf{Z}_i\mathbf{D})^{-1}\mathbf{Z}_i' \\
&= (\mathbf{I} + \mathbf{Z}_i'\mathbf{Z}_i\mathbf{D})^{-1}\mathbf{Z}_i',
\end{aligned}$$

which leads to

$$\widehat{\mathbf{b}}_i = \mathbf{D}(\mathbf{I} + \mathbf{Z}_i'\mathbf{Z}_i\mathbf{D})^{-1}\mathbf{Z}_i'(\mathbf{y}_i - \mathbf{X}_i\widehat{\boldsymbol{\beta}}). \tag{3.52}$$

Interestingly, if $\mathbf{D} = \mathbf{0}$, the estimate is zero. In another extreme situation, when $\mathbf{D} = \rho\mathbf{I} \to \infty$, we have $\widehat{\mathbf{b}}_i = \mathbf{Z}_i^+(\mathbf{y}_i - \mathbf{X}_i\widehat{\boldsymbol{\beta}}_\infty)$, the fixed effects scheme estimator, where $\widehat{\boldsymbol{\beta}}_\infty$ is as defined in (2.31). In practice we estimate the random effect using an estimate of $\mathbf{D}$.

The estimator of the random effect (3.51) or (3.52) is the Best Linear Unbiased Predictor (BLUP); see Henderson (1963) and Robinson (1991). We will show this with a Lagrange function to minimize a quadratic function under linear constraints. For easy presentation, we work with one model equation,

$$\mathbf{y} = \mathbf{X}\boldsymbol{\beta} + \mathbf{Z}\mathbf{b} + \boldsymbol{\varepsilon},$$

where $\mathbf{y}$ is an $N \times 1$ vector, $\mathbf{X}$ is an $N \times m$ full-rank matrix of fixed effects, $\mathbf{Z}$ is an $N \times k$ matrix of random effects, $\mathbf{b}$ is a $k \times 1$ random effect vector and $\boldsymbol{\varepsilon}$ is an $N \times 1$ error term. It is assumed that $\mathbf{b}$ and $\boldsymbol{\varepsilon}$ have zero mean and known covariance matrices $\sigma^2 \mathbf{D}_l$ and $\sigma^2 \mathbf{I}$, respectively (we use the notation $\mathbf{D}_l$ for the covariance matrix of random effect $\mathbf{b}$, not to be confused with the covariance matrix of the random effect $\mathbf{b}_i$ in the LME model). We consider the family of unbiased linear estimators of $\mathbf{b}$, i.e., the predictor for $\mathbf{b}$ has the form $\widehat{\mathbf{b}} = \mathbf{C}\mathbf{y}$, where $\mathbf{C}$ is the $k \times N$ matrix to be found. We seek $\mathbf{C}$ such that $E(\widehat{\mathbf{b}}) = \mathbf{C}(\mathbf{X}\boldsymbol{\beta} + \mathbf{Z}\mathbf{b} + \boldsymbol{\varepsilon}) = \mathbf{C}\mathbf{X}\boldsymbol{\beta} = \mathbf{0}$, which implies that $\mathbf{C}\mathbf{X} = \mathbf{0}$, to provide the unbiasedness of $\widehat{\mathbf{b}}$. Further, we want to choose $\mathbf{C}$ to make

$$\text{cov}(\widehat{\mathbf{b}} - \mathbf{b}) = \sigma^2 \left[\mathbf{C}\mathbf{C}' + (\mathbf{I} - \mathbf{C}\mathbf{Z})\mathbf{D}(\mathbf{I} - \mathbf{C}\mathbf{Z})' \right]$$

as small as possible. Let $\mathbf{p}$ be any $k \times 1$ vector and find the $\mathbf{C}$ that minimizes

$$\mathbf{p}' \left[\mathbf{C}\mathbf{C}' + (\mathbf{C}\mathbf{Z} - \mathbf{I})\mathbf{D}(\mathbf{C}\mathbf{Z} - \mathbf{I})' \right] \mathbf{p}$$

under the restriction $\mathbf{CX} = \mathbf{0}$. The Lagrange function is

$$\mathcal{L}(\mathbf{C}, \mathbf{L}) = \mathbf{p}' \left[\mathbf{CC}' + (\mathbf{CZ} - \mathbf{I})\mathbf{D}(\mathbf{CZ} - \mathbf{I})' \right] \mathbf{p} - \mathrm{tr}(\mathbf{CXL}),$$

where $\mathbf{L}$ is an $m \times k$ Lagrange multiplier matrix. We have

$$\frac{\partial \mathcal{L}}{\partial \mathbf{C}} = 2\mathbf{pp}'\mathbf{C}(\mathbf{I} + \mathbf{ZDZ}') - 2\mathbf{pp}'\mathbf{DZ}' - \mathbf{L}'\mathbf{X}' = \mathbf{0},$$

which implies

$$2\mathbf{pp}'\mathbf{C} = (2\mathbf{pp}'\mathbf{DZ}' + \mathbf{L}'\mathbf{X}')(\mathbf{I} + \mathbf{ZDZ}')^{-1}. \tag{3.53}$$

Multiplying by $\mathbf{X}$, we obtain

$$(2\mathbf{pp}'\mathbf{DZ}' + \mathbf{L}'\mathbf{X}')(\mathbf{I} + \mathbf{ZDZ}')^{-1}\mathbf{X} = \mathbf{0}$$

and consequently,

$$\mathbf{L}' = -2\mathbf{pp}'\mathbf{DZ}'\mathbf{V}^{-1}\mathbf{X}(\mathbf{X}'\mathbf{V}^{-1}\mathbf{X})^{-1}.$$

Substituting for $\mathbf{L}'$ with this, we obtain

$$2\mathbf{pp}'\mathbf{C} = 2\mathbf{pp}'\mathbf{DZ}' \left[\mathbf{V}^{-1} - \mathbf{V}^{-1}\mathbf{X}(\mathbf{X}'\mathbf{V}^{-1}\mathbf{X})^{-1}\mathbf{X}'\mathbf{V}^{-1} \right].$$

Since this is true for all $\mathbf{p}$, we obtain

$$\mathbf{C} = \mathbf{DZ}'\mathbf{V}^{-1} \left[\mathbf{I} - \mathbf{X}(\mathbf{X}'\mathbf{V}^{-1}\mathbf{X})^{-1}\mathbf{X}'\mathbf{V}^{-1} \right].$$

Now we apply this result to the LME model, where $\mathbf{y}, \mathbf{X}, \mathbf{Z}, \boldsymbol{\varepsilon}$, and $\mathbf{b}$ are defined as in (2.9) and $\mathbf{D}_l = \mathbf{I} \otimes \mathbf{D}$. Then the ith block of matrix $\mathbf{C}$ is

$$\begin{aligned}
\mathbf{DZ}_i'\mathbf{V}_i^{-1}(\mathbf{I} - \mathbf{X}_i(\mathbf{X}'\mathbf{V}^{-1}\mathbf{X})^{-1}\mathbf{X}'\mathbf{V}^{-1})\mathbf{y}_i &= \mathbf{DZ}_i'\mathbf{V}_i^{-1}(\mathbf{I} - \mathbf{X}_i\widehat{\boldsymbol{\beta}})\mathbf{y}_i \\
&= \mathbf{DZ}_i'\mathbf{V}_i^{-1}(\mathbf{y}_i - \mathbf{X}_i\widehat{\boldsymbol{\beta}}),
\end{aligned}$$

which agrees with (3.51).

There is another method to estimate random effects and $\boldsymbol{\beta}$ simultaneously that will be used later for nonlinear mixed models. It can be shown that the estimate (3.51) can be derived as the solution to the following optimization problem:

$$\sum_{i=1}^{N} \left[\|\mathbf{y}_i - \mathbf{X}_i\boldsymbol{\beta} - \mathbf{Z}_i\mathbf{b}_i\|^2 + \mathbf{b}_i'\mathbf{D}^{-1}\mathbf{b}_i \right] \Rightarrow \min_{\boldsymbol{\beta}, \mathbf{b}_1, \dots, \mathbf{b}_N}. \tag{3.54}$$

We notice that (3.54) collapses to the sum (2.33) when $\mathbf{D} = \infty$, as in the fixed effects approach. Holding $\boldsymbol{\beta}$ constant, we find the minimum of the sum (3.54) with respect to $\mathbf{b}_i$, which gives $\mathbf{b}_i = (\mathbf{Z}_i'\mathbf{Z}_i + \mathbf{D}^{-1})^{-1}\mathbf{Z}_i'(\mathbf{y}_i - \mathbf{X}_i\boldsymbol{\beta})$. Thus, it suffices to prove that (3.54) gives the solution (2.28). To see this, we find the minimum of (3.54) with respect to $\boldsymbol{\beta}$ using the $\mathbf{b}_i$ above. Combining the terms, we come to the following quadratic form as a function of $\boldsymbol{\beta}$:

$$\sum_{i=1}^{N} (\mathbf{y}_i - \mathbf{X}_i\boldsymbol{\beta})'\mathbf{G}_i(\mathbf{y}_i - \mathbf{X}_i\boldsymbol{\beta}), \tag{3.55}$$

Weight versus Height for 18 families

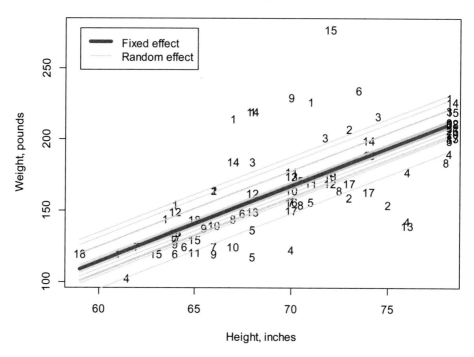

FIGURE 3.4. Estimation of 18 family-specific relationships between weight and height (thin straight lines).

where

$$
\begin{aligned}
\mathbf{G}_i &= \left[(\mathbf{I} - \mathbf{Z}_i(\mathbf{Z}_i'\mathbf{Z}_i + \mathbf{D}^{-1})^{-1}\mathbf{Z}_i')\right]\left[(\mathbf{I} - \mathbf{Z}_i(\mathbf{Z}_i'\mathbf{Z}_i + \mathbf{D}^{-1})^{-1}\mathbf{Z}_i')\right] \\
&\quad + \mathbf{Z}_i(\mathbf{Z}_i'\mathbf{Z}_i + \mathbf{D}^{-1})^{-1}\mathbf{D}^{-1}(\mathbf{Z}_i'\mathbf{Z}_i + \mathbf{D}^{-1})^{-1}\mathbf{Z}_i' \\
&= \mathbf{I} - \mathbf{Z}_i(\mathbf{Z}_i'\mathbf{Z}_i + \mathbf{D}^{-1})^{-1}\left[2(\mathbf{Z}_i'\mathbf{Z}_i + \mathbf{D}^{-1}) - \mathbf{Z}_i'\mathbf{Z}_i - \mathbf{D}^{-1}\right] \\
&\quad \times (\mathbf{Z}_i'\mathbf{Z}_i + \mathbf{D}^{-1})^{-1}\mathbf{Z}_i' \\
&= \mathbf{I} - \mathbf{Z}_i(\mathbf{Z}_i'\mathbf{Z}_i + \mathbf{D}^{-1})^{-1}\mathbf{Z}_i' = (\mathbf{I} + \mathbf{Z}_i\mathbf{D}\mathbf{Z}_i')^{-1} = \mathbf{V}_i^{-1}.
\end{aligned}
$$

Since $\mathbf{G}_i = \mathbf{V}_i^{-1}$, we infer that (3.54) leads to the generalized least squares solution (3.52).

3.7.1 Implementation in R

To illustrate the estimation of random effects in R, we use our previous data on family weight versus height. The function below extracts random intercepts from the lme call and plots the expected family-specific relationship between weight and height shown in Figure 3.4. As we did in our previous R examples, the function is saved as a `txt` file using the `dump` command every time it is executed. This function can be restored using the `source` command.

```
familyI=function()
{
dump("familyI","c:\\MixedModels\\Chapter03\\familyI.r")
library(nlme)
famdat=read.table("c:\\MixedModels\\Chapter02\\Family.txt",
        header=T,stringsAsFactors=F)
lmout=lme(Weight~Height,random=~1|FamilyID,data=famdat,method="ML")
print(summary(lmout))
fam.uniq=unique(famdat$FamilyID)
nfam=length(fam.uniq)
plot(famdat$Height,famdat$Weight,type="n",
        xlab="Height, inches",ylab="Weight, pounds",
main=paste("Weight versus Height for",nfam,"families"))
text(famdat$Height,famdat$W,famdat$FamilyID)
af=lmout$coefficients$fixed
ar=lmout$coefficients$random$FamilyID
lines(famdat$Height,af[1]+af[2]*famdat$Height,col=2,lwd=5)
maxH=max(famdat$Height)+.1
x=range(famdat$Height)
for(i in 1:nfam)
{
    lines(x,af[1]+ar[i]+af[2]*x,col=3,lwd=1)
    text(x[2],af[1]+ar[i]+af[2]*x[2],i,adj=0)
}
legend(x[1],max(famdat$Weight),c("Fixed effect","Random effect"),
lty=1,col=2:3,lwd=c(5,1))
}
```

A few remarks about this code: (1) `af` and `ar` contain the fixed effects estimates (betas) and estimates of the random intercepts respectively; (2) we use the same numbers to plot the weight and the height of relatives from the same family; (3) the family-specific relationships (straight lines) are parallel to each other because they differ by a random intercept/baseline having the same slope; and (4) the family ID is plotted at the right end of the straight line.

Extraction of the matrix $\mathbf{D}$ estimate from the `lme` function is not straightforward. The following R function illustrates how to get this estimate and compares with our function `lmeFS` discussed in Section 2.16. This function generates the random number of observations per cluster, n_i, true $\boldsymbol{\beta}$, true $\mathbf{D}$, and finally, $\mathbf{y}_i$. All data are saved in the dataframe `dL`.

```
lmeD=function(N=100,m=3,rs=434,s2=.02)
{
dump("lmeD","c:\\MixedModels\\Chapter03\\lmeD.r")
library(nlme)
set.seed(rs)
s=sqrt(s2)
k=m+1
b=rnorm(m) # generating random true β
ni=round(runif(n=N,min=80,max=100)) # random nᵢ
NT=sum(ni)
d=matrix(nrow=NT,ncol=2+m+k)
D=matrix(rnorm(k^2),k,k)
D=t(D)%*%D # random true D
TD=t(chol(D))
j <- 1 # the loop generates yᵢ,Xᵢ,Zᵢ and saves in the dataframe
for(i in 1:N) {
n <- ni[i]
d[j:(j + n - 1), 1] <- i
Xi <- matrix(rnorm(n*m),ncol=m)
d[j:(j + n - 1), 3:(2+m)] <- Xi
Zi <- cbind(rep(1,n),Xi)
d[j:(j + n - 1), (3+m):(2+m+k)] <- Zi
d[j:(j + n - 1),2]<-Xi%*%b+Zi%*%TD%*%rnorm(k,0,s))+rnorm(n,0,s))
j <- j + n
}
dL <- as.data.frame(d)
names(dL)<-c("id","y","X1","X2","X3","Zint","Z1","Z2","Z3")
o <- lme(fixed=y~X1+X2+X3,random=~Z1+Z2+Z3|id,data=dL,method="ML")
print(summary(o)) # extracting D̂_{*ML}
os <- matrix(as.numeric(VarCorr(o)),ncol=k+1)
sdb=diag(os[1:k,2],k,k)
LR=os[2:k,3:(k+1)]
Db=matrix(ncol=k,nrow=k)
R=diag(rep(1,k),ncol=k,nrow=k)
for(i in 2:k)
R[i,1:(i-1)]=R[1:(i-1),i]=LR[(i-1),1:(i-1)]
```

```
Db=sdb%*%R%*%sdb
print("Estimate of matrix D from lme:") #matrix $\widehat{\mathbf{D}}_{ML}$
print(Db/o$sigma^2)
dFS=cbind(dL$id,dL$y,rep(1,NT),dL$X1,dL$X2,dL$X3,dL$Zint,
                     dL$Z1,dL$Z2,dL$Z3)
ofs <- lmeFS(d=dFS,m=4,k=4,D=matrix(0,4,4),
       MLRML="ML",MaxIter=25,epspar=0.0001,pr=F) # our function
print("Estimate of matrix D from lmeFS:")
return(ofs[[9]]) #matrix $\widehat{\mathbf{D}}_{ML}$
}
```

In this linear mixed model the slope coefficients are random,

$$\mathbf{y}_i = (\beta_1 + b_1)\mathbf{1}_i + (\beta_2 + b_2)\mathbf{x}_1 + (\beta_3 + b_3)\mathbf{x}_2 + (\beta_4 + b_4)\mathbf{x}_3 + \boldsymbol{\varepsilon}_i$$

with four random effects. As the reader can see, our extraction of the $\mathbf{D}$-estimate needs seven lines of code. For this particular example, the `lme` function took 12 seconds and our function `lmeFS` took only 3 seconds. The estimates of matrix $\mathbf{D}$ from the two codes are practically the same. Note that in the `lme` function the intercept is present by default (for fixed and random effects), but for the function `lmeFS` it must be created (vectors of 1s).

Problems for Section 3.7

1. Demonstrate that estimates of the random effects can be viewed as shrinkage of fixed effects estimates obtained by the dummy variable approach (assume that the matrix $\mathbf{D}$ is positive definite and fixed).

2. Reduce the minimization problem (3.54) to linear least squares. Check your solution by an R code in which random effects are estimated as the coefficients in the `lm` call (the matrix $\mathbf{D}$ is fixed and known).

3. Append the code `lmeD` by computing the estimates of random effects by formula (3.52). Verify that your values coincide with those extracted from the `lme` call.

3.8   Hypothesis and membership testing

Before considering hypothesis testing for the mixed effects model, let us remember the test for a linear hypothesis in a general linear model with known covariance matrix, up to a scalar factor. Let the general linear model be defined as

$$\mathbf{y} = \mathbf{X}\boldsymbol{\beta} + \boldsymbol{\eta}, \quad \boldsymbol{\eta} \sim \mathcal{N}(\mathbf{0}, \sigma^2\mathbf{V}),$$

where σ^2 is unknown but the covariance matrix $\mathbf{V}$ is known and nonsingular, and $\mathbf{X}$ is the $n \times m$ design matrix of full rank. We want to test the linear hypothesis

$$H_0 : \mathbf{C}\boldsymbol{\beta} = \mathbf{0} \tag{3.56}$$

against the alternative $H_A : \mathbf{C}\boldsymbol{\beta} \neq \mathbf{0}$, where $\mathbf{C}$ is a fixed $q \times m$ matrix of full rank, $q \leq m$. Define two residual sums of squares,

$$RSS = (\mathbf{y} - \mathbf{X}\widehat{\boldsymbol{\beta}})'\mathbf{V}^{-1}(\mathbf{y} - \mathbf{X}\widehat{\boldsymbol{\beta}}), \quad RSS_0 = (\mathbf{y} - \mathbf{X}\widehat{\boldsymbol{\beta}}_0)'\mathbf{V}^{-1}(\mathbf{y} - \mathbf{X}\widehat{\boldsymbol{\beta}}_0),$$

where RSS is the absolute minimum of the weighted least squares and $\widehat{\boldsymbol{\beta}}$ is the GLS estimate. RSS_0 is the residual sum of the weighted least squares under restriction $\mathbf{C}\boldsymbol{\beta} = \mathbf{0}$ and $\widehat{\boldsymbol{\beta}}_0$ is the GLS estimate under restriction (3.56). Note that in many instances one can derive RSS_0 by reducing the regression under restriction to a regression with $m - q$ coefficients. Then it is a textbook result that under H_0,

$$\frac{(RSS_0 - RSS)/q}{RSS/(n-m)} \sim F(q, n-m); \tag{3.57}$$

e.g., Searle (1971a), Rao and Toutenburg (1999). The F-test (3.57) is very flexible and allows testing various statistical hypotheses on $\boldsymbol{\beta}$.

In order to test (3.56) through the F-test (3.57) for the linear mixed effects model (2.5), we treat $\mathbf{V}_i = \mathbf{I} + \mathbf{Z}_i\widehat{\mathbf{D}}\mathbf{Z}_i'$ as fixed and as follows from the "long" representation (2.11),

$$RSS = \sum_{i=1}^{N}(\mathbf{y}_i - \mathbf{X}_i\widehat{\boldsymbol{\beta}})'\mathbf{V}_i^{-1}(\mathbf{y}_i - \mathbf{X}_i\widehat{\boldsymbol{\beta}}), \tag{3.58}$$

where $\widehat{\boldsymbol{\beta}}$ is defined by (2.28). Analogously, we define RSS_0. Thus, we straightforwardly apply (3.57) to (2.5) with $n = \sum n_i$. Alternatively, one could apply the likelihood ratio test to (3.56) with $\mathbf{D}$ unknown. However, if $\mathbf{V}$ is known, test (3.57) is better because it is uniformly the most powerful invariant test (Lehmann, 1986). For large samples the tests are equivalent.

Usually, for individual significance testing $H_0 : \beta_l = 0$, one employs the Wald test ($l = 1, ..., m$). Recall that the Wald and likelihood ratio tests are asymptotically equivalent for ordinary linear regression but differ for nonlinear statistical models. Generally the likelihood ratio test outperforms the Wald test (Cox and Hinkley, 1974) although the latter is computationally easier. The same is true for confidence intervals: the profile-likelihood intervals discussed in Section 3.4 outperform Wald intervals but are more time consuming.

3.8.1 Membership test

Here we apply the F-test to the following *membership* problem: let $y_1, y_2, ..., y_n$ be an iid sample from a general population and y_{n+1} be a new observation, independent of the previous n observations. Does y_{n+1} belong to the same population, that is, is y_{n+1} a member? This is a typical question in medical diagnostics, in which case the $\{y_i\}$ are observations of normal patients and y_{n+1} is the observation of a new patient.

To simplify, we assume that observations have a normal distribution and the same variance, or more precisely, $y_i \sim \mathcal{N}(\mu, \sigma^2)$ for $i = 1, 2, ..., n$ and $y_{n+1} \sim \mathcal{N}(\mu_*, \sigma^2)$. Then the question of whether y_{n+1} is a member reduces to the hypothesis $H_0 : \mu = \mu_*$ with the alternative $H_A : \mu \neq \mu_*$. Applying the general test (3.57) it is easy to check that in this case $q = 1$, $RSS = \sum_{i=1}^{n}(y_i - \overline{y})^2$, and $RSS_0 = \sum_{i=1}^{n+1}(y_i - \overline{y}_{n+1})^2$, where $\overline{y} = \sum_{i=1}^{n} y_i/n$ and $\overline{y}_{n+1} = \sum_{i=1}^{n+1} y_i/(n+1)$. After elementary algebra one finds that

$$RSS_0 - RSS = \frac{n}{n+1}(y_{n+1} - \overline{y})^2,$$

and therefore, if y_{n+1} is a member,

$$\frac{n}{n+1}\frac{(y_{n+1}-\overline{y})^2}{s_y^2} \sim F(1, n-1), \qquad (3.59)$$

where $s_y^2 = RSS/(n-1)$. Taking the square root, the F-test (3.59) becomes equivalent to the t-test. Thus, one accepts the membership if

$$|y_{n+1}-\overline{y}| < s_y\sqrt{\frac{n+1}{n}}t_{1-\alpha/2,n-1}, \qquad (3.60)$$

where $t_{1-\alpha/2,n-1}$ is the $(1-\alpha/2)$th quantile of the t-distribution with $n-1$ degrees of freedom (d.f.). As follows from (3.60) for large n, one accepts the membership if y_{n+1} belongs to the $(1-\alpha)$th confidence interval constructed based on the sample $\{y_i, i = 1, ..., n\}$.

Now we generalize the membership test to the LME model (2.5). Again, for clarity we use a patient diagnostic interpretation. Thus, we have N normal patients defined by (2.5) and there is a $(N+1)$th patient who follows the same model but possibly with different fixed effect coefficients,

$$\mathbf{y}_{N+1} = \mathbf{X}_{N+1}\boldsymbol{\beta}_* + \mathbf{Z}_{N+1}\mathbf{b}_{N+1} + \boldsymbol{\varepsilon}_{N+1},$$

where $\mathbf{b}_{N+1} \sim \mathcal{N}(\mathbf{0},\sigma^2\mathbf{D})$ and $\boldsymbol{\varepsilon}_{N+1} \sim \mathcal{N}(\mathbf{0},\sigma^2\mathbf{I})$. Then in hypothesis testing language, the membership problem can be translated into the hypothesis

$$H_0 : \boldsymbol{\beta} = \boldsymbol{\beta}_*. \qquad (3.61)$$

We start with RSS_0. If $\boldsymbol{\beta} = \boldsymbol{\beta}_*$, all $N+1$ patients belong to the same population and, for example, applying maximum likelihood gives the estimates $\widehat{\boldsymbol{\beta}}_{N+1}$ and $\widehat{\mathbf{D}}$. Then the minimal weighted sum of squares under (3.61) is $RSS_0 = \sum_{i=1}^{N+1}(\mathbf{y}_i - \mathbf{X}_i\widehat{\boldsymbol{\beta}}_{N+1})'\mathbf{V}_i^{-1}(\mathbf{y}_i - \mathbf{X}_i\widehat{\boldsymbol{\beta}}_{N+1})$ where $\mathbf{V}_i = \mathbf{I} + \mathbf{Z}_i\mathbf{D}\mathbf{Z}_i'$. Now we find the minimal weighted sum of squares when (3.61) is not true, i.e., $\boldsymbol{\beta}$ and $\boldsymbol{\beta}_*$ are unrelated. Thus, we want to find the minimum of the weighted sum of squares,

$$\sum_{i=1}^{N}(\mathbf{y}_i - \mathbf{X}_i\boldsymbol{\beta})'\mathbf{V}_i^{-1}(\mathbf{y}_i - \mathbf{X}_i\boldsymbol{\beta})$$

$$+(\mathbf{y}_{N+1} - \mathbf{X}_{N+1}\boldsymbol{\beta}_*)'\mathbf{V}_{N+1}^{-1}(\mathbf{y}_{N+1} - \mathbf{X}_{N+1}\boldsymbol{\beta}_*), \qquad (3.62)$$

where $\mathbf{V}_{N+1} = \mathbf{I} + \mathbf{Z}_{N+1}\widehat{\mathbf{D}}\mathbf{Z}_{N+1}'$. Two situations may occur. In the first situation there exists $\widehat{\boldsymbol{\beta}}_*$ such that $\mathbf{y}_{N+1} = \mathbf{X}_{N+1}\widehat{\boldsymbol{\beta}}_*$. In particular, this happens when the length of $\mathbf{y}_{N+1}$ is less then m and matrix $\mathbf{X}_{N+1}$ has full rank. Then the second term of (3.62) vanishes and the minimal sum of squares reduces to $RSS = S_1 = \sum_{i=1}^{N}(\mathbf{y}_i - \mathbf{X}_i\widehat{\boldsymbol{\beta}})'\mathbf{V}_i^{-1}(\mathbf{y}_i - \mathbf{X}_i\widehat{\boldsymbol{\beta}})$, where $\widehat{\boldsymbol{\beta}}$ is defined by (2.28) with $\mathbf{D} = \widehat{\mathbf{D}}$. In the second situation, the minimum of the second term of (3.62) is $S_2 = (\mathbf{y}_{N+1} - \mathbf{X}_{N+1}\widehat{\boldsymbol{\beta}}_*)'\mathbf{V}_{N+1}^{-1}(\mathbf{y}_{N+1} - \mathbf{X}_{N+1}\widehat{\boldsymbol{\beta}}_*)$, where $\widehat{\boldsymbol{\beta}}_* = (\mathbf{X}_{N+1}'\mathbf{V}_{N+1}^{-1}\mathbf{X}_{N+1})^{-1}\mathbf{X}_{N+1}'\mathbf{V}_{N+1}^{-1}\mathbf{y}_{N+1}$, so that $RSS = S_1 + S_2$. Hence, in both situations, according to the F-test, we say that the new patient is normal if

$$\frac{(RSS_0 - RSS)/m}{RSS/(\sum n_i - m)} \sim F(m, \sum n_i - m). \qquad (3.63)$$

Further, we refer to (3.63) as the membership test. Note that as follows from formula (2.52), $RSS_0 = (\sum_{i=1}^{N+1} n_i - m)\widehat{\sigma}_{RML}^2$. Note also that the membership test for the LME model is not exact because we use an estimate of $\mathbf{D}$.

Example (continued). We illustrate the membership test by verifying that family 15 from the motivating example of Section 2.1 belongs to the rest of the population. We refer the reader to Figure 3.4. First, we run the `lme` function of R/S-Plus with the entire sample (family 15 is included). Assuming that the random-intercept model estimated by RML gives $\widehat{\sigma}_{RML}^2 = 25.19$ and $\widehat{\sigma}_d^2 = 13.72$. Then for each family we compute matrix (2.3) with the true value σ_d^2/σ^2 substituted by its estimate $\widehat{\sigma}_d^2/\widehat{\sigma}_{RML}^2 = 13.72/25.19 = 0.545$. Also, we obtain $RSS_0 = 25.19^2 \times (75 - 2) = 46,306.8$. Second, we compute $\widehat{\boldsymbol{\beta}}$ by formula (2.28) with $\mathbf{V}_i$ obtained before for the data excluding family 15; this gives the sum of squares $S_1 = 33887.1$. Third, for family 15 with

$$\mathbf{y}_{15} = \begin{bmatrix} 72 \\ 65 \\ 63 \\ 64 \end{bmatrix}, \quad \mathbf{X}_{15} = \begin{bmatrix} 1 & 278 \\ 1 & 130 \\ 1 & 120 \\ 1 & 135 \end{bmatrix},$$

we compute the minimum sum of squares $S_2 = (\mathbf{y}_{15} - \mathbf{X}_{15}\widehat{\boldsymbol{\beta}}_{15})'\mathbf{V}_{15}^{-1}(\mathbf{y}_{15} - \mathbf{X}_{15}\widehat{\boldsymbol{\beta}}_{15}) = 427.5$ so that $RSS = 33887.1 + 427.5 = 34314.6$. Finally, the value of the F-statistic is 12.7 and the critical value from F-distribution with 12.73 d.f. is 3.12. Thus, we conclude that, indeed, family 15 does not belong to the rest. We may interpret this by saying that this family/cluster is an outlier. In Section 9.9.1 we continue with an influence analysis of this data set. Using a different statistical technique, we will discover that family 15 is indeed influential. Thus, the membership test (3.63) may serve as a test for outliers in the LME model.

The membership test is easy to generalize to a nonlinear mixed effects model. In particular, we apply this test to statistical shape analysis in Chapter 11.

Problems for Section 3.8

1*. Assess how well the F-test (3.57) works in a small sample (N is small) using simulations when matrix $\mathbf{D}$ is unknown and estimated (modify the function `lmeD` from Section 3.7.1). Is there any difference between ML and RML? Estimate the size of the test and the power.

2. Generalize the membership test for the mean to simple linear regression.

3. Test whether family 4 belongs to the rest of the population.

3.9 Ignoring random effects

What if we ignore random effects in the LME model (2.5) and estimate beta parameters using ordinary least squares? This question is especially relevant at the preliminary stage of a mixed model setup. Assume that the beta parameters have been estimated by the OLS method, but we might not be satisfied with the estimation results for two reasons: (a) The OLS estimate has the wrong sign, or (b) the OLS estimate is not statistically significant. Should we go for a random effects model? If "yes," what kind of improvements in terms of (a) or (b) can we expect? In particular, can we expect that after accounting for random effects, the beta coefficients change significantly, or that perhaps their standard errors are reduced? Clearly, to answer these questions we need to investigate the properties of the OLS estimator (2.29) under model (2.5).

(a) The OLS estimator is unbiased in the linear model. Therefore, one may expect that least squares applied to the LME model provides fairly good estimates even in the presence of random effects. Moreover, as we shall learn later, for a balanced growth curve model (i.e., when $\mathbf{X}_i = \mathbf{X}(\mathbf{I} \otimes \mathbf{q}'_i)$ and $\mathbf{Z}_i = \mathbf{X}$) the OLS, GLS and ML estimators coincide, so that estimator (2.28) does not depend on matrix $\mathbf{D}$. Thus, the MLE should not change the OLS estimate dramatically.

(b) Does least squares provide correct standard errors for beta coefficients? The answer to this question is given below: generally, the OLS method inflates standard errors, even for balanced data when beta estimates coincide.

First, we consider the quality (bias) of the OLS estimator σ^2. We have

$$
\widehat{\sigma}^2_{OLS} \;=\; \frac{1}{N_T - m} \sum_{i=1}^{N} \left\| \mathbf{y}_i - \mathbf{X}_i \widehat{\boldsymbol{\beta}}_{OLS} \right\|^2
$$

$$
\;=\; \frac{1}{N_T - m} \sum_{i=1}^{N} \boldsymbol{\eta}'_i (\mathbf{I}_i - \mathbf{X}_i (\sum_{j=1}^{N} \mathbf{X}'_j \mathbf{X}_j)^{-1} \mathbf{X}'_i) \boldsymbol{\eta}_i,
$$

where $\mathrm{cov}(\boldsymbol{\eta}_i) = \sigma^2 \mathbf{V}_i = \sigma^2(\mathbf{I}_i + \mathbf{Z}_i \mathbf{D} \mathbf{Z}'_i)$, $\mathbf{I}_i$ is the $n_i \times n_i$ identity matrix, and $N_T = \sum n_i$ is the total number of observations. Thus, generally, we have

$$
E(\widehat{\sigma}^2_{OLS}) = \frac{1}{N_T - m} \sum_{i=1}^{N} \mathrm{tr} \left\{ \left(\mathbf{I}_i - \mathbf{X}_i (\sum_{j=1}^{N} \mathbf{X}'_j \mathbf{X}_j)^{-1} \mathbf{X}'_i \right) \mathbf{V}_i \right\}. \tag{3.64}
$$

To illustrate the properties of the OLS estimator, we consider the random-intercept model studied in Section 2.4 with $\mathbf{V}_i = \mathbf{I}_i + d\mathbf{1}_i \mathbf{1}'_i$, where $\mathbf{1}_i$ is the $n_i \times 1$ vector of 1's (the first column of $\mathbf{X}_i$ is $\mathbf{1}_i$), and $\sigma^2 d$ is the variance of the random intercept. In this special case, (3.64) takes the form

$$
E(\widehat{\sigma}^2_{OLS}) = \frac{\sigma^2}{N_T - m} \sum_{i=1}^{N} \mathrm{tr} \left\{ (\mathbf{I}_i - \mathbf{X}_i (\sum_{j=1}^{N} \mathbf{X}'_j \mathbf{X}_j)^{-1} \mathbf{X}'_i)(\mathbf{I}_i + d\mathbf{1}_i \mathbf{1}'_i) \right\}.
$$

Combining terms, we yield the bias,

$$
E(\widehat{\sigma}^2_{OLS}) - \sigma^2 = \frac{\sigma^2 d}{N_T - m} K,
$$

where

$$
K = N_T - \sum_{i=1}^{N} (\mathbf{X}'_i \mathbf{1}_i)' \left(\sum_{j=1}^{N} \mathbf{X}'_j \mathbf{X}_j \right)^{-1} (\mathbf{X}'_i \mathbf{1}_i).
$$

We shall prove that $K > 0$ and thus $\widehat{\sigma}^2_{OLS}$ has a positive bias. Indeed, for each i we have $(\sum_{j=1}^N \mathbf{X}'_j \mathbf{X}_j)^{-1} < (\mathbf{X}'_i \mathbf{X}_i)^{-1}$ for all $i = 1, ..., N$, $N > 1$, which implies that

$$N_T - \sum_{i=1}^N (\mathbf{X}'_i \mathbf{1}_i)' \left(\sum_{j=1}^N \mathbf{X}'_j \mathbf{X}_j \right)^{-1} (\mathbf{X}'_i \mathbf{1}_i) > \sum_{i=1}^N \mathbf{1}'_i (\mathbf{I} - \mathbf{X}_i (\mathbf{X}'_i \mathbf{X}_i)^{-1} \mathbf{X}'_i) \mathbf{1}_i = 0.$$

Therefore, we conclude that the OLS estimator of σ^2 is positively biased (inflated) when the random effect is ignored. For example, for VARCOMP model (1.8) we have $\mathbf{X}_i = \mathbf{1}_i$, and it is easy to see that the bias is

$$\frac{\sigma^2 d}{(N_T - m) N_T} (N_T^2 - \sum_{i=1}^N n_i^2).$$

For the balanced random-intercept model with one covariate,

$$\begin{aligned} y_{ij} &= a_i + \beta x_j + \varepsilon_{ij}, \\ a_i &= \alpha + \delta_i, \quad i = 1, ..., N, j = 1, ..., n, \end{aligned} \tag{3.65}$$

we have

$$\left(\sum_{j=1}^N \mathbf{X}'_j \mathbf{X}_j \right)^{-1} = \frac{1}{Nns_x^2} \begin{bmatrix} \sum x_j^2 & -n\overline{x} \\ -n\overline{x} & n \end{bmatrix},$$

where $s_x^2 = \sum_{j=1}^n (x_j - \overline{x})^2$, and the slope is the parameter of interest. Hence,

$$K = Nn - \frac{n}{s_x^2} \begin{bmatrix} 1 \\ \overline{x} \end{bmatrix}' \begin{bmatrix} \sum x_j^2 & -n\overline{x} \\ -n\overline{x} & n \end{bmatrix} \begin{bmatrix} 1 \\ \overline{x} \end{bmatrix} = Nn - n,$$

and the bias is

$$E(\widehat{\sigma}^2_{OLS}) - \sigma^2 = \frac{N(n-1)}{Nn-2} \sigma^2 d.$$

For large N the quantity $N(n-1)/(Nn-2)$ is close to $(n-1)/n$ and we deduce that $\widehat{\sigma}^2_{OLS}$ overestimates σ^2 roughly by the variance of the random effect. Indeed, it has a perfect explanation: since the random effect is not taken into account, it comes out by inflating the variance estimator.

We continue to study the balanced model (3.65) to determine whether the OLS variance,

$$\operatorname{var}(\widehat{\beta}_{OLS}) = \frac{\widehat{\sigma}^2_{OLS}}{Ns_x^2}, \tag{3.66}$$

is unbiased. For model (3.65), using formula (2.69), we have

$$\begin{aligned} \left(\sum \mathbf{X}'_i \mathbf{V}_i^{-1} \mathbf{X}_i \right)^{-1} &= \frac{1}{N} (\mathbf{X}' \mathbf{V}^{-1} \mathbf{X})^{-1} \\ &= \frac{1}{N} \left[\mathbf{X}' \left(\mathbf{I} - \frac{d}{1+nd} \mathbf{1}\mathbf{1}' \right) \mathbf{X} \right]^{-1} = \frac{1}{N} \left[\mathbf{X}'\mathbf{X} - \frac{dn^2}{1+nd} \overline{\mathbf{x}}\overline{\mathbf{x}}' \right]^{-1} \\ &= \frac{1}{N} \begin{bmatrix} \frac{n}{1+nd} & \frac{n}{1+nd}\overline{x} \\ \frac{n}{1+nd}\overline{x} & s_x^2 + \frac{n}{1+nd}\overline{x}^2 \end{bmatrix}^{-1} \\ &= \frac{1+nd}{Nns_x^2} \begin{bmatrix} s_x^2 + \frac{n}{1+nd}\overline{x}^2 & -\frac{n}{1+nd}\overline{x} \\ -\frac{n}{1+nd}\overline{x} & \frac{n}{1+nd} \end{bmatrix}. \end{aligned} \tag{3.67}$$

Denoting $\overline{\mathbf{y}} = N^{-1} \sum_{i=1}^{N} \mathbf{y}_i$ and $\overline{\overline{y}} = (nN)^{-1} \sum_{j=1}^{n} \sum_{i=1}^{N} y_{ij}$ and doing similar algebra, we obtain

$$\sum \mathbf{X}'_i \mathbf{V}_i^{-1} \mathbf{y}_i = N\mathbf{X}' \left(\mathbf{I} - \frac{d}{1+nd} \mathbf{1}\mathbf{1}' \right) \overline{\mathbf{y}} = \frac{nN}{1+nd} \left[\begin{array}{c} n\overline{\overline{y}} \\ \sum x_j \overline{y}_j \end{array} \right].$$

Finally, the GLS estimator for the slope is

$$\widehat{\beta}_{GLS} = \frac{\sum_{j=1}^{n} x_j \overline{y}_j - n\overline{x}\overline{y}}{s_x^2},$$

the OLS estimator. Thus, we proved that the GLS estimator of the slope in model (3.65) does not depend on the variance of the random effect d and coincides with the OLS estimator. We prove a more general result concerning a balanced growth curve model in the next chapter. Taking the $(2,2)$ element of matrix (3.67), we come to the asymptotic variance of the MLE,

$$\mathrm{var}(\widehat{\beta}_{ML}) = \frac{\sigma^2}{Ns_x^2}, \tag{3.68}$$

which is also d independent. Since $\widehat{\sigma}_{ML}^2$ is consistent, the estimate of the MLE variance computed by formula (3.68) is consistent as well, unlike the OLS variance (3.66) which has systematic positive bias. Therefore, we conclude that the variance of the OLS estimator in the LME model (3.65) is incorrect; more precisely, it is inflated, which may result in statistically insignificant OLS estimate. Introducing random effects and doing maximum likelihood estimation would lead to the same estimate but less standard error.

Problems for Section 3.9

1. Prove that the OLS estimate of the beta-coefficient remains unbiased when random effects are ignored.

2. Prove that $(\sum_{j=1}^{N} \mathbf{X}'_j \mathbf{X}_j)^{-1} < (\mathbf{X}'_i \mathbf{X}_i)^{-1}$ when $N > 1$, assuming that matrix $\mathbf{X}_i$ has full rank for all $i = 1, 2, ..., N$.

3*. Use simulations in R to support the conclusion of this section: if random effects are ignored, the OLS estimate of the fixed effects coefficient remains unbiased but has a larger variance (use (3.65) model for simulations).

3.10   MINQUE for variance parameters

Maximum likelihood estimation requires specification of the distribution for the error term and the random effects. Particularly, the MLE for the LME model assumes that both distributions are normal. Therefore, the MLE may not be robust to the distribution specification. Quadratic estimation of variance parameters seems natural in the framework of linear models; it does not require distribution specification and produces noniterative distribution-free estimates. The estimation of variance parameters is crucial for the beta estimation because if an estimate of matrix $\mathbf{D}$ is known, we apply the generalized least squares estimator (2.28). A desirable property of an estimator is the unbiasedness. So, in finding a quadratic estimator, we impose this condition. Further, within the class of quadratic unbiased estimators we want to find the best estimator in a certain sense. Unfortunately, the variance of a quadratic form involves the third and fourth moments, so instead of minimizing the variance, Rao (1973) suggested minimizing the norm of the matrix. The resulting estimator is called the Minimum Norm Quadratic Unbiased Estimator (MINQUE), and for some models, under the normal assumption, it leads to a quadratic unbiased estimator with minimum variance.

In constructing the MINQUE, we start with the general mixed effects model

$$\mathbf{y} = \mathbf{X}\boldsymbol{\beta} + \boldsymbol{\eta}, \quad E(\boldsymbol{\eta}) = \mathbf{0}, \quad \text{cov}(\boldsymbol{\eta}) = \sigma^2\mathbf{I} + \mathbf{Z}\mathbf{D}_*\mathbf{Z}', \tag{3.69}$$

where $\mathbf{y}$ is an $n \times 1$ vector of the dependent variable, $\mathbf{X}$ is an $n \times m$ nonzero design matrix of fixed effects, and $\mathbf{Z}$ is an $n \times k$ nonzero design matrix of random effects. In maximum likelihood theory, we dealt with the scaled variance-covariance matrix $\mathbf{D}$, where $\mathbf{D}_* = \sigma^2\mathbf{D}$. However, use of $\mathbf{D}_*$ makes development of the distribution-free estimation easier. To illustrate the principle of the MINQUE theory, we start with the standard linear model. Then the technique will be extended to the more complicated problem of quadratic estimation in model (3.69) and further to the LME model (2.5) as a special case.

3.10.1   Example: linear regression

It is instructive to illustrate how MINQUE works for the standard linear regression model

$$\mathbf{y} = \mathbf{X}\boldsymbol{\beta} + \boldsymbol{\varepsilon} \quad E(\boldsymbol{\varepsilon}) = \mathbf{0}, \quad \text{cov}(\boldsymbol{\varepsilon}) = \sigma^2\mathbf{I}. \tag{3.70}$$

Here $\mathbf{y}$ is an $n \times 1$ vector of observations of the dependent variable; $\mathbf{X}$ is an $n \times m$ design matrix, not necessarily of full rank; $\boldsymbol{\beta}$ is an $m \times 1$ vector of unknown parameters; and $\boldsymbol{\varepsilon}$ is an $n \times 1$ random error term. It is well known that

$$\widehat{\sigma}^2 = \frac{1}{n-r}\mathbf{y}'\left(\mathbf{I} - \mathbf{X}(\mathbf{X}'\mathbf{X})^-\mathbf{X}'\right)\mathbf{y} = \frac{1}{n-r}\mathbf{y}'\left(\mathbf{I} - \mathbf{X}\mathbf{X}^+\right)\mathbf{y}, \tag{3.71}$$

where $r = \text{rank}(\mathbf{X})$, is an unbiased estimator of σ^2. Now we shall prove that this estimator is the MINQUE. Moreover, we shall prove that estimator (3.71) has a minimum variance among all unbiased quadratic estimators when the distribution of $\boldsymbol{\varepsilon}$ is normal. The technique we use will be employed later to derive the MINQUE for the mixed model (3.69).

Thus, we are looking for a quadratic estimator for σ^2 in model (3.70). Let $\mathbf{A}$ be an $n \times n$ matrix; then a quadratic estimator for σ^2 is defined as

$$\widehat{\sigma}^2 = \mathbf{y}'\mathbf{A}\mathbf{y}. \tag{3.72}$$

First, without loss of generality, we can assume that $\mathbf{A}$ is a symmetric matrix. Second, to make $\widehat{\sigma}^2$ nonnegative for all $\mathbf{y}$, we assume that matrix $\mathbf{A}$ is nonnegative definite. We want the estimator (3.72) to be unbiased. Using the formula $E(\boldsymbol{\varepsilon}'\mathbf{A}\boldsymbol{\varepsilon}) = \text{tr}(\mathbf{A}\text{cov}(\boldsymbol{\varepsilon}))$ yields

$$\begin{aligned} E(\widehat{\sigma}^2) &= E(\mathbf{y}'\mathbf{A}\mathbf{y}) = E\left(\boldsymbol{\beta}'\mathbf{X}'\mathbf{A}\mathbf{X}\boldsymbol{\beta} + 2\boldsymbol{\varepsilon}'\mathbf{A}\mathbf{X}\boldsymbol{\beta} + \boldsymbol{\varepsilon}'\mathbf{A}\boldsymbol{\varepsilon}\right) \\ &= \boldsymbol{\beta}'\mathbf{X}'\mathbf{A}\mathbf{X}\boldsymbol{\beta} + \text{tr}(\mathbf{A}\text{cov}(\boldsymbol{\varepsilon})) = \boldsymbol{\beta}'\mathbf{X}'\mathbf{A}\mathbf{X}\boldsymbol{\beta} + \sigma^2\text{tr}(\mathbf{A}). \end{aligned}$$

The unbiasedness of $\widehat{\sigma}^2$ implies that for all β we need to have $\mathbf{X}'\mathbf{A}\mathbf{X} = \mathbf{0}$ and $\mathrm{tr}(\mathbf{A}) = 1$. Following the MINQUE principle, we find the quadratic unbiased estimator that minimizes the norm of matrix $\mathbf{A}$. This leads to the following quadratic optimization problem:

$$\mathrm{tr}(\mathbf{A}\mathbf{A}') \Rightarrow \min, \tag{3.73}$$

under linear restrictions

$$\mathbf{X}'\mathbf{A}\mathbf{X} = \mathbf{0}, \quad \mathrm{tr}(\mathbf{A}) = 1. \tag{3.74}$$

To solve this problem, we use a matrix version of the Lagrange function. We introduce an $m \times m$ Lagrange multiplier matrix $\mathbf{L}_1$ and a scalar l_2 so that the Lagrange function is written as

$$\mathcal{L}(\mathbf{A}, \mathbf{L}_1, l_2) = \frac{1}{2}\mathrm{tr}(\mathbf{A}\mathbf{A}') + \mathrm{tr}(\mathbf{X}'\mathbf{A}\mathbf{X}\mathbf{L}_1') + (1 - \mathrm{tr}(\mathbf{A}))l_2.$$

Now we differentiate function $\mathcal{L}$ with respect to $\mathbf{A}$ using the formulas

$$\frac{\partial \mathrm{tr}(\mathbf{A})}{\partial \mathbf{A}} = \mathbf{I}, \quad \frac{\partial \mathrm{tr}(\mathbf{A}\mathbf{A}')}{\partial \mathbf{A}} = 2\mathbf{A}, \quad \frac{\partial \mathrm{tr}(\mathbf{C}\mathbf{A}\mathbf{B})}{\partial \mathbf{A}} = \mathbf{C}'\mathbf{B}',$$

for arbitrary matrices $\mathbf{A}, \mathbf{B}, \mathbf{C}$ of appropriate size. The first-order condition for optimization (3.73) under restrictions (3.74) is that the derivative $\partial \mathcal{L}/\partial \mathbf{A}$ must be zero,

$$\frac{\partial \mathcal{L}}{\partial \mathbf{A}} = \mathbf{A} + \mathbf{X}\mathbf{L}_1\mathbf{X}' - l_2\mathbf{I} = \mathbf{0},$$

which gives $\mathbf{A} = l_2\mathbf{I} - \mathbf{X}\mathbf{L}_1\mathbf{X}'$. We find matrix $\mathbf{L}_1$ from the first condition in (3.74), which yields $\mathbf{L}_1 = l_2(\mathbf{X}'\mathbf{X})^+$ and thus

$$\mathbf{A} = l_2(\mathbf{I} - \mathbf{X}(\mathbf{X}'\mathbf{X})^+\mathbf{X}') = l_2(\mathbf{I} - \mathbf{X}\mathbf{X}^+).$$

To satisfy the second condition in (3.74), we take

$$l_2 = \frac{1}{\mathrm{rank}(\mathbf{I} - \mathbf{X}\mathbf{X}^+)}.$$

But matrix $\mathbf{I} - \mathbf{X}\mathbf{X}^+$ is idempotent (Graybill, 1983) and therefore its rank equals its trace, $\mathrm{tr}(\mathbf{I} - \mathbf{X}\mathbf{X}^+) = n - \mathrm{rank}(\mathbf{X})$. This finally yields the estimator (3.71).

The key point of the MINQUE approach is the minimization (3.73). For normally distributed ε, this approach leads to an estimator with minimum variance. Indeed, if ε is normally distributed, then $\mathrm{var}(\mathbf{y}'\mathbf{A}\mathbf{y}) = 2\sigma^4\mathrm{tr}(\mathbf{A}\mathbf{A}')$ so that minimizing $\mathrm{tr}(\mathbf{A}\mathbf{A}')$ is equivalent to minimization of the variance of $\widehat{\sigma}^2$. Hence, for the standard regression model, (3.70), with normally distributed errors, the MINQUE for σ^2 coincides with the minimum variance quadratic unbiased estimator.

If ε is not normally distributed, the variance of $\mathbf{y}'\mathbf{A}\mathbf{y}$ depends on the third and fourth moments. However, we observe that generally, larger elements of $\mathbf{A}$ lead to a larger variance of $\widehat{\sigma}^2$—if all elements of $\mathbf{A}$ would increase by the factor $\rho > 1$, the variance of $\widehat{\sigma}^2$ would increase by ρ^2. Thus, it makes sense to minimize $\sum a_{ij}^2 = \mathrm{tr}(\mathbf{A}\mathbf{A}')$. If the $\{y_i\}$ are normally distributed, then

$$\mathrm{var}(\widehat{\sigma}^2) = \frac{2\sigma^4}{n - r}.$$

Remarkably, the estimator (3.71) is consistent even when the matrix $\mathbf{X}$ does not have full rank—it requires only that $n - r \to \infty$ when $n \to \infty$.

3.10.2   MINQUE for σ^2

Now we employ the MINQUE theory to find a quadratic estimator for σ^2 in the same form (3.72) but for a mixed model (3.69), where again we seek a symmetric nonnegative definite matrix $\mathbf{A}$. We start by taking the expectation

$$E(\widehat{\sigma}^2) = \boldsymbol{\beta}'\mathbf{X}'\mathbf{AX}\boldsymbol{\beta} + \text{tr}(\mathbf{A}\text{cov}(\boldsymbol{\eta})) = \boldsymbol{\beta}'\mathbf{X}'\mathbf{AX}\boldsymbol{\beta} + \sigma^2\text{tr}(\mathbf{A}) + \text{tr}(\mathbf{AZD}_*\mathbf{Z}')$$
$$= \boldsymbol{\beta}'\mathbf{X}'\mathbf{AX}\boldsymbol{\beta} + \sigma^2\text{tr}(\mathbf{A}) + \text{tr}(\mathbf{D}_*\mathbf{Z}'\mathbf{AZ}). \tag{3.75}$$

To make $\widehat{\sigma}^2$ unbiased, we need to have $\mathbf{X}'\mathbf{AX} = \mathbf{0}$ and $\mathbf{Z}'\mathbf{AZ} = \mathbf{0}$, and $\text{tr}(\mathbf{A}) = 1$. By introducing the $n \times (m+k)$ matrix $\mathbf{W} = [\mathbf{X}; \mathbf{Z}]$, the first two linear restrictions are combined as $\mathbf{W}'\mathbf{AW} = \mathbf{0}$. However, we need to show that $\mathbf{X}'\mathbf{AX} = \mathbf{0}$ and $\mathbf{Z}'\mathbf{AZ} = \mathbf{0}$ imply that $\mathbf{W}'\mathbf{AW} = \mathbf{0}$. It suffices to show that the former pair of restrictions imply that $\mathbf{Z}'\mathbf{AX} = \mathbf{0}$. Indeed, since the matrix $\mathbf{A}$ is symmetric and nonnegative definite, there exists the square root, $\mathbf{A}^{1/2}$, which is also a symmetric nonnegative definite matrix. Then $\mathbf{X}'\mathbf{AX} = \mathbf{0}$ may be rewritten as $(\mathbf{A}^{1/2}\mathbf{X})'(\mathbf{A}^{1/2}\mathbf{X}) = \mathbf{0}$, which implies that $\text{tr}[(\mathbf{A}^{1/2}\mathbf{X})'(\mathbf{A}^{1/2}\mathbf{X})] = 0$ and $\mathbf{A}^{1/2}\mathbf{X} = \mathbf{0}$. Multiplying this equation by $\mathbf{A}^{1/2}$ we obtain $\mathbf{AX} = \mathbf{0}$. Finally, multiplying the latter equation by $\mathbf{Z}'$, we obtain $\mathbf{Z}'\mathbf{AX} = \mathbf{0}$. It is worthwhile to note that in the literature on the variance components model, a distinction is made between conditions $\mathbf{AX} = \mathbf{0}$ and $\mathbf{X}'\mathbf{AX} = \mathbf{0}$. The latter condition ensures unbiasedness, and the former ensures unbiasedness and invariance, Rao (1971, 1973). As follows from our proof, the two conditions are equivalent if matrix $\mathbf{A}$ is nonnegative definite.

Following the MINQUE theory, we minimize (3.73) under the restrictions

$$\mathbf{W}'\mathbf{AW} = \mathbf{0}, \quad \text{tr}(\mathbf{A}) = 1. \tag{3.76}$$

But this problem was solved in the previous section when we dealt with the standard linear regression model. The only difference is that now we have $\mathbf{W}$ instead of $\mathbf{X}$. Hence, the MINQUE for σ^2 in model (3.69) is

$$\widehat{\sigma}^2 = \frac{1}{n - \text{rank}(\mathbf{W})}\mathbf{y}'\left(\mathbf{I} - \mathbf{WW}^+\right)\mathbf{y}, \tag{3.77}$$

where for normal $\mathbf{y}$, we have

$$\text{var}(\widehat{\sigma}^2) = \frac{2\sigma^4}{n - r}. \tag{3.78}$$

Now we apply the MINQUE to the LME model (2.5), where matrix $\mathbf{Z}$ is block diagonal and defined by (2.9). Matrix $\mathbf{D}_*$ in model (3.69), admitting some ambiguity of notation, takes the form $(\mathbf{I} \otimes \mathbf{D}_*)$ where $\mathbf{D}_* = \text{cov}(\mathbf{b}_i)$. Note that the size of matrix $\mathbf{A}$ for model (2.5) is $N_T \times N_T$, where $N_T = \sum_{i=1}^{N} n_i$ is the total number of observations. Then, for matrix $\mathbf{W}$ as defined in (2.34), we obtain

$$\mathbf{y}'\left(\mathbf{I} - \mathbf{WW}^+\right)\mathbf{y} = \min_{\boldsymbol{\nu} \in R^{m+Nk}} \|\mathbf{y} - \mathbf{W}\boldsymbol{\nu}\|^2$$
$$= \min_{\boldsymbol{\beta}, \boldsymbol{\gamma}_1, \dots, \boldsymbol{\gamma}_N} \sum_{i=1}^{N} \|\mathbf{y}_i - \mathbf{X}_i\boldsymbol{\beta} - \mathbf{Z}_i\boldsymbol{\gamma}_i\|^2 = S_{\min},$$

as in (2.33). Thus finally the MINQUE estimator for σ^2 in model (2.5) is

$$\widehat{\sigma}^2_{MINQUE} = \frac{S_{\min}}{\sum n_i - \text{rank}(\mathbf{W})}. \tag{3.79}$$

As follows from (3.78), under the normal assumption, this estimator has the variance

$$\text{var}(\widehat{\sigma}^2_{MINQUE}) = \frac{2\sigma^4}{\sum n_i - \text{rank}(\mathbf{W})}. \tag{3.80}$$

To illustrate estimator (3.79), we apply it to the linear growth curve model, where each vector column of matrix $\mathbf{X}_i$ is a linear combination of vector columns of matrix $\mathbf{Z}_i$, or, more precisely, $\mathbf{X}_i = \mathbf{Z}_i \mathbf{A}_i$ for a certain design matrix $\mathbf{A}_i$ (this model is be considered at length in the next chapter). In this case,

$$
\begin{aligned}
S_{\min} &= \min_{\boldsymbol{\beta}, \boldsymbol{\gamma}_i} \sum_{i=1}^N \|\mathbf{y}_i - \mathbf{Z}_i \mathbf{A}_i \boldsymbol{\beta} - \mathbf{Z}_i \boldsymbol{\gamma}_i\|^2 = \min_{\boldsymbol{\beta}, \boldsymbol{\gamma}_i} \sum_{i=1}^N \|\mathbf{y}_i - \mathbf{Z}_i(\mathbf{A}_i \boldsymbol{\beta} + \boldsymbol{\gamma}_i)\|^2 \\
&= \sum_{i=1}^N \min_{\boldsymbol{\tau}_i} \|\mathbf{y}_i - \mathbf{Z}_i \boldsymbol{\tau}_i\|^2 = \sum_{i=1}^N \mathbf{y}_i'(\mathbf{I} - \mathbf{Z}_i \mathbf{Z}_i^+)\mathbf{y}_i.
\end{aligned} \tag{3.81}
$$

Therefore, for the linear growth curve model $S_{\min}$ is equal to the sum of individual residual sum of squares $RSS_i = \mathbf{y}_i'(\mathbf{I} - \mathbf{Z}_i \mathbf{Z}_i^+)\mathbf{y}_i$ and $\text{rank}(\mathbf{W}) = \sum(n_i - k_i)$, where $k_i = \text{rank}(\mathbf{Z}_i)$. Hence if $\mathbf{X}_i = \mathbf{Z}_i \mathbf{A}_i$, the MINQUE estimator of σ^2 is

$$\widehat{\sigma}^2_{MINQUE} = \frac{\sum RSS_i}{\sum(n_i - k)}.$$

This is a well known pooled variance estimator, see Section 4.1.3 for detail.

Now we show that MINQUE=RMLE for the balanced random-intercept model (2.67) with $n_i = n$, $\mathbf{X}_i = \mathbf{X} = [\mathbf{1}, \mathbf{U}]$ of Section 2.4.1, where $\mathbf{1}$ is the $n \times 1$ vector of 1s and matrix $\mathbf{X}$ has full rank. For this model

$$
\mathbf{W} = \begin{bmatrix} \mathbf{1} & \mathbf{0} & \mathbf{0} & \cdots & \mathbf{U} \\ \mathbf{0} & \mathbf{1} & \mathbf{0} & \cdots & \mathbf{U} \\ \mathbf{0} & \mathbf{0} & \vdots & & \vdots \\ \mathbf{0} & \mathbf{0} & \cdots & \mathbf{1} & \mathbf{U} \end{bmatrix}.
$$

It is easy to see that the rank of matrix $\mathbf{W}$ is equal to the number of columns, $N + m - 1$, so that the denominator of (3.79) is $N(n-1) - m + 1$. Next, proceeding as in Section 2.4.1, we obtain

$$
\begin{aligned}
S_{\min} &= \min_{\alpha_i, \gamma} \sum_{i=1}^N \|\mathbf{y}_i - \alpha_i \mathbf{1} - \mathbf{U}\boldsymbol{\gamma}\|^2 = \min_{\alpha_i, \boldsymbol{\beta}} \sum_{i=1}^N \|(\mathbf{y}_i - \alpha_i \mathbf{1}) - \mathbf{X}\boldsymbol{\beta}\|^2 \\
&= \min_{\alpha_i, \overline{\alpha}} \sum_{i=1}^N \left\|(\mathbf{y}_i - \alpha_i \mathbf{1}) - \mathbf{X}(\mathbf{X}'\mathbf{X})^{-1}\mathbf{X}'(\overline{\mathbf{y}} - \overline{\alpha}\mathbf{1})\right\|^2 \\
&= \sum_{i=1}^N \min_{\alpha_i, \overline{\alpha}} \|\widehat{\mathbf{e}} - (\alpha_i - \overline{\alpha})\mathbf{1}\|^2 = \sum_{i=1}^N \|\widehat{\mathbf{e}}\|^2 - \frac{1}{n}\sum_{i=1}^N (\widehat{\mathbf{e}}'\mathbf{1})^2 \\
&= \sum_{i=1}^N \|\widehat{\mathbf{e}}\|^2 - n\sum_{i=1}^N (\overline{y}_i - \overline{\overline{y}})^2.
\end{aligned}
$$

Thus, the numerators for (3.79) and (2.87) coincide and it was shown that they have a common denominator, $\widehat{\sigma}^2_{MINQUE} = \widehat{\sigma}^2_{RML}$ for the balanced random-intercept model.

In another very special case, the VARCOMP model (1.8), the MINQUE (3.79) takes the form

$$\widehat{\sigma}^2_{MINQUE} = \frac{1}{\sum_{i=1}^{N}(n_i - 1)} \sum_{i=1}^{N}\sum_{j=1}^{n}(y_{ij} - \overline{y}_i)^2.$$

This is a well known estimator in the variance components literature (Searle et al., 1992).

3.10.3   MINQUE for $\mathbf{D}_*$

Now we find the MINQUE for matrix $\mathbf{D}_* = \sigma^2\mathbf{D} =\text{cov}(\mathbf{b}_i)$ in the LME model (2.5). In the "long" notation (2.8), the quadratic estimator for $\mathbf{d}_* = \text{vec}(\mathbf{D}_*)$ can be expressed via a $k^2 \times N_T^2$ matrix $\mathbf{A}$,

$$\widehat{\mathbf{d}}_* = \mathbf{A}(\mathbf{y} \otimes \mathbf{y}). \tag{3.82}$$

We require that $\widehat{\mathbf{d}}_*$ be unbiased for all $\boldsymbol{\beta}, \sigma^2$, and $\mathbf{D}_*$, and that matrix $\mathbf{A}$ have minimum norm. We start by calculating the expectation

$$E(\widehat{\mathbf{d}}_*) = \mathbf{A}E(\mathbf{y} \otimes \mathbf{y}) = \mathbf{A}(\mathbf{X}\boldsymbol{\beta} \otimes \mathbf{X}\boldsymbol{\beta}) + \mathbf{A}E(\mathbf{Z}\mathbf{b} \otimes \mathbf{Z}\mathbf{b}) + \mathbf{A}E(\boldsymbol{\varepsilon} \otimes \boldsymbol{\varepsilon}).$$

Using standard formulas for the Kronecker product, we obtain

$$\begin{aligned}
(\mathbf{X}\boldsymbol{\beta} \otimes \mathbf{X}\boldsymbol{\beta}) &= (\mathbf{X} \otimes \mathbf{X})(\boldsymbol{\beta} \otimes \boldsymbol{\beta}), \\
E(\boldsymbol{\varepsilon} \otimes \boldsymbol{\varepsilon}) &= E\text{vec}(\boldsymbol{\varepsilon}\boldsymbol{\varepsilon}') = \sigma^2\text{vec}(\mathbf{I}_{N_T}), \\
E(\mathbf{Z}\mathbf{b} \otimes \mathbf{Z}\mathbf{b}) &= (\mathbf{Z} \otimes \mathbf{Z})E(\mathbf{b} \otimes \mathbf{b}) = (\mathbf{Z} \otimes \mathbf{Z})E(\text{vec}(\mathbf{b}\mathbf{b}')), \\
&= (\mathbf{Z} \otimes \mathbf{Z})\text{vec}(\mathbf{I}_N \otimes \mathbf{D}_*).
\end{aligned}$$

Further, we use the fact that $\text{vec}(\mathbf{I}_N \otimes \mathbf{D}_*)$ can be expressed as a linear function of $\mathbf{d}_*$; namely, $\text{vec}(\mathbf{I}_N \otimes \mathbf{D}_*) = \mathbf{J}\mathbf{d}_*$, where the $(Nk)^2 \times k^2$ matrix $\mathbf{J}$ is defined as $\mathbf{J} = [(\mathbf{I}_N \otimes \mathbf{K}_{k,N})(\text{vec}(\mathbf{I}_N) \otimes \mathbf{I}_k)] \otimes \mathbf{I}_k$ and $\mathbf{K}_{k,N}$ is the $(Nk)^2 \times (Nk)^2$ commutation matrix of the specified order (Magnus, 1988). Thus, to make $\widehat{\mathbf{d}}_*$ unbiased, we need to impose the following linear restrictions on matrix $\mathbf{A}$:

$$\mathbf{A}(\mathbf{X} \otimes \mathbf{X}) = \mathbf{0}, \quad \mathbf{A}\text{vec}(\mathbf{I}_{N_T}) = \mathbf{0}, \quad \mathbf{A}(\mathbf{Z} \otimes \mathbf{Z})\mathbf{J} = \mathbf{I}_{k^2}.$$

Introducing the $N_T^2 \times (m^2 + 1)$ matrix $\mathbf{F} = [\text{vec}(\mathbf{I}_{N_T}), \mathbf{X} \otimes \mathbf{X}]$, we come to the following optimization problem

$$\text{tr}(\mathbf{A}\mathbf{A}') \Rightarrow \min \tag{3.83}$$

under the restrictions

$$\mathbf{A}\mathbf{F} = \mathbf{0}, \quad \mathbf{A}(\mathbf{Z} \otimes \mathbf{Z})\mathbf{J} = \mathbf{I}_{k^2}. \tag{3.84}$$

Notice that the function to minimize is a quadratic function under liner restrictions; hence we can find a closed-form solution. We solve this problem by means of the Lagrange function

$$\mathcal{L}(\mathbf{A}, \mathbf{L}_1, \mathbf{L}_2) = \frac{1}{2}\text{tr}(\mathbf{A}\mathbf{A}') + \text{tr}(\mathbf{A}\mathbf{F}\mathbf{L}_1') + \text{tr}((\mathbf{I}_{k^2} - \mathbf{A}(\mathbf{Z} \otimes \mathbf{Z})\mathbf{J})\mathbf{L}_2'),$$

where $\mathbf{L}_1$ is an $N_T^2 \times (m^2 + 1)$ matrix and $\mathbf{L}_2$ is a $k^2 \times k^2$ matrix. The first-order condition for minimum (3.83) is

$$\frac{\partial \mathcal{L}}{\partial \mathbf{A}} = \mathbf{A} + \mathbf{L}_1\mathbf{F}' - \mathbf{L}_2\mathbf{J}'(\mathbf{Z}' \otimes \mathbf{Z}') = \mathbf{0},$$

which implies that $\mathbf{A} = \mathbf{L}_2\mathbf{J}'(\mathbf{Z}' \otimes \mathbf{Z}') - \mathbf{L}_1\mathbf{F}'$. From the first condition of (3.84), we obtain $\mathbf{L}_2\mathbf{J}'(\mathbf{Z}' \otimes \mathbf{Z}')\mathbf{F} - \mathbf{L}_1\mathbf{F}'\mathbf{F} = 0$ and $\mathbf{L}_1 = \mathbf{L}_2\mathbf{J}'(\mathbf{Z}' \otimes \mathbf{Z}')\mathbf{F}(\mathbf{F}'\mathbf{F})^{-1}$, which gives $\mathbf{A} = \mathbf{L}_2\mathbf{J}'(\mathbf{Z}' \otimes \mathbf{Z}')(\mathbf{I} - \mathbf{M})$, where we denoted $\mathbf{M} = \mathbf{F}(\mathbf{F}'\mathbf{F})^{-1}\mathbf{F}'$. Now we use the second condition of (3.84), which yields $\mathbf{L}_2\mathbf{J}'(\mathbf{Z}' \otimes \mathbf{Z}')(\mathbf{I} - \mathbf{M})(\mathbf{Z} \otimes \mathbf{Z})\mathbf{J} = \mathbf{I}$ and $\mathbf{L}_2 = \left[\mathbf{J}(\mathbf{Z}' \otimes \mathbf{Z}')(\mathbf{I} - \mathbf{M})(\mathbf{Z} \otimes \mathbf{Z})\mathbf{J}\right]^{-1}$. Thus, finally we arrive at

$$\mathbf{A} = [\mathbf{J}'(\mathbf{Z}' \otimes \mathbf{Z}')(\mathbf{I} - \mathbf{M})(\mathbf{Z} \otimes \mathbf{Z})\mathbf{J}]^{-1}\mathbf{J}'(\mathbf{Z}' \otimes \mathbf{Z}')(\mathbf{I} - \mathbf{M}). \qquad (3.85)$$

In the rest of this section we simplify this matrix expression for the LME model (2.5), for which $\mathbf{Z} = \text{diag}(\mathbf{Z}_1, \mathbf{Z}_2, ..., \mathbf{Z}_N)$. In our derivation, we have not used the diagonal structure of $\mathbf{Z}$. We start by simplifying the inverse of the matrix

$$\mathbf{F}'\mathbf{F} = \begin{bmatrix} N_T & \text{vec}'(\mathbf{X}'\mathbf{X}) \\ \text{vec}(\mathbf{X}'\mathbf{X}) & \mathbf{X}'\mathbf{X} \otimes \mathbf{X}'\mathbf{X} \end{bmatrix}, \qquad (3.86)$$

noticing that for the $(1,1)$th block we have $\text{vec}'(\mathbf{I}_{N_T})\text{vec}(\mathbf{I}_{N_T}) = \text{tr}\mathbf{I}_{N_T} = N_T$. Notice that matrix $\mathbf{F}'\mathbf{F}$ takes the form of matrix (3.25). To invert (3.86) we use the matrix block-inverse formula (2.79). For matrix (3.86) we have

$$\begin{aligned} a - \mathbf{b}'\mathbf{H}^{-1}\mathbf{b} &= N_T - \text{vec}'(\mathbf{X}'\mathbf{X})\left[(\mathbf{X}'\mathbf{X})^{-1} \otimes (\mathbf{X}'\mathbf{X})^{-1}\right]\text{vec}(\mathbf{X}'\mathbf{X}) \\ &= N_T - \text{tr}\left[(\mathbf{X}'\mathbf{X})(\mathbf{X}'\mathbf{X})^{-1}(\mathbf{X}'\mathbf{X})^{-1}(\mathbf{X}'\mathbf{X})\right] = N_T - m \end{aligned}$$

and

$$\mathbf{H}^{-1}\mathbf{b} = \left[(\mathbf{X}'\mathbf{X})^{-1} \otimes (\mathbf{X}'\mathbf{X})^{-1}\right]\text{vec}(\mathbf{X}'\mathbf{X}) = \text{vec}(\mathbf{X}'\mathbf{X})^{-1},$$

where hereafter it is denoted

$$\mathbf{N} = (\mathbf{X}'\mathbf{X})^{-1} = \left(\sum_{i=1}^{N} \mathbf{X}_i'\mathbf{X}_i\right)^{-1}. \qquad (3.87)$$

Hence,

$$(\mathbf{F}'\mathbf{F})^{-1} = \frac{1}{N_T - m}\begin{bmatrix} 1 & -\text{vec}'(\mathbf{N}) \\ -\text{vec}(\mathbf{N}) & (N_T - m)\mathbf{N} \otimes \mathbf{N} + \text{vec}(\mathbf{N})\text{vec}'(\mathbf{N}) \end{bmatrix}.$$

After some matrix algebra,

$$(\mathbf{Z}' \otimes \mathbf{Z}')\mathbf{M}(\mathbf{Z} \otimes \mathbf{Z})$$

$$= \frac{1}{N_T - m}[\text{vec}(\mathbf{Z}'\mathbf{Z}), \mathbf{Z}'\mathbf{X} \otimes \mathbf{Z}'\mathbf{X}]$$

$$\times \begin{bmatrix} 1 & -\text{vec}'(\mathbf{N}) \\ -\text{vec}(\mathbf{N}) & (N_T - m)\mathbf{N} \otimes \mathbf{N} + \text{vec}(\mathbf{N})\text{vec}'(\mathbf{N}) \end{bmatrix} \begin{bmatrix} \text{vec}'(\mathbf{Z}'\mathbf{Z}) \\ \mathbf{X}'\mathbf{Z} \otimes \mathbf{X}'\mathbf{Z} \end{bmatrix}$$

$$= \mathbf{R} \otimes \mathbf{R} + \frac{1}{N_T - m}[\text{vec}(\mathbf{R})\text{vec}'(\mathbf{R}) - \text{vec}(\mathbf{R})\text{vec}'(\mathbf{Z}'\mathbf{Z})$$

$$- \text{vec}(\mathbf{Z}'\mathbf{Z})\text{vec}'(\mathbf{R}) + \text{vec}(\mathbf{Z}'\mathbf{Z})\text{vec}'(\mathbf{Z}'\mathbf{Z})]$$

$$= \mathbf{R} \otimes \mathbf{R} + \frac{1}{N_T - m}\text{vec}(\mathbf{Q})\text{vec}'(\mathbf{Q}),$$

where $\mathbf{R} = \mathbf{Z}'\mathbf{P_X}\mathbf{Z}$ and $\mathbf{Q} = \mathbf{Z}'(\mathbf{I} - \mathbf{P_X})\mathbf{Z}$ are $Nk \times Nk$ matrices, and $\mathbf{P_X} = \mathbf{XNX}'$ is the projection matrix. Analogously,

$$\mathbf{F}'(\mathbf{y} \otimes \mathbf{y}) = \begin{bmatrix} \mathbf{y}'\mathbf{y} \\ \mathbf{X}'\mathbf{y} \otimes \mathbf{X}'\mathbf{y} \end{bmatrix},$$

and therefore,

$$(\mathbf{Z}' \otimes \mathbf{Z}')(\mathbf{I} - \mathbf{P_X})(\mathbf{y} \otimes \mathbf{y})$$

$$= \mathbf{Z}'\mathbf{y} \otimes \mathbf{Z}'\mathbf{y} - (\mathbf{Z}' \otimes \mathbf{Z}')\mathbf{M}(\mathbf{y} \otimes \mathbf{y})$$

$$= \mathbf{Z}'\mathbf{y} \otimes \mathbf{Z}'\mathbf{y} - \frac{1}{N_T - m}[\text{vec}(\mathbf{Z}'\mathbf{Z}), \mathbf{Z}'\mathbf{X} \otimes \mathbf{Z}'\mathbf{X}]$$

$$\times \begin{bmatrix} 1 & -\text{vec}'(\mathbf{N}) \\ -\text{vec}(\mathbf{N}) & (N_T - m)\mathbf{N} \otimes \mathbf{N} + \text{vec}(\mathbf{N})\text{vec}'(\mathbf{N}) \end{bmatrix} \begin{bmatrix} \mathbf{y}'\mathbf{y} \\ \mathbf{X}'\mathbf{y} \otimes \mathbf{X}'\mathbf{y} \end{bmatrix}$$

$$= \mathbf{Z}'\mathbf{y} \otimes \mathbf{Z}'\mathbf{y} - \mathbf{Z}'\mathbf{P_X}\mathbf{y} \otimes \mathbf{Z}'\mathbf{P_X}\mathbf{y} - \widehat{\sigma}^2_{OLS}\text{vec}(\mathbf{Q}),$$

where

$$\widehat{\sigma}^2_{OLS} = \frac{1}{N_T - m}\|\mathbf{y} - \widehat{\mathbf{y}}\|^2 = \frac{1}{N_T - m}\mathbf{y}'(\mathbf{I} - \mathbf{P_X})\mathbf{y}$$

can be viewed as the OLS estimator of σ^2. Finally, in terms of matrix $\mathbf{J}$,

$$\text{vec}(\widehat{\mathbf{D}}_{*MINQUE}) =$$

$$\left[\mathbf{J}'\left(\mathbf{Z}'\mathbf{Z} \otimes \mathbf{Z}'\mathbf{Z} - \mathbf{Z}'\mathbf{P_X}\mathbf{Z} \otimes \mathbf{Z}'\mathbf{P_X}\mathbf{Z} - (N_T - m)^{-1}\text{vec}(\mathbf{Q})\text{vec}'(\mathbf{Q})\right)\mathbf{J}\right]^{-1}$$

$$\times \left[\mathbf{J}'\left(\mathbf{Z}'\mathbf{y} \otimes \mathbf{Z}'\mathbf{y} - \mathbf{Z}'\mathbf{P_X}\mathbf{y} \otimes \mathbf{Z}'\mathbf{P_X}\mathbf{y} - \widehat{\sigma}^2_{OLS}\text{vec}(\mathbf{Q})\right)\right].$$

Using the definition for $\mathbf{J}$ above, after some matrix algebra manipulations, one can show that the MINQUE formula is equivalent to

$$\text{vec}(\widehat{\mathbf{D}}_{*MINQUE}) = \mathbf{Q}^{-1}\mathbf{q}, \tag{3.88}$$

where the $k^2 \times 1$ vector and $k^2 \times k^2$ matrix are

$$\mathbf{q} = \sum_{i=1}^{N}(\mathbf{Z}_i'\mathbf{y}_i \otimes \mathbf{Z}_i'\mathbf{y}_i - \mathbf{Z}_i'\widehat{\mathbf{y}}_i \otimes \mathbf{Z}_i'\widehat{\mathbf{y}}_i) - \widehat{\sigma}^2_{OLS}\mathbf{c},$$

$$\mathbf{Q} = \sum_{i=1}^{N}(\mathbf{Z}_i'\mathbf{Z}_i) \otimes (\mathbf{Z}_i'\mathbf{Z}_i) - \mathbf{G}'(\mathbf{N} \otimes \mathbf{N})\mathbf{G} - \frac{1}{N_T - m}\mathbf{cc}',$$

and

$$\mathbf{G} = \sum_{i=1}^{N} \mathbf{X}_i' \mathbf{Z}_i \otimes \mathbf{X}_i' \mathbf{Z}_i, \ \mathbf{c} = \mathrm{vec} \left(\sum_{i=1}^{N} [\mathbf{Z}_i' \mathbf{Z}_i - (\mathbf{Z}_i' \mathbf{X}_i) \mathbf{N} (\mathbf{Z}_i' \mathbf{X}_i)'] \right). \qquad (3.89)$$

It is easy to see that $\widehat{\mathbf{D}}_{*MINQUE}$ is the solution to the following matrix equation:

$$\sum_{i=1}^{N} \mathbf{Z}_i' \mathbf{Z}_i \mathbf{D}_* \mathbf{Z}_i' \mathbf{Z}_i - \sum_{i,j=1}^{N} \mathbf{Z}_i' \mathbf{P}_{ij} \mathbf{Z}_j \mathbf{D}_* \mathbf{Z}_j' \mathbf{P}_{ij}' \mathbf{Z}_i$$

$$- \frac{1}{N_T - m} \sum_{i=1}^{N} \mathbf{Z}_i' (\mathbf{I} - \mathbf{P}_{ii}) \mathbf{Z}_i \mathrm{tr} \left[\mathbf{D}_* \sum_{i=1}^{N} \mathbf{Z}_i' (\mathbf{I} - \mathbf{P}_{ii}) \mathbf{Z}_i \right]$$

$$= \sum_{i=1}^{N} \mathbf{Z}_i' \left[\mathbf{y}_i \mathbf{y}_i' - \widehat{\mathbf{y}}_i \widehat{\mathbf{y}}_i' \right] \mathbf{Z}_i - \widehat{\sigma}_{OLS}^2 \sum_{i=1}^{N} \mathbf{Z}_i' (\mathbf{I} - \mathbf{P}_{ii}) \mathbf{Z}_i, \qquad (3.90)$$

where $\mathbf{P}_{ij} = \mathbf{X}_i \mathbf{N} \mathbf{X}_j'$. Since matrix $\mathbf{D}_*$ is between matrices, one needs to apply the vec operator provided by solution (3.88). In the case of one random effect ($k = 1$) there is no need to use the vec operator, so equation (3.90) can be solved explicitly for $\mathbf{D}_* = d_*$. This case is considered below.

3.10.4 Linear model with random intercepts

Here we derive a special case of the MINQUE (3.90) when the LME model has one random effect, namely, the random-intercept model considered in Section 2.4, where $\mathbf{Z}_i = \mathbf{1}_{n_i}$. For one random effect, vectors $\mathbf{q}$ and $\mathbf{c}$, and matrix $\mathbf{Q}$ collapse to scalars. We have

$$\mathbf{G} = \sum \mathbf{s}_{xi} \otimes \mathbf{s}_{xi}, \ c = \sum (n_i - \mathbf{s}_{xi}' \mathbf{N} \mathbf{s}_{xi}), \ \mathbf{G}'(\mathbf{N} \otimes \mathbf{N}) \mathbf{G} = \mathrm{tr} (\sum \mathbf{s}_{xi} \mathbf{s}_{xi}' \mathbf{N})^2,$$

where $\mathbf{s}_{xi} = \mathbf{X}_i' \mathbf{Z}_i = \sum_{j=1}^{n_i} \mathbf{x}_{ij}$, and thus

$$\widehat{d}_{*MINQUE} = \frac{\sum (s_{yi}^2 - s_{\widehat{y}i}^2) - \widehat{\sigma}_{OLS}^2 c}{\sum n_i^2 - \mathrm{tr} (\sum \mathbf{s}_{xi} \mathbf{s}_{xi}' \mathbf{N})^2 - (N_T - m)^{-1} c^2}, \qquad (3.91)$$

where $s_{yi} = \mathbf{Z}_i' \mathbf{y}_i = \sum_{j=1}^{n_i} y_{ij}$ and $s_{\widehat{y}i} = \sum_{j=1}^{n_i} \widehat{y}_{ij} = \mathbf{s}_{xi}' \widehat{\boldsymbol{\beta}}_{OLS}$.

3.10.5 MINQUE for the balanced model

In this section we apply the MINQUE to the balanced random-coefficient (BRC) model studied in Section 2.3. We will show that the MINQUE for $\mathbf{D}_*$ coincides with the RML estimate derived in Section 2.3. For the balanced random-coefficient model, $\mathbf{Z} = \mathbf{X}_i = \mathbf{Z}_i$ and the left-hand side of equation (3.90) simplifies to

$$(N - 1)(\mathbf{Z}'\mathbf{Z}) \mathbf{D}_* (\mathbf{Z}\mathbf{Z}) - \frac{(N - 1)^2}{Nn - m} (\mathbf{Z}'\mathbf{Z}) \mathrm{tr}(\mathbf{D}_* \mathbf{Z}'\mathbf{Z}).$$

Also for the BRC model $\widehat{\boldsymbol{\beta}}_{OLS} = (\mathbf{Z}'\mathbf{Z})^{-1} \mathbf{Z}' \overline{\mathbf{y}}$ and $\widehat{\mathbf{y}}_i = \widehat{\mathbf{y}} = \mathbf{Z} (\mathbf{Z}'\mathbf{Z})^{-1} \mathbf{Z}' \overline{\mathbf{y}}$. Therefore, $\widehat{\sigma}_{OLS}^2 = (Nn - m)/(N(n - m)) \widehat{\sigma}_{ML}^2$, where $\widehat{\sigma}_{ML}^2$ is given by (2.59). Also, in the notation of Section 2.3, $\widehat{\mathbf{E}}\widehat{\mathbf{E}}' = \sum(\mathbf{y}_i\mathbf{y}_i' - \widehat{\mathbf{y}}_i\widehat{\mathbf{y}}_i')$, so that equation (3.90) takes the form

$$(N-1)(\mathbf{Z}'\mathbf{Z})\mathbf{D}_*(\mathbf{Z}\mathbf{Z}) - \frac{(N-1)^2}{Nn-m}(\mathbf{Z}'\mathbf{Z})\text{tr}(\mathbf{D}_*\mathbf{Z}'\mathbf{Z})$$

$$= \mathbf{Z}'\widehat{\mathbf{E}}\widehat{\mathbf{E}}'\mathbf{Z} - \frac{(Nn-m)(N-1)}{N(n-m)}\widehat{\sigma}_{ML}^2(\mathbf{Z}'\mathbf{Z}). \tag{3.92}$$

Multiplying both sides by $(\mathbf{Z}'\mathbf{Z})^{-1}$ and taking the trace, we obtain the expression for $\text{tr}(\mathbf{D}_*\mathbf{Z}'\mathbf{Z})$, noting that $\text{tr}(\widehat{\mathbf{E}}\widehat{\mathbf{E}}') = (Nn-m)\widehat{\sigma}_{OLS}^2$. Then, multiplying both sides of (3.92) by $(\mathbf{Z}'\mathbf{Z})^{-1}$, we finally find $\mathbf{D}_*$, which leads to (2.61).

3.10.6   lmevarMINQUE function

The R code for MINQUE of σ^2 and $\mathbf{D}_*$ can be downloaded to an R session as

```
source("c:\\MixedModels\\Chapter03\\lmevarMINQUE.r")
```

This function call is `lmevarMINQUE(m,k,d)`, where `m`, `k`, and `d` have the same meaning as in the `lmeFS` function (see Section 2.16). It returns a list with two components: (1) the MINQUE estimate of σ^2, and (2) the MINQUE estimate of $\mathbf{D}_*$. It does not guarantee that the returned matrix is positive definite. The function `lmevarMINQUE` requires the `ginverse.sym` function described in Section 2.2.3.

Problems for Section 3.10

1. Suppose that matrix $\mathbf{X}$ has full rank. Express (3.71) in terms of the residuals $r_i = y_i - \mathbf{x}_i'\widehat{\boldsymbol{\beta}}_{OLS}$.

2. Provide a geometric interpretation of the fact that the variance of $\widehat{\sigma}^2$ does not depend on matrix $\mathbf{X}$, assuming that it has full rank.

3. Show that calculation of $S_{\min}$ can be reduced to the classical linear least squares using the projection values $\widehat{\mathbf{y}}_i = (\mathbf{I} - \mathbf{P}_i)\mathbf{y}_i$ and $\widehat{\mathbf{X}}_i = (\mathbf{I} - \mathbf{P}_i)\mathbf{X}_i$, where $\mathbf{P}_i = \mathbf{Z}_i(\mathbf{Z}_i'\mathbf{Z}_i)^+\mathbf{Z}_i'$. This method is realized in the function `lmevarMINQUE`.

4. Show that $\mathbf{D}_{*MINQUE}$ is the solution to the matrix equation (3.90).

5. Simplify (3.91) when $\mathbf{x}_i - \mathbf{x}$ (balanced LME with random intercepts) and show that it coincides with (2.61).

6*. Conduct a simulation study for the LME model with random intercept and slope to compare the restricted ML with MINQUE in terms of the Mean Square Error (MSE) for the slope of the fixed effects, β, and matrix $\mathbf{D}_*$. Plot the MSEs versus N to demonstrate that MSEs converge for large N. Run the comparison for several true values β, σ^2, and $\mathbf{D}$.

3.11   Method of moments

Here we derive a Method of Moments (MM) estimator for $\mathbf{D}_* = \sigma^2\mathbf{D} = \text{cov}(\mathbf{b}_i)$ in the LME model (2.5) assuming that an unbiased estimator of σ^2 is given; for example, one can take the MINQUE (3.79). In a manner similar to MINQUE derivation, the MM estimator does not require a specification of the distribution for ε_i or for $\mathbf{b}_i$. We will show that the MM estimator is unbiased and consistent. We will also derive a simplified MM estimator which has a nice variance decomposition interpretation. A special case of the MM estimator for the linear growth curve model ($\mathbf{X}_i = \mathbf{Z}_i \mathbf{A}_i$) is considered in Section 4.1.3.

The idea behind deriving a MM estimator for $\mathbf{D}_*$ is as follows: First, we construct the empirical covariance matrix for random effects as the sum of cross-products of residuals, using the OLS estimator. Second, we compute the expectation of that empirical matrix, which is a linear function of the true matrix $\mathbf{D}_*$. Third, we solve the matrix equation for $\mathbf{D}_*$; that is, the MM estimator. We realize our plan below. In fact, this idea of deriving an unbiased quadratic estimation for the variance of random effects is not new and is used widely in the variance components literature (the ANOVA method of estimation). It was introduced by Henderson (1953). Thus, our MM estimator for $\mathbf{D}_*$ can be viewed as a generalization of Henderson's method III (Searle et al., 1992). At that time, this method was considered computationally intensive but most preferable.

First, let $\widehat{\boldsymbol{\beta}}_{OLS}$ be the ordinary least squares estimator in model (2.5), $\widehat{\boldsymbol{\beta}}_{OLS} = (\sum \mathbf{X}_i' \mathbf{X}_i)^{-1} (\sum \mathbf{X}_i' \mathbf{y}_i)$. We calculate the individual OLS residual vector as $\widehat{\mathbf{e}}_i = \mathbf{y}_i - \mathbf{X}_i \widehat{\boldsymbol{\beta}}_{OLS}$ and regress it onto covariates of random effects to obtain an estimate of the random effect. Since matrix $\mathbf{Z}_i$ may not be of full rank, we use the generalized inverse to obtain the random effects prediction, $\widehat{\mathbf{b}}_i = \mathbf{Z}_i^+ \widehat{\mathbf{e}}_i$, where $\mathbf{Z}_i^+$ is the generalized inverse of $\mathbf{Z}_i$ which can be computed as $\mathbf{Z}_i^+ = (\mathbf{Z}_i' \mathbf{Z}_i)^+ \mathbf{Z}_i'$; recall that the generalized inverse of a symmeric matrix can be calculated using the function `ginverse.sym`. Second, we construct the matrix of cross-products, $\sum \widehat{\mathbf{b}}_i \widehat{\mathbf{b}}_i'$, and calculate its expectation,

$$E \sum_{i=1}^N \widehat{\mathbf{b}}_i \widehat{\mathbf{b}}_i' = \sum_{i=1}^N \mathbf{Z}_i^+ E(\widehat{\mathbf{e}}_i \widehat{\mathbf{e}}_i') \mathbf{Z}_i^{+'}. \tag{3.93}$$

Denoting $\boldsymbol{\eta}_i = \mathbf{Z}_i \mathbf{b}_i + \boldsymbol{\varepsilon}_i$ with covariance matrix $\sigma^2 \mathbf{I} + \mathbf{Z}_i \mathbf{D}_* \mathbf{Z}_i'$, we find the expectation of matrix $\widehat{\mathbf{e}}_i \widehat{\mathbf{e}}_i'$,

$$\begin{aligned}
E(\widehat{\mathbf{e}}_i \widehat{\mathbf{e}}_i') &= E(\boldsymbol{\eta}_i - \mathbf{X}_i \mathbf{N} \sum \mathbf{X}_j' \boldsymbol{\eta}_j)(\boldsymbol{\eta}_i - \mathbf{X}_i \mathbf{N} \sum \mathbf{X}_j' \boldsymbol{\eta}_j)' \\
&= \sigma^2 \mathbf{I} - \sigma^2 \mathbf{X}_i \mathbf{N} \mathbf{X}_i' + \mathbf{Z}_i \mathbf{D}_* \mathbf{Z}_i' - \mathbf{Z}_i \mathbf{D}_* \mathbf{Z}_i' \mathbf{X}_i \mathbf{N} \mathbf{X}_i' \\
&\quad - \mathbf{X}_i \mathbf{N} \mathbf{X}_i' \mathbf{Z}_i \mathbf{D}_* \mathbf{Z}_i' + \mathbf{X}_i \mathbf{N} \sum_j [\mathbf{X}_j' \mathbf{Z}_j \mathbf{D}_* \mathbf{Z}_j' \mathbf{X}_j] \mathbf{N} \mathbf{X}_i',
\end{aligned}$$

where matrix $\mathbf{N}$ is defined by (3.87). Substituting this expression into (3.93) yields

$$\begin{aligned}
E \sum \widehat{\mathbf{b}}_i \widehat{\mathbf{b}}_i' &= \sigma^2 \sum_i \mathbf{Z}_i^+ (\mathbf{I} - \mathbf{X}_i \mathbf{N} \mathbf{X}_i') \mathbf{Z}_i^{+'} + \sum_i \mathbf{J}_i \mathbf{D}_* \mathbf{J}_i - \sum_i \mathbf{J}_i \mathbf{D}_* \mathbf{Z}_i' \mathbf{X}_i \mathbf{N} \mathbf{X}_i' \mathbf{Z}_i^{+'} \\
&\quad - \sum_i \mathbf{Z}_i^+ \mathbf{X}_i \mathbf{N} \mathbf{X}_i' \mathbf{Z}_i \mathbf{D}_* \mathbf{J}_i + \sum_{i,j} \mathbf{Z}_i^+ \mathbf{X}_i \mathbf{N} \mathbf{X}_j' \mathbf{Z}_j \mathbf{D}_* \mathbf{Z}_j' \mathbf{X}_j \mathbf{N} \mathbf{X}_i' \mathbf{Z}_i^{+'},
\end{aligned}$$

where we denoted $\mathbf{J}_i = \mathbf{Z}_i^+ \mathbf{Z}_i$. It is easy to prove that $\mathbf{J}_i$ is a $k \times k$ symmetric nonnegative definite idempotent matrix and that $\mathrm{rank}(\mathbf{J}_i) = \mathrm{rank}(\mathbf{Z}_i)$. In fact, if $\mathbf{Z}_i$ has full rank, $\mathbf{J}_i$ is the identity matrix. After denoting

$$\mathbf{L} = \sum \widehat{\mathbf{b}}_i \widehat{\mathbf{b}}_i' - \widehat{\sigma}^2 \sum \mathbf{Z}_i^+ (\mathbf{I} - \mathbf{X}_i \mathbf{N} \mathbf{X}_i') \mathbf{Z}_i^{+'}, \quad \mathbf{R}_{ij} = \mathbf{Z}_i^+ \mathbf{X}_i \mathbf{N} \mathbf{X}_j' \mathbf{Z}_j,$$

where $\widehat{\sigma}^2$ is any unbiased estimator, e.g., the MINQUE (3.79), we come to the following matrix equation for $\mathbf{D}_*$:

$$\mathbf{L} = \sum_{i=1}^{N}(\mathbf{J}_i\mathbf{D}_*\mathbf{J}_i - \mathbf{J}_i\mathbf{D}_*\mathbf{R}'_{ii}\mathbf{J}_i - \mathbf{J}_i\mathbf{R}_{ii}\mathbf{D}_*\mathbf{J}_i) + \sum_{i,j=1}^{N}\mathbf{R}_{ij}\mathbf{D}_*\mathbf{R}'_{ij}. \tag{3.94}$$

We notice that the unknown matrix is between the known matrices, so we apply vec operation to extract $\mathbf{D}_*$ as follows. Let $\mathbf{d}_* =\mathrm{vec}(\mathbf{D}_*)$ be the $k^2 \times 1$ vector of all elements of matrix $\mathbf{D}_*$. Taking the vec operator of both sides of (3.94) and using formula (3.15), we finally obtain the Method of Moments (MM) estimator,

$$\mathrm{vec}(\widehat{\mathbf{D}}_{*MM}) = \mathbf{F}^{-1}\mathrm{vec}(\mathbf{L}), \tag{3.95}$$

where

$$\mathbf{F} = \sum_{i=1}^{N}(\mathbf{J}_i \otimes \mathbf{J}_i - \mathbf{J}_i \otimes \mathbf{J}_i\mathbf{R}_{ii} - \mathbf{J}_i\mathbf{R}_{ii} \otimes \mathbf{J}_i) + \sum_{i,j=1}^{N}\mathbf{R}_{ij} \otimes \mathbf{R}_{ij}. \tag{3.96}$$

The double sum in (3.96) may be replaced by single sums as follows:

$$
\begin{aligned}
\sum_{i,j=1}^{N}\mathbf{R}_{ij} \otimes \mathbf{R}_{ij} &= \sum_{i,j=1}^{N}\mathbf{Z}_i^+\mathbf{X}_i\mathbf{N}\mathbf{X}'_j\mathbf{Z}_j \otimes \mathbf{Z}_i^+\mathbf{X}_i\mathbf{N}\mathbf{X}'_j\mathbf{Z}_j \\
&= \sum_{i,j=1}^{N}(\mathbf{Z}_i^+\mathbf{X}_i\mathbf{N} \otimes \mathbf{Z}_i^+\mathbf{X}_i\mathbf{N})(\mathbf{X}'_j\mathbf{Z}_j \otimes \mathbf{X}'_j\mathbf{Z}_j) \\
&= \left(\sum_{i=1}^{N}\mathbf{Z}_i^+\mathbf{X}_i \otimes \mathbf{Z}_i^+\mathbf{X}_i\right)(\mathbf{N} \otimes \mathbf{N})\left(\sum_{i=1}^{N}\mathbf{X}'_i\mathbf{Z}_i \otimes \mathbf{X}'_i\mathbf{Z}_i\right).
\end{aligned}
$$

Following are a few comments about the MM estimator for $\mathbf{D}_*$. First, this estimator is unbiased because the expectation of the left-hand side of the matrix equation (3.94) is equal to the right-hand side, and $\widehat{\sigma}^2$ is an unbiased estimator. Second, this estimator is a quadratic function of $\{\mathbf{y}_i\}$ since $\widehat{\mathbf{b}}_i\widehat{\mathbf{b}}'_i$ is a quadratic function of $\{\mathbf{y}_i\}$. Third, the estimator (3.95) always exists because the matrix (3.96) is nonsingular. Now we prove the latter statement. To simplify, we shall assume that all the $\mathbf{Z}_i$ have full rank. Let $\mathbf{U}$ be any $k \times k$ nonzero matrix, i.e., $\mathrm{tr}(\mathbf{U}\mathbf{U}') > 0$. We prove that the matrix $\mathbf{F}$ is positive definite by showing that

$$
\begin{aligned}
&\frac{1}{N}\mathrm{vec}'(\mathbf{U})\mathbf{F}\mathrm{vec}(\mathbf{U}) \\
&\geq \mathrm{vec}'(\mathbf{U})\left[\mathbf{I}_{k^2} - \frac{1}{N}\sum_i(\mathbf{R}_{ii} \otimes \mathbf{I}_k + \mathbf{I}_k \otimes \mathbf{R}_{ii})\right]\mathrm{vec}(\mathbf{U}) >0, \tag{3.97}
\end{aligned}
$$

since $\mathrm{vec}'(\mathbf{U})(\sum\mathbf{R}_{ij} \otimes \mathbf{R}_{ij})\mathrm{vec}(\mathbf{U}) \geq 0$. Indeed, using the formula (3.28) and applying the inequality $\mathrm{tr}(\mathbf{A}\mathbf{B}) \leq \mathrm{tr}(\mathbf{A})\mathrm{tr}(\mathbf{B})$ for any nonnegative definite matrices $\mathbf{A}$ and $\mathbf{B}$, one obtains

$$
\begin{aligned}
N^{-1}(\mathrm{vec}'(\mathbf{U})\,(\sum\mathbf{R}_{ii} \otimes \mathbf{I})\,\mathrm{vec}(\mathbf{U})) &= N^{-1}(\mathrm{vec}'(\mathbf{U})\,(\sum\mathbf{R}_{ii} \otimes \mathbf{I})\,\mathrm{vec}(\mathbf{U})) \\
&= N^{-1}\sum\mathrm{tr}(\mathbf{U}\mathbf{R}_{ii}\mathbf{U}') = N^{-1}\sum\mathrm{tr}(\mathbf{R}_{ii}\mathbf{U}'\mathbf{U}) \leq N^{-1}\sum\mathrm{tr}(\mathbf{R}_{ii}) \\
&= N^{-1}\sum_i\mathrm{tr}(\mathbf{X}_i\mathbf{N}\mathbf{X}'_i\mathbf{Z}_i(\mathbf{Z}'_i\mathbf{Z}_i)^{-1}\mathbf{Z}'_i) \leq N^{-1}\sum_i\mathrm{tr}(\mathbf{N}\sum\mathbf{X}'_i\mathbf{X}_i) = m/N.
\end{aligned}
$$

Thus, the left-hand side of inequality (3.97) is greater than $1 - 2m/N$, and therefore matrix $\mathbf{F}$ is nonsingular if $2m < N$.

To get the flavor of (3.95), we derive the MM estimator for a linear model with random coefficients, $\mathbf{Z}_i = \mathbf{X}_i$, where $\mathbf{X}_i$ has full rank; that is,

$$\mathbf{y}_i = \mathbf{X}_i \mathbf{a}_i + \boldsymbol{\varepsilon}_i, \quad \mathbf{a}_i = \boldsymbol{\beta} + \mathbf{b}_i. \tag{3.98}$$

Then $\mathbf{J}_i = \mathbf{I}$ and $\mathbf{R}_{ii} = \mathbf{N}\mathbf{X}_i'\mathbf{X}_i$, and

$$
\begin{aligned}
\sum_{i=1}^{N} \mathbf{R}_{ii} &= \mathbf{N} \sum_{i=1}^{N} \mathbf{X}_i'\mathbf{X}_i = \mathbf{I}, \quad \sum_{i,j=1}^{N} \mathbf{R}_{ij}\mathbf{D}_*\mathbf{R}_{ij}' = \mathbf{N} \sum_{i,j=1}^{N} \mathbf{X}_i'\mathbf{Z}_i\mathbf{D}_*\mathbf{Z}_j'\mathbf{X}_j\mathbf{N} \\
&= \mathbf{N} \left(\sum_{i=1}^{N} \mathbf{X}_i'\mathbf{Z}_i \right) \mathbf{D}_* \left(\sum_{j=1}^{N} \mathbf{Z}_j'\mathbf{X}_j \right) \mathbf{N} = \mathbf{D}_*.
\end{aligned}
$$

Hence, the right-hand side of the matrix equation (3.94) is rewritten as $(N-1)\mathbf{D}_*$. Further,

$$\widehat{\mathbf{b}}_i = \mathbf{Z}_i^+ \widehat{\mathbf{e}}_i = (\mathbf{X}_i'\mathbf{X}_i)^{-1}\mathbf{X}_i(\mathbf{y}_i - \mathbf{X}_i\widehat{\boldsymbol{\beta}}_{OLS}) = \widehat{\mathbf{a}}_i^o - \widehat{\boldsymbol{\beta}}_{OLS},$$

where $\widehat{\mathbf{a}}_i^o$ is the OLS estimator for the ith individual regression. Also, it is easy to see that

$$\sum \mathbf{Z}_i^+ (\mathbf{I} - \mathbf{X}_i\mathbf{N}\mathbf{X}_i')\mathbf{Z}_i^{+'} = \sum (\mathbf{X}_i'\mathbf{X}_i)^{-1} - N\mathbf{N},$$

and finally for model (3.98), we yield

$$
\begin{aligned}
\widehat{\mathbf{D}}_{*MM} = {} & \frac{1}{N-1} \sum_{i=1}^{N} (\widehat{\mathbf{a}}_i^o - \widehat{\boldsymbol{\beta}}_{OLS})(\widehat{\mathbf{a}}_i^o - \widehat{\boldsymbol{\beta}}_{OLS})' \\
& - \frac{\widehat{\sigma}^2}{N-1} \left[\sum (\mathbf{X}_i'\mathbf{X}_i)^{-1} - N \left(\sum \mathbf{X}_i'\mathbf{X}_i \right)^{-1} \right]. \tag{3.99}
\end{aligned}
$$

In particular, for the balanced growth curve model ($\mathbf{Z} = \mathbf{Z}_i = \mathbf{X}_i$, Section 2.3), the MM estimator (3.99) collapses to the unbiased estimator

$$\widehat{\mathbf{D}}_{*MM} = \frac{1}{N-1} \sum_{i=1}^{N} (\widehat{\mathbf{a}}_i^o - \widehat{\boldsymbol{\beta}}_{OLS})(\widehat{\mathbf{a}}_i^o - \widehat{\boldsymbol{\beta}}_{OLS})' - \widehat{\sigma}^2(\mathbf{Z}'\mathbf{Z})^{-1}. \tag{3.100}$$

It is straightforward to show that $\widehat{\sigma}^{-2}\widehat{\mathbf{D}}_{*MM}$ coincides with the RML estimator (2.61). It is not unusual that for the balanced variance components model, the RML is identical to MM (Searle et al., 1992). Also, it is easy to show that for balanced one-way VARCOMP model ($n_i = n$), the estimator (3.100) reduces to

$$\widehat{d}_{*,UMVU} = \frac{1}{N-1} \sum_{i=1}^{N} (\bar{y}_i - \bar{\bar{y}})^2 - \frac{1}{n}\widehat{\sigma}_{UMVU}^2. \tag{3.101}$$

This ANOVA estimator is the Uniformly Minimum Variance Unbiased (UMVU) estimator under the normal assumption, Lehmann and Casella (1998).

In the case of one random effect ($k = 1$), the MM estimator takes the form

$$\widehat{d}_{*MM} = \frac{\sum (\mathbf{z}_i'\widehat{\mathbf{e}}_i)^2 \|\mathbf{z}_i\|^{-4} - \widehat{\sigma}^2 \left(\sum \|\mathbf{z}_i\|^{-2} - q_2 \right)}{N - 2q_1 + \text{tr}(\mathbf{NA}_0\mathbf{NA}_1)}, \tag{3.102}$$

where $\mathbf{z}_i = \mathbf{Z}_i$ is a nonzero $n_i \times 1$ vector, and

$$q_r = \sum (\mathbf{X}_i'\mathbf{z}_i)'\mathbf{N}(\mathbf{X}_i'\mathbf{z}_i) \|\mathbf{z}_i\|^{-2r}, \ r = 1, 2,$$
$$\mathbf{A}_p = \sum \mathbf{X}_i'\mathbf{z}_i\mathbf{z}_i'\mathbf{X}_i \|\mathbf{z}_i\|^{-4p}, \ p = 0, 1.$$

In particular, we derive the MM estimator for the balanced LME model with random intercepts of Section 2.4 as we did in Section 3.10.4. Using Lemma 3, we obtain

$$q_1 = \frac{1}{n}(\mathbf{X}'\mathbf{1})'\mathbf{N}(\mathbf{X}'\mathbf{1}) = 1, \ q_2 = 1/n$$
$$\text{tr}(\mathbf{NA}_0\mathbf{NA}_1) = \frac{1}{n^2} \left(\mathbf{1}'\mathbf{X}(\mathbf{X}'\mathbf{X})^{-1}\mathbf{X1} \right)^2 = 1.$$

We finally obtain for the balanced model with random intercepts, as the generalization of the ANOVA estimator (3.101),

$$\widehat{d}_{*MM} = \frac{1}{N-1} \frac{\sum_{i=1}^{N} \left(\sum_{j=1}^{n} \widehat{e}_{ij} \right)^2}{n^2} - \frac{1}{n}\widehat{\sigma}^2, \tag{3.103}$$

where $\widehat{e}_{ij} = y_{ij} - (\mathbf{X}'\mathbf{X})^{-1}\mathbf{X}'\overline{\mathbf{y}}$ and $\widehat{\sigma}^2$ is the MINQUE/RML estimate defined by (2.87). In the following theorem we obtain a simplified/asymptotic MM estimator.

Theorem 20 *Let all matrices $\{\mathbf{Z}_i\}$ have full rank and, moreover, $\mathbf{Z}_i'\mathbf{Z}_i \geq a\mathbf{I}$ for all $i = 1, 2, ..., N$, where a is a positive number. Then, when $N \to \infty$, the MM estimator (3.95) is equivalent to the Asymptotic MM (AMM) estimator,*

$$\widehat{\mathbf{D}}_{*AMM} = \frac{1}{N} \sum_{i=1}^{N} \widehat{\mathbf{b}}_i\widehat{\mathbf{b}}_i' - \widehat{\sigma}^2 \frac{1}{N} \sum_{i=1}^{N} (\mathbf{Z}_i'\mathbf{Z}_i)^{-1}. \tag{3.104}$$

Proof. Here we give only a sketch of the proof; a rigorous proof may be found in Demidenko and Stukel (2002) for a more general statistical model. Similar to the proof of (3.97), $N^{-1} \sum \mathbf{Z}_i^{+}\mathbf{X}_i\mathbf{NX}_i'\mathbf{Z}_i^{+'} \to \mathbf{0}$, because if $\mathbf{Z}_i$ has full rank then

$$\text{tr} \left(\sum \mathbf{Z}_i^{+}\mathbf{X}_i\mathbf{NX}_i'\mathbf{Z}_i^{+'} \right) = \text{tr} \left(\mathbf{N} \sum \mathbf{X}_i'(\mathbf{Z}_i'\mathbf{Z}_i)^{-1}\mathbf{X}_i \right)$$
$$\leq \frac{1}{a}\text{tr} \left(\mathbf{N} \sum \mathbf{X}_i'\mathbf{X}_i \right) = \frac{m}{a}.$$

Analogously, we can show that matrices $\sum \mathbf{R}_{ii}$ and $\sum \mathbf{R}_{ij}$ are also bounded. Thus, $\mathbf{F} \to N\mathbf{I} \otimes \mathbf{I}$ and we arrive at the estimator (3.104). ∎

The AMM estimator (3.104) has a clear variance decomposition interpretation. Let $\widehat{\sigma}^2$ be fixed, N be sufficiently large, and $\mathbf{Z}_i$ have full rank. Then, since $\widehat{\boldsymbol{\beta}}_{OLS}$ is a consistent estimator, it is close to $\boldsymbol{\beta}$, and therefore

$$E\left(\widehat{\mathbf{b}}_i \widehat{\mathbf{b}}_i'\right) \simeq E(\mathbf{Z}_i^+ \boldsymbol{\eta}_i \boldsymbol{\eta}_i' \mathbf{Z}_i^{+\prime}) = \sigma^2 (\mathbf{Z}_i' \mathbf{Z}_i)^{-1} + \mathbf{D}_*, \ i = 1, ..., N.$$

Summing up these equations and expressing $\mathbf{D}_*$, we come to the estimator (3.104). Note that this estimator is biased for small N. The asymptotic covariance matrix of the MM estimator is derived in Section 4.1.3. This estimator may be used in nonlinear mixed models as well (see Section 6.1).

3.11.1 *lmevarMM function*

The R code for MM estimation of $\mathbf{D}_*$ can be downloaded to an R session as

```
source("c:\\MixedModels\\Chapter03\\lmevarMM.r")
```

The function call is `lmevarMM(m,k,d,s2)`, where `m`, `k`, and `d` have the same meaning as in the previous `lmevarMINQUE` function, and `s2` is the MINQUE estimate as the first component of the `lmevarMINQUE` return. `lmevarMM` returns the MM estimate of $\mathbf{D}_*$ given by formula (3.95). As in the case of MINQUE, it does not gurantee that the returned matrix is positive definite, and it requires the generalized inverse function `ginverse.sym`.

Problems for Section 3.11

1. Simplify (3.96) for the case when all matrices $\mathbf{Z}_i$ have full rank.
2. Prove that the denominator of (3.102) is positive under regular assumptions about the LME model.
3. Derive the AMM estimator for the random intercept model.
4*. Use simulations to compare the MM estimator with RML and MINQUE estimators as in Problem 6 from the previous section.

3.12 Variance least squares estimator

Here we develop another noniterative distribution-free estimator for variance parameters σ^2 and $\mathbf{D}_*$ in the LME model (2.5). We show that this estimator corresponds to the first iteration of the Fisher scoring algorithm under normal assumption. Two versions are considered, biased and unbiased. This method of quadratic estimation of variance parameters will be extended to models with a linear covariance structure. The idea of this method comes from "least squares on squared residuals," suggested by Amemiya (1977) and used widely in the literature on regression with heteroscedastic errors (Jobson and Fuller, 1980; Davidian and Carroll, 1987; Carroll and Ruppert, 1988). The variance least squares is especially useful for generalized linear and nonlinear mixed models (Prentice, 1988). We use this method for variance parameters estimation further in Chapters 6 through 8.

The idea is intuitively appealing. Let $\widehat{\boldsymbol{\beta}}_{OLS}$ be the OLS estimator and we pretend that $\widehat{\boldsymbol{\beta}}_{OLS}$ is the true beta vector. Then $\widehat{\mathbf{e}}_i = \mathbf{y}_i - \mathbf{X}_i \widehat{\boldsymbol{\beta}}_{OLS}$, and the $n \times 1$ residual vector for individual i, might be treated as $\boldsymbol{\eta}_i$. Then, the ith empirical covariance matrix can be assessed as $\widehat{\mathbf{e}}_i\widehat{\mathbf{e}}_i'$. We find an estimator for σ^2 and $\mathbf{D}_*$ by minimizing the sum of traces of squared matrices of the difference between the empirical and theoretical covariance matrix, $\sigma^2\mathbf{I} + \mathbf{Z}_i\mathbf{D}_*\mathbf{Z}_i'$. The resulting estimator will be called Variance Least Squares (VLS) estimator. Precisely, the VLS estimator for σ^2 and $\mathbf{D}_*$ minimizes the sum of traces,

$$\sum_{i=1}^{N} \text{tr}\left(\widehat{\mathbf{e}}_i\widehat{\mathbf{e}}_i' - \sigma^2\mathbf{I} - \mathbf{Z}_i\mathbf{D}_*\mathbf{Z}_i'\right)^2. \tag{3.105}$$

In fact, the minimization of (3.105) can be interpreted as the least squares method applied to the variance parameters because $\text{tr}(\mathbf{A}^2) = \sum A_{ij}^2$ for a symmetric matrix $\mathbf{A}$. To find the minimum of the quadratic form (3.105) we differentiate it with respect to σ^2 and $\mathbf{D}_*$, which leads us to a system of linear equations. After differentiating (3.105) with respect to σ^2, we obtain the equation

$$\sum \text{tr}\left(\widehat{\mathbf{e}}_i\widehat{\mathbf{e}}_i' - \sigma^2\mathbf{I} - \mathbf{Z}_i\mathbf{D}_*\mathbf{Z}_i'\right) = 0. \tag{3.106}$$

After differentiating (3.105) with respect to $\mathbf{D}_*$, we come to

$$\sum \mathbf{Z}_i'\mathbf{Z}_i\mathbf{D}_*\mathbf{Z}_i'\mathbf{Z}_i + \sigma^2 \sum \mathbf{Z}_i'\mathbf{Z}_i = \sum \mathbf{Z}_i'\widehat{\mathbf{e}}_i\widehat{\mathbf{e}}_i'\mathbf{Z}_i. \tag{3.107}$$

As we see, matrix $\mathbf{D}$ appears between two matrices, so to solve (3.106) and (3.107) for σ^2 and $\mathbf{D}$ we need to employ the vector presentation of the matrix using the vec function (Fuller, 1987; Magnus, 1988). First, we represent (3.106) in the vec form as

$$N_T\sigma^2 + \sum \text{vec}'(\mathbf{Z}_i\mathbf{Z}_i)\mathbf{d}_* = \sum \widehat{\mathbf{e}}_i'\widehat{\mathbf{e}}_i,$$

where $\mathbf{d}_* = \text{vec}(\mathbf{D}_*)$. Second, taking the vec operation on both sides of (3.107) and using the formula $\text{vec}(\mathbf{ABC}) = (\mathbf{C}' \otimes \mathbf{A})\text{vec}(\mathbf{B})$, where $\otimes$ denotes the Kronecker product, we come to an equivalent linear equation,

$$\sigma^2\text{vec}(\sum \mathbf{Z}_i'\mathbf{Z}_i) + (\sum \mathbf{Z}_i'\mathbf{Z}_i \otimes \mathbf{Z}_i'\mathbf{Z}_i)\mathbf{d}_* = \sum (\mathbf{Z}_i'\mathbf{e}_i) \otimes (\mathbf{Z}_i'\mathbf{e}_i).$$

Thus, finally, the VLS estimator is

$$\begin{bmatrix} \widehat{\sigma}^2 \\ \widehat{\mathbf{d}}_* \end{bmatrix}_{VLS} = \begin{bmatrix} N_T & \text{vec}'(\sum \mathbf{Z}_i'\mathbf{Z}_i) \\ \text{vec}(\sum \mathbf{Z}_i'\mathbf{Z}_i) & \sum \mathbf{Z}_i'\mathbf{Z}_i \otimes \mathbf{Z}_i'\mathbf{Z}_i \end{bmatrix}^{-1}$$
$$\times \begin{bmatrix} \sum \widehat{\mathbf{e}}_i'\widehat{\mathbf{e}}_i \\ \sum (\mathbf{Z}_i'\widehat{\mathbf{e}}_i) \otimes (\mathbf{Z}_i'\widehat{\mathbf{e}}_i) \end{bmatrix}. \tag{3.108}$$

We can use the block-matrix formula (2.79) to simplify the inverse matrix and to derive separate estimators for σ^2 and $\mathbf{D}_*$. Denoting

$$\mathbf{A} = \sum \mathbf{Z}_i'\mathbf{Z}_i \otimes \mathbf{Z}_i'\mathbf{Z}_i, \quad \mathbf{b} = \sum \text{vec}(\mathbf{Z}_i'\mathbf{Z}_i), \quad c = N_T - \mathbf{b}'\mathbf{A}^{-1}\mathbf{b}$$

we arrive at the VLS estimator for σ^2 and $\mathbf{d}_*$ in the explicit form

$$\widehat{\sigma}^2_{VLS} = c^{-1}\left[\sum \widehat{\mathbf{e}}_i'\widehat{\mathbf{e}}_i - \mathbf{b}'\mathbf{A}^{-1}\sum (\mathbf{Z}_i'\widehat{\mathbf{e}}_i) \otimes (\mathbf{Z}_i'\widehat{\mathbf{e}}_i)\right] \tag{3.109}$$

and

$$\widehat{\mathbf{d}}_{*VLS} = c^{-1} \left\{ \left[c\mathbf{A}^{-1} + \mathbf{A}^{-1}\mathbf{b}\mathbf{b}'\mathbf{A}^{-1}\right] \sum(\mathbf{Z}_i'\widehat{\mathbf{e}}_i) \otimes (\mathbf{Z}_i'\widehat{\mathbf{e}}_i) - \mathbf{A}^{-1}\mathbf{b}\sum\widehat{\mathbf{e}}_i'\widehat{\mathbf{e}}_i \right\}.$$
(3.110)

Note that $\widehat{\sigma}^2$ and $\widehat{\mathbf{d}}_*$ are quadratic functions of $\{\mathbf{y}_i\}$. We have shown in Section 3.3 that if at least one matrix $\mathbf{Z}_i$ has full rank, the inverse matrix in (3.108) is nonsingular. The VLS estimator is easy to generalize to nonlinear mixed models.

3.12.1   Unbiased VLS estimator

The VLS estimator (3.108) is biased. However, we can easily make the bias adjustment by taking the expectation of the VLS estimator. This idea is realized now.

Since the inverse matrix in (3.108) is fixed, it suffices to take the expectation of the vector. Noticing that $\widehat{\mathbf{e}}_i = \boldsymbol{\eta}_i - \mathbf{X}_i\mathbf{N}\sum_j \mathbf{X}_j'\boldsymbol{\eta}_j$, where $\mathbf{N} = (\sum\mathbf{X}_i'\mathbf{X}_i)^{-1}$ and $\{\boldsymbol{\eta}_i\}$ are uncorrelated, $E\boldsymbol{\eta}_i = \mathbf{0}$ and $\mathrm{cov}(\boldsymbol{\eta}_i) = \sigma^2\mathbf{I} + \mathbf{Z}_i\mathbf{D}_*\mathbf{Z}_i'$, we obtain

$$\sum(\mathbf{Z}_i'\widehat{\mathbf{e}}_i) \otimes (\mathbf{Z}_i'\widehat{\mathbf{e}}_i)$$
$$= \sum\mathbf{Z}_i'\boldsymbol{\eta}_i \otimes \mathbf{Z}_i'\boldsymbol{\eta}_i - \sum\mathbf{Z}_i'\mathbf{X}_i\mathbf{N}(\sum\mathbf{X}_j'\boldsymbol{\eta}_j) \otimes \mathbf{Z}_i'\boldsymbol{\eta}_i$$
$$- \sum\mathbf{Z}_i'\boldsymbol{\eta}_i \otimes \mathbf{Z}_i'\mathbf{X}_i\mathbf{N}(\sum\mathbf{X}_j'\boldsymbol{\eta}_j)$$
$$+ \sum\mathbf{Z}_i'\mathbf{X}_i\mathbf{N}(\sum\mathbf{X}_j'\boldsymbol{\eta}_j) \otimes \mathbf{Z}_i'\mathbf{X}_i\mathbf{N}(\sum\mathbf{X}_j'\boldsymbol{\eta}_j). \quad (3.111)$$

Since $E(\boldsymbol{\eta}_i \otimes \boldsymbol{\eta}_i) = E\mathrm{vec}(\boldsymbol{\eta}_i\boldsymbol{\eta}_i') = \sigma^2\mathrm{vec}(\mathbf{I}) + (\mathbf{Z}_i \otimes \mathbf{Z}_i)\mathbf{d}_*$, the expectations of the first through the fourth terms of (3.111) become

$$\sigma^2 \sum\mathrm{vec}(\mathbf{Z}_i'\mathbf{Z}_i) + (\sum\mathbf{Z}_i'\mathbf{Z}_i \otimes \mathbf{Z}_i'\mathbf{Z}_i)\mathbf{d}_*,$$
$$-\sigma^2 \sum\mathrm{vec}(\mathbf{Z}_i'\mathbf{P}_i\mathbf{Z}_i) - (\sum\mathbf{Z}_i'\mathbf{Z}_i \otimes \mathbf{Z}_i'\mathbf{P}_i\mathbf{Z}_i)\mathbf{d}_*,$$
$$-\sigma^2 \sum\mathrm{vec}(\mathbf{Z}_i'\mathbf{P}_i\mathbf{Z}_i) - (\sum\mathbf{Z}_i'\mathbf{P}_i\mathbf{Z}_i \otimes \mathbf{Z}_i'\mathbf{Z}_i)\mathbf{d}_*,$$
$$\sigma^2 \sum\mathrm{vec}(\mathbf{Z}_i'\mathbf{P}_i\mathbf{Z}_i) + (\sum\mathbf{Z}_i'\mathbf{X}_i\mathbf{N} \otimes \mathbf{Z}_i'\mathbf{X}_i\mathbf{N})(\sum\mathbf{X}_i'\mathbf{Z}_i \otimes \mathbf{X}_i'\mathbf{Z}_i)\mathbf{d}_*$$

where $\mathbf{P}_i = \mathbf{X}_i\mathbf{N}\mathbf{X}_i'$. Assembling the terms, we obtain

$$\sigma^2\mathrm{vec}(\sum\mathbf{Z}_i'(\mathbf{I} - \mathbf{P}_i)\mathbf{Z}_i) + \mathbf{H}\mathbf{d}_*,$$

where

$$\mathbf{H} = \sum(\mathbf{Z}_i'\mathbf{Z}_i \otimes \mathbf{Z}_i'\mathbf{Z}_i - \mathbf{Z}_i'\mathbf{Z}_i \otimes \mathbf{Z}_i'\mathbf{P}_i\mathbf{Z}_i - \mathbf{Z}_i'\mathbf{P}_i\mathbf{Z}_i \otimes \mathbf{Z}_i'\mathbf{Z}_i) + \mathbf{G}, \quad (3.112)$$

and for the expectation of the scalar term in the vector of (3.111) we have $\sigma^2(N_T - m) + \mathbf{c}'\mathbf{d}_*$, where $\mathbf{G}$ and $\mathbf{c}$ are as defined in (3.89). Thus, the Unbiased VLS (UVLS) estimator is

$$\left[\begin{array}{c} \widehat{\sigma}^2 \\ \widehat{\mathbf{d}}_* \end{array} \right]_{UVLS} = \left[\begin{array}{cc} N_T - m & \mathbf{c}' \\ \mathbf{c} & \mathbf{H} \end{array} \right]^{-1} \left[\begin{array}{c} \sum\widehat{\mathbf{e}}_i'\widehat{\mathbf{e}}_i \\ \sum(\mathbf{Z}_i'\widehat{\mathbf{e}}_i) \otimes (\mathbf{Z}_i'\widehat{\mathbf{e}}_i) \end{array} \right]. \quad (3.113)$$

One can obtain separate solutions for $\widehat{\sigma}^2$ and $\widehat{\mathbf{d}}_*$ by applying the formula for the matrix inverse (2.79).

3.12.2   Linear model with random intercepts

Using the notation and results of Section 3.10.4 and inverting the 2×2 matrix, we obtain

$$\widehat{\sigma}^2_{UVLS} = \frac{1}{\Delta}[(\sum n_i(n_i - 2\mathbf{s}'_{xi}\mathbf{N}\mathbf{s}_{xi}) + \text{tr}(\sum \mathbf{s}_{xi}\mathbf{s}'_{xi}\mathbf{N})^2)\sum \widehat{\mathbf{e}}'_i\widehat{\mathbf{e}}_i$$
$$- \sum(n_i - \mathbf{s}'_{xi}\mathbf{N}\mathbf{s}_{xi})\sum s^2_{ei}], \tag{3.114}$$

$$\widehat{d}_{*UVLS} = \frac{1}{\Delta}[(N_T - m)\sum s^2_{ei} - \sum(n_i - \mathbf{s}'_{xi}\mathbf{N}\mathbf{s}_{xi})\sum \widehat{\mathbf{e}}'_i\widehat{\mathbf{e}}_i], \tag{3.115}$$

with the determinant

$$\Delta = (N_T - m)[\sum n_i(n_i - 2\mathbf{s}'_{xi}\mathbf{N}\mathbf{s}_{xi}) + \text{tr}(\sum \mathbf{s}_{xi}\mathbf{s}'_{xi}\mathbf{N})^2]$$
$$- [\sum(n_i - \mathbf{s}'_{xi}\mathbf{N}\mathbf{s}_{xi})]^2$$

and $s_{ei} = \sum_{j=1}^{n_i} e_{ij}$.

3.12.3   Balanced design

When matrices $\mathbf{Z}_i$ are the same (balanced design, $n_i = n$, $\mathbf{Z}_i = \mathbf{Z}$) the VLS solutions simplify. Indeed, then

$$c = N_T - N vec'(\mathbf{Z}'\mathbf{Z})\left[(\mathbf{Z}'\mathbf{Z})^{-1} \otimes (\mathbf{Z}'\mathbf{Z})^{-1}\right] \text{vec}(\mathbf{Z}'\mathbf{Z}) = N_T - Nk.$$

Further,

$$\mathbf{b}'\mathbf{A}^{-1}\sum(\mathbf{Z}'_i\widehat{\mathbf{e}}_i) \otimes (\mathbf{Z}'_i\widehat{\mathbf{e}}_i) = \sum \widehat{\mathbf{e}}'_i\mathbf{Z}(\mathbf{Z}'\mathbf{Z})^{-1}\mathbf{Z}'\widehat{\mathbf{e}}'_i$$

and

$$\widehat{\sigma}^2 = \frac{1}{\sum(n_i - k)}\sum \widehat{\mathbf{e}}'_i(\mathbf{I} - \mathbf{Z}(\mathbf{Z}'\mathbf{Z})^{-1}\mathbf{Z}')\widehat{\mathbf{e}}_i.$$

We could derive the solution for $\mathbf{D}_*$ from (3.110), but it is easier to derive it from the matrix equation (3.107). Since $\mathbf{Z}_i = \mathbf{Z}$, we rewrite it as

$$N\mathbf{Z}'\mathbf{Z}\mathbf{D}_*\mathbf{Z}'\mathbf{Z} + N\sigma^2\mathbf{Z}'\mathbf{Z} = \mathbf{Z}'(\sum \widehat{\mathbf{e}}_i\widehat{\mathbf{e}}'_i)\mathbf{Z},$$

so that the VLS estimator for $\mathbf{D}_*$ in this case becomes

$$\widehat{\mathbf{D}}_* = (\mathbf{Z}'\mathbf{Z})^{-1}\mathbf{Z}'\left(\frac{1}{N}\sum \widehat{\mathbf{e}}_i\widehat{\mathbf{e}}'_i\right)\mathbf{Z}(\mathbf{Z}'\mathbf{Z})^{-1} - \widehat{\sigma}^2(\mathbf{Z}'\mathbf{Z})^{-1}.$$

It is obvious that this estimator is equivalent to the simplified MM estimator (3.104), where $(\mathbf{Z}'\mathbf{Z})^{-1}\mathbf{Z}' = \mathbf{Z}^+$ and $\mathbf{b}_i = \mathbf{Z}^+\widehat{\mathbf{e}}_i$.

Now we find the UVLS estimator in case of a balanced random-coefficient (BRC) model, i.e., $\mathbf{Z} = \mathbf{X}_i = \mathbf{Z}_i$. Then

$$\sum \mathbf{Z}'_i(\mathbf{I} - \mathbf{P}_i)\mathbf{Z}_i = (N - 1)\mathbf{Z}'\mathbf{Z}, \quad \mathbf{H} = (N - 1)(\mathbf{Z}'\mathbf{Z}) \otimes (\mathbf{Z}'\mathbf{Z})$$

and using formula (2.79), after some algebra,

$$\begin{bmatrix} Nn - m & (N-1)\mathrm{vec}'(\mathbf{Z}'\mathbf{Z}) \\ (N-1)\mathrm{vec}(\mathbf{Z}'\mathbf{Z}) & (N-1)(\mathbf{Z}'\mathbf{Z}) \otimes (\mathbf{Z}'\mathbf{Z}) \end{bmatrix}^{-1}$$
$$= \frac{1}{N(n-m)} \begin{bmatrix} 1 & -\mathrm{vec}'(\mathbf{M}) \\ -\mathrm{vec}(\mathbf{M}) & \frac{Nn-m}{N-1}\mathbf{M} \otimes \mathbf{M} + \mathrm{vec}(\mathbf{M})\mathrm{vec}'(\mathbf{M}) \end{bmatrix}.$$

where $\mathbf{M} = (\mathbf{Z}'\mathbf{Z})^{-1}$. Thus for the BRC model,

$$\widehat{\sigma}^2_{UVLS} = \frac{1}{N(n-m)} \left[\sum \widehat{\mathbf{e}}'_i \widehat{\mathbf{e}}_i - \mathrm{vec}'(\mathbf{M})(\mathbf{Z} \otimes \mathbf{Z}) \sum \widehat{\mathbf{e}}_i \otimes \widehat{\mathbf{e}}_i \right],$$

$$d_{*UVLS} = \frac{1}{N(n-m)} \left\{ \left[\frac{Nn-m}{N-1}\mathbf{M} \otimes \mathbf{M} + \mathrm{vec}(\mathbf{M})\mathrm{vec}'(\mathbf{M}) \right] \right.$$
$$\left. \times \sum (\mathbf{Z}'\widehat{\mathbf{e}}_i) \otimes (\mathbf{Z}'\widehat{\mathbf{e}}_i) - \mathrm{vec}(\mathbf{Z}'\mathbf{Z})^{-1} \sum \widehat{\mathbf{e}}'_i \widehat{\mathbf{e}}_i \right\}.$$

We prove that $\widehat{\sigma}^2_{UVLS} = \widehat{\sigma}^2_{ML} = \widehat{\sigma}^2_{RML} = \sigma^2_{MINQUE}$. Indeed, $(\mathbf{Z} \otimes \mathbf{Z}) \mathrm{vec}(\mathbf{M}) = \mathrm{vec}(\mathbf{Z}(\mathbf{Z}'\mathbf{Z})^{-1}\mathbf{Z}')$ and the term in brackets is

$$\sum \widehat{\mathbf{e}}'_i [\mathbf{I} - \mathbf{Z}(\mathbf{Z}'\mathbf{Z})^{-1}\mathbf{Z}']\widehat{\mathbf{e}}_i = \sum \mathbf{y}'_i [\mathbf{I} - \mathbf{Z}(\mathbf{Z}'\mathbf{Z})^{-1}\mathbf{Z}']\mathbf{y}_i,$$

which gives (2.59). After some tedious matrix algebra one can show that the UVLS estimator of $\mathbf{D}_*$ coincides with the RMLE, $\widehat{\sigma}^2_{RML}\mathbf{D}_{RML}$, where $\mathbf{D}_{RML}$ is given by (2.61).

3.12.4   VLS as the first iteration of ML

Now we show that (3.109) and (3.110) are derived as the first iteration of the log-likelihood function maximization starting from $\mathbf{D}_0 = \mathbf{0}$. Indeed, assuming that the $\{\mathbf{y}_i\}$ are normally distributed, the log-likelihood function, up to a constant, is written as $l = -0.5 \sum \left(\ln \mid \mathbf{V}_i \mid + \mathbf{e}_i \mathbf{V}_i^{-1} \mathbf{e}_i \right)$, where $\mathbf{V}_i = \sigma^2 \mathbf{I} + \mathbf{Z}_i \mathbf{D}_* \mathbf{Z}'_i$ and $\mathbf{e}_i = \mathbf{y}_i - \mathbf{X}_i \boldsymbol{\beta}$. Differentiating this function with respect to σ^2 and $\mathbf{D}_*$, we come to a pair of estimating equations

$$\sum \mathrm{tr} \left(\mathbf{V}_i^{-1}(\mathbf{e}_i \mathbf{e}'_i - \mathbf{V}_i)\mathbf{V}_i^{-1} \right) = 0, \quad \sum \mathbf{Z}'_i \mathbf{V}_i^{-1} \left(\mathbf{e}_i \mathbf{e}'_i - \mathbf{V}_i \right) \mathbf{V}_i^{-1} \mathbf{Z}_i = \mathbf{0}. \quad (3.116)$$

At the first iteration, $\mathbf{D} = \mathbf{D}_0 = \mathbf{0}$, so that $\mathbf{V}_i = \mathbf{I}$ and $\widehat{\mathbf{e}}_i = \mathbf{y}_i - \mathbf{X}_i \widehat{\boldsymbol{\beta}}$ is the OLS residual vector. But then the first equation of (3.116) is equivalent to (3.106), and the second equation is equivalent to (3.107).

The advantage of the VLS estimator is that it can be applied to more general mixed models, such as the linear model with linear covariance structure of Section 4.3.2 and the nonlinear marginal model, considered in Chapter 8.

3.12.5   lmevarUVLS function

The R code for unbiased VLS estimation for σ^2 and $\mathbf{D}_*$ can be downloaded to an R session as

```
source("c:\\MixedModels\\Chapter03\\lmevarUVLS.r")
```

The function call is `lmevarUVLS(m,k,d)`, where `m`, `k`, and `d` have the same meaning as in our previous codes. Upon completion, this function returns a list with two components: UVLS estimates for σ^2 and $\mathbf{D}_*$.

Problems for Section 3.12

1. Apply the VLS in the form (3.105) to the weighted linear regression model, $y_i = \boldsymbol{\beta}'\mathbf{x}_i + \eta_i$, where $E(\eta_i) = 0$ and $\text{var}(\eta_i) = \sigma^2 + \kappa z_i^2$.

2. Prove that $c = N_T - \mathbf{b}'\mathbf{A}^{-1}\mathbf{b} > 0$.

3. Express $\widehat{\sigma}^2_{VLS}$ and $\widehat{\mathbf{d}}_{*VLS}$ as quadratic functions of the $N_T \times 1$ vector $\mathbf{y}$, defined in (2.9), in the form $g + \mathbf{y}'\mathbf{H}\mathbf{y}$, where g is a constant and $\mathbf{H}$ is a $N_T \times N_T$ fixed matrix.

4. Prove that for linear model with random intercepts we have $\Delta > 0$.

5*. Derive the asymptotic version of the VLS and the unbiased VLS estimators when $N \to \infty$ in the manner of the MM estimator (3.104).

3.13   Projection on $\mathbb{D}_+$ space

The problem of negative estimates of variance parameters in variance components model is common, Searle et al. (1992). If a variance estimate is negative, we set it to zero. However, in the LME model, we estimate the matrix $\mathbf{D}$, and this truncation procedure cannot be generalized in a straightforward manner. If a matrix estimate $\widehat{\mathbf{D}}$ is not nonnegative definite, we project it onto the space of all nonnegative definite matrices $\mathbb{D}_+$ using formula (2.137). Thus, if $\widehat{\mathbf{D}}$ is a noniterative quadratic estimate, we replace it with $\mathbf{P}\boldsymbol{\Lambda}_+\mathbf{P}'$, where $\mathbf{P}$ is the matrix of eigenvectors, $\boldsymbol{\Lambda}$ is the diagonal matrix of eigenvalues, and $\boldsymbol{\Lambda}_+ = \max(0, \boldsymbol{\Lambda})$. If $\widehat{\mathbf{D}}$ is nonnegative definite, this procedure does not change $\widehat{\mathbf{D}}$. Otherwise, $\mathbf{P}\boldsymbol{\Lambda}_+\mathbf{P}'$ is the closest matrix to $\widehat{\mathbf{D}}$ among all nonnegative definite matrices, $\mathbb{D}_+$. It is easy to see that the projection is a singular matrix.

3.14   Comparison of the variance parameter estimation

In this section we compare four estimators of the variance of the random effect d_* in a linear model with random intercepts, Section 2.4. In the next theorem we prove that all four estimates for variance parameters coincide for the balanced random-intercept model of Section 2.4.1, where $n_i = n$ and $\mathbf{X}_i = \mathbf{X}$. Recall that for this model $\widehat{\boldsymbol{\beta}}_{OLS} = (\mathbf{X}'\mathbf{X})^{-1}\mathbf{X}'\overline{\mathbf{y}}$, where $\overline{\mathbf{y}} = N^{-1}\sum_{i=1}^{N}\mathbf{y}_i$.

Theorem 21 *In a balanced random-intercept model, RML=MINQUE= MM=UVLS for variance parameters σ^2 and $d_* = \sigma^2 d$.*

Proof. First we deal with σ^2. The fact that the MINQU estimate=RML estimate in a balanced random-intercept model was proved in Section 3.10.2. Now we prove that UVLS=RML, i.e., (3.114) collapses to (2.87). We start with the calculation of Δ. Since $\mathbf{s}_{xi} = \mathbf{X}'\mathbf{1}$, as follows from Lemma 3 of Section 2.4, we have

$$\sum \mathbf{s}'_{xi}\mathbf{N}\mathbf{s}_{xu} = \text{tr}(\sum \mathbf{s}_{xi}\mathbf{s}'_{xi}\mathbf{N}) = (\mathbf{X}'\mathbf{1})'(\mathbf{X}'\mathbf{X})^{-1}(\mathbf{X}'\mathbf{1}) = n,$$

$$\text{tr}(\sum \mathbf{s}_{xi}\mathbf{s}'_{xi}\mathbf{N})^2 = \text{tr}\left[(\mathbf{X}'\mathbf{1})'(\mathbf{X}'\mathbf{X})^{-1}(\mathbf{X}'\mathbf{1})\right]^2 = n^2,$$

and thus $\Delta = n^2(N-1)[N(n-1)-m+1]$. Using these computations, we obtain

$$\begin{aligned}\widehat{\sigma}^2_{UVLS} &= \frac{n^2(N-1)}{\Delta}\left[\sum \widehat{\mathbf{e}}'_i\widehat{\mathbf{e}}_i - \frac{1}{n}\sum s^2_{ei}\right]\\ &= \frac{1}{N(n-1)-m+1}\left[\sum \|\widehat{\mathbf{e}}_i\|^2 - \frac{1}{n}\sum s^2_{ei}\right].\end{aligned}$$

But due to Lemma 3

$$s_{ei} = \mathbf{1}'\widehat{\mathbf{e}}_i = \mathbf{1}'(\mathbf{y}_i - \mathbf{X}(\mathbf{X}'\mathbf{X})^{-1}\mathbf{X}'\overline{\mathbf{y}}) = n\overline{y}_i - \mathbf{1}'\overline{\mathbf{y}} = n(\overline{y}_i - \overline{\overline{y}}), \qquad (3.117)$$

which leads to estimate (2.87).

Now we deal with d_*. We prove that $\widehat{d}_{*MINQUE} = \widehat{d}_{*RML}$, defined as (3.91) and (2.89). Since $c = n(N-1)$ and

$$\begin{aligned}\sum [s^2_{yi} - s^2_{\overline{y}i}] &= \sum [(\mathbf{1}'\mathbf{y}_i)^2 - (\mathbf{1}'\mathbf{X}(\mathbf{X}'\mathbf{X})^{-1}\mathbf{X}'\overline{\mathbf{y}})^2]\\ &= n^2\sum(\overline{y}^2_i - \overline{\overline{y}}^2) = n^2\sum(\overline{y}_i - \overline{\overline{y}})^2,\end{aligned}$$

(3.91) is reduced to

$$\widehat{d}_{*MINQUE} = \frac{n^2(Nn-m)\sum(\overline{y}_i - \overline{\overline{y}})^2 - n(N-1)\sum \|\widehat{\mathbf{e}}_i\|^2}{n^2(N-1)[N(n-1)-m+1]} = \widehat{d}_{*RML}.$$

MM=RML follows from the fact that $\sum_i(\sum_j \widehat{e}_{ij})^2 = \sum_i s^2_{ei} = n^2\sum(\overline{y}_i - \overline{\overline{y}})^2$ and $\widehat{\sigma}^2 = \widehat{\sigma}^2_{MINQUE} = \widehat{\sigma}^2_{RML}$ in (3.103). For the UVLS estimate of d_* using (3.117) after some elementary algebra we have

$$\begin{aligned}\widehat{d}_{*UVLS} &= \frac{(Nn-m)n^2}{\Delta}\sum(\overline{y}_i - \overline{\overline{y}})^2 - \frac{n(N-1)}{\Delta}\sum \|\widehat{\mathbf{e}}_i\|^2\\ &= \frac{1}{N-1}\sum(\overline{y}_i - \overline{\overline{y}})^2 - \frac{\sum \|\widehat{\mathbf{e}}_i\|^2 - n\sum(\overline{y}_i - \overline{\overline{y}})^2}{n(N(n-1)-m+1)} = \widehat{d}_{*RML}.\end{aligned}$$

∎

Since estimators coincide for balanced data, to compare estimators, we need to consider unbalanced data. Specifically, the following simple random-intercept model with unbalanced data is taken as $y_{ij} = a_i + \beta j + \varepsilon_{ij}$, where $i = 1,...,N, j = 1,...,n_i$, $a_i \sim \mathcal{N}(\alpha, d_*)$ is the random intercept, and $\varepsilon_{ij} \sim \mathcal{N}(0, \sigma^2)$ is the error term. We take two values, $N = 10, 30$, with $\sigma^2 = 0.5$, $\alpha = 1, \beta = 0.5$, and n_i varying from 3 to 7. We compute the variance of $\widehat{d}_*$ for RML, MINQUE (3.91), MM (3.102), and UVLS (3.114) with $\mathbf{Z}_i = \mathbf{z}_i = \mathbf{1}_{n_i}$. The MSE for the restricted ML estimate is assessed via simulations (number of experiments = 3000), and the variance of the other

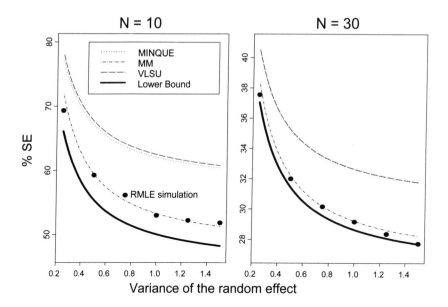

FIGURE 3.5. Comparison of four estimators for the variance of the random effect in a linear model with a random intercept. The variances of the unbiased quadratic estimators are computed exactly, and the MSE of the restricted MLE is assessed via simulations (3000 experiments, dots). % SE is computed as the square root of the variance/MSE divided by the value of d_* times 100. First, the relative SE of $\widehat{d}_*$ decreases with the true value d_* approaching a limit. Second, the SE is about $\sqrt{3}$ less for $N = 30$ than for $N = 10$, in agreement with asymptotic theory. Third, MM outperforms MINQUE and VLSU. Fourth, the restricted maximum likelihood does not outperform the MM estimation. Fifth, when N increases, the SE of the MM/RMLE quickly approaches the lower bound.

three estimates are computed exactly as follows. To compute these variances we use the following fact: $\mathrm{var}(\boldsymbol{\eta}'\mathbf{A}\boldsymbol{\eta}) = 2tr(\mathbf{AV})^2$, where $\boldsymbol{\eta}$ is a random vector normally distributed with zero mean and covariance matrix $\mathbf{V}$ and $\mathbf{A}$ is a fixed matrix of appropriate size. To use this formula, we observe that the three unbiased estimates of d_* may be expressed as a quadratic function $\boldsymbol{\eta}'\mathbf{A}\boldsymbol{\eta}$, where $\boldsymbol{\eta}$ has zero mean and the block diagonal covariance matrix with the ith block $\sigma^2\mathbf{I} + \mathbf{Z}_i\mathbf{D}_*\mathbf{Z}_i'$ is as in equation (2.12). For example, for the MINQUE (3.91) the sum $\sum(s_{yi}^2 - s_{\widehat{y}i}^2)$ can be expressed in terms of $\boldsymbol{\eta}$ as

$$\boldsymbol{\eta}'\mathbf{E}\mathbf{E}'\boldsymbol{\eta} - \boldsymbol{\eta}'(\mathbf{I} - \mathbf{P_X})\mathbf{E}\mathbf{E}'(\mathbf{I} - \mathbf{P_X})\boldsymbol{\eta} = \boldsymbol{\eta}'[\mathbf{E}\mathbf{E}' - (\mathbf{I} - \mathbf{P_X})\mathbf{E}\mathbf{E}'(\mathbf{I} - \mathbf{P_X})]\boldsymbol{\eta},$$

where $\mathbf{P_X}$ is the projection matrix and $\mathbf{E}$ is the $N_T \times N$ block diagonal matrix with $\mathbf{1}_{n_i}$ at the ith block. Similarly, we obtain the exact variance for the MM and UVLS estimates. Since there is no closed solution to the RMLE, when the n_i are different, we use simulations. Also, we compute the lower Cramér–Rao bound for the variance of d_* using formula (3.31).

The results of the comparison are shown in Figure 3.5. We make three major comments: (a) among the three unbiased quadratic estimators, the best is the method of moments estimator; (b) the performance of the MM and RML estimators is very close; and (c) the MM/RML estimators quickly approach the Cramér–Rao bound for the variance of the random effect when N increases.

In summary, we did not get enough evidence beyond a reasonable doubt that the RMLE outperforms the MM estimator for the variance of the random effect, d_*, even when the distribution is normal. Thus, the noniterative distribution-free MM estimator may be a reasonable alternative to the RMLE.

3.14.1   lmesim function

In this section, we compare five methods of estimation of matrix $\mathbf{D}_*$: ML, RML, MINQUE, MM, and UVLS using a simple random intercept and slope model (2.142) with normally distributed errors. The function can be downloaded as

```
source("c:\\MixedModels\\Chapter03\\lmesim.r")
```

The call to this function is as follows:

```
lmesim(N=6,minn=5,maxn=8,betas=c(1,.1),s2=1,
                    D=matrix(c(1,.09,.09,.1),2,2),nExp=100,sr=2)
```

This function depends on other functions to be in the R environment at the time of the execution: `ginverse.sym`, `GLSest`, `lmeFS`, `lmevarMINQUE`, `lmevarMM`, and `lmevarUVLS`. The parameters of `lmesim` have the following meaning:

- `N` is the number of clusters, N.

- `minm` is the minimum number of observations per cluster.

- `maxn` is the maximum number of observations per cluster.

- `betas` is the two-dimensional vector of fixed effects coefficients, $\boldsymbol{\beta}$.

- `s2` is the variance of the error term, σ^2.

- `D` is the 2×2 scaled matrix of the random effects, $\mathbf{D}$.

- `nExp` is the number of simulation experiments.

- `sr` is the seed number.

We make a few remarks: (1) The default value of the number of clusters, $N = 6$, is chosen deliberately small to see whether maximum likelihood works for an extremely low sample size; (2) our function `lmeFS` is used, not `lme`, because in many cases the latter fails with such small sample size; and (3) the figure of merit for the five methods is MSE for $\mathbf{D}_* = \text{cov}(\mathbf{b}_i)$ estimation. With default values, the call `lmesim()` produced the following result:

	MSE
ML	0.8958097
RML	0.9336062
MINQUE	2.2926588
MM	1.0148874
UVLS	1.5529435

As follows from this preliminary simulations, the maximum likelihood estimators slightly outperform the distribution-free estimators of $\mathbf{D}_*$ when errors have normal distribution even for extremely small sample size. It is interesting to know whether MLE remains superior for nonnormal and skewed error distributions such as those suggested in the problem below.

Problems for Section 3.14

1*. Use simulations to compare five estimators of matrix $\mathbf{D}$: ML, RML, MINQUE, MM, and UVLS when error terms do not have a normal distribution; for example, they are distributed as $(\chi_n^2 - n)/\sqrt{2n}$, where χ_n^2 is chi-square distributed with n d.f. (for large n the distribution is close to the standard normal distribution). Use the LME model with random intercepts and slopes (2.142) and compute MSE for β and matrix $\mathbf{D}$ for a sequence of N. State your conclusion.

3.15   Asymptotically efficient estimation for β

The main result of this section is that any of the estimators of $\mathbf{D}$ considered above lead to the same asymptotic and efficient estimation for β applying estimated GLS: For example, when β is estimated by (2.28) with $\mathbf{D}$ substituted by $\widehat{\mathbf{D}}$. The result that the estimated GLS is efficient in linear regression models has been proven by many authors, including Anderson (1973) and Carroll (1982). First, it is necessary to specify what we mean by "asymptotically efficient." In the framework of the LME model, we say that the GLS estimator (2.28) with estimated $\mathbf{D}$ is asymptotically efficient if its limiting/asymptotic distribution coincides with the limiting distribution using the true matrix $\mathbf{D}$. Since, under mild assumptions, both have limiting normal distribution, it suffices to show that the covariance matrices of $\widehat{\beta}(\widehat{\mathbf{D}})$ and $\widehat{\beta}(\mathbf{D})$ are the same in large samples. Second, one needs to prove that all estimators of $\mathbf{D}$ considered above are consistent. The proof of consistency for quadratic estimators is somewhat tedious but principally straightforward, as follows from Demidenko and Stukel (2002), because for a quadratic estimator the variance/covariance matrix may be expressed in closed form. Interestingly, due to the central limit theorem for the asymptotic study, it suffices to assume that the $\{\varepsilon_i\}$ and $\{\mathbf{b}_i\}$ are both iid, and they are independent.

As discussed in Section 3.6, two schema are available when studying the asymptotic behavior of $\widehat{\beta}$: deterministic or stochastic. Let us first consider the *deterministic* scheme. We assume that n_i are uniformly bounded and elements of matrices $\{\mathbf{X}_i\}$

and $\{\mathbf{Z}_i\}$ are uniformly bounded as well when $N \to \infty$. We assume that the limit

$$\mathbf{H} = \mathbf{H}(\mathbf{D}) = \lim_{N \to \infty} \frac{1}{N} \sum_{i=1}^{N} \mathbf{X}_i (\mathbf{I} + \mathbf{Z}_i \mathbf{D} \mathbf{Z}_i')^{-1} \mathbf{X}_i \qquad (3.118)$$

exists for any nonnegative definite matrix $\mathbf{D}$. Using the standard theorem of multivariate calculus, it is easy to prove that $\mathbf{H}$ is a continuous function of $\mathbf{D}$ which belongs to the family of nonnegative definite matrices. Then, if matrix $\mathbf{D}$ was known, the GLS estimator is unbiased, consistent, and asymptotically normally distributed, $\sqrt{N}(\widehat{\boldsymbol{\beta}}(\mathbf{D}) - \boldsymbol{\beta}) \simeq \mathcal{N}(\mathbf{0}, \mathbf{H}^{-1})$, as follows from the multivariate CLT. Since $p\lim_{N \to \infty} \widehat{\mathbf{D}} = \mathbf{D}$ and $p\lim_{N \to \infty} \mathbf{H}(\widehat{\mathbf{D}}) = \mathbf{H}(\mathbf{D})$ from the Slutsky theorem, it follows that $\sqrt{N}(\widehat{\boldsymbol{\beta}}(\widehat{\mathbf{D}}) - \boldsymbol{\beta})$ has the same asymptotic normal distribution. The asymptotic equivalence of $\widehat{\boldsymbol{\beta}}(\mathbf{D})$ and $\widehat{\boldsymbol{\beta}}(\widehat{\mathbf{D}})$ also follows from pseudo-maximum likelihood theory because the information matrix for $\boldsymbol{\beta}$ and $(\sigma^2, \mathbf{D})$ has a block diagonal form.

Under the stochastic scheme, matrix $\mathbf{H}$ in (3.118) is the expectation/integral over $\mathbf{X}_i$ and $\mathbf{Z}_i$, and the asymptotic properties are readily derived from M-estimation theory. See Appendix 13.1 for the basics of the asymptotic theory.

Problems for Section 3.15

1*. Prove that all five (ML, RML, MINQUE, MM, UVLS) estimators of matrix $\mathbf{D}_*$ are consistent under the stochastic scheme when $N \to \infty$. Based on this fact, prove that all five estimators of $\boldsymbol{\beta}$ are asymptotically equivalent using the Slutsky theorem and pseudo-maximum likelihood theory based on the fact that $\widehat{\boldsymbol{\beta}}$ and $\widehat{\mathbf{D}}$ are asymptotically orthogonal, see Appendix 13.1.

3.16   Summary points

- To make the LME model identifiable, one should take either a random or a fixed effects approach. The simultaneous presence of both leads to an unidentifiable statistical model. An example of a poorly defined model is a combination of ANOVA and VARCOMP models, $y_{ij} = \alpha_i + b_i + \varepsilon_{ij}$, where the $\{\alpha_i\}$ are fixed and unknown and b_i is the random effect.

- The information matrix for $\boldsymbol{\beta}$ and $(\sigma^2, \mathbf{D})$ has block diagonal form. There are two consequences of this fact. Numerically, it means that the off-diagonal blocks in the Hessian matrix are close to zero, which justifies separate maximization of the log-likelihood over the beta coefficients and variance parameters. Statistically, the block diagonal structure means asymptotic independence, which implies that *any* consistent estimate of matrix $\mathbf{D}$ leads to an asymptotically efficient estimate of $\boldsymbol{\beta}$.

- Profile-likelihood confidence intervals for beta coefficients are preferable over standard Wald confidence intervals. They are easy to compute using conventional software because the constrained log-likelihood maximum can be obtained via another LME model.

- The likelihood ratio test of the presence of random effects $H_0 : \mathbf{D} = \mathbf{0}$ is not of nominal size. The F-test based on (3.42) is exact, i.e., provides the exact significance level. This test is a generalization of the F-test commonly used in ANOVA and VARCOMP models.

- The restricted and standard maximum likelihood approaches have equivalent statistical properties in large samples. However, one may expect that RML produces less biased estimates of the variance parameters in small samples because for a balanced model, when all design matrices are equal, it gives unbiased estimates for σ^2 and $\mathbf{D}$. RML and ML lead to biased variance estimates for an unbalanced model in small samples.

- An often-forgotten fact is that the maximum likelihood estimator for beta parameters is unbiased in small (and certainly in large) samples. Any estimator of $\mathbf{D}$, as a symmetric function of the error term $\boldsymbol{\eta}$, in generalized least squares leads to an unbiased estimator of $\boldsymbol{\beta}$.

- Random effects may be estimated as posterior means treating the LME model in a Bayesian fashion. For a linear mixed model under normal distribution, there is a closed-form expression. Alternatively, random effects may be derived from penalized least squares, where the penalty is the reciprocal of the scaled matrix of the random effects. The latter approach is used for nonlinear mixed models and for various penalization methods, as described in Chapters 1 and 8.

- Asymptotic properties may be studied under two schema (designs). In the deterministic approach/fixed design, we assume that matrices $\mathbf{X}_i$ and $\mathbf{Z}_i$ are fixed (nonrandom). Then the $\{\mathbf{y}_i\}$ are not identically distributed and special study is required to prove consistency, asymptotic normality, and efficiency because standard ML theory works only for the iid case. In the stochastic approach/random design, we assume that $\{\mathbf{X}_i\}$, $\{\mathbf{Z}_i\}$, and $\{n_i\}$ are random and iid, with certain distributions that may be unknown but that have parameters other than the parameters of the LME model. In this approach the $\{\mathbf{y}_i\}$ are iid, and therefore we can invoke the ML theory, which implies that the estimators are consistent, asymptotically normal, and efficient without additional proof. In particular, this implies that the asymptotic covariance matrix of beta coefficients and variance parameters is obtained as the inverse of the information matrix.

- One cannot expect much difference between the OLS and ML estimates of fixed effects, especially when they have small standard errors and the number of subjects/clusters is large. In particular, the OLS and ML estimates coincide for balanced data. However, the standard error of the OLS estimate in the LME model computed by the standard formula, which ignores random effects, is inflated. Therefore, ML estimation of the LME may lead to statistically significant estimates, whereas the OLS does not. Remember that the difference between standard regression and the mixed effects approach may be considerable in small samples, as pointed out in Section 1.1.

- We develop three noniterative distribution-free quadratic unbiased estimators of the variance parameters in the LME model: MINQUE, Method of Moments (MM), and Unbiased Variance Least Squares (UVLS). In particular, the MM approach may be viewed as a straightforward generalization of Henderson's (1953) method III. For a balanced random-coefficient and random-intercept model, the restricted ML and all unbiased quadratic estimators coincide. One may expect that unbiased quadratic estimation would perform better in a small sample with sparse data. Our simulations demonstrated that the MM estimator is best among three unbiased quadratic estimators of d_* in the random-intercept model. In any event, noniterative estimates can serve as a reasonable starting point for the maximum likelihood iterations considered in Chapter 2, especially when the MLE is on the boundary.

- In a small sample, it is quite possible that an estimate of matrix $\mathbf{D}$ is not non-negative definite. Then a projection on the space of the nonnegative definite matrices should be carried out that is equivalent to the truncation procedure where the negative eigenvalues are replaced by zeros, as follows from Section 2.15.2. Unfortunately, such a procedure destroys the unbiasedness of the estimate.

- In a balanced random-intercept model the variance parameter estimators coincide: restricted MLE = MINQUE = method of moments = variance least squares unbiased. For unbalanced data, RML and MM are closest.

- All estimators of variance parameters considered are consistent. They all lead to the equivalent asymptotic distribution of $\widehat{\boldsymbol{\beta}}$ for large N. This statement follows from the asymptotic independence of $\widehat{\boldsymbol{\beta}}$ and $\widehat{\mathbf{D}}$ (see the details in Appendix 13.1.3).

4

Growth Curve Model and Generalizations

Several special cases and generalizations of the LME model are considered in this chapter. The linear growth curve model may be viewed as a special case of (2.5), where matrix $\mathbf{X}_i$ is a linear combination of vector columns of matrix $\mathbf{Z}_i$. Although all results of Chapters 2 and 3 are applicable, one can simplify the theory and obtain new results, specific to the growth curve model, such as the two-step computation of the GLS estimate. The general growth curve serves as an intermediate model between fixed and random effects. This statistical model is more robust because it does not require specification of all growth curve coefficients in the second-stage model, unlike the standard growth curve model. We also consider the most general linear model with linear covariance structure. This model accommodates well the analysis of longitudinal serially correlated data, a characteristic feature of time series. Another important generalization of the LME model (2.5), the multidimensional mixed model, also has a linear covariance structure. This mixed model is used for our image analysis in Chapter 12. In the last section we consider robust estimation using the Huber function with an estimated threshold. First we illustrate this approach by a simple location problem and then outline its generalization to a mixed effects model.

4.1 Linear growth curve model

The Linear Growth Curve (LGC) model is a special case of the Linear Mixed Effects (LME) model (2.5). Yet it deserves special consideration because of its frequent practical use and the chance to simplify the theory. The model for the LGC is written in hierarchical fashion and is composed of two equations. The first-stage model consists of a set of N independent linear regressions with random coefficients:

$$\mathbf{y}_i = \mathbf{Z}_i\mathbf{a}_i + \boldsymbol{\varepsilon}_i, \quad E(\boldsymbol{\varepsilon}_i) = \mathbf{0},\ \text{cov}(\boldsymbol{\varepsilon}_i) = \sigma^2\mathbf{I}_{n_i}, \tag{4.1}$$

where $\mathbf{y}_i$ is an $n_i \times 1$ vector of the response variable, $\mathbf{Z}_i$ is an $n_i \times k$ design matrix, and $\mathbf{a}_i$ is a $k \times 1$ random vector of individual coefficients, $i = 1, ..., N$. Random vectors $\mathbf{a}_i$ and $\boldsymbol{\varepsilon}_i$ are mutually independent and independent across i. In the second-stage model the individual coefficients are expressed via a linear model as

$$\mathbf{a}_i = \mathbf{A}_i\boldsymbol{\beta} + \mathbf{b}_i, \quad E(\mathbf{b}_i) = \mathbf{0}, \text{cov}(\mathbf{b}_i) = \sigma^2\mathbf{D}, \tag{4.2}$$

where $\mathbf{A}_i$ is a $k \times m$ design matrix and $\boldsymbol{\beta}$ is an $m \times 1$ parameter of interest. Scalar σ^2 and matrix $\mathbf{D}$ are called variance parameters and are unknown. Index i is referred to as the ith subject, so that σ^2 may be interpreted as the within-subject variance and $\mathbf{D}$ may be referred to as the scaled between-subject covariance matrix. The simplest example of the linear growth curve model in a longitudinal setting is given by (2.58). Sometimes we use the notation $\mathbf{D}_* = \text{cov}(\mathbf{b}_i)$ to denote the covariance matrix of random effects. Recall that throughout the book we use the notation $\mathbf{D}_* = \sigma^2\mathbf{D}$. In particular, we estimate $\mathbf{D}_*$ by the method of moments and MINQUE. To avoid the LGC model deficiency, we shall assume that

$$\sum_{i=1}^{N} \mathbf{A}_i'\mathbf{A}_i \text{ is a nonsingular matrix.}$$

Also, in this chapter we assume that *all* matrices $\mathbf{Z}_i$ have full rank:

$$\text{rank}(\mathbf{Z}_i) = k \leq n_i, \quad i = 1, ..., N, \tag{4.3}$$

and that for at least one i, we have $k < n_i$. Note that we do not assume that $m < k$. In a special case when $\mathbf{A}_i = \mathbf{I}$, we come to the growth curve model with random coefficients studied by Swamy (1971) although he assumed that the within-subject variance varies with i.

Substituting (4.2) into (4.1), we come to the LME model $\mathbf{y}_i = \mathbf{X}_i\boldsymbol{\beta} + \mathbf{Z}\mathbf{b}_i + \boldsymbol{\varepsilon}_i$, where

$$\mathbf{X}_i = \mathbf{Z}_i\mathbf{A}_i, \quad i = 1, ..., N. \tag{4.4}$$

Thus, the LGC model is a special case of the LME model when the design matrix of fixed effects is a linear combination of the design matrix of random effects. This observation implies that all results obtained in the previous chapters apply to the LGC model as well. However, the relationship $\mathbf{X}_i = \mathbf{Z}_i\mathbf{A}_i$ brings up something specific—this is the subject of our investigation in this chapter.

When the random variables have a normal distribution, the LGC model may be written compactly as

$$\mathbf{y}_i \sim \mathcal{N}(\mathbf{Z}_i\mathbf{A}_i\boldsymbol{\beta}, \sigma^2(\mathbf{I} + \mathbf{Z}_i\mathbf{D}\mathbf{Z}_i')), \quad i = 1, ..., N. \tag{4.5}$$

As for the linear mixed effects model, matrix $\mathbf{D}$ plays a crucial role in estimation of the beta coefficients because if $\mathbf{D}$ were known, we could apply the generalized least squares, which is efficient. In the next section we start with known $\mathbf{D}$, and in the rest of this chapter we deal with unknown $\mathbf{D}$.

Notice in the LGC model that *all* coefficients of the growth curve (4.1) are assumed random. However, the LME model with random intercepts considered in

Section 2.4 may be treated as a growth curve model with $D_{11} = d$ and the other elements zero. If a part of vector parameter $\mathbf{a}_i$ is specified in the second stage (4.2) but the rest is unspecified, we need to apply the general LGC model considered in the next section.

Sometimes the growth curve model is defined in matrix form as

$$\mathbf{Y} = \mathbf{XBZ} + \boldsymbol{\varepsilon}, \tag{4.6}$$

where $\mathbf{Y}$ is a $p \times n$ matrix of observations, $\mathbf{X}$ and $\mathbf{Z}$ are $p \times m$ and $r \times n$ design matrices, $\mathbf{B}$ is an $m \times r$ matrix of unknown coefficients, and $\boldsymbol{\varepsilon}$ is a $p \times n$ unobserved matrix of random variables (the error term). It is assumed that the error term has zero mean; the columns are independent and have the same $p \times p$ covariance matrix $\boldsymbol{\Omega}$. After taking the vec operator we come to the model $\mathbf{y} = \mathbf{U}\boldsymbol{\beta} + \boldsymbol{\eta}$, where $\text{cov}(\boldsymbol{\eta}) = \mathbf{I} \otimes \boldsymbol{\Omega}$ and $\boldsymbol{\beta} = \text{vec}(\mathbf{B})$. This model was studied initially by Potthoff and Roy (1964) and Rao (1965). A modern discussion of this model can be found in Pan and Fang (2002). The difference between (4.6) and the model defined by (4.1) and (4.2) is that the latter has a more specific covariance structure due to the assumed randomness of the growth curve coefficients although these models share a lot of common statistical properties. Also, in model (4.6) the number of observations for each column is the same. That is, it is a balanced statistical model, unlike our LGC model. For further discussion, see Section 2.3.

4.1.1   Known matrix $\mathbf{D}$

If matrix $\mathbf{D}$ is known, the GLS estimator of $\boldsymbol{\beta}$, as follows from (2.28), takes the form

$$\widehat{\boldsymbol{\beta}}_{GLS} = \left(\sum_{i=1}^{N} \mathbf{A}_i' \mathbf{Z}_i' \mathbf{V}_i^{-1} \mathbf{Z}_i \mathbf{A}_i \right)^{-1} \left(\sum_{i=1}^{N} \mathbf{A}_i' \mathbf{Z}_i' \mathbf{V}_i^{-1} \mathbf{y}_i \right), \tag{4.7}$$

with the covariance matrix

$$\text{cov}(\widehat{\boldsymbol{\beta}}_{GLS}) = \sigma^2 \left(\sum_{i=1}^{N} \mathbf{A}_i' \mathbf{Z}_i' \mathbf{V}_i^{-1} \mathbf{Z}_i \mathbf{A}_i \right)^{-1}.$$

Here we use the earlier notation,

$$\mathbf{V}_i = \mathbf{I} + \mathbf{Z}_i \mathbf{D} \mathbf{Z}_i', \tag{4.8}$$

the $n_i \times n_i$ covariance matrix of the response vector $\mathbf{y}_i$. Letting

$$\mathbf{W}_i = (\mathbf{Z}_i' \mathbf{Z}_i)^{-1} + \mathbf{D}, \quad i = 1, ..., N, \tag{4.9}$$

and applying the dimension-reduction formula (2.25), we obtain

$$
\begin{aligned}
& \mathbf{Z}_i' \mathbf{V}_i^{-1} \mathbf{y}_i \\
=\ & \mathbf{Z}_i'(\mathbf{I} - \mathbf{Z}_i(\mathbf{D}^{-1} + \mathbf{Z}_i'\mathbf{Z}_i)^{-1}\mathbf{Z}_i')\mathbf{y}_i = (\mathbf{Z}_i' - \mathbf{Z}_i'\mathbf{Z}_i(\mathbf{D}^{-1} + \mathbf{Z}_i'\mathbf{Z}_i)^{-1}\mathbf{Z}_i')\mathbf{y}_i \\
=\ & (\mathbf{I} - \mathbf{Z}_i'\mathbf{Z}_i(\mathbf{D}^{-1} + \mathbf{Z}_i'\mathbf{Z}_i)^{-1})\mathbf{Z}_i'\mathbf{y}_i = (\mathbf{D}^{-1} + \mathbf{Z}_i'\mathbf{Z}_i - \mathbf{Z}_i'\mathbf{Z}_i)(\mathbf{D}^{-1} + \mathbf{Z}_i'\mathbf{Z}_i)^{-1}\mathbf{Z}_i'\mathbf{y}_i \\
=\ & \mathbf{D}^{-1}(\mathbf{D}^{-1} + \mathbf{Z}_i'\mathbf{Z}_i)^{-1}\mathbf{Z}_i'\mathbf{y}_i = (\mathbf{I} + \mathbf{Z}_i'\mathbf{Z}_i\mathbf{D})^{-1}\mathbf{Z}_i'\mathbf{y}_i \\
=\ & (\mathbf{I} + \mathbf{Z}_i'\mathbf{Z}_i\mathbf{D})^{-1}(\mathbf{Z}_i'\mathbf{Z}_i)(\mathbf{Z}_i'\mathbf{Z}_i)^{-1}\mathbf{Z}_i'\mathbf{y}_i = \mathbf{W}_i^{-1}\mathbf{a}_i^0.
\end{aligned}
$$

Hence, an economical version of (4.7) takes the form

$$\widehat{\boldsymbol{\beta}}_{GLS} = \left(\sum_{i=1}^{N} \mathbf{A}_i' \mathbf{W}_i^{-1} \mathbf{A}_i \right)^{-1} \left(\sum_{i=1}^{N} \mathbf{A}_i' \mathbf{W}_i^{-1} \mathbf{a}_i^0 \right), \tag{4.10}$$

where

$$\mathbf{a}_i^0 = (\mathbf{Z}_i' \mathbf{Z}_i)^{-1} \mathbf{Z}_i' \mathbf{y}_i \tag{4.11}$$

is the OLS estimator of $\mathbf{a}_i$ in model (4.1). Note that the assumption (4.3) implies that $\mathbf{a}_i^0$ exists for all $i = 1, ..., N$. The covariance matrix simplifies to

$$\mathrm{cov}(\widehat{\boldsymbol{\beta}}_{GLS}) = \sigma^2 \left(\sum_{i=1}^{N} \mathbf{A}_i' \mathbf{W}_i^{-1} \mathbf{A}_i \right)^{-1}.$$

The GLS estimator has the following two-step implementation:

1. Separately estimate (4.1) by the OLS to obtain (4.11) for each $i = 1, ..., N$.

2. Replace $\mathbf{a}_i$ with $\mathbf{a}_i^0$ in (4.2) and apply the weighted least squares with the weight matrix inverse to (4.9).

This interpretation could be called algebraic, however (4.10) can be justified statistically. Indeed, substituting $\mathbf{y}_i$ with $\mathbf{Z}_i \mathbf{A}_i \boldsymbol{\beta} + \mathbf{Z}_i \mathbf{b}_i + \boldsymbol{\varepsilon}_i$ in (4.11) one obtains

$$\mathbf{a}_i^0 = (\mathbf{Z}_i' \mathbf{Z}_i)^{-1} \mathbf{Z}_i' (\mathbf{Z}_i \mathbf{A}_i \boldsymbol{\beta} + \mathbf{Z}_i \mathbf{b}_i + \boldsymbol{\varepsilon}_i) = \mathbf{A}_i \boldsymbol{\beta} + \mathbf{b}_i + (\mathbf{Z}_i' \mathbf{Z}_i)^{-1} \mathbf{Z}_i' \boldsymbol{\varepsilon}_i.$$

Hence, for $\mathbf{a}_i^0$ we have

$$E(\mathbf{a}_i^0) = \mathbf{A}_i \boldsymbol{\beta}, \quad \mathrm{cov}(\mathbf{a}_i^0) = \sigma^2 \mathbf{W}_i = \sigma^2 (\mathbf{D} + (\mathbf{Z}_i' \mathbf{Z}_i)^{-1}),$$

and therefore (4.10) may be derived as an implementation of the weighted least squares to the second-stage model with the weight matrix $\mathbf{W}_i^{-1}$.

Two cases of matrix $\mathbf{D}$ are worthwhile considering. The first case corresponds to the assumption that there are no random effects ($\mathbf{D} = \mathbf{0}$). Then, as follows from (4.10), the GLS estimator collapses to the OLS estimator,

$$\widehat{\boldsymbol{\beta}}_{OLS} = \left(\sum_{i=1}^{N} \mathbf{A}_i' \mathbf{Z}_i' \mathbf{Z}_i \mathbf{\Lambda}_i \right)^{-1} \left(\sum_{i=1}^{N} \mathbf{A}_i' \mathbf{Z}_i' \mathbf{y}_i \right). \tag{4.12}$$

Another extreme case is when $\mathbf{D}$ becomes infinitely large. More precisely, we let $\mathbf{D} = d\mathbf{I}$ and $d \to \infty$, as we did for the LME model in Section 2.2.3. Taking the limit of (4.10), we obtain

$$\lim_{d \to \infty} \left(\sum \mathbf{A}_i' ((\mathbf{Z}_i' \mathbf{Z}_i)^{-1} + d\mathbf{I})^{-1} \mathbf{A}_i \right)^{-1} \left(\sum \mathbf{A}_i' ((\mathbf{Z}_i' \mathbf{Z}_i)^{-1} + d\mathbf{I})^{-1} \mathbf{a}_i^0 \right)$$

$$= \lim_{\delta \to \infty} \left(\sum \mathbf{A}_i' (\delta (\mathbf{Z}_i' \mathbf{Z}_i)^{-1} + \mathbf{I})^{-1} \mathbf{A}_i \right)^{-1} \left(\sum \mathbf{A}_i' (\delta (\mathbf{Z}_i' \mathbf{Z}_i)^{-1} + \mathbf{I})^{-1} \mathbf{a}_i^0 \right)$$

$$= \left(\sum \mathbf{A}_i' \mathbf{A}_i \right)^{-1} \left(\sum \mathbf{A}_i' \mathbf{a}_i^0 \right).$$

Thus, the infinitely large matrix $\mathbf{D}$ leads to the fixed effects estimator

$$\widehat{\boldsymbol{\beta}}_0 = \left(\sum_{i=1}^{N} \mathbf{A}_i' \mathbf{A}_i\right)^{-1} \left(\sum_{i=1}^{N} \mathbf{A}_i' \mathbf{a}_i^0\right). \tag{4.13}$$

This estimator may be interpreted as ordinary least squares applied to the second-stage model ($\mathbf{W}_i = \mathbf{I}$, no weighting). It is elementary to prove that $\widehat{\boldsymbol{\beta}}_0$ and $\widehat{\boldsymbol{\beta}}_{OLS}$ are unbiased. See Section 2.2 for more discussion of the fixed effects model.

4.1.2 Maximum likelihood estimation

Starting from this section it is assumed that matrix $\mathbf{D}$ is unknown and subject to estimation. In this section we apply maximum likelihood assuming that the distributions of $\mathbf{b}_i$ and $\boldsymbol{\varepsilon}_i$ are normal. The log-likelihood function for the LGC model (4.5), up to a constant term, is

$$l(\boldsymbol{\beta}, \sigma^2, \mathbf{D}) = -\frac{1}{2}\left\{ N_T \ln \sigma^2 + \sum \ln |\mathbf{V}_i| \right.$$
$$\left. + \sigma^{-2} \sum (\mathbf{y}_i - \mathbf{Z}_i \mathbf{A}_i \boldsymbol{\beta})' \mathbf{V}_i^{-1} (\mathbf{y}_i - \mathbf{Z}_i \mathbf{A}_i \boldsymbol{\beta}) \right\}, \tag{4.14}$$

where $\mathbf{V}_i$ is the covariance matrix of the response variable defined in (4.8) and $N_T = \sum_{i=1}^{N} n_i$ is the total number of observations. For the linear growth curve model the log-likelihood function may be simplified in the manner in which we derived (4.10). Let $\widehat{\mathbf{e}}_i = \mathbf{y}_i - \mathbf{Z}_i \mathbf{a}_i^0$ be the OLS residual vector. Then

$$\mathbf{y}_i - \mathbf{Z}_i \mathbf{A}_i \boldsymbol{\beta} = (\mathbf{y}_i - \mathbf{Z}_i \mathbf{a}_i^0) + \mathbf{Z}_i (\mathbf{a}_i^0 - \mathbf{A}_i \boldsymbol{\beta}) = \widehat{\mathbf{e}}_i + \mathbf{Z}_i (\mathbf{a}_i^0 - \mathbf{A}_i \boldsymbol{\beta}),$$

and since $\mathbf{Z}_i' \widehat{\mathbf{e}}_i = \mathbf{0}$, we obtain

$$(\mathbf{y}_i - \mathbf{Z}_i \mathbf{A}_i \boldsymbol{\beta})' \mathbf{V}_i^{-1} (\mathbf{y}_i - \mathbf{Z}_i \mathbf{A}_i \boldsymbol{\beta})$$
$$= [\widehat{\mathbf{e}}_i + \mathbf{Z}_i (\mathbf{a}_i^0 - \mathbf{A}_i \boldsymbol{\beta})]' [\mathbf{I} - \mathbf{Z}_i (\mathbf{D}^{-1} + \mathbf{Z}_i' \mathbf{Z}_i)^{-1} \mathbf{Z}_i'] [\widehat{\mathbf{e}}_i + \mathbf{Z}_i (\mathbf{a}_i^0 - \mathbf{A}_i \boldsymbol{\beta})]$$
$$= \|\widehat{\mathbf{e}}_i\|^2 + (\mathbf{a}_i^0 - \mathbf{A}_i \boldsymbol{\beta})' \mathbf{Z}_i' (\mathbf{I} + \mathbf{Z}_i \mathbf{D} \mathbf{Z}_i')^{-1} \mathbf{Z}_i (\mathbf{a}_i^0 - \mathbf{A}_i \boldsymbol{\beta})$$
$$= \|\widehat{\mathbf{e}}_i\|^2 + (\mathbf{a}_i^0 - \mathbf{A}_i \boldsymbol{\beta})' (\mathbf{P}_i + \mathbf{D})^{-1} (\mathbf{a}_i^0 - \mathbf{A}_i \boldsymbol{\beta}),$$

where

$$\mathbf{P}_i = (\mathbf{Z}_i' \mathbf{Z}_i)^{-1}, \quad i = 1, ..., N. \tag{4.15}$$

The determinant of $\mathbf{V}_i$ may be simplified using the dimension-reduction formula (2.22),

$$|\mathbf{V}_i| = |\mathbf{I} + \mathbf{Z}_i \mathbf{D} \mathbf{Z}_i'| = |\mathbf{Z}_i' \mathbf{Z}_i| \cdot |\mathbf{P}_i + \mathbf{D}|.$$

Thus, dropping the constant term $\ln |\mathbf{Z}_i' \mathbf{Z}_i|$, we come to the following economical log-likelihood function

$$l(\boldsymbol{\beta}, \sigma^2, \mathbf{D}) = -\frac{1}{2}\left\{ N_T \ln \sigma^2 + \sum_{i=1}^{N} \ln |\mathbf{P}_i + \mathbf{D}| \right.$$
$$\left. + \sigma^{-2} \left[S_0 + \sum_{i=1}^{N} (\mathbf{a}_i^0 - \mathbf{A}_i \boldsymbol{\beta})' (\mathbf{P}_i + \mathbf{D})^{-1} (\mathbf{a}_i^0 - \mathbf{A}_i \boldsymbol{\beta}) \right] \right\}, \tag{4.16}$$

where the (fixed) total sum

$$S_0 = \sum_{i=1}^{N} \|\widehat{\mathbf{e}}_i\|^2 = \sum_{i=1}^{N} \|\mathbf{y}_i - \mathbf{Z}_i \mathbf{a}_i^0\|^2 \tag{4.17}$$

is the sum of individual sum of squares. As the reader can see, in the original log-likelihood (4.14) one needs to invert $n_i \times n_i$ matrices, whereas in (4.16) one needs to invert $k \times k$ matrices.

Next we show that for the LGC model, we have $S_{\min} = S_0$, where $S_{\min}$ is defined in (2.33). To show this we use the fact that for the LGC model, $\mathbf{X}_i = \mathbf{Z}_i \mathbf{A}_i$, which implies that

$$S_{\min} = \min_{\boldsymbol{\beta}, \mathbf{b}_1, \ldots, \mathbf{b}_N} \sum_{i=1}^{N} \| \mathbf{y}_i - \mathbf{X}_i \boldsymbol{\beta} - \mathbf{Z}_i \mathbf{b}_i \|^2 = \min_{\boldsymbol{\beta}, \mathbf{b}_1, \ldots, \mathbf{b}_N} \sum_{i=1}^{N} \| \mathbf{y}_i - \mathbf{Z}_i \mathbf{A}_i \boldsymbol{\beta} - \mathbf{Z}_i \mathbf{b}_i \|^2$$

$$= \min_{\boldsymbol{\beta}, \mathbf{b}_1, \ldots, \mathbf{b}_N} \sum_{i=1}^{N} \| \mathbf{y}_i - \mathbf{Z}_i (\mathbf{A}_i \boldsymbol{\beta} + \mathbf{b}_i) \|^2 = \min_{\mathbf{a}_1, \ldots, \mathbf{a}_N} \sum_{i=1}^{N} \| \mathbf{y}_i - \mathbf{Z}_i \mathbf{a}_i \|^2 = S_0. \tag{4.18}$$

Consequently, applying Theorem 4 of Section 2.5, we find that the MLE for the LGC model exists if and only if $S_0 > 0$. This means that not all individual fits are perfect. Hence, to avoid nonexistence, we shall assume that $S_0 > 0$. Applying inequality (2.99), we yield the lower bound for the within-subject MLE variance, $\widehat{\sigma}_{ML}^2 \geq S_0/N_T$.

We can also derive the variance-profile log-likelihood function, as we did for the LME model in Section 2.2.4, because the maximum of l over σ^2 is attained at

$$\sigma^2 = \frac{1}{N_T} \sum_{i=1}^{N} (\mathbf{a}_i^0 - \mathbf{A}_i \boldsymbol{\beta})' (\mathbf{P}_i + \mathbf{D})^{-1} (\mathbf{a}_i^0 - \mathbf{A}_i \boldsymbol{\beta}). \tag{4.19}$$

Hence the variance-profile log-likelihood function for the LGC model is

$$l_p(\boldsymbol{\beta}, \mathbf{D}) = -\frac{1}{2} \sum_{i=1}^{N} \Big\{ \ln | \mathbf{P}_i + \mathbf{D} |$$

$$+ N_T \ln \Big[S_0 + \sum_{i=1}^{N} (\mathbf{a}_i^0 - \mathbf{A}_i \boldsymbol{\beta})' (\mathbf{P}_i + \mathbf{D})^{-1} (\mathbf{a}_i^0 - \mathbf{A}_i \boldsymbol{\beta}) \Big] \Big\} \tag{4.20}$$

Further, we can obtain the full-profile log-likelihood function as in Section 2.2 using expression (4.10). We can also apply restricted ML to estimate the LGC model with the augmented term (2.51), where for the LGC model,

$$\sum \mathbf{X}_i' \mathbf{V}_i^{-1} \mathbf{X}_i = \sum \mathbf{A}_i' \mathbf{Z}_i' \mathbf{V}_i^{-1} \mathbf{Z}_i \mathbf{A}_i = \sum \mathbf{A}_i' (\mathbf{P}_i + \mathbf{D})^{-1} \mathbf{A}_i.$$

Maximization algorithms

One can use any algorithm discussed in Chapter 2 to maximize the log-likelihood function for the LGC model (we refer the reader to Appendix 13.2.4 for basic matrix calculus). Here, we derive a simplified version of the variance-profile Newton–Raphson algorithm applying the perturbation formula (2.106). At each iteration, it suffices to obtain an adjustment only for matrix $\mathbf{D}$ because $\boldsymbol{\beta}$ and σ^2 admit closed-form solutions if $\mathbf{D}$ is known. Differentiating (4.20) with respect to $\mathbf{D}$, we obtain

$$\frac{\partial l_p}{\partial \mathbf{D}} = -\frac{1}{2}\left\{\sum(\mathbf{P}_i + \mathbf{D})^{-1} - N_T S^{-1}\sum(\mathbf{P}_i + \mathbf{D})^{-1}\mathbf{r}_i\mathbf{r}_i'(\mathbf{P}_i + \mathbf{D})^{-1}\right\}, \quad (4.21)$$

where

$$S = S(\mathbf{D}) = S_0 + \sum_{i=1}^{N}\mathbf{r}_i'(\mathbf{P}_i + \mathbf{D})^{-1}\mathbf{r}_i, \quad \mathbf{r}_i = \mathbf{a}_i^0 - \mathbf{A}_i\boldsymbol{\beta}.$$

Let $\mathbf{D}_0$ be the current approximation to the MLE; we aim to find the next approximation as $\mathbf{D} = \mathbf{D}_0 + \boldsymbol{\Delta}$, where the increment matrix $\boldsymbol{\Delta}$ is supposed to be small. To approximate the inverse matrix, we use the perturbation formula (2.106),

$$(\mathbf{P}_i + \mathbf{D})^{-1} = (\mathbf{P}_i + \mathbf{D}_0 + \boldsymbol{\Delta})^{-1} \simeq (\mathbf{P}_i + \mathbf{D}_0)^{-1} - (\mathbf{P}_i + \mathbf{D}_0)^{-1}\boldsymbol{\Delta}(\mathbf{P}_i + \mathbf{D}_0)^{-1}.$$

Substituting this approximation into (4.21) and omitting terms of the second order, the estimating/score equation $\partial l_p/\partial \mathbf{D} = \mathbf{0}$ can be approximated as

$$\frac{1}{2}\sum[\mathbf{W}_i^{-1}\boldsymbol{\Delta}\mathbf{W}_i^{-1} - N_T S^{-1}\mathbf{W}_i^{-1}\boldsymbol{\Delta}\mathbf{W}_i^{-1}\mathbf{r}_i\mathbf{r}_i'\mathbf{W}_i^{-1}$$
$$-N_T S^{-1}\mathbf{W}_i^{-1}\mathbf{r}_i\mathbf{r}_i'\mathbf{W}_i^{-1}\boldsymbol{\Delta}\mathbf{W}_i^{-1}] = \mathbf{0},$$

where matrix $\mathbf{W}_i$ is defined by (4.9) and $\mathbf{D} = \mathbf{D}_0$. To find $\boldsymbol{\Delta}$ as the solution to this matrix equation, we employ the vec operator, as we did in Section 2.10. Hence, the increment matrix is given by

$$\text{vec}(\boldsymbol{\Delta}) = \mathbf{J}^{-1}\text{vec}\left(\left.\frac{\partial l}{\partial \mathbf{D}}\right|_{\mathbf{D}=\mathbf{D}_0}\right), \quad (4.22)$$

where the $k^2 \times k^2$ matrix is defined as

$$\mathbf{J} = \frac{1}{2}\sum\left(\mathbf{W}_i^{-1} \otimes \mathbf{W}_i^{-1} + N_T S^{-1}\mathbf{W}_i^{-1}\mathbf{r}_i\mathbf{r}_i'\mathbf{W}_i^{-1} \otimes \mathbf{W}_i^{-1}\right.$$
$$\left. - N_T S^{-1}\mathbf{W}_i^{-1} \otimes \mathbf{W}_i^{-1}\mathbf{r}_i\mathbf{r}_i'\mathbf{W}_i^{-1}\right)$$

and the derivative $\partial l/\partial \mathbf{D}$ is computed by formula (4.21). Thus, the simplified version of the Newton–Raphson algorithm for the LGC model consists of the following steps:

1. Chose an initial matrix $\mathbf{D}_0$ and calculate $\widehat{\boldsymbol{\beta}}_0$ by formula (4.10). Two choices may be used: $\mathbf{D}_0 = \mathbf{0}$ assumes that random effects are small and leads to the estimate (4.12); $\mathbf{D}_0 = \infty$ assumes that random effects are large and leads to the estimate (4.13). Also, any quadratic estimate, such as MM or MINQUE, of matrix $\mathbf{D}$ may be used, see Section 4.1.3.

2. Calculate the increment matrix $\boldsymbol{\Delta}$ by formula (4.22) and compute the next approximation, $\mathbf{D}_1 = \mathbf{D}_0 + \boldsymbol{\Delta}$.

3. Recalculate $\widehat{\boldsymbol{\beta}}$ by formula (4.10), return to step 2, and continue until convergence.

Algorithm (4.22) may be enhanced in different ways following the line of Chapter 2. First, the reduced step length may be used to achieve maximization of l at each iteration. Second, special attention should be paid to matrix $\mathbf{D}$ to arrive at a nonnegative definite solution, see Section 2.15. The Fisher scoring and EM/FP algorithms also apply.

4.1.3 Method of moments for variance parameters

All quadratic estimators developed for the LME model in the previous chapter apply readily to the LGC model with $\mathbf{X}_i = \mathbf{Z}_i\mathbf{A}_i$. Application of the method of moments for the estimation of variance parameters σ^2 and $\mathbf{D}$ seems natural in the LGC model. The advantage of this approach is that it is distribution-free, so that it does not require normal assumptions. Quadratic estimators for variance parameters were developed by several authors for special cases of linear growth curve. For instance, Swamy (1971) proposed the MM estimator of $\mathbf{D}$ for the random-coefficient model ($\mathbf{Z}_i = \mathbf{X}_i$); Reinsel (1985) proposed the MM estimator for the linear growth curve model with $\mathbf{A}_i = \mathbf{I} \otimes \mathbf{q}_i$; Carter and Yang (1986) and Vonesh and Carter (1987) further applied the MM estimator in conjunction with the $\boldsymbol{\beta}$ estimation. In this section we derive the MM estimator of matrix $\mathbf{D}_*$ for the LGC model and show that it collapses to existing estimators in those special cases mentioned.

MM estimator of σ^2

The unbiased and consistent estimator for σ^2, the pooled variance estimator, is well known,

$$\hat{\sigma}^2_{MM} = \frac{1}{\sum_{i=1}^{N}(n_i - k)} \sum_{i=1}^{N} \| \mathbf{y}_i - \mathbf{Z}_i\mathbf{a}_i^0 \|^2, \tag{4.23}$$

where $\mathbf{a}_i^0$ is the OLS estimator of the vector of individual regression coefficients, (4.11). The condition $n_i > k$, for at least one i, guarantees that the denominator is positive. We calculate the variance of $\hat{\sigma}^2_{MM}$ under the normal assumption using the fact that $\text{var}(\mathbf{u}'\mathbf{A}\mathbf{u}) = 2tr(\mathbf{A}\text{cov}(\mathbf{u}))^2$, where $\mathbf{u}$ is a normally distributed vector with zero mean and $\mathbf{A}$ is a fixed symmetric matrix (Graybill, 1983). Then, as follows from this formula,

$$\text{var}(\hat{\sigma}^2_{MM}) = \frac{1}{(\sum(n_i - k))^2} \sum \text{var}(\mathbf{y}_i'(\mathbf{I} - \mathbf{Z}_i(\mathbf{Z}_i'\mathbf{Z}_i)^{-1}\mathbf{Z}_i')\mathbf{y}_i).$$

But

$$\mathbf{y}_i'(\mathbf{I} - \mathbf{Z}_i(\mathbf{Z}_i'\mathbf{Z}_i)^{-1}\mathbf{Z}_i') = (\mathbf{Z}_i\mathbf{A}_i\boldsymbol{\beta} + \mathbf{Z}_i\mathbf{b}_i + \boldsymbol{\varepsilon}_i)'(\mathbf{I} - \mathbf{Z}_i(\mathbf{Z}_i'\mathbf{Z}_i)^{-1}\mathbf{Z}_i')$$
$$= (\mathbf{A}_i\boldsymbol{\beta} + \mathbf{b}_i)\mathbf{Z}_i'(\mathbf{I} - \mathbf{Z}_i(\mathbf{Z}_i'\mathbf{Z}_i)^{-1}\mathbf{Z}_i') + \boldsymbol{\varepsilon}_i'(\mathbf{I} - \mathbf{Z}_i(\mathbf{Z}_i'\mathbf{Z}_i)^{-1}\mathbf{Z}_i')$$
$$= \boldsymbol{\varepsilon}_i'(\mathbf{I} - \mathbf{Z}_i(\mathbf{Z}_i'\mathbf{Z}_i)^{-1}\mathbf{Z}_i'),$$

because $\mathbf{Z}_i'(\mathbf{I} - \mathbf{Z}_i(\mathbf{Z}_i'\mathbf{Z}_i)^{-1}\mathbf{Z}_i') = \mathbf{0}$. Hence, finally

$$\text{var}(\hat{\sigma}^2_{MM}) = \frac{1}{(\sum(n_i - k))^2} \sum \text{var}(\boldsymbol{\varepsilon}_i'(\mathbf{I} - \mathbf{Z}_i(\mathbf{Z}_i'\mathbf{Z}_i)^{-1}\mathbf{Z}_i')\boldsymbol{\varepsilon}_i)$$
$$= \frac{2\sigma^4}{(\sum(n_i - k))^2} \sum tr(\mathbf{I} - \mathbf{Z}_i(\mathbf{Z}_i'\mathbf{Z}_i)^{-1}\mathbf{Z}_i')^2 = \frac{2\sigma^4}{\sum(n_i - k)}. \tag{4.24}$$

As follows from (4.24), the MM estimator of σ^2 is consistent regardless of matrices $\mathbf{Z}_i$ and $\mathbf{A}_i$ because $\mathrm{var}(\hat{\sigma}^2_{MM}) \to 0$ when $\sum(n_i - k) \to \infty$.

Now we show that the pooled variance estimator (4.23) coincides with the MINQUE estimator (3.79) derived for the LME model. Indeed, as follows from (4.18), the denominator of (4.23) is $S_{\min}$; so it suffices to prove that for the linear growth curve model, $\mathrm{rank}(\mathbf{W}) = \sum k_i$. But this equality follows from $\mathbf{X}_i = \mathbf{Z}_i\mathbf{A}_i$, which implies that $\mathrm{rank}(\mathbf{W}) = \mathrm{rank}(\mathbf{Z}) = \sum k_i$, where matrix $\mathbf{Z}$ is defined in (2.9).

MM estimator of $\mathbf{D}_*$

Now we derive the MM unbiased estimator of $\mathbf{D}_* = \mathrm{cov}(\mathbf{b}_i) = \sigma^2\mathbf{D}$, based on the OLS estimator (4.12) and the cross-product residual matrix

$$\mathbf{S} = \sum_{i=1}^{N}(\mathbf{a}_i^0 - \mathbf{A}_i\widehat{\boldsymbol{\beta}}_{OLS})(\mathbf{a}_i^0 - \mathbf{A}_i\widehat{\boldsymbol{\beta}}_{OLS})'. \tag{4.25}$$

We find the MM estimator of $\mathbf{D}_*$ by equating matrix $\mathbf{S}$ to its expectation. Thus, we need to find the expected value of matrix (4.25). To shorten the notation, we introduce the matrices

$$\mathbf{P}_i = (\mathbf{Z}_i'\mathbf{Z}_i)^{-1}, \quad \mathbf{F}_i = (\mathbf{Z}_i'\mathbf{Z}_i)^{-1}\mathbf{A}_i,$$

$$\mathbf{H} = \left(\sum \mathbf{A}_i'(\mathbf{Z}_i'\mathbf{Z}_i)^{-1}\mathbf{A}_i\right)^{-1}, \quad \mathbf{N}_i = \mathbf{F}_i\mathbf{H}\mathbf{A}_i'.$$

Also, we introduce the random vector $\mathbf{u}_i = \mathbf{a}_i^0 - \mathbf{A}_i\widehat{\boldsymbol{\beta}}_{GLS}$, where $\widehat{\boldsymbol{\beta}}_{GLS}$ is calculated by formula (4.10) with $\mathbf{D} = \sigma^{-2}\mathbf{D}_*$. Then it is easy to see that

$$E(\mathbf{u}_i) = \mathbf{0}, \qquad \mathrm{cov}(\mathbf{u}_i) = \mathrm{cov}(\mathbf{b}_i + (\mathbf{Z}_i'\mathbf{Z}_i)^{-1}\mathbf{Z}_i\boldsymbol{\epsilon}_i) = \mathbf{D}_* + \sigma^2\mathbf{P}_i. \tag{4.26}$$

Hence, the residual vector in (4.25) can be rewritten as

$$\mathbf{a}_i^0 - \mathbf{A}_i\widehat{\boldsymbol{\beta}}_{OLS} = (\mathbf{a}_i^0 - \mathbf{A}_i\widehat{\boldsymbol{\beta}}_{GLS}) - \mathbf{A}_i(\widehat{\boldsymbol{\beta}}_{OLS} - \widehat{\boldsymbol{\beta}}_{GLS}) = \mathbf{u}_i - \mathbf{A}_i\mathbf{H}(\sum_j \mathbf{F}_j'\mathbf{u}_j),$$

so that the matrix (4.25) takes the form

$$\sum_i \mathbf{u}_i\mathbf{u}_i' - \sum_i \mathbf{u}_i(\sum_j \mathbf{u}_j'\mathbf{F}_j)\mathbf{H}\mathbf{A}_i' - \sum_i \mathbf{A}_i\mathbf{H}(\sum_j \mathbf{F}_j'\mathbf{u}_j)\mathbf{u}_i'$$

$$+ \sum_i \mathbf{A}_i\mathbf{H}(\sum_j \mathbf{F}_j'\mathbf{u}_j)(\sum_j \mathbf{u}_j'\mathbf{F}_j)\mathbf{H}\mathbf{A}_i'. \tag{4.27}$$

Since $\mathbf{u}_i$ and $\mathbf{u}_j$ are uncorrelated for $i \neq j$, we have

$$E\sum_i \mathbf{u}_i\mathbf{u}_i' = N\mathbf{D}_* + \sigma^2\sum \mathbf{P}_i,$$
$$E\sum_i \mathbf{u}_i(\sum_j \mathbf{u}_j'\mathbf{F}_j)\mathbf{H}\mathbf{A}_i' = \mathbf{D}_*\sum_i \mathbf{N}_i + \sigma^2\sum \mathbf{P}_i\mathbf{N}_i,$$
$$E\sum_i \mathbf{A}_i\mathbf{H}(\sum_j \mathbf{F}_j'\mathbf{u}_j)(\sum_j \mathbf{u}_j'\mathbf{F}_j)\mathbf{H}\mathbf{A}_i'$$
$$= \sum_i \mathbf{A}_i\mathbf{H}[\sum_j \mathbf{F}_j'\mathbf{D}_*\mathbf{F}_j]\mathbf{H}\mathbf{A}_i' + \sigma^2\sum_i \mathbf{A}_i\mathbf{H}(\sum_j \mathbf{F}_j'\mathbf{P}_j\mathbf{F}_j)\mathbf{H}\mathbf{A}_i'.$$

Combining these terms, after some rearrangement, we come to the expectation of $\mathbf{S}$,

$$N\mathbf{D}_* - \mathbf{D}_*\sum_i \mathbf{N}_i - \sum_i \mathbf{N}_i'\mathbf{D}_* + \sum_i \mathbf{A}_i\mathbf{H}(\sum_j \mathbf{F}_j'\mathbf{D}_*\mathbf{F}_j)\mathbf{H}\mathbf{A}_i'$$
$$+ \sigma^2[\sum \mathbf{P}_i - \sum_i \mathbf{P}_i\mathbf{N}_i - \sum_i \mathbf{N}_i'\mathbf{P}_i + \sum_i \mathbf{A}_i\mathbf{H}(\sum_j \mathbf{F}_j'\mathbf{P}_j\mathbf{F}_j)\mathbf{H}\mathbf{A}_i'].$$

$$\tag{4.28}$$

To find matrix $\mathbf{D}_*$, we first calculate the matrix

$$\mathbf{L} = \mathbf{S} - \widehat{\sigma}^2_{MM} \sum_{i=1}^{N} [\mathbf{P}_i - \mathbf{P}_i \mathbf{N}_i - \mathbf{N}'_i \mathbf{P}_i + \mathbf{A}_i \mathbf{H} (\sum_j \mathbf{F}'_j \mathbf{P}_j \mathbf{F}_j) \mathbf{H} \mathbf{A}'_i], \qquad (4.29)$$

with $\widehat{\sigma}^2_{MM}$ as defined by (4.23). Second, we observe that matrix $\mathbf{D}_*$ in (4.28) appears between two matrices. To solve the equation for $\mathbf{D}_*$, we employ the matrix-to-vector transformation, as in Section 3.3. Thus, applying the vec operator to (4.28), we obtain

$$\text{vec}(\mathbf{L}) = \mathbf{d}_* - \left(\frac{1}{N} \sum_i \mathbf{N}'_i \otimes \mathbf{I}_k \right) \mathbf{d}_* - \left(\frac{1}{N} \sum_i \mathbf{I}_k \otimes \mathbf{N}'_i \right) \mathbf{d}_*$$

$$+ \left(\frac{1}{N} \sum_{i,j} \mathbf{K}_{ij} \otimes \mathbf{K}'_{ij} \right) \mathbf{d}_*,$$

where $\mathbf{d}_* = \text{vec}(\mathbf{D}_*)$, $\mathbf{K}_{ij} = \mathbf{A}_i \mathbf{H} \mathbf{F}'_j$ and $i, j = 1, ..., N$. Finally, the MM estimator for $\text{vec}(\mathbf{D}_*)$ is

$$\widehat{\mathbf{d}}_{*MM} = \mathbf{F}^{-1} \text{vec}(\mathbf{L}), \qquad (4.30)$$

where the $k^2 \times k^2$ matrix

$$\mathbf{F} = \mathbf{I}_{k^2} - \frac{1}{N} \sum_i \mathbf{N}'_i \otimes \mathbf{I}_k - \frac{1}{N} \mathbf{I}_k \otimes \sum_i \mathbf{N}'_i + \frac{1}{N} \sum_{i,j} \mathbf{K}_{ij} \otimes \mathbf{K}'_{ij}. \qquad (4.31)$$

Applying the formula $(\mathbf{A} \otimes \mathbf{B})(\mathbf{C} \otimes \mathbf{D}) = (\mathbf{AC} \otimes \mathbf{BD})$, we can reduce the double sum in (4.31) to the product of single sums,

$$\sum_{i,j} \mathbf{K}_{ij} \otimes \mathbf{K}'_{ij} = \sum_i (\mathbf{A}_i \mathbf{H} \otimes \mathbf{I}) \mathbf{E} (\mathbf{I} \otimes \mathbf{H} \mathbf{A}'_i),$$

where $\mathbf{E} = \sum \mathbf{A}'_i \mathbf{P}_i \otimes \mathbf{P}_i \mathbf{A}_i$.

We show that $\mathbf{F}$ is nonsingular in (4.30) if $2k < N$. Let $\mathbf{U}$ be any $k \times k$ matrix. Without loss of generality, we can assume that it is normalized as $\text{tr}(\mathbf{U}'\mathbf{U}) = 1$. We use the formula $\text{vec}'(\mathbf{U})(\mathbf{A} \otimes \mathbf{B})\text{vec}(\mathbf{U}) = \text{tr}(\mathbf{U}\mathbf{A}\mathbf{U}'\mathbf{B}')$. Since for nonnegative definite matrices $\mathbf{A}$ and $\mathbf{B}$ we have $\text{tr}(\mathbf{AB}) \leq \text{tr}(\mathbf{A})\,\text{tr}(\mathbf{B})$ for the second term of (4.31), one obtains

$$(\text{vec}'(\mathbf{U})[\tfrac{1}{N} \sum_i \mathbf{N}'_i \otimes \mathbf{I}]\text{vec}(\mathbf{U}) = \tfrac{1}{N} \sum_i \text{tr}(\mathbf{U}\mathbf{N}'_i\mathbf{U}') =$$
$$\tfrac{1}{N} \sum_i \text{tr}(\mathbf{N}'_i\mathbf{U}'\mathbf{U}) \leq \tfrac{1}{N} \sum_i \text{tr}(\mathbf{N}'_i) = \tfrac{1}{N} \sum_i \text{tr}(\mathbf{A}_i\mathbf{H}\mathbf{A}'_i\mathbf{W}_i^{-1})$$
$$= \tfrac{1}{N} \sum_i \text{tr}(\mathbf{H}\mathbf{A}'_i\mathbf{W}_i^{-1}\mathbf{A}_i) = \tfrac{1}{N}\text{tr}(\mathbf{H} \sum_i \mathbf{A}'_i\mathbf{W}_i^{-1}\mathbf{A}_i) = \tfrac{1}{N}\text{tr}(\mathbf{H}\mathbf{H}^{-1}) = \tfrac{k}{N}.$$

The same holds for the third term of (4.31). Now, since matrix $\sum_{i,j} \mathbf{K}_{ij} \otimes \mathbf{K}'_{ij}$ is nonnegative definite, $\text{vec}'(\mathbf{U})\mathbf{J}\text{vec}(\mathbf{U}) \geq 1 - 2k/N$, which implies that $\mathbf{F}$ is nonsingular.

It is easy to see that the MM estimator (4.30) is a special case of the MM estimator for the LME model derived previously, (3.95). It suffices to prove that the matrix $\sum \widehat{\mathbf{b}}_i\widehat{\mathbf{b}}'_i$, where $\widehat{\mathbf{b}}_i = \mathbf{Z}_i^+\widehat{\mathbf{e}}_i$ for the LME model from Section 3.11, coincides with matrix (4.25). Indeed, since in this section matrix $\mathbf{Z}_i$ is assumed to have full rank, $\mathbf{Z}_i^+ = (\mathbf{Z}_i'\mathbf{Z}_i)^{-1}\mathbf{Z}_i'$, and therefore

$$
\begin{aligned}
\widehat{\mathbf{b}}_i &= (\mathbf{Z}_i'\mathbf{Z}_i)^{-1}\mathbf{Z}_i'(\mathbf{y}_i - \mathbf{X}_i\widehat{\boldsymbol{\beta}}_{OLS}) = (\mathbf{Z}_i'\mathbf{Z}_i)^{-1}\mathbf{Z}_i'(\mathbf{y}_i - \mathbf{Z}_i\mathbf{A}_i\widehat{\boldsymbol{\beta}}_{OLS}) \\
&= \mathbf{a}_i^0 - \mathbf{A}_i\widehat{\boldsymbol{\beta}}_{OLS}.
\end{aligned}
$$

The asymptotic properties of the MM estimator for $\mathbf{D}_*$ are formulated in the following theorem (matrix $\mathcal{D}^+$ was introduced in Section 3.3; see also Appendix 13.2.3).

Theorem 22 *Let $N \to \infty$; then under mild assumptions,*

$$
\widehat{\mathbf{D}}_* = \frac{1}{N}\widehat{\mathbf{S}} - \widehat{\sigma}_{MM}^2 \frac{1}{N}\sum_{i=1}^{N}(\mathbf{Z}_i'\mathbf{Z}_i)^{-1} \tag{4.32}
$$

is asymptotically equivalent to (4.30). Under the normal distribution, the asymptotic covariance matrix for $\mathrm{vech}(\widehat{\mathbf{D}}_*)$ *is*

$$
\frac{2\sigma^4}{N}\mathcal{D}^+\left(\mathbf{D} \otimes \mathbf{D} + \frac{1}{N}\sum_{i=1}^{N}(\mathbf{Z}_i'\mathbf{Z}_i)^{-1} \otimes (\mathbf{Z}_i'\mathbf{Z}_i)^{-1}\right)\mathcal{D}^{+\prime}. \tag{4.33}
$$

The proof is similar to that of Theorem 20.

Some special cases of the MM estimator (4.30) are considered in Section 4.1.5.

MMFE estimator for $\mathbf{D}_*$

Recall that the derivation of the MM estimator (4.30) was based on $\widehat{\boldsymbol{\beta}}_{OLS}$, as an initial estimate of the beta coefficients. This implicitly assumes that $\mathbf{D} = \mathbf{0}$, and therefore one may expect that (4.30) could be a better estimator in a neighborhood of small random effects. However, we can start with $\widehat{\boldsymbol{\beta}}_0$, which implicitly assumes that $\mathbf{D} = \infty$, as in the fixed effects approach of Section 4.1.1. The resulting estimator, called MM Fixed Effects (MMFE), could be a better estimator when $\mathbf{D}_*$ is large.

To derive the MMFE estimator we need to find the expectation of the matrix

$$
\mathbf{S}_0 = \sum_{i=1}^{N}(\mathbf{a}_i^0 - \mathbf{A}_i\widehat{\boldsymbol{\beta}}_0)(\mathbf{a}_i^0 - \mathbf{A}_i\widehat{\boldsymbol{\beta}}_0)'. \tag{4.34}
$$

Similar to the previous derivation, we can express $\mathbf{a}_i^0 - \mathbf{A}_i\widehat{\boldsymbol{\beta}}_0 = \mathbf{u}_i - \mathbf{A}_i\mathbf{H}_0 \times (\sum_j \mathbf{F}_{0j}'\mathbf{u}_j)$, where $\mathbf{H}_0 = (\sum \mathbf{A}_i'\mathbf{A}_i)^{-1}$ and $\mathbf{F}_{0i} = \mathbf{A}_i$. Thus, the expectation of matrix (4.34) is

$$
\begin{aligned}
&N\mathbf{D}_* - \mathbf{D}_*\sum_i \mathbf{N}_i - \sum_i \mathbf{N}_i'\mathbf{D}_* + \sum_i \mathbf{A}_i\mathbf{H}(\sum_j \mathbf{F}_j'\mathbf{D}_*\mathbf{F}_j)\mathbf{H}\mathbf{A}_i' \\
&+\sigma^2[\sum \mathbf{P}_i - \sum_i \mathbf{P}_i\mathbf{N}_i - \sum_i \mathbf{N}_i'\mathbf{P}_i + \sum_i \mathbf{A}_i\mathbf{H}(\sum_j \mathbf{F}_j'\mathbf{P}_j\mathbf{F}_j)\mathbf{H}\mathbf{A}_i'],
\end{aligned}
$$

so that the unbiased MMEF estimator for $\mathbf{d}_* = \mathrm{vec}(\mathbf{D}_*)$ is

$$
\widehat{\mathbf{d}}_{*MMFE} = \mathbf{F}_0^{-1}\mathrm{vec}(\mathbf{L}_0), \tag{4.35}
$$

where $\mathbf{N}_{0i} = \mathbf{A}_i \mathbf{H}_0 \mathbf{A}_i'$ and

$$
\begin{aligned}
\mathbf{L}_0 &= \mathbf{S}_0 - \widehat{\sigma}_{MM}^2 \sum_{i=1}^{N} [\mathbf{P}_i - \mathbf{P}_i \mathbf{N}_{0i} - \mathbf{N}_{0i} \mathbf{P}_i \\
&\quad + \mathbf{A}_i \mathbf{H}_0 (\sum_j \mathbf{A}_j' \mathbf{P}_j \mathbf{A}_j) \mathbf{H}_0 \mathbf{A}_i'],
\end{aligned}
\tag{4.36}
$$

$$
\begin{aligned}
\mathbf{F}_0 &= \mathbf{I}_{k^2} - \frac{1}{N} \sum_i \mathbf{N}_{0i} \otimes \mathbf{I}_k - \frac{1}{N} \mathbf{I}_k \otimes \sum_i \mathbf{N}_{0i} \\
&\quad + \frac{1}{N} \sum_i (\mathbf{A}_i \mathbf{H}_0 \otimes \mathbf{I}) (\sum \mathbf{A}_i' \mathbf{P}_i \otimes \mathbf{P}_i \mathbf{A}_i) (\mathbf{I} \otimes \mathbf{H}_0 \mathbf{A}_i').
\end{aligned}
\tag{4.37}
$$

We illustrate the MM estimators by some special cases of the linear growth curve model.

4.1.4 Two-stage estimation

Due to representation (4.10), estimation of the population parameter $\boldsymbol{\beta}$ may be accomplished in two stages (Davidian and Giltinan, 1995; Stukel and Demidenko, 1997a). At the first stage, we estimate each curve individually by OLS to obtain the subject-specific estimate $\mathbf{a}_i^0$. At the second stage, we apply maximum likelihood in the form (4.20) or use the MM estimator for the variance parameters. Note that the former method gives the MLE of the underlying LME model as follows from representation (4.16).

4.1.5 Special growth curve models

The aim of this subsection is to consider some special cases of the LGC model where the MM and ML estimates simplify. These results may be viewed as an extension of results obtained in Section 2.3. We start with the following definition.

Definition 23 *We say that the LGC model, (4.1) and (4.2), is a rectangular linear growth curve (RLGC) model if matrices $\mathbf{A}_i$ can be represented as*

$$
\mathbf{A}_i = (\mathbf{I} \otimes \mathbf{q}_i'), \qquad i = 1, ..., N,
\tag{4.38}
$$

where $\mathbf{q}_i$ is a $p \times 1$ design vector.

The name *rectangular* comes from the fact that the second-stage model with (4.38) can be written as $\mathbf{a}_i = \mathbf{B}\mathbf{q}_i + \mathbf{b}_i$, where $\mathbf{B}$ is the $k \times p$ matrix of coefficients. Equivalently, we come to (4.38) when each component of the random vector $\mathbf{a}_i = (a_{i1}, ..., a_{ik})'$ has the same set of covariates/explanatory variables, namely,

$$
a_{ij} = \mathbf{q}_i' \boldsymbol{\beta}_j + b_{ij}, \qquad j = 1, ..., k, \quad i = 1, ..., N.
\tag{4.39}
$$

Then in the notation (4.2), $\boldsymbol{\beta}' = (\boldsymbol{\beta}_1', \boldsymbol{\beta}_2', ..., \boldsymbol{\beta}_k')$ and $\mathbf{B} = [\boldsymbol{\beta}_1, \boldsymbol{\beta}_2, ..., \boldsymbol{\beta}_p]$ with $m = kp$. These types of growth curves have been studied by Reinsel (1985), Vonesh and Carter (1987), and Vonesh and Chinchilli (1997). The random-coefficient model where $a_{ij} = \beta_j + b_{ij}$ is a special case of (4.38) with $\mathbf{q}_i = 1$.

Now we apply the MMFE estimator (4.35) to the RLGC model and show that it coincides with the estimator developed by Reinsel (1985). As follows from (4.38),

$$
\begin{aligned}
\mathbf{F}_{0i} &= \mathbf{I} \otimes \mathbf{q}_i', \\
\mathbf{H}_0 &= (\sum (\mathbf{I} \otimes \mathbf{q}_i)(\mathbf{I} \otimes \mathbf{q}_i'))^{-1} = (\sum \mathbf{I} \otimes \mathbf{q}_i \mathbf{q}_i')^{-1} = \mathbf{I} \otimes \mathbf{Q}^{-1}, \\
\mathbf{N}_{0i} &= (\mathbf{I} \otimes \mathbf{q}_i')(\mathbf{I} \otimes \mathbf{Q}^{-1})(\mathbf{I} \otimes \mathbf{q}_i) = \mathbf{q}_i' \mathbf{Q}^{-1} \mathbf{q}_i \mathbf{I},
\end{aligned}
$$

where $\mathbf{Q} = \sum \mathbf{q}_i \mathbf{q}_i'$. Further, for the second and the third terms of expression (4.36), we obtain

$$
\sum_i \mathbf{N}_{0i} = \mathbf{I} \sum_i \mathbf{q}_i' \mathbf{Q}^{-1} \mathbf{q}_i = \mathbf{I} \mathrm{tr}(\sum_i \mathbf{q}_i' \mathbf{Q}^{-1} \mathbf{q}_i) = \mathbf{I}(\mathrm{tr} \mathbf{Q}^{-1} \sum_i \mathbf{q}_i \mathbf{q}_i') = p\mathbf{I}.
$$

For the fourth term of (4.36), we have

$$
\begin{aligned}
&\sum_i \mathbf{A}_i \mathbf{H}_0 (\sum_j \mathbf{F}_{0j}' \mathbf{D}_* \mathbf{F}_{0j}) \mathbf{H}_0 \mathbf{A}_i' \\
&= \sum_{i,j} (\mathbf{I} \otimes \mathbf{q}_i')(\mathbf{I} \otimes \mathbf{Q}^{-1})(\mathbf{I} \otimes \mathbf{q}_j) \mathbf{D}_* (\mathbf{I} \otimes \mathbf{q}_j')(\mathbf{I} \otimes \mathbf{Q}^{-1})(\mathbf{I} \otimes \mathbf{q}_j) \\
&= \mathbf{D}_* \sum_{i,j} (\mathbf{q}_i' \mathbf{Q}^{-1} \mathbf{q}_j)^2 = \mathbf{D}_* \mathrm{tr}(\mathbf{Q}^{-1} \sum_i \mathbf{q}_i \mathbf{q}_i' \mathbf{Q}^{-1} \sum_j \mathbf{q}_j \mathbf{q}_j') \\
&= p\mathbf{D}_*.
\end{aligned}
$$

Analogously,

$$
\sum_i \mathbf{P}_i \mathbf{N}_i = \sum_i \mathbf{N}_i' \mathbf{P}_i = \sum \mathbf{q}_i' \mathbf{Q}^{-1} \mathbf{q}_i (\mathbf{Z}_i' \mathbf{Z}_i)^{-1},
$$

$$
\sum_i \mathbf{A}_i \mathbf{H}(\sum_j \mathbf{F}_j' \mathbf{P}_j \mathbf{F}_j) \mathbf{H} \mathbf{A}_i' = \sum \mathbf{q}_i' \mathbf{Q}^{-1} \mathbf{q}_i (\mathbf{Z}_i' \mathbf{Z}_i)^{-1}.
$$

Combining the terms, we come to the expectation of $\widehat{\mathbf{S}}_0$,

$$
(N - p)\mathbf{D}_* + \sigma^2 \sum \mathbf{q}_i' \mathbf{Q}^{-1} \mathbf{q}_i (\mathbf{Z}_i' \mathbf{Z}_i)^{-1}.
$$

Replacing σ^2 with the unbiased $\widehat{\sigma}_{MM}^2$, we come to the unbiased MMFE estimator of $\mathbf{D}_*$ for the linear growth curve model,

$$
\widehat{\mathbf{D}}_{*MMEF} = \frac{1}{N - p} \widehat{\mathbf{S}} - \frac{\widehat{\sigma}_{MM}^2}{N - p} \sum_i (1 - \mathbf{q}_i' \mathbf{Q}^{-1} \mathbf{q}_i)(\mathbf{Z}_i' \mathbf{Z}_i)^{-1}. \tag{4.40}
$$

This estimator coincides with what has been derived by Reinsel (1985). Thus, the MMFE estimator can be viewed as a generalization of the Reinsel estimator to the linear growth curve model.

Definition 24 *The RLGC with equal $\mathbf{Z}_i$ is called the balanced LGC (BLGC) model.*

For the BLGC model, in addition to (4.38), we have $n_i = n$ and $\mathbf{Z} = \mathbf{Z}_i$ with $kp < n$. When $p = 1$ and $q_1 = 1$, BLGC=BRC, or more precisely, the balanced growth curve model collapses to the balanced random-coefficient model. As was proved in Section 2.3, GLS=OLS for the BRC model. Here, we prove that the same holds for the BLGC model. More precisely, the relevant statement is formulated below.

Theorem 25 *For the BLGC model, $\widehat{\boldsymbol{\beta}}_{GLS}$ does not depend on matrix $\mathbf{D}$ and coincides with the OLS estimator*

$$\widehat{\boldsymbol{\beta}}_j = (\sum_i \mathbf{q}_i \mathbf{q}_i')^{-1} (\sum_i \mathbf{q}_i a_{ij}^0), \quad j = 1, ..., k \tag{4.41}$$

and

$$\text{cov}(\widehat{\boldsymbol{\beta}}_j) = \sigma^2 ((\mathbf{Z}'\mathbf{Z})_{jj}^{-1} + D_{jj})(\sum \mathbf{q}_i \mathbf{q}_i')^{-1}. \tag{4.42}$$

Proof. The following properties of the Kronecker product are used:

$$\begin{aligned}
(\mathbf{A} \otimes \mathbf{B})(\mathbf{C} \otimes \mathbf{D}) &= \mathbf{AC} \otimes \mathbf{BD}, \\
(\mathbf{A} \otimes \mathbf{B})' &= \mathbf{A}' \otimes \mathbf{B}', \quad (\mathbf{A} \otimes \mathbf{B})^{-1} = \mathbf{A}^{-1} \otimes \mathbf{B}^{-1}
\end{aligned}$$

for any suitable matrices $\mathbf{A}$ and $\mathbf{B}$. Applying these formulas and observing that for the BLGC model $\mathbf{W}_i = \mathbf{W} = (\mathbf{Z}'\mathbf{Z})^{-1} + \mathbf{D}$ one obtains

$$\begin{aligned}
\sum \mathbf{A}_i' \mathbf{W}_i^{-1} \mathbf{A}_i &= \sum (\mathbf{I} \otimes \mathbf{q}_i) \mathbf{W}^{-1} (\mathbf{I} \otimes \mathbf{q}_i') = \sum (\mathbf{I} \otimes \mathbf{q}_i)(\mathbf{W}^{-1} \otimes 1)(\mathbf{I} \otimes \mathbf{q}_i') \\
&= \sum (\mathbf{W}^{-1} \otimes \mathbf{q}_i \mathbf{q}_i') = \mathbf{W}^{-1} \otimes (\sum \mathbf{q}_i \mathbf{q}_i'),
\end{aligned}$$

which yields $\left(\sum \mathbf{A}_i' \mathbf{W}_i^{-1} \mathbf{A}_i\right)^{-1} = \mathbf{W} \otimes (\sum \mathbf{q}_i \mathbf{q}_i')^{-1}$. Analogously,

$$\begin{aligned}
\sum \mathbf{A}_i' \mathbf{W}_i^{-1} \mathbf{a}_i^0 &= \sum (\mathbf{I} \otimes \mathbf{q}_i)(\mathbf{W}^{-1} \otimes 1) \mathbf{a}_i^0 = \sum (\mathbf{W}^{-1} \otimes \mathbf{q}_i) \mathbf{a}_i^0 \\
&= \sum (\mathbf{W}^{-1} \otimes \mathbf{I})(\mathbf{I} \otimes \mathbf{q}_i) \mathbf{a}_i^0 = (\mathbf{W}^{-1} \otimes \mathbf{I}) \sum (\mathbf{I} \otimes \mathbf{q}_i) \mathbf{a}_i^0.
\end{aligned}$$

Combing these results, we obtain

$$\begin{aligned}
\widehat{\boldsymbol{\beta}}_{GLS} &= \left(\mathbf{W} \otimes (\sum \mathbf{q}_i \mathbf{q}_i')^{-1}\right) \left((\mathbf{W}^{-1} \otimes \mathbf{I}) \sum (\mathbf{I} \otimes \mathbf{q}_i) \mathbf{a}_i^0\right) \\
&= \left(\mathbf{I} \otimes (\sum \mathbf{q}_i \mathbf{q}_i')^{-1}\right) \sum (\mathbf{I} \otimes \mathbf{q}_i) \mathbf{a}_i^0.
\end{aligned}$$

It can be rewritten as

$$\begin{bmatrix} \widehat{\boldsymbol{\beta}}_1 \\ \widehat{\boldsymbol{\beta}}_2 \\ \vdots \\ \widehat{\boldsymbol{\beta}}_m \end{bmatrix} = \begin{bmatrix} (\sum \mathbf{q}_i \mathbf{q}_i')^{-1} & \mathbf{0} & \mathbf{0} & \mathbf{0} \\ \mathbf{0} & (\sum \mathbf{q}_i \mathbf{q}_i')^{-1} & \mathbf{0} & \mathbf{0} \\ \mathbf{0} & \mathbf{0} & \ddots & \mathbf{0} \\ \mathbf{0} & \mathbf{0} & \mathbf{0} & (\sum \mathbf{q}_i \mathbf{q}_i')^{-1} \end{bmatrix} \begin{bmatrix} \sum \mathbf{q}_i a_{i1}^0 \\ \sum \mathbf{q}_i a_{i2}^0 \\ \vdots \\ \sum \mathbf{q}_i a_{im}^0 \end{bmatrix},$$

which implies (4.41). As follows from the formula above

$$\text{cov}(\widehat{\boldsymbol{\beta}}_{GLS}) = \sigma^2 \left(\mathbf{W} \otimes (\sum \mathbf{q}_i \mathbf{q}_i')^{-1}\right),$$

which gives (4.42). ∎

Comment. Theorem 25 can be applied to balanced growth curves where (4.39) holds for $k' < k$, and for $j = k' + 1, k' + 2, ..., k$ we have $a_{ij'} = \mathbf{q}_i' \boldsymbol{\beta}_{j'}$ (no random effect). Indeed, formally we can say that $D_{i'j'} = 0$ if $i' \geq k'$ or $j' \geq k'$ and apply Theorem 25. In particular, for the balanced linear model with random intercepts studied in Subsections 3.3.1 and 3.10.4, GLS = OLS. The estimate for the variance of the random effect, d_*, is given in Section 3.10.4.

Now we derive the MM and MMFE estimators for the BLGC model. We start with the MMFE estimator. Since $\sum \mathbf{q}_i' \mathbf{Q}^{-1} \mathbf{q}_i = p$ when $\mathbf{Z}_i = \mathbf{Z}$, (4.40) reduces to

$$\widehat{\mathbf{D}}_{*MMEF} = \frac{1}{N - p} \widehat{\mathbf{S}}_0 - \widehat{\sigma}_{MM}^2 (\mathbf{Z}'\mathbf{Z})^{-1}, \qquad (4.43)$$

where matrix $\mathbf{S}_0$ is defined by (4.34). Next we show that the BLGC model estimates (4.12) and (4.13) coincide. Indeed,

$$\widehat{\boldsymbol{\beta}}_{OLS} = \left(\sum (\mathbf{I} \otimes \mathbf{q}_i) \mathbf{Z}' \mathbf{Z} (\mathbf{I} \otimes \mathbf{q}_i') \right)^{-1} \left(\sum (\mathbf{I} \otimes \mathbf{q}_i) \mathbf{Z}' \mathbf{y}_i \right)$$

$$= \left(\mathbf{Q}^{-1} \otimes (\mathbf{Z}'\mathbf{Z})^{-1} \right) \left(\sum (\mathbf{I} \otimes \mathbf{q}_i) \mathbf{Z}' \mathbf{y}_i \right) = \mathbf{Q}^{-1} \otimes \left(\sum (\mathbf{I} \otimes \mathbf{q}_i)(\mathbf{Z}'\mathbf{Z})^{-1} \mathbf{Z}' \mathbf{y}_i \right)$$

$$= \left(\sum \mathbf{A}_i' \mathbf{A}_i \right)^{-1} \left(\sum \mathbf{A}_i' \mathbf{a}_i^0 \right) = \widehat{\boldsymbol{\beta}}_0.$$

Hence, for the BLGC model, $\widehat{\mathbf{D}}_{*MMEF} = \widehat{\mathbf{D}}_{*MM}$.

Maximum likelihood for the BLGC model

Here we derive the closed-form solution to the MLE for variance parameters in the BLGC model, as an extension of the results of Section 2.3. We show that for the BLGC model, results (2.59), (2.60), and (2.61) hold with the following modification. First, in the denominator of (2.59), for the BLGC model we have $m = kp$. Second, $\widehat{\mathbf{D}}_{ML}$ does not change. Third, in the denominator of the first term of (2.61), we have $N - p$. The first two statements follow from the fact that GLS = OLS under the BLGC model and repeating step by step following the line of the proof of Theorem 2. For restricted ML, the estimating equation (2.129) in the case of the BLGC model reduces to

$$N\mathbf{Z}'\mathbf{V}^{-1}\mathbf{Z} - \sigma^{-2} \mathbf{Z}'\mathbf{V}^{-1} \widehat{\mathbf{E}} \widehat{\mathbf{E}}' \mathbf{V}^{-1} \mathbf{Z}$$
$$+ \mathbf{Z}'\mathbf{V}^{-1} \sum_i \mathbf{X}_i \left(\sum_j \mathbf{X}_j' \mathbf{V}^{-1} \mathbf{X}_j \right)^{-1} \mathbf{X}_i' \mathbf{V}^{-1} \mathbf{Z}. \qquad (4.44)$$

But

$$\sum_j \mathbf{X}_j' \mathbf{V}^{-1} \mathbf{X}_j = \sum (\mathbf{I} \otimes \mathbf{q}_j) \mathbf{Z}' \mathbf{V}^{-1} \mathbf{Z} (\mathbf{I} \otimes \mathbf{q}_j') = (\mathbf{Z}' \mathbf{V}^{-1} \mathbf{Z}) \otimes \mathbf{Q},$$

and the third term in (4.44) becomes

$$(\mathbf{Z}'\mathbf{V}^{-1}\mathbf{Z}) \sum_i [(\mathbf{I} \otimes \mathbf{q}_i')((\mathbf{Z}'\mathbf{V}^{-1}\mathbf{Z})^{-1} \otimes \mathbf{Q}^{-1})(\mathbf{I} \otimes \mathbf{q}_i)](\mathbf{Z}'\mathbf{V}^{-1}\mathbf{Z})$$

$$= (\mathbf{Z}'\mathbf{V}^{-1}\mathbf{Z})(\mathbf{Z}'\mathbf{V}^{-1}\mathbf{Z})^{-1}(\mathbf{Z}'\mathbf{V}^{-1}\mathbf{Z}) \sum_i \mathbf{q}_i' \mathbf{Q}^{-1} \mathbf{q}_i = p\mathbf{Z}'\mathbf{V}^{-1}\mathbf{Z}.$$

Finally, equation (4.44) can be rewritten as

$$(N - p)\mathbf{Z}'\mathbf{V}^{-1}\mathbf{Z} - \sigma^{-2} \mathbf{Z}'\mathbf{V}^{-1} \widehat{\mathbf{E}} \widehat{\mathbf{E}}' \mathbf{V}^{-1} \mathbf{Z},$$

which leads to the estimate

$$\widehat{\mathbf{D}}_{*RML} = \frac{1}{N-p}(\mathbf{Z}'\mathbf{Z})^{-1}\mathbf{Z}'\widehat{\mathbf{E}}\widehat{\mathbf{E}}'\mathbf{Z}(\mathbf{Z}'\mathbf{Z})^{-1} - \widehat{\sigma}^2_{ML}(\mathbf{Z}'\mathbf{Z})^{-1}. \qquad (4.45)$$

where, as shown previously, $\widehat{\sigma}^2_{ML} = \widehat{\sigma}^2_{MM} = \widehat{\sigma}^2_{MINQUE}$.

4.1.6 Unbiasedness and efficient estimation for β

Following the line of arguments of Section 3.6, one can easily prove that MLE, RMLE, and any quadratic estimators of $\mathbf{D}$ in the growth curve model considered above are even functions of $\mathbf{b}_i$ and independent of β. Thus, using those $\widehat{\mathbf{D}}$ in the GLS estimator (4.10) will lead to unbiased estimation for β for any N.

Also, as follows from Section 3.15, in the deterministic approach, use of any fixed matrix $\widetilde{\mathbf{D}}$ in (4.10) produces a consistent and asymptotically normally distributed estimator such that $\sqrt{N}(\widetilde{\beta} - \beta) \simeq \mathcal{N}(\mathbf{0}, \sigma^2\mathbf{H})$, where it is assumed that the limit

$$\mathbf{H} = \mathbf{H}(\widetilde{\mathbf{D}}) = \lim_{N\to\infty}\frac{1}{N}\left(\sum_{i=1}^{N}\mathbf{A}'_i\widetilde{\mathbf{W}}^{-1}_i\mathbf{A}_i\right)^{-1}$$

$$\times \left(\sum_{i=1}^{N}\mathbf{A}'_i\mathbf{W}^{-1}_i\mathbf{A}_i\right)\left(\sum_{i=1}^{N}\mathbf{A}'_i\widetilde{\mathbf{W}}^{-1}_i\mathbf{A}_i\right)^{-1} \qquad (4.46)$$

exists and $\widetilde{\mathbf{W}}_i = (\mathbf{Z}'_i\mathbf{Z}_i)^{-1} + \widetilde{\mathbf{D}}$ and $\mathbf{W}_i = (\mathbf{Z}'_i\mathbf{Z}_i)^{-1} + \mathbf{D}$, where $\mathbf{D}$ is the true matrix. Then, by the Slutsky theorem (Appendix 13.1.2), the two-stage procedure, when at the first stage one estimates $\mathbf{D}$ and at the second stage one uses (4.10) with $\mathbf{D}$ replaced by its estimate (estimated GLS), leads to a consistent, asymptotically normally distributed and efficient estimator for β, with the matrix

$$\mathbf{H} = \lim_{N\to\infty}\frac{1}{N}\left(\sum_{i=1}^{N}\mathbf{A}'_i\mathbf{W}^{-1}_i\mathbf{A}_i\right)^{-1} ;$$

Vonesh and Carter (1987). According to our definition, the estimator is asymptotically efficient if its asymptotic distribution coincides with the estimator, which uses the true matrix $\mathbf{D}$ (Section 3.15). We come to the same conclusion in the stochastic approach; then the assumption on the limit (4.46) is not necessary.

Problems for Section 4.1

1. Prove that estimators $\widehat{\beta}_0$ and $\widehat{\beta}_{OLS}$, given by formulas (4.13) and (4.12) respectively, are unbiased when $\mathbf{D}$ is unknown.

2. Simplify $\widehat{\beta}_{GLS}, \widehat{\beta}_0$, and $\widehat{\beta}_{OLS}$ for balanced data.

3. Derive $\widehat{\beta}_0$ when $\mathbf{D} = d\mathbf{D}_0$, where $\mathbf{D}_0$ is a fixed positive definite matrix and $d \to \infty$.

4. Explain why $S_{\min} = S_0$ in equation (4.18).

5. Write an R code for maximization of the function $l_p(\beta, \mathbf{D})$ given by equation (4.20) using algorithm (4.22), and test it through lmeFS.

6. Prove that matrix $\mathbf{J}$ in equation (4.22) is positive definite.

7. Prove that $\hat{\sigma}_{MM}^2$ given by equation (4.23) can be derived from (3.79). Prove that $E(\hat{\sigma}_{MM}^2) = \sigma^2$.

8*. Write an R code for computation of $\widehat{\mathbf{d}}_{*MM}$ defined by equation (4.30) and demonstrate that it coincides with that obtained from the function lmevarMM.

9*. Provide a rigorous proof of Theorem 22.

10. State conditions when estimators $\widehat{\mathbf{d}}_{*MM}$ and $\widehat{\mathbf{d}}_{*MMFE}$ are the same.

11. Derive a special case of estimator (4.45) for the random intercept model and compare it with (3.103).

4.2   General linear growth curve model

Recall that the linear growth curve model is written in two stages. The first-stage model (4.1) consists of N independent linear regression models with random subject-specific coefficients. The second-stage model (4.2) further describes the vector of coefficients $\mathbf{a}_i$ through population covariates (explanatory variables). Importantly, in the LGC model *all* growth curve coefficients are present at the second-stage model. However, sometimes we are interested in only a few components of vector $\mathbf{a}_i$. In the general linear growth curve model, the second-stage model specifies only certain linear combinations of $\mathbf{a}_i$; the rest of the growth curve coefficients are left unspecified (Stukel and Demidenko, 1997a; Demidenko and Stukel, 2002).

The general linear growth curve (GLGC) model is set up as follows. The first-stage model remains the same, (4.1). The second-stage model specifies r linear combinations of $\mathbf{a}_i$ via a linear model of the form

$$\mathbf{Ca}_i = \mathbf{A}_i\boldsymbol{\beta} + \boldsymbol{\delta}_i, \tag{4.47}$$

where $\mathbf{C}$ is a known $r \times k$ matrix of full rank $r \leq k$. Denoting $\mathbf{B} = \mathbf{CDC}'$, we obtain $\text{cov}(\boldsymbol{\delta}_i) = \sigma^2\mathbf{B}$, where $\mathbf{B}$ is called the *scaled covariance matrix* of the random effects $\boldsymbol{\delta}_i$. The design matrix $\mathbf{A}_i$ in (4.47) is $r \times m$, and it is assumed that matrix $\sum \mathbf{A}_i'\mathbf{A}_i$ has full rank. When $r = k$ the GLGC model is equivalent to the usual linear growth curve model.

To illustrate, let us consider the growth as a quadratic function of time $y_{ij} = a_{i1} + a_{i2}t_{ij} + a_{i3}t_{ij}^2 + \varepsilon_{ij}$ for individual $i = 1, ..., N$ at time t_{ij}. Let it be assumed that the rate of growth at time t_0 depends on gender. Thus, the second-stage model is written as

$$a_{i2} + 2a_{i3}t_0 = \beta_1 + \beta_2 gender_i + \delta_i, \tag{4.48}$$

which can be accommodated in the form of the GLGC model (4.47) with $\mathbf{C} = (0, 1, 2t_0)$, the 1×3 vector-row. Sometimes, the left-hand side of (4.47) will be called the growth curve characteristic. Note that we do not specify the coefficients of the quadratic growth function rather than (4.48).

For estimation purposes, it is convenient to rewrite the GLGC model (4.1, 4.47) in the marginal form:

$$\mathbf{y}_i = \mathbf{Z}_i\boldsymbol{\alpha}_i + \boldsymbol{\zeta}_i, \qquad E(\boldsymbol{\zeta}_i) = \mathbf{0}, \quad \text{cov}(\boldsymbol{\zeta}_i) = \sigma^2\mathbf{V}_i, \tag{4.49}$$

where, as in the previous notation,

$$\mathbf{V}_i = \mathbf{I} + \mathbf{Z}_i\mathbf{DZ}_i'$$

is the covariance matrix of the dependent variable $\mathbf{y}_i$. As follows from (4.47) parameters $\boldsymbol{\alpha}_1, ..., \boldsymbol{\alpha}_n, \boldsymbol{\beta}$ are subject to linear constraints

$$\mathbf{C}\boldsymbol{\alpha}_i = \mathbf{A}_i\boldsymbol{\beta}, \qquad i = 1, ..., N \qquad (4.50)$$

where $\boldsymbol{\alpha}_i = E(\mathbf{a}_i)$. We denote $\mathbf{b}_i = \mathbf{a}_i - \boldsymbol{\alpha}_i$ with $E(\mathbf{b}_i) = \mathbf{0}$ and $\text{cov}(\mathbf{b}_i) = \sigma^2\mathbf{D} = \mathbf{D}_*$. The marginal means $\boldsymbol{\alpha}_i$ are not specified completely unless $r = k$. In particular, the number of coefficients/parameters increases with the number of individuals. This feature of the GLGC model makes the study of its statistical properties somewhat complicated because we deal with a large number of nuisance parameters. This was first studied by Neyman and Scott (1948).

Before advancing to methods of estimation for the GLGC model, the following motivating example is suggested, which highlights the advantage of the general linear growth curve model.

4.2.1   Example: Calcium supplementation for bone gain

This example is borrowed from Lloyd et al. (1993) and was considered later in a book by Vonesh and Chinchilli (1997). The objective of this example is to motivate the general growth curve model and to demonstrate that it is less restrictive than the usual LGC model.

The data are from a trial in which healthy adolescent girls were randomized to ingest a daily calcium supplement (500 mg of calcium citrate malate) or a placebo over a two-year period. One of the objectives of the trial was to determine if calcium supplementation improves the rate of bone gain during early adolescence. The girls were scheduled for visits approximately every six months during the two-year follow-up. The placebo group consisted of 53 girls and the calcium group consisted of 52 girls (girls with only one visit have been removed from the analysis). The average age of the girls involved in the study was 11.9 years with a standard deviation of 0.5 year. At each visit, the total body bone mineral density (TBBMD, g/cm^2) was measured. The data for the two groups are shown in Figure 4.1. These graphs reveal a fairly linear growth in time. The question is: Does calcium supplementation improve bone gain? Clearly, to answer this question we have to compare the bone density in the two groups.

In the function below we read and plot the data on two groups. We make a few remarks: (1) as in in our previous codes, the function is saved in ASCII every time it runs; (2) the function plot displays the points and the individual lines (sometimes called a spaghetti line plot) are plotted over the loop based on the girls' id.

```
calcium=function()
{
dump("calcium","c:\\MixedModels\\Chapter04\\calcium.r")
da=read.csv("c:\\MixedModels\\Chapter04\\calcium.txt")
par(mfrow=c(1,2))
grnam=c("Placebo Group","Calcium Group")
```

```
for(tre in c(1,0))
{
  dat=da[da$treat==tre,]
  plot(dat$time,dat$y,xlab="Weeks",ylab="Bone density, g/cm^2",
        xlim=c(0,120),ylim=c(.7,1.1))
  title(grnam[tre+1])
  uid=unique(dat$id)
  nuid=length(uid)
  for(j in 1:nuid)
  lines(dat$time[dat$id==uid[j]],dat$y[dat$id==uid[j]])
}
}
```

To set up the model, we denote the TBBMD of the ith girl at time t_{ij} as y_{ij}. Hence, the first-stage model for this example has the form

$$y_{ij} = a_{i1}t_{ij} + a_{i2} + \varepsilon_{ij}, \quad i = 1,...,N = 105, \ j = 1,...,n_i. \qquad (4.51)$$

The error term ε_{ij} has zero mean and constant variance $\sigma^2 > 0$. Model (4.51) implies that each girl has an individual intercept and slope. The intercept measures the baseline TBBMD and the slope measures the weekly bone density gain. We expect the slope to be affected by the calcium intake, so the second-stage model for the slope takes the form

$$a_{i1} = \beta_1 + \beta_2 C_i + b_{i1}, \qquad (4.52)$$

where the dummy variable C_i is 0 for the placebo and 1 for the calcium group. Random effect b_{i1} has zero mean and variance d_{*11}. If calcium increases the bone density, the coefficient β_2 should be positive and statistically significant.

Following a standard setting of the linear growth curve model, one has to specify the intercept term in the second-stage model as well. The simplest way to do this is to assume a_{i2} to have a common distribution with the mean, regardless of the group:

$$a_{i2} = \beta_3 + b_{i2}, \qquad (4.53)$$

where b_{i2} is the second random effect, $E(b_{i2}) = 0$, $\text{var}(b_{i2}) = d_{*22}$, and $\text{cov}(b_{i1}, b_{i2}) = d_{*12}$. Clearly, while model (4.52) has certain grounds and is relevant to the design of the study, the model for the intercept (4.53) is, in fact, irrelevant and is needed to comply with the assumption that *all* growth curve coefficients must be specified in the second-stage model. In particular, as follows from (4.53), the baseline bone density for all girls (at time zero) belongs to the same general population $\mathcal{N}(\beta_3, d_{*22})$, under the normal assumption.

Furthermore, two kinds of arguments against the model for the intercept (4.53) may be put forward: biological and empirical. From a biological point of view, since TBBMD has a positive trend, the age of the girls at the first visit is critical in determining the intercept. The entire model becomes vulnerable if the baseline TBBMD on May 1, 1990 does not belong to the same general population. To verify

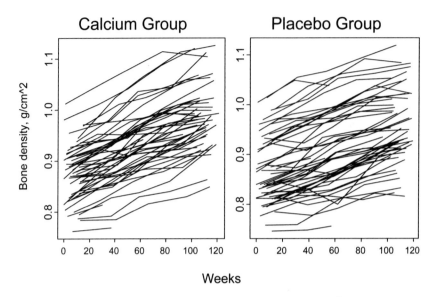

FIGURE 4.1. Total Body Bone Mineral Density (TBBMD), g/cm^2 versus time in two groups of girls, calcium supplementation data. Apparently, bone density increases with time following a linear trend. Does calcium supplementation increase bone density, i.e., is the slope in the calcium group (left) greater?

empirically that the intercepts have the same general population we estimate (4.51) individually by OLS; see the left-hand plot in Figure 4.2. The pair of plots display the estimated densities of the individual intercepts and slopes for the two groups of girls. The slopes for the control and calcium groups have smooth distributions that look very much like normal. In contrast, the left-hand plot reveals that the distributions of the intercept term are not so smooth, and far from normal. In particular, one might suspect that the placebo group consisted of two subgroups with different baseline TBBMD. Therefore, the hypothesis that the TBBMD at May 1, 1990 has the same general population is questionable and may be wrong.

By contrast, the general setting of the growth curve does not require specification of the intercept term: instead of (4.53), we just write

$$a_{i2} = \alpha_{i2} + b_{i2},$$

where α_{i2} is *any* number, treated as a nuisance parameter.

Summing up, the GLGC model is less restrictive because it does not require specification of all growth curve coefficients, particularly coefficients not of interest.

4.2.2 Variance parameters are known

We begin the discussion of estimation for the general linear growth curve model assuming that the variance parameters σ^2 and $\mathbf{D}$ are known in the manner of Section 4.1.1. As follows from the marginal model (4.49), the Generalized Least

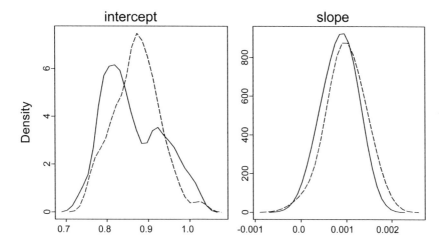

FIGURE 4.2. Densities for individually estimated intercept and slope: solid line, placebo group; dashed line, calcium group. Clearly, the bone density in the placebo group in the initial period may be a mixture of two populations. Consequently, the standard growth curve model, which assumes that subject-specific intercepts have the same mean, is not adequate. The general linear growth curve model would be more appropriate because it allows different subject-specific means for the intercept.

Squares (GLS) estimator for $\boldsymbol{\beta}$ would minimize the weighted sum of squares:

$$\min_{\boldsymbol{\alpha}_i} \sum_i (\mathbf{y}_i - \mathbf{Z}_i\boldsymbol{\alpha}_i)'\mathbf{V}_i^{-1}(\mathbf{y}_i - \mathbf{Z}_i\boldsymbol{\alpha}_i), \tag{4.54}$$

under linear constraints (4.50). To find the solution to this quadratic form, we introduce the Lagrange function

$$\mathcal{L} = \sum_i (\mathbf{y}_i - \mathbf{Z}_i\boldsymbol{\alpha}_i)'\mathbf{V}_i^{-1}(\mathbf{y}_i - \mathbf{Z}_i\boldsymbol{\alpha}_i) + 2\sum_i \boldsymbol{\lambda}_i'(\mathbf{C}\boldsymbol{\alpha}_i - \mathbf{A}_i\boldsymbol{\beta}),$$

where $\boldsymbol{\lambda}_i$ is the $r \times 1$ vector of Lagrange multipliers. Differentiating $\mathcal{L}$ with respect to $\boldsymbol{\alpha}_i$ and $\boldsymbol{\beta}$, we obtain the necessary conditions for the minimum,

$$-\frac{1}{2}\frac{\partial \mathcal{L}}{\partial \boldsymbol{\alpha}_i} = \mathbf{Z}_i\mathbf{V}_i^{-1}(\mathbf{y}_i - \mathbf{Z}_i\boldsymbol{\alpha}_i) - \mathbf{C}'\boldsymbol{\lambda}_i = \mathbf{0}, \; i = 1, ..., N \tag{4.55}$$

and

$$-\frac{1}{2}\frac{\partial \mathcal{L}}{\partial \boldsymbol{\beta}} = \sum \mathbf{A}_i'\boldsymbol{\lambda}_i = \mathbf{0}. \tag{4.56}$$

Define

$$\mathbf{R}_i = \mathbf{Z}_i'\mathbf{V}_i^{-1}\mathbf{Z}_i, \; \mathbf{M}_i = \mathbf{C}\mathbf{R}_i^{-1}\mathbf{C}', \; \mathbf{a}_i^0 = (\mathbf{Z}_i'\mathbf{V}_i^{-1}\mathbf{Z}_i)^{-1}\mathbf{Z}_i'\mathbf{V}_i^{-1}\mathbf{y}_i, \tag{4.57}$$

and notice that matrices $\mathbf{R}_i$ and $\mathbf{M}_i$ are positive definite and $\mathbf{a}_i^0$ is the GLS estimator of $\boldsymbol{\alpha}_i$ in the ith growth curve. Using dimension-reduction formula (2.25), we obtain

$$\mathbf{R}_i^{-1} = (\mathbf{Z}_i'\mathbf{Z}_i)^{-1} + \mathbf{D}, \; \mathbf{M}_i = \mathbf{P}_i + \mathbf{B}, \tag{4.58}$$

where
$$\mathbf{P}_i = \mathbf{C}(\mathbf{Z}_i'\mathbf{Z}_i)^{-1}\mathbf{C}', \ \ \mathbf{B} = \mathbf{CDC}'. \tag{4.59}$$

From (4.55) we obtain $\boldsymbol{\alpha}_i = \mathbf{a}_i^0 - \mathbf{R}_i^{-1}\mathbf{C}'\boldsymbol{\lambda}_i$. Substituting this into $\mathbf{C}\boldsymbol{\alpha}_i - \mathbf{A}_i\boldsymbol{\beta}$, we find that $\boldsymbol{\lambda}_i = (\mathbf{CR}_i^{-1}\mathbf{C}')^{-1}(\mathbf{c}_i^0 - \mathbf{A}_i\boldsymbol{\beta})$, where hereafter it is denoted

$$\mathbf{c}_i^0 = \mathbf{Ca}_i^0, \quad i = 1, ..., N. \tag{4.60}$$

Substituting $\boldsymbol{\lambda}_i$ into (4.56), we arrive at the solution to (4.54),

$$\hat{\boldsymbol{\beta}} = \left(\sum \mathbf{A}_i'\mathbf{M}_i^{-1}\mathbf{A}_i\right)^{-1}\left(\sum \mathbf{A}_i\mathbf{M}_i^{-1}\mathbf{CR}_i^{-1}\mathbf{Z}_i'\mathbf{V}_i^{-1}\mathbf{y}_i\right), \tag{4.61}$$

which is called the Generalized Least Squares under Constraints (GLSC) estimator. This estimator can be simplified noting that

$$\mathbf{R}_i^{-1}\mathbf{Z}_i\mathbf{V}_i^{-1} = (\mathbf{Z}_i'\mathbf{Z}_i)^{-1}\mathbf{Z}_i. \tag{4.62}$$

To prove (4.62), we use the dimension-reduction formula (2.21), which yields

$$\begin{aligned}
&\left[(\mathbf{Z}_i'\mathbf{Z}_i)^{-1} + \mathbf{D}\right]\mathbf{Z}_i'\left[\mathbf{I} - \mathbf{Z}_i(\mathbf{DZ}_i'\mathbf{Z}_i + \mathbf{I})^{-1}\mathbf{DZ}_i'\right] \\
= \ &(\mathbf{Z}_i'\mathbf{Z}_i)^{-1}\mathbf{Z}_i' - (\mathbf{Z}_i'\mathbf{Z}_i)^{-1}\left[(\mathbf{DZ}_i'\mathbf{Z}_i + \mathbf{I})^{-1} + \mathbf{DZ}_i'\mathbf{Z}_i(\mathbf{DZ}_i'\mathbf{Z}_i + \mathbf{I})^{-1}\right]\mathbf{Z}_i' \\
= \ &(\mathbf{Z}_i'\mathbf{Z}_i)^{-1}\mathbf{Z}_i'.
\end{aligned}$$

Hence, the GLSC estimator (4.61) can be simplified as

$$\hat{\boldsymbol{\beta}} = \left(\sum \mathbf{A}_i'\mathbf{M}_i^{-1}\mathbf{A}_i\right)^{-1}\left(\sum \mathbf{A}_i'\mathbf{M}_i^{-1}\mathbf{c}_i^0\right). \tag{4.63}$$

Analogously to the LGC model of Section 4.1.1, two extreme cases can be considered. If there are no random effects ($\mathbf{B} = \mathbf{0}$), the GLSC estimator becomes

$$\hat{\boldsymbol{\beta}}_{OLS} = \left(\sum \mathbf{A}_i'\mathbf{P}_i^{-1}\mathbf{A}_i\right)^{-1}\left(\sum \mathbf{A}_i'\mathbf{P}_i^{-1}\mathbf{c}_i^0\right). \tag{4.64}$$

If matrix $\mathbf{B}$ becomes large (fixed effects approach), i.e., $\mathbf{B} = \rho\mathbf{I}, \rho \to \infty$, the GLSC estimator approaches the OLS estimator applied to the second-stage model,

$$\begin{aligned}
\hat{\boldsymbol{\beta}}_0 &= \lim_{\rho \to \infty}\left(\sum \mathbf{A}_i'(\mathbf{P}_i + \rho\mathbf{I})^{-1}\mathbf{A}_i\right)^{-1}\left(\sum \mathbf{A}_i'(\mathbf{P} + \rho\mathbf{I})^{-1}\mathbf{c}_i^0\right) \\
&= \left(\sum \mathbf{A}_i'\mathbf{A}_i\right)^{-1}\left(\sum \mathbf{A}_i'\mathbf{c}^0_i\right).
\end{aligned} \tag{4.65}$$

The estimator of the subject-specific growth curve coefficients, $\boldsymbol{\alpha}_i$, is

$$\hat{\boldsymbol{\alpha}}_i = \mathbf{a}_i^0 - \mathbf{R}_i^{-1}\mathbf{C}'\mathbf{M}_i^{-1}(\mathbf{c}_i^0 - \mathbf{A}_i\hat{\boldsymbol{\beta}}).$$

Using this expression and denoting the OLS residual as $\mathbf{e}_i^0 = \mathbf{y}_i - \mathbf{Z}_i\mathbf{a}_i^0$ with the sum of squares $S_0 = \sum \| \mathbf{e}_i^0 \|^2$, the minimum (4.54) can be expressed as

$$\begin{aligned}
&\sum (\mathbf{y}_i - \mathbf{Z}_i\boldsymbol{\alpha}_i)'\mathbf{V}_i^{-1}(\mathbf{y}_i - \mathbf{Z}_i\boldsymbol{\alpha}_i) \\
= \ &S_0 + (\boldsymbol{\alpha}_i - \mathbf{a}_i^0)'(\mathbf{Z}_i'\mathbf{V}_i^{-1}\mathbf{Z}_i)(\boldsymbol{\alpha}_i - \mathbf{a}_i^0) \\
= \ &S_0 + (\mathbf{c}_i^0 - \mathbf{A}_i\hat{\boldsymbol{\beta}})'\mathbf{M}_i^{-1}\mathbf{CR}_i^{-1}\mathbf{R}_i\mathbf{R}_i^{-1}\mathbf{C}'\mathbf{M}_i^{-1}(\mathbf{c}_i^0 - \mathbf{A}_i\hat{\boldsymbol{\beta}}) \\
= \ &S_0 + (\mathbf{c}_i^0 - \mathbf{A}_i\hat{\boldsymbol{\beta}})'\mathbf{M}_i^{-1}(\mathbf{c}_i^0 - \mathbf{A}_i\hat{\boldsymbol{\beta}}) \\
= \ &S_0 + (\mathbf{c}_i^0 - \mathbf{A}_i\hat{\boldsymbol{\beta}})'(\mathbf{P}_i + \mathbf{B})^{-1}(\mathbf{c}_i^0 - \mathbf{A}_i\hat{\boldsymbol{\beta}}),
\end{aligned} \tag{4.66}$$

where matrices $\mathbf{P}_i$ and $\mathbf{B}$ are as defined in (4.59). As follows from (4.66), the minimum of the weighted sum of squares can be decomposed into a sum of squares of the OLS residuals plus the weighted sum of squares from the second-stage model (4.47). This decomposition will be used later to simplify the log-likelihood function.

The covariance matrix of the GLSC estimator (4.63) is given by

$$\text{cov}(\hat{\boldsymbol{\beta}}) = \sigma^2 \left(\sum_i \mathbf{A}_i' \mathbf{M}_i^{-1} \mathbf{A}_i \right)^{-1}. \tag{4.67}$$

As follows from formula (4.63), the GLSC estimator can be computed in two steps:

1. Estimate each curve (4.1) individually by OLS.

2. Apply the weighted least squares to (4.47), replacing $\mathbf{Ca}_i$ with $\mathbf{c}_i^0 = \mathbf{Ca}_i^0$ by the weight matrix $\mathbf{M}_i$ defined in (4.58).

Applying the standard theory of linear models with restrictions on parameters (Rao, 1973; Rao and Toutenburg, 1999), it follows that when the variance parameters are known, $\hat{\boldsymbol{\beta}}$ is the best linear unbiased estimator (BLUE). As is shown below, the GLSC estimator does not depend on matrix $\mathbf{B}$ for the balanced GLGC model.

4.2.3 Balanced model

In this section we extend the results of Section 4.1.5 to the GLGC model (4.1, 4.47). We call the GLGC model balanced if $n_i = n$, $\mathbf{Z}_i = \mathbf{Z}$, $\mathbf{A}_i = \mathbf{I} \otimes \mathbf{q}_i'$. For a balanced model, individual random designs are the same and all components of the vector $\mathbf{c}_i = \mathbf{Ca}_i$ have the same set of population explanatory variables. Then in coordinate form, the second-stage model can be written as $c_{ij} = \mathbf{q}_i' \boldsymbol{\beta}_j + b_{ij}$.

Proposition 26 *In the balanced GLGC model, the estimator (4.63) does not depend on the matrix* $\mathbf{B}$. *In particular, for* $j = 1, ..., r$, *we have*

$$\hat{\boldsymbol{\beta}}_j = \left(\sum_{i=1}^N \mathbf{q}_i \mathbf{q}_i' \right)^{-1} \left(\sum_{i=1}^N \mathbf{q}_i c_{ij}^0 \right) \tag{4.68}$$

and

$$\text{cov}(\hat{\boldsymbol{\beta}}_j) = \sigma^2 ((\mathbf{X}'\mathbf{X})_{jj}^{-1} + D_{jj}) \left(\sum_{i=1}^N \mathbf{q}_i \mathbf{q}_i' \right)^{-1}.$$

Proof. The following properties of the Kronecker product are used:

$$(\mathbf{A} \otimes \mathbf{B})(\mathbf{C} \otimes \mathbf{D}) = \mathbf{A}\mathbf{C} \otimes \mathbf{B}\mathbf{D},$$
$$(\mathbf{A} \otimes \mathbf{B})' = \mathbf{A}' \otimes \mathbf{B}', \quad (\mathbf{A} \otimes \mathbf{B})^{-1} = \mathbf{A}^{-1} \otimes \mathbf{B}^{-1}$$

for any suitable matrices $\mathbf{A}$ and $\mathbf{B}$. Applying these formulas and observing that $\mathbf{M}_i = \mathbf{M} = (\mathbf{X}'\mathbf{X})^{-1} + \mathbf{D}$, one obtains

$$\sum \mathbf{A}_i' \mathbf{M}_i^{-1} \mathbf{A}_i = \sum (\mathbf{I} \otimes \mathbf{q}_i) \mathbf{M}^{-1} (\mathbf{I} \otimes \mathbf{q}_i') = \sum (\mathbf{I} \otimes \mathbf{q}_i)(\mathbf{M}^{-1} \otimes 1)(\mathbf{I} \otimes \mathbf{q}_i')$$
$$= \sum (\mathbf{M}^{-1} \otimes \mathbf{q}_i \mathbf{q}_i') = \mathbf{M}^{-1} \otimes \left(\sum \mathbf{q}_i \mathbf{q}_i' \right),$$

which yields $\left(\sum \mathbf{A}_i' \mathbf{M}_i^{-1} \mathbf{A}_i\right)^{-1} = \mathbf{M} \otimes (\sum \mathbf{q}_i \mathbf{q}_i')^{-1}$. Analogously,

$$\sum \mathbf{A}_i' \mathbf{M}_i^{-1} \mathbf{c}_i^0 = \sum (\mathbf{I} \otimes \mathbf{q}_i)(\mathbf{M}^{-1} \otimes 1)\mathbf{c}_i^0 = \sum (\mathbf{M}^{-1} \otimes \mathbf{q}_i)\mathbf{c}_i^0$$
$$= \sum (\mathbf{M}^{-1} \otimes \mathbf{I})(\mathbf{I} \otimes \mathbf{q}_i)\mathbf{c}_i^0 = (\mathbf{M}^{-1} \otimes \mathbf{I}) \sum (\mathbf{I} \otimes \mathbf{q}_i)\mathbf{c}_i^0.$$

Combing these results, we finally obtain

$$
\begin{aligned}
\widehat{\boldsymbol{\beta}} &= \left(\mathbf{M} \otimes (\sum \mathbf{q}_i \mathbf{q}_i')^{-1}\right)\left((\mathbf{M}^{-1} \otimes \mathbf{I}) \sum (\mathbf{I} \otimes \mathbf{q}_i)\mathbf{c}_i^0\right) \\
&= \left(\mathbf{I} \otimes (\sum \mathbf{q}_i \mathbf{q}_i')^{-1}\right) \sum (\mathbf{I} \otimes \mathbf{q}_i)\mathbf{c}_i^0,
\end{aligned}
$$

which immediately implies (4.68). Also, as is easy to see,

$$\operatorname{cov}(\widehat{\boldsymbol{\beta}}) = \sigma^2 (\mathbf{M} \otimes (\sum \mathbf{q}_i \mathbf{q}_i'))^{-1},$$

which gives (4.42).   ∎

In practice, the variance parameters are unknown and the data are seldom balanced, so that to use the GLSC estimator (4.63) we need to estimate $\mathbf{D}$. As follows from formula (4.58), the GLSC estimator depends on $\mathbf{B} = \mathbf{CDC}'$, and consequently, it suffices to estimate $\mathbf{B}$, which is of lesser size. Two types of estimators for variance parameters are considered below: (a) likelihood-based estimators, assuming normal distribution for random terms, and (b) the method of moments estimator.

4.2.4   Likelihood-based estimation

We can apply maximum likelihood to estimate parameters of the general linear growth curve model (4.49), assuming the normal distribution for $\boldsymbol{\zeta}_i$. Thus, the model discussed in this section takes the form

$$\mathbf{y}_i \sim \mathcal{N}\left(\mathbf{Z}_i \boldsymbol{\alpha}_i, \sigma^2 (\mathbf{I} + \mathbf{Z}_i \mathbf{D} \mathbf{Z}_i')\right), \quad i = 1, ..., N \tag{4.69}$$

under constraints (4.50). Two types of likelihood estimates may be considered: full ML and second-stage ML.

Full maximum likelihood estimation

As follows from model (4.69), the log-likelihood function has the form

$$
\begin{aligned}
& l(\boldsymbol{\beta}, \boldsymbol{\alpha}_1, ..., \boldsymbol{\alpha}_N, \sigma^2, \mathbf{D}) \\
&= -\frac{1}{2}\left\{ N_T \ln \sigma^2 + \sum \ln |\mathbf{V}_i| + \sigma^{-2} \sum (\mathbf{y}_i - \mathbf{Z}_i \boldsymbol{\alpha}_i)' \mathbf{V}_i^{-1}(\mathbf{y}_i - \mathbf{Z}_i \boldsymbol{\alpha}_i) \right\},
\end{aligned}
$$

where $\boldsymbol{\beta}$ and $\boldsymbol{\alpha}_1,...,\boldsymbol{\alpha}_N$ are subject to constraints (4.50). To find the maximum of this function over all parameters, we first minimize it over $\boldsymbol{\alpha}_1, ..., \boldsymbol{\alpha}_N$, holding the rest of the parameters fixed, to obtain the profile function. It is easy to see that this optimization problem is equivalent to (4.54). Using the dimension-reduction formula,

$$|\mathbf{V}_i| = |\mathbf{I} + \mathbf{Z}_i \mathbf{D} \mathbf{Z}_i'| = |\mathbf{Z}_i' \mathbf{Z}_i| \cdot |(\mathbf{Z}_i' \mathbf{Z}_i)^{-1} + \mathbf{D}|,$$

and the decomposition (4.66), the profile function, as a function of $\boldsymbol{\beta}$ and the variance parameters, is given by

$$-\frac{1}{2}\{N_T \ln \sigma^2 + \sum \ln |(\mathbf{Z}_i'\mathbf{Z}_i)^{-1} + \mathbf{D}| + \sum \ln |\mathbf{Z}_i'\mathbf{Z}_i|$$

$$+\sigma^{-2}[S_0 + \sum (\mathbf{c}_i^0 - \mathbf{A}_i\boldsymbol{\beta})'(\mathbf{P}_i + \mathbf{CDC}')^{-1}(\mathbf{c}_i^0 - \mathbf{A}_i\boldsymbol{\beta})]\},$$

where $\mathbf{c}_i^0$ is a vector of the OLS characteristics (4.60) and S_0 is the sum of squares of the OLS residuals. Dropping the constant $\sum \ln |\mathbf{Z}_i'\mathbf{Z}_i|$, we come to the following equivalent profile function:

$$l(\boldsymbol{\beta}, \sigma^2, \mathbf{D}) = -\frac{1}{2}\{N_T \ln \sigma^2 + \sum \ln |(\mathbf{Z}_i'\mathbf{Z}_i)^{-1} + \mathbf{D}|$$

$$+\sigma^{-2}[S_0 + \sum (\mathbf{c}_i^0 - \mathbf{A}_i\boldsymbol{\beta})'(\mathbf{P}_i + \mathbf{CDC}')^{-1}(\mathbf{c}_i^0 - \mathbf{A}_i\boldsymbol{\beta})]\}.$$

Given matrix $\mathbf{D}$, $\boldsymbol{\beta}$ maximizes l at

$$\widehat{\boldsymbol{\beta}} = \left(\sum \mathbf{A}_i'(\mathbf{P}_i + \mathbf{CDC}')^{-1}\mathbf{A}_i\right)^{-1} \left(\sum \mathbf{A}_i'(\mathbf{P}_i + \mathbf{CDC}')^{-1}\mathbf{c}_i^0\right). \qquad (4.70)$$

Given $\boldsymbol{\beta}$ and $\mathbf{D}$, σ^2 maximizes l at

$$\widehat{\sigma}^2 = \frac{1}{N_T}\left[S_0 + \sum (\mathbf{c}_i^0 - \mathbf{A}_i\boldsymbol{\beta})'(\mathbf{P}_i + \mathbf{CDC}')^{-1}(\mathbf{c}_i^0 - \mathbf{A}_i\boldsymbol{\beta})\right]. \qquad (4.71)$$

As a consequence, one obtains a lower bound for the MLE of the within-subject variance, $\widehat{\sigma}^2_{ML} \geq S_0/N_T$. We can consider the variance-profile function eliminating σ^2 by (4.71), which gives

$$l_p(\boldsymbol{\beta}, \mathbf{D}) = -\frac{1}{2}\{\sum \ln |(\mathbf{Z}_i'\mathbf{Z}_i)^{-1} + \mathbf{D}|$$

$$+N_T \ln \sum [S_0 + (\mathbf{c}_i^0 - \mathbf{A}_i\boldsymbol{\beta})'(\mathbf{P}_i + \mathbf{CDC}')^{-1}(\mathbf{c}_i^0 - \mathbf{A}_i\boldsymbol{\beta})]\}. \qquad (4.72)$$

We require that $S_0 > 0$ to guarantee the existence of the l-maximum (see Section 2.5).

Maximization of these functions can be accomplished by any algorithm applied in Chapter 2, since the $\mathbf{c}_i^0$ are treated as fixed. Here we develop a simplified version of the Newton–Raphson algorithm using the perturbation formula (2.106) for the variance-profile log-likelihood function (4.72).

First, we need the derivative of l with respect to $\mathbf{D}$. Using standard matrix formulas, as in Section 2.9, we obtain for $\partial l_p/\partial \mathbf{D}$

$$-\frac{1}{2}\{\sum [((\mathbf{Z}_i'\mathbf{Z}_i)^{-1} + \mathbf{D})^{-1} - N_T S^{-1} \mathbf{C}'(\mathbf{P}_i + \mathbf{B})^{-1}\mathbf{r}_i\mathbf{r}_i'(\mathbf{P}_i + \mathbf{B})^{-1}\mathbf{C}]\}, \qquad (4.73)$$

where $S = S_0 + \mathbf{r}_i'(\mathbf{P}_i + \mathbf{B})^{-1}\mathbf{r}_i$ and $\mathbf{r}_i = \mathbf{c}_i^0 - \mathbf{A}_i\boldsymbol{\beta}$. At each iteration we can only adjust matrix $\mathbf{D}$, because $\boldsymbol{\beta}$ is computed by formula (4.70).

Newton–Raphson algorithm. Let $\mathbf{D}_0$ be the current approximation to the MLE for matrix $\mathbf{D}$ in function l_p. We aim to find the next approximation as $\mathbf{D} = \mathbf{D}_0 + \boldsymbol{\Delta}$, where the increment $\boldsymbol{\Delta}$ is supposedly small. Using formula (2.106), as in Section 2.10, we obtain

$$\left((\mathbf{Z}_i'\mathbf{Z}_i)^{-1} + \mathbf{D}_0 + \boldsymbol{\Delta}\right)^{-1} \simeq$$

$$\left((\mathbf{Z}_i'\mathbf{Z}_i)^{-1} + \mathbf{D}_0\right)^{-1} - \left((\mathbf{Z}_i'\mathbf{Z}_i)^{-1} + \mathbf{D}_0\right)^{-1} \boldsymbol{\Delta} \left((\mathbf{Z}_i'\mathbf{Z}_i)^{-1} + \mathbf{D}_0\right)^{-1}$$

$$\times (\mathbf{P}_i + \mathbf{B}_0 + \mathbf{C}\boldsymbol{\Delta}\mathbf{C}')^{-1} \simeq (\mathbf{P}_i + \mathbf{B}_0)^{-1} - (\mathbf{P}_i + \mathbf{B}_0)^{-1}\mathbf{C}\boldsymbol{\Delta}\mathbf{C}'(\mathbf{P}_i + \mathbf{B}_0)^{-1}.$$

Substituting these approximations into (4.73) and omitting terms of the second order, the score equation $\partial l_p/\partial \mathbf{D} = 0$ can be approximated as

$$\frac{1}{2}\sum \left[\mathbf{M}_{i1}\boldsymbol{\Delta}\mathbf{M}_{i1}' - \mathbf{M}_{i2}\boldsymbol{\Delta}\mathbf{M}_{i3} - \mathbf{M}_{i3}\boldsymbol{\Delta}\mathbf{M}_{i2}\right] = \left.\frac{\partial l_p}{\partial \mathbf{D}}\right|_{\mathbf{D}=\mathbf{D}_0}, \qquad (4.74)$$

where

$$\mathbf{M}_{i1} = \left((\mathbf{Z}_i'\mathbf{Z}_i)^{-1} + \mathbf{D}_0\right)^{-1}, \quad \mathbf{M}_{i2} = N_T S^{-1}\mathbf{C}'(\mathbf{P}_i + \mathbf{B}_0)^{-1}\mathbf{C},$$

$$\mathbf{M}_{i3} = \mathbf{C}'(\mathbf{P}_i + \mathbf{B}_0)^{-1}\mathbf{r}_i\mathbf{r}_i'(\mathbf{P}_i + \mathbf{B}_0)^{-1}\mathbf{C}.$$

In order to find $\boldsymbol{\Delta}$ as the solution to the matrix equation (4.74), we again employ the vec function, so that the solution to (4.74) can be rewritten as

$$\mathrm{vec}(\boldsymbol{\Delta}) = \mathbf{J}^{-1}\mathrm{vec}\left(\left.\frac{\partial l_p}{\partial \mathbf{D}}\right|_{\mathbf{D}=\mathbf{D}_0}\right), \qquad (4.75)$$

where

$$\mathbf{J} = \frac{1}{2}\sum_{i=1}^{N}\left[\mathbf{M}_{i1}\otimes\mathbf{M}_{i1} - \mathbf{M}_{i3}'\otimes\mathbf{M}_{i2} - \mathbf{M}_{i2}'\otimes\mathbf{M}_{i3}\right],$$

and the derivative of l_p with respect to $\mathbf{D}$ is defined by (4.73).

Summing up, a simplified Newton–Raphson algorithm for the GLGC model consists of the following steps:

1. Take $\mathbf{D}_0 = \mathbf{0}$ and calculate $\widehat{\boldsymbol{\beta}}_0$ by formula (4.70).

2. Calculate the increment $\boldsymbol{\Delta}$ by formula (4.75) and set the next approximation as $\mathbf{D}_1 = \mathbf{D}_0 + \boldsymbol{\Delta}$.

3. Calculate $\widehat{\boldsymbol{\beta}}_1$ by formula (4.70), return to step 2, and continue until convergence.

One could use another starting point for matrix $\mathbf{D}$ at step 1, such as the method of moments estimate considered in Section 4.2.5. Also, one could use a fraction of step λ to guarantee maximization of l_p from iteration to iteration.

Second-stage maximum likelihood estimation

The second-stage MLE treats individual estimates $\mathbf{c}_i^0 = \mathbf{C}\mathbf{a}_i^0$ as fixed. Furthermore, the following variance decomposition, as a characteristic property of the LME model, takes place:

$$\mathrm{cov}(\mathbf{a}_i^0) - \mathrm{cov}((\mathbf{Z}_i'\mathbf{Z}_i)^{-1}\mathbf{Z}_i'\boldsymbol{\zeta}_i)$$

$$= \sigma^2(\mathbf{Z}_i'\mathbf{Z}_i)^{-1}\mathbf{Z}_i'(\mathbf{I} + \mathbf{Z}_i\mathbf{D}\mathbf{Z}_i')\mathbf{Z}_i(\mathbf{Z}_i'\mathbf{Z}_i)^{-1} = \sigma^2\left((\mathbf{Z}_i'\mathbf{Z}_i)^{-1} + \mathbf{D}\right), \qquad (4.76)$$

which yields $\text{cov}(\mathbf{c}_i^0) = \sigma^2 \mathbf{P}_i + \mathbf{B}_*$, where $\mathbf{B}_* = \sigma^2 \mathbf{B}$. Therefore, the second-stage model becomes equivalent to $\mathbf{c}_i^0 \sim N(\mathbf{A}_i\boldsymbol{\beta}, \sigma^2 \mathbf{P}_i + \mathbf{B}_*)$, with the log-likelihood function

$$l_2(\boldsymbol{\beta}, \sigma^2, \mathbf{B}_*) \tag{4.77}$$
$$= -\frac{1}{2}\sum_{i=1}^{N}\left[\ln|\sigma^2\mathbf{P}_i+\mathbf{B}_*| + (\mathbf{c}_i^0 - \mathbf{A}_i\boldsymbol{\beta})'(\sigma^2\mathbf{P}_i+\mathbf{B}_*)^{-1}(\mathbf{c}_i^0 - \mathbf{A}_i\boldsymbol{\beta})\right].$$

Also, one arrives at this expression considering the conditional likelihood for $\mathbf{y}_i|\mathbf{c}_i^0$ (Demidenko and Stukel, 2002).

Two approaches may be undertaken to estimate $\boldsymbol{\beta}$ from the second-stage model based on the function l_2. In the first approach we replace σ^2 with its estimate (pooled-variance), and therefore l_2 reduces to a function of $\boldsymbol{\beta}$ and $\mathbf{B}_*$. We shall confront the same estimation problem in the meta-analysis model of Chapter 5. In the second approach we estimate σ^2 along with $\mathbf{B}_*$ and $\boldsymbol{\beta}$ (simultaneous estimation).

Approach 1: pooled variance for σ^2. We eliminate σ^2 from l_2 by replacing it with the pooled variance (4.23). We prove that this estimator is unbiased for the general growth curve model as well. As is easy to see, $\mathbf{y}_i - \mathbf{Z}_i\mathbf{a}_i^0 = \mathbf{M}_i\boldsymbol{\zeta}_i$, where $\mathbf{M}_i = \mathbf{I} - \mathbf{Z}_i(\mathbf{Z}_i'\mathbf{Z}_i)^{-1}\mathbf{Z}_i'$ is an idempotent matrix, which implies that $\|\mathbf{y}_i - \mathbf{Z}_i\mathbf{a}_i^0\|^2 = \boldsymbol{\zeta}_i'\mathbf{M}_i\boldsymbol{\zeta}_i$. Now using the fact that $E(\mathbf{u}'\mathbf{A}\mathbf{u}) = \text{tr}(\mathbf{A}\mathbf{C})$ for any random vector $\mathbf{u}$ such that $E(\mathbf{u}) = \mathbf{0}$ and $\text{cov}(\mathbf{u}) = \mathbf{C}$, we obtain

$$E\hat{\sigma}_{MM}^2 = \frac{1}{\sum(n_i - k)}\sum E\|\mathbf{y}_i - \mathbf{Z}_i\mathbf{a}_i^0\|^2 = \frac{1}{\sum(n_i - k)}\sum E(\boldsymbol{\zeta}_i'\mathbf{M}_i\boldsymbol{\zeta}_i)$$
$$= \sigma^2\frac{1}{\sum(n_i - k)}\sum \text{tr}\left(\mathbf{M}_i(\mathbf{I} + \mathbf{Z}_i\mathbf{D}\mathbf{Z}_i')\right)$$
$$= \sigma^2\frac{1}{\sum(n_i - k)}\sum \text{tr}\left(\mathbf{I} - \mathbf{Z}_i(\mathbf{Z}_i'\mathbf{Z}_i)^{-1}\mathbf{Z}_i'\right) = \sigma^2.$$

Further, replacing σ^2 with $\hat{\sigma}_{MM}^2$ in (4.77), we come to a simplified log-likelihood function,

$$l_2(\boldsymbol{\beta}, \mathbf{B}_*) = -\frac{1}{2}\sum_{i=1}^{N}[\ln\left|\hat{\sigma}_{MM}^2\mathbf{P}_i+\mathbf{B}_*\right| \tag{4.78}$$
$$+ (\mathbf{c}_i^0 - \mathbf{A}_i\boldsymbol{\beta})'(\hat{\sigma}_{MM}^2\mathbf{P}_i+\mathbf{B}_*)^{-1}(\mathbf{c}_i^0 - \mathbf{A}_i\boldsymbol{\beta})].$$

with the score equation for $\mathbf{B}_*$ as $\partial l_2/\partial\mathbf{B}_* = \mathbf{0}$, namely,

$$\sum\left[(\hat{\sigma}_{MM}^2\mathbf{P}_i+\mathbf{B}_*)^{-1} - (\hat{\sigma}_{MM}^2\mathbf{P}_i+\mathbf{B}_*)^{-1}\mathbf{r}_i\mathbf{r}_i'(\hat{\sigma}_{MM}^2\mathbf{P}_i+\mathbf{B}_*)^{-1}\right] = \mathbf{0}. \tag{4.79}$$

Generally, this matrix equation must be solved iteratively; however, for the balanced model there is a closed-form solution. Indeed, if $\mathbf{Z}_i = \mathbf{Z}$ then $\mathbf{P}_i = \mathbf{P}$, $\partial l_2/\partial\mathbf{B}_* = \mathbf{0}$ becomes equivalent to $(\hat{\sigma}^2\mathbf{P} + \mathbf{B}_*)^{-1} = \sum\mathbf{r}_i\mathbf{r}_i'/N$, which yields

$$\hat{\mathbf{B}}_* = \left(\frac{1}{N}\sum\mathbf{r}_i\mathbf{r}_i'\right)^{-1} - \hat{\sigma}^2\mathbf{P}. \tag{4.80}$$

Approach 2: simultaneous estimation. Two algorithms for the maximization of the l_2 function, defined by (4.77), are considered briefly below.

Newton–Raphson algorithm. We again use the perturbation formula, which gives the increment for the covariance matrix

$$\text{vec}(\boldsymbol{\Delta}) = \mathbf{J}^{-1} \text{vec}\left(\frac{\partial l_2}{\partial \mathbf{B}_*}\Big|_{\mathbf{B}_*=\mathbf{B}_{*0}} \right), \tag{4.81}$$

where

$$\mathbf{J} = \frac{1}{2}\sum \left[(\widehat{\sigma}^2_{MM}\mathbf{P}_i+\mathbf{B}_*)^{-1} \otimes (\widehat{\sigma}^2\mathbf{P}_i+\mathbf{B}_*)^{-1} - \mathbf{M}'_{i3} \otimes \mathbf{M}_{i2} - \mathbf{M}'_{i2} \otimes \mathbf{M}_{i3} \right].$$

After the next approximation for $\mathbf{B}_*$ is determined, we compute the next approximation for $\boldsymbol{\beta}$ using (4.70).

Fixed-Point algorithm. Pockock et al. (1981) proposed a simple recurrent formula to maximize (4.78) with one random effect, which has a fixed-point form, (2.122). Berkey and Laird (1986) extended that formula to the multivariate case. In the spirit of Section 2.12.1 the Fixed-Point (FP) algorithm can be derived based on rewriting the estimating equation (4.79)

$$\sum (\widehat{\sigma}^2\mathbf{P}_i+\mathbf{B}_*)^{-1}(\mathbf{r}_i\mathbf{r}'_i - \widehat{\sigma}^2\mathbf{P}_i)(\widehat{\sigma}^2\mathbf{P}_i+\mathbf{B}_*)^{-1} + \mathbf{B}_* \sum (\widehat{\sigma}^2\mathbf{P}_i+\mathbf{B}_*)^{-2} = \mathbf{0}$$

Solving for $\mathbf{B}_*$ we come to the fixed-point iterations

$$\mathbf{B}_* = \left(\sum (\widehat{\sigma}^2\mathbf{P}_i+\mathbf{B}_*)^{-2} \right)^{-1} \tag{4.82}$$
$$\times \left(\sum (\widehat{\sigma}^2\mathbf{P}_i+\mathbf{B}_*)^{-1}(\mathbf{r}_i\mathbf{r}'_i - \widehat{\sigma}^2\mathbf{P}_i)(\widehat{\sigma}^2\mathbf{P}_i+\mathbf{B}_*)^{-1} \right)^{-1}.$$

This formula provides a solution to the score equation $\partial l_2/\partial \mathbf{B}_* = \mathbf{0}$ under convergence. At each iteration $\boldsymbol{\beta}$ is recalculated by formula (4.70). For instructive purposes we consider below an important special case when only one growth curve characteristic is specified in the second-stage model.

Second-stage MLE for one characteristic

In this subsection we consider an important case when only one characteristic, as a linear combination of the growth curve coefficients, is specified in the second-stage model ($r = 1$). In this case the second-stage model (4.47) is written as

$$\mathbf{c}'\mathbf{a}_i = \mathbf{A}_i\boldsymbol{\beta} + \delta_i,$$

where $\mathbf{c}$ is a fixed nonzero $k \times 1$ vector, $\mathbf{A}_i$ is a $1 \times m$ design vector and δ_i is the scalar random effect with zero mean and $\text{var}(\delta_i) = b_*$. This model emerges in meta-analysis where c_i^0 are obtained as estimates from individual studies; see Chapter 5 for more detail. Introducing scalars $c_i^0 = \mathbf{c}'\mathbf{a}_i^0$ and $h_i = \widehat{\sigma}^2_{MM}\mathbf{c}'(\mathbf{Z}'_i\mathbf{Z}_i)^{-1}\mathbf{c}$, where $\widehat{\sigma}^2_{MM}$ is the pooled-variance estimate, the second-stage log-likelihood function (4.78) takes the form

$$l_2(\boldsymbol{\beta}, b_*) = -\frac{1}{2}\sum_{i=1}^N \left[\ln(h_i + b_*) + \frac{1}{h_i + b_*}(c_i^0 - \mathbf{A}_i\boldsymbol{\beta})^2 \right]. \tag{4.83}$$

Below we discuss briefly computational aspects of the l_2-maximization.

Holding b_* constant, the maximum of l_2 is attained at the GLS estimator,

$$\widehat{\boldsymbol{\beta}} = \left(\sum_i \frac{1}{h_i + b_*} \mathbf{A}_i \mathbf{A}_i' \right)^{-1} \left(\sum_i \frac{1}{h_i + b_*} \mathbf{A}_i' c_i^0 \right). \tag{4.84}$$

To find the maximum of l_2 for b, we hold $\boldsymbol{\beta}$ fixed and denote residuals as $r_i = c_i^0 - \mathbf{A}_i \boldsymbol{\beta}$. Taking the derivative of l_2 with respect to b_*, we come to the score equation,

$$\sum_i \left[\frac{r_i^2}{(h_i + b_*)^2} - \frac{1}{h_i + b_*} \right] = 0. \tag{4.85}$$

Pockock et al. (1981) suggested the following recurrent formula to solve (4.85), which is the univariate version of algorithm (4.82):

$$b_{*s+1} = \frac{\sum (r_i^2 - h_i)(h_i + b_{*s})^{-2}}{\sum (h_i + b_{*s})^{-2}}, \quad s = 0, 1, ..., \tag{4.86}$$

where s denotes the iteration index, starting from $b_{*0} = 0$. Vector $\widehat{\boldsymbol{\beta}}$ can be re-computed by formula (4.84) after convergence or at each iteration of (4.86). It is easy to verify that at convergence the limit of $\{b_{*s}\}$ satisfies the score equation (4.85), i.e., provides the maximum of l_2 when $\boldsymbol{\beta}$ is fixed. It is worthwhile to note that the nonlinear equation (4.85) may have several positive solutions or may have no positive solutions at all. The following result provides a sufficient condition for the existence of a positive solution; this result is very close to the criterion for the positive definiteness of matrix $\mathbf{D}$ for the LME model of Section 2.6.

Proposition 27 *If $\sum_i r_i^2 h_i^{-2} > \sum_i h_i^{-1}$, the score equation (4.85) has at least one positive solution for a given $\boldsymbol{\beta}$. If $\sum_i (c_i^0 - \mathbf{A}_i \widehat{\boldsymbol{\beta}}_0)^2 h_i^{-2} > \sum_i h_i^{-1}$, where $\widehat{\boldsymbol{\beta}}_0$ is defined as (4.84) with $b_* = 0$, then (4.85) has at least one positive solution for any $\boldsymbol{\beta}$, and the minimum of (4.83) exists.*

Proof. We introduce function $\chi(b_*)$ as the left side of (4.85). By the condition of the proposition, $\chi(0) > 0$. For large b_*, the function $\chi(b_*)$ is negative because

$$\lim_{b_* \to \infty} b_* \chi(b_*) = \lim_{b_* \to \infty} \sum_i \left[\frac{b_* r_i^2}{(h_i + b_*)^2} - \frac{b_*}{h_i + b_*} \right] = -N < 0.$$

This implies that there is at least one positive solution to (4.85). To prove the second statement we notice that

$$\min_{\boldsymbol{\beta}} \chi(0) = \min_{\boldsymbol{\beta}} \sum_i (c_i^0 - \mathbf{A}_i \boldsymbol{\beta})^2 h_i^{-2} - \sum_i h_i^{-1} = \sum_i (c_i^0 - \mathbf{A}_i \widehat{\boldsymbol{\beta}}_0)^2 h_i^{-2} - \sum_i h_i^{-1}$$

and then repeat the previous arguments.

4.2.5   MM estimator for variance parameters

In this section we generalize the method of moments of Section 4.1.3 to the general linear growth curve model. The unbiasedness of the pooled variance estimator (4.23) was proved before. Now we construct the MM estimator for the covariance matrix of the random effects using $\widehat{\sigma}_{MM}^2$.

MMFE estimator for matrix $\mathbf{B}_*$

As follows from Section 4.1.3, there are two variants for the MM estimation of the covariance matrix of random effects. Here we extend the MM estimator to the GLGC model based on the estimator (4.65). Analogously, one can derive another MM estimator based on (4.64). Following the idea of the method of moments, we construct the matrix of cross-products of residuals,

$$\widehat{\mathbf{S}}_0 = \sum (\mathbf{c}_i^0 - \mathbf{A}_i \widehat{\boldsymbol{\beta}}_0)(\mathbf{c}_i^0 - \mathbf{A}_i \widehat{\boldsymbol{\beta}}_0)'. \tag{4.87}$$

Then the MMFE estimator for $\mathbf{B}_*$ is found by equating (4.87) to its mathematical expectation (see Appendix 4.5 for details):

$$\text{vec}(\widehat{\mathbf{B}}_*) = \mathbf{J}^{-1}\text{vec}(\widehat{\mathbf{S}}_0 - \widehat{\sigma}_{MM}^2 \sum_{i=1}^{N}[\mathbf{P}_i - \mathbf{P}_i\mathbf{Q}_i - \mathbf{Q}_i\mathbf{P}_i + \mathbf{Q}_i\mathbf{P}_i\mathbf{Q}_i]), \tag{4.88}$$

where

$$\mathbf{J} = N\mathbf{I}_{r^2} - \sum_{i=1}^{N}(\mathbf{Q}_i \otimes \mathbf{I}_r + \mathbf{I}_r \otimes \mathbf{Q}_i - \mathbf{Q}_i \otimes \mathbf{Q}_i') \tag{4.89}$$

and $\mathbf{Q}_i = \mathbf{A}_i(\sum_j \mathbf{A}_j'\mathbf{A}_j)^{-1}\mathbf{A}_i'$. It is shown in Appendix 4.5 that matrix $\mathbf{J}$ is nonsingular if $2r < N$. Since $\widehat{\mathbf{B}}_*$ is a linear function of (4.87) and $\widehat{\sigma}_{MM}^2$ is unbiased, the estimator (4.88) is unbiased as well. It is not difficult to show that (4.89) collapses to (4.31) and (4.88) collapses to (4.30) when $\mathbf{C} = \mathbf{I}$ and all the $\mathbf{Z}_i$ have full rank.

When N goes to infinity, terms in (4.88) containing $\mathbf{Q}_i$ vanish and we come to a simplified estimator,

$$\widehat{\mathbf{B}}_* = \frac{1}{N}\widehat{\mathbf{S}}_0 - \frac{\widehat{\sigma}^2}{N}\mathbf{C}\sum_i(\mathbf{Z}_i'\mathbf{Z}_i)^{-1}\mathbf{C}', \tag{4.90}$$

which collapses to (4.32) when $\mathbf{C} = \mathbf{I}$. This estimator has a clear variance components interpretation from the formula $\text{cov}(\mathbf{Ca}_i^0 - \mathbf{A}_i\boldsymbol{\beta}) = \text{cov}(\mathbf{Ca}_i^0) + \text{cov}(\boldsymbol{\delta}_i)$.

Under mild assumptions, the estimators (4.88) and (4.90) are consistent and asymptotically equivalent when $N \to \infty$ with the common covariance matrix for $\text{vech}(\widehat{\mathbf{B}}_*)$ as

$$\frac{2\sigma^4}{N}\mathcal{D}^+\left(\mathbf{B} \otimes \mathbf{B} + \frac{1}{N}\sum_{i=1}^{N}\mathbf{P}_i \otimes \mathbf{P}_i\right)\mathcal{D}^{+'}.$$

The proof is given in Demidenko and Stukel (2002).

4.2.6 Two-stage estimator and asymptotic properties

Following the arguments of Section 4.1.6, the estimated GLS leads to $\boldsymbol{\beta}$ estimation that is unbiased for any N. This estimator is consistent, asymptotically normally distributed, and efficient.

4.2.7   Analysis of misspecification

In the general linear growth curve model, coefficients are not specified completely. A natural question arises: What are the consequences of imposing extra restrictions on coefficients when a standard growth curve model is used (overspecification)? Vice versa, what are consequences when the true model is a standard growth curve but we use the general growth curve model, leaving some coefficients unspecified (underspecification)? Below we investigate these two situations.

Overspecification

We start with the case when the true second-stage model is (4.47) with $r < k$ but the standard growth curve model is used to estimate the population parameters $\boldsymbol{\beta}$. To simplify, the variance parameters are assumed known and the true model specifies only the first component of $\mathbf{a}_i$; namely, $r = 1$ and

$$a_{i1} = \mathbf{q}_i\boldsymbol{\beta}+b_{i1}, \quad i = 1, ..., N, \tag{4.91}$$

where $\mathbf{q}_i$ is a $1 \times m$ vector of covariates, $\boldsymbol{\beta}$ is a $k \times 1$ population parameter with $E(b_{i1}) = 0$, and $\text{var}(b_{i1}) = \sigma^2 d_{11}$, where d_{pq} is the (p, q)th element of matrix $\mathbf{D}$. Application of the standard LGC model forces us to make an additional, irrelevant assumption as to the remainder of the components of $\mathbf{a}_i$. This leads to overspecification. Apparently, there are three ways/models to overspecify:

1. Parameters of the growth curve not covered by the specification (4.91) are assumed to be fixed (nonrandom) and unknown,

$$a_{ij} = \tau_j, \quad \text{var}(a_{ij}) = 0, \quad j = 2, ..., k. \tag{4.92}$$

2. The remaining parameters are random with unknown means:

$$a_{ij} = \tau_j + b_{ij}, \quad j = 2, ..., k. \tag{4.93}$$

   where $\mathbf{b}_i = (b_{i1}, ..., b_{ik})'$ and $\text{cov}(\mathbf{b}_i) = \sigma^2\mathbf{D}$.

3. Model (4.91) is applied to all elements of $\mathbf{a}_i$ as in the RLGC model

$$\mathbf{a}_i = (\mathbf{I} \otimes \mathbf{q}_i')\boldsymbol{\nu} + \mathbf{b}_i, \tag{4.94}$$

   where $\boldsymbol{\nu} = (\boldsymbol{\beta}', \boldsymbol{\tau}')'$ is an $mk \times 1$ vector of parameters, $\boldsymbol{\tau} = (\boldsymbol{\beta}_2', ..., \boldsymbol{\beta}_m')'$, and $\text{cov}(\mathbf{b}) = \sigma^2\mathbf{D}$, see Section 4.1.5.

We aim to show that all three models generally lead to a bias in the population parameter. As follows from (4.63), the GLS estimator for all three models can be written in the form

$$\begin{bmatrix} \widehat{\boldsymbol{\beta}} \\ \widehat{\boldsymbol{\tau}} \end{bmatrix} = \left(\sum \mathbf{Q}_i'\mathbf{M}_i^{-1}\mathbf{Q}_i\right)^{-1} \left(\sum \mathbf{Q}_i'\mathbf{M}_i^{-1}\mathbf{a}_i^0\right), \tag{4.95}$$

where $\mathbf{Q}_i = \text{diag}(\mathbf{q}_i, \mathbf{T}_i)$, $\mathbf{T}_i = \mathbf{I}_{k-1}$ for models (4.91) and (4.92), $\mathbf{T}_i = (\mathbf{I}_{k-1} \otimes \mathbf{q}_i)$ for model (4.93), and $\boldsymbol{\tau}$ is the vector of nuisance parameters. Note that the GLSC estimator (4.63) takes the form

$$\widehat{\boldsymbol{\beta}} = \left(\sum \frac{\mathbf{q}_i'\mathbf{q}_i}{(\mathbf{Z}_i'\mathbf{Z}_i)_{11}^{-1}+d_{11}}\right)^{-1} \left(\sum \frac{\mathbf{q}_i'a_{i1}^0}{(\mathbf{Z}_i'\mathbf{Z}_i)_{11}^{-1} + d_{11}}\right) \tag{4.96}$$

and is unbiased.

In the orthogonal case, when $\mathbf{Z}_i'\mathbf{Z}_i$ and $\mathbf{D}$ are diagonal, all four estimators coincide. As shown previously, for balanced data when $\mathbf{Z}_i = \mathbf{Z}$, the estimator (4.95) does not depend on the matrix $\mathbf{D}$ and coincides with the OLS estimator, so that (4.95) and (4.96) coincide. However, in the general case, all three models lead to biased estimates. To show this, we partition $\boldsymbol{\alpha}_i'$ as $(\alpha_{i1}, \boldsymbol{\alpha}_{i2}')$, where $\boldsymbol{\alpha}_{i2}' = (\alpha_{i2}, ..., \alpha_{im})$, and the other quantities are partitioned correspondingly. Then, from (4.95), we find the expectation

$$E\left[\begin{array}{c}\widehat{\beta}\\ \widehat{\tau}\end{array}\right] = \left[\begin{array}{cc}\sum\mathbf{M}_{i11}^{-1}\mathbf{q}_i'\mathbf{q}_i & \sum\mathbf{q}_i'\mathbf{M}_{i12}^{-1}\mathbf{T}_i\\ \sum\mathbf{T}_i'\mathbf{M}_{i12}^{-1\prime}\mathbf{q}_i & \sum\mathbf{T}_i'\mathbf{M}_{i22}^{-1}\mathbf{T}_i\end{array}\right]^{-1}$$
$$\times\left[\begin{array}{c}(\sum\mathbf{M}_{i11}^{-1}\mathbf{q}_i'\mathbf{q}_i)\beta+\sum\mathbf{q}_i'\mathbf{M}_{i12}^{-1}\boldsymbol{\alpha}_{i2}\\ (\sum\mathbf{T}_i'\mathbf{M}_{i12}^{-1\prime}\mathbf{q}_i)\beta+\sum\mathbf{T}_i'\mathbf{M}_{i22}^{-1}\boldsymbol{\alpha}_{i2}\end{array}\right],$$

where, for instance, $\mathbf{M}_{i11}^{-1}$ is the $(1,1)$th element of matrix $\mathbf{M}_i^{-1}$. Denote $\mathbf{U}_{11}=\sum\mathbf{M}_{i11}^{-1}\mathbf{q}_i'\mathbf{q}_i$, $\mathbf{U}_{12}=\sum\mathbf{q}_i'\mathbf{M}_{i12}^{-1}\mathbf{T}_i$, and $\mathbf{U}_{22}=\sum\mathbf{T}_i'\mathbf{M}_{i22}^{-1}\mathbf{T}_i$. Then, using the formula for the partial inverse, we come to the following formula for the bias:

$$E(\widehat{\beta}) - \beta = \mathbf{F}\sum\mathbf{q}_i'\mathbf{M}_{i12}^{-1}\boldsymbol{\alpha}_{i2} - \mathbf{U}_{11}^{-1}\mathbf{U}_{12}\mathbf{E}^{-1}\sum\mathbf{T}_i'\mathbf{M}_{i22}^{-1}\boldsymbol{\alpha}_{i2},$$

where $\mathbf{E} = \mathbf{U}_{22} - \mathbf{U}_{12}'\mathbf{U}_{11}^{-1}\mathbf{U}_{12}$ and $\mathbf{F} = \mathbf{U}_{11}^{-1} + \mathbf{U}_{11}^{-1}\mathbf{U}_{12}\mathbf{E}^{-1}\mathbf{U}_{12}'\mathbf{U}_{11}^{-1}$. Further, it is easy to check that $\mathbf{F}\sum\mathbf{q}_i'\mathbf{M}_{i12}^{-1}\mathbf{T}_i\overline{\boldsymbol{\alpha}} = \mathbf{A}^{-1}\mathbf{B}\mathbf{E}^{-1}\sum\mathbf{T}_i'\mathbf{M}_{i22}^{-1}\mathbf{T}_i\overline{\boldsymbol{\alpha}}$ for any $\overline{\boldsymbol{\alpha}}$. Thus, the above bias can be expressed in terms of the deviation of $\boldsymbol{\alpha}_{i2}$ from its "modeled" value $\mathbf{T}_i\overline{\boldsymbol{\alpha}}$:

$$E(\widehat{\beta}) - \beta = \sum_{i=1}^N(\mathbf{F}\mathbf{q}_i'\mathbf{M}_{i12}^{-1} - \mathbf{U}_{11}^{-1}\mathbf{U}_{12}\mathbf{E}^{-1}\mathbf{T}_i'\mathbf{M}_{i22}^{-1})(\boldsymbol{\alpha}_{i2} - \mathbf{T}_i\overline{\boldsymbol{\alpha}}). \tag{4.97}$$

Thus, the estimate (4.95) is unbiased if either $E(\mathbf{a}_{i2}) = \mathbf{T}_i\overline{\boldsymbol{\alpha}}$ for some $\overline{\boldsymbol{\alpha}}$, or if $\mathbf{F}\mathbf{q}_i'\mathbf{M}_{i12}^{-1} = \mathbf{U}_{11}^{-1}\mathbf{U}_{12}\mathbf{E}^{-1}\mathbf{T}_i'\mathbf{M}_{i22}^{-1}$ for $i = 1, ..., N$. Notice that the latter case occurs when $\mathbf{q}_i'\mathbf{M}_{i12}^{-1}$ and $\mathbf{T}_i'\mathbf{M}_{i22}^{-1}$ are collinear. In particular, for the random-coefficient model when $\mathbf{q}_i = 1$ and $\mathbf{T}_i = \mathbf{I}$, loosely speaking, the magnitude of the bias depends on how unbalanced the data are. However, in general, any irrelevant specification of $\boldsymbol{\alpha}_{i2}$ leads to a bias for the parameter of interest.

We can even compute the maximum bias in terms of the deviation of $\boldsymbol{\alpha}_{i2}$ from $\mathbf{T}_i\overline{\boldsymbol{\alpha}}$. Applying the matrix inequality $\mathbf{Z}'\mathbf{Y}(\mathbf{Y}'\mathbf{Y})^{-1}\mathbf{Y}'\mathbf{Z} \leq \mathbf{Z}'\mathbf{Z}$ (Graybill, 1983) to (4.97), we obtain

$$\parallel E(\widehat{\beta}) - \beta \parallel^2 \leq \sum(\boldsymbol{\alpha}_{i2} - \mathbf{T}_i\overline{\boldsymbol{\alpha}})'(\boldsymbol{\alpha}_{i2} - \mathbf{T}_i\overline{\boldsymbol{\alpha}})\sum\mathrm{tr}(\mathbf{R}_i'\mathbf{R}_i),$$

where $\mathbf{C}_i = \mathbf{F}\mathbf{q}_i'\mathbf{M}_{i12}^{-1} - \mathbf{A}^{-1}\mathbf{B}\mathbf{E}^{-1}\mathbf{T}_i'\mathbf{M}_{i22}^{-1}$. To illustrate, we use the following simple example.

Example. We consider a regression model with random coefficients $y_{ij} = a_{i1}z_{ij} + a_{i2}+\varepsilon_{ij}, j = 1, ..., n_i, i = 1, .., N$, with a second-stage model for the slope $a_{i1} = \beta+b_{i1}$ and no assumption on the intercept rather than $a_{i2} = \alpha_{i2} + b_{i2}$, where the $\{\alpha_{i2}\}$ are nuisance parameters (general linear growth curve model). For all three models (4.92), (4.93), and (4.94), the assumption on the intercept is irrelevant, with $\mathbf{T}_i = 1$

in (4.95). We attempt to find the bias induced by imposing irrelevant specifications (4.92) or (4.93). For these models

$$
\mathbf{Z}_i'\mathbf{Z}_i = \begin{bmatrix} \sum_j z_{ij}^2 & \sum_j z_{ij} \\ \sum_j z_{ij} & n_i \end{bmatrix}, \quad \mathbf{M}_i = \begin{bmatrix} (\mathbf{Z}_i'\mathbf{Z}_i)_{11}^{-1} + d_{11} & (\mathbf{Z}_i'\mathbf{Z}_i)_{12}^{-1} + d_{12} \\ (\mathbf{Z}_i'\mathbf{Z}_i)_{12}^{-1} + d_{12} & (\mathbf{Z}_i'\mathbf{Z}_i)_{22}^{-1} + d_{22} \end{bmatrix},
$$

where $d_{12} = d_{22} = 0$ for model (4.92), and $(\mathbf{Z}_i'\mathbf{Z}_i)_{11}^{-1}$, for instance, denotes the $(1,1)$th element of the inverse matrix. We obtain

$$
\begin{bmatrix} \sum \mathbf{M}_{i11}^{-1}\mathbf{q}_i'\mathbf{q}_i & \sum \mathbf{q}_i'\mathbf{M}_{i12}^{-1}\mathbf{T}_i \\ \sum \mathbf{T}_i'\mathbf{M}_{i12}^{-1}\mathbf{q}_i & \sum \mathbf{T}_i'\mathbf{M}_{i22}^{-1}\mathbf{T}_i \end{bmatrix} = \sum_{i=1}^N \frac{1}{m_{i11}m_{i22} - m_{i12}^2} \begin{bmatrix} m_{i22} & -m_{i12} \\ -m_{i12} & m_{i11} \end{bmatrix},
\tag{4.98}
$$

where m_{ijk} is the (j,k)th element of matrix $\mathbf{M}_i$. Denoting the elements of matrix (4.98) as l_{11}, l_{12}, and l_{22}, and $\Delta = l_{11}l_{22} - l_{12}^2$, the bias from (4.98) can be written as

$$
E(\widehat{\beta}) - \beta = \frac{1}{\Delta} \sum_{i=1}^N \frac{(m_{i12}l_{22} - m_{i11}l_{12})(\alpha_{i2} - \overline{\alpha})}{m_{i11}m_{i22} - m_{i12}^2}.
$$

The maximum bias, as follows from the Cauchy inequality, is

$$
\max_{\|\alpha_{i2} - \overline{\alpha}\| = \delta} | E(\widehat{\beta}) - \beta | = \frac{\delta}{\Delta} \sqrt{\sum \left(\frac{m_{i12}l_{22} - m_{i11}l_{12}}{m_{i11}m_{i22} - m_{i12}^2} \right)^2}.
\tag{4.99}
$$

Surprisingly, simulations reported in Stukel and Demidenko (1997a) demonstrated that when a standard GLS estimator in the form (4.95) is applied to the general growth curve with unknown variance parameters, the bias becomes negligible. This can be explained in the following way. Letting $d_{12} = 0$, we obtain

$$
\mathbf{M}_i^{-1} = \frac{1}{\varphi} \begin{bmatrix} h_{22i} + d_{22} & -h_{12i} \\ -h_{12i} & h_{11i} + d_{11} \end{bmatrix},
$$

where $h_{kli} = (\mathbf{Z}_i'\mathbf{Z}_i)_{kl}^{-1}$, and κ is the determinant of matrix $(\mathbf{Z}_i'\mathbf{Z}_i)^{-1}$, and $\varphi = d_{22}(h_{11i} + d_{11}) + (d_{11}h_{i22} + \kappa)$. Putting $d_{22} \to \infty$, we obtain

$$
\mathbf{M}_i^{-1} \to \begin{bmatrix} ((\mathbf{Z}_i'\mathbf{Z}_i)_{11}^{-1} + d_{11})^{-1} & 0 \\ 0 & 0 \end{bmatrix}, \quad i = 1, ..., N,
$$

so that the estimators $\widehat{\boldsymbol{\beta}}$ from (4.96) and (4.95) coincide, $\mathrm{cov}(\widehat{\beta}, \widehat{\tau}) = (\sum \mathbf{M}_i^{-1})^{-1}$ but $\mathrm{var}(\widehat{\beta})$ is inflated. Therefore, in this example, if the true intercepts were extremely variable (d_{22} is large) but we assumed a population mean model (4.93) or (4.94) for the intercept, one could still obtain nearly unbiased estimates of $\boldsymbol{\beta}$ but with inflated variances. This observation has the following general implication. When a part of the second-stage model is misspecified, the variances of corresponding random effects become inflated (in terms of our example, $d_{22} \to \infty$). As a result of weighting by the inverse of the variances, the contribution of the parameters that are misspecified becomes negligible, and the estimates of parameters that are specified correctly become almost unbiased.

Underspecification

Now it is assumed that the true second-stage model is (4.91), in conjunction with one of (4.92), (4.93), or (4.94), but we use only (4.91) to estimate β by the GLSC estimator (4.63). It is straightforward to show that this estimator remains unbiased with a possible loss of efficiency. The unbiasedness of the GLSC estimator follows directly after taking the expectation of (4.96),

$$\left(\sum \frac{\mathbf{q}_i'\mathbf{q}_i}{(\mathbf{Z}_i'\mathbf{Z}_i)_{11}^{-1}+d_{11}}\right)^{-1}\left(\sum_i \frac{\mathbf{q}_i'\mathbf{q}_i\beta}{(\mathbf{Z}_i'\mathbf{Z}_i)_{11}^{-1}+d_{11}}\right) = \beta,$$

because from (4.91) we have $E(a_{i1}) = \mathbf{q}_i\beta$. However, generally, there is some loss of efficiency, which is illustrated by the following example.

Example (continued). The variance of the GLSC estimator is $\sigma^2/\sum m_{i11}^{-1}$. Denoting $\Delta_i = m_{i11}m_{i22} - m_{i12}^2$, the determinant of $\mathbf{M}_i$, the variance of $\widetilde{\beta}$ from the standard linear growth curve model is

$$\begin{aligned}
\mathrm{var}(\widehat{\beta}) &= \left(\sum m_{i22}\Delta_i^{-1} - (\sum m_{i12}\Delta_i^{-1})^2(\sum m_{i11}\Delta_i^{-1})^{-1}\right)^{-1} \\
&= \left(\sum m_{i11}^{-1} + v\right)^{-1} \leq \mathrm{var}(\widehat{\beta}),
\end{aligned} \tag{4.100}$$

since

$$\begin{aligned}
0 &\leq v = \sum m_{i12}^2 m_{i11}^{-1}\Delta_i^{-1} - (\sum m_{i12}\Delta_i^{-1})^2(\sum m_{i11}\Delta_i^{-1})^{-1} \\
&\leq \sum m_{i12}^2 m_{i11}^{-1}\Delta_i^{-1}.
\end{aligned} \tag{4.101}$$

The left-hand side of this inequality follows from the Cauchy inequality, and the right-hand side is obvious. Based on (4.100) and (4.101), there is no loss in efficiency if and only if for some λ, $m_{i12} = \lambda m_{i22}$ for all $i = 1, ..., N$, which again is true for balanced data. Maximum loss occurs when $m_{i12} = 0$, which is true when the columns of matrix $\mathbf{Z}_i$ are orthogonal and the random effects are uncorrelated, so that we come to estimate (4.96).

Problems for Section 4.2

1. Modify example (4.48) assuming that the intercept depends on the gender as well.

2. Is it true that the classic asymptotic theory does not apply to the general linear growth curve model because the number of parameters grow with the number of clusters (N)?

3. Modify function `calcium` to reproduce Figure 4.2. First, fit an individual TBBMD pattern using the linear model of time, and second, use `density` for the intercept and slope.

4. Prove (4.67).

5. Provide the link between estimator (4.68) and the results from Section 2.3. Can (4.68) be derived from the results of that section?

6. Derive Fisher information matrix for model (4.69), including α_i parameters.

7*. Write an R function for maximization of the log-likelihood (4.72) using algorithm (4.75) and compare its performance against general LME model estimation `lmeFS`. Employ your code for the model specified by equations (4.51) and (4.52) using `calcium.txt` data. Are there any advantages of using specialized software for general linear growth curve model ML estimation?

8*. Similar to the previous problem, write two R functions for the log-likelihood maximization using the Newton-Raphson algorithm (4.81) and Fixed-Point algorithm (4.82). Compare their performance via simulations. Use these codes to estimate the calcium supplementation model with `calcium.txt` data.

9. Prove that the limit point of $\{b_{*s}\}$ defined by (4.86) satisfies the score equation (4.85).

10*. Prove that matrix $\mathbf{J}$ defined by equation (4.89) is positive definite. Prove that (4.89) collapses to (4.31) and (4.88) collapses to (4.30) when $\mathbf{C} = \mathbf{I}$ and all the $\mathbf{Z}_i$ have full rank.

11. Based on the results of Section 4.2.7, describe in a few words whether over-specification is more harmful than underspecification (you may rely on conclusions from the example).

4.3   Linear model with linear covariance structure

A characteristic feature of all mixed models considered earlier is that the covariance matrix of the random term $\boldsymbol{\eta}_i$, in the notation (2.11), can be expressed as a linear combination of fixed symmetric matrices with unknown coefficients/parameters. For example, let the linear mixed effects model be defined by (2.5). We notice that the $n_i \times n_i$ matrix $\mathbf{Z}_i\mathbf{D}\mathbf{Z}_i'$ can be expressed as a linear combination of $k(k+1)/2$ symmetric matrices with coefficients as unique elements of matrix $\mathbf{D}$, namely,

$$\mathbf{Z}_i\mathbf{D}\mathbf{Z}_i' = \sum_{j \leq q}^{k} d_{jq}\mathbf{V}_{i,jq}, \tag{4.102}$$

where $\mathbf{V}_{i,jj} = \mathbf{Z}_{i,\cdot j}\mathbf{Z}_{i,\cdot j}'$, $\mathbf{V}_{i,jq} = \mathbf{Z}_{i,\cdot j}\mathbf{Z}_{i,\cdot q}' + \mathbf{Z}_{i,\cdot q}\mathbf{Z}_{i,\cdot j}'$ for $j \neq q$ and $\mathbf{Z}_{i,\cdot j}$ denotes the jth column of the matrix $\mathbf{Z}_i$ (Stram and Lee, 1994). Representation (4.102) gives a hint to a more general class of Linear Model with Linear Covariance Structure (LMLCS). The LMLCS is defined precisely as

$$\mathbf{y}_i = \mathbf{X}_i\boldsymbol{\beta} + \boldsymbol{\eta}_i, \quad E(\boldsymbol{\eta}_i) = \mathbf{0}, \text{cov}(\boldsymbol{\eta}_i) = \sum_{q=0}^{Q} \theta_q\mathbf{V}_{iq}, \tag{4.103}$$

where the $\{\theta_q\}$ are unknown variance/covariance components, the $\{\mathbf{V}_{iq}\}$ are $n_i \times n_i$ fixed known symmetric matrices, and $\boldsymbol{\theta} = (\theta_0, \theta_1, ..., \theta_Q)'$ is the vector of the variance parameters. Further, we shall assume that $\mathbf{V}_{i0} = \mathbf{I}$, the $n_i \times n_i$ identity matrix, and $\theta_0 > 0$. In this notation the LME model takes the form (4.103), where $\theta_0 = \sigma^2$, $(\theta_1, ..., \theta_Q) = \text{vech}(\mathbf{D}_*)$, and $Q = 1 + k(k+1)/2$. To avoid deficiency, we shall assume that matrix $\sum \mathbf{X}_i'\mathbf{X}_i$ is nonsingular and matrices $\{\mathbf{V}_{iq}\}$ are linearly independent. More precisely, the latter assumption is defined as follows. Let $\widetilde{\mathbf{V}}$ be the $\sum n_i^2 \times (1 + Q)$ matrix with columns comprised of stacked vectors $\{\text{vec}(\mathbf{V}_{iq})\}$. Then it is assumed that the matrix $\widetilde{\mathbf{V}}$ has full rank. An important consequence of this condition is that the $(1 + Q) \times (1 + Q)$ matrix of traces $\{\sum \text{tr}(\mathbf{V}_{iq}\mathbf{V}_{ip})$,

$p, q = 0, 1, ..., Q\}$ is invertible, because it is equal to $\widetilde{\mathbf{V}}'\widetilde{\mathbf{V}}$, due to the identity $\text{tr}(\mathbf{AB}) = \text{vec}'(\mathbf{A})\text{vec}(\mathbf{B})$ for any matrices $\mathbf{A}$ and $\mathbf{B}$ of the same size. One may or may not assume that the error term $\boldsymbol{\eta}_i$ has a normal distribution. If $\boldsymbol{\eta}_i$ is normally distributed ML estimation gives asymptotically efficient estimates, see Section 4.3.1. If the distribution is not normal, a noniterative estimate such as variance least squares may be used, see Section 4.3.2.

A linear model with linear covariance structure was introduced by Anderson (1969, 1971) and was studied extensively by Rao and Kleffé (1988) in the framework of the general variance components model. However, unlike the previous authors, we assume that N independent subjects/clusters are observed (repeated measurements, so loosely speaking we have N independent Anderson models). Maximum likelihood estimation of linear model (4.103) has been discussed by Jennrich and Schluchter (1986). The linear model with linear covariance structure is very flexible and may accommodate the analysis of different types of data, including multilevel, multidimensional, and longitudinal autocorrelated data, which cannot be covered by the basic LME model (2.5). For example, although the LME model (2.5) is often referred to as an adequate model for longitudinal data, it does not reflect the major assumption of the time series analysis, autocorrelation. Indeed, the major feature of longitudinal data is the presence of autocorrelation in serial observations. But as follows from model (2.5), observations are uncorrelated in time. To make the LME model adequate for the analysis of longitudinal data, the covariance structure $\sigma^2 \mathbf{I} + \mathbf{Z}_i \mathbf{D}_* \mathbf{Z}_i'$ has to be augmented by a term that would reflect the time series dependence. In particular, we shall show that model (4.103) is well suited for such time series analysis.

We demonstrate below that many mixed models may be described and analyzed under the umbrella of a linear model with linear covariance structure (4.103). A matter of particular attention is the development of special cases of LMLCS as an extension of the LME model (2.5). This includes the analysis of longitudinal correlated and multidimensional data.

4.3.1 Method of maximum likelihood

If $\boldsymbol{\eta}_i$ are independent and normally distributed, the log-likelihood function for model (4.103) takes the form

$$l(\boldsymbol{\beta}, \boldsymbol{\theta}) = -\frac{1}{2} \sum_{i=1}^{N} \left[\ln|\mathbf{V}_i| + (\mathbf{y}_i - \mathbf{X}_i \boldsymbol{\beta})' \mathbf{V}_i^{-1} (\mathbf{y}_i - \mathbf{X}_i \boldsymbol{\beta}) \right], \qquad (4.104)$$

where $\mathbf{V}_i = \sum_{q=0}^{Q} \theta_q \mathbf{V}_{iq}$ is the $n_i \times n_i$ covariance matrix of $\mathbf{y}_i$, the $\{\mathbf{V}_{iq}\}$ are fixed symmetric matrices, and $\mathbf{V}_{i0} = \mathbf{I}$ with $\theta_0 > 0$. In many instances the parameter space for $(\theta_1, ..., \theta_Q)$ can be well defined based on the specificity of the problem; see the special cases of the LMLCS below. For example, if θ_1 is the correlation coefficient, we impose the restriction $-1 < \theta_1 < 1$. The largest parameter space, as the domain of (4.104), is where all matrices $\{\mathbf{V}_i\}$ are positive definite. However, as we know from Section 2.15.2, this definition may lead to numerical complications.

The restricted log-likelihood function takes the form

$$l_R(\boldsymbol{\beta}, \boldsymbol{\theta}) = -\frac{1}{2} \sum_{i=1}^{N} \left[\ln |\mathbf{V}_i| + (\mathbf{y}_i - \mathbf{X}_i \boldsymbol{\beta})' \mathbf{V}_i^{-1} (\mathbf{y}_i - \mathbf{X}_i \boldsymbol{\beta}) \right] + \ln \left| \sum_{i=1}^{N} \mathbf{X}_i' \mathbf{V}_i^{-1} \mathbf{X}_i \right|.$$

(4.105)

If $\boldsymbol{\theta}$ is known, the GLS estimator for the beta coefficients is given by

$$\widehat{\boldsymbol{\beta}}_{GLS} = \left(\sum \mathbf{X}_i' \mathbf{V}_i^{-1} \mathbf{X}_i \right)^{-1} \left(\sum \mathbf{X}_i' \mathbf{V}_i^{-1} \mathbf{y}_i \right),$$

(4.106)

which maximizes l and l_R when $\boldsymbol{\theta}$ is held. If $\theta_q = 0$ for all $q > 0$, we come to the OLS estimate (2.29). Unfortunately, we cannot use the dimension-reduction formulas to invert $\mathbf{V}_i$ with general $\mathbf{V}_{iq}$. However, as the reader could see, for the special cases considered below, the log-likelihood function can be simplified substantially.

Fisher scoring algorithm

As discussed in Chapter 2, we prefer the Fisher scoring algorithm because it is robust to the starting point of the iteration process. Indeed, since the log-likelihood function is not concave the Hessian matrix $\mathbf{H}$ in the Newton–Raphson (NR) algorithm may not be nonnegative definite, which could lead to algorithm failure. The chances of not getting a matrix that is not nonnegative definite increases when the starting parameter value is far from the ML estimate. Contrary to the NR algorithm, the inverted matrix in the FS algorithm is always positive definite because it is the information matrix. In any case, the information matrix is needed to compute the variances of the ML estimates. Remarkably, the information matrix is even simpler to obtain for the LMLCS than for the LME model (Section 3.3).

We start with the first derivatives with respect to the variance parameters

$$\frac{\partial l}{\partial \theta_q} = -\frac{1}{2} \sum_{i=1}^{N} \left[\text{tr}(\mathbf{V}_i^{-1} \mathbf{V}_{iq}) - \mathbf{e}_i' \mathbf{V}_i^{-1} \mathbf{V}_{iq} \mathbf{V}_i^{-1} \mathbf{e}_i \right]$$

(4.107)

for $q = 0, ..., Q$, where throughout this section

$$\mathbf{e}_i = \mathbf{y}_i - \mathbf{X}_i \boldsymbol{\beta}$$

(4.108)

denotes the $n_i \times 1$ residual vector. For the restricted log-likelihood we have

$$\begin{aligned}
\frac{\partial l_R}{\partial \theta_q} = \ & -\frac{1}{2} \left\{ \sum_{i=1}^{N} \left[\text{tr}(\mathbf{V}_i^{-1} \mathbf{V}_{iq}) - \mathbf{e}_i' \mathbf{V}_i^{-1} \mathbf{V}_{iq} \mathbf{V}_i^{-1} \mathbf{e}_i \right] \right. \\
& \left. -\text{tr} \left(\mathbf{T}^{-1} \sum_{i=1}^{N} \mathbf{X}_i' \mathbf{V}_i^{-1} \mathbf{V}_{iq} \mathbf{V}_i^{-1} \mathbf{X}_i \right) \right\},
\end{aligned}$$

(4.109)

where $\mathbf{T} = \sum \mathbf{X}_i' \mathbf{V}_i^{-1} \mathbf{X}_i$. The second derivatives are

$$\frac{\partial^2 l}{\partial \theta_q \partial \theta_p} = \frac{1}{2} \sum_{i=1}^{N} [\text{tr}(\mathbf{V}_i^{-1} \mathbf{V}_{iq} \mathbf{V}_i^{-1} \mathbf{V}_{ip}) - 2\mathbf{e}_i' \mathbf{V}_i^{-1} \mathbf{V}_{ip} \mathbf{V}_i^{-1} \mathbf{V}_{iq} \mathbf{V}_i^{-1} \mathbf{e}_i],$$

for $p, q = 0, ..., Q$. The information matrix is the negative of the expectation of the second derivative matrix. Using the formula $E(\mathbf{e}'\mathbf{A}\mathbf{e}) = \text{tr}(\mathbf{A}\mathbf{V})$, we obtain

$$\mathcal{I} = \frac{1}{2}\left\{\sum_{i=1}^{N}\text{tr}(\mathbf{V}_i^{-1}\mathbf{V}_{iq}\mathbf{V}_i^{-1}\mathbf{V}_{ip}), \ p, q = 0, 1, ..., Q\right\}, \qquad (4.110)$$

the $Q \times Q$ information matrix for $\boldsymbol{\theta}$. It is easy to see that $\mathcal{I}$ is nonsingular if the $\{\mathbf{V}_{iq}\}$ are linearly independent. Since the information matrix for $(\boldsymbol{\beta}, \boldsymbol{\theta})$ is block diagonal, we can maximize l separately over $\boldsymbol{\beta}$ and $\boldsymbol{\theta}$. Thus, to compute the ML estimates, we proceed as follows: Given starting values $\theta_0, \theta_1, ..., \theta_Q$, we compute $\widehat{\boldsymbol{\beta}}$ using formula (4.106) and residuals (4.108). Then we find the next approximation for $\boldsymbol{\theta}$ using the generic formula (2.103). At the second iteration, we compute the next approximation for the beta coefficients and continue in this fashion until convergence. A good starting value is the OLS, $\theta_0 = \widehat{\sigma}_{OLS}^2$, $\theta_1 = 0, ..., \theta_Q = 0$. Alternatively, one can use the VLS estimate for $\boldsymbol{\theta}$ derived below.

It is straightforward to show that ML = RML asymptotically; that is, the information matrices for the two methods coincide, similar to the case of the LME model of Section 2.14. Therefore, we can use matrix (4.110) with derivatives (4.109) to find the restricted ML estimate.

4.3.2   Variance least squares

In this section we apply the method of variance least squares (Section 3.12) to obtain a noniterative distribution-free unbiased estimator for $\boldsymbol{\theta}$. According to this method, we find $\theta_0, \theta_1, ..., \theta_Q$, which minimize the quadratic function

$$\sum_{i=1}^{N}\text{tr}\left(\widehat{\mathbf{e}}_i\widehat{\mathbf{e}}_i' - \theta_0\mathbf{V}_{i0} - \theta_1\mathbf{V}_{i1} - ... - \theta_Q\mathbf{V}_{iQ}\right)^2,$$

where $\widehat{\mathbf{e}}_i$ is the OLS residual vector. Differentiating with respect to θ_q, we come to a system of linear equations with the solution

$$\widehat{\boldsymbol{\theta}}_{VLS} = \mathbf{M}^{-1}\mathbf{m}, \qquad (4.111)$$

where the elements of the $(Q+1) \times (Q+1)$ matrix $\mathbf{M}$ and the $(Q+1) \times 1$ vector $\mathbf{m}$ are defined as

$$M_{pq} = \sum_{i=1}^{N}\text{tr}(\mathbf{V}_{ip}\mathbf{V}_{iq}), \quad m_q = \sum_{i=1}^{N}\mathbf{e}_i'\mathbf{V}_{iq}\mathbf{e}_i,$$

$p, q = 0, 1, ..., Q$. It is easy to see that in a manner analogous to the LME model, the VLS estimate is obtained at the first iteration of log-likelihood maximization starting from the OLS estimate (Section 3.12.4).

The Variance Least Squares (VLS) estimator (4.111) is biased. To make it unbiased, we take the expectation of $\mathbf{m}$ and solve for $\boldsymbol{\theta}$. Denoting, as in Section 3.12.1,

$$\mathbf{N} = \left(\sum\mathbf{X}_i'\mathbf{X}_i\right)^{-1}, \quad \mathbf{P}_i = \mathbf{X}_i\mathbf{N}\mathbf{X}_i', \quad \mathbf{G}_p = \sum\mathbf{X}_i'\mathbf{V}_{ip}\mathbf{X}_i,$$

and using $E(\boldsymbol{\eta}'\mathbf{A}\boldsymbol{\eta}) = \text{tr}(\mathbf{AV})$ we obtain

$$
\begin{aligned}
&E(m_q) \\
&= E\left[\sum_{i=1}^{N}(\boldsymbol{\eta}_i - \mathbf{X}_i\mathbf{N}\sum_{j=1}^{N}\mathbf{X}_j'\boldsymbol{\eta}_j)'\mathbf{V}_{iq}(\boldsymbol{\eta}_i - \mathbf{X}_i\mathbf{N}\sum_{j=1}^{N}\mathbf{X}_j'\boldsymbol{\eta}_j)\right] \\
&= \sum_{i=1}^{N}\text{tr}(\mathbf{V}_i\mathbf{V}_{iq}) - 2\sum_{i=1}^{N}E(\boldsymbol{\eta}_i'\mathbf{V}_{iq}\mathbf{P}_i\boldsymbol{\eta}_i) + \sum_{i=1}^{N}\sum_{j=1}^{N}E(\boldsymbol{\eta}_j'\mathbf{X}_j\mathbf{N}\mathbf{X}_i'\mathbf{V}_{iq}\mathbf{X}_i\mathbf{N}\mathbf{X}_j'\boldsymbol{\eta}_j) \\
&= \sum_{i=1}^{N}\text{tr}(\mathbf{V}_i\mathbf{V}_{iq}) - 2\sum_{i=1}^{N}\text{tr}(\mathbf{V}_i\mathbf{V}_{iq}\mathbf{P}_i) + \sum_{i=1}^{N}\text{tr}(\mathbf{V}_i\mathbf{X}_i\mathbf{N}\mathbf{G}_q\mathbf{N}\mathbf{X}_i') \\
&= \sum_{p=0}^{Q}\theta_q r_{pq},
\end{aligned}
$$

where

$$
r_{pq} = \text{tr}\left[\sum_{i=1}^{N}(\mathbf{V}_{ip}\mathbf{V}_{iq} - 2\mathbf{V}_{ip}\mathbf{V}_{iq}\mathbf{P}_i)\right] + \text{tr}(\mathbf{N}\mathbf{G}_q\mathbf{N}\mathbf{G}_p). \tag{4.112}
$$

Let $\mathbf{R}$ be the $(Q+1) \times (Q+1)$ matrix with the (p,q)th element defined by (4.112). Then an unbiased quadratic estimator of $\boldsymbol{\theta}$, called the Unbiased VLS (UVLS) estimator, is given by

$$
\widehat{\boldsymbol{\theta}}_{UVLS} = \mathbf{R}^{-1}\mathbf{m}. \tag{4.113}
$$

When $N \to \infty$, the terms $\sum\text{tr}(\mathbf{V}_{ip}\mathbf{V}_{iq}\mathbf{P}_i)$ and $\text{tr}(\mathbf{N}\mathbf{G}_q\mathbf{N}\mathbf{G}_p)$ vanish in (4.112) and matrices $\mathbf{M}$ and $\mathbf{R}$ converge. This means that UVLS is asymptotically equivalent to VLS. It is possible to obtain the MINQUE estimator for $\boldsymbol{\theta}$ following the line of Section 3.10.3. However, our simulations of Section 3.14 suggest that MINQUE and UVLS are similar in performance.

4.3.3 Statistical properties

After the ML/RML iterations converge, we estimate the covariance matrices as

$$
\text{cov}(\widehat{\boldsymbol{\beta}}_{ML}) = \left(\sum\mathbf{X}_i'\widetilde{\mathbf{V}}_i^{-1}\mathbf{X}_i\right)^{-1}, \quad \text{cov}(\widehat{\boldsymbol{\theta}}_{ML}) = \mathcal{I}^{-1}.
$$

The diagonal elements of these matrices may be used to test statistical hypotheses by the Wald test. However, if the null hypothesis is on the boundary of the variance parameter space, we expect the real significance level to be twice as small as the nominal; see Section 3.5 for details. Since the ML/RML estimate of $\boldsymbol{\theta}$ is a symmetric function of $\boldsymbol{\eta}_i$, the estimates for the beta coefficients are unbiased in a small sample (Section 3.6.1). The asymptotic properties of a linear model with linear covariance structure were studied by Anderson (1973). In that paper he assumed that $N = 1$, with the number of observations n_1 going to infinity. On the contrary, we assume that $N \to \infty$ with n_i bounded. However, the principal result is the same: Since the estimated GLS is consistent and efficient, $\widehat{\boldsymbol{\beta}}_{ML}$ is consistent and asymptotically efficient with any consistent estimator of $\boldsymbol{\theta}$, see Section 3.15.

4.3.4   LME model for longitudinal autocorrelated data

Several authors observed that the covariance matrix for autocorrelated longitudinal data may be well represented by a linear combination of fixed matrices, e.g., Vonesh and Chinchilli (1997). Indeed, we make the following two adequate assumptions when modeling autocorrelated data:

- The correlation has maximum lag q; namely, errors ε_t and $\varepsilon_{t'}$ correlate if $|t - t'| \leq q$ but they do not correlate if $|t - t'| > q$.

- The stochastic process $\{\varepsilon_t\}$ is stationary in the wide sense (Anderson, 1971); namely, the correlation ε_t between $\varepsilon_{t'}$ is only a function of $|t - t'|$.

In the theory of time series, it is shown that the process with these properties can be generated by the Moving Average (MA), $\varepsilon_i = \sum_{j=i-q}^{i} c_j \zeta_j$, where $\{\zeta_j\}$ are iid random variables with zero mean and c_j are fixed coefficients, denoted as MA(q). For example, MA(1) has a one-lag correlation, meaning that $\mathrm{cor}(\varepsilon_t, \varepsilon_{t+1}) = \rho$ but $\mathrm{cor}(\varepsilon_t, \varepsilon_{t+k}) = 0$ for $k > 1$. To simplify the notation, we omit the subscript i in the following development.

MA(1) model

If $\mathbf{y}$ is a vector of longitudinal observations, the combination of the random effect $\mathbf{Zb}$ and the MA(1) model for residuals leads to a linear covariance structure,

$$\mathbf{V} = \sigma^2(\mathbf{I} + \rho\mathbf{T}_1 + \mathbf{ZDZ'}), \tag{4.114}$$

where $\mathbf{T}_1$ is an elementary Toeplitz matrix of the first order, which has 1 at the two parallel subdiagonals and zero elsewhere. Model MA(2) accommodates autocorrelation of the second order with a covariance matrix of the form

$$\mathbf{V} = \sigma^2(\mathbf{I} + \rho_1\mathbf{T}_1 + \rho_2\mathbf{T}_2 + \mathbf{ZDZ'}).$$

For example, the 6×6 matrices $\mathbf{T}_1$ and $\mathbf{T}_2$ are

$$\mathbf{T}_1 = \begin{bmatrix} 0 & 1 & 0 & 0 & 0 & 0 \\ 1 & 0 & 1 & 0 & 0 & 0 \\ 0 & 1 & 0 & 1 & 0 & 0 \\ 0 & 0 & 1 & 0 & 1 & 0 \\ 0 & 0 & 0 & 1 & 0 & 1 \\ 0 & 0 & 0 & 0 & 1 & 0 \end{bmatrix}, \quad \mathbf{T}_2 = \begin{bmatrix} 0 & 0 & 1 & 0 & 0 & 0 \\ 0 & 0 & 0 & 1 & 0 & 0 \\ 1 & 0 & 0 & 0 & 1 & 0 \\ 0 & 1 & 0 & 0 & 0 & 1 \\ 0 & 0 & 1 & 0 & 0 & 0 \\ 0 & 0 & 0 & 1 & 0 & 0 \end{bmatrix}. \tag{4.115}$$

Since matrix $\mathbf{V}$ can be expressed as a linear combination of fixed matrices, the theory of LMLCS applies readily. In particular, we can obtain unbiased estimates for ρ and $\mathbf{D}$ using unbiased variance least squares (4.113).

For the simplest and most important case of the MA(1), the log-likelihood function can be simplified by applying the following dimension-reduction formulas. For the determinant,

$$\left|\mathbf{C} + \mathbf{ZDZ'}\right| = |\mathbf{C}| \left|\mathbf{I} + \mathbf{DZ'C}^{-1}\mathbf{Z}\right|, \tag{4.116}$$

and for the inverse matrix,

$$(\mathbf{C} + \mathbf{ZDZ'})^{-1} = \mathbf{C}^{-1} - \mathbf{C}^{-1}\mathbf{Z}(\mathbf{D}^{-1} + \mathbf{Z'C}^{-1}\mathbf{Z})^{-1}\mathbf{Z'C}^{-1}. \tag{4.117}$$

For growth curves another useful formula exists:

$$\mathbf{Z}'(\mathbf{C} + \mathbf{Z}\mathbf{D}\mathbf{Z}')^{-1}\mathbf{Z} = \left(\mathbf{D} + (\mathbf{Z}'\mathbf{C}^{-1}\mathbf{Z})^{-1}\right)^{-1}. \tag{4.118}$$

For $\mathbf{C} = \mathbf{I}$ we obtain formulas (2.22), (2.21), and (2.25), respectively. For the MA(1) model, the $n \times n$ correlation matrix takes the form $\mathbf{C} = \mathbf{I} + \rho\mathbf{T}_1$ with the determinant

$$|\mathbf{C}| = \prod_{k=1}^{n}\left(1 + 2\rho\cos\frac{k\pi}{n+1}\right).$$

The (j,k)th element of matrix $\mathbf{C}^{-1}$ is given by

$$C^{jk} = \frac{(1 - b^{2n_i - 2j + 2})(b^{j+k+1} - b^{k-j+1})}{\rho(1 - b^2)(1 - b^{2n_i+2})},$$

where $b = \frac{1}{2}\rho\left(\sqrt{1 - 4\rho^2} - 1\right)$ for $j \le k$ and $C^{jk} = C^{kj}$ (Graybill, 1983).

We shall use a similar autocorrelation structure for a generalized linear mixed model in Section 7.9.

AR(1) model

Another popular statistical model of a time series is autoregression (Fuller, 1995). The simplest is the first-order autoregression model, denoted AR(1), and it has the form $\varepsilon_t = \rho\varepsilon_{t-1} + \zeta_t$ with the correlation matrix

$$\mathbf{C} = \begin{bmatrix} 1 & \rho & \rho^2 & \rho^3 & \cdots & \rho^{n-1} \\ \rho & 1 & \rho & \rho^2 & \cdots & \rho^{n-2} \\ \rho^2 & \rho & 1 & \rho & \cdots & \rho^{n-3} \\ \rho^3 & \rho^2 & \rho & 1 & \cdots & \rho^{n-4} \\ \vdots & \vdots & \vdots & \vdots & & \vdots \\ \rho^{n-1} & \rho^{n-2} & \rho^{n-3} & \rho^{n-4} & \cdots & 1 \end{bmatrix}.$$

Matrix $\mathbf{C}$ cannot be represented as a linear combination of fixed matrices, so the resulting mixed model does not belong to the class of LMLCS, although the inverse matrix can be represented as a sum of three fixed matrices, (4.119). Chi and Reinsel (1989) consider estimation of the LME model with AR(1) errors in detail; particularly, they develop the score test for the hypothesis $\rho = 0$.

Here we develop a special log-likelihood parameterization based on the dimension-reduction formulas (4.116) and (4.117). We note the advantage of the fact that the inverse and the determinant of matrix $\mathbf{C}$ take simple forms:

$$\mathbf{C}^{-1} = \frac{1}{1 - \rho^2}\begin{bmatrix} 1 & -\rho & 0 & 0 & \cdots & 0 \\ -\rho & 1 + \rho^2 & -\rho & 0 & \cdots & 0 \\ 0 & -\rho & 1 + \rho^2 & -\rho & \cdots & 0 \\ 0 & 0 & -\rho & 1 + \rho^2 & \cdots & 0 \\ \vdots & \vdots & \vdots & \vdots & & \vdots \\ 0 & 0 & 0 & \cdots & -\rho & 1 \end{bmatrix}$$

and

$$|\mathbf{C}| = 1 - \rho^2.$$

Hence, denoting $\mathbf{I}_2$ an $n \times n$ matrix which has 1 on the main diagonal from position 2 to $n-1$ and zero elsewhere, we can write the inverse compactly as a linear combination of three fixed elementary matrices,

$$\mathbf{C}^{-1} = \frac{1}{1 - \rho^2} \mathbf{U},$$

where

$$\mathbf{U} = \mathbf{I} + \rho^2 \mathbf{I}_2 - \rho \mathbf{T}_1. \tag{4.119}$$

The covariance matrix of $\boldsymbol{\eta}$ takes the form $\sigma^2 \mathbf{V} = \sigma^2(\mathbf{C} + \mathbf{ZDZ}')$. First, we simplify the determinant of $\mathbf{V}$ using formula (4.116):

$$|\mathbf{C} + \mathbf{ZDZ}'| = \frac{1 - \rho^2}{|\widetilde{\mathbf{D}}|} \left|\widetilde{\mathbf{D}} + \mathbf{Z}'\mathbf{U}\mathbf{Z}\right| = \frac{1 - \rho^2}{|\widetilde{\mathbf{D}}|} \left|\widetilde{\mathbf{D}} + \mathbf{M}_0 + \rho^2 \mathbf{M}_1 - \rho \mathbf{M}_2\right|,$$

where

$$\begin{aligned} \widetilde{\mathbf{D}} &= (1 - \rho^2)\mathbf{D}^{-1}, \\ \mathbf{M}_0 &= \mathbf{Z}'\mathbf{Z}, \ \mathbf{M}_1 = \mathbf{Z}'\mathbf{I}_2\mathbf{Z}, \ \mathbf{M}_2 = \mathbf{Z}'\mathbf{T}_1\mathbf{Z}. \end{aligned} \tag{4.120}$$

Second, we simplify the inverse matrix using formula (4.117):

$$(\mathbf{C} + \mathbf{ZDZ}')^{-1} = \frac{1}{1 - \rho^2} \left[\mathbf{U} - \mathbf{U}\mathbf{Z}(\widetilde{\mathbf{D}} + \mathbf{Z}'\mathbf{U}\mathbf{Z})^{-1}\mathbf{Z}'\mathbf{U} \right],$$

which can be expressed in terms of matrices (4.120). This finally leads to the *precision-matrix* parameterization, which is analogous to (2.43),

$$\begin{aligned} l_p(\boldsymbol{\beta}, \rho, \widetilde{\mathbf{D}}) = &-\frac{1}{2} \left\{ \ln \left[\sum (\mathbf{e}_i' \mathbf{U}_i \mathbf{e}_i - \mathbf{r}_i'(\widetilde{\mathbf{D}} + \mathbf{Z}_i'\mathbf{U}_i\mathbf{Z}_i)^{-1}\mathbf{r}_i) \right] \right. \\ &+ \left. \sum \ln |\widetilde{\mathbf{D}} + \mathbf{Z}_i'\mathbf{U}_i\mathbf{Z}_i| - N \ln |\widetilde{\mathbf{D}}| - (N_T - N)\ln(1 - \rho^2) \right\}, \end{aligned}$$

where $\mathbf{r}_i = \mathbf{Z}_i'\mathbf{U}_i\mathbf{e}_i$ and matrix $\mathbf{U}_i$ is defined by (4.119).

Now we consider a very special case, a linear model with random intercepts and AR(1) errors, as a generalization of the LME model of Section 2.4.

Linear model with random intercepts and autocorrelated residuals

In this subsection we simplify the log-likelihood function derived earlier for the linear random-intercept model with first-order autocorrelated residuals, which may be considered as an extension of the LME model of Section 2.4 when $\rho = 0$. For this model, $\mathbf{Z}_i = \mathbf{1}_i$ and

$$\begin{aligned} l_p(\boldsymbol{\beta}, \rho, \widetilde{d}) = &-\frac{1}{2} \left\{ N_T \ln \left(s_0 + \rho^2 s_1 - \rho s_2 - \sum_i r_i^2/g_i \right) \right. \\ &+ \left. \sum_i \ln g_i - N \ln \widetilde{d} - (N_T - N)\ln(1 - \rho^2) \right\}, \end{aligned} \tag{4.121}$$

where $\tilde{d} = (1 - \rho^2)/d$ and

$$g_i = \tilde{d} + n_i + \rho^2(n_i - 2) - 2\rho(n_i - 1),$$

$$r_i = \sum_{j=1}^{n_i} e_{ij} + \rho^2 \sum_{j=2}^{n_i-1} e_{ij} - 2\rho \left(2 \sum_{j=2}^{n_i-1} e_{ij} + e_{i1} + e_{i,n_i} \right),$$

$$s_0 = \sum_{j=1}^{n_i} e_{ij}^2, \; s_1 = \sum_{j=2}^{n_i-1} e_{ij}^2, \; s_2 = 2 \sum_{j=1}^{n_i-1} e_{ij}e_{i,j+1}.$$

Example: *growth curve analysis, Potthoff and Roy (1964) data*. This is classical dental growth curve data (see Figure 4.3). As the reader can see, each person has his/her own intercept. Also, boys have a greater distance, which should be taken into account when building the growth model for the combined data. It would be reasonable to accept that there is autocorrelation since we are dealing with time series observations. Since measurements were made at the same time, we have balanced data. An adequate model for these data would be

$$y_{ij} = \alpha + \gamma_1 sex_i + \gamma_2 t_j + b_i + \varepsilon_{ij}, \; i = 1, ..., 27, \; j = 1, 2, 3, 4, \tag{4.122}$$

$t_1 = 8, t_2 = 10, t_3 = 12, t_4 = 14$, where the variance of the random intercept is $\text{var}(b_i) = \sigma^2 d$ and the errors follow an AR(1) model, $\varepsilon_{ij} = \rho \varepsilon_{i,j-1} + \zeta_{ij}$. To find the maximum likelihood estimate, we can use either expression (4.121) or standard software, such as R/S+ or SAS (procedure `mixed`).

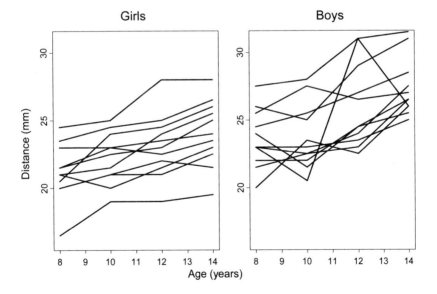

FIGURE 4.3. Distance from the center of the pituitary to the pteryomaxillary fissure for girls and boys (dental growth). Apparently, each person has his/her own intercept and boys are higher. The individual slopes look similar. (Data are from Potthoff and Roy, 1964; see the file `PRdistance.txt`.)

Below we show the R function that estimates the relationship between the distance and kid's age adjusted for sex using the `lme` function with correlation structure AR(1).

```
PRdistance=function()
{
dump("PRdistance", "c:\\MixedModels\\Chapter04\\PRdistance.r")
library(nlme)
da=read.csv(file="c:\\MixedModels\\Chapter04\\PRdistance.txt")
oAR<-lme(fixed=y~ti+sex,random=~1|id,correlation=corAR1(),
         data=da,method="ML")
summary(oAR)
}
```

There are other `correlation` options listed in the `corClasses` function.

Table 4.1. Estimation of model (4.122) by maximum likelihood with and without autocorrelation

Model	Intercept	Slope	Sex	σ^2	d	ρ	l_{max}
ML	15.39	0.66	2.32	2.02	1.48	0	-217.43
SE	0.89	0.06	0.74	0.22			
ML AR(1)	15.39	0.66	2.32	2.07	1.43	0.044	-217.39
SE	0.90	0.06	0.74	0.24		0.18	

In Table 4.1 we present the results of estimation by maximum likelihood assuming that $\rho = 0$ (standard ML) and AR(1) with estimated ρ. As the reader can see, the LME model with autocorrelated residuals does not improve substantially because the autocorrelation parameter is not statistically significant. Since the standard LME model is a submodel (nested) of LME AR(1), we can apply the likelihood ratio test (`anova`) which gives the p-value 0.796. Thus, there is no indication that the growth data are autocorrelated.

The advantage of the profile log-likelihood function (4.121) is that it allows us to construct profile confidence intervals and regions, Section 3.4. For instance, the $(1 - \alpha)$ confidence region for (ρ, d) is the set

$$\left\{\rho, d \in R^2 : l_p(\rho, d) > l_{max} - \frac{1}{2}q_{1-\alpha, \chi^2(2)}\right\},$$

where $l_p(\rho, d)$ is (4.121) with $\boldsymbol{\beta}$ replaced by the GLS estimate given ρ, d, and $q_{1-\alpha, \chi^2(2)}$ is the $(1 - \alpha)$th quantile of the χ^2-distribution with 2 d.f. The 95% confidence region for ρ and d is shown in Figure 4.4, where $q_{0.95, \chi^2(2)} = 5.99$. This region goes beyond positive values of the variance of the random effect/intercept term, but only the positive part is shown.

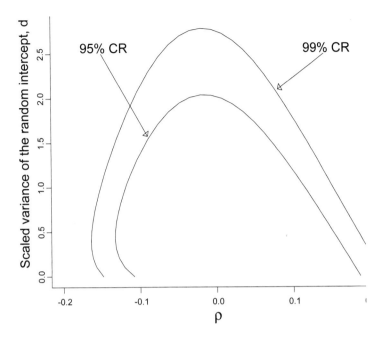

FIGURE 4.4. Ninety-five and 99% profile-likelihood confidence regions for (ρ, d) in a linear growth curve model with random intercept and AR(1) autocorrelated errors (the confidence region is shown for $d > 0$).

4.3.5 Multidimensional LME model

Sometimes we have data on several correlated dependent variables,and each of them follows the linear mixed effects model (2.5). Certainly, we can estimate/analyze these models individually, but it becomes problematic if they share fixed effects coefficients. Even if, in terms of parameters, the models seem to be independent, it would be difficult to accept that the dependent variables or random effects are independent when data come from the same subject/individual/cluster. Although separate estimation would lead to unbiased estimates, the efficiency, generally, would be lost. We prove the relevant statistical result of the advantage of multivariate pooling and illustrate the loss in Section 5.3, where the multivariate meta-analysis model is developed.

To fix the idea, we take our example with Weight and Height of Section 2.1. In addition to the height and weight of each family member, we have the shoe size:

F	H (inches)	W (pounds)	S (shoe size)
1	61	120	8.5
1	64	155	8.5
1	66	165	9.0
1	71	227	11.0
1	63	145	9.5
1	68	220	10.0
1	72	178	10.5

F	H (inches)	W (pounds)	S (shoe size)
$\ldots$	$\ldots$	$\ldots$	$\ldots$
19	66	120	10.0
19	71	220	10.5
19	66	134	9.5
19	68	130	10.00

Then it is reasonable to assume that we have two random-intercept models:

$$\mathbf{W}_i = \alpha_1 + \beta_1 \mathbf{H}_i + b_{i1} + \boldsymbol{\varepsilon}_{i1},$$
$$\mathbf{S}_i = \alpha_2 + \beta_2 \mathbf{H}_i + b_{i2} + \boldsymbol{\varepsilon}_{i2},$$

where $i = 1, ..., 19$ counts family; $\mathbf{W}_i$, $\mathbf{H}_i$, and $\mathbf{S}_i$ are $n_i \times 1$ vectors of weight, height and shoe size of the ith family; and $b_{i1} \sim \mathcal{N}(0, \sigma^2 d_1)$, $b_{i2} \sim \mathcal{N}(0, \sigma^2 d_2)$, $\boldsymbol{\varepsilon}_{i1} \sim \mathcal{N}(\mathbf{0}, \sigma^2 \mathbf{I})$, and $\boldsymbol{\varepsilon}_{i2} \sim \mathcal{N}(\mathbf{0}, \sigma^2 \mathbf{I})$. As we did earlier, we assume that pairs $b_{i1}, \boldsymbol{\varepsilon}_{i1}$ and $b_{i2}, \boldsymbol{\varepsilon}_{i2}$ within a family are independent. Several assumptions on the dependence of the random terms from the two models may be made.

1. The simplest assumption is that the two LME models are independent. In other words, all four random terms are independent. Intuition says that the two models can be analyzed/estimated separately without efficiency loss.

2. $\boldsymbol{\varepsilon}_{i1}$ and $\boldsymbol{\varepsilon}_{i2}$ are correlated but b_{i1} and b_{i2} are not. We can assume that for each family the correlation between the deviation from weight and foot size is the same. If we combine by stacking

$$\boldsymbol{\varepsilon}_i = \begin{bmatrix} \boldsymbol{\varepsilon}_{i1} \\ \boldsymbol{\varepsilon}_{i2} \end{bmatrix} \tag{4.123}$$

into a $2n_i \times 1$ vector, we can write $\operatorname{cov}(\boldsymbol{\varepsilon}_i) = \boldsymbol{\Omega} \otimes \mathbf{I}$, where

$$\boldsymbol{\Omega} = \begin{bmatrix} \omega_{11} & \omega_{12} \\ \omega_{12} & \omega_{22} \end{bmatrix} = \begin{bmatrix} \sigma_1^2 & \rho \sigma_1 \sigma_2 \\ \rho \sigma_1 \sigma_2 & \sigma_2^2 \end{bmatrix}$$

specifies the covariance matrix for the pair (weight, shoe size) and $\mathbf{I}$ is the $n_i \times n_i$ identity matrix.

3. $\boldsymbol{\varepsilon}_{i1}$ and $\boldsymbol{\varepsilon}_{i2}$ are correlated but b_{i1} and b_{i2} are correlated as well. Then in addition to the distribution specification for $\boldsymbol{\varepsilon}_i$ the pair $(b_{i1}, b_{i2})'$ has the two-dimensional normal distribution $\mathcal{N}(\mathbf{0}, \mathbf{D}_*)$, where $\mathbf{0}$ is the 2×1 null vector and

$$\mathbf{D} = \begin{bmatrix} d_{*11} & d_{*12} \\ d_{*12} & d_{*22} \end{bmatrix}.$$

Now we combine the two LME models into one, following the stacking rule (4.123):

$$\mathbf{y}_i = \begin{bmatrix} \mathbf{W}_i \\ \mathbf{S}_i \end{bmatrix}, \quad \mathbf{X}_i = \begin{bmatrix} \mathbf{1} & \mathbf{H}_i & \mathbf{0} & \mathbf{0} \\ \mathbf{0} & \mathbf{0} & \mathbf{1} & \mathbf{H}_i \end{bmatrix}, \quad \boldsymbol{\beta} = \begin{bmatrix} \alpha_1 \\ \beta_1 \\ \alpha_2 \\ \beta_2 \end{bmatrix},$$

$$\mathbf{Z}_i = \begin{bmatrix} \mathbf{1} & \mathbf{0} \\ \mathbf{0} & \mathbf{1} \end{bmatrix}, \quad \mathbf{b}_i = \begin{bmatrix} b_{i1} \\ b_{i2} \end{bmatrix}. \tag{4.124}$$

The combined LME model can be written in the familiar form $\mathbf{y}_i = \mathbf{X}_i\boldsymbol{\beta} + \mathbf{Z}_i\mathbf{b}_i + \boldsymbol{\varepsilon}_i$ with a two-dimensional random effect $\mathbf{b}_i \sim \mathcal{N}(\mathbf{0}, \mathbf{D}_*)$. Thus, we see that the only discrepancy from the standard LME model is the fact that $\boldsymbol{\varepsilon}_i$ has a special covariance structure; namely, $\text{cov}(\boldsymbol{\varepsilon}_i) = \boldsymbol{\Omega} \otimes \mathbf{I}$. In fact, we can combine any number of LME models, stacking the observations as in (4.124). The combined LME models may have common fixed coefficients, matrices $\mathbf{X}_i$ and $\mathbf{Z}_i$ may be arbitrary, and the vector of random effects $\mathbf{b}_i$ may have correlated components. A special case matrix $\mathbf{D}_*$ has a block diagonal form, as in case 2 above.

We showed that after stacking observation vectors, the multidimensional LME (MLME) model can be reduced to the model

$$\mathbf{y}_i = \mathbf{X}_i\boldsymbol{\beta} + \boldsymbol{\eta}_i, \quad \boldsymbol{\eta}_i \sim \mathcal{N}(\mathbf{0}, \boldsymbol{\Omega} \otimes \mathbf{I} + \mathbf{Z}_i\mathbf{D}_*\mathbf{Z}_i'), \quad i = 1, ..., N, \qquad (4.125)$$

with the log-likelihood function

$$l(\boldsymbol{\beta}, \boldsymbol{\Omega}, \mathbf{D}_*) = -\frac{1}{2}\sum[\ln|\boldsymbol{\Omega} \otimes \mathbf{I} + \mathbf{Z}_i\mathbf{D}_*\mathbf{Z}_i'| + \mathbf{e}_i'(\boldsymbol{\Omega} \otimes \mathbf{I} + \mathbf{Z}_i\mathbf{D}_*\mathbf{Z}_i')^{-1}\mathbf{e}_i],$$

where $\mathbf{e}_i = \mathbf{y}_i - \mathbf{X}_i\boldsymbol{\beta}$. Clearly, the Laird and Ware LME model (2.5) is a special case of (4.125) when $\boldsymbol{\Omega} = \sigma^2\mathbf{I}$.

Now we show that given $\boldsymbol{\Omega}$, the MLME model may be reduced to a standard LME model. Indeed, model (4.125) can be rewritten as $\mathbf{y}_i = \mathbf{X}_i\boldsymbol{\beta} + \mathbf{Z}_i\mathbf{b}_i + \boldsymbol{\varepsilon}_i$, where $\mathbf{b}_i \sim \mathcal{N}(\mathbf{0}, \mathbf{D}_*)$ and $\boldsymbol{\varepsilon}_i \sim \mathcal{N}(\mathbf{0}, \boldsymbol{\Omega} \otimes \mathbf{I})$. Let $\mathbf{T}$ be the Cholesky decomposition of matrix $\boldsymbol{\Omega}^{-1}$, i.e., $\mathbf{T}'\mathbf{T} = \boldsymbol{\Omega}^{-1}$. Multiplying both sides by $(\mathbf{T} \otimes \mathbf{I})$ and introducing new variables $\mathbf{y}_{Ti} = (\mathbf{T} \otimes \mathbf{I})\mathbf{y}_i$, $\mathbf{X}_{Ti} = (\mathbf{T} \otimes \mathbf{I})\mathbf{X}_i$, $\mathbf{Z}_{Ti} = (\mathbf{T} \otimes \mathbf{I})\mathbf{Z}_i$, and $\boldsymbol{\varepsilon}_{Ti} = (\mathbf{T} \otimes \mathbf{I})\boldsymbol{\varepsilon}_i$, we come to the standard LME model, $\mathbf{y}_{Ti} = \mathbf{X}_{Ti}\boldsymbol{\beta} + \mathbf{Z}_{Ti}\mathbf{b}_i + \boldsymbol{\varepsilon}_{Ti}$, where $\boldsymbol{\varepsilon}_{Ti} \sim \mathcal{N}(\mathbf{0}, \mathbf{I})$ because $\mathbf{T}\boldsymbol{\Omega}\mathbf{T}' = \mathbf{I}$. Consequently, if an estimate for $\boldsymbol{\Omega}$ is available we could estimate the MLME model by standard software. Such an estimate is developed below in a special case when all individual LME models have the same matrix of random effects.

The dimension-reduction formulas (4.116) and (4.117) apply, leading to the following likelihood simplification. Indeed, since $|\boldsymbol{\Omega} \otimes \mathbf{I}| = |\boldsymbol{\Omega}|$, we obtain

$$|\boldsymbol{\Omega} \otimes \mathbf{I} + \mathbf{Z}_i\mathbf{D}_*\mathbf{Z}_i'| = |\boldsymbol{\Omega}|\,|\mathbf{I} + \mathbf{D}\mathbf{Z}_i'(\boldsymbol{\Omega}^{-1} \otimes \mathbf{I})\mathbf{Z}_i'| = \frac{|\mathbf{I} + \mathbf{D}\mathbf{Z}_i'(\boldsymbol{\Omega}^{-1} \otimes \mathbf{I})\mathbf{Z}_i'|}{|\boldsymbol{\Omega}^{-1}|}$$

and

$$(\boldsymbol{\Omega} \otimes \mathbf{I} + \mathbf{Z}_i\mathbf{D}_*\mathbf{Z}_i')^{-1} = \boldsymbol{\Omega}^{-1} \otimes \mathbf{I} - (\boldsymbol{\Omega}^{-1} \otimes \mathbf{I})\mathbf{Z}_i\left(\mathbf{D}_*^{-1} + \mathbf{Z}_i'(\boldsymbol{\Omega}^{-1} \otimes \mathbf{I})\mathbf{Z}_i\right)^{-1}\mathbf{Z}_i'(\boldsymbol{\Omega}^{-1} \otimes \mathbf{I}).$$

Since both the determinant and the inverse matrix can be expressed in terms of the precision matrix $\boldsymbol{\Omega}^{-1}$, we may use reparameterization $\boldsymbol{\Omega}_* = \boldsymbol{\Omega}^{-1}$. Then the log-likelihood function for the MLME model takes the form

$$l(\boldsymbol{\beta}, \boldsymbol{\Omega}_*, \mathbf{D}_*) = -\frac{1}{2}\left\{-N\ln|\boldsymbol{\Omega}_*| + \sum_{i=1}^{N}[\ln|\mathbf{I} + \mathbf{D}\mathbf{Z}_i'(\boldsymbol{\Omega}_* \otimes \mathbf{I})\mathbf{Z}_i'|\right.$$
$$\left. + \mathbf{e}_i'[\boldsymbol{\Omega}_* \otimes \mathbf{I} - (\boldsymbol{\Omega}_* \otimes \mathbf{I})\mathbf{Z}_i\left(\mathbf{D}_*^{-1} + \mathbf{Z}_i'(\boldsymbol{\Omega}_* \otimes \mathbf{I})\mathbf{Z}_i\right)^{-1}\mathbf{Z}_i'(\boldsymbol{\Omega}_* \otimes \mathbf{I})]\mathbf{e}_i\right\}.$$

Furthermore, we can derive the precision matrix parameterization as in Section 2.2.4,

$$l(\boldsymbol{\beta}, \mathbf{D}_-, \boldsymbol{\Omega}_*) = -\frac{1}{2}\left\{-N\ln|\boldsymbol{\Omega}_*| - N\ln|\mathbf{D}_-| + \sum_{i=1}^{N}[\ln\left|\mathbf{D}_- + \mathbf{Z}_i'(\boldsymbol{\Omega}_* \otimes \mathbf{I})\mathbf{Z}_i'\right|\right.$$
$$\left. + \mathbf{e}_i'[\boldsymbol{\Omega}_* \otimes \mathbf{I} - (\boldsymbol{\Omega}_* \otimes \mathbf{I})\mathbf{Z}_i\left(\mathbf{D}_- + \mathbf{Z}_i'(\boldsymbol{\Omega}_* \otimes \mathbf{I})\mathbf{Z}_i\right)^{-1}\mathbf{Z}_i'(\boldsymbol{\Omega}_* \otimes \mathbf{I})]\mathbf{e}_i\right\}.$$

where $\mathbf{D}_- = \mathbf{D}_*^{-1}$.

To illustrate, we consider the important special case when P models with the same random effects design matrix are combined into the MLME model (4.125). Then $\mathbf{Z}_i = \mathbf{I} \otimes \widetilde{\mathbf{Z}}_i$, where $\mathbf{I}$ is a $P \times P$ identity matrix and $\widetilde{\mathbf{Z}}_i$ is an $n_i \times k$ common random effect design matrix and $\mathbf{Z}_i'(\boldsymbol{\Omega}_* \otimes \mathbf{I})\mathbf{Z}_i = \boldsymbol{\Omega}_* \otimes (\widetilde{\mathbf{Z}}_i'\widetilde{\mathbf{Z}}_i)$. Doing reparameterization $\widetilde{\mathbf{D}} = (\boldsymbol{\Omega}_*^{-1} \otimes \mathbf{I})\mathbf{D}_-$, we obtain

$$\mathbf{D}_- + \mathbf{Z}_i'(\boldsymbol{\Omega}_* \otimes \mathbf{I})\mathbf{Z}_i' = (\boldsymbol{\Omega}_* \otimes \mathbf{I})(\widetilde{\mathbf{D}} + \mathbf{I} \otimes (\widetilde{\mathbf{Z}}_i'\widetilde{\mathbf{Z}}_i)), \ \ln|\mathbf{D}_-| = \ln|\boldsymbol{\Omega}_*| + \ln\left|\widetilde{\mathbf{D}}\right|$$

and therefore as with the variance-profile parameterization, the log-likelihood function can be written as

$$l_p(\boldsymbol{\beta}, \widetilde{\mathbf{D}}, \boldsymbol{\Omega}_*) = -\frac{1}{2}\left\{-N\ln|\boldsymbol{\Omega}_*| - N\ln\left|\widetilde{\mathbf{D}}\right| + \sum_{i=1}^{N}[\ln\left|\widetilde{\mathbf{D}} + \mathbf{I} \otimes \widetilde{\mathbf{Z}}_i'\widetilde{\mathbf{Z}}_i\right|\right.$$
$$\left. + \mathbf{e}_i'[\boldsymbol{\Omega}_* \otimes \mathbf{I} - \widetilde{\mathbf{Z}}_i\left(\widetilde{\mathbf{D}} + \mathbf{I} \otimes (\widetilde{\mathbf{Z}}_i'\widetilde{\mathbf{Z}}_i)\right)^{-1}\widetilde{\mathbf{Z}}_i']\mathbf{e}_i\right\}.$$

Now we find the maximum of this function assuming that matrix $\widetilde{\mathbf{D}}$ and the $n_i P \times 1$ residual vectors $\{\mathbf{e}_i\}$ are known. Then the maximization problem is equivalent to minimization of $-N\ln|\boldsymbol{\Omega}_*| + \text{tr}(\boldsymbol{\Omega}_*\mathbf{S})$, where $\mathbf{S} = \sum \mathbf{E}_i'\mathbf{E}_i$ and $\mathbf{E}_i$ is the $n_i \times p$ matrix with the pth column as the $n_i \times 1$ residual vector from the pth LME model. Differentiating with respect to $\boldsymbol{\Omega}_*$, we come to $\widehat{\boldsymbol{\Omega}}_* = N^{-1}\mathbf{S}^{-1}$. Thus, alternating between estimation of the standard LME model and this estimator for $\boldsymbol{\Omega}_*$, we estimate the MLME model by maximum likelihood.

Problems for Section 4.3

1. Write down matrices $\mathbf{V}_{iq}$ for a linear mixed model $y_{ij} = a_i + b_i x_{ij} + \varepsilon_{ij}$ with independent random intercept and slope, $a_i \sim \mathcal{N}(\alpha, \sigma_a^2)$ and $b_i \sim \mathcal{N}(\beta, \sigma_b^2)$, $j = 1, 2, ..., n_i, i = 1, 2..., N$.

2. Show that ML and RML are asymptotically equivalent by demonstrating that the ln term in (4.105) is $o(N)$ when $N \to \infty$.

3. Prove that the information matrix (4.110) is positive definite if all the $\mathbf{V}_{iq}$ are positive definite, $\theta_q > 0$, and the $\{\mathbf{V}_{iq}\}$ are linearly independent.

4. Do the log-likelihood functions (4.104) and (4.105) go to $-\infty$ when for at least one i we have $|\mathbf{V}_i| \to 0$?

5*. Write an R function for maximization of log-likelihood functions (4.104) and (4.105) using the Fisher scoring algorithm by adopting lmeFS, discussed in Section 2.16. Test your code with model (2.142); the two functions should produce the same result.

6*. Write an R function that implements the variance least squares (biased and unbiased versions).

7*. Prove that VLS and UVLS from Section 4.3.2 are equivalent for LME to VLS and UVLS, respectively, from Sections 3.12.

8. Check the determinant and inverse of matrix $\mathbf{C} = \mathbf{I} + \rho\mathbf{T}_1$ using straightforward calculations for $n = 3$. Do the same for matrix $\mathbf{C}$ with AR(1) model.

9*. Write an R function that implements FS algorithm to maximize the log-likelihood given by equation (4.121). Alternate between $\boldsymbol{\beta}$ estimation via GLS and maximization of (4.121) with fixed e_{ij}. Test this code with model (4.122) using `distance` data.

10. Specify conditions under which the multidimensional LME model collapses to separate LME model estimation.

11*. Write an R function that maximizes the log-likelihood function in the precision matrix parametrization. Test the code through simulations.

4.4   Robust linear mixed effects model

Why the normal distribution? First, this distribution is computationally convenient because for the linear regression model, it leads to sum of squares minimization with a solution to a system of linear equations. Second, the Central Limit Theorem applies if the number of independent factors is large and no factor is dominant. Third, if the density of the error term, $f = f(u)$, has a maximum at zero, $(\ln f)_0' = 0$ and $(\ln f)_0'' < 0$, and expanding $\ln f$ around zero, one obtains $\ln f \simeq \ln f(0) + u(\ln f)_0' + \frac{1}{2}u^2(\ln f)_0'' = \ln f(0) + \frac{1}{2}u^2(\ln f)_0''$. So $\ln f$ may be approximated by a quadratic function that leads to the normal distribution. Thus, the normal distribution may be viewed as a second-order approximation to the original distribution.

However, in a small sample, there may be outliers with a profound effect on the estimate. Then why should the convenience of computation be the main argument, especially when computer power is increasing constantly? Clearly, robust estimation that assumes a non-Gaussian distribution with heavier tails can be an option.

A vast literature exists on robust statistics, the book by Huber (1981) arguably being the earliest classic reference. An easy introduction to robust regression may be found in the books by Montgomery and Peck (1992) and Birkes and Dodge (1993).

The easiest way to introduce robust statistics is through the problem of estimation of the location parameter. Let $y_1, y_2, ..., y_n$ be a random sample (iid) from a general population with the density $f(y - \theta)$, where θ is unknown. If f is the normal density, $f(u) = e^{-u^2/2}/\sqrt{2\pi}$, the standard answer is the average: A well-established theory says that $\overline{y}$ is the efficient unbiased estimator of θ (Lehmann and Casella, 1998). Generally, the maximum likelihood estimator for θ is found as a solution to the equation

$$\sum_{i=1}^{n} \psi(y_i - \theta) = 0, \tag{4.126}$$

where $\psi = f'$. If f is not known, we can use equation (4.126) to define implicitly the estimate for θ via the function ψ. Such an estimator is called the M-estimator, basic

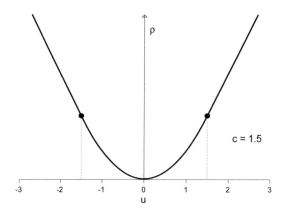

FIGURE 4.5. Huber's ρ function with $c = 1.5$. In the interval $(-c, c)$ this is a quadratic function; outside this interval, this is a linear function. The Huber function is smooth, i.e. the first derivative exists and is continuous.

asymptotic results of M-estimation are given in Appendix 13.1.4. Many functions ψ have been suggested to produce a robust estimate. The main idea is to choose $\psi = \psi(u)$ in such a way that for a small $|u|$ function, ψ is close to $|u|$, but for large $|u|$ function ψ is relatively small (the order is smaller than $|u|$). In particular, one of the first functions was suggested by Huber $(c > 0)$,

$$
\psi(u) = \left\{ \begin{array}{l} u \text{ if } |u| \le c \\ c \text{ if } u > c \\ -c \text{ if } u < c \end{array} \right. .
\tag{4.127}
$$

Equation (4.126) is equivalent to minimization of

$$
\sum_{i=1}^{n} \rho(y_i - \theta),
\tag{4.128}
$$

where the function ρ is defined as

$$
\rho(u) = \left\{ \begin{array}{l} \frac{1}{2}u^2 \text{ if } |u| \le c \\ c|u| - \frac{1}{2}c^2 \text{ if } |u| > c \end{array} \right. .
\tag{4.129}
$$

This function is called the Huber ρ-function with $c > 0$ as a parameter; see Figure 4.5. When $c \to \infty$, the M-estimator approaches $\bar{y}$. When $c \to 0$, the M-estimator approaches the median, a well known robust estimator of the location parameter. This statement comes from a well known result that the minimum of $\sum |y_i - \theta|$ is attained at the median. Thus, the M-estimator with an intermediate c might be a good compromise: in a neighborhood of zero it treats observations as if they come from a normal distribution and outside median-wise.

Equation (4.126) is usually solved by iteratively reweighted least squares (IRLS); see Green (1984) for an overview in the broader contest of generalized linear models. The idea of IRLS is to represent $\psi(y_i - \theta) = (y_i - \theta)w_i$, where $w_i = \psi(y_i - \theta)/(y_i - \theta)$. If $y_i - \theta = 0$, we set $w_i = \psi'(0)$. Then w_i plays the role of the weight, and the iterations take the form

$$\theta_{s+1} = \frac{\sum_{i=1}^{n} y_i w_{i,s}}{\sum_{i=1}^{n} w_{i,s}}, \quad s = 0, 1, ..., \tag{4.130}$$

where the weight $w_{i,s}$ changes from iteration to iteration. For the Huber function, $w_{i,s} = 1$ if $|y_i - \theta| \le c$ and $c/|y_i - \theta|$ elsewhere. Since ρ is a convex function (4.128) is also a convex function and thus there is a unique solution to (4.126). As a word of caution, equation (4.126) does not have a unique solution for all ψ. Demidenko (2000) develops criteria when a local solution that has been found is the global solution.

In the previous literature the threshold c was assumed fixed and known. Clearly, c is the key parameter of robust estimation. In particular, if c is large, we come to the standard normal theory. Although there are ways to come up with an *ad hoc* choice of c (Demidenko, 1981), a desirable solution would be to estimate c from the data. Also, a scale parameter σ should be part of the estimation method, as in standard normal distribution theory. We implement these ideas in the next section.

4.4.1 Robust estimation of the location parameter with estimated σ and c

We estimate c and the scale parameter σ, along with θ, by the maximum likelihood (ML) method. Usually, σ is assessed before IRLS. For example, Montgomery and Peck (1992) use $\hat{\sigma} = \mathcal{M}|e_i - \mathcal{M}|/0.6745$, where $\mathcal{M}$ indicates the median. The problem with this approach is that the OLS residuals e_i may contain outliers, so that ideally, $\hat{\sigma}$ should be a part of the iterative estimation procedure.

Our aim is to find a distribution for which the maximum likelihood estimate for θ is defined as the minimizer of (4.128), where ρ is the Huber function (4.129). Clearly, the density must have the form $f(u) = e^{-\rho(u)}/A(c)$, where the coefficient $A = A(c) = \int_{-\infty}^{\infty} e^{-\rho(u)}$. This integral is elementary to find

$$\int_{-\infty}^{\infty} e^{-\rho(u)} du = 2 \left[\int_0^c e^{-\frac{1}{2}u^2} du + \int_c^{\infty} e^{-cu+\frac{1}{2}c^2} du \right]$$
$$= 2\sqrt{2\pi}[\Phi(c) + \phi(c)/c - 1/2],$$

where ϕ and Φ are the density and the cdf of the standard normal variable. This gives

$$A = 2\sqrt{2\pi}\left[\Phi(c) + \phi(c)/c - 1/2\right]. \tag{4.131}$$

The distribution function is given by

$$F(u) = \frac{1}{A} \begin{cases} \frac{1}{c}e^{\frac{1}{2}c(2u+c)} & \text{if } u < -c \\ \frac{1}{c}e^{-\frac{1}{2}c^2} + \sqrt{2\pi}[\Phi(u) - \Phi(-c)] & \text{if } |u| \le c \\ A - \frac{1}{c}e^{\frac{1}{2}c(-2u+c)} & \text{if } u > c. \end{cases} \tag{4.132}$$

We write $X \sim \mathcal{H}(c)$ if random variable X has this (Huber) distribution. Note that this distribution has heavy tails because when $u \to \infty$, the density approaches zero with the order e^{-cu}, whereas the normal density has the order $e^{-u^2/2}$. Apparently, when c goes to infinity this distribution converges to normal. The formula for the distribution function of $\mathcal{H}$ is useful for simulations because if U is uniformly distributed on $(0, 1)$, the random variable $F^{-1}(U)$ has $\mathcal{H}$, Huber distribution. The variance of the Huber distribution is

$$\frac{2}{A}\left(\int_0^c u^2 e^{-\frac{1}{2}u^2}\, du + \int_c^\infty u^2 e^{-cu+\frac{1}{2}c^2}\, du\right) = 1 + \frac{2(c^2+2)\phi}{c^2(2c\Phi+2\phi-c)}, \quad (4.133)$$

where in the rest of this section we let $\Phi = \Phi(c)$ and $\phi = \phi(c)$, to shorten the notation. Note that variance is a decreasing function of c, and when $c \to \infty$, the variance approaches 1. When c is fixed, the maximum likelihood estimator for θ is found from minimization of (4.128). Now we treat c as an unknown parameter and find it by ML. The model for robust estimation of the location parameter is

$$y_i = \theta + \sigma\varepsilon_i, \quad (4.134)$$

where σ is an unknown scale parameter and the density of iid ε_i is specified by (4.131), or $\varepsilon_i \sim \mathcal{H}(c)$. In the rest of this section we discuss computational issues of log-likelihood maximization.

The log-likelihood function is defined by

$$l(\theta, \sigma^2, c) \quad (4.135)$$
$$= -\left\{n\ln\sigma + n\ln\left[\Phi(c) + \phi(c)/c - 0.5\right] + \sum_{i=1}^n \rho\left(\frac{y_i - \theta}{\sigma}\right)\right\}.$$

When c and σ are held, we find θ via iterations (4.130). Now we find the Fisher information matrix and develop the Fisher scoring algorithm to find the MLEs for θ and σ. Letting $u_i = (y_i - \theta)/\sigma$, the standardized residual, we obtain

$$\frac{\partial l}{\partial c} = \frac{n\phi}{c^2\Phi + c\phi - 0.5c^2} - \sum_{|u_i|>c}(|u_i| - c), \quad (4.136)$$

$$\frac{\partial l}{\partial \sigma} = -\frac{n}{\sigma} + \frac{1}{\sigma}\left[\sum_{|u_i|\le c}u_i^2 + c\sum_{|u_i|>c}|u_i|\right], \quad (4.137)$$

where to shorten the notation we use $\phi = \phi(c)$ and $\Phi = \Phi(c)$. After some algebra we obtain the Fisher information,

$$I_c = \frac{4\phi(2c\Phi + \phi - c)}{c^2(2c\Phi + 2\phi - c)^2}, \quad I_{c\sigma} = -\frac{2\phi(1+c^2)}{(2c\Phi+2\phi-c)c\sigma},$$

$$I_\sigma = \frac{2}{\sigma^2}\left[1 - \frac{(1+c^2)\phi}{2c\Phi+2\phi-c}\right]. \quad (4.138)$$

Information about θ is

$$I_\theta = \frac{1}{\sigma^2}\Pr(|u| < c) = \frac{1}{\sigma^2}\left[1 - \frac{2\phi}{2\Phi c + 2\phi - c}\right]. \quad (4.139)$$

Combining all quantities, we come to 3×3 information matrix for (θ, c, σ):

$$\mathcal{I} = \begin{bmatrix} \frac{c}{\sigma^2}\frac{2\Phi-1}{2\Phi c+2\phi-c} & 0 & 0 \\ 0 & \frac{4\phi(2c\Phi+\phi-c)}{c^2(2c\Phi+2\phi-c)^2} & -\frac{2\phi(1+c^2)}{(2c\Phi+2\phi-c)c\sigma} \\ 0 & -\frac{2\phi(1+c^2)}{(2c\Phi+2\phi-c)c\sigma} & \frac{2}{\sigma^2}\left[1 - \frac{(1+c^2)\phi}{2c\Phi+2\phi-c}\right] \end{bmatrix}. \quad (4.140)$$

As the reader can see, the MLE for θ and (c, σ) are independent. Similar to the LME model, we can infer that (a) any consistent estimates of c and σ would lead to an asymptotically efficient estimate of θ, and (b) the likelihood may be maximized separately over θ and (c, σ). According to the general maximum likelihood theory, the distribution of the MLE is asymptotically normal with covariance matrix $n^{-1} \mathcal{I}^{-1}$. It is easy to prove that I_θ is an increasing function of c with $I_\theta(0) = 0$. Indeed, if we denote $\Psi = \Phi - 1/2$ ($\Psi' = \phi$), then I_θ is proportional to $\Psi/(\Psi + \phi/c)$ with derivative

$$\frac{d\Psi}{dc} = \frac{\phi(\Psi + \phi/c) - \Psi(\phi - \phi - \phi/c^2)}{(\Psi + \phi/c)^2} = \frac{\phi(\Psi + \phi/c) + \Psi\phi/c^2}{(\Psi + \phi/c)^2} > 0.$$

Also, when $c \to \infty$, we have $\Psi \to 1/2$ and $\phi/c \to 0$, so that $I_\theta \to 1/\sigma^2$. It means that when c is large, we come to the normal distribution with the variance for the mean as σ^2/n, the standard result. However, for $c > 0$ we lose precision, which may be interpreted as a trade-off with robustness. The asymptotic variance for the robust M-estimator of θ is

$$\mathrm{var}(\widehat{\theta}_{ML}) = \frac{1}{nI_\theta} = \frac{\sigma^2}{n}\left[1 + \frac{2\phi(c)}{c(2\Phi(c) - 1)}\right]. \qquad (4.141)$$

Note that when $c \to \infty$ we have $\Phi(c) \to 1$ and $\phi(c)/c \to 0$, so that $\mathrm{var}(\widehat{\theta}_{ML}) \to \sigma^2/n$, which was expected because when $c \to \infty$, the distribution approaches normal.

Why robust statistics?

Robust statistics copes with outliers. But how exactly do outliers affect estimation? Why does the MLE under the normal assumption deteriorate when the true distribution, in fact, is not normal and has heavy tails? We can illustrate the point by the location parameter model (4.126) with Huber distribution; see also Section 8.12. Indeed, if we assume that the $\{\varepsilon_i\}$ are normally distributed, the estimate for θ would be the least squares estimate (LSE), $\widehat{\theta}_{LS} = \overline{y}$, with the variance $\sigma^2\mathrm{var}(\varepsilon)/n$. If the true distribution function is (4.126), as follows from (4.133), we have the representation

$$\mathrm{var}(\widehat{\theta}_{LS}) = \frac{\sigma^2}{n}\left[1 + \frac{2(c^2 + 2)\phi(c)}{c^2(2c\Phi(c) + 2\phi(c) - c)}\right]. \qquad (4.142)$$

We compare this variance to the variance of the robust M-estimate, (4.141). Note that (4.142) is the exact variance of the LSE while (4.141) is the asymptotic variance. It is possible to prove that $\mathrm{var}(\widehat{\theta}_{LS}) > \mathrm{var}(\widehat{\theta}_{ML})$. We plot the two variances in Figure 4.6. The lower the c the less variance the M-estimate has relative to the least squares estimate. However, when $c > 2$, robust estimation does not improve the least squares.

Computational issues

To find the MLE, we use separate maximization of the log-likelihood function for θ and (c, σ). When c and σ are held, we can use either IRLS (4.130) or the FS

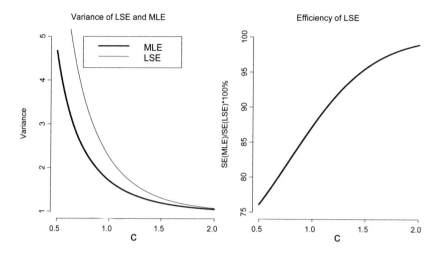

FIGURE 4.6. Comparison of least squares and the robust M-estimate of θ via asymptotic variances (4.142) and (4.141) assuming that $\sigma^2 = 1$ and $n = 1$. A heavy tail distribution such as $\mathcal{H}$ makes the LSE less efficient. For example, if $c = 1$, the standard error of the robust estimate is 86% of the standard error of the LSE. However, when c is sufficiently large ($c > 2$), the two estimators perform almost equally well.

algorithm with total information nI_θ. When θ is held, we use the FS algorithm:

$$\begin{bmatrix} c \\ \sigma \end{bmatrix}_{s+1} = \begin{bmatrix} c \\ \sigma \end{bmatrix}_s + \lambda_s \frac{1}{n} \begin{bmatrix} I_c & I_{c\sigma} \\ I_{c\sigma} & I_\sigma \end{bmatrix}_s^{-1} \begin{bmatrix} \frac{\partial l}{\partial c} \\ \frac{\partial l}{\partial \sigma} \end{bmatrix}_s, \tag{4.143}$$

where $s = 0, 1, \ldots$ is the iteration index and $0 < \lambda_s \le 1$ is the step length. The step length should provide positiveness of c and σ and the log-likelihood increase from iteration to iteration. A good starting point is to let $\sigma_0 = c_0 = \hat{\sigma}$, where $\hat{\sigma}$ is the median estimate presented at the beginning of the section. Only several iterations (two or three) may be sufficient, because we alternate the maximization over θ and (c, σ) until convergence.

4.4.2 Robust linear regression with estimated threshold

We can readily extend the location parameter model (4.134) to the linear regression model

$$y_i = \boldsymbol{\beta}' \mathbf{x}_i + \sigma \varepsilon_i, \tag{4.144}$$

where n vectors $\{\mathbf{x}_i, i = 1, \ldots, n\}$ have full rank and iid $\varepsilon_i \sim \mathcal{H}(c)$. The IRLS algorithm to estimate $\boldsymbol{\beta}$ when the threshold, c and SD, σ are held fixed takes the form

$$\boldsymbol{\beta}_{s+1} = \left(\sum_{i-1}^n w_{i,s} \mathbf{x}_i \mathbf{x}_i' \right)^{-1} \left(\sum_{i=1}^n y_i w_{i,s} \mathbf{x}_i \right),$$

where $w_{i,s} = 1$ if $\left| y_i - \boldsymbol{\beta}_s' \mathbf{x}_i \right| \le \sigma c$ and $\sigma c / \left| y_i - \boldsymbol{\beta}_s' \mathbf{x}_i \right|$ otherwise (as before, we set $w_{i,s} = 1$ if $y_i = \boldsymbol{\beta}_s' \mathbf{x}_i$). The derivatives (4.136) and (4.137) and the information matrices (4.138) do not change. As follows from (4.139),

$$\text{cov}(\widehat{\boldsymbol{\beta}}_{ML}) = \sigma^2 \left[1 + \frac{2\phi}{c(2\Phi - 1)} \right] \left(\sum_{i=1}^{n} \mathbf{x}_i \mathbf{x}_i' \right)^{-1}$$

in a large sample. Further computational detail on robust regression with known c is given by Huber (1981).

4.4.3 Robust LME model

Several authors have attempted to develop a robust theory for a mixed effects model. For example, Lange et al. (1989), and Pinheiro et al. (2001) take the t-distribution with few degrees of freedom as a distribution with heavy tails. The problem with this approach is that one needs to know the degrees of freedom, the key parameter, because if the degree-of-freedom value is large, the t-distribution is very close to normal. Gill (2000) uses the Huber function with known c. Huggins (1993) uses Tukey's bisquare function, which is constant outside a predefined interval. The problem with this approach is that one needs to know c. In our approach outlined below, the robustness parameter is estimated along with the parameters of interest.

We can write the LME model (2.5) as

$$\mathbf{y}_i = \mathbf{X}_i \boldsymbol{\beta} + \mathbf{Z}_i \mathbf{D}^{1/2} \mathbf{b}_i + \sigma \boldsymbol{\varepsilon}_i, \quad i = 1, 2, ..., N, \tag{4.145}$$

so that the components of the $n_i \times 1$ vector

$$\boldsymbol{\eta}_i = \frac{1}{\sigma} (\mathbf{I} + \mathbf{Z}_i \mathbf{D} \mathbf{Z}_i')^{-1/2} (\mathbf{y}_i - \mathbf{X}_i \boldsymbol{\beta})$$

are iid with the distribution $\mathcal{H}(c)$. Let u_{ij} denote the jth component of vector $(\mathbf{I} + \mathbf{Z}_i \mathbf{D} \mathbf{Z}_i')^{-1/2} (\mathbf{y}_i - \mathbf{X}_i \boldsymbol{\beta})$. Then the model (4.145) is rewritten as

$$\begin{aligned} l(\boldsymbol{\beta}, \sigma, \mathbf{D}, c) &= -N_T \left\{ \ln \left[\Phi(c) + \phi(c)/c - 1/2 \right] + \ln \sigma \right\} \\ &\quad - \sum_{i=1}^{N} \left\{ \frac{1}{2} \ln \left| \mathbf{I} + \mathbf{Z}_i \mathbf{D} \mathbf{Z}_i' \right| + \sum_{j=1}^{n_i} \rho \left(\frac{u_{ij}}{\sigma} \right) \right\}. \end{aligned} \tag{4.146}$$

When $c \to \infty$ we obtain the standard log-likelihood function (2.15). A separate maximization over $(\boldsymbol{\beta}, \mathbf{D})$ and (σ, c) may be used. When σ and c are held constant, we maximize l using the FS or IRLS algorithm, as indicated by Gill (2000). When $\boldsymbol{\beta}$ and $\mathbf{D}$ are held constant, we use the FS algorithm, similar to (4.143).

4.4.4 Alternative robust functions

Several alternatives to the Huber ρ function can be considered. Unfortunately, they require a numerical quadrature solution. If y has a symmetric distribution around zero, it makes sense to consider symmetric robust functions as well. For, example, instead of (4.129), one can take $\frac{1}{2} u^2/(1 + c|u|)$ or $\frac{1}{2} u^2/(1 + cu^2)$, where $c > 0$ (Demidenko, 2000). Like ρ, this function is close to quadratic when $|u|$ is small, but for large $|u|$ the function is proportional to $|u|$. Parameter c controls how close this function is to quadratic. Robust functions of different kinds have asymptotes when $|u|$ goes to infinity. For example, Tukey's bisquare function considered by Huggins (1993) in the framework of the LME model is given by

$$\rho_b = \frac{1}{6} \begin{cases} -b^2 \left[\left(1 - \left(\frac{x}{b}\right)^2\right)^3 - 1 \right] & \text{if } |x| \le b \\ b^2 \text{ elsewhere} \end{cases},$$

where b is a positive parameter. The censoring for robust functions with asymptotes is stronger because observations with an absolute value of residuals greater than b are not involved at all in the estimation procedure, as follows from the estimating equation.

4.4.5   Robust random effect model

In the work cited above, no distinction has been made between the distribution of the random effect $\mathbf{b}_i$ and the error term $\boldsymbol{\varepsilon}_i$. In fact, in many applications it is more probable to expect a cluster outlier rather than an outlier within a cluster. To address this phenomenon, we model the distribution of the error term as Gaussian and the distribution of the random effect as Huber. Then the problem of modeling of robust random effect reduces to the convolution of the Huber distribution $\mathcal{H}$ and the normal distribution $\mathcal{N}$. More precisely, given positive scale coefficients σ_1 and σ_2, we want to find the density of the random variable $Z = \sigma_1 X + \sigma_2 Y$, where $X \sim \mathcal{N}(0,1)$ and $Y \sim \mathcal{H}(c)$ are independent. It is well known that the density of Z is the convolution of densities of $\sigma_1 X$ and $\sigma_2 Y$ and is given by $\int_{-\infty}^{\infty} f_1(y) f_2(x-y) dy$ (Rice, 1995). Since the density of $\sigma_2 Y$ is given by $f_2(z) = (A\sigma_2)^{-1} \exp(-z^2/(2\sigma_2^2))$ if $|z| \le c\sigma_2$ and by $(A\sigma_2)^{-1} \exp(-c|z|/\sigma_2 + c^2/2)$ otherwise, the convolution is proportional to

$$\int_{|y-x| \le \sigma_2 c} e^{-\frac{1}{2}\left(\frac{y^2}{\sigma_1^2} + \frac{(y-x)^2}{\sigma_2^2}\right)} dy + \int_{|y-x| > \sigma_2 c} e^{-\frac{y^2}{2\sigma_1^2} - \frac{c|y-x|}{\sigma_2} + \frac{1}{2}c^2} dy$$

with the coefficient reciprocal of $A\sigma_1\sigma_2\sqrt{2\pi}$. It is possible to express this integral via functions Φ and ϕ to obtain the log-likelihood function for the robust MLE, although we do not pursue this approach here.

Problems for Section 4.4

1. Prove that the IRLS algorithm converges to the median in a simple model $y_i - \theta \sim f(y)$, where f is the density of the double-exponential (Laplace) distribution.

2*. Write an R function that estimates a linear model using Huber loss function (4.129) with c as a parameter. Test your code using simulations. Compare properties of the robust estimation versus LS estimation, estimating the probability $\Pr(|\widehat{\beta} - \beta| < \delta)$ as a function of δ using simulations.

3*. Write an R function that finds the MLE of θ for model (4.134) when c is fixed.

4*. Write an R function that finds the MLE of θ for model (4.134) using the FS algorithm, when c is unknown and is subject to estimation.

5*. Using the Fisher information matrix, compare asymptotic variances of $\widehat{\theta}_{ML}$ when c is fixed and known versus when c is estimated. Plot these variances as a function of c (reproduce Figure 4.6). Prove that the variance is larger when c is unknown.

6. How can separate log-likelihood maximization for θ and (c, σ) be justified?

7*. Write an R function that estimates a robust linear regression (4.144) with the Huber function by modifying the code in problem 4.

8*. Write an R function that estimates a robust LME model by maximizing the log-likelihood function (4.146) using algorithm alternation as suggested. Test the properties of robust estimation via simulation for a sequence of c.

9*. Develop robust random effect model estimation as discussed in the last section.

4.5 Appendix: derivation of the MM estimator

The aim of this section is to derive the Method of Moments (MM) estimator for matrix $\mathbf{B}_* = \mathbf{C}\mathbf{D}_*\mathbf{C}'$ in the general linear growth curve model of Section 4.2.5. The proof follows that of a paper by Demidenko and Stukel (2002).

Following the general idea of Henderson (1953), we find an estimator for the variance parameter by equating the empirical sum of squares to its expectation. Let $\mathbf{u}_i = \mathbf{C}\mathbf{a}_i^0 - \mathbf{A}_i\boldsymbol{\beta} = \mathbf{C}(\mathbf{Z}_i'\mathbf{Z}_i)^{-1}\mathbf{Z}_i'\boldsymbol{\zeta}_i$, where $\boldsymbol{\beta}$ is the true parameter vector and $\boldsymbol{\zeta}_i$ is an $n_i \times 1$ random vector with zero mean and covariance matrix $\sigma^2\mathbf{I} + \mathbf{Z}_i\mathbf{D}_*\mathbf{Z}_i'$. Then the $\{\mathbf{u}_i\}$ are independent and $\text{cov}(\mathbf{u}_i) = \sigma^2\mathbf{P}_i + \mathbf{B}_*$, where $\mathbf{P}_i = \mathbf{C}(\mathbf{Z}_i'\mathbf{Z}_i)^{-1}\mathbf{C}'$. Matrix (4.87) can be rewritten as

$$\sum_i \mathbf{u}_i\mathbf{u}_i' - \sum_i \mathbf{u}_i(\sum_j \mathbf{u}_j'\mathbf{A}_j)\mathbf{H}\mathbf{A}_i' - \sum_i \mathbf{A}_i\mathbf{H}(\sum_j \mathbf{A}_j'\mathbf{u}_j)\mathbf{u}_i'$$
$$+ \sum_i \mathbf{A}_i\mathbf{H}(\sum_j \mathbf{A}_j'\mathbf{u}_j)(\sum_j \mathbf{u}_j'\mathbf{A}_j)\mathbf{H}\mathbf{A}_i',$$

where $\mathbf{H} = (\sum \mathbf{A}_i'\mathbf{A}_i)^{-1}$. Our aim is to find its expectation. Since $\mathbf{u}_i$ and $\mathbf{u}_j$ are independent for $i \neq j$, we obtain

$$E\sum_i \mathbf{u}_i\mathbf{u}_i' = N\mathbf{B}_* + \sigma^2\sum \mathbf{P}_i,$$
$$E(\sum_i \mathbf{u}_i(\sum_j \mathbf{u}_j'\mathbf{A}_j)\mathbf{H}\mathbf{A}_i') = E(\sum_i \mathbf{u}_i\mathbf{u}_i'\mathbf{A}_i\mathbf{H}\mathbf{A}_i') = \sigma^2\sum_i \mathbf{P}_i\mathbf{Q}_i + \mathbf{B}_*\sum \mathbf{Q}_i,$$
$$E(\sum_i \mathbf{A}_i\mathbf{H}(\sum_j \mathbf{A}_j'\mathbf{u}_j)\mathbf{u}_i') = \sigma^2\sum_i \mathbf{Q}_i\mathbf{P}_i + \sum \mathbf{Q}_i\mathbf{B}_*,$$
$$E(\sum_i \mathbf{A}_i\mathbf{H}(\sum_j \mathbf{A}_j'\mathbf{u}_j)(\sum_j \mathbf{u}_j'\mathbf{A}_j)\mathbf{H}\mathbf{A}_i') = E(\sum_i \mathbf{A}_i\mathbf{H}\mathbf{A}_i'\mathbf{u}_i\mathbf{u}_i'\mathbf{A}_i\mathbf{H}\mathbf{A}_i')$$
$$= \sigma^2\sum \mathbf{Q}_i\mathbf{P}_i\mathbf{Q}_i + \sum \mathbf{Q}_i\mathbf{B}_*\mathbf{Q}_i.$$

By definition, $\widehat{\mathbf{B}}_*$ is the solution to the matrix equation

$$N\mathbf{B}_* - \mathbf{B}_*\sum \mathbf{Q}_i - \sum \mathbf{Q}_i\mathbf{B}_* + \sum \mathbf{Q}_i\mathbf{B}_*\mathbf{Q}_i = \mathbf{L}, \qquad (4.147)$$

where σ^2 is replaced by the pooled variance (4.23) and is denoted $\mathbf{L} = \widehat{\mathbf{S}}_0 - \widehat{\sigma}_{MM}^2[\mathbf{P}_i - \mathbf{P}_i\mathbf{Q}_i - \mathbf{Q}_i\mathbf{P}_i + \mathbf{Q}_i\mathbf{P}_i\mathbf{Q}_i]$. To solve (4.147) for $\mathbf{B}$, we employ the vec operator and the formula $\text{vec}(\mathbf{A}\mathbf{B}\mathbf{F}) = (\mathbf{F}' \otimes \mathbf{A})\text{vec}(\mathbf{B})$, which yields (4.88). To be valid, we need to show that the matrix $\mathbf{J}$ in (4.88) is nonsingular. We show that this is true if $2r < N$. Indeed, let $\mathbf{U}$ be any $r \times r$ matrix. Without loss of generality we can assume that it is normalized, i.e., $\text{tr}(\mathbf{U}'\mathbf{U}) = 1$. It suffices to show that

$$\text{vec}'(\mathbf{U})\left[\mathbf{I}_{r^2} - \frac{1}{N}\sum_{i=1}^{N}(\mathbf{Q}_i \otimes \mathbf{I}_r + \mathbf{I}_r \otimes \mathbf{Q}_i - \mathbf{Q}_i \otimes \mathbf{Q}_i')\right]\text{vec}(\mathbf{U}) > 0. \qquad (4.148)$$

Using the formula $\text{vec}'(\mathbf{U})(\mathbf{A} \otimes \mathbf{B})\text{vec}(\mathbf{U}) = \text{tr}(\mathbf{U}\mathbf{A}\mathbf{U}'\mathbf{B}')$ and applying the inequality $\text{tr}(\mathbf{A}\mathbf{B}) \leq \text{tr}(\mathbf{A})\text{tr}(\mathbf{B})$ for any nonnegative definite matrices $\mathbf{A}$ and $\mathbf{B}$, one obtains

$$\frac{1}{N}(\text{vec}'(\mathbf{U})\left(\sum_i \mathbf{Q}_i \otimes \mathbf{I}\right)\text{vec}(\mathbf{U}) = \frac{1}{N}(\text{vec}'(\mathbf{U})\left(\sum_i \mathbf{Q}_i \otimes \mathbf{I}\right)\text{vec}(\mathbf{U})$$
$$= \frac{1}{N}\sum_i \text{tr}(\mathbf{U}\mathbf{Q}_i\mathbf{U}') = \frac{1}{N}\sum_i \text{tr}(\mathbf{Q}_i\mathbf{U}'\mathbf{U}) \leq \frac{1}{N}\sum_i \text{tr}(\mathbf{Q}_i)$$
$$= \frac{1}{N}\sum_i \text{tr}(\mathbf{A}_i\mathbf{H}\mathbf{A}_i') = \frac{1}{N}\sum_i \text{tr}(\mathbf{H}\sum \mathbf{A}_i'\mathbf{A}_i) = \frac{r}{N}.$$

Since $\text{vec}'(\mathbf{U})(\mathbf{Q}_i \otimes \mathbf{Q}_i)\text{vec}(\mathbf{U}) \geq 0$, the left-hand side of the inequality (4.148) is greater than $1 - 2r/N$. Therefore, if $2r < N$, the matrix $\mathbf{J}$ is nonsingular.

4.6   Summary points

- The linear growth curve model is a special case of the standard Laird and Ware LME model where the matrix of fixed effects can be represented as a linear combination of the columns of the matrix of random effects. A special case of the linear growth curve model is the random-coefficient model. All numerical algorithms and statistical properties of the LME model discussed in Chapters 2 and 3 apply to the linear growth curve model.

- The general least squares estimator for the linear growth curve model may be computed in two steps: In the first step, individual data are processed separately to obtain ordinary least squares estimates; in the second step, the weighted least squares is applied to the OLS estimates from the first step.

- The log-likelihood function for the growth curve model may be simplified using dimension-reduction formulas. One can apply the Newton–Raphson or Fisher scoring algorithms to maximize the function.

- The MINQU estimator of σ^2 developed for the LME model in Chapter 3 coincides with the method of moments (MM) estimator for the linear growth curve model, the pooled variance estimator.

- Two method of moments unbiased estimators for the covariance matrix of random effects are developed with regard to two extreme cases of matrix $\mathbf{D}$, the scaled covariance matrix of random effects. The first one uses the least squares estimator applied to all data ($\mathbf{D} = \mathbf{0}$), and the second uses the least squares applied to the second-stage model ($\mathbf{D} = \infty$), as in the fixed effects approach. A simplified version of the MM estimator has a clear variance decomposition interpretation.

- In some special growth curve models the estimates are simplified. We call a growth curve rectangular if all coefficients in the second stage are expressed via the same set of covariates, so the second-stage model may be written in a matrix (rectangular) form. It is shown that for a rectangular growth curve the fixed effects approach estimator coincides with the estimator suggested by Reinsel (1985).

- The balanced growth curve model is the rectangular growth curve with the same matrix in the first-stage model. Then generalized and ordinary least squares estimators coincide. For this model, the method of moments and restricted maximum likelihood estimates coincide.

- Likelihood-based and two-stage estimators for beta coefficients are unbiased in small samples and are asymptotically equivalent in large samples: when the number of people tends to infinity and the number of observations per person remains bounded.

- Often only some of the growth curve coefficients or, generally, some linear combinations of coefficients are of interest. A standard setting of the linear growth curve model forces us to model all coefficients. On the contrary, the general growth curve model does not require specification of all parameters and leaves the unspecified parameters free.

- The general growth curve model may be estimated by the maximum likelihood method. Two versions of log-likelihood are available: full and second stage maximum likelihood. For the second-stage maximization, one can use the Newton–Raphson or fixed-point algorithm. The method of moments is generalized to the general linear growth curve model.

- The general growth curve model is robust to misspecification of the second-stage model. The standard linear growth curve model does not include this feature. In particular, population parameters are systematically biased when the second-stage model is misspecified. Models under the general growth curve setting lose some efficiency but retain parameter unbiasedness.

- Many covariance structures may be well specified by a linear combination of fixed matrices with coefficients as parameters (to be estimated from the data). This class of linear models was developed by T.W. Anderson. For example, the covariance matrix in the LME model may be represented as a linear combination with coefficients as unique elements of matrix $\mathbf{D}$. The Hessian matrix for variance/covariance parameters takes a simple form with elements as traces of certain matrices. Thus, implementation of the Fisher scoring algorithm seems relevant.

- Variance and unbiased variance least squares is extended to LMLCS. The estimates for beta coefficients are unbiased because the estimate of the covariance matrix is an even function of the error term.

- Although many authors suggest the standard LME model (2.5) for longitudinal data analysis, this requires one to account for serial correlation to model the data adequately. The covariance matrix generated by the moving average can be represented by a linear covariance structure, and therefore the analysis of longitudinal data can be performed under the umbrella of linear models with linear covariance structure. The log-likelihood function for the autoregression error term in the LME model can be well simplified and allows fast profile confidence region/interval construction.

- Another example of LMLCS is the multidimensional mixed model when several correlated dependent variables are available and each of them follows the

LME model. Each model can be studied/estimated separately, but simultaneous estimation gains efficiency. If each model has the same set of random effects covariates, maximum likelihood estimation of multidimensional LME can be accomplished with standard LME software.

- A compromise between the least squares estimate (average) and the median can be achieved using the Huber ρ-function, which is quadratic within the interval $(-c, c)$ and linear elsewhere. In previous work the threshold c, the key parameter of robust estimation, was assumed known. We estimate c by maximum likelihood along with the location (θ) and scale (σ) parameters introducing a distribution $\mathcal{H}$, which yields the standard estimate of θ when c is fixed. The robust regression techniques may be extended to mixed models. We estimate parameters of the model along with the threshold c by maximum likelihood. In many applications one may expect cluster outliers that may be modeled via a convolution of the Huber and normal distribution.

5
Meta-analysis Model

The meta-analysis model is probably the simplest random effects model, yet it has important applications for pooling studies, especially in medicine and epidemiology. Thus, to be specific, we talk about the common treatment effect that synthesizes the results of several studies. There exist an enormous number of papers on application of the meta-analysis model. However, fewer papers cover statistical issues of the model; DerSimonian and Laird (1986), Whitehead and Whitehead (1991), Berkey et al. (1995), Hardy and Thompson (1998), Aitken (1999), and Brockwell and Gordon (2001). The strength of the meta-analysis model is that we do not care how the estimate of the study-specific treatment effect in each study has been obtained unless the estimate and its variance are available. For example, in one study, Cox logistic regression may be used, in another study the characteristic of interest might be adjusted for the patient's age, etc. Usually, the sample size in each study is fairly large, so the Central Limit Theorem applies. Thus, the estimate from each study should have a distribution close to normal. However, the distribution of the random effect may not be normal and. particularly, may have heavy tails. We develop a theory for robust/median meta-analysis assuming that the random effect has double-exponential (Laplace) distribution.

The key parameter of the meta-analysis model is the variance of the random effect σ^2, which reflects the variation between studies. Fortunately, a homogeneity test is available with an exact confidence level, the Q-test. Generally, there are two approaches to estimating σ^2: maximum likelihood, which assumes normal distribution, and quadratic unbiased estimation.

This chapter comprises three sections. In the first section a simple meta-analysis model is considered where likelihood and quadratic unbiased estimation methods are described at length. In the second section we consider the meta-analysis model with study-specific covariates to adjust the common treatment effect. In the third section a general multivariate meta-analysis model is introduced. Some efficiency may be gained if the treatment effect is observed along with other, correlated estimates.

5.1 Simple meta-analysis model

In the meta-analysis model it is assumed that each study $i = 1, ..., n$ provides a value (estimate) of the characteristic of interest y_i along with its variance σ_i^2. For example, a new surgical operation has been tested in n hospitals on a different number of patients and the treatment effect y_i; for example, as the coefficient of a logistic regression model. How can we combine studies and come up with an overall (common) treatment effect? A naive approach would be to take simple average $\bar{y}$ but then we do not take into account that in different studies y_i has different precision (SE) because of the difference in the number of patients involved. A better approach is to take a weighted average with weights equal to the reciprocal of the variances. However, a risk is that if the variance in one study is close to zero, the resulting estimate will be determined only by that study. The meta-analysis model based on the random effect approach provides something of a compromise assuming that the studies are heterogeneous, i.e., there is a random effect.

In the meta-analysis model, y_i is treated as an observation and the within-study variance σ_i^2 is treated as a fixed (given) number. Following the line of the random effect approach, it is assumed that besides the variation within the study, there exists a variation between studies, and this variation is represented by the random effect b_i with an unknown variance σ^2. Clearly, without variation between studies the best estimator would be the weighted average, $(\sum y_i/\sigma_i^2)/(\sum 1/\sigma_i^2)$. Since σ^2 is unknown, we need to estimate it first and then apply the weighted average. A hypothetical situation with and without extra variation between studies (heterogeneity) is depicted in Figure 5.1. Characteristically, if σ^2 is considerable, there is little or no overlap among the 95% confidence intervals.

The simplest meta-analysis model has no covariates and is written as

$$y_i = \beta + b_i + \varepsilon_i, \tag{5.1}$$

where b_i is a random effect with unknown variance σ^2 and ε_i is an error term with known positive variance σ_i^2. In the next section we consider a more general model where in addition to the intercept term, there are explanatory variables/covariates. The random terms have zero means and are independent across studies $i = 1, ..., n$. If b_i and ε_i have normal distribution, the meta-analysis model (5.1) can be written as

$$y_i \sim \mathcal{N}(\beta, \sigma^2 + \sigma_i^2), \qquad i = 1, ..., n. \tag{5.2}$$

Strictly speaking, the meta-analysis model (5.1) is not a special case of the linear mixed effects model (2.5) because the $\{\sigma_i^2\}$ are known. However, as we shall learn, the model (5.1) shares many properties with the LME model, and we will consistently refer the reader to our previous theory.

To be specific, hereafter the y_i will be called study-specific treatments, β will be called the common treatment effect, and the variance of the random effect σ^2 will be called the heterogeneity (variance) parameter. The flexibility of the meta-analysis

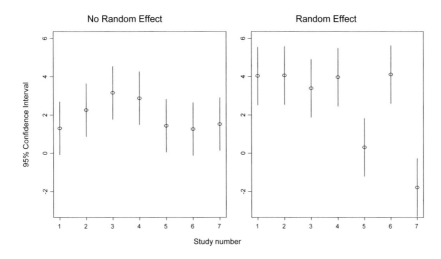

FIGURE 5.1. Two hypothetical situations in the meta-analysis model. Left: There is no random effect (studies are homogeneous) and the 95% CI overlap. Right: Studies are hetero-geneous because there is an extra variation among studies and the CI do not overlap—the meta-analysis model is valid.

model comes from the fact that we do not specify how y_i and its variance σ_i^2 have been calculated. In particular, different study-specific statistical models could be used, with different (study-specific) adjustments, confounders, and so on.

The heterogeneity variance is the key parameter in the meta-analysis model. Indeed, as follows from the Gauss–Markov theorem, if the variance of the random effect were known, the weighted average

$$\widehat{\beta} = \frac{\sum_{i=1}^n y_i(\sigma^2 + \sigma_i^2)^{-1}}{\sum_{i=1}^n (\sigma^2 + \sigma_i^2)^{-1}} \tag{5.3}$$

would be unbiased with minimum variance among all linear unbiased estimators,

$$\mathrm{var}(\widehat{\beta}) = \frac{1}{\sum_{i=1}^n (\sigma^2 + \sigma_i^2)^{-1}}. \tag{5.4}$$

Also, we know that if the $\{y_i\}$ had normal distribution, $\widehat{\beta}$ would have the minimum variance among *all* (linear and nonlinear) unbiased estimators, as follows from the Cramér–Rao inequality (Rao, 1973; Bickel and Doksum, 2001). It is interesting to note that for any σ^2, the weighted least squares estimate (5.3) lies in the range $(\min y_i, \max y_i)$. In practice we never know σ^2, so that (5.3) will be used with $\widehat{\sigma}^2$ in place of σ^2. Then we call that estimator the estimated weighted least squares estimator.

Two extreme cases of σ^2 are important in formula (5.3). When $\sigma^2 = 0$ we come to the weighted least squares estimator,

$$\widehat{\beta}_0 = \widehat{\beta}\Big|_{\sigma^2=0} = \frac{\sum y_i/\sigma_i^2}{\sum 1/\sigma_i^2}. \tag{5.5}$$

When the variance of the random effect becomes large, we approach the simple average,

$$\widehat{\beta}_{OLS} = \widehat{\beta}\Big|_{\sigma^2=\infty} = \lim_{\sigma^2\to\infty} \frac{\sum y_i(\sigma^2 + \sigma_i^2)^{-1}}{\sum(\sigma^2 + \sigma_i^2)^{-1}} = \frac{1}{n}\sum y_i = \overline{y}. \tag{5.6}$$

In the balanced case, when all within-study variances are the same ($\sigma_i^2 = $const), the estimator (5.3) does not depend on σ^2 and collapses to the simple average $\overline{y}$. A similar phenomenon was observed earlier for the balanced growth curve model, see Section 4.1.5. It is easy to see that both estimators are unbiased regardless of σ^2. In the rest of the chapter we deal with the meta-analysis model under unknown heterogeneity variance σ^2.

5.1.1   Estimation of random effects

The random effects or better stated the cluster-specific deviations can be 'estimated' in the framework of a mixed model. In Section 3.7, we provide the general theory and respective formulas. In this section we apply that theory to the meta-analysis model with the goal to estimate random effects b_i. The difference with the general linear mixed model is that the y_i are heterogeneous even in the absence of the random effect (due to presence of σ_i^2) but this fact changes the theory just slightly.

In the notation of Section 3.7 we have $\mathbf{X}_i = \mathbf{Z}_i = 1$ and $\mathbf{D} = \sigma^2$, so that the penalized sum of squares, as the counterpart of (3.54), takes the form

$$S = \sum_{i=1}^{n} \frac{(y_i - \beta - b_i)^2}{\sigma_i^2} + \frac{1}{\sigma^2}\sum_{i=1}^{n} b_i^2, \tag{5.7}$$

where b_i is the estimate of the random effect sought for study i. It is easy to verify that minimization of S over μ and $\{b_1, ..., b_n\}$, with fixed σ^2, leads to $\widehat{\beta}$ given by (5.3) and random effects estimates given by

$$\widehat{b}_i = \frac{\sigma^2}{\sigma^2 + \sigma_i^2}(y_i - \widehat{\beta}) \tag{5.8}$$

with the minimum

$$\min S = \sum_{i=1}^{n} \frac{(y_i - \widehat{\beta})^2}{\sigma^2 + \sigma_i^2}. \tag{5.9}$$

When the heterogeneity variance, σ^2, is large, the random effects estimates are close to the deviation of the data from the mean; when σ^2 is close to zero, the estimates, $\widehat{b}_i$, are close to zero as well. We employ these estimates in Section 5.1.6 for the random effect coefficient of determination and illustrate them with an example.

5.1.2   Maximum likelihood estimation

Here it is assumed that random variables have a normal distribution, so that the model under consideration is (5.2) with the log-likelihood function (up to a constant term)

$$l(\beta, \sigma^2) = -\frac{1}{2}\sum_{i=1}^{n}\left[\ln(\sigma^2 + \sigma_i^2) + \frac{(y_i - \beta)^2}{\sigma^2 + \sigma_i^2}\right]. \tag{5.10}$$

For a balanced model, $\sigma_i^2 = \sigma_1^2 =$const, the maximum of this log-likelihood function admits a closed-form solution

$$\widehat{\beta} = \overline{y}, \quad \widehat{\sigma}^2 = \frac{1}{n}\sum(y_i - \overline{y})^2 - \sigma_1^2. \tag{5.11}$$

If σ^2 is known, l attains a maximum at (5.3); and if $\sigma_i^2 \neq$const, we have to use an iterative algorithm to find the maximum of l. To maximize this function, we need the first and second derivatives:

$$\frac{\partial l}{\partial \beta} = \sum_{i=1}^{n} \frac{y_i - \beta}{\sigma^2 + \sigma_i^2}, \quad \frac{\partial l}{\partial \sigma^2} = -\frac{1}{2}\sum_{i=1}^{n}\left[\frac{1}{\sigma^2 + \sigma_i^2} - \frac{(y_i - \beta)^2}{(\sigma^2 + \sigma_i^2)^2}\right],$$

$$\frac{\partial^2 l}{\partial \beta^2} = -\sum_{i=1}^{n}\frac{1}{\sigma^2 + \sigma_i^2}, \quad \frac{\partial^2 l}{\partial \beta \partial \sigma^2} = -\sum_{i=1}^{n}\frac{y_i - \beta}{(\sigma^2 + \sigma_i^2)^2},$$

$$\frac{\partial^2 l}{\partial \sigma^4} = \frac{1}{2}\sum_{i=1}^{n}\left[\frac{1}{(\sigma^2 + \sigma_i^2)^2} - \frac{2(y_i - \beta)^2}{(\sigma^2 + \sigma_i^2)^3}\right].$$

The Hessian matrix for l is the 2×2 matrix

$$\mathbf{H} = -\begin{bmatrix} \sum_{i=1}^{n}\frac{1}{\sigma^2+\sigma_i^2} & \sum_{i=1}^{n}\frac{y_i-\beta}{(\sigma^2+\sigma_i^2)^2} \\ \sum_{i=1}^{n}\frac{y_i-\beta}{(\sigma^2+\sigma_i^2)^2} & \frac{1}{2}\sum_{i=1}^{n}\left[\frac{2(y_i-\beta)^2}{(\sigma^2+\sigma_i^2)^3} - \frac{1}{(\sigma^2+\sigma_i^2)^2}\right] \end{bmatrix}.$$

As we see, the log-likelihood function (5.10) is not a concave function of (β, σ^2) because the $(2,2)$th element of matrix $\mathbf{H}$ may be positive. This means that the Newton–Raphson algorithm may fail if the starting point is far from the maximum. As a word of caution, the log-likelihood function (5.10) may have several local maxima. Indeed, substituting (5.3) into $\partial l/\partial \sigma^2 = 0$, we come to an equivalent equation for σ^2. Getting rid of the denominators, one can show that the latter equation is equivalent to a polynomial of σ^2, which may have several roots.

Another comment pertains to the domain of maximization. Following the idea of Section 2.15.2, we could maximize l over its entire domain, which is $\sigma^2 > -\min\sigma_i^2$, and then after maximization is complete, take $\max(0, \widehat{\sigma}^2)$, where $\widehat{\sigma}^2$ is the point of its absolute maximum, but this does not work for function (5.10). Indeed, without loss of generality (after re-indexing) we can assume that $\sigma_1^2 \leq \sigma_2^2 \leq \ldots \leq \sigma_n^2$. Let $\sigma_1^2 = \min\sigma_i^2 < \sigma_2^2$, so that the domain of l is $\{\beta \in R^1\} \times \{\sigma^2 > -\sigma_1^2\}$. Then, letting $\sigma^2 \to -\sigma_1^2$ and $\beta = y_1$, we find that $l \to +\infty$, and therefore the maximum cannot be achieved. Thus, during the maximization procedure, one has to be sure that at each iteration σ^2 stays nonnegative.

The negative expected Hessian matrix for the log-likelihood function, called the information matrix, is given by

$$\mathcal{I} = -E(\mathbf{H}) = \begin{bmatrix} \sum_{i=1}^{n}\frac{1}{\sigma^2+\sigma_i^2} & 0 \\ 0 & \frac{1}{2}\sum_{i=1}^{n}\frac{1}{(\sigma^2+\sigma_i^2)^2} \end{bmatrix}.$$

Unlike the Hessian matrix $\mathbf{H}$, the information matrix, $\mathcal{I}$ is always positive definite, and therefore the Fisher scoring (FS) algorithm is more reliable than the Newton–Raphson algorithm.

By inverting the information matrix $\mathcal{I}$, we obtain an asymptotic covariance matrix with a large-sample approximation to the variance of the heterogeneity parameter,

$$\text{var}(\widehat{\sigma}^2_{ML}) = 2 \left(\sum_{i=1}^{n} \frac{1}{(\sigma^2 + \sigma_i^2)^2} \right)^{-1}. \tag{5.12}$$

We notice that for the meta-analysis model, as for the LME model, the expected value of the cross-derivative is zero, and therefore the MLEs for β and σ^2 are asymptotically independent for large n. As follows from the general theory presented in Chapter 3, there are two consequences of this fact:

1. Maximization of the log-likelihood function may be accomplished separately for β and σ^2.

2. All consistent estimators of σ^2 lead to an asymptotically equivalent and efficient estimation for β, as the weighted average,

$$\widehat{\beta} = \frac{\sum_{i=1}^{n} y_i (\widehat{\sigma}^2 + \sigma_i^2)^{-1}}{\sum_{i=1}^{n} (\widehat{\sigma}^2 + \sigma_i^2)^{-1}}. \tag{5.13}$$

Another property of the MLE is that $\widehat{\beta}_{ML}$ is unbiased, even in small samples, following the outline of Section 3.6, an apparently overlooked fact. Indeed, the unbiasedness of the MLE follows from the observation that $\widehat{\sigma}^2_{ML}$ is a symmetric function of $\eta_i = b_i + \varepsilon_i$ and therefore that

$$\widehat{\beta}_{ML} - \beta = \frac{\sum_{i=1}^{n} \eta_i (\widehat{\sigma}^2_{ML} + \sigma_i^2)^{-1}}{\sum_{i=1}^{n} (\widehat{\sigma}^2_{ML} + \sigma_i^2)^{-1}}$$

has zero mean.

As follows from the information matrix, the lower Cramér–Rao bound for an unbiased $\widehat{\beta}$ is $1/\sum_{i=1}^{n}(\sigma^2 + \sigma_i^2)^{-1}$. Although we are not able to prove that estimates considered below reach this bound, there is empirical evidence that $\widehat{\beta}$ is quite efficient (see Section 5.1.4).

Algorithms of log-likelihood maximization

Now we discuss computational issues of the log-likelihood maximization. As mentioned above, since the information matrix is block diagonal, the FS algorithm leads to separate maximization over β and σ^2 :

$$\widehat{\beta}_{s+1} = \widehat{\beta}_s + \left(\sum_{i=1}^{n} \frac{1}{\widehat{\sigma}_s^2 + \sigma_i^2} \right)^{-1} \sum_{i=1}^{n} \frac{y_i - \widehat{\beta}_s}{\widehat{\sigma}_s^2 + \sigma_i^2}, \tag{5.14}$$

$$\widehat{\sigma}_{s+1}^2 = \widehat{\sigma}_s^2 + \left(\sum_{i=1}^{n} \frac{1}{(\widehat{\sigma}_s^2 + \sigma_i^2)^2} \right)^{-1} \sum_{i=1}^{n} \left[\frac{(y_i - \widehat{\beta}_s)^2}{(\widehat{\sigma}_s^2 + \sigma_i^2)^2} - \frac{1}{\widehat{\sigma}_s^2 + \sigma_i^2} \right], \tag{5.15}$$

where s is the iteration index. Equation (5.14) can be rewritten as

$$
\begin{aligned}
\widehat{\beta}_{s+1} &= \left(\sum_{i=1}^{n} \frac{1}{\widehat{\sigma}_s^2 + \sigma_i^2} \right)^{-1} \sum_{i=1}^{n} \left(\frac{\widehat{\beta}_s}{\widehat{\sigma}_s^2 + \sigma_i^2} + \frac{y_i - \widehat{\beta}_s}{\widehat{\sigma}_s^2 + \sigma_i^2} \right) \\
&= \left(\sum_{i=1}^{n} \frac{1}{\widehat{\sigma}_s^2 + \sigma_i^2} \right)^{-1} \sum_{i=1}^{n} \frac{y_i}{\widehat{\sigma}_s^2 + \sigma_i^2},
\end{aligned}
\tag{5.16}
$$

which takes the form of the weighted average (5.3) for $\sigma^2 = \widehat{\sigma}_s^2$. Equation (5.15) takes the form

$$
\begin{aligned}
\widehat{\sigma}_{s+1}^2 &= \left(\sum_{i=1}^{n} \frac{1}{(\widehat{\sigma}_s^2 + \sigma_i^2)^2} \right)^{-1} \sum_{i=1}^{n} \left[\frac{\widehat{\sigma}_s^2}{(\widehat{\sigma}_s^2 + \sigma_i^2)^2} + \frac{(y_i - \widehat{\beta}_s)^2}{(\widehat{\sigma}_s^2 + \sigma_i^2)^2} - \frac{1}{\widehat{\sigma}_s^2 + \sigma_i^2} \right] \\
&= \left(\sum_{i=1}^{n} \frac{1}{(\widehat{\sigma}_s^2 + \sigma_i^2)^2} \right)^{-1} \sum_{i=1}^{n} \left[\frac{(y_i - \widehat{\beta}_s)^2 - \sigma_i^2}{(\widehat{\sigma}_s^2 + \sigma_i^2)^2} \right],
\end{aligned}
\tag{5.17}
$$

with a good start $\widehat{\sigma}_0^2 = 0$. Iterations (5.15) and (5.17) may use the updated value $\widehat{\beta}_{s+1}$ instead.

It is easy to prove that function l attains its maximum at $\beta \in R^1, \sigma^2 \geq 0$ if and only if $y_i \neq \text{const}$, in compliance with Theorem 4 in Section 2.5. However, a positive solution for σ^2 may not exist. Below we formulate a sufficient condition that the MLE for σ^2 is positive. It is similar to Theorem 5 in Section 2.6.

Theorem 28 *The MLE for σ^2 in a meta-analysis model (5.2) is positive if*

$$
\sum_{i=1}^{n} \frac{(y_i - \widehat{\beta}_0)^2}{\sigma_i^4} > \sum_{i=1}^{n} \frac{1}{\sigma_i^2}.
\tag{5.18}
$$

Proof. Following the line of the proof of Theorem 5, we notice that the MLE is positive if the derivative $\partial l / \partial \sigma^2$ is positive at $\sigma^2 = 0$, that is, when (5.18) holds. Since the minimum of l at $\sigma^2 = 0$ is attained at $\beta = \beta_0$, there exists a $\sigma_1^2 > 0$ that makes the log-likelihood function greater than that at $\sigma^2 = 0$. Therefore, the maximum of l is attained at an inner point of the set $\{\beta \in (-\infty, \infty), \sigma^2 \in [0, \infty)\}$, i.e., $\widehat{\sigma}_{ML}^2$ is positive. ∎

One of the first methods used to maximize function (5.10), suggested by Pockock et al. (1981), has the fixed-point form (2.122),

$$
\widehat{\sigma}_{s+1}^2 = \widehat{\sigma}_s^2 \frac{\sum_{i=1}^{n} (\sigma_i^2 + \widehat{\sigma}_s^2)^{-2} (y_i - \widehat{\beta}_s)^2}{\sum_{i=1}^{n} (\sigma_i^2 + \widehat{\sigma}_s^2)^{-1}}, \quad s = 0, 1, ...,
\tag{5.19}
$$

where $\widehat{\beta}_s$ is recalculated by formula (5.16). Berkey and Laird (1986) showed that this algorithm can be derived via the EM algorithm. If we denote $R(\widehat{\sigma}_s^2)$ as the right-hand side of equation (5.19), we can see that $R(0) = 0$, and using (5.6), we obtain $R(\infty) = n^{-1} \sum_{i=1}^{n} (y_i - \overline{y})^2$. Hence, in view of Section 2.12.1, for the Pockock algorithm (5.19) it is reasonable to start from $\widehat{\sigma}_0^2 = \sum(y_i - \overline{y})^2/n$. Note that we cannot start from zero in (5.19) as in the FS algorithm (5.15), because zero is a fixed point of R. As follows from Chapter 2, the Pockock algorithm converges slowly if the MLE for the random effect variance is close to zero. For this reason, we prefer the FS algorithm (5.17).

The R code below computes the ML estimates for β and σ^2 using Fisher scoring iterations (5.17); array y contains values y_i and array sigma2i contains values σ_i^2. It does not restrict the variance to be positive. Of course, if the output sigma2ML is negative, we set the estimate to zero.

```
metaMLFS=function(y, sigma2i,maxiter=10,eps=10^-7)
{
#Fisher scoring algorithm for simple meta-analysis model
n = length(y)
w <- 1/sigma2i
sw <- sum(w)
beta0 <- sum(y * w)/sw
sigma2ML <- 0
for(iter in 1:maxiter)
{
w <- 1/(sigma2i + sigma2ML)
sw <- sum(w)
sw2 <- sum(w^2)
betaML <- sum(y * w)/sw
sigma2ML.new <- sum(((y - betaML)^2 - sigma2ML) * w^2)/sw2
if(abs(sigma2ML - sigma2ML.new) < eps) break
sigma2ML=sigma2ML.new
}
return(c(betaML, sigma2ML))
}
```

Restricted maximum likelihood

As follows from Section 2.2.6 for the RML estimation the augmented term has the general form $-0.5 \ln |\mathbf{X}'\mathbf{V}^{-1}\mathbf{X}|$, which for the meta-analysis model takes the specific form $-0.5 \ln \sum(\sigma^2 + \sigma_i^2)^{-1}$. Thus, the log-likelihood function for the restricted ML is

$$l_R(\beta, \sigma^2) = -\frac{1}{2}\left\{\sum_{i=1}^{n}\left[\ln(\sigma^2 + \sigma_i^2) + \frac{(y_i - \beta)^2}{\sigma^2 + \sigma_i^2}\right] + \ln\sum_{i=1}^{n}(\sigma^2 + \sigma_i^2)^{-1}\right\}. \tag{5.20}$$

For the balanced model ($\sigma_i^2 = \sigma_1^2 =$const), we again have $\widehat{\beta} = \overline{y}$ and

$$\widehat{\sigma}^2 = \frac{1}{n-1}\sum(y_i - \overline{y})^2 - \sigma_1^2. \tag{5.21}$$

Characteristically, the RML estimator of the variance parameter in the balanced model is unbiased, unlike the ML estimator (5.11). However, in the unbalanced model, RML is biased. We will prove that for the balanced model the estimator (5.21) coincides with the method of moments and MINQUE.

To maximize function (5.20), we need its derivatives,

$$\frac{\partial l_R}{\partial \sigma^2} = -\frac{1}{2} \sum_{i=1}^{n} \left[\frac{1}{\sigma^2 + \sigma_i^2} - \frac{(y_i - \beta)^2}{(\sigma^2 + \sigma_i^2)^2} \right] + \frac{1}{2} \frac{\sum(\sigma^2 + \sigma_i^2)^{-2}}{\sum(\sigma^2 + \sigma_i^2)^{-1}}.$$

Since the information matrices for ML and RML coincide, the FS algorithm takes the form

$$\widehat{\sigma}_{s+1}^2 = \left(\sum_{i=1}^{n} \frac{1}{(\widehat{\sigma}_s^2 + \sigma_i^2)^2} \right)^{-1} \sum_{i=1}^{n} \frac{(y_i - \widehat{\beta}_s)^2 - \sigma_i^2}{(\widehat{\sigma}_s^2 + \sigma_i^2)^2} + \frac{1}{\sum(\widehat{\sigma}_s^2 + \sigma_i^2)^{-1}}, \qquad (5.22)$$

with a good start, $\widehat{\sigma}_0^2 = 0$.

To derive a fixed-point version of the solution to $\partial l_R / \partial \sigma^2 = 0$, we rewrite this equation as

$$\sum_{i=1}^{n} (\sigma^2 + \sigma_i^2)^{-1} - \frac{\sum(\sigma^2 + \sigma_i^2)^{-2}}{\sum(\sigma^2 + \sigma_i^2)^{-1}} = \sum (y_i - \beta)^2 (\sigma^2 + \sigma_i^2)^{-2}.$$

Multiplying by σ^2, we come to the following fixed-point iteration:

$$\widehat{\sigma}_{s+1}^2 = \widehat{\sigma}_s^2 \frac{\sum_{i=1}^{n} (\sigma_i^2 + \widehat{\sigma}_s^2)^{-2} (y_i - \widehat{\beta}_s)^2}{\sum_{i=1}^{n} (\sigma_i^2 + \widehat{\sigma}_s^2)^{-1} - \frac{\sum(\widehat{\sigma}_s^2 + \sigma_i^2)^{-2}}{\sum(\widehat{\sigma}_s^2 + \sigma_i^2)^{-1}}}, \qquad s = 0, 1, \ldots \qquad (5.23)$$

The iterations always lead to a positive solution because the denominator is positive ($y_i \neq$const). Again, we cannot start iterations from zero; a good start is $\widehat{\sigma}_0^2 = R(\infty)$, where R is the right-hand side of (5.23) as a function of $\widehat{\sigma}_s^2$. It is trivial to show that $R(\infty) = \sum_{i=1}^{n} (y_i - \overline{y})^2 / (n-1)$. Repeating the arguments of the proof in Theorem 28, we come to a sufficient condition on the existence of positive $\widehat{\sigma}_{RML}^2$.

Theorem 29 *The RML estimate for σ^2 in meta-analysis model (5.2) is positive if*

$$\sum_{i=1}^{n} \sigma_i^{-4} (y_i - \widehat{\beta}_0)^2 > \sum_{i=1}^{n} \sigma_i^{-2} - \frac{\sum_{i=1}^{n} \sigma_i^{-4}}{\sum_{i=1}^{n} \sigma_i^{-2}}.$$

Since the number of studies is usually small, we prefer RML over ML estimation.

5.1.3   Quadratic unbiased estimation for σ^2

In this section we consider several quadratic unbiased estimations of the random effect variance. Estimation of σ^2 plays the central role in the meta-analysis model because once $\widehat{\sigma}^2$ is available, we apply the weighted least squares estimator (5.13). A characteristic property of the quadratic unbiased estimation is that it is distribution-free: a very attractive property, especially for a small number of studies.

Further, it will be easier to handle the meta-analysis model by rewriting it in vector notation as

$$\mathbf{y} = \beta\mathbf{1} + \boldsymbol{\eta}, \quad E(\boldsymbol{\eta}) = \mathbf{0}, \quad \text{cov}(\boldsymbol{\eta}) = \sigma^2\mathbf{I} + \boldsymbol{\Lambda} = \mathbf{V}, \tag{5.24}$$

where $\boldsymbol{\Lambda} = \text{diag}(\sigma_1^2, ..., \sigma_n^2)$ and $\mathbf{1} = (1, ..., 1)'$.

Variance least squares estimator

The VLS estimator, introduced in Section 3.12, is perhaps the easiest way to estimate variance parameters, particularly the heterogeneity parameter in the meta-analysis model. Following the outline of that method, we estimate β by (5.5) or (5.6) and find residuals $e_i = y_i - \hat{\beta}$. The empirical variance is e_i^2 and the theoretical variance is $\sigma_i^2 + \sigma^2$. Therefore, to find σ^2 we minimize the sum of squares of residuals between empirical and theoretical values, the same as in the ordinary least squares approach but applied to variances using squared residuals. Hence, according to this method, σ^2 minimizes the sum of squares $\sum(e_i^2 - \sigma_i^2 - \sigma^2)^2$, which leads to

$$\hat{\sigma}_{VLS}^2 = \frac{1}{n}\sum_{i=1}^{n} e_i^2 - \frac{1}{n}\sum_{i=1}^{n} \sigma_i^2. \tag{5.25}$$

This estimator is a quadratic function of y_i but a biased estimator of σ^2. Unbiased estimation is described below.

Method of moments

Following the line of the method of moments (MM) estimation theory, earlier applied to the LME model in Chapter 3, we proceed as follows:

1. Take an unbiased estimator, $\hat{\beta}_0$ or $\hat{\beta}_1$, as the weighted or unweighted MM estimator, respectively.

2. Construct the sum of squares of residuals.

3. Take the expectation of the sum from step 2.

4. Solve for σ^2, equating the empirical sum to its expected value.

It is important that we not assume a distribution of the error term since we deal only with the first two moments. We start with the unweighted version of MM and take the simple average estimator $\bar{y} = \hat{\beta}_1 = \sum_{i=1}^{n} y_i/n$ with the empirical sum of squares $\sum(y_i - \bar{y})^2$. It is easy to see that in matrix notation

$$\sum_{i=1}^{n}(y_i - \bar{y})^2 = \mathbf{y}'\left(\mathbf{I} - \frac{1}{n}\mathbf{1}\mathbf{1}'\right)\mathbf{y}.$$

Now we calculate the expected value of this sum of squares using the formula for the expected value of the quadratic form (Graybill, 1983; Schott, 1997), $E(\boldsymbol{\eta}'\mathbf{A}\boldsymbol{\eta}) =$

$\text{tr}(\mathbf{A}\text{cov}(\boldsymbol{\eta}))$. We have

$$
\begin{aligned}
& E\sum(y_i - \bar{y})^2 \\
= & E\mathbf{y}'\left(\mathbf{I} - \frac{1}{n}\mathbf{1}\mathbf{1}'\right)\mathbf{y} = E\left[(\beta\mathbf{1} + \boldsymbol{\eta})'\left(\mathbf{I} - n^{-1}\mathbf{1}\mathbf{1}'\right)(\beta\mathbf{1} + \boldsymbol{\eta})\right] \\
= & E\boldsymbol{\eta}'\left(\mathbf{I} - n^{-1}\mathbf{1}\mathbf{1}'\right)\boldsymbol{\eta} = \text{tr}\left[\left(\mathbf{I} - n^{-1}\mathbf{1}\mathbf{1}'\right)\text{cov}(\boldsymbol{\eta})\right] \\
= & tr cov(\boldsymbol{\eta}) - n^{-1}\mathbf{1}'\text{cov}(\boldsymbol{\eta})\mathbf{1} = n\sigma^2 + \sum\sigma_i^2 - n^{-1}(n\sigma^2 + \sum\sigma_i^2) \\
= & (1 - n^{-1})(n\sigma^2 + \sum\sigma_i^2).
\end{aligned}
$$

Next, we equate the empirical sum to its expected value,

$$
\sum(y_i - \bar{y})^2 = (1 - n^{-1})(n\sigma^2 + \sum\sigma_i^2)
$$

and solve for σ^2, which yields the Unweighted MM (UMM) unbiased estimator of the random effect variance,

$$
\widehat{\sigma}_{UMM}^2 = \frac{1}{n-1}\sum_{i=1}^n(y_i - \bar{y})^2 - \frac{1}{n}\sum_{i=1}^n\sigma_i^2. \tag{5.26}
$$

The UMM estimator is close to the VLS estimator with $\widehat{\beta} = \bar{y}$, but the former is unbiased, unlike the latter, because $n - 1$ is used in the denominator.

Now we derive the weighted MM estimator based on the weighted least squares estimator $\widehat{\beta}_0$. The weighted sum of squared residuals is

$$
\sum_{i=1}^n\sigma_i^{-2}(y_i - \widehat{\beta}_0)^2, \tag{5.27}
$$

where $\widehat{\beta}_0$ is defined in (5.5). We can write (5.27) in matrix form by denoting $\mathbf{w} = (\sigma_1^{-2}, ..., \sigma_n^{-2})'$; then $\widehat{\beta}_0 = \mathbf{w}'\mathbf{y}/\mathbf{w}'\mathbf{1}$ and

$$
\sum\sigma_i^{-2}(y_i - \widehat{\beta}_0)^2 = \mathbf{y}'\left(\mathbf{I} - \frac{1}{\mathbf{w}'\mathbf{1}}\mathbf{w}\mathbf{1}'\right)\boldsymbol{\Lambda}^{-1}\left(\mathbf{I} - \frac{1}{\mathbf{w}'\mathbf{1}}\mathbf{1}\mathbf{w}'\right)\mathbf{y}.
$$

Since $\left(\mathbf{I} - \frac{1}{\mathbf{w}'\mathbf{1}}\mathbf{1}\mathbf{w}'\right)\mathbf{1} = \mathbf{0}$, the expectation of (5.27) becomes

$$
\begin{aligned}
& E(\beta\mathbf{1} + \boldsymbol{\eta})'\left(\mathbf{I} - \frac{1}{\mathbf{w}'\mathbf{1}}\mathbf{1}\mathbf{w}'\right)\boldsymbol{\Lambda}^{-1}\left(\mathbf{I} - \frac{1}{\mathbf{w}'\mathbf{1}}\mathbf{w}\mathbf{1}'\right)(\beta\mathbf{1} + \boldsymbol{\eta}) \\
= & E\left[\boldsymbol{\eta}'\left(\mathbf{I} - \frac{1}{\mathbf{w}'\mathbf{1}}\mathbf{1}\mathbf{w}'\right)\boldsymbol{\Lambda}^{-1}\left(\mathbf{I} - \frac{1}{\mathbf{w}'\mathbf{1}}\mathbf{w}\mathbf{1}'\right)\boldsymbol{\eta}\right] \\
= & \text{tr}\left[\left(\mathbf{I} - \frac{1}{\mathbf{w}'\mathbf{1}}\mathbf{w}\mathbf{1}'\right)\boldsymbol{\Lambda}^{-1}\left(\mathbf{I} - \frac{1}{\mathbf{w}'\mathbf{1}}\mathbf{1}\mathbf{w}'\right)\mathbf{V}\right] \\
= & \sum\frac{\sigma_i^2 + \sigma^2}{\sigma_i^2} - \frac{1}{\sum 1/\sigma_i^2}\sum\frac{\sigma_i^2 + \sigma^2}{\sigma_i^4} \\
= & (n-1) + \sigma^2\left(\sum\sigma_i^{-2} - \frac{\sum\sigma_i^{-4}}{\sum\sigma_i^{-2}}\right).
\end{aligned}
$$

Equating it to the empirical sum of squares, we come to the weighted MM unbiased estimator,

$$\widehat{\sigma}^2_{WMM} = \frac{\sum_{i=1}^n \sigma_i^{-2}(y_i - \widehat{\beta}_0)^2 - (n-1)}{\sum_{i=1}^n \sigma_i^{-2} - \frac{\sum_{i=1}^n \sigma_i^{-4}}{\sum_{i=1}^n \sigma_i^{-2}}}, \tag{5.28}$$

as derived by DerSimonian and Laird (1986) and later used by Berlin et al. (1989) and Hardy and Thompson (1998), among others. The denominator is always positive for positive σ_i^2, as follows from the elementary inequality $(\sum a_i)^2 > \sum a_i^2$ for positive $\{a_i\}$.

MINQUE

The Minimum Norm Quadratic Unbiased Estimation (MINQUE) theory was applied to the LME model in Chapter 3 to estimate variance parameters. We can apply this theory to the meta-analysis model. Thus, we seek an unbiased quadratic estimator for σ^2 in the form

$$\widehat{\sigma}^2 = \mathbf{y}'\mathbf{A}\mathbf{y} - c, \tag{5.29}$$

where the $n \times n$ symmetric matrix $\mathbf{A}$ and scalar c are found to make this estimator unbiased, with matrix $\mathbf{A}$ having minimum norm. We start with the calculation of the expectation,

$$
\begin{aligned}
E(\mathbf{y}'\mathbf{A}\mathbf{y}) &= E\left[(\beta\mathbf{1} + \boldsymbol{\eta})'\mathbf{A}(\beta\mathbf{1} + \boldsymbol{\eta})\right] = \beta^2 \mathbf{1}'\mathbf{A}\mathbf{1} + \mathrm{tr}(\mathbf{A}\,\mathrm{cov}(\boldsymbol{\eta})) \\
&= \beta^2 \sum_{i,j=1}^n A_{ij} + \sigma^2 \mathrm{tr}(\mathbf{A}) + \sum_{i=1}^n A_{ii}\sigma_i^2.
\end{aligned}
$$

After matrix $\mathbf{A}$ is found, we set

$$c = \sum_{i=1}^n A_{ii}\sigma_i^2. \tag{5.30}$$

To make $\widehat{\sigma}^2$ unbiased, we need to chose matrix $\mathbf{A}$ such that

$$\mathrm{tr}(\mathbf{A}) = 1, \quad \sum_{i,j=1}^n A_{ij} = 0. \tag{5.31}$$

Following the outline of the MINQUE theory, we find an $\mathbf{A}$ that minimizes the norm of the matrix, $\mathrm{tr}(\mathbf{A}^2) = \min$. To solve this optimization problem, we introduce the Lagrange function as we did in Section 3.10,

$$\mathcal{L}(\mathbf{A}, l_1, l_2) = \frac{1}{2}\mathrm{tr}(\mathbf{A}^2) - l_1(\mathrm{tr}(\mathbf{A}) - 1) - l_2 \mathbf{1}'\mathbf{A}\mathbf{1},$$

where l_1 and l_2 are Lagrange multipliers. The first-order condition for the minimum is

$$\frac{\partial \mathcal{L}}{\partial \mathbf{A}} = \mathbf{A} - l_1\mathbf{I} - l_2\mathbf{1}\mathbf{1}' = \mathbf{0},$$

which gives

$$\mathbf{A} = l_1\mathbf{I} + l_2\mathbf{1}\mathbf{1}'. \tag{5.32}$$

The first condition of (5.31) gives a linear equation

$$\text{tr}(l_1\mathbf{I}+l_2\mathbf{11}') = l_1 n + l_2 n = 1.$$

The second condition of (5.31) gives $l_1 n + l_2 n^2 = 0$. Solving the system of two linear equations for l_1 and l_2 yields $l_1 = 1/(n-1)$ and $l_2 = -1/(n(n-1))$. Substituting these values back into (5.32) finally gives the MINQUE matrix,

$$\mathbf{A} = \frac{1}{n-1}\left(\mathbf{I}-\frac{1}{n}\mathbf{11}'\right).$$

Noting that for this matrix $A_{ii} = 1/n$, we finally find the MINQUE for the variance of the random effect,

$$\widehat{\sigma}^2 = \frac{1}{n-1}\sum_{i=1}^{n}(y_i - \bar{y})^2 - \frac{1}{n}\sum_{i=1}^{n}\sigma_i^2.$$

As the reader can see, the MINQUE coincides with the unweighted MM estimator, (5.26).

There is a general problem with estimation of variance components—the estimates may be negative; e.g., Searle et al. (1992). When using maximum likelihood we set $\sigma^2 = 0$ if an iteration leads to a negative number. We do the same with quadratic estimation truncating as

$$\widetilde{\sigma}^2_{UMM} = \max(0, \widehat{\sigma}^2_{UMM}), \quad \widetilde{\sigma}^2_{WMM} = \max(0, \widehat{\sigma}^2_{WMM}). \tag{5.33}$$

The problem with these estimators is that they lose unbiasedness! Indeed, they become slightly positively biased; in particular, this bias is seen for small σ^2 (see the simulations below).

Variance estimation comparison

Which MM estimator of σ^2, unweighted or weighted, is better? Unfortunately, it is impossible to answer this question categorically because there is no estimator that is uniformly better, in terms of the MSE, over the entire range of σ^2 even if the distribution is known (normal). In particular, as shown in this section, the WMM estimator is preferable for minor heterogeneity and the UMM estimator is better when studies vary significantly. To compare the estimators it is convenient to specify the distribution; namely, it is assumed that the distribution of y_i is normal.

First, we compare the Mean Square Error (MSE) of the two quadratic unbiased estimators (5.26) and (5.28). Since these estimators are unbiased, the MSE is equal to the variance. We use the following fact on the variance of the quadratic form (Graybill 1983, p. 367): If $\mathbf{y} \sim \mathcal{N}(\boldsymbol{\mu}, \mathbf{V})$ then

$$\text{var}(\mathbf{y}'\mathbf{A}\mathbf{y}) = 2tr(\mathbf{A}\mathbf{V})^2 + 4\boldsymbol{\mu}'\mathbf{A}\mathbf{V}\mathbf{A}\boldsymbol{\mu}. \tag{5.34}$$

For model (5.2) $\boldsymbol{\mu} = \beta\mathbf{1}$, $\mathbf{V} = \sigma^2\mathbf{I} + \boldsymbol{\Lambda}$, and

$$\mathbf{A}_{UMM} = \frac{1}{n-1}\left(\mathbf{I}-\frac{1}{n}\mathbf{11}'\right), \quad \mathbf{A}_{WMM} = C\left(\boldsymbol{\Lambda}^{-1} - \frac{1}{\mathbf{w}'\mathbf{1}}\mathbf{ww}'\right), \tag{5.35}$$

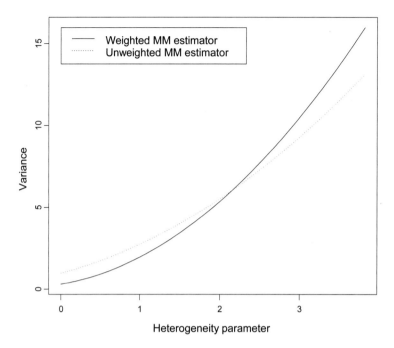

FIGURE 5.2. Variances of the weighted and unweighted MM estimators of the hetero-geneity parameter σ^2 in a typical meta-analysis model. As we see, the WMM is better for small σ^2; however, for large σ^2, the unweighted version outperforms. The estimators peform equally around $\sigma^2 = 2$ in this particular example.

where

$$C = \left(\sum \sigma_i^{-2} - \frac{\sum \sigma_i^{-4}}{\sum \sigma_i^{-2}} \right)^{-1}.$$

It is easy to see that $(\sum \sigma_i^{-2})^2 > \sum \sigma_i^{-4}$ for any positive $\{\sigma_i\}$. Since for both estimators $\mathbf{A1} = \mathbf{0}$, the second term in (5.34) vanishes so that the variance is a quadratic function of the heterogeneity parameter,

$$
\begin{aligned}
\frac{1}{2}\mathrm{var}(\mathbf{y}'\mathbf{Ay}) &= \mathrm{tr}\left[(\mathbf{A\Lambda}+\sigma^2\mathbf{A})(\mathbf{A\Lambda}+\sigma^2\mathbf{A})\right] \\
&= \mathrm{tr}(\mathbf{A\Lambda A\Lambda})+2\sigma^2\mathrm{tr}(\mathbf{A}^2\mathbf{\Lambda}) + \sigma^4\mathrm{tr}(\mathbf{A}^2) \\
&= q_0 + 2q_1\sigma^2 + q_2\sigma^4.
\end{aligned}
$$

Straightforward algebra gives

$$
\begin{aligned}
q_0 &= \frac{n-2}{n(n-1)^2} \sum \sigma_i^2 + \frac{1}{n^2(n-1)^2}\left(\sum \sigma_i^2\right)^2, \\
q_1 &= \frac{1}{n(n-1)} \sum \sigma_i^2, \\
q_2 &= \frac{1}{n-1},
\end{aligned}
\qquad (5.36)
$$

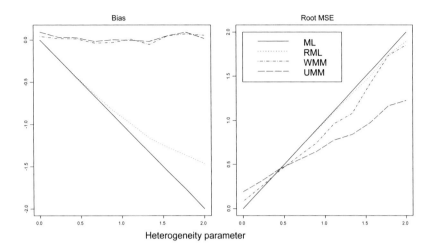

FIGURE 5.3. Comparison of four estimators for σ^2 via Monte Carlo (100,000 simulations). RML and WMM are very close. The slight positive bias for small heterogeneity parameter, σ^2 is due to the restriction $\widehat{\sigma}^2 \geq 0$. For relatively large heterogeneity the bias vanishes. Interestingly, ML MSE is less despite the bias.

for the UMM estimator, and

$$
\begin{aligned}
q_0 &= C^2(n-1), \\
q_1 &= C^2 \left(\sum \sigma_i^{-2} - \frac{\sum \sigma_i^{-4}}{\sum \sigma_i^{-2}} \right) = C, \\
q_2 &= C^2 \left(\sum \sigma_i^{-4} - \frac{2 \sum \sigma_i^{-6}}{\sum \sigma_i^{-2}} + \frac{(\sum \sigma_i^{-4})^2}{(\sum \sigma_i^{-2})^2} \right),
\end{aligned}
\tag{5.37}
$$

for the WMM estimator. In Figure 5.2 the variances of WMM and UMM estimators are shown as functions of the heterogeneity parameter σ^2. The graph confirms MINQUE theory: For large σ^2, the unweighted version is better, but for small σ^2 the estimator $\widehat{\sigma}^2_{WMM}$ outperforms $\widehat{\sigma}^2_{UMM}$. Since we do not expect that studies are very heterogeneous (otherwise, pooling would be quite questionable), we prefer the weighted version.

Second, we compare quadratic against maximum likelihood estimation. Since there are no closed-form formulas for the variance of MLEs in a small sample, we need to use simulation. In Figure 5.3 one can see the comparison of four estimators of the heterogeneity parameter σ^2 (the number of studies is $n = 10$, and σ_i^2 are in the range $(0,1)$). As was mentioned above, the MLE is generally negatively biased. A slight positive bias for small σ^2 is due to the censoring procedure (5.33); this is also true for ML (we force σ^2 to stay nonnegative during likelihood maximization). Also, we notice that RML and WMM estimators are very close. Our choice is to estimate the variance of the random effect by weighted MM because it is close to RML for normal distribution and probably would perform well for a nonnormal distribution as well (it is at least unbiased or slightly biased for small σ^2 if the censored version is used).

5.1.4 Statistical inference

There are two major statistical questions in the framework of the meta-analysis model:

- Are studies homogeneous, $\sigma^2 = 0$?

- Is the common treatment effect statistically significant, $\beta = 0$?

If the $\{\varepsilon_i\}$ are normally distributed, there is a test for $\sigma^2 = 0$ with the exact significance level suggested by DerSimonian and Laird (1986). If random terms are not normally distributed, we use kurtosis to provided a test for homogeneity when the number of studies is relatively large. To test $\beta = 0$ and construct a confidence interval with the confidence level specified, calculation of the variance for $\widehat{\beta}$ is crucial.

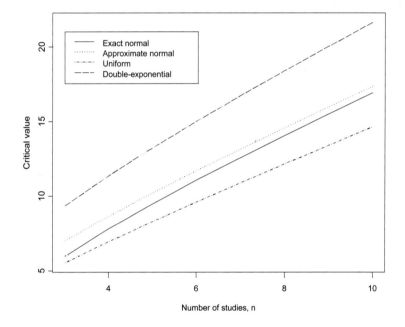

FIGURE 5.4. Four critical values versus number of studies, n in the meta-analysis model. Normal asymptotic approximation is fairly good. The higher the kurtosis, the greater the critical value. The highest critical values have the double-exponential distribution, which is not surprising because it has heavier tails. Approximately, conservative critical values are 50% higher than for the DerSimonian and Laird test.

Test for homogeneity

The importance of this test is obvious: If studies are homogeneous ($\sigma^2 = 0$), there is no statistical problem in estimating β because (5.5) would be the best estimator.

The χ^2-test is based on the observation that if $\sigma^2 = 0$, then, under model (5.2), $y_i \sim \mathcal{N}(\beta, \sigma_i^2)$ and, consequently,

$$Q = \sum_{i=1}^{n} \sigma_i^{-2}(y_i - \widehat{\beta}_0)^2 \sim \chi^2(n-1), \qquad (5.38)$$

where $\widehat{\beta}_0$ is the weighted mean, (5.5). This test, based on the Q-statistic (5.38), was suggested by DerSimonian and Laird (1986). Indeed, under the null hypothesis, $H_0 : \sigma^2 = 0$, we can rewrite the meta-analysis model as $z \sim \mathcal{N}(\beta x_i, 1)$, where $z_i = y_i \sigma_i^{-1}$ and $x_i = \sigma_i^{-1}$. Therefore, statistic (5.38) can be represented as

$$Q = \sum_{i=1}^{n}(z_i - \widehat{\beta}_0 x_i)^2 = \varepsilon' \left(\mathbf{I} - \frac{1}{\|\mathbf{x}\|} \mathbf{x}\mathbf{x}' \right) \varepsilon, \qquad (5.39)$$

where $\widehat{\beta}_0$ is the OLS in regression z on x, $\varepsilon \sim \mathcal{N}(0, \mathbf{I})$ and $\mathbf{x} = (x_1, ..., x_n)'$. It is a standard result of regression theory that the quadratic form Q has χ^2-distribution with $n-1$ degrees of freedom, e.g., Searle (1971a). If there is a random effect, the value of the sum will be greater than the critical value of the χ^2-distribution and we reject the hypothesis $H_0 : \sigma^2 = 0$. Thus, the χ^2-test works as follows: If $\chi^2_{1-\alpha}$ is the $(1 - \alpha)$th quantile of the χ^2-distribution with $n-1$ degrees of freedom, one rejects H_0 if $Q > \chi^2_{1-\alpha}$, where α is the significance level, e.g., $\alpha = 0.05$. There are two merits of this test. First, it has the exact probability of the type I error (size), α. Second, it does not depend on the distribution of the random effect–an attractive feature, keeping in mind that the number of studies (n) is usually not large. However, as indicated by Hardy and Thompson (1998), this test may have low power. Several other tests on homogeneity have been compared by Takkouche et al. (1999), but it was concluded that (5.38) is the overall best choice if the underlying distribution is normal. Biggerstaff and Tweedie (1997) compute the variance of Q and approximate it with gamma distribution.

Now we investigate the distribution of the Q-statistic when the distribution of y_i is not normal, which may happen when the sample size in each study is not big enough to apply the Central Limit Theorem (CLT). We derive the asymptotic distribution assuming that the number of studies is large. Assuming that the $\{\varepsilon_i\}$ are iid with common distribution and have kurtosis κ for large n, we have

$$Q \simeq \mathcal{N}(n, (\kappa - 1)n). \qquad (5.40)$$

Recall that the kurtosis of a random variable X is defined as $E(X^4)/\mathrm{var}^2(X)$. For example, for normal distribution kurtosis it is 3, for uniform distribution kurtosis it is 1.8 and for double-exponential distribution kurtosis it is 6. The kurtosis for symmetric distribution characterizes how sharp the density is around zero. The sharper the density at zero, the heavier the tails are. Thus, using (5.40) and providing κ, one rejects $H_0 : \sigma^2 = 0$ if Q is greater than the $(1 - \alpha)$th quantile of the normal distribution $\mathcal{N}(n, (\kappa - 1)n)$. To see how the critical value depends on the kurtosis, we plot it versus the number of studies in Figure 5.4. The first critical value is for Q-test (5.38), $\chi^2_{1-\alpha}$, assuming that the $\{\varepsilon_i\}$ have normal distribution. The rest is based on the distribution approximation (5.40); the second critical value is the $(1 - \alpha)$th quantile of $\mathcal{N}(0, 1)$; the third and fourth critical values are for uniform and double-exponential distributions with kurtosis 1.8 and 6, respectively. As follows from this graph, the critical value for Q may be 50% higher for a nonnormal distribution. Hence one may infer that, conservatively, if the value Q is greater than $1.5\chi^2_{1-\alpha}$ in test (5.38), the studies are heterogeneous even for distribution with heavy tails.

Exact confidence interval for σ^2

The exact CI for σ^2 can be found using the pivotal quantity, Shao (2010, p. 471),

$$P(\sigma^2) = \sum_{i=1}^{n} \frac{(y_i - \widehat{\beta}(\sigma^2))^2}{\sigma^2 + \sigma_i^2}, \tag{5.41}$$

where $\widehat{\beta} = \widehat{\beta}(\sigma^2)$ is given by (5.3). A function of the data and the true parameter is called pivotal if its distribution does not depend on the true parameter. The exact confidence interval is obtained as the quantile inverse.

As follows from the previous considerations, $P(\sigma^2) \sim \chi^2(n-1)$ for the true σ^2, i.e. does not depend on σ^2. Thus, the interval $(0, \widehat{\sigma}_u^2)$ will cover the true σ^2 with probability $1 - \alpha$, where $\widehat{\sigma}_u^2$ is the solution to the equation $P(\sigma^2) = \chi^2_\alpha(n-1)$, the $100\alpha\%$ quantile of the chi-distribution with $n-1$ d.f. We set $\widehat{\sigma}_u^2 = 0$ if $P(0) \le \chi^2_\alpha(n-1)$. The latter equation can be solved iteratively using the Newton algorithm starting from $\sigma^2 = 0$. Usually, the convergency is fast and requires 3-4 iterations.

Below we display the R code for computation of the upper bound $\widehat{\sigma}_u^2$ as the solution to the equation $P(\sigma^2) = \chi^2_\alpha(n-1)$ using Newton's algorithm. In this code, y contains array y_i and s2i contains array σ_i^2. The exact double-sided CI for σ^2 is found from equations $P(\sigma^2) = \chi^2_{1-\alpha/2}(n-1)$ and $P(\sigma^2) = \chi^2_{\alpha/2}(n-1)$; the same R code ups2 can be used for this purpose.

```
ups2=function(y,s2i,alpha=0.05,maxit=10,eps=0.0001)
{
m0=sum(y/s2i)/sum(1/s2i) # β(0)
cff0=sum((y-m0)^2/s2i) # P(0)
n=length(s2i)
qc=qchisq(alpha,df=n-1) #χ²ₐ(n − 1)
if(cff0<=qc) return(0)
TL=0
for(iter in 1:maxit)
{
mut=sum(y/(TL+s2i))/sum(1/(TL+s2i)) # β(σ²)
dbd1=-1/sum(1/(TL+s2i))*sum(y/(TL+s2i)^2)
dbd2=sum(y/(TL+s2i))*sum(1/(TL+s2i)^2)/sum(1/(TL+s2i))^2
dbd=dbd1+dbd2 # derivative β'
```

```
p1=-2*dbd*sum((y-mut)/(TL+s2i))-sum((y-mut)^2/(TL+s2i)^2)
# derivative P'(σ²)
PS2=sum((y-mut)^2/(TL+s2i)) # P(σ²)
TLL=TL-(PS2-qc)/p1 # Newton's iteration
if(abs(TLL-TL)<eps) break
TL=TLL
}
return(TL) # σ̂²_u
}
```

Efficiency and estimation of the variance of $\widehat{\beta}$

As mentioned before, the ML, RML, or MM estimators of the heterogeneity variance, σ^2, lead to unbiased estimation of the common treatment effect,

$$\widehat{\beta} = \frac{\sum_{i=1}^{n} y_i(\widehat{\sigma}^2 + \sigma_i^2)^{-1}}{\sum_{i=1}^{n}(\widehat{\sigma}^2 + \sigma_i^2)^{-1}} = \beta + \frac{\sum_{i=1}^{n} \eta_i(\widehat{\sigma}^2 + \sigma_i^2)^{-1}}{\sum_{i=1}^{n}(\widehat{\sigma}^2 + \sigma_i^2)^{-1}}. \tag{5.42}$$

Indeed, since these estimators of σ^2 are symmetric functions of $\boldsymbol{\eta} = (\eta_1, ..., \eta_n)'$, we deduce that the second term in (5.42) has zero mean, and therefore $\widehat{\beta}$ is an unbiased estimator of β for any n. Is $\widehat{\beta}$ efficient; that is, does its variance reach the Cramér–Rao bound $1/\sum(\sigma_i^2 + \sigma^2)^{-1}$? We are not able to prove or disprove the efficiency, but the following simulations demonstrate that the efficiency is quite high. In Figure 5.5 we show the results of 100,000 simulations with real-life data from Berkey et al. (1995) on skin cancer, $n = 13$. For each value of the heterogeneity variance σ^2, we generated 100,000 data with 13 points $\{y_i, i = 1, 2, ..., 13\}$, where $\beta = -0.74$ and σ_i^2 ranges from 0.004 to 0.54. For each data set, we computed $\widehat{\sigma}^2_{WMM}$ and $\widehat{\beta}$. The theoretical value/variance is the Cramér–Rao bound $1/\sum(\sigma_i^2 + \sigma^2)^{-1}$, the empirical value is the sample variance of $\widehat{\beta}$, and the estimated value is the average of $1/\sum(\sigma_i^2 + \widehat{\sigma}^2_{WMM})^{-1}$. As follows from the left-hand graph, the variances are almost indistinguishable. On the right-hand graph we show the percent difference from $1/\sum(\sigma_i^2 + \sigma^2)^{-1}$. As we see, the empirical variance is slightly higher and the estimated variance is slightly lower than those of the Cramér–Rao bound, within $\pm 3\%$.

Theorem 30 *Let $\widehat{\sigma}^2$ be any unbiased estimate of the heterogeneity variance σ^2 in the meta-analysis model (5.2). Then $1/\sum(\sigma_i^2 + \widehat{\sigma}^2)^{-1}$ underestimates the Cramér–Rao lower bound $1/\sum(\sigma_i^2 + \sigma^2)^{-1}$ if $\sigma_i^2 \neq const.$*

Proof. We need to show that

$$E\frac{1}{\sum_{i=1}^{n}(\sigma_i^2 + \widehat{\sigma}^2)^{-1}} < \frac{1}{\sum_{i=1}^{n}(\sigma_i^2 + \sigma^2)^{-1}}.$$

We shall show that $\Psi(\sigma^2) = 1/\sum_{i=1}^{n}(\sigma_i^2 + \sigma^2)^{-1}$ is a concave function of σ^2, i.e., the second derivative is negative. It is elementary to take the second derivative,

$$\frac{d^2\Psi}{d\sigma^2} = \frac{2}{(\sum w_i)^3}\left[\left(\sum w_i^2\right)^2 - \left(\sum w_i\right)\left(\sum w_i^3\right)\right], \tag{5.43}$$

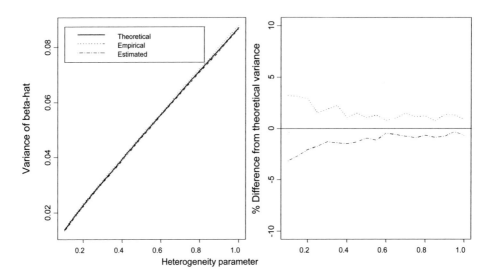

FIGURE 5.5. Estimation of the variance of $\widehat{\beta}$ based on the weighted MM estimator for the heterogeneity parameter/variance σ^2 for Berkey et al. (1995) data (the number of simulations is 100,000). The empirical variance is slightly higher than the theoretical variance (Cramér–Rao bound).

where $w_i = 1/(\sigma_i^2 + \sigma^2)^{-1}$, $i = 1, 2, ..., n$. But the right-hand side of (5.43) is nonnegative due to the Cauchy inequality,

$$\left(\sum w_i^2\right)^2 = \left(\sum w_i^{1/2} w_i^{3/2}\right)^2 \leq \left(\sum w_i^2\right)\left(\sum w_i^3\right).$$

We note that the equality takes place if and only if w_i =const, i.e., when σ_i^2 =const. Then, by the Jensen inequality for a concave function,

$$E \frac{1}{\sum_{i=1}^n (\widehat{\sigma}^2 + \sigma_i^2)^{-1}} < \frac{1}{\sum_{i=1}^n (E\widehat{\sigma}^2 + \sigma_i^2)^{-1}} = \frac{1}{\sum_{i=1}^n (\sigma^2 + \sigma_i^2)^{-1}},$$

which proves our statement.

∎

Our simulations confirm the underestimation of the Cramér–Rao bound; see the right-hand graph in Figure 5.5, where the dashed curve is below the zero line.

Hypothesis testing for the common effect, β

We aim to test the hypothesis $H_0 : \beta = 0$ and construct the confidence interval for β. The situation with this statistical inference is more complex. Assuming that n is large, we use the Wald test and take the ratio

$$Z = \frac{\widehat{\beta}}{\sqrt{v}} = \frac{\sum y_i (\widehat{\sigma}^2 + \sigma_i^2)^{-1}}{\sqrt{\sum (\widehat{\sigma}^2 + \sigma_i^2)^{-1}}} \simeq \mathcal{N}(0, 1). \tag{5.44}$$

The Z-test works as follows: if $|Z| > Z_{1-\alpha/2}$, where $Z_{1-\alpha/2}$ is the $(1 - \alpha/2)$th quantile of standard normal distribution, $H_0 : \beta = 0$ is rejected with significance

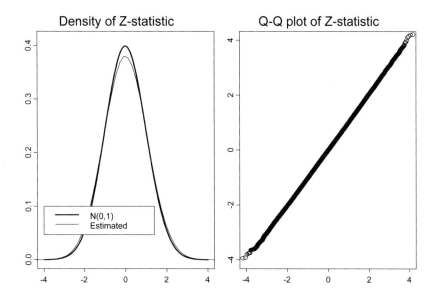

FIGURE 5.6. Distribution of Z-statistic in a meta-analysis model with real-life data (Berkey et al., 1995). $n = 13$; based on 100,000 simulations; weighted method of moments (WMM) as the estimator of σ^2. The distribution is close to normal.

level α. In particular, an approximate 95% CI for β is $(\widehat{\beta} - 1.96\sqrt{v}, \widehat{\beta} + 1.96\sqrt{v})$, where

$$v = \frac{1}{\sum(\widehat{\sigma}^2 + \sigma_i^2)^{-1}}$$

is the estimated variance of $\widehat{\beta}$. Note that the Z-test may be applied with any estimator of σ^2, such as RMLE or WMM. A natural question is whether Z has a normal distribution. In Figure 5.6 we plot the estimated and $\mathcal{N}(0,1)$ density with the Q-Q plot for the Berkey et al. (1995) data from 100,000 simulations. As we see, the normal approximation is quite accurate.

The power function for testing the beta-parameter is reported in the paper by Jackson (2006).

Profile-likelihood confidence intervals

Several authors have demonstrated that a profile-likelihood confidence interval (CI) performs better than the Wald CI: Its coverage probability is closer to the nominal and its CI is more narrow, e.g., a profile-likelihood CI in nonlinear regression was used by Bates and Watts (1988). The reader is referred to Section 3.4 for a general discussion of the profile-likelihood CI construction. We can easily adopt a profile-likelihood CI to meta-analysis by considering the profile log-likelihood,

$$l_p(\beta) = -\frac{1}{2}\sum_{i=1}^{n}\left[\ln(\sigma^2(\beta) + \sigma_i^2) + \frac{(y_i - \beta)^2}{\sigma^2(\beta) + \sigma_i^2}\right],$$

where $\sigma^2(\beta)$ maximizes the log-likelihood (5.10) holding β constant (Hardy and Thompson, 1996; Brockwell and Gordon, 2001). Then the left and right bounds for the $(1-\alpha)100\%$ CI are the pair of solutions to the equation $l_p(\beta) = l_{\max} - 0.5\chi^2_{1-\alpha}(1)$, where $\chi^2_{1-\alpha}(1)$ is the $(1-\alpha)$th quantile of the chi-squared distribution with 1 degree of freedom. Simulations reported by Brockwell and Gordon (2001) show that profile-likelihood CIs are closer to nominal probabilities, although for small n and large σ^2 it may be a few percent off.

Asymptotic equivalence

We know that for the LME model all GLS estimates are asymptotically equivalent and efficient if a consistent estimator for the covariance matrix of random effects is used, see Section 3.15. The same holds for the meta-analysis model: All consistent estimators of σ^2 in place of σ^2 in (5.13) lead to the same asymptotic distribution,

$$\widehat{\beta}_n \simeq \mathcal{N}\left(\beta, \frac{1}{\sum_{i=1}^n (\sigma^2 + \sigma_i^2)^{-1}}\right), \quad n \to \infty, \tag{5.45}$$

where the subscript n is used to emphasize its dependence on the number of studies. It is assumed that for the meta-analysis model (5.1), $\{\varepsilon_i\}$ and $\{b_i\}$ are iid (they may have different distribution). Probably the easiest way to prove (5.45) is to employ the Slutsky theorem, see Appendix 13.1.2. Under the deterministic scheme of Section 3.6.2, we assume the following conditions on $\{\sigma_i^2\}$: (a) there are two positive constants $a \le A$ such that $a \le \sigma_i^2 \le A$ for all $i = 1, 2, \ldots$ and (b) for any nonnegative σ^2 there exists a limit $\lim n^{-1} \sum_{i=1}^n (\sigma^2 + \sigma_i^2)^{-1} = T(\sigma^2)$. Then, since η_i are independent from the CLT Theorem (see Appendix 13.1.1), it follows that for any fixed nonnegative σ_*^2,

$$\sqrt{n}(\widehat{\beta}(\sigma_*^2) - \beta) = \sqrt{n}\frac{\sum_{i=1}^n \eta_i(\sigma_*^2 + \sigma_i^2)^{-1}}{\sum_{i=1}^n (\sigma_*^2 + \sigma_i^2)^{-1}} \simeq \mathcal{N}\left(0, \frac{T(\sigma^2)}{T^2(\sigma_*^2)}\right).$$

Thus, using any consistent estimator $\widehat{\sigma}_n^2$ will lead to the same distribution. Under the stochastic scheme we assume that σ_i^2 are random, then the asymptotic properties follow from the M-estimation theory.

5.1.5 Robust/median meta-analysis

There is a controversy as to what studies can or cannot be included in meta-analysis (Davey-Smith, 2001). This is partly explained by the fact that some studies may be so different from the bulk that an outlier effect can happen. Indeed, when the number of studies (n) is fairly small, one or two outliers may dramatically change the outcome of the meta-analysis. Although random effect accounts for heterogeneity, in the presence of an outlier the estimate $\widehat{\sigma}^2$ becomes inflated and statistical significance drops. In this section we develop a robust meta-analysis that copes with outliers. The theme of robust estimation for a linear mixed effect model was discussed in Section 4.4. Here we take a more specific approach, which leads to convolution of the double–exponential and normal distributions.

The motivation of the robust/median meta-analysis is as follows. In many situations, individual studies are accomplished based on a large sample, and therefore we

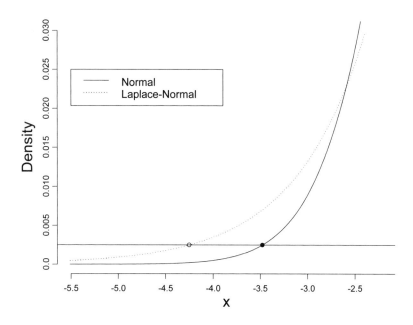

FIGURE 5.7. Left tail of the normal and Laplace–normal distributions with the same variance. The latter has a heavier tail. For instance, the difference on the x-axis is more than 1 for the density value 0.0025. Thus, the Laplace–normal distribution is more robust to outlier studies.

can expect normal distribution for the ε_i in model (5.1), due to the CLT. However, there is no indication that random effect b_i also has normal distribution (this is just a convenient assumption). In particular, the distribution of the random effect may have heavy tails. A well known distribution with heavy tails is the double–exponential, or Laplace distribution with density $0.5\nu e^{-\nu|x-\mu|}$. Also, it is known that the maximum likelihood estimate of μ in Laplace distribution is the median, a robust estimate of the location parameter (Huber, 1981; Lehmann and Casella, 1998). Thus, a reasonable distribution for the random term in the meta-analysis model is the convolution of the normal and Laplace distributions. This distribution, called *Laplace–normal*, has heavier tails and therefore will be less sensitive to outlier studies. In Figure 5.7 we depict the left tail of two distributions with the same variance (since the Laplace–normal distribution is symmetric, it is sufficient to depict only the left tail). The Laplace-normal distribution has a heavier tail and the difference on the x-axis is greater than 1 for the density value 0.0025 (horizontal line).

Now we specify the Laplace–normal distribution density. As discussed above, it is assumed that the study-specific error term ε_i has normal distribution and the random effect b_i has Laplace (double-exponential) distribution,

$$\varepsilon_i \sim \mathcal{N}(0, \sigma_i^2), \quad b_i \sim \mathcal{L}(0, \nu),$$

where the latter means that the density of b_i is $\nu e^{-\nu|x|}/2$ with variance $2/\nu^2$. It is assumed that the random effect and study-specific errors are independent, and therefore the density of the sum $\eta_i = \varepsilon_i + b_i$ is the convolution,

$$p_{\eta_i}(x) = \int_{-\infty}^{\infty} p_{b_i}(u) p_{\varepsilon_i}(x-u) du = \frac{\nu}{2\sigma_i\sqrt{2\pi}}(I_1 + I_2),$$

where

$$I_1 = \int_{-\infty}^{0} \exp\left(\nu u - \frac{(x-u)^2}{2\sigma_i^2}\right) du, \quad I_2 = \int_{0}^{\infty} \exp\left(-\nu u - \frac{(x-u)^2}{2\sigma_i^2}\right) du.$$

After some algebra we arrive at the following density for the combined error term

$$p_{\eta_i}(x) = \frac{\nu}{2} e^{0.5\sigma_i^2\nu^2} \left[e^{x\nu} \Phi\left(-\frac{x+\nu\sigma_i^2}{\sigma_i}\right) + e^{-x\nu} \Phi\left(\frac{x-\nu\sigma_i^2}{\sigma_i}\right)\right], \qquad (5.46)$$

where Φ denotes the cdf of $\mathcal{N}(0,1)$. Notice that this density is symmetric around zero and has continuous first and second derivatives, unlike the Laplace density, with the variance $\sigma_i^2 + 2/\nu^2$. The log-likelihood function for model (5.1) with the error term $b_i + \varepsilon_i$ distributed as (5.46) takes the form

$$
\begin{aligned}
l(\beta,\nu) &= n\ln\nu + \frac{1}{2}\nu^2\sum_{i=1}^{n}\sigma_i^2 + \sum_{i=1}^{n}\ln\{e^{\nu(y_i-\beta)}\Phi[-\nu\sigma_i - \sigma_i^{-1}(y_i-\beta)] \\
&\quad + e^{-\nu(y_i-\beta)}\Phi[\sigma_i^{-1}(y_i-\beta) - \nu\sigma_i]\}.
\end{aligned}
\qquad (5.47)
$$

To maximize this function, we need first derivatives. To shorten the notation, we introduce

$$
\begin{aligned}
E_i &= e^{\nu(y_i-\beta)}, \quad G_i = E_i\Phi_{i1} + E_i^{-1}\Phi_{i2} \\
\Phi_{i1} &= \Phi[-\nu\sigma_i - \sigma_i^{-1}(y_i-\beta)], \quad \Phi_{i2} = \Phi[\sigma_i^{-1}(y_i-\beta) - \nu\sigma_i],
\end{aligned}
$$

so that the log-likelihood (5.47) can be rewritten as

$$l(\beta,\nu) = n\ln\nu + \frac{1}{2}\nu^2\sum_{i=1}^{n}\sigma_i^2 + \sum_{i=1}^{n}\ln\left(E_i\Phi_{i1} + E_i^{-1}\Phi_{i2}\right). \qquad (5.48)$$

It is easy to derive

$$
\begin{aligned}
\frac{\partial E_i}{\partial\beta} &= -\nu E_i, \quad \frac{\partial E_i}{\partial\nu} = (y_i-\beta)E_i, \\
\frac{\partial\Phi_{i1}}{\partial\beta} &- \sigma_i^{-1}\phi_{i1}, \quad \frac{\partial\Phi_{i1}}{\partial\nu} - -\sigma_i\phi_{i1}, \\
\frac{\partial\Phi_{i2}}{\partial\beta} &= -\sigma_i^{-1}\phi_{i2}, \quad \frac{\partial\Phi_{i2}}{\partial\nu} = -\sigma_i\phi_{i2},
\end{aligned}
$$

where ϕ is the density of the standard normal variable. The first derivatives are

$$
\frac{\partial l}{\partial \beta} = \sum_{i=1}^{n} [\sigma_i^{-1} \phi_{i1} e^{\nu(y_i - \beta)} - \nu e^{\nu(y_i - \beta)} \Phi_{i1}
$$
$$
+ \nu e^{-\nu(y_i - \beta)} \Phi_{i2} - \sigma_i^{-1} \phi_{i2} e^{-\nu(y_i - \beta)}] G_i^{-1}, \qquad (5.49)
$$

$$
\frac{\partial l}{\partial \nu} = \frac{n}{\nu} + \nu \sum_{i=1}^{n} \sigma_i^2 - \sum_{i=1}^{n} [\sigma_i E_i \phi_{i1} - (y_i - \beta) E_i \Phi_{i1}
$$
$$
+ (y_i - \beta) E_i^{-1} \Phi_{i2} + \sigma_i E_i^{-1} \phi_{i2}] G_i^{-1}. \qquad (5.50)
$$

Principally, the log-likelihood function (5.48) can be maximized by any algorithm described in Chapter 2. We will use the Empirical Fisher scoring (EFS) algorithm where the information matrix is approximated by the sum of first-order derivatives (see also Appendix 13.3.4),

$$
\begin{bmatrix} \beta \\ \nu \end{bmatrix}_{s+1} = \begin{bmatrix} \beta \\ \nu \end{bmatrix}_s + \lambda_s \left(\begin{bmatrix} \frac{\partial l}{\partial \beta} \\ \frac{\partial l}{\partial \nu} \end{bmatrix} \begin{bmatrix} \frac{\partial l}{\partial \beta} \\ \frac{\partial l}{\partial \nu} \end{bmatrix}' \right)^{-1} \begin{bmatrix} \frac{\partial l}{\partial \beta} \\ \frac{\partial l}{\partial \nu} \end{bmatrix}.
$$

The derivatives are evaluated at (β_s, ν_s) and λ_s is chosen such that the log-likelihood function increases at each iteration, $s = 0, 1, 2, \ldots$. A good starting point for μ is the median and $\nu_0 = \sqrt{2}/\hat{\sigma}$, where $\hat{\sigma}$ is an estimate from the standard meta-analysis model.

The robust/median maximum likelihood maximization algorithm described above is realized in R as function

```
RobustMedianML(b,y,si,nu,maxiter=100,eps=0.0001)
```

The arguments of this function are: b is the initial value of the beta-estimate (can be taken as the regular ML estimate), y is the array of y_i values, si is the array of σ_i values, and nu is the initial value for ν (can be taken as ν_0). Use

```
source("c:\\MixedModels\\Chapter05\\RobustMedianML.r")
```

to download the function.

Tuberculosis example

We use the data from Berkey et al. (1995) on the efficacy of the BCG vaccine for the prevention of tuberculosis from 13 studies, see Figure 5.8. The data are in the file BerkeyMeta.txt; use the command

```
read.table("c:\\MixedModels\\Chapter05\\BerkeyMeta.txt")
```

to open the file (it contains 13 values of y_i as the LOG odds ratios and σ_i). As one can see from this graph, studies are quite heterogeneous, and thus the robust/median approach may be appropriate. These data will also be used in the next section to illustrate the meta-analysis model with covariates. The results of ML estimation of the robust/median meta-analysis model and restricted ML are presented in Table 5.1. RMLE is obtained by applying iterations (5.22).

Table 5.1. Results of estimation of the meta-analysis model by the restricted ML and robust/median method using the data on the efficacy of the BCG vaccine for the prevention of tuberculosis (Berkey et al., 1995).

	RML		Robust/Median		
	μ	σ^2	μ	ν	$2/\nu^2$
Parameter	-0.716	0.314	-0.679	2.321	0.186
SE	0.180	0.159	0.150	1.594	
Z-statistic	3.978	1.976	4.527	1.456	

As follows from Table 5.1, the robust/median meta-analysis model gives a slightly higher value for the common treatment effect (μ). However, the Z-statistic, as the ratio of the estimate to its standard error, is higher for the robust/median model. Parameter $2/\nu^2$ gives an estimate of the variance of the random effect. One could explain the relatively better precision of the estimation in the robust/median meta-analysis model by the fact that this model substantially reduces the random effect, 0.186 versus 0.314. We speculate that this might be a common feature of the two models: When studies are heterogeneous, the standard meta-analysis model, which assumes a normal distribution for the random effect, inflates the variance of the random effect, whereas the robust/median model, which accounts for possible outliers and heavy tails, estimates the variance moderately. This results in more efficient estimation of the common treatment effect, μ.

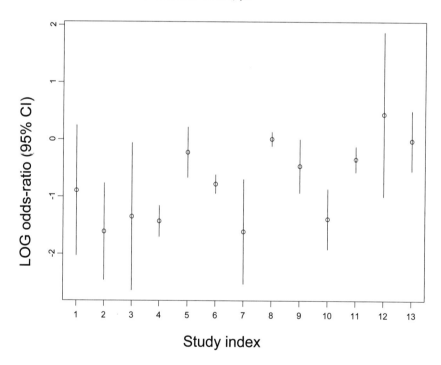

FIGURE 5.8. Data on efficacy of a vaccine from Berkey et al. (1995), 13 studies.

5.1.6   Random effect coefficient of determination

The heterogeneity of the studies is reflected in the variance σ^2. Unfortunately, this quantity cannot be used to compare different meta-analyses because it depends on the unit of measurements. Moreover, it is difficult to judge on the strength of studies heterogeneity because σ^2 does not have the upper limit. In regression analysis, the coefficient of determination is a widely popular goodness-of-fit measure as the proportion of the variance of the dependent variable explained by the independent variable. An important property of the coefficient of determination is that its values are in the interval $[0, 1]$. The aim of this section is to develop a measure for the meta-analysis model which takes zero value when $\sigma^2 = 0$ and is closed to 1 when σ^2 is large. The discussion in this section follows recent paper by Demidenko et al. (2012).

The basis for construction of the measure for studies heterogeneity is the minimum of the sum of squares (5.9) as a function of σ^2. When $\sigma^2 = 0$ we have

$$Q = \sum_{i=1}^{n} \frac{(y_i - \widehat{\beta}_0)^2}{\sigma_i^2},$$

the Q-statistic (5.38), and when $\sigma^2 \to \infty$ we have $\min S \to 0$. Therefore, the random effect coefficient of determination can be defined as

$$R_r^2 = 1 - \frac{\widehat{S}_{\min}}{Q}, \tag{5.51}$$

where $\widehat{S}_{\min}$ is the minimum sum of squares with the estimated heterogeneity variance, $\widehat{\sigma}^2$; in other words, (5.9) evaluated at $\sigma^2 = \widehat{\sigma}^2$. As the standard coefficient of determination, R_r^2 refers to the sum of squares comparison with the values in the interval $[0, 1]$. Indeed, the inequality $R_r^2 \leq 1$ follows from the fact that the sum of squares is non-negative. To prove that $R_r^2 \geq 0$ it suffices to prove that $S_{\min}(\sigma^2)$ defined by (5.9) is a decreasing function. Applying the chain rule for the derivative we obtain

$$\frac{dS_{\min}(\sigma^2)}{d\sigma^2} = -\sum_{i=1}^{n} \frac{(y_i - \widehat{\beta})^2}{(\sigma^2 + \sigma_i^2)^2} - \sum_{i=1}^{n} \frac{y_i - \widehat{\beta}}{\sigma^2 + \sigma_i^2} \times \frac{d\widehat{\beta}}{d\sigma^2}.$$

But the second term vanishes due to (5.3), which implies that $S_{\min}(\sigma^2)$ is a decreasing function of σ^2. We interpret R_r^2 as the proportion of the variance of y explained by the heterogeneity of studies reflected in the random effect. When studies are homogeneous (the heterogeneity variance is zero), $R_r^2 = 0$. When studies are highly heterogeneous, R_r^2 is close to 1. This coefficient can be used to compare the heterogeneity of different meta-analysis studies.

Tuberculosis example (continued)

We continue with the meta-analysis for tuberculosis vaccine studies reported by Berkey et al. (1995). The treatment effect with the 95% confidence intervals (horizontal segments) is shown in Figure 5.9; note that the study index is on the y-axis compared to Figure 5.8. We start with resting the homogeneity of the studies using the Q-statistic (5.38). In our case $Q = 152$ with the critical value 22 from the chi-square distribution with 12 degrees of freedom; the p-value $= 0$. There is a strong indication of the presence of random effects.

Now we turn our attention to computation of the random effect coefficient of determination. The original data ($y = \log OR$) for each study are depicted in Figure 5.9 by a circle, and the data adjusted by the random effect are depicted by a cross, computed as $y_i - \widehat{b}_i$, an 'estimate' of ε_i. The maximum likelihood estimate of the overall vaccine effect is $\widehat{\beta} = -0.71$ (OR $= e^{-0.71} = 0.49$) with the heterogeneity variance $\widehat{\sigma}^2_{ML} = 0.28$ ($\widehat{\sigma}_{ML} = SE = 0.53$) and $\widehat{S}_{\min} = 13.7$ that yields $R^2_r = 0.91$. The 95% confidence band for the overall vaccine effect is shown as a shaded rectangle. We conclude that studies are quite heterogeneous because 91% of the variance of log OR can be explained by the random effect. The strong presence of a random effect is also seen from the figure—the LOG OR adjusted for the random effect substantially moves toward ero. This means that the deviation of studies from the mean is explained primarily by the studies' heterogeneity.

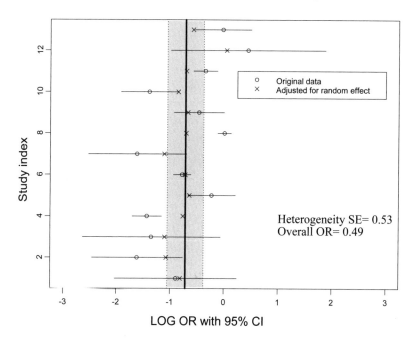

FIGURE 5.9. Log odds ratios from 13 studies of the tuberculosis vaccine effect with estimation of the overall effect using the meta-analysis model. The studies are highly heterogeneous because $R^2_r = 0.91$.

Problems for Section 5.1

1. Under what conditions on $\{\sigma^2_i, i = 1, ..., n\}$ does not the estimator $\widehat{\beta}$ depend on the heterogeneity variance, σ^2?

2. Find the ML estimator for σ^2 when $\sigma^2_i = $const.

3. Plot contours of the log-likelihood function (5.10) for several n using the contour function in R (generate σ^2_i using the chi-square distribution and compute

the log-likelihood function values on the grid of β and σ^2). Display the points with the true parameter value (β, σ^2) and the ML estimates where the log-likelihood function takes the maximum.

4*. Reduce the ML estimation to finding roots of a polynomial, as suggested in Section 5.1. Find conditions under which the ML score equation has multiple solutions. Using simulations, assess the chance to get multiple solutions as a function of n and σ^2 (use the chi-square distribution to generate σ_i^2). Compare the criterion (5.18) with the exact computation of the number of different real roots of the polynomial.

5. Does the reverse statement (5.18) hold, namely, if $\widehat{\sigma}_{ML}^2 > 0$, does (5.18) hold?

6. Assess the probability of (5.18) either analytically or via simulations for several n as a function of σ^2.

7. Which algorithm, the FS iterations (5.17) or Pockock (5.19), is better in terms of time to converge? Use simulated values for y_i to write an R program for the comparison.

8*. Is it true that the RML estimator of σ^2 is always unbiased, i.e. is unbiased for unequal σ_i^2 as well? Is it true that the RML estimator for σ^2 is less biased than the ML estimator? Use simulations if this question is difficult to answer analytically.

9*. Reduce the RML estimation to finding roots of a polynomial. Find conditions under which the RML score equation has multiple solutions. Using simulations, assess the chance to get multiple solutions as a function of n and σ^2 (use the chi-square distribution to generate σ_i^2). Compare the criterion in Theorem (29) with the exact computation of the number of real roots of the polynomial (`polyroot`).

10. Derive (5.37) in analogy with (5.36).

11*. Compare the weighted and unweighted estimators of σ^2 in terms of their variances assuming that the σ_i^2 belong to a chi-square distribution. Compute or estimate via simulations the expected values for q_0, q_1, and q_2 in (5.36) and (5.37).

12. Reproduce Figure 5.3 via simulations (use the chi-square distribution to generate σ_i^2).

13. Reproduce Figure 5.5 via simulations.

14*. Write an R function that computes the profile CI for β based on $l_p(\beta)$ using Newton's iterations. Compute the derivative of $\sigma^2(\beta)$ as an implicit function. Start iterations with the Wald CI. Is the profile-likelihood CI better than the usual one based on the Z-score? Compare the coverage probability and the width using simulations.

15. Reproduce Table 5.1 using the function `RobustMedianML`. Use `contour` to verify that the values returned by this function are the ML estimates.

5.2 Meta-analysis model with covariates

Sometimes we want to make study-specific adjustments. For example, if one deals with epidemiology of skin cancer and several studies have been conducted at different sites, the number of sunny days per year z_i (covariate) may play an important role as a general cause of cancer. Therefore, in combining those studies, an adequate meta-analysis model would be $y_i = \beta_0 + \beta_1 z_i + b_i + \varepsilon_i$. Berkey et al. (1995) consider an example of the meta-analysis model where the latitude of the study site is taken into account, see Figure 5.10. As the reader can learn from this plot the presence of a covariate may change the common treatment effect considerably.

The goal of this section is to extend the results of the previous section to the meta-analysis model with covariates, namely,

$$y_i = \beta_0 + \boldsymbol{\beta}_1' \mathbf{z}_i + b_i + \varepsilon_i, \quad i = 1, ..., n$$

where β_0 is interpreted as the common treatment effect, $\boldsymbol{\beta}_1$ is the $m \times 1$ vector of adjusted coefficients, $\mathbf{z}_i$ is the $m \times 1$ vector of study-specific covariates, b_i is the random effect with unknown variance σ^2, and ε_i is an error term with known study-specific variance σ_i^2. According to this setting, we are interested in parameter β_0, and vector $\boldsymbol{\beta}_1$ may be treated as a nuisance parameter. To shorten the notation, we combine β_0 and $\boldsymbol{\beta}_1$ into one $(m+1) \times 1$ vector $\boldsymbol{\beta}$ and do the same with 1 and $\mathbf{z}_i$ to obtain the $(m+1) \times 1$ vector $\mathbf{x}_i = (1, \mathbf{z}_i')'$. Thus, the meta-analysis model we study in this section takes the form

$$y_i = \boldsymbol{\beta}' \mathbf{x}_i + b_i + \varepsilon_i, \quad i = 1, ..., n. \tag{5.52}$$

Further it is assumed that the system of vectors $\{\mathbf{x}_i\}$ has full rank. Assuming that the distribution of the random terms is normal, we can write compactly

$$y_i \sim \mathcal{N}(\boldsymbol{\beta}' \mathbf{x}_i, \sigma^2 + \sigma_i^2). \tag{5.53}$$

If σ^2 is known, we apply weighted least squares with

$$\widehat{\boldsymbol{\beta}} = \left[\sum_{i=1}^n (\sigma^2 + \sigma_i^2)^{-1} \mathbf{x}_i \mathbf{x}_i' \right]^{-1} \left[\sum_{i=1}^n (\sigma^2 + \sigma_i^2)^{-1} \mathbf{x}_i y_i \right].$$

Letting $\sigma^2 = 0$, we obtain the weighted LS estimator, and for large σ^2 we come to the OLS estimator,

$$\widehat{\boldsymbol{\beta}}_0 = \left[\sum_{i=1}^n \sigma_i^{-2} \mathbf{x}_i \mathbf{x}_i' \right]^{-1} \left[\sum_{i=1}^n \sigma_i^{-2} \mathbf{x}_i y_i \right], \quad \widehat{\boldsymbol{\beta}}_{OLS} = \left[\sum_{i=1}^n \mathbf{x}_i \mathbf{x}_i' \right]^{-1} \left[\sum_{i=1}^n \mathbf{x}_i y_i \right]. \tag{5.54}$$

Matrices in these formulas are invertible because the $\mathbf{x}_i$ have full rank.

Model (5.53) may be viewed as the weighted regression where the y_i come from other studies with known variance σ_i^2. The reader can learn more about weighted regression from the book by Carroll and Ruppert (1988).

5.2.1 Maximum likelihood estimation

The log-likelihood function for model (5.53) is

$$l(\boldsymbol{\beta}, \sigma^2) = -\frac{1}{2} \sum_{i=1}^n \left[\ln(\sigma^2 + \sigma_i^2) + \frac{(y_i - \boldsymbol{\beta}' \mathbf{x}_i)^2}{\sigma^2 + \sigma_i^2} \right]. \tag{5.55}$$

Only for balanced data ($\sigma_i^2 = \sigma_1^2 = $const) does the MLE have a closed-form solution,

$$\widehat{\boldsymbol{\beta}} = \widehat{\boldsymbol{\beta}}_{OLS}, \quad \widehat{\sigma}^2 = \frac{1}{n} \sum_{i=1}^n (y_i - \widehat{\boldsymbol{\beta}}_{OLS}' \mathbf{x}_i)^2 - \sigma_1^2,$$

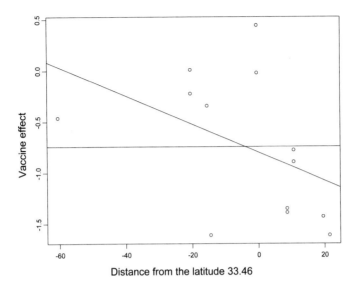

FIGURE 5.10. Meta-analysis model for the efficacy of the BCG vaccine adjusted for the lattitude, Berkey et al. (1995). The horizontal line corresponds to a simple meta-analysis model and the line with negative slope corresponds to a meta-analysis model with latitude as a covariate. As we see, the effect of latitude is significant. In particular, the vaccine effect becomes zero if the latitude is about -60^0.

otherwise, one needs to use an iterative algorithm. For this purpose we need the derivatives of (5.55),

$$\frac{\partial l}{\partial \boldsymbol{\beta}} = \sum_{i=1}^{n} \frac{y_i - \boldsymbol{\beta}' \mathbf{x}_i}{\sigma^2 + \sigma_i^2} \mathbf{x}_i, \quad \frac{\partial l}{\partial \sigma^2} = -\frac{1}{2} \sum_{i=1}^{n} \left[\frac{1}{\sigma^2 + \sigma_i^2} - \frac{(y_i - \boldsymbol{\beta}' \mathbf{x}_i)^2}{(\sigma^2 + \sigma_i^2)^2} \right],$$

$$\frac{\partial^2 l}{\partial \boldsymbol{\beta}^2} = -\sum_{i=1}^{n} \frac{1}{\sigma^2 + \sigma_i^2} \mathbf{x}_i \mathbf{x}_i', \quad \frac{\partial^2 l}{\partial \boldsymbol{\beta} \partial \sigma^2} = -\sum_{i=1}^{n} \frac{y_i - \boldsymbol{\beta}' \mathbf{x}_i}{(\sigma^2 + \sigma_i^2)^2} \mathbf{x}_i,$$

$$\frac{\partial^2 l}{\partial \sigma^4} = \frac{1}{2} \sum_{i=1}^{n} \left[\frac{1}{(\sigma^2 + \sigma_i^2)^2} - \frac{2(y_i - \boldsymbol{\beta}' \mathbf{x}_i)^2}{(\sigma^2 + \sigma_i^2)^3} \right].$$

The information matrix is the negative of the expected Hessian matrix,

$$\mathcal{I} = \begin{bmatrix} \sum_{i=1}^{n} \frac{1}{\sigma^2 + \sigma_i^2} \mathbf{x}_i \mathbf{x}_i' & \mathbf{0} \\ \mathbf{0} & \frac{1}{2} \sum_{i=1}^{n} \frac{1}{(\sigma^2 + \sigma_i^2)^2} \end{bmatrix}.$$

Interestingly, the asymptotic variance of the heterogeneity parameter is not affected by the presence of covariates and is defined by the expression (5.12).

The generalization of the FS and FP algorithms defined by recursive equations (5.17) and (5.19) is straightforward: instead of $\widehat{\boldsymbol{\beta}}_s$, one uses $\mathbf{x}_i' \widehat{\boldsymbol{\beta}}_s$, where

$$\widehat{\boldsymbol{\beta}}_s = \left[\sum_{i=1}^{n} \frac{1}{\widehat{\sigma}_s^2 + \sigma_i^2} \mathbf{x}_i \mathbf{x}_i' \right]^{-1} \left[\sum_{i=1}^{n} \frac{1}{\widehat{\sigma}_s^2 + \sigma_i^2} \mathbf{x}_i y_i \right],$$

the weighted least squares estimate at iteration s. Analogously, one reformulates the criterion for positiveness of $\widehat{\sigma}^2_{ML}$.

Restricted MLE maximizes the function

$$l_R(\boldsymbol{\beta}, \sigma^2) = -\frac{1}{2}\left\{\sum_{i=1}^{n}\left[\ln(\sigma^2 + \sigma_i^2) + \frac{(y_i - \boldsymbol{\beta}'\mathbf{x}_i)^2}{\sigma^2 + \sigma_i^2}\right] + \ln\left|\sum_{i=1}^{n}\frac{1}{\sigma^2 + \sigma_i^2}\mathbf{x}_i\mathbf{x}_i'\right|\right\}.$$

The derivative with respect to $\boldsymbol{\beta}$ is the same as for standard ML, but with respect to σ^2 we obtain

$$\frac{\partial l}{\partial \sigma^2} = -\frac{1}{2}\left[\sum\left(\frac{1}{\sigma^2 + \sigma_i^2} - \frac{(y_i - \boldsymbol{\beta}'\mathbf{x}_i)^2}{(\sigma^2 + \sigma_i^2)^2}\right) - G(\sigma^2)\right],$$

where

$$G(\sigma^2) = \operatorname{tr}\left(\sum\frac{1}{\sigma^2 + \sigma_i^2}\mathbf{x}_i\mathbf{x}_i'\right)^{-1}\left(\sum\frac{1}{(\sigma^2 + \sigma_i^2)^2}\mathbf{x}_i\mathbf{x}_i'\right).$$

Therefore, the FS algorithm is

$$\widehat{\sigma}^2_{s+1} = \left(\sum\frac{1}{(\widehat{\sigma}^2_s + \sigma_i^2)^2}\right)^{-1}\left[\sum\frac{(y_i - \widehat{\boldsymbol{\beta}}'_s\mathbf{x}_i)^2 - \sigma_i^2}{(\widehat{\sigma}^2_s + \sigma_i^2)^2} + G(\widehat{\sigma}^2_s)\right],$$

where again we may start with $\widehat{\sigma}^2_0 = 0$. The FP algorithm is derived from the following equation, which is equivalent to $\partial l_R/\partial\sigma^2 = 0$:

$$\sum\frac{1}{\sigma^2 + \sigma_i^2} - G(\sigma^2) = \sum\frac{(y_i - \boldsymbol{\beta}'\mathbf{x}_i)^2}{(\sigma^2 + \sigma_i^2)^2}.$$

Multiplying it by σ^2, we come to the recursive formula,

$$\widehat{\sigma}^2_{s+1} = \widehat{\sigma}^2_s\frac{\sum_{i=1}^{n}(\sigma_i^2 + \widehat{\sigma}^2_s)^{-2}(y_i - \widehat{\boldsymbol{\beta}}'_s\mathbf{x}_i)^2}{\sum_{i=1}^{n}(\sigma_i^2 + \widehat{\sigma}^2_s)^{-1} - G(\widehat{\sigma}^2_s)}.$$

To start, we set

$$\widehat{\sigma}^2_0 = \frac{\sum_{i=1}^{n}(y_i - \widehat{\boldsymbol{\beta}}'_{OLS}\mathbf{x}_i)^2}{n - (m+1)},$$

where $\lim_{\sigma^2\to\infty} G(\sigma^2)\sigma^2 = m + 1$ is the number of columns of matrix $\mathbf{X}$. Theorem 29 reformulates as follows: if

$$\sum_{i=1}^{n}\sigma_i^{-4}(y_i - \widehat{\boldsymbol{\beta}}'_{OLS}\mathbf{x}_i)^2 > \sum_{i=1}^{n}\sigma_i^{-2} - G(0),$$

then $\widehat{\sigma}^2_{RML} > 0$, where

$$G(0) = \operatorname{tr}\left[\left(\sum\sigma_i^{-2}\mathbf{x}_i\mathbf{x}_i'\right)^{-1}\left(\sum\upsilon_i^{-4}\mathbf{x}_i\mathbf{x}_i'\right)\right]. \tag{5.56}$$

Again, we prefer RML over ML, particularly if the number of studies is small.

5.2.2 Quadratic unbiased estimation for σ^2

In matrix notation, the meta-analysis model (5.52) is written as

$$\mathbf{y} = \mathbf{X}\boldsymbol{\beta} + \boldsymbol{\eta}, \quad E(\boldsymbol{\eta}) = \mathbf{0}, \quad \text{cov}(\boldsymbol{\eta}) = \sigma^2\mathbf{I} + \boldsymbol{\Lambda} = \mathbf{V},$$

where $\mathbf{X}$ is an $n \times (m+1)$ matrix with vector rows $\{\mathbf{x}_i, i = 1, ..., n\}$ and as before $\boldsymbol{\Lambda} = \text{diag}(\sigma_1^2, ..., \sigma_n^2)$. The VLS estimator remains the same, (5.25), where $e_i = y_i - \mathbf{x}_i'\widehat{\boldsymbol{\beta}}$ is the ith residual and $\widehat{\boldsymbol{\beta}}$ is estimated as in (5.54).

Method of moments

We start from unweighted MM with a sum of squares:

$$\sum(y_i - \widehat{y}_i)^2 = \sum(y_i - \widehat{\boldsymbol{\beta}}_{OLS}'\mathbf{x}_i)^2 = \mathbf{y}(\mathbf{I} - \mathbf{X}(\mathbf{X}'\mathbf{X})^{-1}\mathbf{X}')\mathbf{y}.$$

Using previous formulas, we obtain

$$E\sum(y_i - \widehat{y}_i)^2$$

$$= E\boldsymbol{\eta}'(\mathbf{I} - \mathbf{X}(\mathbf{X}'\mathbf{X})^{-1}\mathbf{X}')\boldsymbol{\eta} = \text{tr}\left[(\mathbf{I} - \mathbf{X}(\mathbf{X}'\mathbf{X})^{-1}\mathbf{X}')(\sigma^2\mathbf{I} + \boldsymbol{\Lambda})\right]$$

$$= \sigma^2(n - m) + \sum\sigma_i^2 - \text{tr}((\mathbf{X}'\mathbf{X})^{-1}\mathbf{X}'\boldsymbol{\Lambda}\mathbf{X})$$

$$= \sigma^2(n - m) + \sum\sigma_i^2 - \text{tr}\left[(\mathbf{X}'\mathbf{X})^{-1}(\mathbf{X}'\boldsymbol{\Lambda}\mathbf{X})\right].$$

Thus, the UMM unbiased estimator is

$$\widehat{\sigma}_{UMM}^2 = \frac{1}{n-m}\left\{\sum(y_i - \widehat{y}_i)^2 - \sum\sigma_i^2 + \text{tr}\left[(\mathbf{X}'\mathbf{X})^{-1}(\mathbf{X}'\boldsymbol{\Lambda}\mathbf{X})\right]\right\}.$$

The expectation of the weighted sum of squares is

$$E\sum\sigma_i^{-2}(y_i - \widehat{\boldsymbol{\beta}}_0'\mathbf{x}_i)^2 = E\left\{\mathbf{y}'\left(\boldsymbol{\Lambda}^{-1} - \boldsymbol{\Lambda}^{-1}\mathbf{X}(\mathbf{X}'\boldsymbol{\Lambda}^{-1}\mathbf{X})^{-1}\mathbf{X}'\boldsymbol{\Lambda}^{-1}\right)\mathbf{y}\right\}$$

$$= \text{tr}\left[\left(\boldsymbol{\Lambda}^{-1} - \boldsymbol{\Lambda}^{-1}\mathbf{X}(\mathbf{X}'\boldsymbol{\Lambda}^{-1}\mathbf{X})^{-1}\mathbf{X}'\boldsymbol{\Lambda}^{-1}\right)(\sigma^2\mathbf{I} + \boldsymbol{\Lambda})\right]$$

$$= \sigma^2\text{tr}\left(\boldsymbol{\Lambda}^{-1} - \boldsymbol{\Lambda}^{-1}\mathbf{X}(\mathbf{X}'\boldsymbol{\Lambda}^{-1}\mathbf{X})^{-1}\mathbf{X}'\boldsymbol{\Lambda}^{-1}\right) + n - m$$

$$= \sigma^2\sum\sigma_i^{-2} - G(0) + (n - m).$$

Thus, the weighted MM unbiased estimator has the form

$$\widehat{\sigma}_{WMM}^2 = \frac{1}{\sum\sigma_i^{-2} - G(0)}\left[\sum\sigma_i^{-2}(y_i - \widehat{\boldsymbol{\beta}}_0'\mathbf{x}_i)^2 - (n - m)\right], \tag{5.57}$$

where $G(0)$ is as defined in (5.56). This estimator in the case of a single covariate was derived by Thompson and Sharp (1999).

MINQUE

We are looking for quadratic estimator of σ^2 in the form (5.29), where now

$$E(\mathbf{y}'\mathbf{A}\mathbf{y}) = E\left[(\mathbf{X}\boldsymbol{\beta} + \boldsymbol{\eta})'\mathbf{A}(\mathbf{X}\boldsymbol{\beta} + \boldsymbol{\eta})\right] = \boldsymbol{\beta}'\mathbf{X}'\mathbf{A}\mathbf{X}\boldsymbol{\beta} + \text{tr}(\mathbf{A}\text{cov}(\boldsymbol{\eta}))$$

$$= \boldsymbol{\beta}'\mathbf{X}'\mathbf{A}\mathbf{X}\boldsymbol{\beta} + \sigma^2\text{tr}(\mathbf{A}) + \text{tr}(\mathbf{A}\boldsymbol{\Lambda}).$$

To make $\widehat{\sigma}^2$ unbiased, we let $c = \text{tr}(\mathbf{A}\mathbf{\Lambda})$ and $\mathbf{X}'\mathbf{A}\mathbf{X} = \mathbf{0}$, $\text{tr}(\mathbf{A}) = 1$. According to MINQUE, matrix $\mathbf{A}$ has to have a minimal norm, so that the Lagrange function is

$$\mathcal{L}(\mathbf{A}, l_1, l_2) = \frac{1}{2}\text{tr}(\mathbf{A}^2) - l_1(\text{tr}(\mathbf{A}) - 1) + \text{tr}(\mathbf{X}'\mathbf{A}\mathbf{X}\mathbf{L}_2'),$$

where $\mathbf{L}_2$ is an $(m+1) \times (m+1)$ matrix. The first-order condition for the minimum is

$$\frac{\partial \mathcal{L}}{\partial \mathbf{A}} = \mathbf{A} - l_1 \mathbf{I} + \mathbf{X}\mathbf{L}_2\mathbf{X}' = \mathbf{0}.$$

From condition $\mathbf{X}'\mathbf{A}\mathbf{X} = \mathbf{0}$, we obtain $\mathbf{L}_2 = l_1(\mathbf{X}'\mathbf{X})^{-1}$ and $\sigma^2_{MINQUE} = \sigma^2_{UMM}$ as before.

5.2.3   Hypothesis testing

The analog for the Q-statistic (5.38) is

$$Q = \sum_{i=1}^{n} \sigma_i^{-2}(y_i - \widehat{\boldsymbol{\beta}}_0'\mathbf{x}_i)^2,$$

and under $H_0 : \sigma^2 = 0$, we have $y_i \sim \mathcal{N}(\boldsymbol{\beta}'\mathbf{x}_i, \sigma_i^2)$. Then

$$y_i\sigma_i^{-1} \sim \mathcal{N}(\boldsymbol{\beta}'(\sigma_i^{-1}\mathbf{x}_i), 1),$$

and thus under the null hypothesis, using a standard technique, it follows that

$$Q \sim \chi^2(n - m - 1), \tag{5.58}$$

where m is the number of covariates in the meta-analysis model. If the number of studies is large and the ε_i are iid with kurtosis κ, we approximate $Q \simeq \mathcal{N}(n, (\kappa - 1)n)$. Hypothesis testing regarding the coefficient and the intercept (common treatment effect) can be done using a standard linear regression technique.

Problems for Section 5.2

1. Write an R code for the log-likelihood maximization as an adoptation of the code metaMLFS.

2. Derive an expression for $G(0)$ defined by equation (5.56) for the case when there is only one x $(m = 2)$.

3*. Derive the profile CI for the coefficient at x in case $m = 2$.

4*. Compare the performance of $\widehat{\sigma}^2_{UMM}$ and $\widehat{\sigma}^2_{WMM}$ using simulations. Compare the bias and the standard error of the beta-coefficient using these variance estimators.

5.3   Multivariate meta-analysis model

Sometimes, in addition to the main characteristic of interest, such as treatment effect, one can collect several other characteristics with a complete covariance matrix from each study. Certainly, one can ignore the auxiliary data and estimate the common treatment effect using a (univariate) meta-analysis model. Another approach is to estimate the entire vector of characteristics using a multivariate meta-analysis model and then take the component of interest from the estimated vector. We shall demonstrate that the univariate approach is, in fact, efficient if the precision of the estimation in each study is the same (covariance matrices are the same) or if the characteristic of interest is independent of others (the covariance matrix has a block diagonal form). The results of this section may be applied to the multiresponse weighted regression model. The reader is referred to a recent paper by Jackson et al. (2011) to learn more about application of the multivariate meta-analysis model.

To illustrate the point we start with the following simplified statistical problem. Let $\mathbf{y}_i$ be the $p \times 1$ vector derived from the ith study. It is assumed that it has an unknown mean $\boldsymbol{\mu}$ and known covariance matrix $\mathbf{V}_i$. We are interested in estimating the first component of vector $\boldsymbol{\mu}$ (treatment effect); the data on components $2, 3, ..., p$ are auxiliary. Also, we shall assume that the distribution of $\mathbf{y}_i$ is normal ($\mathbf{y}_i$ are iid). If the rest of the observations are ignored (i.e., one deals with the standard univariate model), the unbiased estimator for μ_1 is

$$\frac{\sum_{i=1}^{n} y_{i1}/V_{i11}}{\sum_{i=1}^{n} 1/V_{i11}}, \tag{5.59}$$

where V_{i11} is the $(1,1)$th element of matrix $\mathbf{V}_i$. Can we beat this estimator by considering the entire vector of observations? Since the $\mathbf{V}_i$ are known, the best estimator for $\boldsymbol{\mu}$ minimizes the sum of squares

$$\sum_{i=1}^{n} (\mathbf{y}_i - \boldsymbol{\mu})' \mathbf{V}_i^{-1} (\mathbf{y}_i - \boldsymbol{\mu}).$$

Taking the derivative with respect to $\boldsymbol{\mu}$, we come to a multivariate weighted least squares,

$$\widehat{\boldsymbol{\mu}} = \left(\sum_{i=1}^{n} \mathbf{V}_i^{-1} \right)^{-1} \left(\sum_{i=1}^{n} \mathbf{V}_i^{-1} \mathbf{y}_i \right), \tag{5.60}$$

with covariance matrix

$$\text{cov}(\widehat{\boldsymbol{\mu}}) = \left(\sum_{i=1}^{n} \mathbf{V}_i^{-1} \right)^{-1}.$$

Interestingly, if all $\mathbf{V}_i$ are the same, then $\widehat{\boldsymbol{\mu}} = \sum_{i=1}^{n} \mathbf{y}_i/n$ and $\mu_1 = \bar{y}_1$, the same as if we had ignored the rest of the $\mathbf{y}$ components. Now, to answer the question of whether the estimator (5.59) is better than the first component of vector (5.60), we compare univariate and multivariate variances,

$$Var_U = \frac{1}{\sum_{i=1}^{n} 1/V_{i11}}, \quad Var_M = \left[\left(\sum_{i=1}^{n} \mathbf{V}_i^{-1} \right)^{-1} \right]_{11}. \tag{5.61}$$

It is easy to see that the two quantities are the same when $\mathbf{V}_i = \mathbf{V}$ (it also follows from the fact that the two estimators coincide). Another case in which univariate and multivariate meta-analysis models have the same precision is when the first component of vector $\mathbf{y}$ is independent of the others. In other words, when the first row/column of matrices $\mathbf{V}_i$ except the first element, is zero. Otherwise, $Var_U > Var_M$. For the sake of simplicity we consider the case $p = 2$. If

$$\mathbf{V}_i = \begin{bmatrix} a_i & b_i \\ b_i & c_i \end{bmatrix},$$

then

$$\mathbf{V}_i^{-1} = \begin{bmatrix} c_i/\Delta_i & -b_i/\Delta_i \\ -b_i/\Delta_i & a_i/\Delta_i \end{bmatrix}, \quad \Delta_i = a_i c_i - b_i^2$$

and

$$\sum_{i=1}^{n} \mathbf{V}_i^{-1} = \begin{bmatrix} \sum c_i/\Delta_i & -\sum b_i/\Delta_i \\ -\sum b_i/\Delta_i & \sum a_i/\Delta_i \end{bmatrix},$$

with the $(1,1)$th element of the inverted matrix as

$$\frac{\sum a_i/\Delta_i}{(\sum c_i/\Delta_i)(\sum a_i/\Delta_i) - (\sum b_i/\Delta_i)^2}.$$

We need to prove that $1/Var_U \leq 1/Var_M$, that is,

$$\frac{(\sum c_i/\Delta_i)(\sum a_i/\Delta_i) - (\sum b_i/\Delta_i)^2}{\sum a_i/\Delta_i} \geq \sum 1/a_i. \qquad (5.62)$$

We rewrite the left-hand side of this inequality as

$$\frac{(\sum c_i/\Delta_i)(\sum a_i/\Delta_i) - (\sum b_i/\Delta_i)^2}{\sum a_i/\Delta_i} = \sum c_i/\Delta_i - \frac{(\sum b_i/\Delta_i)^2}{\sum a_i/\Delta_i}$$

and apply the Cauchy inequality $(\sum x_i y_i)^2 \leq (\sum x_i^2)(\sum y_i^2)$, letting $x_i = \sqrt{a_i}/\sqrt{\Delta_i}$ and $y_i = b_i/\sqrt{a_i \Delta_i}$. Then finally,

$$\sum c_i/\Delta_i - \frac{(\sum b_i/\Delta_i)^2}{\sum a_i/\Delta_i} \geq \sum c_i/\Delta_i - \sum b_i^2/(a_i \Delta_i)$$

$$= \sum (a_i c_i - b_i^2)/(a_i \Delta_i) = \sum 1/a_i,$$

which we intended to prove. As follows from the Cauchy inequality, the inequality (5.62) turns into an equality when $b_i = 0$ or $a_i = \lambda b_i$ for all $i = 1, ..., n$. ∎

In Figure 5.11 we simulated V_{i11} with values in the range 1 to 3 and took $V_{i22} = 2$, $V_{i12} = \rho V_{i11} V_{i22}$, where $i = 1, ..., n = 10$. As the reader can see, the multivariate estimate beats the univariate on the entire range of the correlation coefficient, ρ. Particularly, Var_M decreases dramatically when ρ approaches 1. Variance comparison of the multivariate and univariate approaches in a more general setting is discussed in a paper by Ritz et al. (2008).

5.3.1   The model

The data in multivariate meta-analysis models comprise n multidimensional vectors $\mathbf{y}_1, \mathbf{y}_2, ..., \mathbf{y}_n$ with covariance matrices $\mathbf{C}_1, \mathbf{C}_2, ..., \mathbf{C}_n$. Vectors $\mathbf{y}_i$ may have a different dimension $p_1, p_2, ..., p_n$. For example, treatment effect y_i may be estimated in n

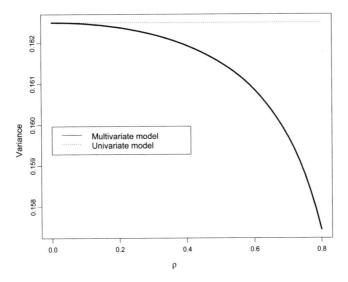

FIGURE 5.11. Variances Var_U and Var_M are the functions of the correlation coefficient ρ between the first and second components of vector $\mathbf{y}$. The number of studies $n = 10$, and the dimension of $\mathbf{y}$ is 2; the variance of the first component of $\mathbf{y}$ varies from 1 to 3 and the variance of the second component is constant, 2. The variance of the multivariate estimate decreases when ρ approaches 1. Thus, the multivariate estimation is more efficient when there is a positive correlation between components.

studies along with other estimates, such as smoking status, s_i and age, a_i. We postulate that for the first study one may have only y_i; for the second study the treatment effect might be adjusted for smoking status so that we have in our possession a pair of estimates (y_i, s_i) with their 2×2 covariance matrix, for the third study one might have (y_i, s_i, a_i), etc. The following multivariate meta-analysis model accommodates study-specific covariates and the possibility of estimating the main characteristic along with augmented correlated estimates:

$$\mathbf{y}_i = \mathbf{X}_i \boldsymbol{\beta} + \mathbf{b}_i + \boldsymbol{\varepsilon}_i, \quad i = 1, ..., n, \tag{5.63}$$

where

$$E(\mathbf{b}_i) = \mathbf{0}, \quad E(\boldsymbol{\varepsilon}_i) = \mathbf{0}, \quad \text{cov}(\mathbf{b}_i) = \mathbf{H}_i \boldsymbol{\Omega} \mathbf{H}'_i, \quad \text{cov}(\boldsymbol{\varepsilon}_i) = \mathbf{C}_i. \tag{5.64}$$

In model (5.63), $\mathbf{y}_i$ is a $p_i \times 1$ vector of study outcomes, including the treatment effect or other characteristics of interest (without loss of generality, we can assume that the characteristic of interest is the first component of the vector); $\mathbf{X}_i$ is a $p_i \times m$ matrix of study-specific covariates; $\boldsymbol{\beta}$ is an $m \times 1$ vector of coefficients; $\mathbf{b}_i$ is a vector of random effects, where matrices $\mathbf{H}_i$ are given design matrices $p_i \times k$ with full rank $p_i \leq k$; $\boldsymbol{\Omega}$ is an unknown $k \times k$ covariance matrix; the positive definite matrix $\mathbf{C}_i$ comes from study i and represents the study-specific covariance matrix of $\mathbf{y}_i$ with the total $\mathbf{C}_i + \mathbf{H}_i \boldsymbol{\Omega} \mathbf{H}'_i$. We call $\boldsymbol{\Omega}$ the heterogeneity matrix.

We illustrate this model with three studies ($p_1 = 1$, $p_2 = 2$, $p_3 = 3$):

$$\mathbf{y}_1 = y_1, \quad \mathbf{y}_2 = \begin{bmatrix} y_2 \\ s_2 \end{bmatrix}, \quad \mathbf{y}_3 = \begin{bmatrix} y_3 \\ s_3 \\ a_3 \end{bmatrix}.$$

For this model,

$$\mathbf{H}_1 = (1, 0, 0), \quad \mathbf{H}_2 = \begin{bmatrix} 1 & 0 & 0 \\ 0 & 1 & 0 \end{bmatrix}, \quad \mathbf{H}_3 = \begin{bmatrix} 1 & 0 & 0 \\ 0 & 1 & 0 \\ 0 & 0 & 1 \end{bmatrix}$$

and

$$\mathrm{var}(\varepsilon_1) = C_{1,11}, \quad \mathrm{cov}(\boldsymbol{\varepsilon}_2) = \mathbf{C}_2 = \begin{bmatrix} C_{2,11} & C_{2,12} \\ C_{2,12} & C_{2,22} \end{bmatrix},$$

$$\mathrm{cov}(\boldsymbol{\varepsilon}_3) = \mathbf{C}_3 = \begin{bmatrix} C_{3,11} & C_{3,12} & C_{3,13} \\ C_{3,12} & C_{3,22} & C_{3,23} \\ C_{3,13} & C_{3,23} & C_{3,33} \end{bmatrix}.$$

Then it is easy to see

$$\mathrm{var}(y_1) = C_{1,11} + \Omega_{11}, \quad \mathrm{cov}(\mathbf{y}_2) = \begin{bmatrix} C_{2,11} & C_{2,12} \\ C_{2,12} & C_{2,22} \end{bmatrix} + \begin{bmatrix} \Omega_{11} & \Omega_{12} \\ \Omega_{12} & \Omega_{22} \end{bmatrix},$$

$$\mathrm{cov}(\mathbf{y}_3) = \begin{bmatrix} C_{3,11} & C_{3,12} & C_{3,13} \\ C_{3,12} & C_{3,22} & C_{3,23} \\ C_{3,13} & C_{3,23} & C_{3,33} \end{bmatrix} + \begin{bmatrix} \Omega_{11} & \Omega_{12} & \Omega_{13} \\ \Omega_{12} & \Omega_{22} & \Omega_{23} \\ \Omega_{13} & \Omega_{23} & \Omega_{33} \end{bmatrix}.$$

If the dimension of $\mathbf{y}_i$ is the same, we set $\mathbf{H}_i = \mathbf{I}$; if there are no covariates $\mathbf{X}_i = 1$ and β is one-dimensional.

If $\boldsymbol{\Omega}$ was known, the best estimator would be the Weighted Least Squares (WLS) estimator,

$$\widehat{\boldsymbol{\beta}} = \left[\sum_{i=1}^{n} \mathbf{X}_i' \mathbf{V}_i^{-1} \mathbf{X}_i \right]^{-1} \left[\sum_{i=1}^{n} \mathbf{X}_i' \mathbf{V}_i^{-1} \mathbf{y}_i \right], \tag{5.65}$$

where to shorten the notation we denoted $\mathbf{V}_i = \mathbf{C}_i + \mathbf{H}_i \boldsymbol{\Omega} \mathbf{H}_i'$. Two extreme cases in formula (5.65) are important. If there are no random effects, $\boldsymbol{\Omega} = \mathbf{0}$ and we obtain

$$\widehat{\boldsymbol{\beta}}_0 = \left[\sum_{i=1}^{n} \mathbf{X}_i' \mathbf{C}_i^{-1} \mathbf{X}_i \right]^{-1} \left[\sum_{i=1}^{n} \mathbf{X}_i' \mathbf{C}_i^{-1} \mathbf{y}_i \right]. \tag{5.66}$$

If $\boldsymbol{\Omega}$ becomes large, $\widehat{\boldsymbol{\beta}}$ converges to

$$\widehat{\boldsymbol{\beta}}_{OLS} = \left[\sum_{i=1}^{n} \mathbf{X}_i' (\mathbf{H}_i \mathbf{H}_i')^{-1} \mathbf{X}_i \right]^{-1} \left[\sum_{i=1}^{n} \mathbf{X}_i' (\mathbf{H}_i \mathbf{H}_i')^{-1} \mathbf{y}_i \right], \tag{5.67}$$

noting that $\mathbf{H}_i \mathbf{H}_i'$ is nonsingular. Thus, the WLS estimator is somewhat in between.

5.3.2   Maximum likelihood estimation

In this section we assume that $\mathbf{y}_i$ has normal distribution; then the multivariate meta-analysis model can be simplified to

$$\mathbf{y}_i \sim \mathcal{N}(\mathbf{X}_i\boldsymbol{\beta}, \mathbf{C}_i + \mathbf{H}_i\boldsymbol{\Omega}\mathbf{H}_i'). \tag{5.68}$$

The log-likelihood function for model (5.68) takes the form

$$
\begin{aligned}
l(\boldsymbol{\beta}, \boldsymbol{\Omega}) \;=\; & -\frac{1}{2}\sum_{i=1}^{n}\{\ln\left|\mathbf{C}_i + \mathbf{H}_i\boldsymbol{\Omega}\mathbf{H}_i'\right| \\
& + (\mathbf{y}_i - \mathbf{X}_i\boldsymbol{\beta})'(\mathbf{C}_i + \mathbf{H}_i\boldsymbol{\Omega}\mathbf{H}_i')^{-1}(\mathbf{y}_i - \mathbf{X}_i\boldsymbol{\beta})\}.
\end{aligned}
\tag{5.69}
$$

The MLE maximizes l over $\boldsymbol{\beta} \in R^m$ and $k \times k$ nonnegative definite matrix $\boldsymbol{\Omega}$. Holding $\boldsymbol{\Omega}$ constant, the log-likelihood maximizes at the WLS estimator (5.65). We use the previously developed theory for the LME model from Chapter 2 to derive the Newton–Raphson (NR) algorithm for (5.69). Using familiar matrix formulas, we obtain the estimating (score) equation for heterogeneity matrix $\boldsymbol{\Omega}$:

$$\frac{\partial l}{\partial \boldsymbol{\Omega}} = -\frac{1}{2}\sum_{i=1}^{n}\left[\mathbf{H}_i'\mathbf{V}_i^{-1}\mathbf{H}_i - \mathbf{H}_i'\mathbf{V}_i^{-1}\mathbf{e}_i\mathbf{e}_i'\mathbf{V}_i^{-1}\mathbf{H}_i\right] = \mathbf{0}. \tag{5.70}$$

Only when all $\mathbf{C}_i$ and $\mathbf{H}_i$ are the same can this equation be solved explicitly via $\{\mathbf{e}_i\}$. Indeed, if $\mathbf{C}_i = \mathbf{C}$ and $\mathbf{H}_i = \mathbf{I}$, then

$$\widehat{\boldsymbol{\Omega}} = \frac{1}{n}\sum_{i=1}^{n}\mathbf{e}_i\mathbf{e}_i' - \mathbf{C}.$$

Otherwise, one needs to apply some iterative procedure to find the solution to (5.70). We solve this equation using perturbation formula (2.106). Let $\boldsymbol{\Delta}$ denote the $k \times k$ adjustment matrix for $\boldsymbol{\Omega}$, and let $\mathbf{V}_i$ be the current matrix. Then using the perturbation formula, one obtains the first-order approximation for the inverse as

$$\mathbf{V}_{i,new}^{-1} = (\mathbf{V}_i + \mathbf{H}_i\boldsymbol{\Delta}\mathbf{H}_i')^{-1} \simeq \mathbf{V}_i^{-1} - \mathbf{V}_i^{-1}\mathbf{H}_i\boldsymbol{\Delta}\mathbf{H}_i'\mathbf{V}_i^{-1}.$$

Replacing $\mathbf{V}_i^{-1}$ with $\mathbf{V}_{i,new}^{-1}$ in (5.70) and leaving only adjustments of the first order, we come to a linear matrix equation for adjustments $\boldsymbol{\Delta}$:

$$\frac{1}{2}\sum_{i=1}^{n}[\mathbf{R}_i\boldsymbol{\Delta}\mathbf{r}_i\mathbf{r}_i' + \mathbf{r}_i\mathbf{r}_i'\boldsymbol{\Delta}\mathbf{R}_i - \mathbf{R}_i\boldsymbol{\Delta}\mathbf{R}_i] = \left.\frac{\partial l}{\partial \boldsymbol{\Omega}}\right|_{\boldsymbol{\Omega}=\boldsymbol{\Omega}_s}, \tag{5.71}$$

where $\mathbf{r}_i = \mathbf{H}_i'\mathbf{V}_i^{-1}\mathbf{e}_i$ and $\mathbf{R}_i = \mathbf{H}_i'\mathbf{V}_i^{-1}\mathbf{H}_i$. We notice that the matrix $\boldsymbol{\Delta}$ appears between matrices and generally cannot be expressed explicitly from (5.71). Therefore, we apply the vec operator to (5.71) as we did in Section 2.10 to extract $\text{vec}(\boldsymbol{\Omega})$. Hence, recalling the formula $\text{vec}(\mathbf{ABC}) = (\mathbf{C}' \otimes \mathbf{A})\text{vec}(\mathbf{B})$ and denoting

$$\mathbf{H}_s = \frac{1}{2}\sum[\mathbf{r}_i\mathbf{r}_i' \otimes \mathbf{R}_i + \mathbf{R}_i \otimes \mathbf{r}_i\mathbf{r}_i' - \mathbf{R}_i \otimes \mathbf{R}_i]\bigg|_{\boldsymbol{\Omega}=\boldsymbol{\Omega}_s}, \tag{5.72}$$

the NR algorithm for (5.69) takes the form

$$\text{vec}(\mathbf{\Omega}_{s+1}) = \text{vec}(\mathbf{\Omega}_s) + \lambda_s \mathbf{H}_s^{-1} \text{vec} \left(\left. \frac{\partial l}{\partial \mathbf{\Omega}} \right|_{\mathbf{\Omega}=\mathbf{\Omega}_s} \right), \quad s = 0, 1, \ldots \quad (5.73)$$

where λ_s is the step length. We start with $\lambda_s = 1$ and halve it until $l_{s+1} > l_s$, provided that the gradient is not zero. As in the univariate case, we can start the iterative process (5.73) with zero approximation, $\mathbf{\Omega}_0 = \mathbf{0}$. The next approximation to $\widehat{\boldsymbol{\beta}}_{ML}$ is found from formula (5.65) with $\mathbf{V}_i = \mathbf{C}_i + \mathbf{H}_i \mathbf{\Omega}_{s+1} \mathbf{H}_i'$, continuing in this fashion until convergence. Following the line of arguments in Section 2.10, we can show that (5.72) is the Hessian of l with respect to $\text{vec}(\mathbf{\Omega})$. The disadvantage of the NR algorithm was discussed earlier: it may fail because matrix $\mathbf{H}_s$ may not be positive definite and therefore there does not exist a positive step length that maximizes the log-likelihood function.

We derive the Fisher scoring (FS) algorithm if the expected value of matrix $\mathbf{H}_s$ is used. Since $E(\mathbf{r}_i \mathbf{r}_i') = \mathbf{H}_i' \mathbf{V}_i^{-1} \mathbf{H}_i = \mathbf{R}_i$, equation (5.71) simplifies to

$$\frac{1}{2} \sum_{i=1}^n \mathbf{R}_i \mathbf{\Delta} \mathbf{R}_i = \left. \frac{\partial l}{\partial \mathbf{\Omega}} \right|_{\mathbf{\Omega}=\mathbf{\Omega}_s}$$

and therefore the FS algorithm takes the form

$$\text{vec}(\mathbf{\Omega}_{s+1}) = \text{vec}(\mathbf{\Omega}_s) + 2\lambda_s \left(\sum_{i=1}^n \mathbf{R}_{is} \otimes \mathbf{R}_{is} \right)^{-1} \text{vec} \left(\left. \frac{\partial l}{\partial \mathbf{\Omega}} \right|_{\mathbf{\Omega}=\mathbf{\Omega}_s} \right), \quad (5.74)$$

where $\mathbf{R}_{is}$ means that $\mathbf{R}_i$ computed at iteration s. There is another way to derive the FS algorithm based on a fixed-point approach from Section 2.12. In this case, we derive the algorithm directly from the score equation (5.70). The idea is to express $\mathbf{\Omega}$ in linear form. Indeed, for the first term, we can write

$$\begin{aligned}
\mathbf{H}_i' \mathbf{V}_i^{-1} \mathbf{H}_i &= \mathbf{H}_i' \mathbf{V}_i^{-1} \mathbf{V}_i \mathbf{V}_i^{-1} \mathbf{H}_i = \mathbf{H}_i' \mathbf{V}_i^{-1} (\mathbf{C}_i + \mathbf{H}_i \mathbf{\Omega} \mathbf{H}_i') \mathbf{V}_i^{-1} \mathbf{H}_i \\
&= \mathbf{H}_i' \mathbf{V}_i^{-1} \mathbf{C}_i \mathbf{V}_i^{-1} \mathbf{H}_i + \mathbf{R}_i \mathbf{\Omega} \mathbf{R}_i.
\end{aligned}$$

Substituting this into (5.70), we come to a matrix equation

$$\sum_{i=1}^n \mathbf{R}_i \mathbf{\Omega} \mathbf{R}_i = \sum_{i=1}^n \mathbf{H}_i' \mathbf{V}_i^{-1} (\mathbf{e}_i \mathbf{e}_i' - \mathbf{C}_i) \mathbf{V}_i^{-1} \mathbf{H}_i,$$

which is again solved using the vec operator,

$$\begin{aligned}
\text{vec}(\mathbf{\Omega}_{s+1}) &= \left(\sum_{i=1}^n \mathbf{R}_{is} \otimes \mathbf{R}_{is} \right)^{-1} \quad (5.75) \\
&\times \text{vec} \left(\left. \sum_{i=1}^n \mathbf{H}_i' \mathbf{V}_i^{-1} (\mathbf{e}_i \mathbf{e}_i' - \mathbf{C}_i) \mathbf{V}_i^{-1} \mathbf{H}_i \right|_{\mathbf{\Omega}=\mathbf{\Omega}_s} \right).
\end{aligned}$$

It is straightforward to show that (5.74) with $\lambda_k = 1$ and (5.75) are equivalent. Also, it is a good exercise to check that for the one-dimensional meta-analysis model, (5.75) collapses to (5.17).

The advantage of the FS over the NR algorithm is that the inverted matrix is always positive definite.

Analogously to the LME model, the expected cross-derivative of l is zero, and therefore any consistent estimator of $\mathbf{\Omega}$ in (5.65) leads to an asymptotically efficient estimator.

Restricted MLE

For restricted MLE the log-likelihood function is augmented by the term

$$-\frac{1}{2}\ln\left|\sum_{i=1}^{n}\mathbf{X}_i'\mathbf{V}_i^{-1}\mathbf{X}_i\right|,$$

with derivative analogous to (2.129),

$$\frac{\partial l_R}{\partial \mathbf{\Omega}} = -\frac{1}{2}\sum_{i=1}^{n}\left[\mathbf{H}_i'\mathbf{V}_i^{-1}\mathbf{H}_i - \mathbf{H}_i'\mathbf{V}_i^{-1}\mathbf{e}_i\mathbf{e}_i'\mathbf{V}_i^{-1}\mathbf{H}_i + \mathbf{H}_i'\mathbf{X}_i\mathbf{G}^{-1}\mathbf{X}_i'\mathbf{H}_i\right],$$

where $\mathbf{G} = \sum_{i=1}^{n}\mathbf{X}_i'\mathbf{V}_i^{-1}\mathbf{X}_i$. Algorithms of l_R maximization are straightforward to generalize. Our favorite FS algorithm can be written as

$$\text{vec}(\mathbf{\Omega}_{s+1}) = \left(\sum_{i=1}^{n}\mathbf{R}_{is}\otimes\mathbf{R}_{is}\right)^{-1} \tag{5.76}$$

$$\times\text{vec}\left(\left.\sum_{i=1}^{n}(\mathbf{H}_i'\mathbf{V}_i^{-1}(\mathbf{e}_i\mathbf{e}_i' - \mathbf{C}_i - \mathbf{V}_i\mathbf{X}_i\mathbf{G}^{-1}\mathbf{X}_i'\mathbf{V}_i)\mathbf{V}_i^{-1}\mathbf{H}_i\right|_{\mathbf{\Omega}=\mathbf{\Omega}_s}\right).$$

As usual, we start with $\mathbf{\Omega}_0 = \mathbf{0}$, compute $\widehat{\boldsymbol{\beta}}_0$ by formula (5.65), and recalculate $\mathbf{\Omega}$ to find $\mathbf{\Omega}_1$, proceeding in this manner until there is convergence.

An important issue of the likelihood maximization is to ensure that the heterogeneity matrix remains nonnegative definite at any iteration. The reader is referred to Section 2.15, where this problem is discussed at length. In particular, one has to be sure that the stopping criteria hold and the Kuhn–Tucker condition is fulfilled. Anyway, if iteration produces a singular $\widehat{\mathbf{\Omega}}$, it is a good practice to repeat iterations from another starting value to see that iterations converge to the same $\widehat{\mathbf{\Omega}}$. Several starting values for NR and FS are given in the next section.

5.3.3   Quadratic estimation of the heterogeneity matrix

Estimation of variances and covariances of random effects in a linear model is the key because then we apply weighted least squares to estimate the beta coefficients (fixed effects). The use of likelihood methods assumes normal distribution. Since the meta-analysis model is a linear model, we may apply quadratic estimation for $\mathbf{\Omega}$ as we did for the linear mixed effects model in earlier chapters. Those estimators do not require a distribution assumption and therefore are distribution-free. The problem with quadratic estimation is that the estimate may not be a nonnegative definite matrix. Then we take its projection on the set of all nonnegative matrices, which may be viewed as a generalization of the censoring procedure in the one-dimensional case (5.33). For a discussion at length, see Section 2.15.

Variance least squares estimation

Let $\boldsymbol{\beta}$ be estimated by either (5.66) or (5.67), and let $\mathbf{e}_i$ denote the vector of residuals for study i; precisely, $\mathbf{e}_i = \mathbf{y}_i - \mathbf{X}_i\boldsymbol{\beta}$. The empirical covariance matrix is $\mathbf{e}_i\mathbf{e}_i'$, and it should be close to the theoretical $\mathbf{C}_i + \mathbf{H}_i\boldsymbol{\Omega}\mathbf{H}_i'$. Thus, it is logical to find $\boldsymbol{\Omega}$ that minimizes the sum of squares of residuals between empirical and theoretical matrices. This leads to VLS estimation,

$$\sum_{i=1}^{n} \operatorname{tr}\left(\mathbf{e}_i\mathbf{e}_i' - \mathbf{C}_i - \mathbf{H}_i\boldsymbol{\Omega}\mathbf{H}_i'\right)^2 \Rightarrow \min_{\boldsymbol{\Omega}}.$$

Differentiating with respect to $\boldsymbol{\Omega}$, we come to a linear matrix (estimating) equation

$$\sum_{i=1}^{n} \mathbf{H}_i'\left(\mathbf{e}_i\mathbf{e}_i' - \mathbf{C}_i - \mathbf{H}_i\boldsymbol{\Omega}\mathbf{H}_i'\right)\mathbf{H}_i = \mathbf{0}, \tag{5.77}$$

with the solution

$$\operatorname{vec}(\widehat{\boldsymbol{\Omega}}) = \left[\sum_{i=1}^{n}(\mathbf{H}_i'\mathbf{H}_i) \otimes (\mathbf{H}_i'\mathbf{H}_i)\right]^{-1} \operatorname{vec}\left[\sum_{i=1}^{n}\mathbf{H}_i'(\mathbf{e}_i\mathbf{e}_i' - \mathbf{C}_i)\mathbf{H}_i\right]. \tag{5.78}$$

If vectors the $\mathbf{y}_i$ in each study have the same length $(\mathbf{H}_i = \mathbf{I})$, from (5.77) we obtain

$$\widehat{\boldsymbol{\Omega}} = \frac{1}{n}\sum_{i=1}^{n}\mathbf{e}_i\mathbf{e}_i' - \frac{1}{n}\sum_{i=1}^{n}\mathbf{C}_i, \tag{5.79}$$

an obvious analog of the one-dimensional model (5.25).

Unweighted Method of Moments

Let $\mathbf{e}_i$ be the residual vector as above using the estimator $\widehat{\boldsymbol{\beta}}_{OLS}$, i.e., $\mathbf{e}_i = \mathbf{y}_i - \mathbf{X}_i\widehat{\boldsymbol{\beta}}_{OLS}$. We create the empirical $k \times k$ matrix $\sum \mathbf{H}_i'\mathbf{e}_i\mathbf{e}_i'\mathbf{H}_i$ and compute its expectation. It turns out that the expectation is a linear function of $\boldsymbol{\Omega}$ so that we find the Unweighted Method of Moments (UMM) estimator by equating the empirical matrix to its expected value (the reader should be prepared for some fairly heavy matrix algebra). First, we need the expectation

$$\begin{aligned} E\sum \mathbf{H}_i'\mathbf{e}_i\mathbf{e}_i'\mathbf{H}_i &= E\sum \mathbf{H}_i'(\mathbf{y}_i - \mathbf{X}_i\widehat{\boldsymbol{\beta}}_{OLS})(\mathbf{y}_i - \mathbf{X}_i\widehat{\boldsymbol{\beta}}_{OLS})'\mathbf{H}_i \\ &= \sum \mathbf{H}_i'(\mathbf{C}_i + \mathbf{H}_i\boldsymbol{\Omega}\mathbf{H}_i')\mathbf{H}_i - \sum \mathbf{H}_i'\mathbf{X}_i\operatorname{cov}(\widehat{\boldsymbol{\beta}}_{OLS})\mathbf{X}_i'\mathbf{H}_i. \end{aligned}$$

Denoting $\mathbf{Q}_U = \sum_{i=1}^{n} \mathbf{X}_i'(\mathbf{H}_i\mathbf{H}_i')^{-1}\mathbf{X}_i$, we can write

$$\operatorname{cov}(\widehat{\boldsymbol{\beta}}_{OLS}) = \mathbf{A}_U + \sum_{j=1}^{n}\mathbf{Q}_U^{-1}\mathbf{X}_j'(\mathbf{H}_j\mathbf{H}_j')^{-1}\mathbf{H}_j\boldsymbol{\Omega}\mathbf{H}_j'(\mathbf{H}_j\mathbf{H}_j')^{-1}\mathbf{X}_j\mathbf{Q}_U^{-1},$$

where

$$\mathbf{A}_U = \mathbf{Q}_U^{-1}\left[\sum_{j=1}^{n}\mathbf{X}_j'(\mathbf{H}_j\mathbf{H}_j')^{-1}\mathbf{C}_j(\mathbf{H}_j\mathbf{H}_j')^{-1}\mathbf{X}_j\right]\mathbf{Q}_U^{-1};$$

we use the subscript $_U$ to indicate that the unweighted MM is used (below we consider the weighted version using the subscript $_W$). Second, we split the expectation above into two pieces; one doesn't contain the heterogeneity matrix, and the other does. This leads us to the following equation for the heterogeneity matrix:

$$\sum H_i' e_i e_i' H_i = \sum_{i=1}^{n} H_i'(C_i - X_i A_U X_i') H_i$$

$$+ \sum_{i=1}^{n} H_i' H_i \Omega H_i' H_i - \sum_{i,j=1}^{n} H_i' X_i T_{jU} \Omega T_{jU}' X_i' H_i, \qquad (5.80)$$

where we denoted $T_{jU} = Q_U^{-1} X_j'(H_j H_j')^{-1} H_j$. Finally, we solve equation (5.80) for Ω by applying the vec operator,

$$\text{vec}(\widehat{\Omega}_{UMM}) = \left[\sum_{i=1}^{n} H_i' H_i \otimes H_i' H_i - \sum_{i,j=1}^{n} H_i' X_i T_{jU} \otimes H_i' X_i T_{jU} \right]^{-1}$$

$$\times \text{vec} \left\{ \sum H_i'(e_i e_i' - C_i + X_i A_U X_i') H_i \right\}, \qquad (5.81)$$

the UMM estimator for the heterogeneity matrix.

It is instructive to derive the UMM estimator for the special case when there are no covariates ($X_i = I$), and in all studies outcome characteristics have the same dimension ($H_i = I$). Then, $Q_U = nI$, $T_{jU} = n^{-1}I$, $A_U = n^{-2} \sum_{j=1}^{n} C_j$, and equation (5.80) is rewritten as

$$\sum_i (y_i - \overline{y})(y_i - \overline{y})' = \sum_i C_i - \frac{1}{n^2} \sum_{i,j} C_j + n\Omega - \Omega,$$

which leads to the familiar unbiased estimator

$$\widehat{\Omega}_{UMM} = \frac{1}{n-1} \sum_{i=1}^{n} (y_i - \overline{y})(y_i - \overline{y})' - \frac{1}{n} \sum_{i=1}^{n} C_i.$$

Notice the difference with the VLS estimator (5.79): $n - 1$ appears instead of n in the denominator, which adjusts for degrees of freedom to make $\widehat{\Omega}_{UMM}$ unbiased.

Weighted method of moments

For the weighted version, we take $\widehat{\beta}_0$ with residual vector $e_i = y_i - X_i \widehat{\beta}_0$ and compute the weighted sum $\sum H_i C_i^{-1/2} e_i e_i' C_i^{-1/2} H_i'$, where $C_i^{-1/2}$ is the square root matrix of C_i. Taking the expectation of this sum and denoting

$$A_W = \left(\sum X_i' C_i^{-1} X_i \right)^{-1}, \quad T_{jW} = A_W X_j' C_j^{-1} H_j,$$

one can show that the WMM estimator for the heterogeneity matrix is the solution to the following matrix equation:

$$F = \sum_{i=1}^{n} S_i \Omega S_i' - \sum_{i,j=1}^{n} G_{ij} \Omega G_{ij}', \qquad (5.82)$$

where

$$\mathbf{F} = \sum_{i=1}^{n} \mathbf{H}_i' \mathbf{C}_i^{-1/2} \left[\mathbf{e}_i \mathbf{e}_i' - \mathbf{C}_i + \mathbf{X}_i \mathbf{A}_W \mathbf{X}_i' \right] \mathbf{C}_i^{-1/2} \mathbf{H}_i,$$
$$\mathbf{S}_i = \mathbf{H}_i' \mathbf{C}_i^{-1/2} \mathbf{H}_i, \quad \mathbf{G}_{ij} = \mathbf{H}_i' \mathbf{C}_i^{-1/2} \mathbf{X}_i \mathbf{T}_{jW}.$$

Taking the vec operator of both sides, we finally obtain

$$\text{vec}(\widehat{\boldsymbol{\Omega}}_{WMM}) = \left(\sum_{i=1}^{n} \mathbf{S}_i \otimes \mathbf{S}_i - \sum_{i,j=1}^{n} \mathbf{G}_{ij} \otimes \mathbf{G}_{ij} \right)^{-1} \text{vec}(\mathbf{F}). \qquad (5.83)$$

We illustrate this estimator by the previous example with $\mathbf{H}_i = \mathbf{X}_i = \mathbf{I}$. Then $\mathbf{A}_W = \mathbf{J}^{-1}$, $\mathbf{T}_{jW} = \mathbf{J}^{-1} \mathbf{C}_j^{-1}$, $\mathbf{S}_i = \mathbf{C}_i^{-1/2}$, and $\mathbf{G}_{ij} = \mathbf{C}_i^{-1/2} \mathbf{J}^{-1} \mathbf{C}_j^{-1/2}$, where we denoted $\mathbf{J} = \sum \mathbf{C}_i^{-1}$. Hence, according to (5.82), the WMM estimator for $\boldsymbol{\Omega}$ is the solution to the matrix equation

$$\sum \mathbf{C}_i^{-1/2} [(\mathbf{y}_i - \overline{\mathbf{y}}_W)(\mathbf{y}_i - \overline{\mathbf{y}}_W)' - \mathbf{C}_i + \mathbf{J}^{-1}] \mathbf{C}_i^{-1/2}$$
$$= \sum \mathbf{C}_i^{-1/2} \boldsymbol{\Omega} \mathbf{C}_i^{-1/2} - \sum_{i,j} \mathbf{C}_i^{-1/2} \mathbf{J}^{-1} \mathbf{C}_j^{-1/2} \boldsymbol{\Omega} \mathbf{C}_j^{-1/2} \mathbf{J}^{-1} \mathbf{C}_i^{-1/2},$$

where the weighted average is $\overline{\mathbf{y}}_W = \mathbf{J}^{-1}(\sum \mathbf{C}_i^{-1} \mathbf{y}_i)$. As we see, even for this simple model the solution cannot be expressed without the vec operator and is provided by (5.83). It is a good exercise to check that for the one-dimensional case, this estimator collapses to (5.57).

What if the estimate is not a nonnegative definite matrix?

Unfortunately, there is no guarantee that the quadratic estimator of the heterogeneity matrix is nonnegative definite (it should be because it is an estimate of the covariance matrix). In the one-dimensional case we set the estimate to zero, (5.33). How can we generalize this procedure to the multivariate case? As a word of caution, it is not sufficient to check the nonnegativeness of the diagonal elements of matrix $\widehat{\boldsymbol{\Omega}}$ because it does not apply nonnegative definiteness of the matrix. A symmetric matrix is nonnegative definite if and only if all eigenvalues are nonnegative. When some eigenvalues of $\widehat{\boldsymbol{\Omega}}$ are negative, we advocate for taking a projection on the set of all nonnegative definite matrix $\mathbb{D}_+$, as we did in Section 2.15.2. Thus, if $\widehat{\boldsymbol{\Omega}}$ is not a nonnegative definite matrix, we set $\widetilde{\boldsymbol{\Omega}} = \mathbf{P}\boldsymbol{\Lambda}_+ \mathbf{P}'$, where $\mathbf{P}$ is the $k \times k$ matrix of eigenvectors and $\boldsymbol{\Lambda}_+$ is the diagonal matrix of $\max(0, \lambda_i)$, where λ_i is the eigenvalue of matrix $\widehat{\boldsymbol{\Omega}}$. As shown in Section 2.15.2, matrix $\widetilde{\boldsymbol{\Omega}}$ is the closest to $\widehat{\boldsymbol{\Omega}}$ among all nonnegative definite matrices. However, the reader should realize that $\widetilde{\boldsymbol{\Omega}}$ receives a slight positive bias.

5.3.4 Test for homogeneity

It is fairly straightforward to generalize Q-tests (5.38) and (5.58) to the multivariate meta-analysis model (5.68). Indeed, under the hypothesis

$$H_0 : \boldsymbol{\Omega} = \mathbf{0}, \qquad (5.84)$$

the model becomes $\mathbf{y}_i \sim \mathcal{N}(\mathbf{X}_i \boldsymbol{\beta}, \mathbf{C}_i)$, which is equivalent to $\mathbf{C}_i^{-1} \mathbf{y}_i \sim \mathcal{N}(\mathbf{C}_i^{-1} \mathbf{X}_i \boldsymbol{\beta}, \mathbf{I})$. This implies (e.g., Searle, 1971) that, under the null (5.84), the weighted sum of squares has χ^2-distribution, namely,

$$Q = \sum_{i=1}^{n} (\mathbf{y}_i - \mathbf{X}_i\widehat{\boldsymbol{\beta}}_0)'\mathbf{C}_i^{-1}(\mathbf{y}_i - \mathbf{X}_i\widehat{\boldsymbol{\beta}}_0) \sim \chi^2(\sum_{i=1}^{n} p_i - m).$$

Here $\sum_{i=1}^{n} p_i$ is the total number of observations and m is the dimension of beta coefficients.

Is the Q-test robust to the normality assumption? Here we derive the asymptotic distribution of the Q-statistic when $n \to \infty$, assuming that (a) components of vector $\mathbf{C}_i^{-1/2}\boldsymbol{\varepsilon}_i$ are independent and have identical symmetrical distributions with kurtosis κ, and (b) there exist positive a and A such that $a\mathbf{I} \le \mathbf{C}_i \le A\mathbf{I}$ for all $i = 1, 2, ...n \to \infty$. Then, as follows from Appendix 13.1.4, $Q \simeq \mathcal{N}\left(\sum_{i=1}^{n} p_i, (\kappa - 1)\sum_{i=1}^{n} p_i\right)$ when $n \to \infty$. The reader is referred to Figure 5.4, where critical values of the Q-statistic are shown for different values of kurtosis.

Problems for Section 5.3

1. Find the limit of the variance as a function of ρ in Figure 5.11 when $\rho \to 1$.

2. Prove that $\widehat{\boldsymbol{\beta}}$ converges to (5.65) when $\boldsymbol{\Omega} \to \infty$. Define the latter limit for $\boldsymbol{\Omega} = \eta\mathbf{D}$, where $\mathbf{D}$ is an arbitrary positive definite matrix and $\eta \to \infty$.

3*. Derive a sufficient condition for positive definiteness of the ML estimate for matrix $\boldsymbol{\Omega}$ similar to that for condition (5.18).

4. Derive the FS algorithms (5.75) and (5.76) for a special case when the multivariate model reduces to the univariate meta-analysis model and compare the formulas with (5.17) and (5.22), respectively.

5*. Write an R code for FS algorithms (5.75) and (5.76), and test them via simulations.

6. Prove that the multivariate meta-analysis formulas for the weighted and unweighted method of moments coincide with the estimators for the univariate meta-analysis model derived previously.

7*. Compare the performance of ML, RML, and MM estimators of $\boldsymbol{\Omega}$ and implied $\widehat{\boldsymbol{\beta}}$ using simulations. Is any of the methods superior to others in terms of beta estimation?

5.4   Summary points

- The meta-analysis model is perhaps the simplest random effects model designed to combine studies, provided that the outcome characteristic (such as treatment effect) and its variance are known from each study. Although strictly speaking, the meta-analysis model is not a special case of the linear mixed effects model because study-specific variances are known, it shares many properties.

- The key parameter in the meta-analysis model is the heterogeneity variance (parameter) σ^2. If studies estimate the treatment effect with the same precision (study-specific variances are the same) or studies are very heterogeneous (σ^2 is large), the best estimate is a simple average. If heterogeneity is small, the weighted average is better. The meta-analysis model (with a random effect) provides a compromise between those extreme estimates.

- One can use standard or restricted maximum likelihood estimation for σ^2 if it is believed that error terms have a normal distribution. Otherwise, distribution-free unbiased quadratic estimation can be used. It is shown that MINQUE for σ^2 is equivalent to the weighted method of moments estimator. It is assumed that the $\{y_i\}$ are normally distributed. We suggest the use of the restricted MLE if the number of studies is relatively small (say, $n < 20$).

- The estimator of the treatment effect is unbiased for any number of studies if an estimate of the heterogeneity variance is used, such as weighted or unweighted MM, ML, or RML. However, the distribution of the estimator is neither normal nor t. Although simulation studies confirm that the variance of the estimator is assessed fairly well, in a very small samples, say $n < 10$, one may find a better variance assessment that leads to a more precise coverage probability for confidence intervals and the significance level for hypothesis testing.

- The Q-test for homogeneity suggested by DerSimonian and Laird (1986) preforms well. This test is modified for nonnormal distributions, with a relatively large number of studies, using kurtosis. The homogeneity test is generalized to the multivariate meta-analysis model.

- The robust/median meta-analysis model assumes that the random effect has Laplace distribution with heavy tails. This model may be useful when studies are heterogeneous or in the presence of outlier(s). One may expect that this model increases the efficiency of estimation of the common treatment effect.

- The common treatment effect may be adjusted for study-specific covariates such as study latitude. This should be done with care because covariates can easily "eat up" the common treatment effect.

- The multivariate meta-analysis model may be applied when additional information on other characteristics with a complete covariance matrix for each study is available. If the characteristic of interest has considerable correlation with others and studies have different precision, some efficiency may be gained.

6
Nonlinear Marginal Model

In this chapter we generalize the linear mixed effects model to a nonlinear mixed model in which random effects enter the model in a linear fashion. This type of mixed model will be called *marginal*. Zeger et al. (1988) call such a model *population-averaged*. In a nonlinear marginal model, the mean and covariance matrix of the dependent variable are expressed *explicitly* through the parameter vector. Thus, unlike the nonlinear mixed effects model considered in the later chapters, estimation of the marginal model does not require integration.

A marginal model is suitable for a continuous dependent variable with the normal distribution as an obvious candidate. The marginal model may emerge in two situations: (a) when linear coefficients in a nonlinear model are random or (b) after an originally nonlinear random effects model is linearized (see the following chapters for detail). A marginal model can be viewed as a multivariate generalization of a regression model with heteroscedastic errors and a parametrically defined variance-covariance function, as described by Goldfeld and Quandt (1972), Davidian and Carroll (1987), Gallant (1987), and Carroll and Ruppert (1988). We distinguish two important types of nonlinear marginal models: (a) the matrix of random effects, $\mathbf{Z}_i$ is constant (does not depend on $\boldsymbol{\beta}$), and (b) the matrix $\mathbf{Z}_i$ is a function of $\boldsymbol{\beta}$. For the former model, *any* consistent estimator of the variance-covariance matrix of random effects produces an asymptotically efficient estimator of $\boldsymbol{\beta}$. For the latter model, however, this statement is not true, and only the straightforward maximum likelihood is efficient. Particularly in case (b), when the distribution is normal, iteratively reweighted nonlinear least squares, also known as extended generalized least squares, is less efficient than MLE. On the other hand, some authors have cautioned that MLE is not robust to a distribution misspecification—arguably a common objection against maximum likelihood. We compute the efficiency of the iteratively reweighted nonlinear least squares in logistic and Gompertz growth curve models with random parameters.

In this chapter we assume that the components of the error term, ε_i, are independent and have the same variance. First, it is quite straightforward to generalize the analysis to the case when components correlate (Section 4.3). Second, we caution the reader against overcomplication in the framework of nonlinear statistical models, especially in the presence of random effects.

Three types of nonlinear marginal models of increasing complexity are studied: the matrix of random effects is constant (type I), the matrix of random effects is parameter dependent (type II), and the most general case, the mean and covariance matrix are functions of the parameter vector (type III). At the end of the chapter we consider the total generalized estimating equations approach, which may be especially useful for estimation of the type III model.

6.1   Fixed matrix of random effects

A straightforward generalization of the linear mixed effects (LME) model in the Laird and Ware (1982) formulation, as defined by equation (2.5), would be to assume that the fixed effects are nonlinear functions of the population parameter $\boldsymbol{\beta}$; namely,

$$\mathbf{y}_i = \mathbf{f}_i(\boldsymbol{\beta}) + \mathbf{Z}_i \mathbf{b}_i + \boldsymbol{\varepsilon}_i, \quad i = 1, ..., N, \tag{6.1}$$

where $\mathbf{f}_i(\boldsymbol{\beta})$ is an $n_i \times 1$ nonlinear vector function. As in the LME model, we assume that the $k \times 1$ vector of random effects, $\mathbf{b}_i$, has a zero mean and a $k \times k$ covariance matrix, $\mathbf{D}_* = \sigma^2 \mathbf{D}$, and that the error term ε_i has a zero mean and a covariance matrix proportional to the $n_i \times n_i$ identity matrix, $\text{cov}(\boldsymbol{\varepsilon}_i) = \sigma^2 \mathbf{I}$. As before, we call σ^2 and $\mathbf{D}$ variance parameters. Note that for this model, the $n_i \times k$ matrix $\mathbf{Z}_i$ does not depend on parameter $\boldsymbol{\beta}$ and is fixed. In practice, explanatory variables/covariates, combined in matrix $\mathbf{X}_i$, are involved in the function $\mathbf{f}$, so we let $\mathbf{f}_i(\boldsymbol{\beta}) = \mathbf{f}(\mathbf{X}_i, \boldsymbol{\beta})$—a conventional notation of the nonlinear regression model (Gallant, 1987; Bates and Watts, 1988; Seber and Wild, 1989). Estimation of a nonlinear regression with variance components, which is a special case of model (6.1), was studied by Gumpertz and Pantula (1992). Clearly, the mixed model (6.1) collapses to (2.5) when $\mathbf{f}_i(\boldsymbol{\beta}) = \mathbf{X}_i \boldsymbol{\beta}$. We require model (6.1) to be mean identifiable: $\mathbf{f}_i(\boldsymbol{\beta}_1) = \mathbf{f}_i(\boldsymbol{\beta}_2)$ for all $i = 1, ..., N$ implies that $\boldsymbol{\beta}_1 = \boldsymbol{\beta}_2$. The LME is identifiable if the matrix composed of $\{\mathbf{X}_i\}$ has full rank.

The key characteristic of model (6.1) is that the random effects enter the model in a linear fashion. This model is called *marginal* because the marginal expected value of the response variable, $\mathbf{y}_i$ can be expressed in closed-form as a function of the population parameter $\boldsymbol{\beta}$, namely, $E(\mathbf{y}_i) = \mathbf{f}_i(\boldsymbol{\beta})$. Consequently, even a straightforward Nonlinear Least Squares (NLS), which minimizes the sum of squares

$$\sum_{i=1}^{N} \|\mathbf{y}_i - \mathbf{f}_i(\boldsymbol{\beta})\|^2, \tag{6.2}$$

produces a consistent estimator of $\boldsymbol{\beta}$ when $N \rightarrow \infty$ and $\{n_i\}$ are bounded. This follows from the fact that the corresponding estimating equation is unbiased,

$$E\left[\sum (\partial \mathbf{f}_i / \partial \boldsymbol{\beta})' (\mathbf{y}_i - \mathbf{f}_i(\boldsymbol{\beta}))\right] = \sum (\partial \mathbf{f}_i / \partial \boldsymbol{\beta})' E(\mathbf{y}_i - \mathbf{f}_i(\boldsymbol{\beta})) = \mathbf{0};$$

see Appendix 13.1.4 for detail.

In view of Section 3.6.2, we can take either a deterministic or a stochastic approach to the study of the asymptotic properties of mixed models. In the latter approach, we assume that $\mathbf{X}_i, \mathbf{Z}_i$,and n_i are random and identically distributed, so that the marginal model is written in conditional form as $\mathbf{y}_i|(\mathbf{X}_i, \mathbf{Z}_i, \mathbf{b}_i) = \mathbf{f}(\mathbf{X}_i, \boldsymbol{\beta}) + \mathbf{Z}_i\mathbf{b}_i + \boldsymbol{\varepsilon}_i$. The advantage of the stochastic approach is that we can refer to the standard theory of maximum likelihood, or M-estimation, and thus we do not have to prove that the estimates are consistent and asymptotically normally distributed. See detail in Section 3.6.2.

We apply marginal model (6.1) to data with a continuous dependent variable, $\mathbf{y}_i$, where the normal distribution of $\mathbf{b}_i$ and $\boldsymbol{\varepsilon}_i$, possibly after an appropriate transformation such as log, is a good candidate. Although the normal assumption is not necessary, estimates that are found from the weighted NLS would have optimal statistical properties (at least asymptotically) if the $\{\mathbf{y}_i\}$ have a normal distribution.

6.1.1 Log-likelihood function

If $\boldsymbol{\varepsilon}_i$ and $\mathbf{b}_i$ are normally distributed, the marginal model (6.1) can be written compactly as

$$\mathbf{y}_i \sim \mathcal{N}\left(\mathbf{f}_i(\boldsymbol{\beta}),\sigma^2(\mathbf{I} + \mathbf{Z}_i\mathbf{D}\mathbf{Z}_i')\right), \quad i = 1, ..., N \tag{6.3}$$

with the log-likelihood function, up to a constant term $-(N_T/2)\ln(2\pi)$,

$$l(\boldsymbol{\theta}) = -\frac{1}{2}\left\{N_T \ln\sigma^2 + \sum_{i=1}^{N}\left[\ln|\mathbf{I} + \mathbf{Z}_i\mathbf{D}\mathbf{Z}_i'|\right.\right.$$
$$\left.\left.+\sigma^{-2}(\mathbf{y}_i - \mathbf{f}_i(\boldsymbol{\beta}))'(\mathbf{I} + \mathbf{Z}_i\mathbf{D}\mathbf{Z}_i')^{-1}(\mathbf{y}_i - \mathbf{f}_i(\boldsymbol{\beta}))\right]\right\}, \tag{6.4}$$

where, similar to (2.15), $\boldsymbol{\theta} = (\boldsymbol{\beta}, \sigma^2, \text{vech}(\mathbf{D}))$ is the complete vector of parameters. The information matrix for the nonlinear model (6.3) for $\boldsymbol{\theta}$ has a block diagonal form,

$$\mathcal{I} = \begin{bmatrix} \sum_{i=1}^{N}\left(\frac{\partial\mathbf{f}_i}{\partial\boldsymbol{\beta}}\right)'\mathbf{V}_i^{-1}\left(\frac{\partial\mathbf{f}_i}{\partial\boldsymbol{\beta}}\right) & \mathbf{0} \\ \mathbf{0} & \mathbf{H} \end{bmatrix},$$

where the $(1 + k(k+1)/2) \times (1 + k(k+1)/2)$ matrix,

$$\mathbf{H} = \frac{1}{2}\sum_{i=1}^{N}\begin{bmatrix} n_i\sigma^{-4} & \sigma^{-2}\text{vec}'(\mathbf{R}_i)\mathcal{D}^{+'} \\ \sigma^{-2}\mathcal{D}^+\text{vec}(\mathbf{R}_i) & \mathcal{D}^+(\mathbf{R}_i \otimes \mathbf{R}_i)\mathcal{D}^{+'} \end{bmatrix}, \tag{6.5}$$

is the expected Hessian (information) matrix for variance parameters, and the dimension-reduction formulas of Section 2.2.3 apply:

$$\mathbf{V}_i = \mathbf{I} + \mathbf{Z}_i\mathbf{D}\mathbf{Z}_i', \quad \mathbf{V}_i^{-1} = \mathbf{I} - \mathbf{Z}_i(\mathbf{D}^{-1}+\mathbf{Z}_i'\mathbf{Z}_i)^{-1}\mathbf{Z}_i',$$
$$\mathbf{R}_i = \mathbf{Z}_i(\mathbf{I} + \mathbf{Z}_i\mathbf{D}\mathbf{Z}_i')^{-1}\mathbf{Z}_i' = \left((\mathbf{Z}_i'\mathbf{Z}_i)^{-1} + \mathbf{D}\right)^{-1}.$$

Note that the right-hand sides are valid if the matrices $\mathbf{D}$ and $\mathbf{Z}_i'\mathbf{Z}_i$ are invertible. The asymptotic covariance matrix for $\boldsymbol{\theta}$ is the inverse of $\mathcal{I}$.

One may obtain a variance-profile likelihood, as in Section 2.2.4,

$$l_p(\boldsymbol{\beta}, \mathbf{D}) = -0.5\{N_T \ln\sum(\mathbf{y}_i - \mathbf{f}_i(\boldsymbol{\beta}))'\mathbf{V}_i^{-1}(\mathbf{y}_i - \mathbf{f}_i(\boldsymbol{\beta})) + \sum\ln|\mathbf{V}_i|\} \tag{6.6}$$

because when $\boldsymbol{\beta}$ and $\mathbf{D}$ are held fixed, the log-likelihood maximum is attained at $\sigma^2 = (N_T)^{-1} \sum (\mathbf{y}_i - \mathbf{f}_i(\boldsymbol{\beta}))' \mathbf{V}_i^{-1} (\mathbf{y}_i - \mathbf{f}_i(\boldsymbol{\beta}))$. Since the information matrix, $\mathcal{I}$, has a block diagonal form, we may maximize l over $\boldsymbol{\beta}$ and the variance parameters separately (at least in a large sample the cross-derivatives of l are close to zero). Thus, the maximum likelihood estimate can be found using the following algorithm:

1. Set $\mathbf{D}_0 = \mathbf{0}$ and apply nonlinear least squares, (6.2), to find $\widehat{\boldsymbol{\beta}}_0$ and compute the residuals $\widehat{\mathbf{e}}_i = \mathbf{y}_i - \mathbf{f}_i(\widehat{\boldsymbol{\beta}}_0)$.

2. Find estimates for σ^2 and $\mathbf{D}$ by iterating until convergence,

$$\left[\begin{array}{c} \sigma^2 \\ \text{vech}(\mathbf{D}) \end{array} \right]_{s+1} = \left[\begin{array}{c} \sigma^2 \\ \text{vech}(\mathbf{D}) \end{array} \right]_s + \lambda_s \mathbf{H}_s^{-1} \left[\begin{array}{c} \partial l / \partial \sigma^2 \\ \text{vech}(\partial l / \partial \mathbf{D}) \end{array} \right],$$

where s is the iteration index and λ_s is a positive step length (typically $\lambda_s = 1$). Matrix $\mathbf{H}$ is defined by (6.5), and the derivatives of l with respect to the variance parameters are given by

$$\frac{\partial l}{\partial \sigma^2} = -\frac{1}{2} N_T \sigma^{-2} + \frac{1}{2} \sigma^{-4} \sum \mathbf{e}_i' \mathbf{V}_i^{-1} \mathbf{e}_i, \tag{6.7}$$

$$\frac{\partial l}{\partial \mathbf{D}} = -\frac{1}{2} \sum [\mathbf{Z}_i' \mathbf{V}_i^{-1} \mathbf{Z}_i - \sigma^{-2} \mathbf{Z}_i' \mathbf{V}_i^{-1} \mathbf{e}_i \mathbf{e}_i' \mathbf{V}_i^{-1} \mathbf{Z}_i] \tag{6.8}$$

for $\mathbf{e}_i = \widehat{\mathbf{e}}_i$, as in Section 2.9.

3. Find the weighted NLS solution, $\widehat{\boldsymbol{\beta}}_1$, to

$$\sum_{i=1}^{N} (\mathbf{y}_i - \mathbf{f}_i(\boldsymbol{\beta}))' (\mathbf{I} + \mathbf{Z}_i \mathbf{D} \mathbf{Z}_i')^{-1} (\mathbf{y}_i - \mathbf{f}_i(\boldsymbol{\beta})) = \min_{\boldsymbol{\beta}} \tag{6.9}$$

where $\mathbf{D} = \widehat{\mathbf{D}}$ from step 2. Compute $\widehat{\mathbf{e}}_i = \mathbf{y}_i - \mathbf{f}_i(\widehat{\boldsymbol{\beta}}_1)$.

4. Return to step 2 if the convergence criterion is not met.

We make several comments. First, we may start not from zero ($\mathbf{D}_0 = \mathbf{0}$) but from some other reasonable estimate of $\mathbf{D}$, such as the method of moments or variance least squares estimate of $\mathbf{D}$, considered in the next section. Second, we may try several step lengths, λ_s, to ensure that the log-likelihood function increases from iteration to iteration. We know that if the gradient is not zero, a positive λ exists that increases the log-likelihood function value since matrix $\mathbf{H}^{-1}$ is positive definite (Ortega and Rheinboldt, 1970). Third, the weighted nonlinear least squares, (6.9), may be reduced to standard nonlinear least squares by replacing $\widetilde{\mathbf{y}}_i = \mathbf{R}_i \mathbf{y}_i$ and $\widetilde{\mathbf{f}}_i(\boldsymbol{\beta}) = \mathbf{R}_i \mathbf{f}_i(\boldsymbol{\beta})$, where $\mathbf{R}_i$ is the $n_i \times n_i$ Cholesky decomposition matrix, $\mathbf{R}_i' \mathbf{R}_i = (\mathbf{I} + \mathbf{Z}_i \widehat{\mathbf{D}}_s \mathbf{Z}_i')^{-1}$. Fourth, step 2 may be accomplished using standard LME software, i.e., lme with zero fixed effects. Finally, the MLE may be obtained by calling the R function nlme because it uses the Laplace approximation, which is exact for linear random effects with a fixed matrix $\mathbf{Z}_i$. See detail in Section 8.8. We discuss the maximum likelihood estimation within a more general framework of total GEE in Section 6.4.

6.1.2   nls function in R

In this section we describe how to run nonlinear regression using the `nls` function in R. The purpose of the code below is to illustrate how the weighted NLS problem can be reduced to the regular NLS problem and how to keep running R in the case on an error returned by the `nls` function.

We are concerned with estimation of the Michaelis-Menten nonlinear regression problem (Bates and Watts, 1988),

$$y_i = \frac{\beta_1 x_i}{\beta_2 + x_i} + \varepsilon_i, \quad i = 1, 2, ..., n \tag{6.10}$$

where the ε_i have zero mean and constant variance. As we know, the choice of the starting values for parameters may be crucial. For model (6.10), we can derive starting values by multiplying both sides of the equation by $\beta_2 + x_i$ and dividing by x_i to reduce the heterogeneity. Specifically, the starting values for β_1 and β_2 are found from the linear least squares by regressing y_i on $-y_i/x_i$ with the estimate of β_1 as the intercept and the estimate of β_2 as the slope.

The function `nlsMM` runs `nExp` simulations with the starting values specified above; the true parameter values are `b1=1` and `b2`. It is assumed that errors are correlated with the $n \times n$ covariance matrix $\mathbf{W} = \mathbf{I} + \theta \mathbf{1} \mathbf{1}'$, where $\mathbf{1}$ is the $n \times 1$ vector of ones. The criterion to minimize with respect to β_1 and β_2 is the weighted nonlinear least squares,

$$\left(\mathbf{y} - \frac{\beta_1}{\beta_2 + \mathbf{x}} \right)' (\mathbf{I} + \theta \mathbf{1} \mathbf{1}')^{-1} \left(\mathbf{y} - \frac{\beta_1}{\beta_2 + \mathbf{x}} \right), \tag{6.11}$$

where θ is a fixed parameter ($\theta + 1/n > 0$). The function returns a matrix of estimates with `nExp` rows and two columns. When iterations do not converge, the row is `NA`. The condition on the lack of convergency is extracted via `attr` to the output of the `nls` call.

```
nlsMM=function(b1=1,b2=2,n=10,sigma=.5,theta=.3,nExp=1000)
{
dump("nlsMM","c:\\MixedModels\\Chapter06\\nlsMM.r")
MMw=function(x,a1,a2,chW) # weighted Michaelis-Menten model
{
    fx=a1*x/(a2+x)
    return(chW%*%fx)
}
x=1:n; un=rep(1,n)
W=diag(rep(1,n),n,n)+theta*un%*%t(un)
iW=solve(W); chW=chol(W) # Cholesky decomposition
apar=matrix(ncol=2,nrow=nExp)
```

```
for(iexp in 1:nExp)
{
    y=b1*x/(b2+x)+rnorm(n,mean=0,sd=sigma)
    z=-y/x
    olm=lm(y~z) # starting values
    yc=chW%*%y # transform y vector
    onls <- try(nls(yc~MMw(x=x,b1,b2,chW=chW),
        start=list(b1=coef(olm)[1],b2=coef(olm)[2]),
        control = list(maxiter = 500))))
    if(attr(onls,"class")!="try-error")
        apar[iexp,]=summary(onls)$coefficients[,1]
}
return(apar)
}
```

The `nls` function has several parameters to control. In this particular example, only the maximum number of iterations is specified; other parameters for controls are the tolerance criterion, `tol`, and `minFactor` which specifies the minimum reduction step length in the Gauss-Newton algorithm, λ_s, in the equation below. The key to the weighted nonlinear least squares is factorization of matrix $(\mathbf{I}+\theta\mathbf{1}\mathbf{1}')^{-1}$ via the product of two triangular matrices using Cholesky decomposition, $(\mathbf{I}+\theta\mathbf{1}\mathbf{1}')^{-1} = \mathbf{C}'\mathbf{C}$, where $\mathbf{C}$ is the upper triangular matrix (the function `chol`). Indeed, criterion (6.11) can be rewritten as the regular sum of squares $\left\|\widetilde{\mathbf{y}} - \widetilde{\mathbf{f}}(\beta_1,\beta_2)\right\|^2$, where $\widetilde{\mathbf{y}} = \mathbf{C}\mathbf{y}$ and $\widetilde{\mathbf{f}}(\beta_1,\beta_2) = \mathbf{C}\mathbf{f}(\beta_1,\beta_2)$.

6.1.3 Computational issues of nonlinear least squares

Unweighted (6.2) or weighted (6.9) nonlinear least squares may lead to a difficult numerical problem. In this subsection we discuss briefly possible complications that may be encountered in practice.

The main minimization algorithm for (6.9) takes the form

$$
\beta_{s+1} = \beta_s + \lambda_s \left(\sum_{i=1}^{N} \mathbf{F}_i' \mathbf{V}_i^{-1} \mathbf{F}_i + \mu_s \mathbf{J}_s \right)^{-1} \left(\sum_{i=1}^{N} \mathbf{F}_i' \mathbf{V}_i^{-1} (\mathbf{y}_i - \mathbf{f}_i(\beta_s)) \right),
$$

where λ_s is the step length, μ_s is a positive regularization parameter, $\mathbf{J}_s$ is a positive definite regularization matrix, and $\mathbf{F}_i = \partial\mathbf{f}_i/\partial\beta$ is the $n_i \times m$ matrix of derivatives. When $\lambda_s = 1$ and $\mu_s = 0$, we come to the popular Gauss–Newton algorithm (Seber and Wild, 1989). Sometimes the unit step does not reduce the sum of squares and a lesser value should be tried. A popular procedure is to halve the step length until the sum of squares becomes less than at the previous iteration, as discussed in Section 2.8. Hartley (1961) suggested using a quadratic interpolation to find λ. Due to multicollinearity, the optimization problem may become ill-conditioned and the matrix $\sum \mathbf{F}_i' \mathbf{V}_i^{-1} \mathbf{F}_i$ may become deficient. To avoid the ill-conditioned matrix inversion

Levenberg (1944) and Marquardt (1963) suggested a positive regularization parameter, μ_s. Levenberg takes $\mathbf{J}_s = \mathbf{I}$, and Marquardt takes $\mathbf{J}_s = \text{diag}(\sum \mathbf{F}_i' \mathbf{V}_i^{-1} \mathbf{F}_i)$. According to Marquardt, the regularization parameter should approach zero as the iterations converge.

Two major problems may emerge in nonlinear least squares and, generally, in nonquadratic optimization:

- *Nonexistence of the minimum.* The absolute minimum may not be attainable if the optimization problem has no solution. The necessary and sufficient condition for the existence of the MLE in the LME model is developed in Section 2.5 and for the binary model in Section 7.10. Demidenko (1989, 1996) provided a general approach for the construction of sufficient criteria for the least squares estimate in a nonlinear regression model that may also be applied to NLS, (6.2), or weighted NLS, (6.9).

- *Many local minima.* Nonlinear least squares may find only one local minimum among several. To construct a criterion that would determine whether the minimum found is the global one is a difficult mathematical problem. Demidenko (2000) outlined several approaches to this problem. Good practical advice is to start iterations from a different value to see whether they converge to the same solution.

See Appendix 13.3 for a general discussion of the optimization problem, including criteria for convergence.

6.1.4 Distribution-free estimation

Here we generalize the method of moments (MM) of Section 3.11 and the variance least squares of Section 3.12 to the nonlinear marginal model (6.1). Recall that MM does not require the normal assumption.

Pooled variance estimator for σ^2

Since for model (6.1) $\mathbf{f}_i(\boldsymbol{\beta})$ plays the role of $\mathbf{X}_i\boldsymbol{\beta}$, to generalize the pooled variance estimator/MINQUE (3.81), we find the minimum,

$$S_{\min} = \min_{\boldsymbol{\beta}, \boldsymbol{\gamma}_1, \dots, \boldsymbol{\gamma}_N} \sum_{i=1}^{N} \|\mathbf{y}_i - \mathbf{f}_i(\boldsymbol{\beta}) - \mathbf{Z}_i \boldsymbol{\gamma}_i\|^2, \qquad (6.12)$$

treating $\{\boldsymbol{\gamma}_i\}$ as nuisance parameters, as in the fixed effects approach. See Section 2.2.3 for details. This minimum may be reduced to a standard nonlinear regression problem after the residual transformation

$$\widetilde{\mathbf{y}}_i = (\mathbf{I} - \mathbf{Z}_i \mathbf{Z}_i^+)\mathbf{y}_i, \quad \widetilde{\mathbf{f}}_i(\boldsymbol{\beta}) = (\mathbf{I} - \mathbf{Z}_i \mathbf{Z}_i^+)\mathbf{f}_i(\boldsymbol{\beta}),$$

where $\mathbf{Z}_i^+$ is the general matrix inverse to $\mathbf{Z}_i$. If $\mathbf{Z}_i$ has full rank, then $\mathbf{Z}_i^+ = (\mathbf{Z}_i'\mathbf{Z})^{-1}\mathbf{Z}_i'$. Then, in terms of residuals,

$$S_{\min} = \min_{\boldsymbol{\beta}} \sum_{i=1}^{N} \left\|\widetilde{\mathbf{y}}_i - \widetilde{\mathbf{f}}_i(\boldsymbol{\beta})\right\|^2 = \min_{\boldsymbol{\beta}} \left\|\widetilde{\mathbf{y}} - \widetilde{\mathbf{f}}(\boldsymbol{\beta})\right\|^2, \qquad (6.13)$$

where $\widetilde{\mathbf{y}} = (\widetilde{\mathbf{y}}_1, ..., \widetilde{\mathbf{y}}_N)'$ and $\widetilde{\mathbf{f}} = (\widetilde{\mathbf{f}}_1, ..., \widetilde{\mathbf{f}}_N)'$. Now we need to find the degrees of freedom (d.f.), the denominator of (3.79). There is no unique way to do this for a nonlinear model. First, we may set d.f. $= N_T - m - \mathrm{rank}(\mathbf{Z})$, where the $N_T \times Nk$ block diagonal matrix $\mathbf{Z}$ is defined as in (2.9), and in the previous notation $N_T = \sum_{i=1}^{N} n_i$, the total number of observations. Second, we may set d.f. $= N_T - \mathrm{rank}(\mathbf{W})$, where the matrix $\mathbf{X}$ is replaced by $\partial \mathbf{f}/\partial \boldsymbol{\beta}$ evaluated at $\widehat{\boldsymbol{\beta}}_0$ or where $S_{\min}$ is attained, and the matrix $\mathbf{W}$ is defined as in (2.34). Finally, the pooled variance for model (6.1) is given by

$$\widehat{\sigma}^2 = \frac{S_{\min}}{\mathrm{d.f.}}. \tag{6.14}$$

Obviously, this estimator is not unbiased for a nonlinear model. However, it collapses to its linear prototype if the $\{\mathbf{f}_i\}$ are linear functions.

Method of moments for $\mathbf{D}$

Now we generalize the method of moments of Section 3.11 to the nonlinear marginal model (6.1). We use the asymptotic MM (AMM) estimator (3.104) because the unbiased MM estimator essentially requires linearity of $\mathbf{f}_i$. As before, we start with the nonlinear least squares (6.2) and residuals $\widehat{\mathbf{e}}_i = \mathbf{y} - \mathbf{f}_i(\widehat{\boldsymbol{\beta}}_0)$. Then we "estimate" the random effects as $\widehat{\mathbf{b}}_i = \mathbf{Z}_i^+ \mathbf{e}_i$, and using the estimator (6.14), we arrive at

$$\widehat{\mathbf{D}}_{*AMM} = \frac{1}{N} \sum_{i=1}^{N} \widehat{\mathbf{b}}_i \widehat{\mathbf{b}}_i' - \widehat{\sigma}^2 \frac{1}{N} \sum_{i=1}^{N} (\mathbf{Z}_i' \mathbf{Z}_i)^{-1}. \tag{6.15}$$

Under mild assumptions it is possible to prove that this estimator is consistent and asymptotically normally distributed. Vonesh and Carter (1992) used a special MM estimator of matrix $\mathbf{D}$ for model (6.1) in the form (4.40).

Variance least squares for $\mathbf{D}$

It is straightforward to apply the variance least squares (VLS) of Section 3.12 to a nonlinear model. Indeed, if $\widehat{\mathbf{e}}_i$ is the residual vector, we use the same formula, (3.108), which gives an estimate for σ^2 and $\mathrm{vec}(\mathbf{D}_*)$.

6.1.5 Testing for the presence of random effects

This essential type of testing translates into the statistical hypothesis $H_0 : \mathbf{D} = \mathbf{0}$. In Section 3.5 an exact F-test based on statistic (3.42) was developed for the linear mixed effects model. Although we cannot generalize that result to the nonlinear model (6.1), we may compute analogs of S_{OLS} and $S_{\min}$ and apply (3.42), where r may be set to either $m - \mathrm{rank}(\mathbf{Z})$ or $\mathrm{rank}(\mathbf{W})$, as in Section 6.1.4. For model (6.1), S_{OLS} is the minimum of (6.2), and $S_{\min}$ is given by (6.12) or (6.13). Apparently, the test should work well if the $\mathbf{f}_i$ are not too nonlinear. We illustrate this test in Section 6.1.7.

6.1.6 Asymptotic properties

Unlike in the LME model, $\boldsymbol{\beta}$-estimates of model (6.1) are biased in small samples even if matrix $\mathbf{D}$ is known due to the nonlinearity of the $\mathbf{f}_i$. However, they are asymptotically unbiased, and the bias vanishes when the sample size increases to infinity. Furthermore, the asymptotic properties of the nonlinear marginal mixed effects model with a fixed matrix of random effects, (6.1), are similar to those of the LME model (2.5):

- Nonlinear least squares, which minimizes (6.2), leads to a consistent and asymptotically normally distributed estimate.

- Any weighted nonlinear least squares estimate (6.9), with a fixed matrix $\mathbf{D}$, is consistent and asymptotically normally distributed.

- The MM and VLS estimators of matrix $\mathbf{D}$ in the weighted least squares estimate, (6.9), both produce an asymptotic distribution of $\widehat{\boldsymbol{\beta}}$ equivalent to that produced using the true matrix $\mathbf{D}$.

In addition, if $\boldsymbol{\varepsilon}_i$ and $\mathbf{b}_i$ are normally distributed:

- The maximum likelihood estimates of $\boldsymbol{\beta}$ and the variance parameters are asymptotically independent because the information matrix has a block diagonal form.

- Use of MM or VLS estimates of matrix $\mathbf{D}$ in (6.9) leads to $\boldsymbol{\beta}$ estimates asymptotically equivalent to the MLE.

Again, these properties are particularly easy to prove under the stochastic scheme because then the $\{\mathbf{y}_i\}$ are iid and we can use M-estimation theory. Asymptotic study of $\widehat{\boldsymbol{\beta}}$ under the deterministic scheme, when n_i is bounded and $N \to \infty$, was conducted by Vonesh and Carter (1992).

6.1.7   Example: log-Gompertz growth curve

In this subsection we illustrate estimation of the nonlinear marginal model with a fixed matrix of random effects by the Gompertz growth curve, $Y(t) = Ae^{-e^{b-ct}}$, where t denotes time and Y is the growth characteristic, such as height or volume. With a Gompertzian growth curve, the growth is limited (with exponential growth there is no such limitation). Parameter A is the maximum limit of $Y(t)$ when t increases to infinity. Parameter b determines the value of Y at $t = 0$, namely, $Y(0) = Ae^{-e^{-b}}$, and parameter c determines the rate at which $Y(t)$ approaches A.

There is a well-established theory of *monotonic* growth modeled via growth curves, such as exponential, logistic, or Gompertz. For a complete review of growth curves in a statistical framework, the reader is referred to Seber and Wild (1989). For numerous mathematical derivations based on differential equation theory, the reader is referred to Banks (1994). Specifically, in this section, we are concerned with the modeling of *tumor growth*. Many studies indicate that the Gompertz curve introduced in 1825 is an adequate model for tumor size/volume growth of untreated tumors *in vitro* and *in vivo* (Norton and Simon, 1977; Heitjan, 1991; Bassukas, 1994; Bajzer and Vuk-Pavlovic, 1997; Ferrante et al., 2000). Note, in Chapter 10 we develop a theory of regrowth for treated tumors that describes nonmonotonic growth.

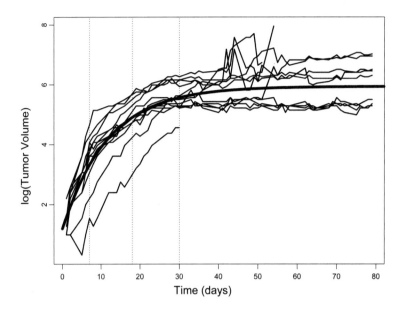

FIGURE 6.1. Growth trajectories of 12 polyclonal unperturbed multicellular tumor spheroids, Chignola et al. (1999). Apparently, each spheroid has its own growth pattern. Clearly, the tumor volume limit is a tumor-specific parameter. Thus, the log-Gompertz random intercept model would be appropriate. The bold curve is derived from maximum likelihood; the three vertical dotted lines correspond to three critical points of Gompertzian growth.

We use data on the growth of multicellular tumor spheroids (MTSs) that comprise three-dimensional aggregates of cancer cells, that have been grown under controlled conditions, as described by Chignola et al. (1999). See Figure 6.1. MTS represent a tumor model with an intermediate complexity between standard two-dimensional monolayer cultures *in vitro* and tumors *in vivo*. They approximate many biological characteristics of micrometastasis regions of larger cancer tumors. In previous work, the parameters of the Gompertzian curve were estimated by nonlinear least squares, either applied to individual growth data, as in Chignola et al. (1999), or averaged over individuals. In the former case, it is hard to come to a conclusive decision because the number of estimates is equal to the number of individual tumors. In the latter case one implicitly assumes that all tumors have the same parameters. A mixed effects model, where some parameters may be tumor-specific (random), seems to be a good compromise between these two approaches.

To set up a statistical model for the Gompertz curve, we use equivalent parameterization in the form $Y(t) = e^{\beta_1 - \beta_2 e^{-\beta_3 t}}$, where $A = e^{\beta_1}, b = \ln \beta_2$ and $c = \beta_3$. It is reasonable to assume that the accuracy of the tumor volume measurements is proportional to the value of the tumor volume. Therefore, a multiplicative error leads to the statistical model $y = \beta_1 - \beta_2 e^{-\beta_3 t} + \varepsilon$, where $y = \ln Y$ and ε is the error term. As shown in Figure 6.1, spheroids have different volume limits, so it is adequate to assume that parameter β_1 is tumor-specific but that $\beta_2 > 0$ and $\beta_3 > 0$ are constant across spheroids (population-averaged parameters). These assumptions lead to the *log-Gompertz random intercept* growth curve model,

$$y_{ij} = (\beta_1 + b_i) - \beta_2 e^{-\beta_3 t_{ij}} + \varepsilon_{ij}, \ j = 1, ..., n_i, \tag{6.16}$$

where the $\{\varepsilon_{ij}\}$ are iid normally distributed random variables with zero mean and constant variance σ^2, and the $\{b_i\}$ are iid normally distributed random effects with zero mean and variance $d_* = \sigma^2 d$, $i = 1, ..., N$. In this model $\beta_1 + b_i$ corresponds to the individual tumor volume limit, $\beta_1 + b_i - \beta_2$ corresponds to the ith spheroid initial tumor volume (at time zero, on the log scale), and β_3 is the rate at which tumor volume approaches its limit. Denoting $\mathbf{t}_i = (t_{i1}, t_{i2}, ..., t_{in_i})'$, model (6.16) takes the form (6.1) with $\boldsymbol{\beta} = (\beta_1, \beta_2, \beta_3)'$, $\mathbf{f}_i(\boldsymbol{\beta}) = \beta_1 - \beta_2 e^{-\beta_3 \mathbf{t}_i}$, and $\mathbf{Z}_i = \mathbf{1}_i$, so that $\text{cov}(\mathbf{y}_i) = \sigma^2(\mathbf{I} + d\mathbf{1}_i\mathbf{1}_i')$. It is of great interest to test whether other parameters do not change from spheroid to spheroid (population-averaged) due to genetic inheritance. In Section 6.4.5, we continue this example with a more complicated model that involves a subject-specific/random coefficient at $e^{-\beta_3 t_{ij}}$ without assuming that the distribution is normal.

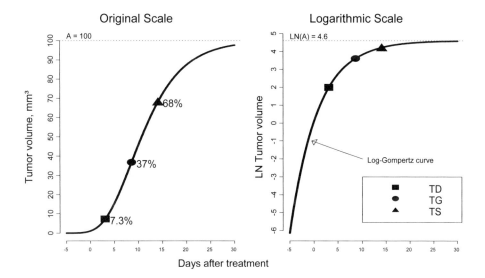

FIGURE 6.2. Three critical points on the Gompertz curve for tumor spheroids. The Gompertz curve on the original scale is S-shaped and has a regular increasing-concave character on the logarithmic scale. By day 3, when the tumor volume is 7.3% of the maximum, the tumor vasculature is completed and the tumor starts growing rapidly with the maximum rate at 37% of the maximum volume. When the tumor reaches 68%, the growth slows down.

In the R function that floows we show the R function `logG`, which reads the data on 12 tumor spheroids and runs nlme using a log-Gompertz curve with random intercept (6.16). This function requires two libraries: `nlme` and `lattice`. The former is needed for nonlinear mixed effects model estimation, and the latter, for individual log tumor volume spheroid plots.

```
logG=function()
{
dump("logG","c:\\MixedModels\\Chapter06\\logG.r")
library(nlme);library(lattice)
dat=read.csv("c:\\MixedModels\\Chapter06\\TUMspher.txt")
xyplot(lntumvol~day|id,type="b",data=dat)
out.nlme<-nlme(lntumvol~a1-a2*exp(-a3*day),fixed=a1+a2+a3~1,
    random=a1~1|id, data=dat,start=c(6,5,0.07))
summary(out.nlme)
}
```

This function is used in one of the problems at the end of this section.

Three critical points on the Gompertz curve

Three critical time points on the Gompertz curve and corresponding growth phases of the tumor growth *in vivo* may be distinguished: (a) tumor development/slow growth that covers the period from when the first clonogenic cell divides until the tumor vasculature is completed, T_D; (b) aggressive tumor growth, T_G; and (c) slowed growth due to the limited supply of oxygen, nutrients, and space, T_S (see Figure 6.2). Below, we define these three time points mathematically via derivatives.

Derivation of T_D, T_G, and T_S. The time of maximum growth occurs when the first derivative, dY/dt, attains its maximum, i.e., when the second derivative vanishes. Since $d^2Y/dt^2 = Ac^2e^{b-ct-e^{b-ct}}(e^{b-ct} - 1)$, we find that the second derivative turns zero when $b - ct = 0$, which means that the maximum rate of growth occurs at time $T_G = b/c$. Evaluating $Y(T_G)$, we infer that the maximum growth occurs when the tumor reaches 37% of its maximum limit, A, because $Y(b/c) = A/e = 0.37A$. The times when slow growth changes to rapid growth and when rapid growth changes back to slow growth correspond to time points where the third derivative of the Gompertz curve vanishes. Since

$$\frac{d^3Y}{dt^3} = Ac^3e^{b-ct-e^{b-ct}}(1 - 3e^{b-ct} + e^{2(b-ct)}),$$

denoting $z = e^{b-ct}$, we conclude that the third derivative turns zero (inflection point) when the quadratic equation $1 - 3z + z^2 = 0$. Thus we obtain $z_{1,2} = (3 \pm \sqrt{5})/2$. Solving for t, we infer that $d^3Y/dt^3 = 0$ when $T_D = (b - \ln[(3 + \sqrt{5})/2])/c = (b - 0.962)/c$, which occurs when the tumor volume reaches $Y(T_D) = 0.073A$, and $T_S = (b - \ln[(3 - \sqrt{5})/2])/c = (b + 0.962)/c$ when the tumor volume reaches $0.68A$.

The tumor grows relatively slowly before reaching about 7.3% of its maximum limit, A. From day T_D to day $T_S = (b + 0.962)/c$, the Gompertzian tumor grows rapidly before reaching 68% of its maximum, which corresponds to the second inflection point of the growth. Maximum growth occurs at day $T_G = b/c$ when the tumor reaches 37% of its maximum, which corresponds mathematically to the inflection point of the tumor volume (second derivative is zero). These three critical time points of Gompertzian growth (especially T_D) may provide a guideline for treatment timing. Modeling of a post-treatment tumor is covered in Chapter 10.

Starting values for the Gompertz curve

Every iterative nonlinear optimization problem requires a starting value. A bad starting value may lead to computer overflow and failure to converge. Here we provide a three-point solution to the log-Gompertz curve $y_t = \beta_1 - \beta_2 e^{-\beta_3 t}$, $t = 1, 2, ..., n$. We divide the observation period into three equal-length intervals so that p is the average time point of the first interval, $p + a$ is the average time point of the second interval, and $p + 2a$ is the average time point of the third interval, where $a = n/3$ is the length of each interval. Then we compute y-averages within each interval, $\overline{y}_1, \overline{y}_2, \overline{y}_3$. We find rough estimates of the beta parameters from the condition that the log-Gompertz curve passes through three points $(p + ka, \overline{y}_{k+1})$, $k = 0, 1, 2$. Solving these three equations yields

$$\widehat{\beta}_3 = \frac{1}{a} \ln \frac{\overline{y}_2 - \overline{y}_1}{\overline{y}_3 - \overline{y}_2}, \ \widehat{\beta}_2 = \frac{\overline{y}_2 - \overline{y}_1}{e^{-\widehat{\beta}_3 p} - e^{-\widehat{\beta}_3 (p+a)}}, \ \widehat{\beta}_1 = \frac{\overline{y}_2 - \overline{y}_1 e^{-\widehat{\beta}_3 a}}{1 - e^{-\widehat{\beta}_3 a}}.$$

If all observation points fall on a log-Gompertz curve, these formulas give the exact solution. Otherwise, these starting values may fail, e.g., one may get a negative value under the logarithm or negative parameters, and these starting values do not guarantee convergence. These starting values, applied to the average growth, $\overline{y}_t$ are presented in Table 6.1. The maximum likelihood estimation by the expected Newton–Raphson algorithm is described in Section 6.4.5.

Method of moments

We start computing the pooled variance estimate by finding the minimum, (6.13). Since $\mathbf{Z}_i = \mathbf{1}_i$, we have $\widetilde{\mathbf{y}}_i = \mathbf{y}_i - \overline{y}_i$ and $\widetilde{\mathbf{f}}_i = \widetilde{\mathbf{f}}_i(\beta_2, \beta_3) = \beta_2 (\sum_{j=1}^{n_i} e^{-\beta_3 t_{ij}} - e^{-\beta_3 \mathbf{t}_i})$. Applying nonlinear least squares to these data, we obtain $S_{\min} = 93.56$. We use the second way to compute the degrees of freedom, which gives $\widehat{\sigma}^2 = 0.16$. The AMM estimate for d_* is defined by formula (6.15), where for the log-Gompertz random-intercept model, $\widehat{\mathbf{b}}_i = n_i^{-1} \sum_{j=1}^{n_i} \widehat{e}_{ij}$ and $\mathbf{Z}_i' \mathbf{Z}_i = n_i$. Knowing that $\widehat{d} = \widehat{d}_*/\widehat{\sigma}^2$, we apply the weighted nonlinear least squares (6.9) with the weight matrix $(\mathbf{I} + \widehat{d} \mathbf{1}_i \mathbf{1}_i')^{-1} = \mathbf{I} - \widehat{d}/(1 + n_i \widehat{d}) \mathbf{1}_i \mathbf{1}_i'$.

Variance least squares

Let $\widehat{\mathbf{e}}_i$ be the nonlinear least squares residuals. Then according to (3.108), the estimates for σ^2 and d_* are the solution to

$$\begin{bmatrix} \sum n_i & \sum n_i \\ \sum n_i & \sum n_i^2 \end{bmatrix} \begin{bmatrix} \sigma^2 \\ d \end{bmatrix} = \begin{bmatrix} \sum \|\widehat{\mathbf{e}}_i\|^2 \\ \sum (\widehat{\mathbf{e}}_i' \mathbf{1}_i)^2 \end{bmatrix}.$$

Statistical testing of the random effect

For our example, the left-hand side of (3.42) is 93, and the critical value of the F-statistic with $\alpha = 5\%$, and $14 - 3 = 11$ and $590 - 14 = 576$ degrees of freedom is $2.28 < 93$. Thus, there is statistical evidence that the maximum tumor volume is spheroid-specific ($d > 0$).

Table 6.1. Estimation results for the log-Gompertz random-intercept model with tumor spheroids data from Chignola et al. (1999).

Estimation method	β_1	β_2	β_3	σ^2	d
Starting values	5.24	6.84	0.081		
Nonlinear least squares	6.03	4.83	0.082	0.19	0
(SE)	(0.045)	(0.141)	(0.0044)		
Method of moments	5.94	4.75	0.085	0.16	2.43
(SE)	(0.182)	(0.087)	(0.0028)		
Variance least squares	5.94	4.75	0.085	0.22	1.00
(SE)	(0.139)	(0.101)	(0.0033)		
Maximum likelihood	5.94	4.75	0.085	0.16	2.45
(SE)	(0.184)	(0.088)	(0.0029)		

Estimation methods comparison

Estimates of the beta coefficients are quite close except for the nonlinear least squares, Table 6.1. This means that the presence of the random effect/intercept for these data is important. This is because for model (6.1), the information matrix for beta and the variance parameters is block diagonal, and therefore the asymptotic efficiency of the beta estimates is not affected by estimates of matrix $\mathbf{D}$. However, the efficiency for $\mathbf{D}$ is different for different methods, and the most efficient estimation method is maximum likelihood. The MM estimator is very close to the MLE, which is not surprising, as follows from our simulation study for the linear model of Section 3.14.

Three critical time points

We compute the three critical time points of tumor spheroid growth as defined above. Principally, any estimate may be used to compute T_D, T_G, and T_S; we use the MLE of Table 6.1. We obtain $T_G = \ln \beta_2 / \beta_3 \simeq 18$, $T_D = (\ln \beta_2 - 0.962)/\beta_3 \simeq 3$, $T_S = (\ln \beta_2 + 0.962)/\beta_3 \simeq 30$ days. Thus, until day 3, spheroids grow relatively slowly; at day 18 they have the maximum rate of growth; and after day 30 the growth slows down, see Figure 6.1. One can obtain approximate standard errors of these quantities by the delta-method (Rao, 1973; Rice, 1995).

Problems for Section 6.1

1. Suppose that repeated measurements follow the model $y_{ij} = f(x_i; \boldsymbol{\beta}) + \eta_j + \varepsilon_{ij}$, where $i = 1, 2, ..., N$ and $j = 1, 2, ..., n_i$ is the index for measurement repetitions (for each x_i, several repeated measurements, n_i, are available). Assume that $\eta_j \sim \mathcal{N}(0, \sigma_0^2)$ and $\varepsilon_{ij} \sim \mathcal{N}(0, \sigma^2)$, where the variances σ_0^2 and σ^2 are subject to estimation. Express this model in the form (6.3). Find $\mathbf{V}_i^{-1}$ and $\mathbf{H}$ in closed form. Simplify algorithm 1-4 on page 294 (reduce matrix $\mathbf{D}$ to scalar).

2. Prove that the NLS estimate does not exist for the nonlinear regression model $y_i \sim \mathcal{N}(e^{-\beta i}, \sigma^2)$ with a positive probability. (Hint: Prove that the estimate does not exist when $y_i < 0$ for all $i = 1, 2, ..., n$ and then prove that this probability is not zero; express the probability as a function of Φ.) Plot the probability against n for different σ and β.

3*. Estimate the probability that the normal equation for the NLS estimation has multiple solutions for the model $y_i \sim \mathcal{N}(e^{-\beta i}, \sigma^2)$. Simulate $y_1, ..., y_n$ and express the normal equation as a polynomial with the argument $x = e^{-\beta}$. Use function `polyroot` to find all roots including complex roots. Then find only positive real roots.

4. Modify the function `nlsMM` to estimate the probability that the `nls` function does not converge, starting from the linear least squares values specified in Section 6.1.2. Compute and plot this probability for several σ.

5*. Write R code that implements algorithm 1-4 for maximization of function (6.4). Modify the function `nlsMM` to solve minimization problem (6.9). Test the code through simulations using Michaelis-Menten regression function.

6*. Write and R function that estimates σ^2 and $\mathbf{D}$ by method of moments as in Section 6.1.4. Compare the properties of the beta-estimates using maximum likelihood from problem 5 with nonlinear least squares which uses distribution-free estimates of σ^2 and $\mathbf{D}$ via simulations (use the log-Gompertz growth curve and the data from `logG` to specify the true parameters). Demonstrate that the log-likelihood (6.4) maximization yields the same results as `nlme` from the function `logG`.

7. Estimate the variances of three critical points on the Gompertz curve using the delta-method assuming that the beta-estimates and their covariance matrix are known.

6.2   Varied matrix of random effects

A straightforward generalization of model (6.1) is to assume that the matrix of the random effects, $\mathbf{Z}_i$, depends on the population parameter $\boldsymbol{\beta}$. This leads to a mixed model:

$$\mathbf{y}_i = \mathbf{f}_i(\boldsymbol{\beta}) + \mathbf{Z}_i(\boldsymbol{\beta})\mathbf{b}_i + \boldsymbol{\varepsilon}_i, \quad i = 1, ..., N. \tag{6.17}$$

Other assumptions of Section 6.1 remain the same. Although models (6.1) and (6.17) seem similar, they have quite different statistical properties. The major difference is that for model (6.1), *any* consistent estimator of matrix $\mathbf{D}$ in the reweighted nonlinear least squares, formula (6.9) produces an asymptotically efficient and normally distributed estimator of $\boldsymbol{\beta}$, asymptotically equivalent to the maximum likelihood estimate. On the contrary, in model (6.17), one loses efficiency compared to maximum likelihood, if the least squares, formula (6.9) is applied, even if the true matrix $\mathbf{D}$ is known. In particular, under the normal assumption, the iteratively reweighted nonlinear least squares based on (6.17) with estimated matrix $\mathbf{Z}_i = \mathbf{Z}_i(\boldsymbol{\beta})$ leads to an asymptotically normal, but less efficient, $\boldsymbol{\beta}$ estimate. We illustrate the efficiency loss in this section with an example; in the following section, we provide comprehensive theoretical development. We shall arrive at model (6.17) taking the first-order approximation of the original nonlinear mixed effects model (see Section 8.6 for details).

6.2.1   Maximum likelihood estimation

In this subsection we consider the maximum likelihood estimation of mixed model (6.17) assuming that $\mathbf{b}_i$ and $\boldsymbol{\varepsilon}_i$ are normally distributed. We find the information matrix and develop a computational algorithm. The information matrix will be used later for an efficiency comparison.

The log-likelihood function, up to a constant term, takes the form

$$l(\boldsymbol{\beta}, \sigma^2, \mathbf{D}) = -\frac{1}{2} \left\{ N \ln \sigma^2 + \sum_{i=1}^{N} \left[\ln |\mathbf{V}_i(\boldsymbol{\beta})| + \sigma^{-2} \mathbf{e}_i'(\boldsymbol{\beta}) \mathbf{V}_i^{-1}(\boldsymbol{\beta}) \mathbf{e}_i(\boldsymbol{\beta}) \right] \right\}, \quad (6.18)$$

where

$$\mathbf{V}_i(\boldsymbol{\beta}) = \mathbf{I} + \mathbf{Z}_i(\boldsymbol{\beta}) \mathbf{D} \mathbf{Z}_i'(\boldsymbol{\beta}), \quad \mathbf{e}_i(\boldsymbol{\beta}) = \mathbf{y}_i - \mathbf{f}_i(\boldsymbol{\beta}).$$

Since the MLE is asymptotically efficient (when $N \to \infty$), we start by computing the information matrix as the benchmark to compare the efficiency of different estimation methods. Also, the information matrix may be used for computational purposes in the Fisher scoring algorithm. The derivatives of (6.18) with respect to σ^2 and $\mathbf{D}$ are the same as before, (6.7) and (6.8), and therefore the respective block of the information matrix does not change, (6.5). To compute the blocks with $\boldsymbol{\beta}$, we need the derivatives of the log-likelihood function. To shorten the notation, we omit i, as in Section 3.3, where the information matrix for the LME model was derived. Let the lth component of vector $\boldsymbol{\beta}$ be fixed; then $\dot{\mathbf{f}}_l = \partial \mathbf{f}/\partial \beta_l$ denotes an $n \times 1$ vector and $\dot{\mathbf{Z}}_l$ denotes an $n \times k$ matrix $\partial \mathbf{Z}/\partial \beta_l$, $l = 1, ..., m$. Using the standard chain rule for the ith cluster/log-likelihood contribution, we obtain

$$\begin{aligned}
\frac{\partial l}{\partial \beta_l} &= -\frac{1}{2} \left\{ -2\sigma^{-2} \dot{\mathbf{f}}_l' \mathbf{V}^{-1} \mathbf{e} + \mathrm{tr}[\mathbf{V}^{-1}(\dot{\mathbf{Z}}_l \mathbf{D} \mathbf{Z}' + \mathbf{Z} \mathbf{D} \dot{\mathbf{Z}}_l')] \right. \\
&\quad \left. -\sigma^{-2} \mathbf{e}' \mathbf{V}^{-1}(\dot{\mathbf{Z}}_l \mathbf{D} \mathbf{Z}' + \mathbf{Z} \mathbf{D} \dot{\mathbf{Z}}_l') \mathbf{V}^{-1} \mathbf{e} \right\}.
\end{aligned} \quad (6.19)$$

To compute the covariance matrix of this vector, we use the following fact.

Lemma 31 *If* $\mathbf{e} \sim \mathcal{N}(\mathbf{0}, \sigma^2 \mathbf{V})$, *then*

$$\mathrm{cov}(\mathbf{a}'\mathbf{e} + \mathbf{e}'\mathbf{A}\mathbf{e}, \mathbf{b}'\mathbf{e} + \mathbf{e}'\mathbf{B}\mathbf{e}) = \sigma^2 \mathbf{a}'\mathbf{V}\mathbf{b} + 2\sigma^4 \mathrm{tr}(\mathbf{A}\mathbf{V}\mathbf{B}\mathbf{V})$$

for any fixed vectors $\mathbf{a}, \mathbf{b}$ *and matrices* $\mathbf{A}, \mathbf{B}$ *of appropriate size.*

Proof. We have

$$\begin{aligned}
&\mathrm{cov}(\mathbf{a}'\mathbf{e} + \mathbf{e}'\mathbf{A}\mathbf{e}, \mathbf{b}'\mathbf{e} + \mathbf{e}'\mathbf{B}\mathbf{e}) \\
= \ &\mathrm{cov}(\mathbf{a}'\mathbf{e}, \mathbf{b}'\mathbf{e}) + \mathrm{cov}(\mathbf{a}'\mathbf{e}, \mathbf{e}'\mathbf{B}\mathbf{e}) + \mathrm{cov}(\mathbf{e}'\mathbf{A}\mathbf{e}, \mathbf{b}'\mathbf{e}) + \mathrm{cov}(\mathbf{e}'\mathbf{A}\mathbf{e}, \mathbf{e}'\mathbf{B}\mathbf{e}).
\end{aligned}$$

For the first term, $\mathrm{cov}(\mathbf{a}'\mathbf{e}, \mathbf{b}'\mathbf{e}) = E(\mathbf{e}'\mathbf{a}\mathbf{b}'\mathbf{e}) = \sigma^2 \mathrm{tr}(\mathbf{V}\mathbf{a}\mathbf{b}') = \sigma^2 \mathbf{a}'\mathbf{V}\mathbf{b}$. The second and third terms vanish because the third moment is zero; for the fourth term, we apply the result from Graybill (1983, p. 367). ∎

Denoting $\mathbf{G}_l = \dot{\mathbf{Z}}_l \mathbf{D} \mathbf{Z}' + \mathbf{Z} \mathbf{D} \dot{\mathbf{Z}}_l'$ in the notation of Lemma 31, we let

$$\begin{aligned}
\mathbf{a} &= \sigma^{-2} \mathbf{V}^{-1} \dot{\mathbf{f}}_l, \quad \mathbf{A} = \frac{1}{2} \sigma^{-2} \mathbf{V}^{-1} \mathbf{G}_l \mathbf{V}^{-1}, \\
\mathbf{b} &= \sigma^{-2} \mathbf{V}^{-1} \dot{\mathbf{f}}_h, \quad \mathbf{B} = \frac{1}{2} \sigma^{-2} \mathbf{V}^{-1} \mathbf{G}_h \mathbf{V}^{-1},
\end{aligned}$$

yielding

$$\mathrm{cov}\left(\frac{\partial l}{\partial \beta_l}, \frac{\partial l}{\partial \beta_h}\right) = \sigma^{-2}\dot{\mathbf{f}}_l'\mathbf{V}^{-1}\dot{\mathbf{f}}_h + \frac{1}{2}\mathrm{tr}(\mathbf{V}^{-1}\mathbf{G}_l\mathbf{V}^{-1}\mathbf{G}_h).$$

Note that if matrix $\mathbf{Z}$ does not depend on $\boldsymbol{\beta}$, the second term vanishes. Let vector $\partial l/\partial \mathbf{D}$ be multiplied by any $k \times 1$ vectors $\mathbf{q}'$ and $\mathbf{w}$. Then, as follows from (6.8), we obtain

$$\mathrm{cov}\left(\frac{\partial l}{\partial \beta_l}, \mathbf{q}'\frac{\partial l}{\partial \mathrm{vec}(\mathbf{D})}\mathbf{w}\right) = \frac{1}{4\sigma^4}\mathrm{cov}\left(\mathbf{q}'\mathbf{Z}'\mathbf{V}^{-1}\mathbf{e}\mathbf{e}'\mathbf{V}^{-1}\mathbf{Z}\mathbf{w}, \mathbf{e}'\mathbf{V}^{-1}\mathbf{G}_l\mathbf{V}^{-1}\mathbf{e}\right)$$

$$= \frac{1}{4\sigma^4}\mathrm{cov}\left(\mathbf{e}'\mathbf{V}^{-1}\mathbf{Z}\mathbf{w}\mathbf{q}'\mathbf{Z}'\mathbf{V}^{-1}\mathbf{e}, \mathbf{e}'\mathbf{V}^{-1}\mathbf{G}_l\mathbf{V}^{-1}\mathbf{e}\right).$$

Again, applying Lemma 31 with $\mathbf{a} = \mathbf{b} = \mathbf{0}$ and

$$\mathbf{A} = \mathbf{V}^{-1}\mathbf{Z}\mathbf{w}\mathbf{q}'\mathbf{Z}'\mathbf{V}^{-1}, \qquad \mathbf{B} = \mathbf{V}^{-1}\mathbf{G}_l\mathbf{V}^{-1},$$

we obtain

$$\mathrm{cov}\left(\frac{\partial l}{\partial \beta_l}, \frac{\partial l}{\partial \mathrm{vech}(\mathbf{D})}\right) = \frac{1}{2}\mathrm{vech}(\mathbf{Z}'\mathbf{V}^{-1}\mathbf{G}_l\mathbf{V}^{-1}\mathbf{Z}).$$

Analogously,

$$\mathrm{cov}\left(\frac{\partial l}{\partial \beta_l}, \frac{\partial l}{\partial \sigma^2}\right) = \frac{1}{4\sigma^4}\mathrm{cov}(\mathbf{e}'\mathbf{V}^{-1}\mathbf{e}, \mathbf{e}'\mathbf{V}^{-1}\mathbf{G}_l\mathbf{V}^{-1}\mathbf{e}) = \frac{1}{2\sigma^2}\mathrm{tr}(\mathbf{V}^{-1}\mathbf{G}_l).$$

Combining the results, we come to the information matrix for $\boldsymbol{\theta}$:

$$\mathcal{I} = \begin{bmatrix} \mathbf{I}_{\boldsymbol{\beta}} & \mathbf{I}'_{\boldsymbol{\beta},\sigma^2} & \mathbf{I}'_{\boldsymbol{\beta},\mathrm{vech}(\mathbf{D})} \\ \mathbf{I}_{\boldsymbol{\beta},\sigma^2} & \mathbf{I}_{\sigma^2} & \mathbf{I}'_{\sigma^2,\mathrm{vech}(\mathbf{D})} \\ \mathbf{I}_{\boldsymbol{\beta},\mathrm{vech}(\mathbf{D})} & \mathbf{I}_{\sigma^2,\mathrm{vech}(\mathbf{D})} & \mathbf{I}_{\mathrm{vech}(\mathbf{D})} \end{bmatrix}, \tag{6.20}$$

where the $m \times m$, $m \times 1$, and $m \times (k(k+1)/2)$ information matrix blocks are

$$\mathbf{I}_{\boldsymbol{\beta}} = \sum_{i=1}^N \left\{\sigma^{-2}\dot{\mathbf{f}}_{il}'\mathbf{V}_i^{-1}\dot{\mathbf{f}}_{ih} + \frac{1}{2}\mathrm{tr}(\mathbf{V}_i^{-1}\mathbf{G}_{il}\mathbf{V}_i^{-1}\mathbf{G}_{ih})\right\}, \tag{6.21}$$

$$\mathbf{I}_{\boldsymbol{\beta},\sigma^2} = \frac{1}{2\sigma^2}\sum_{i=1}^N \{\mathrm{tr}(\mathbf{V}_i^{-1}\mathbf{G}_{il})\}, \tag{6.22}$$

$$\mathbf{I}_{\boldsymbol{\beta},\mathrm{vech}(\mathbf{D})} = \frac{1}{2}\sum_{i=1}^N \{\mathrm{vech}(\mathbf{Z}_i'\mathbf{V}_i^{-1}\mathbf{G}_{il}\mathbf{V}_i^{-1}\mathbf{Z}_i)\}. \tag{6.23}$$

Here $l, h = 1, 2, ..., m$, and the $(1 + k(k+1)/2) \times (1 + k(k+1)/2)$ information matrix for $(\sigma^2, \mathrm{vech}(\mathbf{D}))$,

$$\mathbf{H} = \begin{bmatrix} \mathbf{I}_{\sigma^2} & \mathbf{I}'_{\sigma^2,\mathrm{vech}(\mathbf{D})} \\ \mathbf{I}_{\sigma^2,\mathrm{vech}(\mathbf{D})} & \mathbf{I}_{\mathrm{vech}(\mathbf{D})} \end{bmatrix}$$

is defined by (6.5).

Comments. First, the matrix block $\mathbf{I}_{\boldsymbol{\beta}}$ defines the information matrix when variance parameters are known. Consequently, if σ^2 and $\mathbf{D}$ were known, the asymptotic covariance matrix of the beta-MLE would be $\mathbf{I}_\beta^{-1}$. Second, if the matrix $\mathbf{Z}_i$ does not depend on the population-averaged parameter β, we have $\dot{\mathbf{Z}}_l = \mathbf{0}$ and $\mathbf{G}_l = \mathbf{0}$. Then, the information matrix becomes block diagonal and the information matrix reduces to that of the previous section. Otherwise, matrix $\mathcal{I}$ is not block diagonal, meaning that the MLE for β and the variance parameters are correlated, even in a large sample. This property makes the mixed model with *varied* matrix $\mathbf{Z}_i$ different from the mixed model with *fixed* matrix $\mathbf{Z}_i$.

Two algorithms for ML computation

We consider two algorithms for maximization of the log-likelihood function (6.18).

First, Fisher scoring (FS) can be readily applied since the information matrix and first derivatives are available; see Section 2.8 for a general discussion. The advantages of this algorithm are that (a) the matrix is always invertible if the model is well specified (the relevant conditions for the LME model are provided in Section 3.3), and (b) all parameters are adjusted simultaneously, and therefore fast convergence may be expected.

Second, since for fixed β the optimization problem reduces to the LME model with zero fixed effects, one may use standard software to estimate the variance parameters by standard or restricted maximum likelihood. Thus, one needs only to have an algorithm for (6.18) optimization over β when σ^2 and $\mathbf{D}$ are held. Again, we can use the information matrix to generate beta iterations as follows:

$$\beta_{s+1} = \beta_s + \lambda_s \mathbf{I}_\beta^{-1} \left(\sum_{i=1}^N \frac{\partial l_i}{\partial \beta} \right), \quad s = 0, 1, ..., \tag{6.24}$$

where $\mathbf{I}_\beta$ is the $m \times m$ information block for β and $\partial l_i / \partial \beta_l$ is given by (6.17). When $\lambda_s = 1$ and σ^2 is relatively small, iterations (6.24) are reduced to the well known Gauss–Newton algorithm. See Section 6.1.3 for a general discussion.

6.2.2 Distribution-free variance parameter estimation

Instead of applying maximum likelihood to estimate the variance parameters when β is held, we may apply the distribution-free noniterative estimate of Section 6.1.4. Indeed, let $\widehat{\beta}$ be an estimate, the limit point of iterations (6.24). We compute residuals $\widehat{\mathbf{e}}_i = \mathbf{y}_i - \mathbf{f}_i(\widehat{\beta})$ and $\widehat{\mathbf{Z}}_i = \mathbf{Z}_i(\widehat{\beta})$. Then the pooled variance estimate of σ^2 is defined as

$$\widehat{\sigma}^2 = \frac{1}{N_T - Nk} \sum_{i=1}^N \widehat{\mathbf{e}}_i'(\mathbf{I} - \widehat{\mathbf{Z}}_i \widehat{\mathbf{Z}}_i^+) \widehat{\mathbf{e}}_i.$$

The AMM estimator for matrix $\mathbf{D}_*$ is defined by (6.15) with $\mathbf{Z}_i = \widehat{\mathbf{Z}}_i$. The variance least squares estimation is readily applicable as well. After the estimate of $\mathbf{D}$ is computed, we return to iterations (6.24). Note that the distribution-free estimation of variance parameters does not produce estimates asymptotically equivalent to the MLE.

6.2.3   GEE and iteratively reweighted least squares

A popular method to estimate (6.17) is to reduce the model to (6.1) by replacing $\mathbf{Z}_i(\boldsymbol{\beta})$ with $\mathbf{Z}_i(\widehat{\boldsymbol{\beta}})$, where $\widehat{\boldsymbol{\beta}}$ is derived from the weighted NLS. More precisely, we start with nonlinear least squares (6.2) and compute $\mathbf{Z}_{i0} = \mathbf{Z}_i(\widehat{\boldsymbol{\beta}}_0)$ after convergence. Replace model (6.17) with $\mathbf{y}_i = \mathbf{f}_i(\boldsymbol{\beta}) + \mathbf{Z}_{i0}\mathbf{b}_i + \boldsymbol{\varepsilon}_i$, and treating $\mathbf{Z}_{i0}$ as fixed and using the algorithm of Section 6.1, to find the next estimate, $\widehat{\boldsymbol{\beta}}_1$. Then compute $\mathbf{Z}_{i1} = \mathbf{Z}_i(\widehat{\boldsymbol{\beta}}_1)$ and estimate the model $\mathbf{y}_i = \mathbf{f}_i(\boldsymbol{\beta}) + \mathbf{Z}_{i1}\mathbf{b}_i + \boldsymbol{\varepsilon}_i$, iterating in such a fashion until convergence. Clearly, this method of estimation is equivalent to solving m nonlinear estimating equations for $\boldsymbol{\beta}$,

$$\sum_{i=1}^{N} \mathbf{F}_i'(\boldsymbol{\beta})[\mathbf{I} + \mathbf{Z}_i(\boldsymbol{\beta})\widehat{\mathbf{D}}\mathbf{Z}_i'(\boldsymbol{\beta})]^{-1}(\mathbf{y}_i - \mathbf{f}_i(\boldsymbol{\beta})) = \mathbf{0}, \qquad (6.25)$$

where $\mathbf{F}_i = \mathbf{F}_i(\boldsymbol{\beta})$ is an $n_i \times m$ matrix of first derivatives, $\mathbf{F}_i = \{\dot{\mathbf{f}}_l, l = 1, ..., m\}$, and $\widehat{\mathbf{D}}$ is a consistent estimate of $\mathbf{D}$. This estimate may be found by solving the score equations (6.7) and (6.8) or by using distribution-free estimation based on variance least squares. Equations (6.25) are called generalized estimating equations (GEEs) because an estimate of $\mathbf{D}$ is used. General information on GEE is presented in Appendix 13.1.5. The algorithm to solve (6.25) is widely used and has several names. Perhaps the most common name is Iteratively Reweighted Least Squares (IRLS). Carroll and Ruppert (1988) call this algorithm extended nonlinear least squares within the framework of nonlinear regression and with heteroscedastic errors defined by a variance function. In Chapter 8, we show that IRLS, with variance parameters derived from score equations (6.7) and (6.8), is equivalent to the Lindstrom–Bates procedure (1990) and therefore may be obtained in R using the function `nlme`.

Asymptotic properties and efficiency considerations

Either a deterministic or a stochastic scheme may be chosen to study asymptotic properties, Section 3.6.2. Typically, the deterministic scheme is taken in the literature although the stochastic scheme is easier to handle because it reduces to the iid case. To prove the consistency of the GEE (6.25), under the stochastic scheme the standard Slutsky theorem can be used. Under the deterministic scheme, the generalized Slutsky theorem can be used, as shown in Appendix 13.1.2. As follows from the general theory of GEE, Appendix 13.1.5, use of a consistent estimate in (6.25) does not increase the asymptotic variance of $\widehat{\boldsymbol{\beta}}$ because the expectation of the derivative of an estimating equations with respect to $\mathbf{D}$ is zero.

Since equations (6.19) and (6.25) differ, the GEE is less efficient than the ML. Our current aim is to find the asymptotic covariance matrix for GEE using the sandwich formula of Appendix 13.1.4. As follows from the previous comment, we can assume that the variance parameters are known. To shorten the notation, we omit the subscript i; the estimating equation for $\boldsymbol{\beta}$ takes the form

$$\mathbf{F}'[\mathbf{I} + \mathbf{Z}(\boldsymbol{\beta})\mathbf{D}\mathbf{Z}'(\boldsymbol{\beta})]^{-1}(\mathbf{y} - \mathbf{f}(\boldsymbol{\beta})) = \mathbf{0}. \qquad (6.26)$$

This equation can be represented as $\boldsymbol{\Psi}(\boldsymbol{\beta}) = \mathbf{0}$, where $\boldsymbol{\Psi}$ is the left-hand side of (6.26). We want to find the expected value of the derivative of $\boldsymbol{\Psi}$ with respect to $\boldsymbol{\beta}$. Since $E(\mathbf{y} - \mathbf{f}(\boldsymbol{\beta})) = \mathbf{0}$, we obtain that an estimating equation that is unbiased and therefore the GEE is consistent and asymptotically normally distributed. Further, since $\text{cov}(\mathbf{y}) = \sigma^2 \mathbf{V} = \sigma^2(\mathbf{I} + \mathbf{Z}(\boldsymbol{\beta})\mathbf{D}\mathbf{Z}'(\boldsymbol{\beta}))$, it is easy to see that

$$E\left(\frac{\partial \boldsymbol{\Psi}}{\partial \boldsymbol{\beta}}\right) = -\mathbf{F}'\mathbf{V}^{-1}\mathbf{F}, \quad E\left(\boldsymbol{\Psi}\boldsymbol{\Psi}'\right) = \mathbf{F}'\mathbf{V}^{-1}\mathbf{F}.$$

Therefore, in a large sample,

$$\text{cov}(\widehat{\boldsymbol{\beta}}_{IRLS}) = \sigma^2 \left(\sum \mathbf{F}_i' \mathbf{V}_i^{-1} \mathbf{F}_i\right)^{-1}. \tag{6.27}$$

As follows from (6.21), the covariance matrix of the MLE is represented as the sum of two matrices,

$$\text{cov}(\widehat{\boldsymbol{\beta}}_{ML}) = \sigma^2 \left(\sum \mathbf{F}_i' \mathbf{V}_i^{-1} \mathbf{F}_i + \frac{1}{2}\sigma^2 \sum \mathbf{T}_i\right)^{-1}, \tag{6.28}$$

where the (l, h)th element of matrix $\mathbf{T}_i$ is $\text{tr}(\mathbf{V}_i^{-1}\mathbf{G}_{il}\mathbf{V}_i^{-1}\mathbf{G}_{ih})$. Comparing the two matrices, we infer that under the normal assumption, the GEE is less efficient than the ML estimator. However, for small σ^2, there is not much gain in relative efficiency (the second term in (6.28) is small). Again, one cannot expect much efficiency gain when the matrices $\mathbf{Z}_i$ are not highly nonlinear in $\boldsymbol{\beta}$ because then the matrices $\mathbf{T}_i$ are small. When the variance of random effects is zero, ML = GEE. Thus, one can speculate that the difference between the two estimation methods may be considerable for large random effects.

The GEE and ML methods are consistent, even if the distribution is misspecified. Moreover, unlike maximum likelihood, GEE produces consistent and asymptotically normal estimates, even if the covariance matrix is misspecified. Rigorous analysis is deferred to the next section.

6.2.4   Example: logistic curve with random asymptote

One of the first examples of a nonlinear random effects model was considered by Lindstrom and Bates (1990). The same model has since been studied by Pinheiro and Bates (1995). The data consist of the trunk circumference (in millimeters) of five orange trees as a function of time, where measurements are taken on the same day for each tree. Days are counted from January 1, 1969 so that the data are balanced; the data are given in Draper and Smith (1998, p. 524), see Figure 6.3. Here y_{ij} denotes the trunk circumference of the ith tree, $i = 1, 2, 3, 4, 5 = N$ (the number of trees) at the jth measurement, $j = 1, ..., 7 = n$ (the number of measurements). By the assumption, the trunk circumference grows according to a logistic curve with the random effect in the numerator,

$$y_{ij} = \frac{\beta_1 + b_i}{1 + \exp(\beta_2 - \beta_3 t_j)} + \varepsilon_{ij}, \tag{6.29}$$

where $\varepsilon_{ij} \sim \mathcal{N}(0, \sigma^2)$ with the random effect $b_i \sim \mathcal{N}(0, \sigma^2 d)$; all random terms are independent. Using our conventional notation, $d_* = \sigma^2 d$ denotes the variance of the random effect and d denotes the scaled variance (as the proportion of σ^2). In this mixed model only the asymptote $\beta_1 + b_i$, the trunk circumference of the

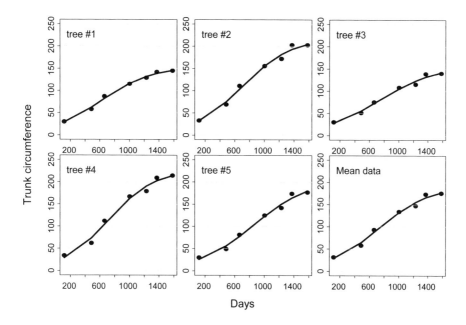

FIGURE 6.3. Trunk circumference of five orange trees ($N = 5$, $n = 7$). It is assumed that only the circumference of the adult tree (asymptote) is tree-specific (random). All other parameters of the logistic curve are the same for all trees (population averaged). The line shows the individual NLS fit (see Table 5.2 for parameter values).

adult tree, is random and tree-specific. Parameters β_2 and β_3 are common to all five trees (fixed and unknown). Model (6.29) can be called logistic regression with a random asymptote. Lindstrom and Bates (1990) applied their procedure to estimate parameters and the scaled variance of the random effect d, see Chapter 8. In this section we provide a comprehensive estimation analysis and efficiency comparison for model (6.29) .

Table 6.2. Individual and mean logistic growth curves for the tree data (SE), separate nonlinear least squares fit, see Figure 6.3.

Tree	β_1	β_2	β_3	SS
1	154.3 (6.10)	1.80 (.14)	.0029 (.00031)	63.1
2	219.0 (14.3)	2.11 (.23)	.0030 (.00048)	290.7
3	158.8 (15.1)	1.83 (.19)	.0025 (.00046)	156.7
4	226.8 (15.6)	2.30 (.29)	.0032 (.00056)	407.7
5	207.3 (22.2)	2.26 (.22)	.0026 (.00047)	259.7
Mean	192.77 (13.6)	2.07 (.21)	.0028 (.00044)	202.5
SD/mean	15.9%	10.2%	9.3%	

We start our analysis with an individual (separate) Nonlinear Least Squares (NLS) fit applied to each tree and the mean group data in Table 6.2. As the reader can see, individual fits are quite satisfactory and the estimates are highly significant

(Mean estimates are derived from the fit to the mean group data). The last row of the table indicates the relative variability of the estimates around the mean estimate and is calculated as the ratio of the empirical deviation of individual estimates from the mean to the mean group. These computations show that the asymptote is the most variable parameter, and therefore model (6.29) seems adequate.

Next, we notice that since the random effect is in the numerator, measurement y_{ij} is also normally distributed with the marginal expectation

$$E(y_{ij}) = \frac{\beta_1}{1 + \exp(\beta_2 - \beta_3 t_j)}, \qquad i = 1, ..., N, j = 1, ..., n,$$

so that the mean circumference, $\bar{y}_j = N^{-1} \sum_{i=1}^{N} y_{ij}$, follows the logistic curve,

$$E(\bar{y}_j) = \frac{\beta_1}{1 + \exp(\beta_2 - \beta_3 t_j)}, \qquad j = 1, ..., n. \tag{6.30}$$

Consequently, parameters of the logistic curve may be estimated consistently (for large n) by NLS applied to the mean data in Table 6.2. However, the presence of the random effect induces tree heterogeneity and a correlation between serial measurements of the circumference. Indeed, as is easy to see,

$$\text{var}(y_{ij}) = \sigma^2(1 + dh_j^2), \quad \text{cov}(y_{ij}, y_{ik}) = \sigma^2 dh_j h_k, \quad j \neq k,$$

where $h_j = (1 + e^{\beta_2 - \beta_3 t_j})^{-1}$. If adult trees were of the same thickness ($d = 0$), we would come to the standard nonlinear regression problem because $\text{var}(y_{ij}) =$ const and $\text{cov}(y_{ij}, y_{ik}) = 0$. Then the best way to estimate the parameters (at least asymptotically) would be nonlinear least squares, which minimizes the total sum of squares,

$$\sum_{ij} \left(y_{ij} - \frac{\beta_1}{1 + \exp(\beta_2 - \beta_3 t_j)} \right)^2. \tag{6.31}$$

Now we show that minimization of (6.31) is equivalent to the nonlinear regression fit to the mean data/tree thickness. Indeed, after elementary algebra, we obtain

$$\sum_{ij} (y_{ij} - \beta_1 h_j)^2 = \sum_{ij} (y_{ij} - \bar{y}_j)^2 + N \sum_j (\bar{y}_j - \beta_1 h_j)^2. \tag{6.32}$$

Thus, the minimization of the total sum of squares (6.31) is equivalent to the minimization of $\sum_j (\bar{y}_j - \beta_1 h_j)^2$ because the first term in expression (6.32) is parameter independent. Note that this feature is a consequence of the fact that the data are balanced because the thickness of each tree has been measured at the same time points. Although the logistic regression applied to the mean group data produces consistent estimates, (a) more efficient parameter estimates can be obtained by maximum likelihood, and (b) we need an estimate of d to provide satisfactory standard errors for the parameters. Our analysis for the linear mixed effects model of Section 3.9 suggests that the standard errors of Table 6.2 underestimate the true standard errors.

In the following R function we read the data on five orange trees and plot individual trunk circumferences versus days of growth. As in the previous function, logG, two libraries are required.

```
logtree=function()
{
dump("logtree","c:\\MixedModels\\Chapter06\\logtree.r")
library(nlme);library(lattice)
dat=read.csv("c:\\MixedModels\\Chapter06\\trunktree.txt")
xyplot(trunk~day|id,data=dat,type="b")
out.nlme<-nlme(trunk~a1/(1+exp(a2-a3*day)),fixed=a1+a2+a3~1,
    random=a1~1|id, data=dat,start=c(200,2,0.003))
summary(out.nlme)
}
```

Maximum likelihood estimation

Now we estimate the parameters of the logistic curve by maximum likelihood. Importantly, it does not involve the integration problem, as in the general nonlinear mixed effects model of Chapter 8, because model (6.29) is marginal. Denote $\boldsymbol{\beta} = (\beta_1, \beta_2, \beta_3)'$, $\mathbf{t} = (t_1, t_2, ..., t_7)'$, $\mathbf{y}_i = (y_{i1}, y_{i2}, ..., y_{i7})'$, and $\mathbf{h} = \mathbf{h}(\beta_2, \beta_3)$ $=(h_1, ..., h_7)'$. Then, in vector notation, we can rewrite statistical model (6.29) as $\mathbf{y}_i = \beta_1\mathbf{h}+b_i\mathbf{h} + \boldsymbol{\varepsilon}_i$ with normally distributed b_i and $\boldsymbol{\varepsilon}_i$, or compactly,

$$\mathbf{y}_i \sim \mathcal{N}\left(\beta_1\mathbf{h}, \sigma^2(\mathbf{I}+d\mathbf{h}\mathbf{h}')\right), \qquad i = 1, ..., N = 5. \tag{6.33}$$

This model is a special case of a nonlinear marginal model with a varied matrix of random effects (6.17). The log-likelihood function for this model is

$$\begin{aligned} l(\boldsymbol{\beta}, \sigma^2, d) &= -\frac{1}{2}\{N\ln|\mathbf{I}+d\mathbf{h}\mathbf{h}'| + Nn\ln\sigma^2 \\ &\quad + \frac{1}{\sigma^2}\sum_{i=1}^{N}(\mathbf{y}_i - \beta_1\mathbf{h})'(\mathbf{I}+d\mathbf{h}\mathbf{h}')^{-1}(\mathbf{y}_i - \beta_1\mathbf{h})\}. \end{aligned} \tag{6.34}$$

We can eliminate σ^2 and come to the variance-profile log-likelihood function. Also, applying decomposition (6.32), we can reduce the above sum to $\overline{\mathbf{y}}$. Further applying the dimension-reduction formulas $|\mathbf{I}+d\mathbf{h}\mathbf{h}'| = 1 + d\|\mathbf{h}\|^2$ and $(\mathbf{I}+d\mathbf{h}\mathbf{h}')^{-1} = \mathbf{I}-d\mathbf{h}\mathbf{h}'/(1 + d\|\mathbf{h}\|^2)$, we can simplify the log-likelihood function substantially, especially when the number of observations in each cluster is large.

Iteratively reweighted least squares

The initial step is to fit standard nonlinear regression (no weighting, $d = 0$), then estimate the variance parameters σ^2 and d based on the NLS residuals and apply weighted NLS, iterating in such a manner until convergence. Below we provide some technical details.

1. Since the tree data are balanced, as follows from (6.32), NLS applied to all the data is equivalent to NLS applied to the mean data, $\overline{\mathbf{y}}$, which produce $\widehat{\boldsymbol{\beta}}_0$.

2. There are several ways to estimate σ^2 and d given residuals $\mathbf{e}_i = \mathbf{y}_i - \mathbf{f}_i(\widehat{\boldsymbol{\beta}}_0)$. First, we can solve the ML equations (6.7) and (6.8) when $\{\mathbf{e}_i\}$ are held.

Second, we can use the distribution-free estimate of Section 6.2.2. Third, we can apply the variance least squares of Section 3.12. We illustrate the latter approach. Thus, treating $\{e_i\}$ and $\mathbf{h}$ as fixed, we want to minimize the sum of squares between empirical and theoretical squared values

$$T(\sigma^2, d) = \sum_{i=1}^{n} \text{tr} \left(e_i e_i' - \sigma^2 \mathbf{I} - d_* \mathbf{h} \mathbf{h}' \right)^2,$$

where $d_* = \sigma^2 d$. Taking the derivative with respect to σ^2 and d and solving the system of linear equations, we come to the variance least squares solution,

$$\widehat{\sigma}^2 = \frac{\|\mathbf{h}\|^2 \sum \|e_i\|^2 - \sum (e_i' \mathbf{h})^2}{N(n-1)\|\mathbf{h}\|^2}, \quad \widehat{d}_* = \frac{n \sum (e_i' \mathbf{h})^2 - \|\mathbf{h}\|^2 \sum \|e_i\|^2}{N(n-1)\|\mathbf{h}\|^4}.$$

We observe that $\widehat{\sigma}^2 \geq 0$ because by the Cauchy inequality, $\sum (e_i' \mathbf{h})^2 \leq \sum \|e_i\|^2 \|\mathbf{h}\|^2 = \|\mathbf{h}\|^2 \sum \|e_i\|^2$. On the other hand, $\widehat{d}_*$ may be negative, although we may expect it to be positive for a large n (if $\widehat{d}_* < 0$, we set $\widehat{d}_* = 0$); then $\widehat{d} = \widehat{d}_*/\widehat{\sigma}^2$.

3. When $\mathbf{V} = \mathbf{I} + \widehat{d}\mathbf{h}\mathbf{h}'$ is held, we apply the weighted nonlinear least squares $(\overline{\mathbf{y}} - \mathbf{f}(\boldsymbol{\beta}))' \mathbf{V}^{-1}(\overline{\mathbf{y}} - \mathbf{f}(\boldsymbol{\beta}))$ to obtain the next approximation of $\widehat{\boldsymbol{\beta}}$. Then we recompute residuals and $\mathbf{h}$ and return to the variance least squares, iterating until convergence.

This method produced beta estimates close to the mean NLS with $\widehat{\sigma}_{IRLS}^2 = 56.96$ and $\widehat{d}_{IRLS} = 17.18$. As mentioned before, the IRLS estimates with the MLE for variance parameters can be obtained via the R (or S+) function nlme; it yields $\widehat{s}_{ML}^2 = 56.96$ and $\widehat{d}_{ML} = 16.97$. Recall that these estimates are obtained from maximum likelihood estimation of the LME model with zero fixed effects.

Efficiency comparison

Here we compare the efficiency of IRLS and ML using formulas (6.27) and (6.28). Since the tree data are balanced, we ignore index i. Also we assume that variance parameters are known; we set $\sigma = 7.5$ and compute the asymptotic variances of $\widehat{\beta}_1, \widehat{\beta}_2$, and $\widehat{\beta}_3$ for d in the range 0 to 20. In our computations we assume that the true values are $\beta_1 = 193$, $\beta_2 = 2$, and $\beta_3 = 0.003$. As follows from formula (6.27),

$$\text{cov}_{IRLS} = \frac{\sigma^2}{N}(\mathbf{F}'\mathbf{V}^{-1}\mathbf{F})^{-1},$$

where $\mathbf{F} = (\partial \mathbf{f}/\partial \beta_1, \partial \mathbf{f}/\partial \beta_2, \partial \mathbf{f}/\partial \beta_3)$ is an $n \times 3$ matrix of derivatives of the logistic growth curve model. To compute the covariance matrix for the ML, we introduce the notation $\mathbf{h}_2 = \partial \mathbf{h}/\partial \beta_2$ and $\mathbf{h}_3 = \partial \mathbf{h}/\partial \beta_3$. Then the $n \times n$ matrix $\mathbf{G}_l = (\mathbf{h}_l \mathbf{h}' + \mathbf{h} \mathbf{h}_l')d$ for $l = 2, 3$ and $\mathbf{G}_1 = \mathbf{0}$, in the notation of formula (6.21). The (h, l)th element of matrix $\mathbf{T}$ for $2 \leq h, l \leq 3$ is

$$\begin{aligned}
T_{lh} &= \text{tr}(\mathbf{V}^{-1}\mathbf{G}_l \mathbf{V}^{-1}\mathbf{G}_h) = d^2 \text{tr}\left(\mathbf{V}^{-1}(\mathbf{h}_l \mathbf{h}' + \mathbf{h} \mathbf{h}_l')\mathbf{V}^{-1}(\mathbf{h}_h \mathbf{h}' + \mathbf{h} \mathbf{h}_h')\right) \\
&= d^2 \text{tr}\left(\mathbf{V}^{-1}(\mathbf{h}_l \mathbf{h}' + \mathbf{h} \mathbf{h}_l')\mathbf{V}^{-1}(\mathbf{h}_h \mathbf{h}' + \mathbf{h} \mathbf{h}_h')\right) \\
&= 2d^2(\mathbf{h}'\mathbf{V}^{-1}\mathbf{h}_l \mathbf{h}'\mathbf{V}^{-1}\mathbf{h}_h + \mathbf{h}_h'\mathbf{V}^{-1}\mathbf{h}_l \mathbf{h}'\mathbf{V}^{-1}\mathbf{h}),
\end{aligned}$$

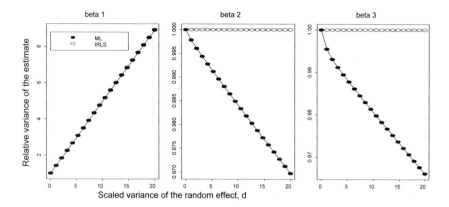

FIGURE 6.4. Relative efficiency comparison for ML versus IRLS in logistic regression with a random asymptote (orange tree example). The two methods produce the same variance for the β_1 estimate, which increases linearly with the variance of the random effect, D. The variances of $\widehat{\beta}_2$ and $\widehat{\beta}_3$ of IRLS are invariant with respect to D, but the variances of the MLE drop slightly, so that one may expect the MLE to be more efficient by 3%.

so that

$$\text{cov}_{ML} = \frac{\sigma^2}{N}\left(\mathbf{F}'\mathbf{V}^{-1}\mathbf{F} + \frac{\sigma^2}{2}\mathbf{T}\right)^{-1}.$$

Clearly, $\text{cov}_{ML} \leq \text{cov}_{IRLS}$, which implies that the MLE has equal or lesser variances than the IRLS estimates. We investigate how these asymptotic variances behave as a function of the scaled variance of the random effect, d in Figure 6.4. When $d = 0$, MLE = IRLS = NLS and therefore the variances of all parameters as functions of d start from the same point. In this figure, we show the relative variance of the estimates as $\text{var}(d)/\text{var}(0)$, which means that all curves start from $(0,1)$. Interestingly, the variance of the trunk circumference of the adult tree (β_1) increases linearly with d, whereas the variance for the other two parameters does not. Since d is around 17, we conclude that the tree variation increases the variance of $\widehat{\beta}_1$ by a factor of 8. Basically, IRLS and ML are very close due to the fact that the data are balanced (recall that ML = GLS = OLS for the balanced random-coefficient LME model described in Section 2.3). The variance of the ML is just slightly less than the variance of IRLS (by less than 3%).

Problems for Section 6.2

1^*. Modify the function `logtree` to compute the ML estimates that maximize the function l given by (6.34), following the dimension-reduction formula. Write an R code for iteratively reweigted least squares using suggestions 1 to 3.

2. Prove that $\text{cov}_{ML} \leq \text{cov}_{IRLS}$. Under what conditions does the inequality turn into an equality?

3^*. Carry out a relative efficiency comparison as in Figure 6.4 for a Michaelis-Menten model; namely, $y_{ij} = (\beta_1 + b_i)x_j/(\beta_2 + x_j) + \varepsilon_{ij}$, where $b_i \sim \mathcal{N}(0, \sigma^2 d)$.

4^*. Develop the ML estimation for a special varied matrix random effects model $y_{ij} = (\gamma + b_i)h_j(\boldsymbol{\beta}) + \varepsilon_{ij}$, where $b_i \sim \mathcal{N}(0, d_*)$, as a generalization of logistic growth curve model with random asymptote (6.29). Derive the information matrix (6.20) and simplify the distribution-free estimation of σ^2 and d_*. Write an R code to test your derivations and estimation algorithm against nlme. Use Michaelis-Menten and the logistic growth curve model in the test examples.

6.3   Three types of nonlinear marginal models

So far, we have considered two types of nonlinear marginal models for repeated measurements. In both models, random effects are linear, but in model (6.1) the matrix of the random effects is fixed, and in model (6.17) this matrix depends on the beta parameters. In other words, for model (6.1), the mean, $E(\mathbf{y}) = \mathbf{f}$, and the covariance matrix, $\mathrm{cov}(\mathbf{y}) = \sigma^2 \mathbf{V}$, do not share parameters, but in model (6.17), matrix $\mathbf{V}$ depends on parameters from $\mathbf{f}$. However, there is an important, more general class of nonlinear marginal models when $\mathbf{f}$ and $\mathbf{V}$ *share* parameters, particularly when some variance parameters enter the mean function $\mathbf{f}$. To illustrate this possibility, we recall the log-Gompertz model, (6.16), but now assuming that the rate parameter is also subject-specific. Then the log-Gompertz model takes the form $y_{ij} = (\beta_1 + b_i) - \beta_2 e^{-(\beta_3 + \delta_i)t_{ij}} + \varepsilon_{ij}$, where $\delta_i \sim \mathcal{N}(0, \sigma_\delta^2)$. The marginal expectation for y_{ij} can be expressed in closed form as $E(y_{ij}) = \beta_1 - \beta_2 e^{-\beta_3 t_{ij} + .5\sigma_\delta^2 t_{ij}^2}$, and therefore, as we see, the mean depends on the variance σ_δ^2.

To facilitate the study of nonlinear marginal models, we define the following three *generic* nonlinear models. These models can be viewed as a generalization of the nonlinear regression model, $\mathbf{y} = \mathbf{f}(\boldsymbol{\beta}) + \boldsymbol{\eta}$, where $\mathbf{y} = (y_1, ..., y_N)'$ is a vector of observations of the dependent variable, $\boldsymbol{\beta} = (\beta_1, ..., \beta_m)'$ is a vector of unknown parameters, $\mathbf{f} = (f_1, ..., f_N): R^m \to R^N$ is an $N \times 1$ vector function of the vector argument $\boldsymbol{\beta}$, and $\boldsymbol{\eta} = (\eta_1, ..., \eta_N)$ is a vector of errors. Computational issues associated with the use of nonlinear least squares are well covered in books by Bard (1974), Nash and Walker-Smith (1987), Gallant (1987), Bates and Watts (1988), Seber and Wild (1989), and Demidenko (1981, 1989). Although some authors have attempted to study the small-sample properties of the Nonlinear Least Squares (NLS) estimate (Beale, 1960; Gallant, 1975), asymptotic study is fairly general and widely used in the framework of nonlinear estimation. It is especially easy to study the asymptotic properties under the stochastic scheme, discussed in Section 3.6.2, assuming that $f_i(\boldsymbol{\beta}) = f(\boldsymbol{\beta}; \mathbf{x}_i)$, so that the nonlinear regression model is written in a hierarchical fashion as $y_i | \mathbf{x}_i = f(\boldsymbol{\beta}; \mathbf{x}_i) + \eta_i$, where the $\{\mathbf{x}_i\}$ are iid random vectors. Then the $\{y_i\}$ are iid random variables, and application of the estimating equations theory becomes straightforward. See Appendix 13.1.4.

We require the nonlinear models to be identifiable, meaning that if the mean and variance coincide, the parameters coincide as well. For instance, for standard nonlinear regression, the model is identifiable if $\mathbf{f}(\boldsymbol{\beta}_1) = \mathbf{f}(\boldsymbol{\beta}_2)$ implies that $\boldsymbol{\beta}_1 = \boldsymbol{\beta}_2$.

The common feature of the following three models is that they define the first two moments via nonlinear functions of unknown parameters. To complete the specification, the distribution is required. For a continuous response variable, the normal distribution is a good candidate, although these models may be helpful for modeling discrete data as well.

The three general nonlinear models differ by the degree to which the mean and the variance/covariance share their parameters:

1. Type I nonlinear marginal model:

$$\mathbf{y} = \mathbf{f}(\boldsymbol{\beta}) + \boldsymbol{\eta}, \quad \mathrm{cov}(\boldsymbol{\eta}) = \mathbf{V}(\boldsymbol{\gamma}). \tag{6.35}$$

A characteristic feature of this model is that the regression and variance parameters do not overlap; in other words, vectors $\boldsymbol{\beta}$ and $\boldsymbol{\gamma}$ have different components. VARCOMP model (1.8) and LME model (2.5) are special cases, as can be seen after combining data as in (2.9), where $\boldsymbol{\gamma} = (\sigma^2, \mathrm{vech}(\mathbf{D}))$ and $\mathbf{V} = \sigma^2(\mathbf{I} + \mathbf{Z}\mathbf{D}\mathbf{Z}')$. The LME model with the linear covariance structure of Section 4.3 and autocorrelated errors of Section 4.3.4 are also special cases of (6.35). The nonlinear marginal model (6.1) belongs to this type with covariance matrix $\mathbf{V}$. Model (6.35) is identifiable if $\mathbf{f}(\boldsymbol{\beta}_1) = \mathbf{f}(\boldsymbol{\beta}_2)$ implies that $\boldsymbol{\beta}_1 = \boldsymbol{\beta}_2$ and $\mathbf{V}(\boldsymbol{\gamma}_1) = \mathbf{V}(\boldsymbol{\gamma}_2)$ implies that $\boldsymbol{\gamma}_1 = \boldsymbol{\gamma}_2$. Also, it is assumed that matrices $\mathbf{F} = \partial \mathbf{f}/\partial\boldsymbol{\beta}$ and $\mathbf{V}$ have full rank for all $\boldsymbol{\beta}$ and $\boldsymbol{\gamma}$.

2. Type II nonlinear marginal model:

$$\mathbf{y} = \mathbf{f}(\boldsymbol{\beta}) + \boldsymbol{\eta}, \quad \mathrm{cov}(\boldsymbol{\eta}) = \mathbf{V}(\boldsymbol{\beta}, \boldsymbol{\gamma}). \tag{6.36}$$

In this model, parameters of the mean are part of the covariance matrix. Model (6.17) is of this type, with $\mathbf{V} = \sigma^2(\mathbf{I} + \mathbf{Z}(\boldsymbol{\beta})\mathbf{D}\mathbf{Z}'(\boldsymbol{\beta}))$. This model is identifiable if $\mathbf{f}(\boldsymbol{\beta}_1) = \mathbf{f}(\boldsymbol{\beta}_2)$ and $\mathbf{V}(\boldsymbol{\beta}_1, \boldsymbol{\gamma}_1) = \mathbf{V}(\boldsymbol{\beta}_2, \boldsymbol{\gamma}_2)$ imply $\boldsymbol{\beta}_1 = \boldsymbol{\beta}_2$ and $\boldsymbol{\gamma}_1 = \boldsymbol{\gamma}_2$. Note that for this model, it may be that $\mathbf{f}(\boldsymbol{\beta}_1) = \mathbf{f}(\boldsymbol{\beta}_2)$ for $\boldsymbol{\beta}_1 \neq \boldsymbol{\beta}_2$ but that the model is still identifiable. We call the type II model *mean-identifiable* if $\mathbf{f}(\boldsymbol{\beta}_1) = \mathbf{f}(\boldsymbol{\beta}_2)$ implies that $\boldsymbol{\beta}_1 = \boldsymbol{\beta}_2$.

3. Type III nonlinear marginal model:

$$\mathbf{y} = \mathbf{f}(\boldsymbol{\theta}) + \boldsymbol{\eta}, \quad \mathrm{cov}(\boldsymbol{\eta}) = \mathbf{V}(\boldsymbol{\theta}). \tag{6.37}$$

For this model, the mean and variance parameters are common and generally indistinguishable. This is the most general nonlinear model, and models types I and II are special cases of (6.37). This model is identifiable if $\mathbf{f}(\boldsymbol{\theta}_1) = \mathbf{f}(\boldsymbol{\theta}_2)$ and $\mathbf{V}(\boldsymbol{\theta}_1) = \mathbf{V}(\boldsymbol{\theta}_2)$ imply that $\boldsymbol{\theta}_1 = \boldsymbol{\theta}_2$. We call this model *mean-identifiable* if $\mathbf{f}(\boldsymbol{\theta}_1) = \mathbf{f}(\boldsymbol{\theta}_2)$ implies that $\boldsymbol{\theta}_1 = \boldsymbol{\theta}_2$.

Below we apply maximum likelihood for each model to estimate parameters, assuming normal distribution. We derive the Fisher information matrix for further efficiency analysis to compare with Iteratively Reweighted Least Squares (IRLS).

6.3.1 Type I nonlinear marginal model

As mentioned before, one trivial example of this type of model is the LME model, (2.5). The log-Gompertz growth curve with random intercept of Section 6.1.7 is another example.

Assuming that $\mathbf{y} \sim \mathcal{N}(\mathbf{f}(\boldsymbol{\beta}), \mathbf{V}(\boldsymbol{\gamma}))$, the log-likelihood function, up to a constant term, takes the form $l(\boldsymbol{\beta}, \boldsymbol{\gamma}) = -\frac{1}{2}(\ln|\mathbf{V}| + (\mathbf{y} - \mathbf{f})'\mathbf{V}^{-1}(\mathbf{y} - \mathbf{f}))$. We derive the score equations for $\boldsymbol{\beta}$ and $\boldsymbol{\gamma}$ and the Fisher information matrix using the Kronecker product and matrix differentiation formulas of Appendix 13.2. We have

$$\begin{aligned}
\frac{\partial(\mathbf{y} - \mathbf{f})'\mathbf{V}^{-1}(\mathbf{y} - \mathbf{f})}{\partial\boldsymbol{\gamma}} &= -\mathbf{G}'\left(\mathbf{V}^{-1} \otimes \mathbf{V}^{-1}\right)[(\mathbf{y} - \mathbf{f}) \otimes (\mathbf{y} - \mathbf{f})] \\
&= -\mathbf{G}'[\mathbf{V}^{-1}(\mathbf{y} - \mathbf{f}) \otimes \mathbf{V}^{-1}(\mathbf{y} - \mathbf{f})]
\end{aligned}$$

and $\partial \ln |\mathbf{V}(\boldsymbol{\gamma})| / \partial \boldsymbol{\gamma} = \mathbf{G}' \left(\mathbf{V}^{-1} \otimes \mathbf{I}\right) \mathrm{vec}(\mathbf{I}) = \mathbf{G}' \mathrm{vec}(\mathbf{V}^{-1})$, where $\mathbf{F} = \partial \mathbf{f} / \partial \boldsymbol{\beta}$ and $\mathbf{G} = \partial \mathrm{vec}(\mathbf{V}) / \partial \boldsymbol{\gamma}$ are $n \times m$ and $n^2 \times p$ matrices, respectively (the dimension of $\boldsymbol{\gamma}$ is p). The first derivatives of the log-likelihood function are

$$\frac{\partial l}{\partial \boldsymbol{\beta}} = \mathbf{F}' \mathbf{V}^{-1} (\mathbf{y} - \mathbf{f}), \qquad (6.38)$$

$$\frac{\partial l}{\partial \boldsymbol{\gamma}} = \frac{1}{2} \mathbf{G}' \left[\mathbf{V}^{-1} (\mathbf{y} - \mathbf{f}) \otimes \mathbf{V}^{-1} (\mathbf{y} - \mathbf{f}) - \mathrm{vec}(\mathbf{V}^{-1}) \right]. \qquad (6.39)$$

The maximum likelihood estimate solves the $m + p$ score (estimating) equations $\partial l / \partial \boldsymbol{\beta} = \mathbf{0}$ and $\partial l / \partial \boldsymbol{\gamma} = \mathbf{0}$ for $(\boldsymbol{\beta}, \boldsymbol{\gamma})$. Now we find the information matrix, following the outline in Section 3.3. The complete $(m+p) \times (m+p)$ Fisher information matrix takes the form

$$\mathcal{I} = \begin{bmatrix} \mathbf{F}' \mathbf{V}^{-1} \mathbf{F} & \mathbf{0} \\ \mathbf{0}' & \frac{1}{2} \mathbf{G}'(\mathbf{V}^{-1} \otimes \mathbf{V}^{-1}) \mathbf{G} \end{bmatrix}, \qquad (6.40)$$

where the (h, l)th element of the second-block matrix is $0.5 tr(\dot{\mathbf{V}}_h \mathbf{V}^{-1} \dot{\mathbf{V}}_l \mathbf{V}^{-1})$ and $\dot{\mathbf{V}}_h = \partial \mathbf{V} / \partial \gamma_h$ is the $n \times n$ derivative matrix $(h, l = 1, 2, ..., p)$. For instance, as follows from (6.40), $\mathrm{cov}(\widehat{\boldsymbol{\beta}}_{ML}) = (\mathbf{F}' \mathbf{V}^{-1} \mathbf{F})^{-1}$.

Notice that the estimates for $\boldsymbol{\beta}$ and $\boldsymbol{\gamma}$ are asymptotically independent because the information matrix has a block diagonal structure. This implies that if $\boldsymbol{\beta}$ are obtained from $\partial l / \partial \boldsymbol{\beta} = \mathbf{0}$, where instead of solving (6.39), one uses a $O(1/\sqrt{N})$-consistent estimate $\widetilde{\boldsymbol{\gamma}}$, the resulting estimate for $\boldsymbol{\beta}$ will still be consistent with the covariance matrix $(\mathbf{F}' \mathbf{V}^{-1} \mathbf{F})^{-1}$. This estimator is called pseudo-MLE; see Appendix 13.1.3. The pseudo-MLE for this type of model is asymptotically equivalent to MLE. For the linear model, this result was discussed in Section 3.15 and the same result holds for model (6.1). The MM estimator for $\mathbf{D}$, in generalized/weighted least squares, leads to an estimator asymptotically equivalent to the MLE.

Another feature of model (6.35) is that *any* fixed matrix $\mathbf{V}_0$ produces a consistent and asymptotically normally distributed estimate in the weighted least squares, $(\mathbf{y} - \mathbf{f})' \mathbf{V}_0 (\mathbf{y} - \mathbf{f}) = \min$. In particular, it is instructive to show that the ordinary LS ($\mathbf{V}_0 = \mathbf{I}$) is less efficient than maximum likelihood.

Proof. We use the sandwich formula of Appendix 13.1.4 to show that asymptotically $\mathrm{var}_{LS} \geq \mathrm{var}_{ML}$. Indeed, for the ordinary LS, the estimating equation is $\mathbf{F}'(\mathbf{y} - \mathbf{f}) = 0$, and therefore, in the notation of Appendix 13.1.4, $\boldsymbol{\Psi} = \mathbf{F}'(\mathbf{y} - \mathbf{f})$ with $E(\partial \boldsymbol{\Psi} / \partial \boldsymbol{\beta}) = -\mathbf{F}' \mathbf{F}$ and $E(\boldsymbol{\Psi} \boldsymbol{\Psi}') = \mathbf{F}' \mathbf{V} \mathbf{F}$, where $\mathbf{V} = \mathrm{cov}(\mathbf{y})$. Thus, the asymptotic covariance matrix of the LSE is $(\mathbf{F}' \mathbf{F})^{-1} (\mathbf{F}' \mathbf{V} \mathbf{F}) (\mathbf{F}' \mathbf{F})^{-1}$. We need to prove that $(\mathbf{F}' \mathbf{V}^{-1} \mathbf{F})^{-1} \leq (\mathbf{F}' \mathbf{F})^{-1} (\mathbf{F}' \mathbf{V} \mathbf{F}) (\mathbf{F}' \mathbf{F})^{-1}$, the difference between the right- and left-hand sides, is a nonnegative definite matrix. To prove this inequality, we note that it is equivalent to $\mathbf{F}' \mathbf{V}^{-1} \mathbf{F} \geq (\mathbf{F}' \mathbf{F})(\mathbf{F}' \mathbf{V} \mathbf{F})^{-1}(\mathbf{F}' \mathbf{F})$. We prove the latter matrix inequality using $\mathbf{Q}(\mathbf{Q}' \mathbf{Q})^{-1} \mathbf{Q}' \leq \mathbf{I}$ for any matrix $\mathbf{Q}$ of full rank, Rao (1973), Graybill (1983). Indeed, let $\mathbf{x}$ be any $m \times 1$ vector and $\mathbf{y} = \mathbf{V}^{-1/2} \mathbf{F} \mathbf{x}$. Then $\mathbf{x}' \mathbf{F}' \mathbf{V}^{-1} \mathbf{F} \mathbf{x} = \|\mathbf{y}\|^2$, and denoting $\mathbf{Q} = \mathbf{V}^{1/2} \mathbf{F}$, we obtain $\mathbf{x}'(\mathbf{F}' \mathbf{F})(\mathbf{F}' \mathbf{V} \mathbf{F})^{-1}(\mathbf{F}' \mathbf{F}) \mathbf{x} = \mathbf{y}' \mathbf{Q}(\mathbf{Q}' \mathbf{Q})^{-1} \mathbf{Q}' \mathbf{y}$.

6.3.2   Type II nonlinear marginal model

An example of this model is the logistic curve with a random asymptote of Section 6.2.4. For this model, $\mathbf{y} \sim \mathcal{N}\left(\mathbf{f}(\boldsymbol{\beta}), \mathbf{V}(\boldsymbol{\beta}, \boldsymbol{\gamma})\right)$ and the score equation is $\partial l/\partial\boldsymbol{\theta} = \mathbf{0}$, where $\boldsymbol{\theta} = (\boldsymbol{\beta}', \boldsymbol{\gamma}')'$ and $\partial l/\partial\boldsymbol{\theta}$ takes the form

$$\mathbf{F}'\mathbf{V}^{-1}(\mathbf{y} - \mathbf{f}) + 0.5\left\{\mathbf{G}'_\beta[(\mathbf{V}^{-1}(\mathbf{y} - \mathbf{f}) \otimes \mathbf{V}^{-1}(\mathbf{y} - \mathbf{f})) - \mathrm{vec}(\mathbf{V}^{-1})]\right\}$$
$$-0.5\mathbf{G}'_\gamma[\mathbf{V}^{-1}(\mathbf{y} - \mathbf{f}) \otimes \mathbf{V}^{-1}(\mathbf{y} - \mathbf{f}) - \mathrm{vec}(\mathbf{V}^{-1})] = \mathbf{0}, \tag{6.41}$$

where

$$\mathbf{G}_\beta = \frac{\partial\mathrm{vec}(\mathbf{V})}{\partial\boldsymbol{\beta}}, \quad \mathbf{G}_\gamma = \frac{\partial\mathrm{vec}(\mathbf{V})}{\partial\boldsymbol{\gamma}}$$

are $n^2 \times m$ and $n^2 \times p$ matrices. Now we find the information matrix with estimating equations (6.41) by obtaining

$$\mathrm{cov}\left(\frac{\partial l}{\partial\boldsymbol{\gamma}}\right) = \frac{1}{4}\mathrm{cov}(\mathbf{G}'_\gamma\left(\mathbf{V}^{-1}(\mathbf{y} - \mathbf{f}) \otimes \mathbf{V}^{-1}(\mathbf{y} - \mathbf{f})\right))$$

$$= \frac{1}{4}\mathbf{G}'_\gamma(\mathbf{V}^{-1/2} \otimes \mathbf{V}^{-1/2}) \times \mathrm{cov}((\mathbf{y} - \mathbf{f}) \otimes (\mathbf{y} - \mathbf{f}))(\mathbf{V}^{-1/2} \otimes \mathbf{V}^{-1/2})\mathbf{G}_\gamma$$

$$= \frac{1}{2}\mathbf{G}'_\gamma(\mathbf{V}^{-1} \otimes \mathbf{V}^{-1})\mathbf{G}_\gamma.$$

Finally, the complete Fisher information matrix is given by

$$\mathcal{I} = \left[\begin{array}{cc} \mathbf{F}'\mathbf{V}^{-1}\mathbf{F} + \frac{1}{2}\mathbf{G}'_\beta(\mathbf{V}^{-1} \otimes \mathbf{V}^{-1})\mathbf{G}_\beta & \frac{1}{2}\mathbf{G}'_\beta(\mathbf{V}^{-1} \otimes \mathbf{V}^{-1})\mathbf{G}_\gamma \\ \frac{1}{2}\mathbf{G}'_\gamma(\mathbf{V}^{-1} \otimes \mathbf{V}^{-1})\mathbf{G}_\beta & \frac{1}{2}\mathbf{G}'_\gamma(\mathbf{V}^{-1} \otimes \mathbf{V}^{-1})\mathbf{G}_\gamma \end{array}\right]. \tag{6.42}$$

We can derive (6.40) from (6.42) because for the type I model, $\mathbf{G}_\gamma = \mathbf{G}$ and $\mathbf{G}_\beta = \mathbf{0}$.

If model (6.36) is mean-identifiable, we can apply IRLS: (a) to find an estimate of $\boldsymbol{\beta}$ by minimizing $(\mathbf{y} - \mathbf{f}(\boldsymbol{\beta}))'\mathbf{V}_0^{-1}(\mathbf{y} - \mathbf{f}(\boldsymbol{\beta}))$, where $\mathbf{V}_0$ is fixed; (b) having an estimate of $\boldsymbol{\beta}$, we can find an estimate of $\boldsymbol{\gamma}$, iterating until convergence. In Section 6.2.3, we showed that even when $\boldsymbol{\gamma}$ is known, IRLS leads to an estimate with covariance matrix $(\mathbf{F}'\mathbf{V}^{-1}\mathbf{F})^{-1}$, while the MLE produces estimates with covariance matrix $[\mathbf{F}'\mathbf{V}^{-1}\mathbf{F} + \frac{1}{2}\mathbf{G}'_\beta(\mathbf{V}^{-1} \otimes \mathbf{V}^{-1})\mathbf{G}_\beta]^{-1}$. We see that the two matrices coincide if and only if $\mathbf{G}_\beta = \mathbf{0}$, which means that matrix $\mathbf{V}$ is beta independent.

6.3.3   Type III nonlinear marginal model

An example of this model is the exponential model with a random rate, $y_{ij} = \exp(\alpha + b_i x_{ij}) + \varepsilon_{ij}$, where the rate b_i is subject-specific and random or more precisely $b_i \sim \mathcal{N}(\beta, \sigma_b^2)$. Then, if the error term is also normally distributed, $E(y_{ij}) = \exp(\alpha + \beta x_{ij} + \frac{1}{2}\beta^2 x_{ij}^2 \sigma_b^2)$ and $\mathrm{cov}(\mathbf{y}_i) = \sigma^2 \mathbf{I} + e^{\sigma_b^2}(e^{\sigma_b^2} - 1)\mathbf{1}_i\mathbf{1}_i'$, where $\mathbf{y}_i = (y_{i1}, ..., y_{in_i})'$ and $\mathbf{1}_i$ is the $n_i \times 1$ vector of 1's. Since the marginal mean depends on σ_b^2, this is a type III model. However, this model can be reduced to a type I model by reparameterizing $\gamma = \frac{1}{2}\beta^2\sigma_b^2$ so that $E(y_{ij}) = \exp(\alpha + \beta x_{ij} + \gamma x_{ij}^2)$. After $\widehat{\gamma}$ and $\widehat{\sigma}_b$ are obtained, one derives an estimate of β as $\sqrt{2\widehat{\gamma}}/\widehat{\sigma}_b$.

For the type III model, $\mathbf{y} \sim \mathcal{N}\left(\mathbf{f}(\boldsymbol{\theta}), \mathbf{V}(\boldsymbol{\theta})\right)$ and the score equation $\partial l/\partial\boldsymbol{\theta} = \mathbf{0}$ takes the form

$$\mathbf{F}'\mathbf{V}^{-1}(\mathbf{y} - \mathbf{f}) + \frac{1}{2}\mathbf{G}'[(\mathbf{V}^{-1}(\mathbf{y} - \mathbf{f}) \otimes \mathbf{V}^{-1}(\mathbf{y} - \mathbf{f})) - \mathrm{vec}(\mathbf{V}^{-1})] = \mathbf{0}, \tag{6.43}$$

where $\mathbf{F} = \partial \mathbf{f}/\partial \boldsymbol{\theta}$ and $\mathbf{G} = \partial \text{vec}(\mathbf{V})/\partial \boldsymbol{\theta}$. The Fisher information matrix is given by

$$\mathcal{I} = \mathbf{F}'\mathbf{V}^{-1}\mathbf{F} + \frac{1}{2}\mathbf{G}'(\mathbf{V}^{-1} \otimes \mathbf{V}^{-1})\mathbf{G}. \tag{6.44}$$

The type III model is the most general nonlinear marginal model, and the estimating equations and information matrices obtained previously may be derived from (6.43) and (6.44). Strictly speaking, we cannot apply IRLS to this type of model because the mean and variance parameters are indistinguishable. A new method of estimation, as a generalization of IRLS and MLE, is considered in Section 6.4.

6.3.4   Asymptotic properties under distribution misspecification

When the distribution is normal, the solution to the score/estimating equations leads to the ML estimator. Therefore, when $N \to \infty$, it is consistent, asymptotically normally distributed, and efficient with a covariance matrix equal to the inverse of the Fisher information matrix, $\mathcal{I}$. Now we investigate what happens if the same estimating equations are used but the distribution of $\mathbf{y}$ is, in fact, not normal. The estimator will still be consistent because the estimating equations for all three types are unbiased. Indeed, for the type I model, as follows from (6.38), $E(\partial l/\partial \boldsymbol{\beta}) = \mathbf{F}'\mathbf{V}^{-1}E(\mathbf{y} - \mathbf{f}) = \mathbf{0}$. The estimating equation for $\boldsymbol{\gamma}$ is also unbiased because, as follows from (6.39),

$$
\begin{aligned}
E\left(\frac{\partial l}{\partial \boldsymbol{\gamma}}\right) &= \frac{1}{2}\mathbf{G}'\left[E\left\{\mathbf{V}^{-1}(\mathbf{y} - \mathbf{f}) \otimes \mathbf{V}^{-1}(\mathbf{y} - \mathbf{f})\right\} - \text{vec}(\mathbf{V}^{-1})\right] \\
&= \frac{1}{2}\mathbf{G}'\left[(\mathbf{V}^{-1} \otimes \mathbf{V}^{-1})E\left\{(\mathbf{y} - \mathbf{f}) \otimes (\mathbf{y} - \mathbf{f})\right\} - \text{vec}(\mathbf{V}^{-1})\right] \\
&= \frac{1}{2}\mathbf{G}'\left[(\mathbf{V}^{-1} \otimes \mathbf{V}^{-1})\text{vec}(\mathbf{V}) - \text{vec}(\mathbf{V}^{-1})\right] = \mathbf{0}.
\end{aligned}
$$

See Appendix 13.2 for relevant formulas. The same proof is valid for estimating equations (6.41) and (6.43).

However, when the distribution is not normal, the MLE estimating equations will not lead to efficient estimators. In the next section we develop a general method that can also be applied to non-Gaussian distributions, particularly for distributions with long tails.

Problems for Section 6.3

1. Prove that the linear mixed model belongs to the type I nonlinear marginal model.

2. Prove that the logistic regresion with random asympote belongs to the type II nonlinear marginal model.

3. Check that the (2,2) block of the Fisher information matrix (6.40) reduces to (3.17) for the linear mixed effect model.

4. Prove that IRLS converges to the score equations (to be rigorous, each limit point of the IRLS sequence is the solution to the score equation).

5. Prove that the information matrix (6.42) is nonnegative definite. Specify conditions under which the matrix is positive definite.

6. Consider an exponential model with random intercept, $y_{ij} = \exp(a_i + \beta x_{ij}) + \varepsilon_{ij}$, where $a_i \sim \mathcal{N}(\beta, \sigma_a^2)$. To what type of nonlinear marginal model does it belong to? Find the information matrix.

7. Consider an exponential model with random intercept and slope, $y_{ij} = \exp(a_i + b_i x_{ij}) + \varepsilon_{ij}$, where $a_i \sim \mathcal{N}(\beta, \sigma_a^2)$ and $b_i \sim \mathcal{N}(\beta, \sigma_b^2)$ are independent. To what type of nonlinear marginal model does it belong? Find the information matrix.

8. For what type of nonlinear marginal model is the ML estimator not consistent, when in fact the distribution is not normal but the first two moments are the same as in the normal distribution?

6.4 Total generalized estimating equations approach

As shown above, if the mean and variance functions do not share parameters, the IRLS is asymptotically equivalent to the MLE. If the mean and variance do share parameters, the IRLS is easier to implement but less efficient. On the other hand, the IRLS is robust to the distribution misspecification but the MLE is not. As a word of caution, IRLS cannot be applied to a type III model when the mean and variance parameters are indistinguishable. The goal of this section is to combine the IRLS and MLE under one umbrella, with one control parameter, which specifies a distribution-free estimation method.

We concentrate our attention on the most general estimating equations, (6.43). The key observation for our approach, called the *total generalized estimating equations approach*, is that the estimating equations will stay unbiased if factor $\frac{1}{2}$ is replaced by any positive coefficient (we will provide an interpretation for that coefficient later). Thus, we come to the total generalized estimating equations (Total GEE or TGEE) approach, which gives estimates for $\boldsymbol{\theta}$ as the solution to the vector equation

$$\mathbf{F}'\mathbf{V}^{-1}(\mathbf{y} - \mathbf{f}) + \nu \mathbf{G}'[\mathbf{V}^{-1}(\mathbf{y} - \mathbf{f}) \otimes \mathbf{V}^{-1}(\mathbf{y} - \mathbf{f}) - \text{vec}(\mathbf{V}^{-1})] = \mathbf{0}, \qquad (6.45)$$

where ν is a positive constant. The left-hand side of (6.45) is called the estimating function and, following the notation of Appendix 13.1.4, is denoted $\boldsymbol{\Psi} = \boldsymbol{\Psi}(\boldsymbol{\theta})$. This estimating equation may be viewed as a linear combination of two estimating equations, one for the mean and another for the variance. Parameter ν may be viewed as the weight coefficient of the variance part. If $\mathbf{y}$ is normally distributed and $\nu = \frac{1}{2}$, we come to maximum likelihood. Thus, maximum likelihood is a special case of TGEE. For a type I marginal model, Total GEE collapses to $\partial l / \partial \boldsymbol{\beta} = \mathbf{0}$ and $\partial l / \partial \boldsymbol{\gamma} = \mathbf{0}$ defined by (6.38) and (6.39), and ν does not matter. For a type II marginal model (6.45) collapses to (6.41). However, now we do not assume that $\mathbf{y}$ is normally distributed.

One comment on the terminology. The estimating equations (EE) approach is a general method to obtain an estimate by solving the vector equation $\sum_{i=1}^{N} \boldsymbol{\Psi}(\mathbf{y}_i, \boldsymbol{\gamma}) = 0$, where $\boldsymbol{\gamma}$ is the m-dimensional parameter and $\boldsymbol{\Psi}$ is the m-dimensional vector function; see Appendix 13.1.4. The Generalized estimating equations (GEE) approach is a special case of EE when the estimating equation is expressed in terms of the mean and variance of $\mathbf{y}_i$, particularly for the generalized linear model (Zeger and Liang, 1986; Liang and Zeger, 1986). Since (6.45) is expressed in terms of the first two moments, we call it TGEE. The GEE approach, applied to binary and count data, is considered in the next chapter.

In the next theorem, we formulate the general properties of the TGEE approach. For model (6.37), we introduce the normalized vector $\boldsymbol{\zeta} = \mathbf{V}^{-1/2}(\mathbf{y} - \mathbf{f})$. Notice that all components of this vector $\zeta_1, ..., \zeta_N$ have zero mean and unit variance. Then we have $\text{var}(\zeta_i^2) = E(\zeta_i^4) - 1 = \kappa - 1$, where κ is the kurtosis; see Section 5.1.4. For a normally distributed $\boldsymbol{\eta}$, the kurtosis is 3. A greater kurtosis indicates a flatter distribution around the mean; typically, distributions with large kurtosis have long tails.

Now we formulate the main result.

Theorem 32 *The TGEE estimator $\widehat{\boldsymbol{\theta}}_{TGEE}$, as the solution to estimating equations (6.45), is consistent and asymptotically normally distributed for any positive ν. If the third moment of ζ_i is zero, then*

$$\text{cov}(\widehat{\boldsymbol{\theta}}_{TGEE}) = (\mathbf{P} + \nu\mathbf{Q})^{-1}(\mathbf{P} + \nu^2(\kappa - 1)\mathbf{Q})(\mathbf{P} + \nu\mathbf{Q})^{-1}, \qquad (6.46)$$

where the $p \times p$ matrices $\mathbf{P}$ and $\mathbf{Q}$ are defined as

$$\mathbf{P} = \mathbf{F}'\mathbf{V}^{-1}\mathbf{F}, \quad \mathbf{Q} = \mathbf{G}'(\mathbf{V}^{-1} \otimes \mathbf{V}^{-1})\mathbf{G}. \qquad (6.47)$$

Furthermore: (a) The covariance matrix (6.46) attains its minimum at $\nu = 1/(\kappa - 1)$. (b) If $\mathbf{y}$ is normally distributed, then $\nu = \frac{1}{2}$ produces an MLE with $\text{cov}(\widehat{\boldsymbol{\theta}}_{TGEE})$ $= \text{cov}(\widehat{\boldsymbol{\theta}}_{ML}) = (\mathbf{P} + \mathbf{Q})^{-1}$. (c) For any distribution of $\mathbf{y}$, there exists a sufficiently small positive ν that $\text{cov}(\widehat{\boldsymbol{\theta}}_{TGEE}) \leq \mathbf{P}^{-1}$.

Proof. First, we see that the estimating equation (6.45) is unbiased because $E(\mathbf{y} - \mathbf{f}) = \mathbf{0}$ and $E\left[\mathbf{V}^{-1}(\mathbf{y} - \mathbf{f}) \otimes \mathbf{V}^{-1}(\mathbf{y} - \mathbf{f})\right] = \mathbf{V}^{-1}\mathbf{V}\mathbf{V}^{-1} = \mathbf{V}^{-1}$, so that the expected value of the second term of (6.45) is zero. Second, we use the sandwich formula of Appendix 13.1.4 to obtain the asymptotic covariance matrix of $\widehat{\boldsymbol{\theta}}_{TGEE}$. For this we need to find the expected value of the derivative of (6.45) with respect to $\boldsymbol{\theta}$. The expected value of the first term is $-\mathbf{G}'\mathbf{V}^{-1}\mathbf{G}'$. For the second term, we use formula (13.31), which yields

$$E\frac{\mathbf{V}^{-1}(\mathbf{y} - \mathbf{f}) \otimes \mathbf{V}^{-1}(\mathbf{y} - \mathbf{f})}{\partial\boldsymbol{\theta}} = E\frac{\text{vec}\left[\mathbf{V}^{-1}(\mathbf{y} - \mathbf{f})(\mathbf{y} - \mathbf{f})'\mathbf{V}^{-1}\right]}{\partial\boldsymbol{\theta}}$$
$$= -E\{\left[\mathbf{V}^{-1}(\mathbf{y} - \mathbf{f})(\mathbf{y} - \mathbf{f})' \otimes \mathbf{I}\right](\mathbf{V}^{-1} \otimes \mathbf{V}^{-1})\mathbf{G}$$
$$+ \left[\mathbf{I} \otimes \mathbf{V}^{-1}(\mathbf{y} - \mathbf{f})(\mathbf{y} - \mathbf{f})'\right](\mathbf{V}^{-1} \otimes \mathbf{V}^{-1})\mathbf{G}\} = -2(\mathbf{V}^{-1} \otimes \mathbf{V}^{-1})\mathbf{G}.$$

Thus we obtain

$$E\frac{\partial\mathbf{G}'[\mathbf{V}^{-1}(\mathbf{y} - \mathbf{f}) \otimes \mathbf{V}^{-1}(\mathbf{y} - \mathbf{f}) - \text{vec}(\mathbf{V}^{-1})]}{\partial\boldsymbol{\theta}}$$
$$= \mathbf{G}'\left[-2(\mathbf{V}^{-1} \otimes \mathbf{V}^{-1})\mathbf{G} + (\mathbf{V}^{-1} \otimes \mathbf{V}^{-1})\mathbf{G}\right] = -\mathbf{Q},$$

and we finally obtain $E(\partial\boldsymbol{\Psi}/\partial\boldsymbol{\theta}) - -(\mathbf{P} + \nu\mathbf{Q})$, where $\boldsymbol{\Psi}$ is the left-hand side of (6.45). If $E(\zeta_i) = 0$, the expectation between the first and second terms of (6.45) is zero and $E(\boldsymbol{\Psi}\boldsymbol{\Psi}') = \mathbf{P} + \nu^2(\kappa - 1)\mathbf{Q}$. Formula (6.46) is proved. Now we prove statement (a) that the minimum of $\text{cov}(\widehat{\boldsymbol{\theta}}_{TGEE})$ is attained at $\nu = 1/(\kappa - 1)$. Denoting $\mathbf{R} = \mathbf{Q}^{-1/2}\mathbf{P}\mathbf{Q}^{-1/2}$, we obtain

$$\mathbf{Q}^{1/2}\text{cov}(\widehat{\boldsymbol{\theta}}_{TGEE})\mathbf{Q}^{1/2} = (\mathbf{R}+\nu\mathbf{I})^{-1}(\mathbf{R}+\nu^2(\kappa - 1)\mathbf{I})(\mathbf{R}+\nu\mathbf{I})^{-1}. \qquad (6.48)$$

Taking the spectral decomposition of matrix $\mathbf{R} = \sum \lambda_i\mathbf{p}_i\mathbf{p}_i'$, where $\{\lambda_i\}$ are positive eigenvalues and the $\{\mathbf{p}_i\}$ are eigenvectors, we may write $(\mathbf{R}+\nu\mathbf{I})^{-1} = \sum(\lambda_i + \nu)^{-1}\mathbf{p}_i\mathbf{p}_i'$, $\mathbf{R}+\nu^2(\kappa - 1)\mathbf{I} = \sum(\lambda_i + \nu^2(\kappa - 1))\mathbf{p}_i\mathbf{p}_i'$ so that the right-hand side of (6.48) can be written as $\mathbf{L}(\nu) = \sum(\lambda_i + \nu^2(\kappa - 1))(\lambda_i + \nu)^{-2}\mathbf{p}_i\mathbf{p}_i'$. Let $\mathbf{c}$ be any nonzero vector. Then function $L_c(\nu) = \mathbf{c}'\mathbf{L}(\nu)\mathbf{c} = \sum(\lambda_i + \nu^2(\kappa - 1))(\lambda_i + \nu)^{-2}h_i^2$, where $h_i = \mathbf{p}_i'\mathbf{c}$, takes the minimum where $dL_c/d\kappa = 0$. But $dL_c/d\nu = 2(\nu(\kappa - 1) - 1)\sum \lambda_i h_i^2(\lambda_i + \nu)^{-3}$, which becomes zero if and only if $\nu = 1/(\kappa - 1)$. Thus the minimum of $\mathbf{r}'\text{cov}(\widehat{\boldsymbol{\theta}}_{TGEE})\mathbf{r}$ for any vector $\mathbf{r}$ takes its minimum at $\nu = 1/(\kappa - 1)$. Statement (a) is proved. For $0 < \nu < 1/(\kappa - 1)$ we have $dL_c/d\nu < 0$ for all $\mathbf{c} \neq \mathbf{0}$ regardless of $\mathbf{y}$ distribution; this proves (c) because if the derivative is negative, we can find ν_0 such that $L_c(0) > L_c(\nu_0)$. Statement (b) follows from the fact that for the normal distribution, $\kappa - 1 = 2$ and $(\kappa - 1)^2\nu = \kappa - 1$.

6.4.1 Robust feature of total GEE

Total GEE is controlled by parameter ν. For the Gaussian distribution, the optimal $\nu = 1/2$; for a distribution with kurtosis κ, the optimal parameter is $\nu = 1/(\kappa - 1)$. For example, for the Laplace (double–exponential) distribution, $\kappa = 6$, and therefore the optimal $\nu = 1/5$. Since a larger kurtosis typically implies a heavier tail, we conclude that a smaller coefficient ν in the estimating equation (6.45) leads to a more robust estimate. In Table 6.3 we show kurtosis and the respective optimal ν for several symmetric distributions with heavy tails. (The positive coefficient C is such that the area under the curve is 1.) As follows from this table, $\nu = 1/5$ or smaller may be a good choice if a distribution with a heavy tail is suspected. Estimation with several ν (including $\nu = 1/2$) may shed light on how sensitive the estimates are to the normal distribution assumption (see the example in Section 6.4.5).

Table 6.3. Optimal values for ν for different distributions

Distribution of η_i	Density	Kurtosis κ $E(X^4)/\sigma^4$	Optimal ν $1/(\kappa - 1)$
Normal	$Ce^{-x^2/2\sigma^2}$	3	0.50
Normal×Power2	$C(1 + x^6)e^{-4x^2}$	3.76	0.36
Normal×Power10	$C(1 + x^{20})e^{-10x^2}$	5.39	0.23
Laplace	$Ce^{-\lambda|x|}$	6	0.20
t-distr. with k d.f.	$C\left(1 + \frac{x^2}{k}\right)^{-\frac{k+1}{2}}$	$\frac{3(k-2)}{k-4}$	$\frac{k-4}{2(k+2)}$

6.4.2 Expected Newton–Raphson algorithm for total GEE

To solve the estimating equation (6.45), we may use the linear approximation, as in the Newton algorithm. If $\boldsymbol{\theta}_0$ is the initial approximation to the solution of $\boldsymbol{\Psi}(\boldsymbol{\theta}) = \mathbf{0}$ after linearization, $\boldsymbol{\Psi}(\boldsymbol{\theta}) \simeq \boldsymbol{\Psi}_0 + (\partial\boldsymbol{\Psi}/\partial\boldsymbol{\theta})_0(\boldsymbol{\theta} - \boldsymbol{\theta}_0)$, we come to the next approximation, $\boldsymbol{\theta}_1 = \boldsymbol{\theta}_0 - (\partial\boldsymbol{\Psi}/\partial\boldsymbol{\theta})_0^{-1}\boldsymbol{\Psi}_0$, where $\boldsymbol{\Psi}_0 = \boldsymbol{\Psi}(\boldsymbol{\theta}_0)$ and $(\partial\boldsymbol{\Psi}/\partial\boldsymbol{\theta})_0 =$

$\partial\boldsymbol{\Psi}(\boldsymbol{\theta} = \boldsymbol{\theta}_0)/\partial\boldsymbol{\theta}$. Now we observe that instead of $(\partial\boldsymbol{\Psi}/\partial\boldsymbol{\theta})_0$, one may use any other number fairly close to $(\partial\boldsymbol{\Psi}/\partial\boldsymbol{\theta})_0$, so that we may take the expectation of $\partial\boldsymbol{\Psi}/\partial\boldsymbol{\theta}$, which is $-(\mathbf{P}_s + \nu\mathbf{Q}_s)$. This leads to iterations

$$\boldsymbol{\theta}_{s+1} = \boldsymbol{\theta}_s + (\mathbf{P}_s + \nu\mathbf{Q}_s)^{-1}\boldsymbol{\Psi}_s, \tag{6.49}$$

where s is the iteration index, $\boldsymbol{\Psi}_s$ is the estimating function, and $\mathbf{P}_s$ and $\mathbf{Q}_s$ are matrices defined in (6.47), all computed at $\boldsymbol{\theta} = \boldsymbol{\theta}_s$. We call this algorithm the Expected Newton–Raphson (ENR) algorithm. The word *expected* comes from the fact that $-(\mathbf{P}_s + \nu\mathbf{Q}_s)$ is the expected value of the Jacobian used in the standard Newton–Raphson algorithm. Below we show that for the linear mixed effects model, this algorithm is Fisher scoring.

6.4.3 Total GEE for the mixed effects model

It is straightforward to apply the formulas for the mixed model with repeated measurements in the form $\mathbf{y}_i = \mathbf{f}_i(\boldsymbol{\theta}) + \boldsymbol{\eta}_i$, where $\text{cov}(\boldsymbol{\eta}_i) = \mathbf{V}_i(\boldsymbol{\theta})$ and $i = 1, 2, ..., N$ denotes cluster/subject. (It merely requires the subindex i.) As always, we assume that observations between clusters are independent. Due to this independence, the estimating equation takes the form of the sum over all clusters,

$$\sum_{i=1}^{N}\left\{\mathbf{F}_i'\mathbf{V}_i^{-1}(\mathbf{y}_i-\mathbf{f}_i)+\nu\mathbf{G}_i'[\mathbf{V}_i^{-1}(\mathbf{y}_i-\mathbf{f}_i)\otimes\mathbf{V}_i^{-1}(\mathbf{y}_i-\mathbf{f}_i)-\text{vec}(\mathbf{V}_i^{-1})]\right\} = \mathbf{0}. \tag{6.50}$$

To solve this equation, we use the ENR algorithm (6.49), where $\boldsymbol{\Psi}$ is the left-hand side of the estimating equation above and

$$\mathbf{P} = \sum_{i=1}^{N}\mathbf{F}_i'\mathbf{V}_i^{-1}\mathbf{F}_i, \quad \mathbf{Q} = \sum_{i=1}^{N}\mathbf{G}_i'(\mathbf{V}_i^{-1}\otimes\mathbf{V}_i^{-1})\mathbf{G}_i. \tag{6.51}$$

As follows from (6.49), if iterations converge, the limit is the solution to (6.50) because then $\lim_{s\to\infty}(\boldsymbol{\theta}_{s+1} - \boldsymbol{\theta}_s) = \mathbf{0}$, and multiplying by $\mathbf{P}_s + \nu\mathbf{Q}_s$ we obtain $\lim_{s\to\infty}\boldsymbol{\Psi}_s = \mathbf{0}$. Below we illustrate TGEE by two examples. Also, we shall apply this approach to the Poisson model with random effects, where the covariance matrix can be computed exactly, Section 7.5.

6.4.4 Total GEE for the LME model

To illustrate, we apply Total GEE to the LME model (2.14). Since the parameters of the mean and covariance matrix do not overlap, we conclude that model (2.14) is a type I marginal model. For this model, TGEE (6.45) collapses to two separate equations, for $\boldsymbol{\beta}$ and $(\sigma^2, \mathbf{D}_*)$, defined by (6.38) and (6.39), respectively, where the covariance matrix of the ith cluster is $\mathbf{V}_i = \sigma^2\mathbf{I} + \mathbf{Z}_i\mathbf{D}_*\mathbf{Z}_i'$. Note here that we use matrix $\mathbf{D}_*$ as the parameter matrix (in the previous notation, $\mathbf{D}_* = \sigma^2\mathbf{D}$). The estimating equation for $\boldsymbol{\beta}$ is given by (6.38) and leads to the GLS estimator, $(\sum\mathbf{X}_i'\mathbf{V}_i^{-1}\mathbf{X}_i)\sum\mathbf{X}_i'\mathbf{V}_i^{-1}\mathbf{y}_i$. Now we derive the estimating equation for the variance parameters using (6.39). In particular, our current aim is to obtain an explicit expression for the derivative matrix $\mathbf{G}$. Using the properties of the matrix

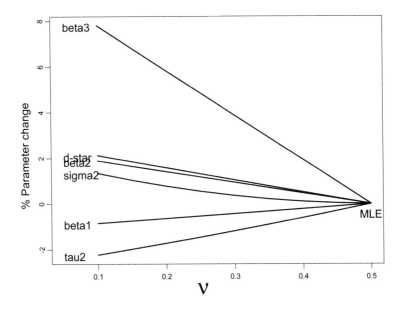

FIGURE 6.5. Six parameter estimates of the log-Gompertz curve with two random effects/parameters, as a function of ν in total GEE. When $\nu = 1/2$, all curves start from MLE assuming normal distribution. The most sensitive parameter to the distribution specification is β_3. However, when the kurtosis of the distribution is $1/0.1 + 1 = 11$ (very flat), this parameter changes from the MLE by only 8%. Thus, the MLE for these data and model is robust to the distribution specification.

Kronecker product (see Appendix 13.2.3), we have vec$(\mathbf{V})$ =vec$(\sigma^2\mathbf{I} + \mathbf{Z}_i\mathbf{D}_*\mathbf{Z}_i')$ = σ^2vec$(\mathbf{I}) + (\mathbf{Z}_i \otimes \mathbf{Z}_i)vec(\mathbf{D}_*)$, and therefore $\mathbf{G} = [\text{vec}(\mathbf{I}), \mathbf{Z}_i \otimes \mathbf{Z}_i]$. Hence, the estimating equation (6.39) can be rewritten as

$$\sum_{i=1}^{N}\left[\begin{array}{c} \text{vec}'(\mathbf{I})\left[\mathbf{V}_i^{-1}(\mathbf{y}_i-\mathbf{X}_i\boldsymbol{\beta}) \otimes \mathbf{V}_i^{-1}(\mathbf{y}_i-\mathbf{X}_i\boldsymbol{\beta})-\text{vec}(\mathbf{V}_i^{-1})\right] \\ (\mathbf{Z}_i' \otimes \mathbf{Z}_i')\left[\mathbf{V}_i^{-1}(\mathbf{y}_i-\mathbf{X}_i\boldsymbol{\beta}) \otimes \mathbf{V}_i^{-1}(\mathbf{y}_i-\mathbf{X}_i\boldsymbol{\beta})-\text{vec}(\mathbf{V}_i^{-1})\right] \end{array}\right] = \mathbf{0}.$$

Using further properties of the Kronecker product, we find that this system is equivalent to

$$\sum\left[(\mathbf{y}_i-\mathbf{X}_i\boldsymbol{\beta})'\mathbf{V}_i^{-2}(\mathbf{y}_i-\mathbf{X}_i\boldsymbol{\beta}) - \text{tr}(\mathbf{V}_i^{-1})\right] = 0,$$
$$\sum\left[\mathbf{Z}_i'\mathbf{V}_i^{-1}(\mathbf{y}_i-\mathbf{X}_i\boldsymbol{\beta})(\mathbf{y}_i-\mathbf{X}_i\boldsymbol{\beta})'\mathbf{V}_i^{-1}\mathbf{Z}_i - \mathbf{Z}_i'\mathbf{V}_i^{-1}\mathbf{Z}_i\right] = 0, \qquad (6.52)$$

where $\boldsymbol{\beta} = (\sum\mathbf{X}_i'\mathbf{V}_i^{-1}\mathbf{X}_i)^{-1}(\sum\mathbf{X}_i'\mathbf{V}_i^{-1}\mathbf{y}_i)$. These are the score equations for the log-likelihood function under parameterization $(\sigma^2, \mathbf{D}_*)$, see Section 2.2.4.

6.4.5   Example (continued): log-Gompertz curve

We illustrate the TGEE approach by the log-Gompertz growth curve (6.16) studied in Section 6.1.7. This model is a type I nonlinear model because the mean and the covariance matrix depend on different parameters. Now we provide formulas for the maximum likelihood estimation by the ENR algorithm based on

(6.49). In the notation of the TGEE approach, $\mathbf{V}_i = \sigma^2\mathbf{I} + d_*\mathbf{1}_i\mathbf{1}_i'$ and $\mathbf{G}_{i\beta} = \partial\mathrm{vec}(\mathbf{V}_i)/\partial\boldsymbol{\beta} = \mathbf{0}$ because $\mathbf{V}_i$ does not contain components of the $\boldsymbol{\beta}$ vector. Further, $\mathbf{G}_{i\gamma} = \partial\mathrm{vec}(\mathbf{V}_i)/\partial\boldsymbol{\gamma} = [\mathrm{vec}(\mathbf{I}), \mathbf{1}_i \otimes \mathbf{1}_i]$, where $\boldsymbol{\gamma} = (\sigma^2, d_*)$ is the variance parameter vector, so that $\mathbf{G}_i = [\mathbf{0}, \mathrm{vec}(\mathbf{I}), \mathbf{1}_i \otimes \mathbf{1}_i]$. The total parameter vector of dimension $3 + 2 = 5$ is $\boldsymbol{\theta} = (\boldsymbol{\beta}, \boldsymbol{\gamma})$. The $n_i \times 5$ matrix of the first derivatives of the mean is $\mathbf{F}_i = \partial\mathbf{f}_i/\partial\boldsymbol{\theta} = [\mathbf{1}_i, -\mathbf{e}_i, \beta_2(\mathbf{t}_i\mathbf{e}_i), \mathbf{0}, \mathbf{0}]$, where $\mathbf{e}_i = e^{-\beta_3\mathbf{t}_i}$, and $(\mathbf{t}_i\mathbf{e}_i)$ is an $n_i \times 1$ vector with the jth component $t_{ij}e^{-\beta_3 t_{ij}}$. Now, application of the ENR algorithm defined by (6.49), where matrices $\mathbf{P}$ and $\mathbf{Q}$ are given by (6.51), is straightforward. One can even yield closed forms for matrices $\mathbf{P}$ and $\mathbf{Q}$ using the matrix inverse formula (2.69). The ENR algorithm required three or four iterations to converge to the MLE regardless of the initial value of the parameters.

Next we complicate the model by assuming that the second parameter of the log-Gompertz curve is also spheroid-specific and random, namely, $y_{ij} = (\beta_1 + b_i) - (\beta_2 + \delta_i)e^{-\beta_3 t_{ij}} + \varepsilon_{ij}$. In addition to the previous assumptions, we assume that the $\{\delta_i\}$ are iid with zero mean and unknown variance τ^2. However, unlike the previous log-Gompertz model, we do not assume that the distribution is normal, but symmetric with kurtosis κ. To simplify, we assume that b_i and δ_i are uncorrelated. The matrix $\mathbf{V}_i = \sigma^2\mathbf{I} + d_*\mathbf{1}_i\mathbf{1}_i' + \tau^2\mathbf{e}_i\mathbf{e}_i'$ is the $n_i \times n_i$ covariance matrix of $\mathbf{y}_i$. This model is of type II and belongs to the family of marginal mixed models with a varied matrix of random effects, (6.17). Since the mean function does not depend on the variance parameter $\boldsymbol{\gamma} = (\sigma^2, d_*, \tau^2)'$, we have $\mathbf{F}_i = [\mathbf{1}_i, -\mathbf{e}_i, \beta_2(\mathbf{t}_i\mathbf{e}_i); \mathbf{0}]$ where $\mathbf{0}$ is an $n_i \times 3$ zero matrix. Noting that in vector form $\mathrm{vec}(\mathbf{V}_i) = \sigma^2\mathrm{vec}(\mathbf{I}) + d_*(\mathbf{1}_i \otimes \mathbf{1}_i) + \tau^2(\mathbf{e}_i \otimes \mathbf{e}_i)$, we find that

$$\mathbf{G}_{i\beta} = \frac{\partial\mathrm{vec}(\mathbf{V}_i)}{\partial\boldsymbol{\beta}} = [\mathbf{0}, \mathbf{0}, -\tau^2(\mathbf{e}_i \otimes (\mathbf{t}_i\mathbf{e}_i) + (\mathbf{t}_i\mathbf{e}_i) \otimes \mathbf{e}_i)],$$

$$\mathbf{G}_{i\gamma} = \frac{\partial\mathrm{vec}(\mathbf{V}_i)}{\partial\boldsymbol{\gamma}} = [\mathrm{vec}(\mathbf{I}), \mathbf{1}_i \otimes \mathbf{1}_i, \mathbf{e}_i \otimes \mathbf{e}_i].$$

The combined matrix of the derivatives is $\mathbf{G}_i = [\mathbf{G}_{i\beta}, \mathbf{G}_{i\gamma}]$. We apply the ENR algorithm to find estimates with different ν (it required a few iterations to converge). The results are displayed graphically in Figure 6.5. $\nu = 0.5$ produces the MLE under a normal distribution; $\nu = 0.1$ is optimal if the kurtosis of the distribution is $1/0.1 + 1 = 11$ (very flat). Parameter β_3 is the most sensitive to deviation from the normal distribution, although the difference is small (maximum 8%). One may conclude that for these data (parameter values) and this model, the normal assumption is fairly adequate.

6.4.6   Photodynamic tumor therapy

In this section we present the data for an application of the total GEE aproach to model the mouse response to tumor treatment (Demidenko, 2006a). PhotoDynamic Therapy (PDT) is an alternative to the standard radiation tumor treatment (Pogue et al., 2003). An advantage of PDT over the traditional gamma-ray therapy is that the light is less harmful to normal tissue, although penetration is limited. The data are in the file `phototumdat.csv` and the R function below reads and plots the data using the `xyplot` function from the library `lattice` (see Figure 6.6) and estimates the tumor response by the `nlme` function using the LINEXP tumor regrowth model.

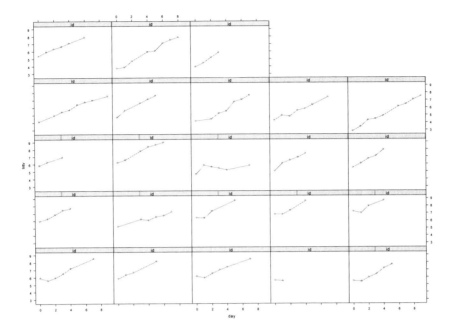

FIGURE 6.6. Post-PDT tumor volume growth in 31 mice on the log scale.

```
phototum=function(){
library(lattice);library(nlme)
dump("phototum","c:\\MixedModels\\Chapter06\\phototum.r")
datpt=read.csv("c:\\MixedModels\\Chapter06\\phototumdat.csv")
xyplot(lntv~day|id,type="b",data=datpt)
outnlme<-nlme(lntv~alpha+gamma*day+beta*(exp(-delta*day)-1),
        fixed=alpha+gamma+beta+delta~1, random=pdDiag(alpha+beta~1),
        groups=~id,data=datpt,start=c(5,0.5,2.7,0.23))
summary(outnlme)
}
```

We model the response of mouse tumor to PDT using the following nonmonotonic function of time on the log scale:

$$y(t) = \alpha + \gamma t + \beta(e^{-\delta t} - 1), \quad t \geq 0, \tag{6.53}$$

where $y(t) = \ln V(t)$, the logarithm of the tumor volume. This function, called the LINEXP function (Demidenko, 2006a), has easily interpretable parameters: parameter α determines the initial log tumor volume, parameter γ is the rate of growth of the untreated tumor volume, parameter δ is the rate at which killed cells are washing out from the tumor, and $e^{-\beta}$ is the fraction of cancer cells surviving treatment. A statistical model that describes the tumor dynamics after PDT takes the form

$$y_{ij} = a_i + \gamma t_{ij} + b_i(e^{-\delta t_{ij}} - 1) + \varepsilon_{ij},$$

where $i = 1, 2, ..., N = 31$ is the number of mice and $j = 1, 2, ..., n_i$ are indices of observations within the mouse. We assume that γ and δ are fixed unknown parameters and that a_i and b_i are mouse-specific and random. To make the statistical model easier, we shall assume that a_i and b_i are independent. This assumption has been confirmed empirically—the correlation coefficient was -0.11 with the p-value=0.45. Moreover, the results of the estimation with an unstructured covariance matrix for a_i and b_i using the `nlme` function were practically identical to the results based on the independence assumption.

Of course, the normal assumption is questionable and we ask you to apply the total GEE with different ν to these data in the Problem 4 below.

Problems for Section 6.4

1*. Apply TGEE and the results of the theorem to regression with a symmetric but not normal distribution, $(y_i - \boldsymbol{\beta}'\mathbf{x}_i)/\sigma = \eta_i \sim f$, as in Table 6.3. Use simulations to confirm the superiority of TGEE compared to the linear least squares. Apply the ENR algorithm for estimate computation.

2. Develop an algorithm to solve the $(1 + k^2)$ score equations (6.52) for σ^2 and $\mathbf{D}_*$. Rewrite $\mathbf{V}_i = \mathbf{V}_{i0} + (\sigma^2 - \sigma_0^2)\mathbf{I} + \mathbf{Z}_i(\mathbf{D}_* - \mathbf{D}_{*0})\mathbf{Z}_i'$ and use approximation (2.108) to obtain adjustments for σ^2 and $\mathbf{D}_*$. Write an R function that estimates a linear mixed model using the GEE approach. Run simulations with normally distributed errors to test the code. Run simulations with nonnormal errors, such as those presented in Table 6.3, and compare with the maximum likelihood estimation (use `lme` or our own `lmeFS`).

3. Reproduce the efficiency computation in Figure 6.5 for the log-Gompertz curve using `TUMspher.txt` data.

4*. Apply the total GEE approach to the `photutumdat.csv` data set using the LINEXP model described above. Use the ENR algorithm and construct the derivative matrices similar to those in Section 6.4.5. Plot all seven parameters as a function of ν in the range 0.2 to 0.5. Consult Demidenko (2006a).

6.5   Summary points

- In this chapter, nonlinear marginal mixed models are considered in which the mean and variance/covariance functions are explicit functions of the population-averaged parameters. Models in which the regression function/marginal mean cannot be expressed in closed form, therefore requiring integration, are studied in the subsequent chapters. A marginal model is suitable for a continuous dependent variable where the normal distribution (perhaps after taking the log transformation) is a good candidate.

- A straightforward generalization of the linear mixed effects model is the model in which fixed effects/mean is a nonlinear function of the population-averaged parameter $\boldsymbol{\beta}$ with a fixed matrix of random effects, (6.1). Two kinds of estimation methods can be applied: maximum likelihood and distribution-free. In the latter we borrow estimates for the variance parameters from the linear model. A characteristic property of this model is that one comes to an asymptotically efficient estimate for β if any consistent estimate for the matrix of random effects, $\mathbf{D}$, is used in the weighted nonlinear least squares.

- Estimation of a nonlinear regression and a nonlinear mixed model may lead to difficult optimization problems that involve the absence of a solution (minimum of sum of squares), nonuniqueness (several local minima), and nonconvergence of the iterative minimization procedure. At least two initial points for iterations should be tried to ensure that iterations converge to the same value.

- The next generalization of the linear mixed effects model is to assume that the variance/covariance function is a nonlinear function and contains parameters of the mean, (6.17). The model with a varied matrix of random effects principally differs from the model with a fixed matrix of random effects in that use of a consistent matrix $\mathbf{D}$ no longer leads to asymptotically efficient estimates for β. Particularly, a popular iterated reweighted least squares (IRLS) method yields consistent but less efficient estimates for β. The maximum likelihood estimator is more efficient but loses consistency if the distribution is misspecified. On the contrary, IRLS remains consistent even if the distribution is misspecified. If the data are balanced, the advantage of the MLE over IRLS may be slim even if the distribution is normal.

- Generally, three types of nonlinear models of increasing complexity, as a generalization of the regression model with variance function, can be considered. In the type I model, the mean/regression and variance parameters are different. In the type II model, the variance function depends on the mean parameters. Finally, in the type III model, the mean and variance share parameters. Thus, the marginal model with a fixed matrix of random effects, (6.1), belongs to type I, and with a varied matrix of random effects, (6.17), to type II.

- For a type I nonlinear model, any consistent estimate of the variance parameters leads to an asymptotically efficient estimate of β. For the mean-identifiable type II model, IRLS leads to a consistent estimate of β regardless of distribution. If the distribution is normal, MLE is more efficient, but it loses its consistency if the distribution is misspecified. Strictly speaking, IRLS cannot be applied to a type III model because variance parameters are involved.

- The Total Generalized Estimating Equations (TGEE) approach combines the MLE and IRLS under one umbrella. The estimating equation is a linear combination of the estimating equation for the mean and variance with the weight coefficient ν, assuming that the distribution has a zero third moment (true for symmetric distribution). For a type I model, TGEE reduces to maximum likelihood; for a type II model, $\nu = 0$ corresponds to IRLS and $\nu = 1/2$ to the ML.

- A smaller ν gives a more robust estimation that is less efficient if the distribution is normal. For example, if the distribution is double–exponential (Laplace), the optimal $\nu = 1/5$. Computation of the TGEE estimates with several ν (including $\nu = 1/2$) may shed light on how sensitive estimates are to the normal distribution assumption.

- The expected Newton–Raphson algorithm is developed to solve TGEE. For a linear mixed effects model, this algorithm collapses to Fisher scoring and usually requires a few iterations to converge, provided that there is a good initial value/starting point.

- The three types of nonlinear models require gradually increasing complexity of methods of estimation. For a type I model, GEE and MLE for β are asymptotically equivalent. For a type II model, GEE/IRLS is consistent and asymptotically distributed with variances larger then MLE. Use of any consistent estimate of the variance parameters γ in the estimating equation for β leads to the same distribution as that when the true variance parameters are used. For type III model, no distinction between parameters (such as model coefficients β and the variance parameters γ) can be made to facilitate the estimation. Parameters may be estimated by either TGEE or maximum likelihood.

7
Generalized Linear Mixed Models

In this chapter we continue studying nonlinear mixed models. In the preceding chapter we dealt with marginal mixed models where the dependent variable is the sum of nonlinear fixed effects and linear random effects. Starting with this chapter, random effects are nonlinear as well. Consequently, we cannot express the marginal mean of $\mathbf{y}$ in closed form, and integration is required. The Generalized Linear Mixed Model (GLMM) is an extension of the generalized linear model (GLM) complicated by random effects. The marginal mixed model of Chapter 6 plays an important role in nonlinear random effects methodology because, after approximation, the latter model is reduced to the former. GLMM takes an intermediate position between the marginal model and the nonlinear mixed effects model. In recent years it has gained significant popularity in modeling binary/count clustered and longitudinal data.

Usually, the GLMM is introduced in general terms via an exponential distribution family. Then special cases of GLMM, such as logistic or Poisson regressions, are *deduced* as specific forms of the link function. We take an alternative, *inductive* route. First we discuss in detail the most important special cases, such as logistic and probit regression for binary data and Poisson regression for count data. Second, we illustrate how GLMM, generally, may be derived from the exponential family convoluted with random effects. Although an inductive approach may seem repetitive (the models have common features), it is more powerful because the specificity of the model is taken into account. We consider in detail *special* generalized linear mixed models. For example, for binomial observations with beta distribution for the probability, probit, and Poisson regression models with normally distributed random effects admit an elegant solution that avoids integration.

First, we study an important special case: clustered/panel data with a cluster-specific intercept. Intercepts may be fixed or random, and we develop estimation methods under both assumptions. The advantage of the model with a random intercept (one random effect) is that the ideas can be presented in a concise way, so that further generalization to several random effects becomes straightforward. Second, we generalize the GLM by allowing several correlated random effects. At the end of the chapter we discuss limitations of the generalized estimating equations (GEE) approach.

Usually, estimation of the nonlinear mixed effects model is computationally intensive and requires advanced numerical procedures. Thus, discussion of the appropriate algorithms constitutes a substantial part of the chapter.

Several excellent texts are available on the topic. The book by McCullagh and Nelder (1989) is a classic reference for GLM. A broad discussion of GLMM may be found in books by McCulloch and Searle (2001), Fahrmeir and Tutz (2001), and Agresti (2002).

7.1   Regression models for binary data

In this section, we briefly review statistical modeling with a binary dependent variable. A binary regression model (more precisely, a logistic regression model) is a special case of GLM. Classic reference books on the subject are those of Cox and Snell (1989) and McCullagh and Nelder (1989). The binary regression model can be specified as follows. Let y_i be a binary dependent variable and $\mathbf{x}_i$ the corresponding $m \times 1$ vector of covariates (explanatory variables or predictors), $i = 1, ..., n$. It is assumed that the number of observations is equal to or greater than the number of covariates ($n \geq m$) and that n vectors $\{\mathbf{x}_i\}$ have full rank,

$$\text{rank}(\mathbf{x}_1, ..., \mathbf{x}_n) = m. \tag{7.1}$$

The probability of the event $y_i = 1$ in the binary model is specified via a strictly increasing function $\mu = \mu(s)$, the *inverse link* function in the language of GLM, namely,

$$\Pr(y_i = 1) = \mu(\boldsymbol{\beta}'\mathbf{x}_i), \quad i = 1, ..., n, \tag{7.2}$$

where $\boldsymbol{\beta}$ is the $m \times 1$ vector of parameters to be estimated using the data $(y_i, \mathbf{x}_i)$. It is assumed that the n random binary variables, $y_1, ..., y_n$, are independent. Also, it is assumed that μ is a continuous, twice-differentiable strictly increasing function. The inverse function, $\eta = \mu^{-1}$, is called the *link* function. We prefer the term *probability function* for μ because it models the probability of y. Typically, the first component of vector $\mathbf{x}_i$ is 1, so that the first component of vector $\boldsymbol{\beta}$ is the intercept term. Model (7.2) may be rewritten as $E(y_i|\mathbf{x}_i) = \mu(\boldsymbol{\beta}'\mathbf{x}_i)$, and it is therefore called a regression model for binary data. Equivalently, in terms of the link function, $\eta(E(y_i)) = \boldsymbol{\beta}'\mathbf{x}_i$. For binary data,

$$\text{var}(y_i) = \Pr(y_i = 1)\Pr(y_i = 0) = \mu(\boldsymbol{\beta}'\mathbf{x}_i)(1 - \mu(\boldsymbol{\beta}'\mathbf{x}_i)).$$

The following properties usually hold for the probability function μ:

1. The function $\mu = \mu(s)$ is defined for all $s \in (-\infty, \infty)$.

2. $0 < \mu(s) < 1$, $\lim_{s \to -\infty} \mu(s) = 0$, $\lim_{s \to \infty} \mu(s) = 1$.

3. $d\mu/ds = \mu' = \dot{\mu} > 0$.

4. $d^2(\ln \mu)/ds^2 < 0$.

5. Many probability functions are symmetric,

$$\mu(s) = 1 - \mu(-s). \tag{7.3}$$

The symmetry holds if μ' is an even function.

The second property complies with the fact that μ models the probability. The probability function is a strictly increasing function, as follows from the third property. The fourth property ensures that the log-likelihood is a concave function of parameters, see Section 7.1.4. This property, in conjunction with (7.3), implies that $\ln \mu$ and $\ln(1 - \mu)$ are concave functions. Indeed, the concavity of $\ln \mu$ follows directly from it. The concavity of $\ln(1 - \mu)$ under (7.3) follows from the fact that $\ln(1 - \mu(s)) = \ln \mu(-s)$ and $d^2(\ln \mu(-s))/ds^2 = d^2(\ln \mu(s))/ds^2 < 0$. The concavity is needed for uniqueness of the maximum likelihood estimate, see Section 7.1.4 for details.

The popular choices of probability function μ and respective regressions have their own names:

$\mu(s) = e^s/(1 + e^s)$, logistic regression.

$\mu(s) = \Phi(s) = (1/\sqrt{2\pi}) \int_{-\infty}^{s} e^{-0.5t^2} dt$, probit regression.

$\mu(s) = 1 - e^{-e^s}$, complementary log-log regression.

Each of the three binary models has its domain of applications (see Figure 7.1 with these functions). Formally, any cumulative distribution function may be used as μ.

Logistic regression. All five properties hold for this regression. The second property is easy to see. The third and fourth properties follow readily from

$$\frac{d\mu}{ds} = \frac{e^s}{(1 + e^s)^2} > 0, \quad \frac{d^2 \ln \mu}{ds^2} = -\frac{e^s}{(1 + e^s)^2} < 0.$$

Symmetry (7.3) is also easy to check,

$$\mu(-s) = \frac{e^{-s}}{1 + e^{-s}} = \frac{1}{1 + e^s} = 1 - \frac{e^s}{1 + e^s} = 1 - \mu(s).$$

Logistic regression is popular in epidemiological and biomedical studies where the strength of association between the dependent variable and covariate (exposure or risk factor) is measured by e^β, the odds ratio. For example, if y codes the occurrence of cancer and x codes the smoking status ($x = 1$ for smoker and $x = 0$ for nonsmoker), e^β is the ratio of two odds. The first odd is the ratio of probabilities of cancer to noncancer within the smoker group,

$$O_1 = \frac{\Pr(y_i = 1|x = 1)}{\Pr(y_i = 0|x = 1)} = e^{\alpha+\beta}.$$

The second odd is the ratio of probabilities of cancer to noncancer within the nonsmoker group,

$$O_0 = \frac{\Pr(y_i = 1|x = 0)}{\Pr(y_i = 0|x = 0)} = e^{\alpha}.$$

Then the odds ratio (OR) is

$$\frac{O_1}{O_0} = e^{\beta}.$$

This relationship does not hold for the probit or complementary log-log function. The fact that the odds ratio in logistic regression is expressed easily through coefficients is the major reason for using this binary model in epidemiology.

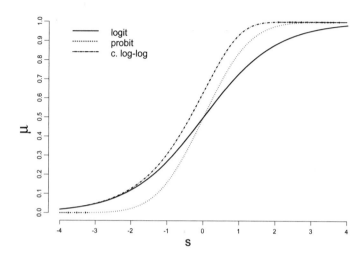

FIGURE 7.1. Three probability functions $\mu = \mu(s)$ to model binary data. The logit and probit functions are symmetric and take value $1/2$ at $s = 0$. The complementary log-log link, $\mu(s) = 1 - e^{-e^{s}}$, is not symmetric. Generally, any distribution function may be used to model binary data.

Probit regression. All five properties hold for this probability function. The third and fourth properties follow from the inequalities

$$\frac{d\Phi}{ds} = \frac{1}{\sqrt{2\pi}} e^{-\frac{1}{2}s^2} > 0, \quad \frac{d^2 \ln \Phi}{ds^2} = -(s\Phi(s) + \phi(s)) < 0,$$

where Φ is the cumulative distribution function (cdf) of the standard normal variable $\mathcal{N}(0, 1)$ and $\phi = \Phi'$ is the density. The second inequality is given by Feller (1966). The probit model is popular in engineering and econometric studies. For example, let z_i be a continuous measure related to a set of explanatory variables $\mathbf{x}_i$ via the standard linear regression model

$$z_i = \beta_0 + \boldsymbol{\beta}'\mathbf{x}_i + \varepsilon_i, \tag{7.4}$$

where $\varepsilon_i \sim \mathcal{N}(0, \sigma^2)$. However, let the z_i be unobservable (latent variable); instead we observe a binary variable

$$y_i = \begin{cases} 0 \text{ if } z_i < c \\ 1 \text{ if } z_i \geq c \end{cases}, \tag{7.5}$$

where c is a cut-off point/threshold (McCulloch and Searle, 2001). Then, an appropriate binary model for the binary y_i is the probit regression because

$$\Pr(y_i = 1) = \frac{1}{\sqrt{2\pi\sigma^2}} \int_c^\infty e^{-\frac{1}{2\sigma^2}(z-\beta_0-\boldsymbol{\beta}'\mathbf{x}_i)^2} dz$$

$$= 1 - \Phi\left(\frac{c-\beta_0-\boldsymbol{\beta}'\mathbf{x}_i}{\sigma}\right) = \Phi\left(\beta_* + \boldsymbol{\beta}'_*\mathbf{x}_i\right),$$

where $\beta_* = (\beta_0 - c)/\sigma$ and $\boldsymbol{\beta}_* = \boldsymbol{\beta}/\sigma$. In a dose–response framework, x_{i1} may be poison/drug concentration (or radioactive dose) and x_{i2} may be age or gender. For example, let z_i be a continuous measure of the health damage due to poisoning. Then we may assume that if poison concentration exceeds a certain threshold, c, death occurs ($y_i = 1$). The question is whether the coefficients β_1 and β_2 can be determined by observing a binary event, in our case, death. Unfortunately, we cannot identify the coefficients of the original model (7.4) having binary truncation observations (7.5). However, we can identify the ratio of the coefficients. For example, if we are interested in the *relative* strength of the association in the linear regression model $z_i = \beta_0 + \beta_1 x_{i1} + \beta_2 x_{i2} + \varepsilon_i$, which can be expressed as β_1/β_2, we can estimate this ratio using binary data (7.5) with the probit model because the common factor σ^{-1} is eliminated, namely,

$$\frac{\beta_{1*}}{\beta_{2*}} = \frac{\beta_1/\sigma}{\beta_2/\sigma} = \frac{\beta_1}{\beta_2}.$$

To identify $\boldsymbol{\beta}$ and σ, one has to have repeated measurements for the binary y and has to apply a random effects methodology, a mixed model.

Complementary log-log regression. For this regression

$$\frac{d\mu}{ds} = e^{s-e^s} > 0, \quad \frac{d^2 \ln\mu}{ds^2} = e^{s-e^s}\frac{1-e^{-e^s}-e^s}{(1-e^{-e^s})^2} < 0. \tag{7.6}$$

To prove the second inequality, we notice that $e^{-x} > 1 - x$ for $x \neq 0$ and therefore $e^{-e^s} > 1 - e^s$ for all s, implying that the numerator of the second inequality (7.6) is negative. The log-log function is not symmetric, $\mu(s) \neq 1 - \mu(-s)$. The name of this regression comes from the fact that the inverse link contains two logs: $\eta = \ln(-\ln(1-\mu))$.

The log-log link function emerges in connection with Poisson regression. If a random variable, z_i, takes nonnegative values $0, 1, 2, \dots$ and has a Poisson distribution,

$$\Pr(z_i = k) = \frac{1}{k!} e^{k(\boldsymbol{\beta}'\mathbf{x}_i)-e^{\boldsymbol{\beta}'\mathbf{x}_i}}, \tag{7.7}$$

then $E(z_i) = e^{\boldsymbol{\beta}'\mathbf{x}_i}$. Now, we are interested in modeling $\Pr(z_i > 0)$ as a function of $\mathbf{x}_i$. Some authors apply logistic regression to the binary (or truncated) count variable

$$y_i = \min(z_i, 1) = \begin{cases} 0 \text{ if } z_i = 0 \\ 1 \text{ if } z_i > 0 \end{cases}. \tag{7.8}$$

But it is easy to see that Poisson regression (7.7) implies the log-log probability because

$$\Pr(y_i = 1) = 1 - \Pr(y_i = 0) = 1 - \frac{1}{0!}e^{0(\boldsymbol{\beta}'\mathbf{x}_i)-e^{\boldsymbol{\beta}'\mathbf{x}_i}} = 1 - e^{-e^{\boldsymbol{\beta}'\mathbf{x}_i}}.$$

Summing up, if the original count variable, z, follows a Poisson distribution: (a) applying logistic regression to the binary variable (7.8) leads to a misspecified model with a systematic bias, and (b) the complementary log-log regression with the probability function $1 - e^{-e^s}$ is an adequate model.

The three probability functions are shown in Figure 7.1. The logit and probit are symmetric and pass the point $(0, 1/2)$. The probit function approaches the zero asymptote with a quadratic exponential rate, $O(e^{-x^2/2})$, and the logit with an exponential rate, $O(e^{-x})$. Thus, one may conclude that the probit is less affected by outliers in the covariate space. This phenomenon was confirmed empirically by McCullagh and Nelder (1989).

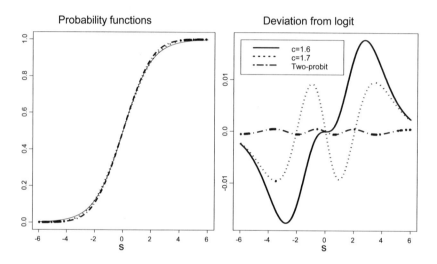

FIGURE 7.2. Logit approximation by probit(s). One-probit approximation (7.9) uses $c = 1.6$ and $c = 1.7$. The latter c gives an absolute error of approximation of less than 0.01. The two-probit approximation (7.11) yields an absolute error of 0.000526.

7.1.1 Approximate relationship between logit and probit

The phenomenon of the close relationship between logit and probit was discovered in early work: Chambers and Cox (1967), Finney (1971), and Cox and Snell (1989). In particular, Chambers and Cox came to the conclusion that a sample of over 1000 observations is necessary to distinguish the two functions by statistical means. Cox and Snell (pp. 20–23) noticed that logit can be well approximated by stretching probit, that is, with the appropriate scale transformation on the s-axis. Liang and Liu (1991) used the relationship between the two probability functions to demonstrate the attenuation in the logistic model with covariate measurement error. The fact behind the idea of approximating logit by probit is that the expectation of probit over a normally distributed argument is again a probit that eliminates the integration problem in logistic regression with normally distributed measurement error (the proof is given in the next subsection). This fact is well known in the literature on measurement error, and several authors have made use of it (Carroll et al., 1984,

1995; Burr, 1988; Tosteson et al., 1989). Zeger et al. (1988) used this approximation to demonstrate the impact of the random effect in logistic regression. We will also use this approximation for logistic regression with random effects. In this section we consider one- and two-probit approximations.

There are several approaches to approximate logit by Φ. Following the idea of stretching, we look for a coefficient, $c > 1$, such that uniformly over s,

$$\mu_L(s) \simeq \Phi\left(\frac{s}{c}\right), \tag{7.9}$$

where $\mu_L(s) = e^s/(1 + e^s)$ is the probability function. This approximation will be called the *one-probit approximation*. Perhaps the easiest way to obtain coefficient c is to approximate μ_L by Φ in the neighborhood of zero. Notice that for all c the left- and right-hand sides of (7.9) equal $1/2$ at $s = 0$. Thus, we can find c that makes the first derivatives equal. To realize this idea, we compute

$$\left.\frac{d\mu_L}{ds}\right|_{s=0} = \frac{1}{4}, \quad \left.\frac{d\Phi(s)}{ds}\right|_{s=0} = \phi(0) = \frac{1}{\sqrt{2\pi}}.$$

Therefore, to make the first derivatives equal, we take $c = \sqrt{8/\pi} \simeq 1.6$, as suggested by Amemiya (1981), see Figure 7.2.

Another one-probit approximation seeks c such that the maximum absolute difference between inverse logit and probit is minimum (minimax criterion),

$$\max_{-\infty < s < \infty}\left|\frac{e^s}{1 + e^s} - \Phi\left(\frac{s}{c}\right)\right| \Rightarrow \min_c.$$

Using numerical computation, one can show that $c = 16\sqrt{3}/(15\pi) \simeq 1.7$ gives the accuracy

$$\max_{-\infty < s < \infty}\left|\frac{e^s}{1 + e^s} - \Phi\left(\frac{s}{1.7}\right)\right| = 0.00946 < 0.01;$$

Johnson and Kotz (1970, p. 6) and Carroll et al. (1995, p. 64).

Now we consider a two-probit approximation as a linear combination of two probits with the sum of the coefficients equal to 1. Thus, we want to approximate

$$\mu_L(s) \simeq p\Phi\left(\frac{s}{c_1}\right) + (1 - p)\Phi\left(\frac{s}{c_2}\right),$$

where $0 < p < 1$ and positive c_1 and c_2 are to be found based on some criteria of discrepancy between the left- and right-hand sides. In the case of two or more probits, from a computational point of view, it is more convenient to use the integral quadratic error,

$$\int_{-\infty}^{\infty}\left(\mu_L(s) - p\Phi\left(\frac{s}{c_1}\right) + (1 - p)\Phi\left(\frac{s}{c_2}\right)\right)^2 ds \Rightarrow \min_{p, c_1, c_2}. \tag{7.10}$$

The advantage of this criterion is that the left-hand side of (7.10) is a differentiable function of p, c_1, and c_2, and consequently, its minimum can be found by a standard optimization technique, such as the Newton–Raphson algorithm. The solution to optimization problem (7.10) leads to the *two-probit approximation*

$$\mu_L(s) \simeq 0.4353\Phi\left(\frac{s}{2.2967}\right) + 0.5647\Phi\left(\frac{s}{1.3017}\right). \tag{7.11}$$

This approximation works very well—the maximum absolute error is as little as 0.000526. Three approximations with $c = 1.6$, $c = 1.7$, and the two-probit approximation (7.11) are shown in Figure 7.2.

We illustrate numerical integration in R using the function `integrate`. First, we need to specify the integrand,

```
SSlogprob=function(s,p,c1,c2)
{
    muL=1/(1+exp(-s))
    appr=p*pnorm(s/c1)+(1-p)*pnorm(s/c2)
    return((muL-appr)^2)
}
```

Second, we call `integrate` with specific values of p, c_1, and c_2,

```
integrate(f=SSlogprob,lower=-Inf,upper=Inf,p=.43,c1=2.3,c2=1.3)
```

This call produces the output `4.54087e-06 with absolute error < 4.4e-06`.

More accurate approximations, based on a linear combination of an arbitrary number of probits, were suggested by Monahan and Stefanski (1991). However, they did not impose the restriction that the sum of the coefficients at Φ be 1. Approximation (7.11) has the advantage that the right-hand side is again a distribution function.

7.1.2 Computation of the logistic-normal integral

The logistic-normal integral plays an important role in statistics. In particular, this integral is central to logistic regression with a normally distributed covariate measurement error, see the literature cited in the previous subsection. Also, we encounter this integral in the framework of logistic regression with a normally distributed random effects and, as a special case, with a normally distributed intercept term. Approximations discussed in this section are used later for the generalized linear mixed model and nonlinear mixed effects model of the next chapter. For example, the link-approximation will give rise to new methods of estimation for probit and logistic regression with normally distributed random effects, VARLINK; see Section 7.3.5.

The logistic-normal integral is an improper integral defined as

$$I = I(s, \sigma^2) = \frac{1}{\sigma\sqrt{2\pi}} \int_{-\infty}^{\infty} \frac{e^x}{1 + e^x} e^{-\frac{1}{2\sigma^2}(x-s)^2} dx. \tag{7.12}$$

After a change of variable, we can represent this integral as

$$I = \frac{1}{\sqrt{2\pi}} \int_{-\infty}^{\infty} \frac{e^{s+\sigma x}}{1 + e^{s+\sigma x}} e^{-\frac{1}{2}x^2} dx. \tag{7.13}$$

The logistic-normal integral can be interpreted as the expected value of the probability function contaminated with a normally distributed error,

$$I = E_{u \sim \mathcal{N}(0,1)} \frac{e^{s+\sigma u}}{1 + e^{s+\sigma u}}. \tag{7.14}$$

We find the first approximation to I via Φ using the following important fact

$$E_{u \sim \mathcal{N}(0,\sigma^2)} \Phi(s+u) = \Phi\left(\frac{s}{\sqrt{1+\sigma^2}}\right). \qquad (7.15)$$

Proof. As follows from its definition,

$$
\begin{aligned}
E_{u \sim \mathcal{N}(0,\sigma^2)} \Phi(s+u) &= \frac{1}{\sqrt{2\pi}\sigma} \int_{-\infty}^{\infty} \Phi(s+u) e^{-\frac{1}{2\sigma^2}u^2} du \\
&= \frac{1}{2\pi\sigma} \int_{-\infty}^{\infty} \int_{-\infty}^{s+u} e^{-\frac{1}{2}z^2 - \frac{1}{2\sigma^2}u^2} dz\,du.
\end{aligned}
$$

The two-dimensional integral may be viewed as the probability that the difference between two independent normally distributed random variables, w and u, is less than s, where $u \sim \mathcal{N}(0,\sigma^2)$ and $w \sim \mathcal{N}(0,1)$. But $w - u \sim \mathcal{N}(0, 1+\sigma^2)$, and therefore

$$E_{u \sim \mathcal{N}(0,\sigma^2)} \Phi(s+u) = \Pr(w - u < s) = \Phi\left(\frac{s}{\sqrt{1+\sigma^2}}\right),$$

and formula (7.15) is established.

Probit approximation

Now we apply formula (7.15) to approximate the logistic-normal integral (7.12) using the one-probit approximation (7.9). We have

$$
\begin{aligned}
I(s,\sigma^2) &\simeq E_{u \sim \mathcal{N}(0,1)} \Phi\left(\frac{s+\sigma u}{c}\right) = E_{u \sim \mathcal{N}(0,\sigma^2/c^2)} \Phi\left(c^{-1}s + u\right) \\
&= \Phi\left(\frac{s}{\sqrt{c^2 + \sigma^2}}\right) = \Phi\left(\frac{s}{\sqrt{1.7^2 + \sigma^2}}\right), \qquad (7.16)
\end{aligned}
$$

where we used $c = 1.7$. Employing the two-probit approximation (7.11), we obtain

$$I(s,\sigma^2) \simeq 0.4353\Phi\left(\frac{s}{\sqrt{2.2967^2 + \sigma^2}}\right) + 0.5647\Phi\left(\frac{s}{\sqrt{1.3017^2 + \sigma^2}}\right). \qquad (7.17)$$

Since the integrand of I is positive and less than 1, the maximum absolute error of the integral approximation (7.17) is about 0.000526, uniformly over the range of s and σ.

Link-approximation

In this section we consider another approximation to the logistic-normal integral (7.12), or equivalently (7.14). The idea is to approximate the link function and then apply the back transformation. Thus, instead of approximating integral (7.14) we approximate the corresponding link function; therefore, we call this *link-approximation*. Since the link function is $\ln[\mu_L/(1-\mu_L)]$, where $\mu_L(s) = e^s/(1+e^s)$ is the probability function, we introduce a function of σ,

$$R(\sigma) = \ln \frac{E_u \frac{e^{s+\sigma u}}{1+e^{s+\sigma u}}}{E_u \frac{1}{1+e^{s+\sigma u}}} = \ln E_u \frac{e^{s+\sigma u}}{1+e^{s+\sigma u}} - \ln E_u \frac{1}{1+e^{s+\sigma u}}, \qquad (7.18)$$

where E_u indicates the expectation over $u \sim \mathcal{N}(0,1)$. It is easy to see that $R(0) = s$. Now we find the first two derivatives of R at zero. The first derivative is

$$\frac{d}{d\sigma}R(\sigma) = \left[\left(E_u \frac{e^{s+\sigma u}}{1 + e^{s+\sigma u}}\right)^{-1} + \left(E_u \frac{1}{1 + e^{s+\sigma u}}\right)^{-1}\right] E_u \left[\frac{e^{s+\sigma u}}{(1 + e^{s+\sigma u})^2} u\right].$$

But $E(u) = 0$, which implies that the second factor on the right-hand side is zero and $\frac{d}{d\sigma}R(\sigma)\big|_{\sigma=0} = 0$. Next we find the second derivative at $\sigma = 0$,

$$\frac{d^2}{d\sigma^2}R(\sigma)\bigg|_{\sigma=0} = \left[\frac{1 + e^s}{e^s} + 1 + e^s\right] E_u \left[\frac{e^s(1 - e^s)}{(1 + e^s)^3} u^2\right]$$

$$= \left[\frac{1 + e^s}{e^s} + 1 + e^s\right] \frac{e^s(1 - e^s)}{(1 + e^s)^3} = \frac{1 - e^s}{1 + e^s},$$

since $E(u^2) = 1$. This means that if σ^2 were treated as an argument of R, we would have

$$\frac{d}{d(\sigma^2)}R(\sigma)\bigg|_{\sigma^2=0} = \frac{1}{2}\frac{1 - e^s}{1 + e^s}. \tag{7.19}$$

Next, inspired by the relationship for the probit model, (7.15), we seek an approximation of the form $R(\sigma^2) \simeq S(\sigma^2)$, where $S(\sigma^2) = s/\sqrt{1 + A\sigma^2}$ with the coefficient A to be determined. We find coefficient A such that for small σ^2, functions $R(\sigma^2)$ and $S(\sigma^2)$ are close meaning that the first derivatives at $\sigma^2 = 0$ are equal. Hence, from (7.19) one finds that

$$A = \frac{e^s - 1}{s(1 + e^s)}. \tag{7.20}$$

Since $\lim_{s\to 0}(e^s - 1)/s = 1$ we set $A = 1/2$ when $s = 0$. It is elementary to prove that A is always positive and attains its maximum $1/2$ at $s = 0$. After back transformation, we finally arrive at the link-approximation of the logistic-normal integral,

$$I(s, \sigma^2) \simeq \frac{\exp\left(s\left(1 + \frac{e^s - 1}{s(1 + e^s)}\sigma^2\right)^{-1/2}\right)}{1 + \exp\left(s\left(1 + \frac{e^s - 1}{s(1 + e^s)}\sigma^2\right)^{-1/2}\right)}. \tag{7.21}$$

An advantage of this link-approximation over the two-probit approximation is that for $\sigma^2 = 0$, (7.21) gives the exact value, although the two-probit approximation has a uniform error of 0.000526. We compare this to other methods at the end of this section.

Another link-approximation (tanh approximation) was suggested by McCullagh and Nelder (1989, p. 452):

$$I(s, \sigma^2) \simeq \frac{\exp\left(s - \frac{1}{2}\tanh\left[s(1 + 2e^{-\sigma^2/2})/6\right]\right)}{1 + \exp\left(s - \frac{1}{2}\tanh\left[s(1 + 2e^{-\sigma^2/2})/6\right]\right)}, \tag{7.22}$$

where $\tanh(x) = (e^x - e^{-x})/(e^x + e^{-x})$.

First-order approximation

Perhaps the easiest way to approximate the logistic-normal integral is to apply the Taylor series expansion. Here we consider the first- and second-order approximations. The accuracy of the first-order approximation is not satisfactory; we present it only for instructive purposes.

We write $e^{s+\sigma x}/(1+e^{s+\sigma x})$ as $e^{l(x)}$, where $l(x) = s + \sigma x - \ln(1 + e^{s+\sigma x})$ and find the first-order approximation to $l(x)$ at $x = 0$ as $l(x) \simeq s - \ln(1 + e^s) + x\sigma/(1 + e^s)$. Then using the identity

$$\frac{1}{\sqrt{2\pi}} \int_{-\infty}^{\infty} e^{ax-bx^2} dx = \frac{1}{\sqrt{2b}} e^{\frac{a^2}{4b}}, \tag{7.23}$$

we have

$$I(s, \sigma^2) \simeq \frac{e^s}{1 + e^s} e^{\frac{\sigma^2}{2(1+e^s)^2}}. \tag{7.24}$$

This approximation should be accurate for small σ.

Second-order approximation

Here we use the same idea but expand the function $l(x)$ in a Taylor series up to the second order,

$$l(x) \simeq s - \ln(1 + e^s) + x\frac{\sigma}{1 + e^s} - x^2\frac{\sigma^2 e^s}{2(1 + e^s)^2}. \tag{7.25}$$

Again using the identity (7.23), we obtain

$$I(s, \sigma^2) \simeq \frac{e^s}{1 + e^s} \frac{1}{\sqrt{1 + \frac{\sigma^2 e^s}{(1+e^s)^2}}} e^{\frac{\sigma^2}{2((1+e^s)^2 + \sigma^2 e^s)}}. \tag{7.26}$$

An improvement in the quadratic approximation is the following Laplace approximation.

Laplace approximation

This is the major approximation for the nonlinear mixed effects models and will be used extensively later. Here we apply this method to the approximation of the logistic-normal integral. The idea of the Laplace approximation (LA) is again to use a quadratic approximation, but at the point where the integrand takes its maximum. Indeed, since the integral can be interpreted as the area under the curve, the best coverage will be in the neighborhood of the maximum. Thus, instead of taking $x = 0$ as in the quadratic approximation above, we approximate

$$h(x) = l(x) - \frac{1}{2}x^2 = s + \sigma x - \ln(1 + e^{s+\sigma x}) - \frac{1}{2}x^2 \tag{7.27}$$

around $x_{\max}$, the maximum point of $h(x)$. Generally, if we want to approximate the integral $\int_{-\infty}^{\infty} e^{h(x)} dx$, we first need to find $\max h(x)$. Since the first derivative of $h(x)$ at $x_{\max}$ vanishes, we come to the second-order approximation,

$$h(x) \simeq h_{\max} + \frac{1}{2}(x - x_{\max})^2 \left(-\frac{d^2 h}{dx^2}\bigg|_{x=x_{\max}} \right). \tag{7.28}$$

Hence, applying the identity (7.23), we arrive at the Laplace approximation,

$$\int_{-\infty}^{\infty} e^{h(x)} dx \simeq \sqrt{2\pi} e^{h_{\max}} \left(-\frac{d^2 h}{dx^2} \bigg|_{x=x_{\max}} \right)^{-1/2}. \tag{7.29}$$

It is assumed that the second derivative of h at the maximum is negative. In fact, one can guarantee that this derivative is at least nonpositive because $x_{\max}$ gives the maximum of h. This approximation requires finding the maximum, which usually involves some iterative process. The LA, (7.29), is general and applies to any function $h(x)$, not necessarily defined by (7.27). Approximation (7.29) turns into an equality when $h(x)$ is a quadratic function. A multivariate version of the LA is considered in Section 7.7.1.

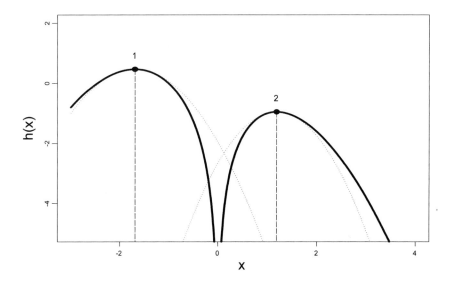

FIGURE 7.3. The function $h(x) = -0.5x(x+1) + 2\ln|x|$ has two local maxima (the dotted lines are quadratic approximations). If LA is based on the first local maximum, the integral is 3.06. If LA is based on the second local maximum, the integral is 0.62. The improved LA yields 3.67; the exact value is 3.55.

Improved Laplace approximation

An implicit assumption of the Laplace approximation is that the function $h(x)$ is unimodal, i.e., its maximum is attained at one point. For example, if function h has two maxima, approximation (7.29) may be poor whichever maximum point is taken, especially if the maximum values are close. One can improve the Laplace approximation by splitting the domain $(-\infty, \infty)$ into two intervals. Specifically, let $h(x)$ have two maximum points, x_1 and x_2, and let c be any point between x_1 and x_2 (a good choice is to let c be the point of local minimum). Then we split $(-\infty, \infty)$ into $(-\infty, c)$ and (c, ∞), so that

$$\int_{-\infty}^{\infty} e^{h(x)} dx = \int_{-\infty}^{c} e^{h(x)} dx + \int_{c}^{\infty} e^{h(x)} dx.$$

Applying quadratic approximation (7.28) at x_1 and x_2, we obtain an integral approximation expressed through the standard normal cdf:

$$\int_{-\infty}^{\infty} e^{h(x)}dx \simeq \sqrt{2\pi}\left[e^{h_1}\frac{\Phi\left(\sqrt{D_1}(c-x_1)\right)}{\sqrt{D_1}} + e^{h_2}\frac{1-\Phi\left(\sqrt{D_2}(c-x_2)\right)}{\sqrt{D_2}}\right], \quad (7.30)$$

where $D_j = -\left.\frac{d^2h}{dx^2}\right|_{x=x_j}$ and h_j is the maximum value, $j=1,2$.

Example. We illustrate approximation (7.30) by approximating the integral $\int_{-\infty}^{\infty} x^2 e^{-\frac{1}{2}x^2+x}dx$ for which $h(x) = -\frac{1}{2}x(x+1) + 2\ln|x|$, see Figure 7.3. This function has two local maxima, $x_1 = -1.686$ and $x_2 = 1.186$ with $h_1 = 0.4664$, $h_2 = -.9551$ (for this integral it is natural to chose $c = 0$). If the standard LA is based on the first maximum, the integral is 3.06. If the LA is based on the second local maximum, the integral is 0.62. The improved LA yields 3.67; the exact value is 3.55.

Another application of the improved LA is an approximation for a nonpositive integrand. For example, to approximate the integral $\int_{-\infty}^{\infty} xe^{h(x)}dx$, we represent

$$\int_{-\infty}^{\infty} xe^{h(x)}dx = -\int_{-\infty}^{0} e^{h(x)+\ln(-x)}dx + \int_{0}^{\infty} e^{h(x)+\ln(x)}dx$$

and apply the quadratic approximation to $h(x)+\ln(-x)$ and $h(x)+\ln(x)$ at the respective maximum points. Generalization of the improved LA with several local maxima is straightforward.

Approximation of some other integrals

Laplace approximation can easily be generalized to approximate integrals of the form $\int_{-\infty}^{\infty} g(x)e^{h(x)}dx$, assuming that the maximum point of h is known. Indeed, using the Taylor series expansion of the second order, we approximate

$$g(x) \simeq g(x_{\max}) + (x - x_{\max})g'(x_{\max}) + \frac{1}{2}(x-x_{\max})^2 g''(x_{\max}).$$

Hence,

$$\int_{-\infty}^{\infty} g(x)e^{h(x)}dx \simeq \sqrt{2\pi}\frac{e^{h_{\max}}}{\sqrt{-\left.\frac{d^2h}{dx^2}\right|_{x=x_{\max}}}}\left(g(x_{\max}) + \frac{g''(x_{\max})}{-2h''_{\max}}\right).$$

This approximation is especially useful when the ratio of the integrals is sought, as follows:

$$\frac{\int_{-\infty}^{\infty} g(x)e^{h(x)}dx}{\int_{-\infty}^{\infty} e^{h(x)}dx} \simeq g(x_{\max}) + \frac{g''(x_{\max})}{-2h''_{\max}}.$$

In the special case $g(x) = x^2$, we find that

$$\frac{\int_{-\infty}^{\infty} x^2 e^{h(x)}dx}{\int_{-\infty}^{\infty} e^{h(x)}dx} \simeq x_{\max}^2 + \frac{1}{-h''_{\max}}. \quad (7.31)$$

These kinds of approximations will be used in the next section for estimation of logistic regression with random effects.

Laplace approximation for the logistic-normal integral

Now we apply LA to the logistic-normal integral, rewriting (7.12) as

$$I = \frac{1}{\sqrt{2\pi}} \int_{-\infty}^{\infty} e^{h(x)} dx,$$

where h is as defined by (7.27). It is elementary to prove that $h \to -\infty$ when $x \to \infty$ or $x \to -\infty$ for any $s, \sigma > 0$, and thus the maximum of h exists. The first and second derivatives are

$$\frac{dh}{dx} = \frac{\sigma}{1 + e^{s+\sigma x}} - x, \quad \frac{d^2 h}{dx^2} = -\left[\frac{\sigma^2 e^{s+\sigma x}}{(1 + e^{s+\sigma x})^2} + 1\right]. \tag{7.32}$$

Since the second derivative is negative, the function h is concave. The Newton algorithm

$$x_{s+1} = x_s + \frac{[\sigma - x(1 + e^{s+\sigma x_s})](1 + e^{s+\sigma x_s})}{\sigma^2 e^{s+\sigma x_s} + (1 + e^{s+\sigma x_s})^2}, \quad s = 0, 1, 2, \ldots$$

quickly converges to the maximum point from $x_0 = 0$ (see Appendix 13.3). Let $x_{\max}$ be the limit point of the iterations, then due to the LA, (7.29),

$$I(s, \sigma^2) \simeq \frac{e^{s+\sigma x_{\max} - \frac{1}{2}x_{\max}^2}}{\sqrt{\sigma^2 e^{s+\sigma x_{\max}} + (1 + e^{s+\sigma x_{\max}})^2}}. \tag{7.33}$$

Practice shows that the first iteration,

$$x_1 = \frac{\sigma(1 + e^s)}{\sigma^2 e^s + (1 + e^s)^2}, \tag{7.34}$$

already provides a good approximation to the maximum, $x_{\max}$. Hence, using x_1 instead of $x_{\max}$, we obtain Laplace approximation 1 (LA1):

$$I(s, \sigma^2) \sim \frac{e^{s+\sigma x_1 - \frac{1}{2}x_1^2}}{\sqrt{\sigma^2 e^{s+\sigma x_1} + (1 + e^{s+\sigma x_1})^2}}. \tag{7.35}$$

Approximation comparison

We divide the approximations to the logistic-normal integral into two groups. The first four approximations are shown in Figure 7.4; the first-order approximation (7.24) is not shown because of its poor quality. The approximations are compared with the exact value (computed with precision 10^{-8}) for s in the interval $(0, 4)$ for small (0.5) and large (1.5) values of σ. The link-approximation is the best in this group with an absolute error of less than 0.01, even for large σ. The second group involves more sophisticated approximations, with the link-approximation among them, see Figure 7.5. When σ becomes large, the approximations deteriorate, except the two-probit approximation. This is easy to explain because the maximum error of this approximation is 0.000526 regardless of σ. Thus, this approximation is robust. Interestingly, the link-approximation is better than the LA. Also, LA1 is very close to the original LA.

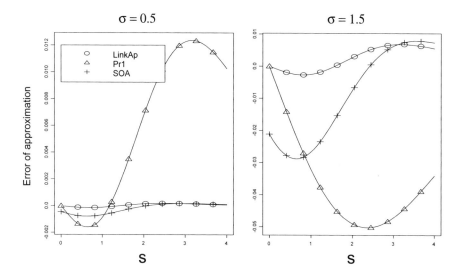

FIGURE 7.4. Three approximations to the logistic-normal integral for two values of σ: the link-approximation, LinkAp (7.21); the one-probit approximation, Pr1 (7.16), and the second-order approximation, SOA (7.26). The error of the approximation is the difference between the approximate and true values. The link-approximation is the best in this group and will be considered in the second group of approximations (see Figure 7.5).

Numerical integration

It is well known that a proper integral (over a finite interval) can be approximated by a finite sum with any predefined precision $\varepsilon > 0$,

$$\int_{-\infty}^{\infty} f(x)dx \simeq \int_{A}^{B} f(x)dx \simeq \sum_{k=1}^{K} w_k f(x_x) = S_K, \qquad (7.36)$$

where $A = x_1 < x_2 < ... < x_K = B$ are the nodes (knots or abscissas) and w_k are the positive weights. A and B are called the lower and upper limits of the integration. For a general introduction to the methods of numerical quadrature, we refer the reader to a book by Evans and Swartz (2000), which has plenty of statistical applications. There is a great deal of choice in A and B, nodes and weights. A comprehensive treatment of the logistic-normal integral based on the Gaussian quadrature is given by Crouch and Spiegelman (1990).

In the Gauss–Hermite (GH) quadrature, nodes and weights are available for the case when function f is proportional to e^{-x^2}, Abramowitz and Stegun (1972). The closer f is to e^{-x^2}, the better the precision of the Gauss–Hermite quadrature. Abscissas and weights, $\{x_k, w_k, k = 1, ..., K\}$, are given by Abramowitz and Stegun (1972, p. 924) up to $K = 20$ as a part of Gauss–Hermite quadrature for evaluating an integral of the form $\int_{-\infty}^{\infty} f(x) e^{-x^2} dx$ (sometimes this type of integral is called an intergral with a Gaussian kernel). After (x_k, w_k) are determined, the integral is approximated as a simple sum,

$$\int_{-\infty}^{\infty} f(x)e^{-x^2}dx = \sum_{k=1}^{K} w_k f(x_x). \tag{7.37}$$

The GH method of integral approximation is especially useful for normally distributed random effects. We illustrate this method with computation of the logistic-normal integral below.

An algorithm to compute the abscissas and weights for any K is given by Press et al. (1992, p. 154). In Table 7.1, we show $\{x_k, w_k\}$ for $K = 11$ and $K = 13$ (an odd K gives the first abscissa at zero).

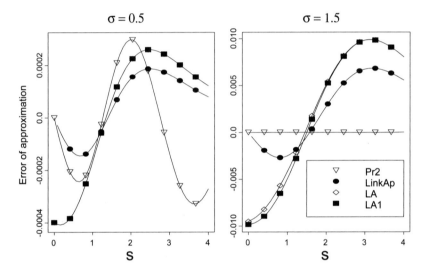

FIGURE 7.5. Four best approximations to the logistic-normal integral: two-probit approximation Pr2, (7.17); the link-approximation LinkAp (7.21); the LA (7.33); and the LA1 (7.35).

Table 7.1. Abscissas and weights for the Gauss–Hermite quadrature with 11 and 13 nodes

$K = 11$		$K = 13$	
x	w	x	w
0	0.6547592869	0	0.6043931879
±0.6568095669	0.4293597524	±0.6057638792	0.4216162969
±1.326557084	0.1172278752	±1.220055037	0.1403233207
±2.025948016	0.0119113954	±1.853107652	0.0208627753
±2.783290100	0.0003468195	±2.519735686	0.0012074600
±3.668470847	0.0000014396	±3.246608978	0.0000204304
		±4.101337596	0.0000000483

We make several comments. First, the farther the value is from zero, the lower the weight. Second, abscissas are symmetrical around zero and have the same weight. Third, the number of abscissas greater than 13 is unlikely to improve the precision because the weights approach zero rapidly with $K \to \infty$.

Our R function gauher computes the x coordinates and respective weights w based on the algorithm presented by Press et al. (1992). It is called

```
gauher(K,EPS=3e-014,PIM4=0.75112554446494295,MAXIT=100)
```

For example, gauher(K=13) returns

```
              x             w
 [1,]  4.101338e+00  4.825732e-08
 [2,]  3.246609e+00  2.043036e-05
 [3,]  2.519736e+00  1.207460e-03
 [4,]  1.853108e+00  2.086278e-02
 [5,]  1.220055e+00  1.403233e-01
 [6,]  6.057639e-01  4.216163e-01
 [7,] -1.972152e-31  6.043932e-01
 [8,] -6.057639e-01  4.216163e-01
 [9,] -1.220055e+00  1.403233e-01
[10,] -1.853108e+00  2.086278e-02
[11,] -2.519736e+00  1.207460e-03
[12,] -3.246609e+00  2.043036e-05
[13,] -4.101338e+00  4.825732e-08
```

We compare computation of the logistic-normal integral using the built-in function integrate with GH quadrature. Representing (7.13) as

$$I = \frac{1}{\sqrt{\pi}} \int_{-\infty}^{\infty} \frac{e^{s+\sqrt{2}\sigma x}}{1 + e^{s+\sqrt{2}\sigma x}} e^{-x^2} dx,$$

we obtain

$$I \simeq \frac{1}{\sqrt{\pi}} \sum_{k=1}^{K} \frac{e^{s+\sqrt{2}\sigma x_k}}{1 + e^{s+\sqrt{2}\sigma x_k}} w_k$$

where (x_k, w_k) are computed using gauher. Below we show the R function.

```
LNGHint=function(K=13)
{
dump("LNGHint","c:\\MixedModels\\Chapter07\\LNGHint.r")
LNint=function(x,s,sigma)
{
  ex1=exp(-(x-s)^2/2/sigma^2)
  ex2=1/sigma/sqrt(2*pi)*exp(x)/(1+exp(x))
  return(ex1*ex2)
}
```

```
xw=gauher(K)
out=as.data.frame(matrix(ncol=4,nrow=6))
names(out)=c("s","sigma","GH quadrature","integrate")
j=0
for(s in c(-1,0,1))
for(sigma in c(1,2))
{
j=j+1
ex=exp(s+sqrt(2)*sigma*xw[,1])
out[j,1]=s;out[j,2]=sigma
out[j,3]=sum(ex/(1+ex)*xw[,2])/sqrt(pi)
out[j,4]=integrate(f=LNint,s=s,sigma=sigma,low=s-5*sigma,
        up=s+5*sigma)$value
}
print(paste("K =",K))
return(out)
}
```

This function can be downloaded to the R session as

```
source("c:\\MixedModels\\Chapter07\\\\LNGHint.r")
```

The results of integrate and GH quadrature are basically identical. Note that low=-Inf,up=Inf in the function integrate does not work in this case, so we need to specify the lower and upper limits of integration manually; $\pm\sigma$ works satisfactory. The GH quadrature can be easily generalized to multidimensional integrals, see Section 7.1.3.

In the *adaptive* integral approximation/evaluation the Gauss–Hermite quadrature is carried out around the maximum value of the integrand, as in the Laplace approximation (Liu and Pierce, 1994; Pinheiro and Bates, 1995). Thus, if $x_{\max}$ is the maximum point of $h(x)$, then in Gauss–Hermite quadrature, we approximate

$$\int_{-\infty}^{\infty} e^{h(x)}\,dx \simeq \sqrt{2}\widehat{\sigma}_h \sum_{k=1}^{K} w_k \exp\left[x_k^2 + h(x_{\max} + \sqrt{2}\widehat{\sigma}_h x_k)\right], \qquad (7.38)$$

where

$$\widehat{\sigma}_h = \left(-\left.\frac{d^2h}{dx^2}\right|_{x=x_{\max}}\right)^{-1/2}.$$

Obviously, one has to assume that the second derivative at the maximum is negative. When the function $h(x)$ is bimodal, we need to approximate the integral with two sums around each maximum (as in the improved LA). For example, we apply the Gauss–Hermite quadrature to logistic regression with random effects in Section 7.3.1.

We make several comments regarding numerical integration:

- It is important not only to approximate an integral but to know the error of the approximation. The error of approximation requires an estimate of the upper bound of the absolute value of the second derivative of the integrand.

- Complicated numerical integration rules and quadratures take more time for integral evaluation; thus, simpler integration rules may be preferable.

- There does not exist a universal numerical integration method for all integrands over the entire range of parameters; thus, a separate study is required.

- Gauss–Hermite quadrature with 11 or 13 nodes is satisfactory for the logistic-normal integral over a wide range of parameters.

Keeping these guidelines in mind, one may prefer simple integration rules with the approximation error under control. In particular, below we provide such an approximation based on the trapezoid rule, with any predefined accuracy $\varepsilon > 0$.

In the trapezoid rule, nodes are equally spaced, $x_k = A + (k-1)h$, where $k = 1, 2, ..., K$ with the step $h = (B-A)/(K-1)$ and the integration sum

$$S_K = h \left[\frac{1}{2} f(A) + \sum_{k=2}^{K-1} f(x_k) + \frac{1}{2} f(B) \right]. \tag{7.39}$$

This rule has the absolute error of approximation

$$\left| \int_A^B f(x)dx - S_K \right| \leq \frac{(B-A)^2}{12K^2} \max \left\{ |f''(x)|, A \leq x \leq B \right\}. \tag{7.40}$$

To apply the trapezoid rule to the logistic-normal integral in the form (7.13), we need to solve two problems: (a) approximate the improper integral by a proper integral, and (b) find an upper bound for the second derivative of the integrand to determine the K that gives the integration approximation with accuracy $0 < \varepsilon < 1$.

To solve problem (a), we find $A < B$ such that

$$\frac{1}{\sqrt{2\pi}} \int_{-\infty}^A \frac{e^{s+\sigma x}}{1 + e^{s+\sigma x}} e^{-x^2/2} dx + \frac{1}{\sqrt{2\pi}} \int_B^\infty \frac{e^{s+\sigma x}}{1 + e^{s+\sigma x}} e^{-x^2/2} dx < \frac{\varepsilon}{2}.$$

It suffices to find A and B such the first and second integrals are less than $\varepsilon/4$. Using the inequality $e^{s+\sigma x}/(1 + e^{s+\sigma x}) < e^{s+\sigma x}$, we find the lower and upper limits,

$$A = \sigma + \Phi^{-1}(0.25\varepsilon e^{-s-0.5\sigma^2}), \quad B = \sigma + \Phi^{-1}(1 - 0.25\varepsilon e^{-s-0.5\sigma^2}). \tag{7.41}$$

A more general result is formulated in Lemma 35 of Section 7.3.1. To solve the second problem, we find an upper bound for the absolute value of the second derivative, $e^{h(x)} = E - F$, where

$$E = \frac{qe^{-x^2/2}}{1+q} \left(\frac{\sigma}{1+q} - x \right)^2, \quad F = \left(1 + \frac{\sigma^2 q}{(1+q)^2} \right) \frac{qe^{-x^2/2}}{1+q},$$

and $q = e^{s+\sigma x}$. Since for positive E and F we have $|E - F| \leq \max(E, F)$, it suffices to find the upper bound for each term separately. Applying elementary inequalities, we obtain

$$\sqrt{E} \leq \sigma \frac{\sqrt{q}}{\sqrt{(1+q)^3}} + \max \left(xe^{-x^2/4} \right) \leq \frac{2\sigma}{9} \sqrt{3} + \sqrt{2}e^{-\frac{1}{2}}$$

and

$$F \leq \frac{qe^{-x^2/2}}{1+q} + \frac{\sigma^2 z^2 e^{-x^2/2}}{(1+z)^3} \leq \frac{1}{2} + \frac{4}{27}\sigma^2.$$

Combing all inequalities, we finally obtain the upper bound for the second derivative in (7.40),

$$|f''(x)| \leq \frac{1}{\sqrt{2\pi}} \left(\sigma \frac{2}{9}\sqrt{3} + \sqrt{2}e^{-\frac{1}{2}} \right)^2.$$

Thus, if the number of nodes in the trapezoid rule (7.39) is greater that or equal to

$$K = \frac{-\Phi^{-1}(0.25\varepsilon e^{-s-0.5\sigma^2})(2\sigma\sqrt{3}/9 + \sqrt{2/e})}{\sqrt{3\pi\varepsilon}}, \qquad (7.42)$$

the difference between S_K and (7.12) in absolute value is less than ε. Although the number of nodes computed by this formula may be very large, it requires less time to evaluate the logistic-normal integral than some sophisticated algorithms of numerical integration for the same accuracy. For example, to evaluate 500 logistic-normal integrals using the adaptive 15-point Gauss–Kronrod quadrature with $\varepsilon = 10^{-7}$, S-Plus 6 requires 33 seconds; for the trapezoid rule with the same accuracy and the number of nodes chosen by formula (7.42), 12 seconds is required.

As a final comment, despite tremendous effort and the extensive literature on numerical quadrature, the integrals in statistical applications cannot be evaluated *exactly*. Only integrals in closed form are exact; otherwise, we want to approximate the integral with a predefined, small enough tolerance ε. One faces two major problems when controlling for quadrature error: (a) replacing an improper integral with the proper one, and (b) controlling for error over the entire range of parameters involved (such as σ in the logistic-normal integral). Although some general guidance from numerical mathematics is available, one needs to provide a detailed analytical investigation of the integrand on a case-by-case basis to control for the error in numerical integration.

7.1.3   Gauss-Hermite numerical quadrature for multidimensional integrals in R

The GH quadrature for two-dimensional (double) integrals with the Gaussian kernel takes the form

$$\int_{-\infty}^{\infty} \int_{-\infty}^{\infty} f(x,y)e^{-x^2-y^2} dx dy \simeq \sum_{k=1}^{K} \sum_{k'=1}^{K} w_k w_{k'} f(x_k, y_{k'}), \qquad (7.43)$$

where w_k, $w_{k'}$ and $x_k, y_{k'}$ are the same as before. This method of integral approximation can be used for estimation of the generalized linear and nonlinear mixed models studied in this and following chapters. In particular, it will be used for the fixed sample likelihood approximation method in Section 7.3.2.

The R code that follow illustrates numerical quadrature (7.43) to compute

$$\int_{-\infty}^{\infty} \int_{-\infty}^{\infty} (x^2 + y^2)e^{-x^2-y^2} dx dy. \qquad (7.44)$$

```
twoint=function (K=13)
{
dump("twoint","c:\\MixedModels\\Chapter07\\twoint.r")
xw=gauher(K)
x=rep(xw[, 1],times=K)
y=rep(xw[, 1],each=K)
wx=rep(xw[, 2],times=K)
wy=rep(xw[, 2],each=K)
INT=sum((x^2+y^2)*wx*wy)
INT
}
```

It is elementary to show that integral (7.44) is π; the function `twoint()` returns 3.141593 exactly as `pi`.

It is straightforward to generalize the GH quadrature to multidimensional integrals. For example, for a three-dimensional integral with Gaussian kernel, we have

$$\int_{-\infty}^{\infty}\int_{-\infty}^{\infty}\int_{-\infty}^{\infty} f(x,y,z)e^{-x^2-y^2-z^2}\,dxdy \simeq \sum_{k=1}^{K}\sum_{k'=1}^{K}\sum_{k''=1}^{K} w_k w_{k'} w_{k''} f(x_k, y_{k'}, z_{k''}).$$

The R function below approximates the integral

$$\int_{-\infty}^{\infty}\int_{-\infty}^{\infty} (x^2+y^2+z^2)e^{-x^2-y^2-z^2}\,dxdydz.$$

```
threeint=function (K=13)
{
dump("twoint","c:\\MixedModels\\Chapter07\\threeint.r")
xw=gauher(K)
x=rep(rep(xw[, 1],times=K),times=K)
y=rep(rep(xw[, 1],each=K),times=K)
z=rep(rep(xw[, 1],each=K),each=K)
wx=rep(rep(xw[, 2],times=K),times=K)
wy=rep(rep(xw[, 2],each=K),times=K)
wz=rep(rep(xw[, 2],each=K),each=K)
INT=sum((x^2+y^2+z^2)*wx*wy*wz)
INT
}
```

It is possible to show that the exact integral is $(3/2)\pi^{3/2} = 8.352492$. The function `threeint` returns the same number. We draw the readers' attention to how x,y, and z (and respective weights) are constructed from original values produced by `gauher`. Shortly, we use permutations of the options `times` and `each` in the `rep` function. With this rule, one can proceed to integrals with fourth, fifth, and higher dimensions. Of course, it should be remembered that summation requires K^M terms for the integral of dimension M.

The GH quadrature is very convenient for numerical integration when the domain is specified by another function $g(x, y)$, say,

$$\int_{g(x,y)>h} f(x,y)e^{-x^2-y^2}\,dxdy$$

where h is a constant. Then, using approximation (7.43), we obtain

$$\int_{g(x,y)>h} f(x,y)e^{-x^2-y^2}\,dxdy \simeq \sum_{(k,k'):g(x_k,y_{k'})>h} w_k w_{k'} f(x_k, y_{k'}).$$

In short, the summation is over indices where the function g takes values greater than h. In R, this means that the summation operator in the code above should be replaced by `INT=sum(((x^2+y^2)*wx*wy)[g(x,y)>h])`, where `g(x,y)` is a user-defined function. Additional examples of using this method of numerical integration appear in Section 8.9.

7.1.4 Log-likelihood and its numerical properties

The log-likelihood function for the binary model with probability function μ is given by

$$\begin{aligned}
l(\boldsymbol{\beta}) &= \sum_{y_i=1} \ln \mu(\boldsymbol{\beta}'\mathbf{x}_i) + \sum_{y_i=0} \ln(1 - \mu(\boldsymbol{\beta}'\mathbf{x}_i)) \\
&= \sum_{i=1}^{n} \left[y_i \ln \mu(\boldsymbol{\beta}'\mathbf{x}_i) + (1 - y_i)\ln(1 - \mu(\boldsymbol{\beta}'\mathbf{x}_i)) \right]. \quad (7.45)
\end{aligned}$$

Assuming that μ satisfies the conditions formulated at the beginning of this section, it is easy to prove that the log-likelihood function is nonpositive, $l(\boldsymbol{\beta}) \leq 0$. To prove this, we use the fact that ln is a concave function so that $y \ln A + (1 - y) \ln B \leq \ln [yA + (1 - y)B]$ for any $y \in [0, 1]$ and positive A and B. Using this inequality with $y = y_i$, $A = \mu(\boldsymbol{\beta}'\mathbf{x}_i)$, and $B = 1 - \mu(\boldsymbol{\beta}'\mathbf{x}_i)$, we obtain

$$l(\boldsymbol{\beta}) \leq \sum_{i=1}^{n} \ln \left[y_i\mu(\boldsymbol{\beta}'\mathbf{x}_i) + (1 - y_i)(1 - \mu(\boldsymbol{\beta}'\mathbf{x}_i)) \right] = \sum_{i=1}^{n} \ln 1 = 0.$$

Thus, zero is the absolute upper bound of the log-likelihood function for any binary model. This absolute maximum is attained when $\mu(\boldsymbol{\beta}'\mathbf{x}_i) \to 1$ for $y_i = 1$ and when $\mu(\boldsymbol{\beta}'\mathbf{x}_i) \to 0$ for $y_i = 0$.

The Maximum Likelihood Estimate (MLE) is found as the solution to the system of nonlinear (score) equations

$$\frac{\partial l}{\partial \boldsymbol{\beta}} = \sum_{i=1}^{N} (y_i - \mu_i) \frac{\dot{\mu}_i}{\mu_i(1 - \mu_i)} \mathbf{x}_i = \mathbf{0}, \quad (7.46)$$

where $\dot{\mu}_i$ denotes the derivative of μ evaluated at $\boldsymbol{\beta}'\mathbf{x}_i$. The Hessian matrix of the log-likelihood function is given by

$$\frac{\partial^2 l}{\partial \boldsymbol{\beta}^2} = -\sum_{i=1}^{n} \left[y_i \frac{\dot{\mu}_i^2 - \ddot{\mu}_i \mu_i}{\mu_i^2} + (1 - y_i) \frac{\ddot{\mu}_i(1 - \mu_i) + \dot{\mu}_i^2}{(1 - \mu_i)^2} \right] \mathbf{x}_i \mathbf{x}_i'. \qquad (7.47)$$

The information matrix is the negative expected Hessian,

$$\mathbf{H} = -E \left(\frac{\partial^2 l}{\partial \boldsymbol{\beta}^2} \right) = \sum_{i=1}^{n} \frac{\dot{\mu}_i^2}{\mu_i(1 - \mu_i)} \mathbf{x}_i \mathbf{x}_i'. \qquad (7.48)$$

The Hessian is a negative definite matrix and the log-likelihood function is strictly concave ($\cap$-shaped) because the functions $\ln \mu$ and $\ln(1-\mu)$ are concave. This statement follows from a well known fact of optimization theory: a nonnegative linear combination of concave functions is a concave function, Ortega and Rheinboldt (1970). This property of (7.45) implies that the MLE is unique, if it exists, Haberman (1974, p. 309). Note that for linear regression, condition (7.1) is sufficient for the existence of the ML/OLS estimate. Binary model (7.2) is a nonlinear statistical model and therefore special criteria are needed to establish the MLE existence, Demidenko (2000). Several authors have addressed the problem of the MLE existence with logit and probit links: Weddenburn (1976), Haberman (1979), Silvapulle (1981), Albert and Anderson (1984), Lesaffre and Kaufmann (1992). It has been found that the MLE exists if and only if the two sets of points $\{\mathbf{x}_i\}$ with $y = 1$ and $y = 0$ can be separated by a plane. In Section 7.10 we suggest some constructive criteria to determine if such a plane exists.

Two algorithms can be used to maximize the log-likelihood function, (7.45), the Newton–Raphson (NR) and Fisher scoring (FS) in generic form

$$\widehat{\boldsymbol{\beta}}_{s+1} = \widehat{\boldsymbol{\beta}}_{s+1} + \lambda_s \mathbf{H}_s^{-1} \left(\left. \frac{\partial l}{\partial \boldsymbol{\beta}} \right|_{\boldsymbol{\beta}=\boldsymbol{\beta}_s} \right), \qquad (7.49)$$

where $0 < \lambda_s \leq 1$ is a step length to provide a decrease of l. For the NR algorithm, $\mathbf{H}$ is the negative Hessian, for the FS $\mathbf{H}$ is the expected negative Hessian. At the final iteration, $\mathbf{H}^{-1}$ gives the asymptotic covariance matrix of the MLE. For this purpose, we prefer the expected Hessian over the observed one, (7.47). It is possible to rewrite the FS algorithm in iterated reweighted least squares (IRLS, Section 6.2.3) fashion, Green (1984). Indeed, taking the linear approximation of $\mu_i = \mu(\mathbf{x}_i'\boldsymbol{\beta})$ at $\widehat{\boldsymbol{\beta}}_s$, we obtain $\mu_i \simeq \mu_i^s + \dot{\mu}_i^s(\boldsymbol{\beta} - \widehat{\boldsymbol{\beta}}_s)'\mathbf{x}_i$. Next replacing μ_i in (7.46), we solve for $\boldsymbol{\beta}$ and get the FS algorithm, in other words, FS=IRLS. Computational issues of the probit model are discussed in Demidenko (2001).

A general discussion of optimization problems in statistics, including criteria for convergence, is given in Appendix 13.3.

7.1.5 Unit step algorithm

In both the NR and FS algorithms, it may require several trials to find a step length (λ) that increases the likelihood value. Here we describe a unit step algorithm, introduced by Demidenko (2001), that increases the log-likelihood function from iteration to iteration and needs only one matrix inverse.

The key point of the algorithm is the observation that for popular binary models such as logistic or probit, the scalar coefficient in (7.47) for each i admits an upper bound. Indeed, for $\mu(s) = e^s/(1 + e^s)$, this scalar takes the form $e^s/(1 + e^s)^2$, and it is elementary to prove that $e^s/(1 + e^s)^2 \leq 1/4$. For probit regression, it is possible to prove that this scalar is less than 1. This follows from the two inequalities $s\Phi(s) + \phi(s) > 0$ and $\phi(s) - s(1 - \Phi(s)) > 0$ (Feller, 1957). Thus, it is assumed that there exists a positive constant τ that $\partial^2 l/\partial\beta^2 \geq -\tau\mathbf{X}'\mathbf{X}$ ($\tau = 1/4$ for the logistic model and $\tau = 1$ for the probit regression model). Iterations in the unit step algorithm take the form

$$\widehat{\boldsymbol{\beta}}_{s+1} = \widehat{\boldsymbol{\beta}}_s + \tau^{-1}(\mathbf{X}'\mathbf{X})^{-1}\mathbf{g}_s, \tag{7.50}$$

where $\mathbf{g}_s$ denotes the gradient of l evaluated at $\boldsymbol{\beta} = \widehat{\boldsymbol{\beta}}_s$. Hence one may interpret (7.50) as a maximization algorithm with a fixed step, $\lambda = 1/\tau$. Matrix $\mathbf{X}'\mathbf{X}$ can be inverted once before iterations begin (it is nonsingular due to (7.1)).

The properties of the unit step algorithm are formulated below.

Theorem 33 *Iterations (7.50) decrease the log-likelihood function (7.45) from iteration to iteration, where $\tau > 0$ is such that $\partial^2 l/\partial\beta^2 \geq -\tau\mathbf{X}'\mathbf{X}$. If the MLE exists, the unit step algorithm converges to it from any starting point.*

Proof. If $l_s = l(\widehat{\boldsymbol{\beta}}_s)$, by the Taylor theorem there exists $\boldsymbol{\beta}_*$ such that

$$
\begin{aligned}
l(\widehat{\boldsymbol{\beta}}_{s+1}) - l_s &= (\widehat{\boldsymbol{\beta}}_{s+1} - \widehat{\boldsymbol{\beta}}_s)'\mathbf{g}_s + \frac{1}{2}(\widehat{\boldsymbol{\beta}}_{s+1} - \widehat{\boldsymbol{\beta}}_s)'\left(\left.\frac{\partial^2 l}{\partial\boldsymbol{\beta}^2}\right|_{\beta=\beta_*}\right)(\widehat{\boldsymbol{\beta}}_{s+1} - \widehat{\boldsymbol{\beta}}_s) \\
&\geq (\widehat{\boldsymbol{\beta}}_{s+1} - \widehat{\boldsymbol{\beta}}_s)'\mathbf{g}_s - \frac{\tau}{2}(\widehat{\boldsymbol{\beta}}_{s+1} - \widehat{\boldsymbol{\beta}}_s)'(\mathbf{X}'\mathbf{X})(\widehat{\boldsymbol{\beta}}_{s+1} - \widehat{\boldsymbol{\beta}}_s) \\
&= \frac{1}{\tau}\mathbf{g}_s'(\mathbf{X}'\mathbf{X})^{-1}\mathbf{g}_s > 0,
\end{aligned}
$$

assuming that at iteration s we did not reach the maximum and $\mathbf{g}_s$ is not zero. Further, since $l(\boldsymbol{\beta}) \to -\infty$ when $\|\boldsymbol{\beta}\| \to \infty$, the sequence $\{\widehat{\boldsymbol{\beta}}_s\}$ is bounded and therefore there exists at least one limit point. At the limit point $\boldsymbol{\beta}_*$, the gradient vanishes because $\widehat{\boldsymbol{\beta}}_* = \widehat{\boldsymbol{\beta}}_* + \tau^{-1}(\mathbf{X}'\mathbf{X})^{-1}\mathbf{g}_*$ implies that $\mathbf{g}_* = \mathbf{0}$. Since the log-likelihood is a strictly concave function, there is only one point, the MLE, where the gradient is zero. Hence, $\{\widehat{\boldsymbol{\beta}}_s\}$ converges to the MLE regardless of the starting point, $\widehat{\boldsymbol{\beta}}_0$.

Problems for Section 7.1

1. Reproduce Figure 7.1.

2*. Use the Gauss-Newton algorithm for the minimization of (7.10) to arrive at an approximation of logit with two probits based on the integral quadratic criterion. Use the `integrate` function in R with `low=-Inf` and `upper=Inf` to compute the left-hand side of (7.10).

3. Derive the exact absolute error of approximation for (7.17) on the array of values for s and σ^2. For example, you may choose `sseq=rep(seq(from=-10,to=10,`

length=1000),1000) and `ssigma2=rep(seq(from=0,to=10,length=1000),each=` 1000) and then compute the absolute difference between the left- and the right-hand sides.

4. Use `integrate` command to plot (7.13) and (7.17) on one graph for a sequence of s with σ held at a specific value.

5. Similar to the previous problem, compare other logistic-normal integral approximations.

6. Using abscissas and weights from Table 7.1, compare the Gauss-Hermite quadrature with other logistic-normal integral approximations, plotting them on the same graph against s. Use the `gauher` program with larger K to determine whether there is a substantial improvement (use $K = 300$ or `integrate` as the gold standard).

7. Evaluate how precisely the minimum number of nodes given by formula (7.42) yields the absolute error ε.

8*. Write an `R` function that maximizes the log-likelihood (7.45) using the FS algorithm (7.49) with $\lambda_s = 1$. The function μ, along with its derivative, should be user-defined. Apply your algorithm to the probit and logistic regressions to verify if they produce the same result as the `glm` function in `R`. Compare the FS algorithm with the unit step algorithm defined by formula (7.50) through simulations.

9. Find the MLE of β in logistic regression when x_i is a binary variable.

7.2   Binary model with subject-specific intercept

The simplest linear mixed effects model is the model with random intercepts considered in Section 2.4. This model imposes an exchangeable (compound symmetry) correlation structure. Similarly, the binary model with varied (subject/cluster/stratum specific) intercepts is the simplest and perhaps the most important generalized linear mixed model. To motivate this model, we continue our example on the relationship between cancer occurrence (e.g., lung cancer) and smoking status as one of the prominent risk factors. Let us assume that the sample consists of N subsamples/surveys conducted in different parts of the country (states) or even worldwide; to be concrete we shall assume states. Let i code the state and j code the person. Then the binary variable y_{ij} codes the presence or absence of cancer ($y_{ij} = 1$, cancer; $y_{ij} = 0$, cancer-free) and x_{ij} codes the smoking status of the jth person in the ith state ($x_{ij} = 1$, smoker; $x_{ij} = 0$, nonsmoker). Let n_i denote the number of people surveyed in the ith state. Standard logistic regression applied to $\{y_{ij}, x_{ij}\}$ implicitly assumes that the lung cancer incidence (the probability for nonsmokers to get cancer) is constant across states. Clearly, this assumption may be wrong because states may have different environmental conditions, antismoking campaigns, traditions, health policy, population age, etc. These factors can lead to different cancer incidences in different states. Therefore, assuming that this incidence is the same would lead to improper conclusions regarding the effect of smoking (see Section 7.2.1 for the statistical consequence of ignoring a random effect). It is better to assume that intercepts differ from state to state, so an appropriate model would be

$$\Pr(y_{ij} = 1) = \mu(a_i + \boldsymbol{\beta}'\mathbf{x}_{ij}), \tag{7.51}$$

where $\mathbf{x}_{ij}$ is the $m \times 1$ covariate vector, which along with smoking status may include other relevant risk factors, such as age and gender, with the coefficient at the smoking status variable of interest. Since a_i is the intercept term, we assume in this section that $\mathbf{x}_{ij}$ does not have a constant component. In fact, the intercept term also may be a parameter of interest if we are interested in comparing cancer occurrence across the states, adjusted by risk factors.

In model (7.51), there is no room for cluster-specific covariates such as in the model $\Pr(y_{ij} = 1) = \mu(a_i + \boldsymbol{\gamma}'\mathbf{z}_i + \boldsymbol{\beta}'\mathbf{x}_{ij})$. More precisely, the latter model is not identifiable because the cluster-specific intercept, a_i consumes all variation due to the presence of cluster-specific covariates, $\mathbf{z}_i$.

Another example in which intercepts vary from stratum to stratum is the case-control study of Breslow and Day (1980). Indeed, if an epidemiologist wants to exclude the effect of age, he/she would collect data within an age group (frequency matched study) assuming that there is an age-specific incidence rate reflected in the intercept a_i. Then, y_{ij} codes the presence of disease for the jth person in the ith age group.

Regarding intercept term a_i, similar to the LME model, we may take one of two assumptions, leading to two different statistical models:

1. *Fixed effects model/fixed intercepts*: $\{a_i\}$ are fixed unknown parameters to be estimated along with $\boldsymbol{\beta}$. Sometimes parameters $\{a_i\}$ are called nuisance or incidental parameters, after a pioneering work by Neyman and Scott (1948).

2. *Random effects model/random intercepts*: $\{a_i\}$ are random, $a_i = \alpha + u_i$, where $\{u_i\}$ are iid random variables with zero mean and variance σ^2 and α is the population-averaged parameter. It is assumed that $\{y_{ij}\}$ are independent conditional on u_i.

These models have both advantages and disadvantages. The fixed effects model leads to increasing the number of additional parameters equal to the number of states in our example. The advantage of this model is that it does not require special methods of estimation because the introduction of dummy variables (equal to the number of states) reduces the model to standard logistic regression. However, if the number of clusters/strata is large, one faces the problem of a large number of nuisance intercepts. An elegant solution, bypassing a large number of dummy variables, is suggested in Section 7.2.3. In contrast, the random effects model has only two parameters (α and σ^2) in addition to $\boldsymbol{\beta}$, however, standard logistic regression is not applicable and more complicated methods should be applied (the consequences of ignoring the random effect are considered in the next subsection).

The advantage of the random effects model is that it is more flexible and includes the fixed effects model as an extreme case when the variance of the random effect, σ^2, goes to infinity. This was proved for the LME model in Section 2.2.3 using the closed form for the fixed effects estimator (2.31). Now we demonstrate it for model (7.51) with a normally distributed random intercept, $a_i \sim \mathcal{N}(\alpha, \sigma^2)$. Let σ^2 be fixed and known. We want to show that when σ^2 goes to infinity, the MLE for $\boldsymbol{\beta}$ approaches the MLE of the fixed effects model assuming that the a_i are fixed and unknown. Indeed, the MLE of the random effects model maximizes the function

$$l(\alpha, \boldsymbol{\beta}) = -\frac{N \ln(2\pi\sigma^2)}{2} + \sum_{i=1}^{N} l_i(\alpha, \boldsymbol{\beta}), \qquad (7.52)$$

where the individual log-likelihood is

$$l_i(\alpha, \boldsymbol{\beta}) = \ln \int_{-\infty}^{\infty} \exp \left\{ \tilde{l}_i(a_i, \boldsymbol{\beta}) - \frac{1}{2\sigma^2}(a_i - \alpha)^2 \right\} da_i \qquad (7.53)$$

and $\tilde{l}_i$ is the conditional log-likelihood function (assuming that a_i is fixed),

$$\tilde{l}_i(a_i, \boldsymbol{\beta}) = \sum_{y_{ij}=1} \ln \mu(a_i + \boldsymbol{\beta}'\mathbf{x}_{ij}) + \sum_{y_{ij}=0} \ln[1 - \mu(a_i + \boldsymbol{\beta}'\mathbf{x}_{ij})].$$

Since σ^2 is known the first term in (7.53) may be omitted. When $\sigma^2 \to \infty$, the term $(a_i - \alpha)^2/(2\sigma^2)$ in (7.53) vanishes and we come to the maximization of the log-likelihood $\sum_{i=1}^{N} \tilde{l}_i(a_i, \boldsymbol{\beta})$, which corresponds to the fixed effects model. This result is true for a linear model with random intercepts, Section 2.4.

Criteria for MLE existence

The absolute upper bound of the joint log-likelihood function (7.52) is zero. Indeed, in Section 7.1.4 we proved that $\tilde{l}_i(a_i, \boldsymbol{\beta}) \leq 0$, which implies that

$$l(\alpha, \boldsymbol{\beta}) \leq \sum_{i=1}^{N} \ln \frac{1}{\sqrt{2\pi\sigma^2}} \int_{-\infty}^{\infty} e^{-\frac{1}{2\sigma^2}(a_i - \alpha)^2} da_i = 0.$$

As follows from Section 7.10, the MLE does not exist if there exists a vector $(a, \boldsymbol{\beta}')$ that separates $\sum n_i$ vectors $(1, \mathbf{x}'_{ij})$ into two groups, corresponding to $y_{ij} = 1$ and $y_{ij} = 0$, or symbolically,

$$\begin{aligned} a + \boldsymbol{\beta}'\mathbf{x}_{ij} &< \ 0 \text{ if } y_{ij} = 0, \\ a + \boldsymbol{\beta}'\mathbf{x}_{ij} &> \ 0 \text{ if } y_{ij} = 1. \end{aligned} \qquad (7.54)$$

If (7.54) holds, then, technically, the MLE $= \infty$ and iterations of any maximization algorithm diverge. Some algorithms to check (7.54) are described in Section 7.10.

7.2.1   Consequences of ignoring a random effect

As noted in Section 3.9, ignoring a random effect in a linear model and applying ordinary least squares leaves the estimate unbiased. The aim of this subsection is to demonstrate that this is not true for a binary model. Generally, ignoring random effects in a *nonlinear* mixed model leads to attenuation and inconsistent estimation, Zeger et al. (1988). We illustrate the systematic bias for the probit model with a normally distributed intercept using the identity (7.15). If the random effect is ignored, the estimated model is $E(y_{ij}) = \Phi\left(\alpha_* + \boldsymbol{\beta}'_*\mathbf{x}_{ij}\right)$, but the true model is

$$E(y_{ij}) = E_{u_i \sim \mathcal{N}(0,\sigma^2)} \Phi\left(\alpha + \boldsymbol{\beta}'\mathbf{x}_{ij} + u_i\right) = \Phi\left(\frac{\alpha + \boldsymbol{\beta}'\mathbf{x}_{ij}}{\sqrt{1 + \sigma^2}}\right). \qquad (7.55)$$

Thus, by ignoring the random effect, u_i, one obtains estimates of α_* and $\boldsymbol{\beta}_*$ that converge to the true values α and β *attenuated* by $1/\sqrt{1 + \sigma^2}$. The phenomenon of attenuation, or bias toward the null, is well known in the measurement error literature and is associated with the fact that the measurement error flattens out the regression, Carroll et al. (1995). To assess the attenuation for logistic regression, we can use logit link approximation, discussed in Section 7.1. For example, using (7.15) and (7.9) with $c = 1.7$, we find that ignoring the randomness of the intercept in logistic regression would attenuate the coefficients by the factor $1/\sqrt{1 + 1.7^2\sigma^2}$, Breslow and Clayton (1993). Coming back to our example with smoking, we infer that ignoring the state-specific cancer incidence rate diminishes the estimated effect of smoking by $\sqrt{1 + 2.89\sigma^2}$.

7.2.2 ML logistic regression with a fixed subject-specific intercept

The model is (7.51), where all $\{y_{ij}, i = 1, ..., N, j = 1, .., n_i\}$ are independent and $\mu(s) = e^s/(1 + e^s)$. The intercepts $\{a_i\}$ are assumed fixed and unknown. Sometimes we call this model the fixed effects model. If the number of observations per cluster (n_i) is fairly large (the data are not sparse), this approach may work well. Then the log-likelihood function takes the form

$$
\begin{aligned}
l(a_1, ..., a_N, \boldsymbol{\beta}) &= \sum_{i=1}^{N}\left\{\sum_{y_{ij}=1}(a_i + \boldsymbol{\beta}'\mathbf{x}_{ij}) - \sum_{j=1}^{n_i}\ln(1 + e^{a_i + \boldsymbol{\beta}'\mathbf{x}_{ij}})\right\} \\
&= \boldsymbol{\beta}'\mathbf{u} + \sum_{i=1}^{N}p_i a_i - \sum_{i=1}^{N}\sum_{j=1}^{n_i}\ln(1 + e^{a_i + \boldsymbol{\beta}'\mathbf{x}_{ij}}), \qquad (7.56)
\end{aligned}
$$

where $\mathbf{u} = \sum_{i=1}^{N}\sum_{y_{ij}=1}\mathbf{x}_{ij}$ and $p_i = \sum_{j=1}^{n_i}y_{ij}$. The $N + m$ estimating equations for the MLE are:

$$
\frac{\partial l}{\partial a_i} = m_i - \sum_{j=1}^{n_i}\frac{e^{a_i + \boldsymbol{\beta}'\mathbf{x}_{ij}}}{1 + e^{a_i + \boldsymbol{\beta}'\mathbf{x}_{ij}}} = 0, \; i = 1, ..., N \qquad (7.57)
$$

$$
\frac{\partial l}{\partial \boldsymbol{\beta}} = \mathbf{u} - \sum_{i=1}^{N}\sum_{j=1}^{n_i}\frac{e^{a_i + \boldsymbol{\beta}'\mathbf{x}_{ij}}}{1 + e^{a_i + \boldsymbol{\beta}'\mathbf{x}_{ij}}} = 0. \qquad (7.58)
$$

As mentioned above, this system may be solved using standard logistic regression software by introducing N dummy variables. However, if N is large, one can alternate between (7.57) and (7.58) to avoid a large matrix inverse. zIndeed, denoting $B_{ij} = \exp(\boldsymbol{\beta}'\mathbf{x}_{ij})$ and $h_i = \exp(-a_i)$, equation (7.57) can be rewritten as

$$
\sum_{j=1}^{n_i}\frac{B_{ij}}{h_i + B_{ij}} = p_i. \qquad (7.59)
$$

To solve (7.59) safely, Newton's iterations should start from

$$
h_i = \frac{n_i(n_i/p_i - 1)}{\sum_{j=1}^{n_i}1/B_{ij}}, \quad i = 1, ..., N.
$$

This approximation provides a monotonic convergence of the Newton algorithm because, by harmonic-mean inequality, $\sum_{j=1}^{n_i}B_{ij}/(h_i + B_{ij}) \geq n_i^2/(n_i + \sum_{j=1}^{n_i}1/B_{ij})$,

Ortega and Rheinboldt (1970). If $p_i = 0$, we set $h_i = \infty$, and if $p_i = n_i$, we set $h_i = 0$. After making a few Newton steps to approximate the solution to (7.59), we come to $\mathbf{u} = \sum_{i,j} e^{\boldsymbol{\beta}'\mathbf{x}_{ij}}/(h_i + e^{\boldsymbol{\beta}'\mathbf{x}_{ij}})$ for $\boldsymbol{\beta}$, which is also easy to solve by the Newton algorithm.

When N is fixed and n_i goes to infinity, the MLE holds all its optimal properties. However, if N goes to infinity and the $\{n_i\}$ are uniformly bounded, the logistic regression model with fixed intercepts suffers from inconsistency. The problem with a large number of nuisance parameters has been encountered in the general linear growth curve model of Section 4.2, where we proved that the MLE is consistent. Neyman and Scott (1948) call this problem an incidental-parameter problem. While the MLE is consistent for the linear model with fixed intercepts studied in Section 2.4, it is *inconsistent* for logistic regression. In particular, Andersen (1970, 1980) proved that when $n_i = 2$ and x_{ij} is binary $\widehat{\beta}_{ML}$ converges to 2β. The proof can also be found in Hsiao (2003). To eliminate nuisance intercepts, a conditional likelihood approach has been suggested. We shall apply a generalization of this model to an ensemble of gray images in Section 12.6.1.

7.2.3 Conditional logistic regression

There is an elegant solution to the problem of the large number of nuisance intercepts in logistic regression based on conditional likelihood (this approach does not work for other link functions, such as probit). Originally the conditional likelihood approach was suggested by Cox (1972), Cox and Snell (1989) within the framework of proportional hazards model in survival analysis. The trick is that conditional likelihood eliminates nuisance intercepts, Prentice (1988). Although here we treat $\{a_i\}$ as fixed, one can apply this approach for random intercepts as well (see the next section).

Let index i be fixed, so it will be omitted for awhile to simplify the notation. The idea of conditional logistic regression is to consider the probability of obtaining binary outcomes $y_1, y_2, ..., y_n$ conditioned by the number of "successes," the sufficient statistic for a_i, $k = \sum_{j=1}^{n} y_j$. More precisely, let y_j be a binary variable such that $\Pr(y_j = 1) = p_j$, assuming that observations $\{y_j, j = 1, ..., n\}$ are independent. If $z_1, z_2, ..., z_n$ is a sequence of 0's or 1's such that $\sum_{j=1}^{n} z_j = k$, the probability

$$\Pr(y_1 = z_1, ..., y_n = z_n) = \prod_{j=1}^{n} p_j^{z_j}(1 - p_j)^{1-z_j}. \tag{7.60}$$

The conditional probability of $y_1 = z_1, ..., y_n = z_n$ under $\sum_{j=1}^{n} z_j = k$ is the ratio of (7.60) to the sum of *all* possible probabilities to obtain $\sum_{j=1}^{n} y_j = k$,

$$\frac{\prod_{j=1}^{n} p_j^{y_j}(1 - p_j)^{1-y_j}}{\sum_{\mathbf{z} \in \mathbf{Z}_k^n} \prod_{j=1}^{n} p_j^{z_j}(1 - p_j)^{1-z_j}}, \tag{7.61}$$

where $\mathbf{z} = (z_1, z_2, ..., z_n)$ is a vector with binary components 0 or 1 such that $\sum z_j = k$ and $\mathbf{Z}_k^n$ is a set of all possible n-dimensional vectors $\mathbf{z}$ with the sum of elements

k. Apparently, $\mathbf{Z}_k^n$ contains $\binom{n}{k}$ elements (the number of ways to pick k elements out of n (the number of combinations of n distinct objects taken k at a time). For example, if $n = 3$ and $k = 2$, the set $\mathbf{Z}_k^n$ contains three elements as three-dimensional binary vectors, $\mathbf{Z}_k^n = \{(1,1,0),(1,0,1),(0,1,1)\}$. For logistic regression, $p_j = e^{a+\beta \mathbf{x}_j}/(1 + e^{a+\beta \mathbf{x}_j})$, so that the probability (7.60) takes the form

$$\prod_{j=1}^n \frac{e^{z_j(\alpha+\beta'\mathbf{x}_j)}}{(1+e^{\alpha+\beta'\mathbf{x}_j})} = \frac{1}{\prod_{j=1}^n(1+e^{\alpha+\beta'\mathbf{x}_j})} e^{\alpha k+\beta'\sum_{j=1}^n \mathbf{x}_j z_j}$$

because $\sum z_j = k$. Substituting this quantity into (7.61), one finds that $\prod_{j=1}^n(1 + e^{\alpha+\beta'\mathbf{x}_j})$ and $e^{\alpha k}$ cancel out so that the conditional probability (7.61) simplifies to

$$\frac{e^{\alpha k+\beta'\sum_{j=1}^n \mathbf{x}_j y_j}}{\sum_{\mathbf{z}\in\mathbf{Z}_k^n} e^{\alpha k+\beta'\sum_{j=1}^n \mathbf{x}_j z_j}} = \frac{e^{\beta'\sum_{j=1}^n \mathbf{x}_j y_j}}{\sum_{\mathbf{z}\in\mathbf{Z}_k^n} e^{\beta'\sum_{j=1}^n \mathbf{x}_j z_j}}$$

as a function of β only. In the denominator z_j are components of vector $\mathbf{z}$ such that $\sum_{j=1}^n z_j = \sum_{j=1}^n y_j = k$. Putting back the subindex i, we obtain the joint conditional log-likelihood function as a function of β only,

$$l_c(\beta) = \beta'\mathbf{r} - \sum_{i=1}^N \ln\left(\sum_{\mathbf{z}\in\mathbf{Z}_{k_i}^{n_i}} e^{\beta'\sum_{j=1}^{n_i} \mathbf{x}_{ij} z_j}\right), \tag{7.62}$$

in which the vector $\mathbf{r} = \sum_{i=1}^N \sum_{j=1}^n \mathbf{x}_{ij}y_{ij}$ is fixed (notice that k_i varies with i because it is equal to the sum of the y's in cluster i). The conditional MLE, $\widehat{\beta}_{CML}$, maximizes (7.62). Andersen (1970) proved that the conditional ML estimator of β is consistent under mild assumptions, when N goes to infinity and the $\{n_i\}$ are bounded. Moreover, he proved that the minus inverse Hessian of l_c is a consistent estimator of the asymptotic covariance matrix of $\widehat{\beta}_{CML}$; see also Chamberlain (1980).

Now we discuss some computational issues of l_c maximization. To find the conditional MLE, we apply the Newton–Raphson algorithm, $\widehat{\beta}_{s+1} = \widehat{\beta}_s + \mathbf{H}_s^{-1}\mathbf{g}_s$. Here s is the iteration index, and $\mathbf{H}_s$ and $\mathbf{g}_s$ are the minus Hessian matrix and the gradient evaluated at $\beta = \widehat{\beta}_s$,

$$\mathbf{g} = \mathbf{r} - \sum_{i=1}^N \frac{1}{S_i}\mathbf{t}_i, \quad \mathbf{H} = \sum_{i=1}^N \frac{1}{S_i}\left[\sum_{\mathbf{z}\in\mathbf{Z}_{k_i}^{n_i}} e^{\beta'\sum_{j=1}^{n_i} \mathbf{x}_{ij} z_j}\mathbf{w}_{ij}\mathbf{w}_{ij}'\right] - \sum_{i=1}^N \frac{1}{S_i^2}\mathbf{t}_i\mathbf{t}_i',$$

where

$$S_i = \sum_{\mathbf{z}\in\mathbf{Z}_{k_i}^{n_i}} e^{\beta'\sum_{j=1}^{n_i} \mathbf{x}_{ij} z_j}, \quad \mathbf{t}_i = \sum_{\mathbf{z}\in\mathbf{Z}_{k_i}^{n_i}} e^{\beta'\sum_{j=1}^{n_i} \mathbf{x}_{ij} z_j}\mathbf{w}_i, \quad \mathbf{w}_i = \sum_{j=1}^{n_i}\mathbf{x}_{ij}z_j.$$

The variance-covariance matrix of the conditional MLE is estimated as the inverse of $\mathbf{H}$ at the final iteration. When the number of observations per cluster is large, the number of elements in the set $\mathbf{Z}_{k_i}^{n_i}$ may be large as well and computation may slow down. There exists, however, an efficient way to enumerate possible combinations with $\sum_{j=1}^{n} y_{ij} = k_i$ (Krailo and Pike, 1984). With that programming trick, the time of computation is comparable to that of standard logistic regression.

Now we prove that function l_c is concave, or more specifically, the minus Hessian matrix is nonnegative definite.

Lemma 34 *Let $\mathbf{a}, \mathbf{u}_1, \mathbf{u}_2, ..., \mathbf{u}_K$ be $m \times 1$ vectors and $b_k > 0$ for $k = 1, 2, ..., K$. Then the negative Hessian of the function $\mathbf{a}'\boldsymbol{\beta} - \ln \sum_{k=1}^{K} b_k e^{\boldsymbol{\beta}' \mathbf{u}_k}$, as a function of $\boldsymbol{\beta}$, is a nonnegative definite matrix for all $\boldsymbol{\beta} \in R^m$.*

Proof. We use the following matrix form of the Cauchy inequality. Let $\{\mathbf{u}_k, k = 1, ..., K\}$ be $m \times 1$ vectors and q_k positive numbers; then

$$\left(\sum q_k \mathbf{u}_k \right) \left(\sum q_k \mathbf{u}_k \right)' \le \sum q_k^2 \sum \mathbf{u}_k \mathbf{u}_k', \tag{7.63}$$

meaning that the difference between the right- and left-hand sides is a nonnegative definite matrix (Rao, 1973). Twice differentiating the function $g(\boldsymbol{\beta}) = \mathbf{a}'\boldsymbol{\beta} - \ln \sum_{k=1}^{K} b_k e^{\boldsymbol{\beta}' \mathbf{u}_k}$, we obtain the Hessian,

$$\frac{\left(\sum \mathbf{u}_k b_k e_k \right) \left(\sum \mathbf{u}_k b_k e_k \right)'}{\left(\sum b_k e_k \right)^2} - \frac{\sum \mathbf{u}_k \mathbf{u}_k' b_k e_k}{\sum b_k e_k},$$

where $e_k = e^{\boldsymbol{\beta}' \mathbf{u}_k}$ to shorten the notation. Then the lemma follows from (7.63), letting $q_k = b_k e_k > 0$. ∎

The method of conditional logistic regression is realized in the R code `logric` (it can be downloaded as `source("c:\\MixedModels\\Chapter07\\logric.r")`. The call to this function has the form

```
logric(dat,maxiter=20,eps=1e-005,silent=1)
```

where the `dat` matrix contains the data (the first column is cluster id, the second column is y_i, and the remaining columns are $\mathbf{x}_i$); `maxiter` specifies the maximum number of iterations, and `silent` is the flag variable (0=print iterations, 1=no print). The output is a list with three components: (1) the beta estimate, (2) the covariance of the beta-estimate ($\mathbf{H}^{-1}$), and (3) the number of iterations done. The `logric` function can be used when the number of observations in each cluster is small; say, $n_i \le 15$.

Problems for Section 7.2

1. Does the MLE exist with the log-likelihood function (7.52) when all $y_i = 0$? Does the answer depend on the choice of μ? Does the MLE for the binary model with m-dimensional $\mathbf{x}$ exist if the number of observations with $y_i = 0$ is less than m?

2. Illustrate the effect of the cluster-specific intercept on the slope estimate by plotting the individual (cluster-specific) probabilities as functions of x and the

population-averaged probability function defined by (7.55). What conclusion can you draw?

3*. Maximize the log-likelihood function (7.56) by reducing the estimation problem to N dummy variables, and subsequently use glm. Write an R function that solves equations (7.59) by Newton's algorithm. Check if the two approaches produce the same solutions. Generate data with N clusters and random intercepts with variance σ^2 and estimate the slope using the fixed subject-specific intercept approach to show that the slope estimates converge when σ^2 becomes large. Explain the result.

4*. Generate N clusters as in the previous problem with $n_i \leq 15$ and estimate the beta-coefficients using conditional regression (modify the function asN). Repeat the calculations nExp times and assess the bias and the variance produced by $\mathbf{H}^{-1}$. Make conclusions regarding the performance of this method.

5*. Estimate the cluster-specific intercept separately for each i after the slope coefficients are obtained from conditional logistic regression. Derive a closed-form expression.

7.3   Logistic regression with random intercept

Several methods of estimation for logistic regression with a normally distributed random intercept are considered in this section. The model remains the same, (7.51), but now it is assumed that the $\{a_i\}$ are iid random variables, $a_i \sim \mathcal{N}(\alpha, \sigma^2)$, where the population-averaged intercept α and the intercept variance σ^2 are unknown and subject to estimation. Denoting $b_i = a_i - \alpha \sim \mathcal{N}(0, \sigma^2)$, the model with random intercept can be rewritten as a conditional probability, $\Pr(y_{ij} = 1|b_i) = \mu(b_i + \boldsymbol{\beta}'\mathbf{x}_{ij})$, where the first component of the $m \times 1$ vector $\mathbf{x}_{ij}$ is 1 and the first component of the $m \times 1$ vector $\boldsymbol{\beta}$ is the population-averaged intercept. This model implies that observations y_{ij} and y_{ik} are dependent within a cluster. If the number of observations per cluster (n_i) is not large, one can apply the conditional logistic regression that eliminates random a_i. An advantage of this approach is that it does not involve specification of the distribution, b_i. However, if n_i is fairly large, this approach is prohibitive because for each cluster i it involves $n_i!/[k_i!(n_i - k_i)!]$ terms, where $k_i = \sum_{j=1}^{n_i} y_{ij}$. For example, if $n_i = 20$ and $k_i = 10$, this number is 184,756.

Three approaches to estimation are considered in this section. First, we discuss maximum likelihood estimation, involving several computations of one-dimensional integration for each cluster. Second, likelihood approximation, such as the quadratic of the Laplace, avoid integration. Third, the link approximations of Section 7.1.2 may be applied, also avoiding integration with the variance of the random intercepts estimated from individual logistic regressions (VARLINK).

7.3.1   Maximum likelihood

In this section we consider the maximum likelihood estimation that involves one-dimensional integration. The log-likelihood function takes the form

$$l(\boldsymbol{\beta}, \sigma^2) = -\frac{N}{2}\ln(2\pi\sigma^2) + \boldsymbol{\beta}'\mathbf{r} + \sum_{i=1}^{N}\ln\int_{-\infty}^{\infty} e^{h_i(\boldsymbol{\beta};u)}du, \qquad (7.64)$$

where

$$h_i(\boldsymbol{\beta};u) = k_i u - \frac{u^2}{2\sigma^2} - \sum_{j=1}^{n_i} \ln(1 + e^{\boldsymbol{\beta}'\mathbf{x}_{ij}+u}). \tag{7.65}$$

where $k_i = \sum_{j=1}^{n_i} y_{ij}$ and $\mathbf{r} = \sum_{i=1}^{N} \sum_{j=1}^{n_i} y_{ij}\mathbf{x}_{ij}$ are a fixed scalar and an $m \times 1$ vector. It is assumed that the first component of vector $\mathbf{x}_{ij}$ is 1. We observe that sufficient statistics are $\mathbf{r}$ and $\{k_i\}$.

We are concerned with maximization of (7.64) over $\boldsymbol{\beta}$ and σ^2. The first derivatives are

$$\frac{\partial l}{\partial \boldsymbol{\beta}} = \mathbf{r} - \sum_{i=1}^{N} \frac{\mathbf{I}_{i3}}{I_{i1}}, \quad \frac{\partial l}{\partial \sigma^2} = -\frac{N}{2\sigma^2} + \frac{1}{2\sigma^4} \sum_{i=1}^{N} \frac{I_{i2}}{I_{i1}}, \tag{7.66}$$

with the three integrals defined as

$$I_{i1} = \int_{-\infty}^{\infty} e^{h_i(\boldsymbol{\beta};u)} du, \quad I_{i2} = \int_{-\infty}^{\infty} u^2 e^{h_i(\boldsymbol{\beta};u)} du,$$

$$\mathbf{I}_{i3} = \int_{-\infty}^{\infty} \left[\sum_{j=1}^{n_i} \mathbf{x}_{ij} \frac{e^{\boldsymbol{\beta}'\mathbf{x}_{ij}+u}}{1 + e^{\boldsymbol{\beta}'\mathbf{x}_{ij}+u}} e^{h_i(\boldsymbol{\beta};u)} \right] du, \tag{7.67}$$

where the latter is an $m \times 1$ vector. The information matrix for $\boldsymbol{\beta}$ can be approximated as

$$-E\left(\frac{\partial^2 l}{\partial \boldsymbol{\beta}^2}\right) \simeq \mathbf{H} = \sum_{i=1}^{N} \left(\frac{1}{I_{i1}} \mathbf{I}_{i4} - \frac{1}{I_{i1}^2} \mathbf{I}_{i3}\mathbf{I}_{i3}'\right), \tag{7.68}$$

where

$$\mathbf{I}_{i4} = \int_{-\infty}^{\infty} \left[\sum_{j=1}^{n_i} \mathbf{x}_{ij}\mathbf{x}_{ij}' \frac{e^{\boldsymbol{\beta}'\mathbf{x}_{ij}+u}}{(1 + e^{\boldsymbol{\beta}'\mathbf{x}_{ij}+u})^2} e^{h_i(\boldsymbol{\beta},u)} \right] du \tag{7.69}$$

is an $m \times m$ matrix. To maximize (7.64), we may iterate as

$$\widehat{\boldsymbol{\beta}}_{s+1} = \widehat{\boldsymbol{\beta}}_s + \lambda_s \mathbf{H}^{-1}\left(\frac{\partial l}{\partial \boldsymbol{\beta}}\bigg|_{\boldsymbol{\beta}=\boldsymbol{\beta}_s}\right), \quad \widehat{\sigma}_{s+1}^2 = \frac{1}{N} \sum_{i=1}^{N} \frac{I_{i2}}{I_{i1}}, \tag{7.70}$$

assuming that $\mathbf{H}$ and $\{I_{ik}, k = 1, 2, 3, 4; i = 1, 2, ..., N\}$ are computed at the current values, $\boldsymbol{\beta} = \boldsymbol{\beta}_s$ and $\sigma = \sigma_s$. One can avoid computation of the integral matrix $\mathbf{I}_{i4}$ by applying the unit step algorithm of Section 7.1.5. Indeed, since for all $-\infty < s < \infty$ we have $e^s/(1+e^s)^2 < 1/4$, it is elementary to show that $\mathbf{H} \le \frac{1}{4}\sum_{j=1}^{n_i} \mathbf{x}_{ij}\mathbf{x}_{ij}' \equiv \mathbf{K}$, a constant matrix. Thus, instead of $\mathbf{H}$ in (7.70), we can use $\mathbf{K}$, which can be computed once at the beginning of the iteration procedure. Using Lemma 34, one can prove that matrix $\mathbf{H}$ is positive definite if the vectors $\{\mathbf{x}_{i1}, ..., \mathbf{x}_{in_i}\}$ have full rank at least for one i.

Another, simpler way to maximize the log-likelihood function is to use the Empirical Fisher scoring (EFS) algorithm, where the $(m+1) \times (m+1)$ information matrix for $\boldsymbol{\theta} = (\boldsymbol{\beta}', \sigma^2)'$ is estimated as the sum of cross-product derivatives, $\mathbf{H} = \sum \mathbf{d}_i\mathbf{d}_i'$, where

$$\mathbf{d}_i = \begin{bmatrix} \sum_{j=1}^{n_i} y_{ij}\mathbf{x}_{ij} - I_{i1}^{-1}\mathbf{I}_{i3} \\ -0.5\sigma^{-2} + 0.5\sigma^{-4}I_{i1}^{-1}I_{i2} \end{bmatrix}$$

is the derivative of the ith log-likelihood function $(i = 1, ..., N)$. Then iterations $\widehat{\boldsymbol{\theta}}_{s+1} = \widehat{\boldsymbol{\theta}}_s + \lambda_s \left(\sum \mathbf{d}_i \mathbf{d}_i'\right)^{-1} \sum \mathbf{d}_i$ approximate $\boldsymbol{\beta}$ and σ^2 simultaneously. An advantage of the EFS algorithm is that $\mathbf{H}^{-1}$, evaluated at the final iteration, provides a consistent estimate for the asymptotic covariance matrix of $\boldsymbol{\theta}$. Usually, $\lambda_s = 1$ leads to an increase in l from iteration to iteration, but sometimes we need to decrease the step length to avoid divergence.

The expectation of the cross-derivative vector, $\partial^2 l / \partial \boldsymbol{\beta} \partial \sigma^2$, is not zero, unlike the linear mixed effects model or the marginal model with a fixed matrix of random effects of Section 6.1. This means that we cannot use *any* estimate of σ^2 and still gain 100% efficiency—only maximum likelihood is asymptotically efficient. In particular, an asymptotically biased $\widehat{\sigma}^2$ will yield an asymptotically biased $\widehat{\boldsymbol{\beta}}$.

We refer the reader to Section 2.15.5, where criteria for convergence were discussed, and to Appendix 13.3 for general facts on optimization. Below we discuss how to evaluate the integrals involved.

Integrals approximation

We notice that to find the MLE using iterations (7.70), we actually do not need to compute the value of the log-likelihood function unless the length step λ_s is different from 1. Also, we do not need the exact information matrix and associated integrals, such as $\mathbf{I}_{i4}$, because EFS may be used. However, the derivatives (7.66) that involve integrals (7.67) should be computed as precisely as possible to be sure that maximum likelihood estimates are obtained, because the MLE is the solution to the score equations, $\partial l / \boldsymbol{\beta} = \mathbf{0}$ and $\partial l / \sigma^2 = 0$.

The main problem of the deterministic integral approximation is finding where the integrand values are sampled (Evans and Swartz, 2000). In the adaptive/Laplace approximation approach, values are sampled in the neighborhood where the integrand has its maximum (Liu and Pierce, 1994; Pinheiro and Bates, 1996). In the sum approach, we sample in the interval where the integrand is greater than a predefined small number. In the Monte Carlo approach, we rely on a random sample. Each of these three approaches has advantages and disadvantages, which we discuss later.

Adaptive Gauss–Hermite quadrature for integrals (7.67). From Section 7.1.2, it follows that one achieves better precision when the integral is approximated around the point where the integrand attains its maximum.

We start with an approximation/evaluation of I_{i1}, requiring us to find the minimum of the function

$$h(u) = -ku + u^2/(2\sigma^2) + \sum_{j=1}^{n} \ln(1 + B_j e^u), \qquad (7.71)$$

where the subindex i is omitted, and we let $B_j = e^{\boldsymbol{\beta}' \mathbf{x}_{ij}}$. To find its minimum we need the derivatives,

$$\frac{dh}{du} = -k + u/\sigma^2 + e^u \sum_{j=1}^{n} \frac{B_j}{1 + B_j e^u}, \quad \frac{d^2 h}{du^2} = 1/\sigma^2 + e^u \sum_{j=1}^{n} \frac{B_j}{(1 + B_j e^u)^2}.$$

First, since the second derivative is positive, this function has a unique minimum. Second, since $h \to \infty$ when $u \to \pm\infty$, the minimum of h on $(-\infty, \infty)$

exists. To solve $dh/du = 0$, we apply the Newton–Raphson algorithm, $u_{s+1} = u_s - (dh/du) \left(d^2h/du^2 \right)^{-1}$, starting from zero. Then, if u_* is the limiting point of the iterations, we approximate I_{i1} by (7.38).

To approximate integral I_{i2}, we need to apply the *improved* Laplace approximation because the integrand is not a unimodal function. A typical integrand function $u^2 e^{h_i(\beta;u)}$ is shown in Figure 7.6. Standard adaptive quadrature may fail because the function is bimodal, so the integration should be carried out with care. According to the improved Laplace approximation, the integral should be split into two intervals: $(-\infty, 0)$ and $(0, \infty)$.

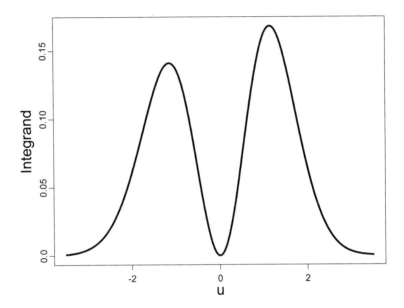

FIGURE 7.6. Typical integrand function for the integral I_{i2}. Since the function is bimodal, the integration should be carried out with care.

Referring to Section 7.1.2, we set the threshold $c = 0$, as in the example. Hence, we first need to minimize functions $h(u) - 2\ln u$ for $u > 0$ and $h(u) - 2\ln(-u)$ for $u < 0$. Again, the minimum can be found by the Newton algorithm. For the positive part, we start with $u_0 = 0.5\sigma[\sqrt{(n-k)^2\sigma^2 + 8} - (n-k)\sigma]$, and for the negative part, $u_0 = -0.5\sigma[\sqrt{(n-k)^2\sigma^2 + 8} + (n-k)\sigma]$. Similarly, one can obtain the maximum of the integrand for I_{i3}.

Integral approximation by sum. In Section 7.1.2 we argued that numerical integration should not be too complex because the time of computation is important and one might achieve the same precision by a simple sum with a large enough number of terms. In particular, it was suggested that we approximate the logistic-normal integral by a simple sum on the interval where the proper and improper integrals differ by a small $\varepsilon/2$. The same idea can be applied to approximate integrals $I_{ik}, k = 1, 2, 3, 4$. The main task is to find $A < B$ so that the proper integral approximates the improper one with a given, small enough precision. We illustrate this approach by evaluating I_1, where the subindex i is omitted for simplicity of notation. Since the negative function h is bounded from below by a quadratic function, $-h \geq u^2/(2\sigma^2) + nu + \beta' \sum_{j=1}^{n} \mathbf{x}_j$. Following the outline of the logistic-normal integral, we can find A and B such that the improper integral can be replaced by a proper one with any given precision. The lower and upper limits are given in the following lemma.

Lemma 35 *Let function $h(u)$ be defined on $(-\infty, \infty)$ and for some σ, D, and E have a quadratic lower bound, $h(u) \leq -u^2/(2\sigma^2) + Du + E$. Let ε be any positive sufficiently small number. Then for $A = \sigma C + \sigma^2 D$ and $B = -\sigma C + \sigma^2 D$, where $C = \Phi^{-1}(\varepsilon e^{-E-\sigma^2 D^2/2}/(\sigma\sqrt{8\pi}))$, the difference between the improper and proper integrals of $e^{h(u)}$ on (A, B) is less than ε, or more precisely, $\int_{-\infty}^{\infty} e^{h(u)} du - \int_A^B e^{h(u)} du < \varepsilon$.*

Proof. Since $-u^2/(2\sigma^2) + Du + E = -(u - \sigma^2 D)^2/(2\sigma^2) + (\sigma^2 D^2/2 + E)$ for any $A < B$ we have

$$
\int_{-\infty}^{\infty} e^{h(u)} du - \int_A^B e^{h(u)} du = \int_{-\infty}^{A} e^{h(u)} du + \int_B^{\infty} e^{h(u)} du
$$
$$
\leq \int_{-\infty}^{A} e^{-\frac{1}{2\sigma^2}u^2 + Du + E} du + \int_B^{\infty} e^{-\frac{1}{2\sigma^2}u^2 + Du + E} du
$$
$$
= \sigma\sqrt{2\pi} e^{(\sigma^2 D^2/2 + E)} \left[\Phi\left(\frac{A - \sigma^2 D}{\sigma}\right) + \Phi\left(-\frac{B - \sigma^2 D}{\sigma}\right) \right].
$$

The lower and upper limits are found by equating the first and second terms in the last expression to $\varepsilon/2$. ∎

Clearly, a sufficiently small number ε means that $\varepsilon e^{-E-\sigma^2 D^2/2}/(\sigma\sqrt{8\pi}) < 1/2$, so that $C < 0$.

We illustrate this lemma by computing A and B such that the proper integral $\int_A^B e^{h(u)} du$ differs from the improper integral $\int_{-\infty}^{\infty} e^{h(u)} du$ by ε, where $h = ku - u^2/(2\sigma^2) - \sum \ln(1 + e^{\beta' \mathbf{x}_j + u})$. First, we use a trivial inequality $\ln(1 + e^{\beta' \mathbf{x}_j + u}) \geq 0$, which in the notation of Lemma 35 means that $D = k$ and $E = 0$, implying that $A = \sigma^2 k + \sigma C$ and $B = \sigma^2 k - \sigma C$, where $C = \Phi^{-1}(\varepsilon e^{-\sigma^2 k^2/2}/(\sigma\sqrt{8\pi}))$. Second, the inequality $\ln(1 + e^{\beta' \mathbf{x}_j + u}) \geq u + \beta' \mathbf{x}_j$ means that $D = -(n - k)$ and $E = \beta' \sum \mathbf{x}_j$, with the appropriate limits A and B. Apparently, one can take the maximum of A's and the minimum of B's. After A and B are determined, we approximate $\int_{-\infty}^{\infty} e^{h(u)} du$ by the sum $\sum_{k=1}^{K} e^{h(u_k)}(B - A)/K$, where $u_k = A + k(B - A)/K$.

To replace the improper integral $\int_{-\infty}^{\infty} u^2 e^{h(u)} du = \int_{-\infty}^{\infty} e^{h(u) + 2\ln|u|} du$, we use inequality $\ln|u| \leq |u| - 1$, so that we find $A < 0$ and $B > 0$ using Lemma 35 such that

$$
\int_{-\infty}^{\infty} u^2 e^{h(u)} du - \left(\int_A^0 u^2 e^{h(u)} du + \int_0^B u^2 e^{h(u)} du \right) < \varepsilon.
$$

Then the improper integral is approximated by two sums with $u_k = A(1 - (k-1)/K)$ and $u_k = kB/K$.

Monte Carlo simulations. The integrals involved can be evaluated by statistical simulations. We refer the reader to books by Robert and Casella (1999) and Evans and Swartz (2000) for detail. The advantage of this approach is that it is quite general and easy to implement. The disadvantage is that it may require very large K to achieve a satisfactory approximation. Also, when using statistical simulations, one should remember that with any precision there is an assigned probability to achieve the integral precision. For example, to approximate integral I_{i1}, one generates a presumably large number (say, $K = 1000$) normally distributed $u_k \sim \mathcal{N}(0, \sigma^2)$ and then approximates $I_{i1} \simeq K^{-1} \sigma \sqrt{2\pi} \sum_{k=1}^{K} e^{k_i u_k - \sum_{j=1}^{n_i} \ln(1 + e^{\beta' \mathbf{x}_{ij} + u_k})}$. Typically, the number of simulations are picked out of convenience and are rarely justified. A better way to do simulations involves three steps: (1) estimate SD with a relatively small number of simulations, (2) compute the number of simulations, K, to make SE smaller than, say, 10^{-4}, which implies that $10^{-4} =$ SD$/\sqrt{K}$ or $K =$ SD $\times 10^8$; and (3) do K simulations, see Problem 4.

Discussion of the integral approximation techniques

Most numerical methods approximate the integral $\int_{-\infty}^{\infty} f(x) dx$ by a sum, $\sum_{k=1}^{K} w_k$ $f(x_x)$. Specifically, we discuss advantages and disadvantages of several integration techniques when the integrand takes the form $f(x) = g(x) e^{-x^2/(2\sigma^2)}$, where the function g is nonnegative. Three integration parameters are involved: (a) the number of nodes, K; (b) the specific nodes, $\{x_k, k = 1, 2, ..., K\}$ and (c) the weights, $\{w_k, k = 1, 2, ..., K\}$.

Generally, the higher the value of K, the better the approximation. It is not necessary to keep K constant during iterations. Actually, K should increase with convergence/number of iterations. Neither Gauss–Hermite nor Monte Carlo provide accuracy analysis and appropriate choice of K. When integrals are approximated by a sum (say, using the trapezoid rule), a more sophisticated analysis of the second derivative of the integrand should be carried out to yield the number of nodes required to approximate the integral with a specified precision. Such an analysis was done for the logistic-normal integral in Section 7.1.2. A big advantage of this approach is that the precision of integration is under control. However, it involves (a) finding A and B such that the improper integral can be replaced with the proper one with the specified epsilon, and (b) assessing the upper bound for the second derivative of the integrand.

In order to choose nodes we need to determine the neighborhood/interval from which the integrand values are sampled. There are at least three ways to chose $\{x_k\}$ and the corresponding positive weights $\{w_k\}$. The easiest way to choose $\{x_k\}$ is to sample randomly from $\mathcal{N}(0, \sigma^2)$, and then the integral is approximated by the empirical mean with $w_k = 1/K$. This is the Monte Carlo method or statistical simulation. Although this method is quite general and easy to realize, it gives a poor approximation when the maximum of g is far from zero. For example, Monte Carlo may give poor integral approximation for I_{i2} because the integrand is sampled in the neighborhood of zero where the integrand is zero. This problem with the Monte Carlo technique is well known and there is an improved technique, called *importance sampling*, discussed thoroughly by Robert and Casella (1999). The idea of this technique is to sample the integrand from an "important" neighborhood, where the integrand takes maximum values. This means that before statistical simulation, we need to find the maximum point of $f(x)$ and compute its second derivative, as in adaptive Gauss–Hermite quadrature. If x_* is the point of maximum and $\hat{\sigma}$ is the square root of the reciprocal of the second derivative, we represent $f(x) =$

$g(x)e^{-(x-x_*)^2/(2\hat{\sigma}^2)}$, where $g(x) = f(x)e^{(x-x_*)^2/(2\hat{\sigma}^2)}$. Hence, if $\{x_k\}$ is a sample from $\mathcal{N}(x_*, \hat{\sigma}^2)$, we estimate $\int_{-\infty}^{\infty} f(x)dx$ as $\hat{\sigma}\sqrt{2\pi}$ times the empirical mean of g. Particularly, this technique would require approximating I_{i2} by two samples.

Implementation in R

Two maximum likelihood estimation functions can be found in the directory `"c:\\`
`MixedModels\\Chapter07\\"`. The first R function, `logMLE1` uses the built-in function `integrate` for integral evaluation, and the second function, `logMLgh`, uses the Gauss–Hermite quadrature with the user-defined number of nodes based on the `gauher` function presented above. The calls to the two function are:

```
logMLE1(dat,b,s2,maxiter=20,eps=1e-010,silent=1)

logMLEgh(dat,b,s2,maxiter=20,ngh=13,eps=1e-010,silent=1)
```

The data are supplied via the argument `dat`; this matrix has the same format as in the `logric` function above. The starting values for the beta-coefficients are in array `b`; `s2` passes the starting value for σ^2. The starting values can be obtained using the fixed subject-specific intercept approach discussed in the previous section (`s2` is the variance of the intercepts). The parameter `ngh` passes the number of Gauss-Hermite nodes. It is a great deal of research to find out what `ngh` value is optimal: a small value will result in the large error of the integral approximation, and a large value will prolong computation. Examples of calls to these functions can be found in function `logsim`, which compares several methods and algorithms for logistic regression with random intercept.

In the following subsections we consider several estimators that avoid integration. They are all derived via approximation of the original log-likelihood function (7.64).

7.3.2   Fixed sample likelihood approximation

We have noticed before that the majority of integral approximations have the generic form $\sum_{s=1}^{S} w_s f(x_s)$, where x_s is the abscissa and w_s is the weight. For example, by the trapezoid rule the integral $\int_{A}^{B} f(x)dx$ is approximated by the sum with $x_s = A + (s-1)h$ and $w_1 = w_S = h/2$, $w_s = h = (B-A)/(S-1)$ for $1 < s < S$, see (7.39). In Gauss–Hermite quadrature, given the number of nodes S, the pairs $\{x_s, w_s\}$ are defined, for example, as in Table 7.1. We deliberately use notation s for nodes, rather than k, because in this section $\{x_s\}$ will be given a different interpretation as a sample at which the integrand values are computed. In Monte Carlo, the integral $\int f(x)\phi(x)dx = E_{x \sim \mathcal{N}(0,1)} f(x)$ is again approximated by the sum $\sum_{s=1}^{S} w_s f(x_s)$, where the x_s are randomly chosen from $\mathcal{N}(0,1)$ and the weights are $w_s = 1/S$.

A different sort of observation is that up to a constant term, the likelihood (7.64) can be parameterized as

$$l(\boldsymbol{\beta}, \sigma) = \sum_{i=1}^{N} \ln \int_{-\infty}^{\infty} e^{\sum_{j=1}^{n_i} l_{ij}(\boldsymbol{\beta}, \sigma)} e^{-u^2/2} du, \tag{7.72}$$

where

$$l_{ij}(\boldsymbol{\beta}, \boldsymbol{\sigma}) = y_{ij} \ln \mu(\boldsymbol{\beta}' \mathbf{x}_{ij} + \sigma u) + (1 - y_{ij}) \ln(1 - \mu(\boldsymbol{\beta}' \mathbf{x}_{ij} + \sigma u))$$

and μ is the logit probability function. Notice that we express the log-likelihood in terms of a general probability function μ that facilitates application with other probability functions, such as probit. An advantage of (7.72) parameterization is that the kernel of the integration, $e^{-u^2/2}$, is a fixed function and σ acts as a parameter. In Fixed Sample Likelihood (FSL) approximation we couple the previous idea of approximating the integral as a sum with parameterization (7.72). So let S pairs be given $\{u_s, w_s\}$. We combine $\boldsymbol{\beta}$ with σ into an $(m+1) \times 1$ vector $\boldsymbol{\theta} = (\boldsymbol{\beta}', \sigma)'$ and construct the respective $(m+1) \times 1$ data vector $\mathbf{g}_{ijs} = (\mathbf{x}'_{ij}, u_s)'$. Then the log-likelihood (7.72) can be approximated as

$$l_{FSL}(\boldsymbol{\theta}) = \sum_{i=1}^{N} \ln \sum_{s=1}^{S} w_s e^{\sum_{j=1}^{n_i} l_{ijs}(\boldsymbol{\theta})}, \qquad (7.73)$$

where

$$l_{ijs}(\boldsymbol{\theta}) = y_{ij} \ln \mu(\boldsymbol{\theta}' \mathbf{g}_{ijs}) + (1 - y_{ij}) \ln(1 - \mu(\boldsymbol{\theta}' \mathbf{g}_{ijs})).$$

Now we treat (7.73) as a new log-likelihood function and find the $\boldsymbol{\theta}$ value that maximizes l_{FSL}. The derivatives needed are

$$\frac{\partial l_{FSL}}{\partial \boldsymbol{\theta}} = \sum_{i=1}^{N} \frac{1}{\sum_{s=1}^{S} w_s e_{is}} \sum_{s=1}^{S} w_s e_{is} \mathbf{q}_{is}, \qquad (7.74)$$

$$\mathbf{H} = \sum_{i=1}^{N} \left[\frac{\left(\sum_{s=1}^{S} w_s e_{is} \mathbf{q}_{is} \right) \left(\sum_{s=1}^{S} w_s e_{is} \mathbf{q}_{is} \right)'}{\left(\sum_{s=1}^{S} w_s e_{is} \right)^2} \right. \qquad (7.75)$$

$$\left. - \frac{\sum_{s=1}^{S} w_s e_{is} (\mathbf{Q}_{is} + \mathbf{q}_{is} \mathbf{q}'_{is})}{\sum_{s=1}^{S} w_s e_{is}} \right],$$

where $\mathbf{H} = -\partial^2 l / \partial \boldsymbol{\theta}^2$ is the negative Hessian, and

$$e_{is} = e^{\sum_{j=1}^{n_i} l_{ijs}}, \quad \mathbf{q}_{is} = \sum_{j=1}^{n_i} \dot{l}_{ijs} \mathbf{g}_{ijs}, \quad \mathbf{Q}_{is} = \sum_{j=1}^{n_i} \ddot{l}_{ijs} \mathbf{g}_{ijs} \mathbf{g}'_{ijs}. \qquad (7.76)$$

The first and second derivatives of the log-likelihood are similar to what was given before in Section 7.1.4; namely,

$$\dot{l}_{ijs} = (y_{ij} - \mu_{ijs}) \frac{\dot{\mu}_{ijs}}{\mu_{ijs}(1 - \mu_{ijs})},$$

$$\ddot{l}_{ijs} = y_{ij} \frac{\dot{\mu}_{ijs}^2 - \ddot{\mu}_{ijs} \mu_{ijs}}{\mu_{ijs}^2} + (1 - y_{ij}) \frac{\ddot{\mu}_{ijs}(1 - \mu_{ijs}) + \dot{\mu}_{ijs}^2}{(1 - \mu_{ijs})^2}.$$

Then the NR algorithm has the form

$$\boldsymbol{\theta}_{new} = \boldsymbol{\theta} + \lambda \mathbf{H}^{-1} \frac{\partial l_{FSL}}{\partial \boldsymbol{\theta}}, \qquad (7.77)$$

where λ is a positive step length (typically, $\lambda = 1$).

We emphasize that the difference between FSL and exact ML is that in the latter we use numerical integration for each integral (7.67) and (7.70) whereas in the FSL approach we approximate only the integral of the log-likelihood function. The FSL approach covers Gauss–Hermite quadrature and Monte Carlo under one methodological umbrella.

An important advantage of FSL approximation is that it produces the joint covariance matrix of β and σ. For LME and nonlinear marginal models with the fixed matrix of random effects, the ML estimates do not correlate. But for a nonlinear mixed model, including logistic regression with random intercepts, the estimates correlate asymptotically. This means that the variance of $\widehat{\beta}$ computed under the assumption that σ is known would have a systematic bias (one may expect a negative bias, i.e., variances will be underestimated). Also, one can test the hypothesis $H_0 : \sigma = 0$, treating σ as just one of the coefficients using the one-tailed test with the alternative $H_A : \sigma > 0$. It is straightforward to generalize this method to multivariate random effects in GLMM (Section 7.8.3) and the nonlinear mixed effects model of the next chapter.

Implementation in R

The calls to two R functions that implement the fixed sample likelihood approximation method are

```
logFS(dat,nSim=100,bsigma,maxiter=20,eps=0.001,silent =1)
logFSL(dat,xwFSL=gauher(13),bsigma,maxiter=20,eps=0.001,silent=1)
```

The parameter nSim specifies the sample size, S. The $(m+1)$ array bsigma specifies the starting values for (β,σ). In the first function, the sample is generated within the function, and in the second function it is generated outside the function and is passed through the argument xwFSL; a good choice is to take the Gauss–Hermite nodes from gauher. The second function can be viewed as a fast version of the first. In both cases the output is a list with four components: (1) b=β estimate, (2) sigma^2=σ^2 estimate, (3) iH=the $(m+1) \times (m+1)$ information matrix inverse (covariance matrix for $\widehat{\theta}$), and (4) iter=number of iterations done (if iter=maxiter then the number of iterations reached maximum without convergence). In short, logFS uses random and logFSL used Gauss-Hermite nodes. Also we offer two simplified versions of the functions, logFS1 and logFSL1 that use $\lambda = 1$ (it was noticed that for many iterations $\lambda = 1$ lead to a log-likelihood function increase). Note that in these functions matrix $\mathbf{H}$ is not computed by formula (7.75) but approximated using the cross-derivatives: namely,

$$\mathbf{H} \sim \sum_{i=1}^{N} \left(\frac{\partial l_{iFSL}}{\partial \boldsymbol{\theta}} \right) \left(\frac{\partial l_{iFSL}}{\partial \boldsymbol{\theta}} \right)',$$

where the derivative of l_{iFSL} is the ith term in expression (7.74).

7.3.3   Quadratic approximation

We note that the main obstacle in obtaining the exact integral in (7.64) is the nonlinear function $\sum_{j=1}^{n_i} \ln(1 + e^{\boldsymbol{\beta}' \mathbf{x}_{ij}+u})$. However, we can take the exact integral after approximating this function by a quadratic function around zero after Taylor's series expansion, $\sum_{j=1}^{n_i} \ln(1 + e^{\boldsymbol{\beta}' \mathbf{x}_{ij}+u}) \simeq C_0 + C_1 u + 0.5 C_2 u^2$, where

$$C_0 = \sum_{j=1}^{n_i} \ln(1 + e^{\boldsymbol{\beta}' \mathbf{x}_{ij}}), \ C_1 = \sum_{j=1}^{n_i} \frac{e^{\boldsymbol{\beta}' \mathbf{x}_{ij}}}{1 + e^{\boldsymbol{\beta}' \mathbf{x}_{ij}}}, \ C_2 = \sum_{j=1}^{n_i} \frac{e^{\boldsymbol{\beta}' \mathbf{x}_{ij}}}{(1 + e^{\boldsymbol{\beta}' \mathbf{x}_{ij}})^2}.$$

The fact that the function is approximated around zero is important. In fact, one may expect a satisfactory approximation if the deviation of the subject-specific intercept from the population-based intercept is not large. In the next section we approximate the function around the subject-specific intercept. This approximation also follows from the Laplace approximation. Early authors considered a first-order (linear) approximation around zero (Goldstein 1991; Rodriguez and Goldman, 1995), but we will not discuss it here, due to poor performance.

Using the formula

$$\int_{-\infty}^{\infty} e^{-Au^2/2-Bu-C} du = \exp\left(0.5B^2/A - C\right) \sqrt{2\pi/A}$$

for positive A, we approximate $\int_{-\infty}^{\infty} e^{h_i(\boldsymbol{\beta}, u)} du$ as

$$\int_{-\infty}^{\infty} e^{-\frac{1}{2}(\sigma^{-2}+C_2)u^2 - (C_1 - k_i)u - C_0} du$$

$$= \sqrt{2\pi} \exp\left(\frac{1}{2}(C_1 - k_i)^2 (\sigma^{-2} + C_2)^{-1} - C_0\right) / \sqrt{\sigma^{-2} + C_2}.$$

This leads to the approximated log-likelihood function (7.64), up to a constant term,

$$
\begin{aligned}
l_2(\boldsymbol{\beta}, \sigma^2) = & -\frac{N \ln 2\pi \sigma^2}{2} + \boldsymbol{\beta}' \mathbf{r} \\
& + \frac{1}{2} \sum_{i=1}^{N} \left\{ \frac{(L_i - k_i)^2}{L_i + \sigma^{-2}} - 2 \sum_{j=1}^{n_i} \ln(1 + e_{ij}) - \ln(L_i + \sigma^{-2}) \right\},
\end{aligned}
$$

where to shorten the notation we let $e_{ij} = e^{\boldsymbol{\beta}' \mathbf{x}_{ij}}$ and $L_i = \sum_{j=1}^{n_i} e_{ij}(1 + e_{ij})^{-2}$. The subscript 2 indicates quadratic approximation. We need to maximize l_2 over $\boldsymbol{\beta}$ and σ^2 to obtain an approximation to the MLE. The first (and second) derivatives of l_2 are straightforward to obtain; then we apply either the empirical FS or Newton–Raphson algorithm to maximize l_2.

7.3.4   Laplace approximation to the likelihood

In Subsections 7.1.2 and 7.3.1 we applied the Laplace approximation to evaluate integrals around the maximum point of the integrand. One can also apply the Laplace approximation to the likelihood and maximize the resulting function to obtain an approximation to the MLE that avoids integration.

Let u_{*i} be the maximum of $h_i(\boldsymbol{\beta};u)$, assuming that $\boldsymbol{\beta}$ is fixed, say at the value of the previous iteration (algorithms to find this maximum were discussed in the previous subsection). Applying the Laplace approximation (7.29) to (7.64), we obtain, up to a constant term, an approximated log-likelihood function

$$l_{LA}(\boldsymbol{\beta},\sigma^2) = \boldsymbol{\beta}'\mathbf{r} - \frac{1}{2\sigma^2}\sum_{i=1}^{N}u_{*i}^2 - \sum_{i=1}^{N}\sum_{j=1}^{n_i}\ln(1+e^{\boldsymbol{\beta}'\mathbf{x}_{ij}+u_{*i}})$$

$$-\frac{1}{2}\sum_{i=1}^{N}\ln\left(\frac{1}{\sigma^2}+\sum_{j=1}^{n_i}\frac{e^{\boldsymbol{\beta}'\mathbf{x}_{ij}+u_{*i}}}{(1+e^{\boldsymbol{\beta}'\mathbf{x}_{ij}+u_{*i}})^2}\right) - \frac{N\ln\sigma^2}{2}. \qquad (7.78)$$

Note that we omitted the terms that do not depend on $\boldsymbol{\beta}$ or σ^2; namely, $N\ln(2\pi)$ $/2+\sum k_i u_{*i}$. Now we treat this function as a log-likelihood-function, expecting that the maximum point will be close to the MLE as the maximum point of the original function (7.64). Maximization of l_{LA} involves finding individual u_{*i} when $\boldsymbol{\beta}$ and σ^2 are held constant, for $i = 1, 2, ..., N$. To maximize l_{LA}, we need the first derivatives,

$$\frac{\partial l_{LA}}{\partial \boldsymbol{\beta}} = \mathbf{r} - \sum_{i=1}^{N}\sum_{j=1}^{n_i}q_{ij1}\mathbf{x}_{ij} - \frac{1}{2}\sum_{i=1}^{N}\frac{\sum_{j=1}^{n_i}q_{ij3}\mathbf{x}_{ij}}{\sigma^{-2}+\sum_{j=1}^{n_i}q_{ij2}}, \qquad (7.79)$$

$$\frac{\partial l_{LA}}{\partial \sigma^2} = -\frac{N}{2\sigma^2} + \frac{1}{2\sigma^4}\sum_{i=1}^{N}\left(u_{*i}^2 + \frac{1}{\sigma^{-2}+\sum_{j=1}^{n_i}q_{ij2}}\right), \qquad (7.80)$$

where $e_{ij} = e^{\boldsymbol{\beta}'\mathbf{x}_{ij}+u_{*i}}$, and

$$q_{ij1} = \frac{e_{ij}}{1+e_{ij}}, \quad q_{ij2} = \frac{e_{ij}}{(1+e_{ij})^2}, \quad q_{ij3} = \frac{e_{ij}(1-e_{ij})}{(1+e_{ij})^3}.$$

Equating $\partial l_{LA}/\partial \sigma^2 = 0$ and applying the fixed-point algorithm of Chapter 2, we obtain a recursive formula for the variance,

$$\widehat{\sigma}_{s+1}^2 = \frac{1}{N}\sum_{i=1}^{N}\left(u_{*i}^2 + \frac{1}{\widehat{\sigma}_s^{-2}+\sum_{j=1}^{n_i}q_{ij2}}\right). \qquad (7.81)$$

The estimate of σ^2 will be greater than the "sample variance" of the estimated random effects. The right-hand side of (7.81), as a function of $\widehat{\sigma}_s^2$, is an increasing function with positive values at zero and infinity. Thus, as follows from Appendix 13.3.4, the FP iterations converge for any $\{u_{*i}, q_{ij2}\}$. For $\boldsymbol{\beta}$ we use the Newton–Raphson algorithm, which requires the second-order derivative $\mathbf{H} = \partial^2 l_{LA}/\partial\boldsymbol{\beta}^2 = -\sum_{i=1}^{N}\mathbf{H}_i$, where

$$\mathbf{H}_i = \sum_{j=1}^{n_i}q_{ij2}\mathbf{x}_{ij}\mathbf{x}_{ij}' + \frac{1}{2}\frac{\sum_{j=1}^{n_i}q_{ij4}\mathbf{x}_{ij}\mathbf{x}_{ij}'}{\sigma^{-2}+\sum_{j=1}^{n_i}q_{ij2}} - \frac{1}{2}\frac{(\sum_{j=1}^{n_i}q_{ij3}\mathbf{x}_{ij})(\sum_{j=1}^{n_i}q_{ij3}\mathbf{x}_{ij})'}{(\sigma^{-2}+\sum_{j=1}^{n_i}q_{ij2})^2}$$

and $g_{ij4} = (e_{ij} - 4e_{ij}^2 + e_{ij}^3)/(1+e_{ij})^4$. Numerically, the alternation between maximization of $h_i(\boldsymbol{\beta};u)$ and (7.78) is equivalent to simultaneous maximization of (7.78) over $(\boldsymbol{\beta},u_1,...,u_N)$ when σ^2 is fixed.

Penalized quasi-likelihood

Breslow and Clayton (1993) omit the last term in (7.78). The resulting method is called Penalized Quasi-Likelihood (PQL). We justify the omission by an observation that when N and n_i approach infinity, the contribution of the last term vanishes. To simplify, we let $n_i = n$ and $\lim_{N \to \infty} N/n = p$, a finite positive number. Dividing l_{LA} by Nn, we see that the first term has the order $O(n^{-1})$, the second term has the order $O(1)$, the third term has the order $O(n^{-1})$, and the fourth term has the order $O(1)$. For the last term, $\sum_{j=1}^{n_i} e^{\boldsymbol{\beta}' \mathbf{x}_{ij} + u_{*i}} (1 + e^{\boldsymbol{\beta}' \mathbf{x}_{ij} + u_{*i}})^{-2} \sim An$, where A is a positive constant. But elementary calculus shows that $\lim_{n \to \infty} n^{-1} \ln(\sigma^{-2} + An) = 0$ because by L'Hospital's rule, this limit is equal to $\lim_{n \to \infty} A(\sigma^{-2} + An)^{-1} = 0$. Thus the last term has the order $O(N^{-1})$. This means that only the second and fourth terms of $(Nn)^{-1} l_{LA}$ do not vanish; in particular, the last term may be omitted if $\min n_i$ goes to infinity when $N \to \infty$. After omitting the last term in (7.78), we arrive at the PQL function

$$
\begin{aligned}
l_{PQL}(\boldsymbol{\beta}, \sigma^2) &= \boldsymbol{\beta}' \mathbf{r} - \sum_{i=1}^{N} \sum_{j=1}^{n_i} \ln(1 + e^{\boldsymbol{\beta}' \mathbf{x}_{ij} + u_{*i}}) - \frac{N}{2} \ln 2\pi\sigma^2 - \frac{1}{2\sigma^2} \sum_{i=1}^{N} u_{*i}^2 \\
&= \sum_{i=1}^{N} \left[l_i(\boldsymbol{\beta}, u_{*i}) - \frac{1}{2\sigma^2} u_{*i}^2 \right] - \frac{N}{2} \ln 2\pi\sigma^2,
\end{aligned}
\tag{7.82}
$$

where l_i is the individual (subject-specific) log-likelihood function. The expression in brackets is interpreted as a penalized log-likelihood where the penalty has the form of the squared distance of subject-specific intercepts from the population-based intercept ($u_i = a_i - \alpha$), adjusted by their variance. Moreover, since u_{*i} is the maximum point of $l_i(\boldsymbol{\beta}, u_i) - u_i^2/(2\sigma^2)$, maximization of l_{PQL} is equivalent to maximization of

$$
l_{PQL}(\boldsymbol{\beta}, u_1, ..., u_N, \sigma^2) = \sum_{i=1}^{N} l_i(\boldsymbol{\beta}, u_i) - \frac{1}{2\sigma^2} \sum_{i=1}^{N} u_i^2 - \frac{N}{2} \ln 2\pi\sigma^2.
\tag{7.83}
$$

However, the maximum of this function occurs at $u_i = 0$ and $\sigma^2 = 0$, and $\boldsymbol{\beta}$ is the standard MLE (fixed parameters). Indeed, differentiating with respect to σ^2, we find that the optimum $\sigma^2 = \sum u_i^2/N$. Substituting this back into (7.83), we come to an equivalent function to maximize, $\sum l_i(\boldsymbol{\beta}, u_i) - 0.5N \ln \sum u_i^2$. But this function takes a maximum $+\infty$ when $u_i \to 0$ for all $i = 1, ..., N$. To avoid such a degeneration, we suggest updating σ^2 by formula (7.81). Thus, in the PQL method for fixed σ^2, we maximize the penalized log-likelihood function

$$
l_{PQL}(\boldsymbol{\beta}, u_1, ..., u_N) = \sum_{i=1}^{N} l_i(\boldsymbol{\beta}, u_i) - \frac{1}{2\sigma^2} \sum_{i=1}^{N} u_i^2,
\tag{7.84}
$$

updating σ^2 at each iteration as

$$
\widehat{\sigma}_{s+1}^2 = \frac{1}{N} \sum_{i=1}^{N} \left(u_{*i}^2 + \frac{1}{\widehat{\sigma}_s^{-2} + \sum_{j=1}^{n_i} e^{\widehat{\boldsymbol{\beta}}_s' \mathbf{x}_{ij} + u_{*i}} (1 + e^{\widehat{\boldsymbol{\beta}}_s' \mathbf{x}_{ij} + u_{*i}})^{-2}} \right).
\tag{7.85}
$$

This is equivalent to omitting the third term in estimating equation (7.79) and leaving (7.80) the same. If N is relatively small, one can update $\boldsymbol{\beta}$ and u_i from l_{PQL} by solving $N + m$ equations simultaneously.

Log-likelihood (7.84) has a clear "penalized" interpretation: the first term is the standard log-likelihood assuming that $\{u_i\}$ are fixed as in Section 7.2.2 and $-(2\sigma^2)^{-1}\sum u_i^2$ is the penalty term. The penalized log-likelihood function is a characteristic feature of the mixed effects methodology.

Variance update formulas (7.81) and (7.85) have a nice interpretation as a Laplace approximation of the maximum likelihood update formula (7.70). Indeed, applying formula (7.31) to (7.70), we come to (7.81):

$$\widehat{\sigma}_{s+1}^2 = \frac{1}{N}\sum_{i=1}^N \frac{I_{i2}}{I_{i1}} = \frac{1}{N}\sum_{i=1}^N \frac{\int_{-\infty}^{\infty} u^2 e^{h_i(\boldsymbol{\beta},u)}\,du}{\int_{-\infty}^{\infty} e^{h_i(\boldsymbol{\beta},u)}\,du} \simeq \frac{1}{N}\sum_{i=1}^N \left[u_{*i}^2 + \frac{1}{\widehat{\sigma}_s^{-2} + \sum_{j=1}^{n_i} q_{ij2}} \right].$$
(7.86)

This interpretation, along with the penalized log-likelihood (7.84), will be generalized to generalized linear mixed models in the following sections and to nonlinear mixed models in the next chapter. The u_{*i} computed at the final iteration may serve as an estimate of the random effect, the deviation of the subject-specific from the population-averaged intercept.

glmmPQL function from library MASS

The library `MASS` offers the `glmmPQL` function , which a estimates GLM mixed model with random effects; it has the same syntax as `lme`. This function is very flexible and handles different links, as in the `glm` function, and multiple random effects as in `lme`. For example, to run a logistic regression with two covariates and a random intercept, you have to issue

```
glmmPQL(y~x1+x2,random=~1|id,family=binomial,data=da,verbose=F)
```

See an example of the call to this function in our `logsim` function.

7.3.5 VARLINK estimation

In this section we develop a simplified method for estimation of a logistic regression with a random intercept, VARLINK. This method can be applied to any link where the marginal binary model admits a closed-form solution or has a satisfactory approximation. The key to this estimation method is the link approximation developed in Section 7.1.2, which approximates marginal probability and thus avoids integration. VARLINK alternates between estimation of the subject-specific regression coefficients, holding the population-averaged parameters constant, and estimation of a binary model using link approximation. The idea of such two-stage estimation was originally suggested by Stiratelli et al. (1984) and described at length by Davidian and Giltinan (1995). The authors, however, assumed that *each* coefficient of the logistic regression is subject-specific, with the mean specified in the second-stage model (4.2) of Section 4.1. More details on the two-stage estimation in the framework of a more general nonlinear mixed model may be found in Section 8.5.

However, often the model contains population-averaged parameters that must be estimated jointly. Then, even knowing the variance parameters of random effects, one cannot eliminate an integration problem, and therefore the two-stage method cannot be applied. Thus, VARLINK may be viewed as a generalization of the two-stage method to situations when population-averaged parameters are present. We call this procedure VARLINK because it consists of two steps, variance estimation and link approximation. As any two-stage procedure, it requires a sufficient number of observations per cluster to estimate the subject-specific parameters satisfactorily. It is particularly easy to estimate the probit regression with a normally distributed random intercept because the marginal model is again a probit regression with attenuated coefficients, see the next section.

The VARLINK estimation procedure for logistic regression with random intercepts consists of two alternating steps.

1. *Estimation of the subject-specific intercept and its variance.* We want to estimate the deviation of the subject-specific intercept from the population-averaged intercept, u_i assuming that $\boldsymbol{\beta}$ is held constant for each cluster $i = 1, ..., N$. As before, it is assumed that the first component of vector $\boldsymbol{\beta}$ is the intercept. Omitting i and letting $B_j = \exp(\boldsymbol{\beta}'\mathbf{x}_j)$ and $k = \sum_{j=1}^n y_j$, the individual maximum likelihood reduces to maximization of the function $ku - \sum_{j=1}^n \ln(1 + B_j e^u)$. Equivalently, we need to solve the equation $\sum_{j=1}^n (1 + B_j w)^{-1} = n - k$ for positive $w = e^u$. Note that if $k = 0$ or $k = n$, there is no solution for u, so we take only clusters where $0 < k < n$. The latter equation has a unique positive solution, which can be obtained by Newton's iterations $w_{s+1} = w_s + [\sum_{j=1}^n (1 + B_j w)^{-1} - (n - k)]/\sum_{j=1}^n B_j (1 + B_j w)^{-2}$. A good start can be obtained from the inequality $\sum (1 + B_j w)^{-1} \geq n^2/(n + w \sum B_j)$, which gives $w_0 = (\sum B_j)^{-1} nk/(n - 1)$. Then the sequence $\{w_s\}$ is increasing and converges to a positive w_*. At the final iteration we let $u_i = \ln w_*$. After the subject-specific $\{u_i\}$ are obtained, we estimate σ^2. If u_i were estimated exactly then an estimator for σ^2 would be the mean of $\{u_i^2\}$. But since the $\{u_i\}$ are estimated from an individual logistic regression fit, it has the variance $v_i = [\sum_{j=1}^{n_i} B_{ij} (1 + B_{ij})^{-2}]^{-1}$. Thus, generalizing (4.32), we obtain an estimate $\sigma^2 = N^{-1} \sum_{i=1}^N (u_i^2 - v_i)$. Unfortunately, it can produce negative values (then we let $\sigma^2 = 0$), a common drawback of noniterative variance estimation. This type of estimator for the random effect variance will be used for general nonlinear mixed effects model in the next chapter.

2. *Estimation of the binary model using link approximation.* After σ^2 is estimated from the preceding step, we can use several logit approximations with the normally distributed intercept derived in Section 7.1.2. If $\mu = \mu(s, \sigma^2)$ denotes an approximation to $E_{u \sim \mathcal{N}(0,\sigma^2)} e^{u+s}/(1 + e^{u+s})$, as a function of s and σ^2, we come to a log-likelihood function similar to that one we considered in Section 7.1.4,

$$l(\boldsymbol{\beta}) = \sum_{i=1}^N \sum_{j=1}^{n_i} [y_{ij} \ln \mu(s_{ij}) + (1 - y_{ij}) \ln(1 - \mu(s_{ij}))],$$

where $s_{ij} = \boldsymbol{\beta}'\mathbf{x}_{ij}$ and $\mu = \mu(s)$ is the right-hand side of the marginal link approximations, such as (7.17) or (7.21), with σ^2 estimated from step 1. Clearly,

$\{y_{ij}\}$ are treated as independent random variables and the FS/IRLS algorithm of Section 7.1.4 yields an update formula

$$\boldsymbol{\beta}_{s+1} = \boldsymbol{\beta}_s + \lambda_s \left(\sum_{i,j} w_{ij} \dot{\mu}_{ij}^2 \mathbf{x}_{ij} \mathbf{x}_{ij}' \right)^{-1} \left(\sum_{i,j} w_{ij}(y_{ij} - \mu_{ij}) \dot{\mu}_{ij} \mathbf{x}_{ij} \right),$$

where $\dot{\mu}_{ij} = d\mu/ds$ evaluated at s_{ij} and λ_s is the step length (typically, $\lambda_s = 1$ suffices). After convergence, we return to step 1.

As mentioned above, this procedure is especially appealing for probit regression with normally distributed random effects because then the marginal model admits a closed-form solution (see Section 7.4).

The VARLINK method is implemented in the function

```
logVARLINK1(dat,b,s2,maxiter=20,eps=0.001,silent =1)
```

This function has the same arguments and output as in our previous R functions.

7.3.6   Beta-binomial model

The combination of the binomial distribution with probability distributed as the beta distribution leads again to the beta distribution. This fact was observed more than 50 years ago, and many authors suggested a beta-binomial model to describe the binomial data with overdispersion avoiding integration. Concise coverage of the beta-binomial model without covariates is found in the book by McCulloch and Searle (2001, pp. 57–64). It is worthwhile to remember that in the beta-binomial model, the values of the dependent variable are nonnegative integers (counts), not 0 or 1 as in logistic regression, considered earlier. Equivalently, one may assume that the covariates, $\{\mathbf{x}_i\}$, are only cluster-, not subject-specific.

For each cluster $i = 1, 2, ..., N$, we observe count data $y_i = \sum_{j=1}^{n_i} y_{ij}$, where the $\{y_{ij}\}$ are the iid binary data with probability p_i. We do not observe p_i, but instead assume that p_i is also a random variable with beta distribution on $(0, 1)$ with parameters α and β. The beta distribution is quite flexible and may produce uniform, bell-shaped, or even delta-function/constant p_i distribution. Thus, the beta-binomial model is specified as a hierarchical model,

$$y_i|p_i \sim \text{Binomial}(n_i, p_i), \quad p_i \sim B(\alpha, \beta). \tag{7.87}$$

The beta distribution for p_i is given by $p_i^{\alpha-1}(1 - p_i)^{\beta-1}/B(\alpha, \beta)$, where $B(\alpha, \beta) = \int_0^1 x^{\alpha-1}(1-x)^{\beta-1}dx$ is the beta function. Recall that $B(\alpha, \beta) = \Gamma(\alpha+\beta)/[\Gamma(\alpha)\Gamma(\beta)]$, where Γ is the gamma function (many software packages have a built-in $\ln\Gamma$). The key observation is that the hierarchical model (7.87) implies the marginal distribution of y_i also like a beta distribution, specifically omitting the constant coefficient, $\int_0^1 p_i^{y_i}(1 - p_i)^{n_i-y_i}p_i^{\alpha-1}(1 - p_i)^{\beta-1}dp_i = B(\alpha + y_i, \beta + n_i - y_i)$. The binomial coefficient can be expressed as $\binom{n}{y} = n!/(y!(n - y)!)$. Allowing α or β to vary across clusters after reparameterization $\mu_i = \alpha/(\alpha + \beta)$ and $\tau = 1/(\alpha + \beta) =$const$> 0$, we come to the log-likelihood up to a constant term,

$$l(\boldsymbol{\beta},\tau)$$
$$= \sum_{i=1}^{N} \left[\sum_{h=0}^{y_i-1} \ln{(h\tau + \mu_i)} + \sum_{h=0}^{n_i-y_i-1} \ln{(h\tau + (1 - \mu_i))} - \sum_{h=0}^{n_i-1} \ln{(1 + h\tau)} \right].$$

For example, in the case of a logit link, we let $\mu_i = \mu_i(\boldsymbol{\beta}) = e^{\boldsymbol{\beta}'\mathbf{x}_i}/(1 + e^{\boldsymbol{\beta}'\mathbf{x}_i})$, where $\mathbf{x}_i$ is the $m \times 1$ cluster covariate. The derivatives are

$$\frac{\partial l}{\partial \boldsymbol{\beta}} = \sum_{i=1}^{N} \left[\sum_{h=0}^{y_i-1} \frac{1}{h\tau + \mu_i} - \sum_{h=0}^{n_i-y_i-1} \frac{1}{h\tau + (1 - \mu_i)} \right] \dot{\mu}_i \mathbf{x}_i,$$

$$\frac{\partial l}{\partial \tau} = \sum_{i=1}^{N} \left[\sum_{h=0}^{y_i-1} \frac{h}{h\tau + \mu_i} - \sum_{h=0}^{n_i-y_i-1} \frac{h}{h\tau + (1 - \mu_i)} - \sum_{h=0}^{n_i-1} \frac{h}{1 + h\tau} \right].$$

The $(m+1) \times (m+1)$ information matrix for $(\boldsymbol{\beta},\tau)$ is given by

$$\mathcal{I} = \left[\begin{array}{cc} \mathcal{I}_{\boldsymbol{\beta}} & \mathcal{I}'_{\tau\boldsymbol{\beta}} \\ \mathcal{I}_{\tau\boldsymbol{\beta}} & \mathcal{I}_{\tau} \end{array} \right],$$

where the blocks are

$$\mathcal{I}_{\boldsymbol{\beta}} = \sum_{i=1}^{N} \left[\sum_{h=0}^{n_i} p_{ih} \left(\sum_{h=0}^{k-1} \frac{1}{(h\tau + \mu_i)^2} - \sum_{h=0}^{n_i-k-1} \frac{1}{(h\tau + (1 - \mu_i))^2} \right) \right] \ddot{\mu}_i \mathbf{x}_i \mathbf{x}'_i$$

$$\mathcal{I}_{\tau\boldsymbol{\beta}} = \sum_{i=1}^{N} \left[\sum_{h=0}^{n_i} p_{ih} \left(\sum_{h=0}^{k-1} \frac{h}{(h\tau + \mu_i)^2} - \sum_{h=0}^{n_i-k-1} \frac{h}{(h\tau + (1 - \mu_i))^2} \right) \right] \dot{\mu}_i \mathbf{x}_i,$$

$$\mathcal{I}_{\tau} = \sum_{i=1}^{N} \left[\sum_{h=0}^{n_i} p_{ih} \left(\sum_{h=0}^{k-1} \frac{h^2}{(h\tau + \mu_i)^2} - \sum_{h=0}^{n_i-k-1} \frac{h^2}{(h\tau + (1 - \mu_i))^2} \right) \right],$$

and

$$p_{ih} = \Pr(y_i = h) = \binom{n_i}{h} \frac{B(\mu_i/\tau + h, n_i + (1 - \mu_i)/\tau - h)}{B(\mu_i/\tau, (1 - \mu_i)/\tau)}.$$

The log-likelihood can be maximized by the FS algorithm since the derivatives and the information matrix are available. $\mathcal{I}^{-1}$ at the final iteration gives an asymptotic covariance matrix for $(\boldsymbol{\beta},\tau)$. It is easy to check that, marginally,

$$E(y_i) = n_i\mu_i,$$
$$\text{var}(y_i) = n_i\mu_i(1 - \mu_i) + \frac{\tau}{2(1 + \tau)}n_i(n_i - 1)\mu_i(1 - \mu_i),$$

and $\text{cor}(y_{ij}, y_{ik}) = \text{const} = \tau/(1+\tau)$. The latter means that the beta-binomial model implies the intracluster equi correlation structure, and $0.5\tau/(1+\tau)n_i(n_i-1)\mu_i(1-\mu_i)$ is the overdispersion. Although standard logistic regression or GEE (Moore and Tsiatis, 1991) would lead to consistent estimates, the described likelihood approach is asymptotically efficient.

7.3.7 Statistical test of homogeneity

The question of homogeneity of the intercepts is essential. For the linear mixed model we have developed an exact F-test for $H_0 : \mathbf{D} = \mathbf{0}$, see Section 3.5. For the meta-analysis model the homogeneity test, $\sigma^2 = 0$, is based on the Q-statistic, see Section (5.1.4). In Section 6.1.5, we applied the F-test to a nonlinear mixed model with normally distributed random effects. In this section we want to test the homogeneity of the intercepts: whether the intercepts are constant $H_0 : \sigma^2 = 0$. Two tests will be considered: the first is a straightforward generalization of the F-test (3.42), and the second is the score test developed in the framework of the generalized linear mixed model (Breslow and Lin, 1995; Lin, 1997). An important feature of these tests is that they do not require estimation of the random effects. At the end of this subsection we present a small simulation study.

F-test

It is well known that the deviance, twice the negative log-likelihood function, behaves asymptotically as the sum of squares (McCullagh and Nelder, 1989). Thus, we just mimic the test statistic (3.42), replacing S by $-2l$ to get

$$\frac{(l_0 - l_{\min})/(N - m)}{l_{\min}/(N_T - N)} \simeq F(N - m, N_T - N). \qquad (7.88)$$

Here l_0 is the maximum value of the log-likelihood function from the ordinary logistic regression and $l_{\min}$ is the maximum value of the log-likelihood function assuming fixed intercepts, see Section 7.2.2. The hypothesis $H_0 : \sigma^2 = 0$ is rejected if the left-hand side of (7.88) is greater than the critical value of the F-statistic with $N - m$ and $N_T - N$ degrees of freedom.

Score test

Generally, the score test statistic has the form $(\partial l/\partial \boldsymbol{\theta})'\mathbf{I}^{-1}(\partial l/\partial \boldsymbol{\theta})$, where $\mathbf{I}$ is the information matrix for the k-dimensional parameter $\boldsymbol{\theta}$. Then, under the null, this quantity can be approximated by a $\chi^2(k)$ distribution. We argue that when the alternative is one-sided, as in the homogeneity test, an adequate test statistic would be proportional to $\partial l/\partial \boldsymbol{\theta}$, not $(\partial l/\partial \boldsymbol{\theta})^2$. The score test for the LME model is developed in Verbeke and Molenberghs (2003). The score test for logistic regression with random intercepts is developed below.

One may expect that the random effect exists ($\sigma^2 > 0$) if the derivative of the log-likelihood function with respect to σ^2, evaluated at the ordinary MLE, is positive. Indeed, if $\partial l/\partial \sigma^2 > 0$, there exists $\sigma_0^2 > 0$ that the value of the log-likelihood function will be greater than at zero. We refer the reader to Section 2.6, where a numerical test on the positiveness of the variance of the random effect is developed. In fact, even if $\sigma^2 = 0$, this derivative may be positive but takes small values. Thus, we need to find a positive threshold for $\partial l/\partial \sigma^2$ at which the null hypothesis is rejected. To do this, we need to obtain the derivative $\partial l/\partial \sigma^2$ at the null ($\sigma^2 = 0$) and find its asymptotic distribution as $N \to \infty$.

To find the derivative at zero, it is more convenient to write the log-likelihood function as a function of σ, not σ^2, in a slightly different form, namely,

$$l(\boldsymbol{\beta}, \sigma) = \sum_{i=1}^{N} \ln \int_{-\infty}^{\infty} e^{l_i} \phi(u) du, \qquad (7.89)$$

where $u \sim \mathcal{N}(0, 1)$ and $\phi(\cdot)$ is the standard normal density. The ith log-likelihood function takes the familiar form

$$l_i = l_i(\boldsymbol{\beta}, u; \sigma) = \sigma u \sum_{j=1}^{n_i} y_{ij} + \sum_{j=1}^{n_i} y_{ij} \boldsymbol{\beta}' \mathbf{x}_{ij} - \sum_{j=1}^{n_i} \ln(1 + e^{\sigma u + \boldsymbol{\beta}' \mathbf{x}_{ij}}).$$

Notice that $l(\boldsymbol{\beta}; \sigma = 0)$ is the joint log-likelihood function of the ordinary logistic regression assuming that all $\{y_{ij}\}$ are independent. Further, noting that $\int_{-\infty}^{\infty} e^{l_i} \phi(u) du = E_{u \sim \mathcal{N}(0,1)}(e^{l_i})$, we simplify (7.89) as $l = \sum \ln E_u(e^{l_i})$. The first derivative is $\partial l / \partial \sigma = \sum E_u(e^{l_i} l_i') / E_u(e^{l_i})$, where

$$l_i' = \frac{\partial l_i}{\partial \sigma} = u \sum \left(y_{ij} - \frac{e^{\sigma u + \boldsymbol{\beta}' \mathbf{x}_{ij}}}{1 + e^{\sigma u + \boldsymbol{\beta}' \mathbf{x}_{ij}}} \right).$$

The expected value of the first derivative is zero, symbolically $E(l_i(u; \sigma = 0)) = 0$, because $E(u) = 0$. Take the second derivative,

$$\frac{\partial^2 l}{\partial \sigma^2} = \sum \left[\frac{E_u[e^{l_i}(l_i'^2 + l_i'')]}{E_u e^{l_i}} - \frac{E_u^2(e^{l_i} l_i')}{E_u^2 e^{l_i}} \right], \qquad (7.90)$$

where $l_i'' = -u^2 \sum p_{ij}(1 - p_{ij})$ and $p_{ij} = e^{\boldsymbol{\beta}' \mathbf{x}_{ij}} / (1 + e^{\boldsymbol{\beta}' \mathbf{x}_{ij}})$. Since $E_u(l_i') = 0$, the second term in (7.90) vanishes and we obtain

$$\frac{\partial^2 l}{\partial \sigma^2} \bigg|_{\sigma=0} = \sum_{i=1}^{N} E_u(l_i'^2 + l_i'') = \sum_{i=1}^{N} \left(\sum_{j=1}^{n} (y_{ij} - p_{ij}) \right)^2 - \sum_{i=1}^{N} \sum_{j=1}^{n_i} p_{ij}(1 - p_{ij}).$$

Now, observing that $\partial l / \partial(\sigma^2) = 2 \partial^2 l / \partial \sigma^2$, we infer that the sign of $\partial^2 l / \partial \sigma^2$ is determined by the statistic

$$S = \sum_{i=1}^{N} \left[\left(\sum_{j=1}^{n} (y_{ij} - \widehat{p}_{ij}) \right)^2 - \sum_{j=1}^{n_i} \widehat{p}_{ij}(1 - \widehat{p}_{ij}) \right], \qquad (7.91)$$

where $\widehat{p}_{ij} = e^{\widehat{\boldsymbol{\beta}}' \mathbf{x}_{ij}} / (1 + e^{\widehat{\boldsymbol{\beta}}' \mathbf{x}_{ij}})$ is the predicted probability from the ordinary logistic regression. Statistic S has a nice interpretation. The first term measures the variance from the data, and the second term measures the variance from the model. If there is an overdispersion, S should be positive. To find the positive threshold above which the homogeneity is rejected, we need to find the asymptotic distribution of S under the null. Under mild assumptions, $p \lim_{N \to \infty} S/N = 0$; if there is no overdispersion, the variance from data and model should be the same. To yield the variance of S, the following fact is used; the proof is similar to that given by Graybill (1969, p. 362).

Lemma 36 *Let $z_1, z_2, ..., z_n$ be independent random variables with zero mean and $E(z_i^2) = v_i$, $E(z_i^4) = h_i$. Then*

$$\text{var} \left(\sum_{i=1}^{n} z_i \right)^2 = \sum_{i=1}^{n} h_i + 2 \left(\sum_{i=1}^{n} v_i \right)^2 - 3 \sum_{i=1}^{n} v_i^2.$$

Denoting $z_{ij} = y_{ij} - p_{ij}$, we find that $v_i = p_{ij}(1 - p_{ij})$ and $h_i = p_{ij} - 4p_{ij}^2 + 6p_{ij}^3 - 3p_{ij}^4$, and finally,

$$\text{var}(S) \simeq \sum_{i=1}^{N} \left[2 \left(\sum_{j=1}^{n} \widehat{p}_{ij}(1 - \widehat{p}_{ij}) \right)^2 + \sum_{j=1}^{n} (\widehat{p}_{ij} - 6\widehat{p}_{ij}^2 + 12\widehat{p}_{ij}^3 - 6\widehat{p}_{ij}^4) \right].$$

Thus, by the score test we reject $H_0 : \sigma^2 = 0$ if $D > \sqrt{v} Z_{1-\alpha}$, where $Z_{1-\alpha}$ is the $(1 - \alpha)$th quantile of the normal distribution and α is the size, say 5%.

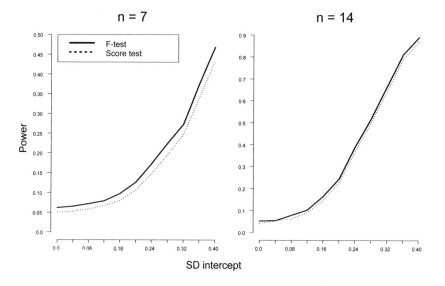

FIGURE 7.7. Empirical power of F and score tests for intercept homogeneity in logistic regression. The true values are $\beta_0 = -1$ and $\beta_1 = 0.1$, the nominal size 5%, and $N = 100$.

Test comparison by statistical simulation

We present a small simulation study to compare the F and score tests. The true value for the intercept $\beta_0 = -1$ and the slope $\beta_1 = 0.1$ with $x_{ij} = j$ for $j = 1, 2, ..., n$, where $n = 7$ or $n = 14$ and $i = 1, 2, ..., N = 100$. The power function is estimated as the proportion of runs at which the hypothesis $\sigma = 0$ is rejected for $\sigma = 0, ..., 0.4$. At $\sigma = 0$ the probability should be close to the nominal size, $\alpha = 0.05$, see Figure 7.7. The two tests are close in terms of the empirical versus nominal significance level and power.

7.3.8 Asymptotic properties

In cluster or tabular data, there are three interpretations of "large sample": (a) N is fixed and $\min n_i \to \infty$, (b) $N \to \infty$ and $\{n_i\}$ are bounded/finite, and (c) $N \to \infty$ and $\min n_i \to \infty$. See further discussion of asymptotics in Chapter 8. In the first case, the fixed intercepts model is adequate (say, when the number of observations per cluster is greater than the number of clusters). In case (a), the asymptotic theory does take place and one deals with finite sample properties. We refer the reader to Section 3.6.2 for a general discussion.

In case (b) or (c) the MLE is asymptotically unbiased and consistent, asymptotically normal, and efficient. It is especially easy to prove these properties using the stochastic approach of Section 3.6.2. Then we assume that n_i is a random number picked from a discrete distribution defined by $\Pr(n = k) = p_k$. Apparently, the bounded case, (b), is when $p_k = 0$ after $k \geq K$. Conditional logistic regression also leads to the same asymptotic properties under (b), but with a slight efficiency loss. However, when the $\{n_i\}$ are large, this method becomes computationally prohibitive. Our practice shows that when $\{n_i\}$ are relatively small ($n \leq 15$), conditional likelihood gives estimates very close to the MLE.

There is a price for approximations—all those estimation methods require both N and $\min n_i$ to be large, to provide an asymptotically unbiased estimation. More details on the asymptotic properties of the Laplace and PQL approximation methods are given in Chapter 8. Some efficiency comparisons for the logistic regression model with random intercepts are discussed by Neuhaus and Lesperance (1996).

Problems for Section 7.3

1. Prove that all four integrals $I_1, ..., I_4$ from Section 7.3.1 exist.

2. Why is (7.68) true?

3. Assess how precise the upper error bound from Lemma 35 is by comparing the approximate integral with the 'exact' value using the `integrate` function in R.

4*. Estimate the number of experiments in Monte Carlo logistic-normal integral approximation using the rule described on page 367: First, use a small number of experiments to estimate SD and then use a large/estimated number of experiments. Test your algorithm via simulations with the exact integral computed using the `integrate` function. Generalize your experience to other integral approximations.

5. Investigate how the number of nodes in the Gauss-Hermite quadrature affects the performance of the `logMLEgh` algorithm (use function the `logsim`). Use `silent=0` to see the iterations printout.

6. Derive the FSL algorithm for logistic and probit regressions (find the derivatives of μ). Write an R function and test it.

7. Using simulations, investigate how the number of simulated values and the number of nodes in `gauher` affect the performance of `logFS` and `logFSL` (modify the function `logsim`).

8*. Write R programs that implement Quadratic and Laplace algorithms. Compare their performance via simulations with `glmmPQL` (modify the function `logsim`).

9*. Write an R program that implements the beta-binomial model estimation. Test your program via simulations (generate the overdispersed data and run your program).

10. Reproduce Figure 7.7.

11*. Use simulations to illustrate the three cases of asymptotics. Is there a method that outperforms others for each case?

7.4 Probit model with random intercept

The binary model is defined as $\Pr(y_{ij} = 1|u_i) = \Phi\left(u_i + \boldsymbol{\beta}'\mathbf{x}_{ij}\right)$, where $\{u_i, i = 1, ..., N\}$ are independent and normally distributed random variables with zero mean and unknown variance σ^2, and Φ is the cdf $\mathcal{N}(0,1)$. It is assumed that the first component of vector $\mathbf{x}_{ij}$ is 1, so that the first component of vector $\boldsymbol{\beta}$ is the population-averaged intercept. The subject-specific (conditional on u_i) log-likelihood is given by

$$l_i(\boldsymbol{\beta}, u_i) = \sum_{j=1}^{n_i} \left\{ y_{ij} \ln \Phi\left(u_i + \boldsymbol{\beta}'\mathbf{x}_{ij}\right) + (1 - y_{ij}) \ln[1 - \Phi\left(u_i + \boldsymbol{\beta}'\mathbf{x}_{ij}\right)] \right\}. \quad (7.92)$$

If N is small and $\{n_i\}$ are relatively large, one can assume that $\{u_i\}$ are fixed and unknown (nuisance parameters). Then, by maximizing the joint log-likelihood function, $\sum_{i=1}^{N} l_i(\boldsymbol{\beta}, u_i)$, we estimate $\boldsymbol{\beta}$ and $\{u_i\}$ simultaneously. If N is large and $\{n_i\}$ are relatively small, the model with random intercept is more appropriate, $u_i \sim \mathcal{N}(0, 1)$. ML leads to maximization of the function with the intercept integrated out,

$$l(\boldsymbol{\beta}) = -\frac{N}{2} \ln 2\pi\sigma^2 + \sum_{i=1}^{N} \ln \int_{-\infty}^{\infty} e^{h_i(\boldsymbol{\beta};u)} du, \quad (7.93)$$

where $h_i(\boldsymbol{\beta};u) = l_i(\boldsymbol{\beta}, u_i) - u^2/(2\sigma^2)$, using notation similar to (7.64). The formulas and results of Section 7.3.1 are readily modified.

7.4.1 Laplace and PQL approximations

The Laplace and PQL approximations applied previously to logistic regression can be easily modified for the probit model. First, we need to find the maximum of the penalized subject-specific log-likelihood function, $l_i(\boldsymbol{\beta}, u) - u^2/(2\sigma^2)$. Assuming that $\boldsymbol{\beta}$ and σ^2 are being held constant (the subscript i is omitted to shorten the notation), we find u_i by the FS algorithm:

$$u_{s+1} = u_s + \frac{\sum_{j=1}^{n}(y_j - \Phi_j)\phi_j w_j - u_s/\sigma^2}{\sum_{j=1}^{n} \phi_j^2 w_j + 1/\sigma^2}, \quad s = 0, 1, ...,$$

where $\Phi_j = \Phi(u_s + \boldsymbol{\beta}'\mathbf{x}_{ij})$, ϕ is the density of the normal cdf, and $w_j = 1/(\Phi_j(1-\Phi_j))$ is the weight, starting from zero ($u_0 = 0$). Second, if u_{*i} is the limit point from previous iterations, the Laplace approximation to (7.93) gives

$$l_{LA}(\boldsymbol{\beta}, \sigma^2) = -\frac{N \ln \sigma^2}{2} - \frac{1}{2\sigma^2} \sum_{i=1}^{N} u_{*i}^2$$

$$+ \sum_{i=1}^{N} \left\{ l_i(\boldsymbol{\beta}, u_{*i}) - 0.5 \ln[\sigma^{-2} + \sum_{j=1}^{n_i} H_i(\boldsymbol{\beta}, u_{*i})] \right\},$$

where H_i is the negative second derivative of l_i, namely,

$$H_i(\boldsymbol{\beta}, u_{*i}) = \sum_{j=1}^{n_i} \phi_{ij}^2 w_{ij} + \sum_{j=1}^{n_i} (y_{ij} - \Phi_{ij})[s_{ij}\Phi_{ij}(1 - \Phi_{ij}) + \phi_{ij}(1 - 2\Phi_{ij})]w_{ij}^2,$$

$s_{ij} = u_{*i} + \boldsymbol{\beta}'\mathbf{x}_{ij}$ and $\Phi_{ij} = \Phi(s_{ij}), \phi_{ij} = \phi(s_{ij})$. We come to the PQL log-likelihood (7.84), ignoring the second term in the brakcts as we did for logistic regression. The updated variance is computed via the recursive relation

$$\widehat{\sigma}_{s+1}^2 = \frac{1}{N} \sum_{i=1}^{N} \left(u_{*i}^2 + \frac{1}{\widehat{\sigma}_s^{-2} + H_i(\widehat{\boldsymbol{\beta}}, u_{*i})} \right). \tag{7.94}$$

Another variant of this formula can be obtained by replacing H_i with its expected value, $\sum_{j=1}^{n_i} \phi_{ij}^2 w_{ij}$.

7.4.2   VARLINK estimation

The advantage of this method is that due to (7.15), if σ^2 were known, we could estimate $\boldsymbol{\beta}$ from ordinary probit regression. It suffices to run the probit regression only once because for any $\widehat{\sigma}^2$, the joint probit model gives $\widehat{\boldsymbol{\beta}} = \widehat{\boldsymbol{\beta}}_0 \sqrt{1 + \widehat{\sigma}^2}$, where $\widehat{\boldsymbol{\beta}}_0$ is the MLE from the ordinary probit model, $\Pr(y_{ij} = 1) = \Phi(\boldsymbol{\beta}'\mathbf{x}_{ij})$. Thus, as in Section 7.3.5, we alternate between (a) estimating u_i by the FS algorithm, $u_{s+1} = u_s + [\sum(y_j - \Phi_j)\phi_j w_j][\sum \phi_j^2 w_j]^{-1}$, with $\boldsymbol{\beta}$ held, and (b) updating the variance, $\sigma_{s+1}^2 = N^{-1} \sum_{i=1}^{N}(u_{*i}^2 - v_i)$, where v_i is the variance estimate of u_{*i} from the individual probit model, $v_i = (\sum_{j=1}^{n} \phi_j^2 w_j)^{-1}$. When computing an estimate for σ^2, only successful iterations from (a) are used.

7.4.3   Heckman method for the probit model

As mentioned above, we can consistently estimate the probit model coefficients as $\widehat{\boldsymbol{\beta}}_0 \sqrt{1 + \sigma^2}$, if σ^2 is known. Heckman (1981) suggested plugging this estimate back into the log-likelihood function and maximizing it over σ^2. The resulting estimate for σ^2 can be called pseudo-MLE because it is derived from the log-likelihood after substituting the true beta parameter by its consistent estimate, see Appendix 13.1.3. To facilitate the maximization, we write the log-likelihood as

$$l(\sigma^2) = \sum_{i=1}^{N} \ln E_{u \sim \mathcal{N}(0,1)} \left[\exp \left(\sum_{j=1}^{n_i} [y_{ij} \ln \Phi_{ij} + (1 - y_{ij}) \ln(1 - \Phi_{ij})] \right) \right], \tag{7.95}$$

where $\Phi_{ij} = \Phi(\sigma u + z_{ij}\sqrt{1 + \sigma^2})$ and $z_{ij} = \widehat{\boldsymbol{\beta}}_0'\mathbf{x}_{ij}$ is fixed. The maximum of this function may be found by standard optimization techniques such as quadratic interpolation or golden search (Press et al., 1992). Although this method still requires quadrature problem solving, it may be less time consuming because it requires only one integral for each i.

7.4.4 Generalized estimating equations approach

The presence of the random intercept makes observations stochastically dependent within cluster. In the method described above, parameter $\boldsymbol{\beta}$ was estimated assuming that the $\{y_{ij}\}$, with the marginal probability $\Phi(\boldsymbol{\beta}'\mathbf{x}_{ij}/\sqrt{1+\sigma^2})$, are independent. Although this assumption leaves the estimation equation unbiased, one may expect better efficiency when the intracluster correlation is addressed. To account for this correlation, we need to assess the covariance matrix of $\{y_{i1}, ..., y_{in_i}\}$. A method to estimate parameters of the generalized linear model with cluster-dependent data by the generalized estimating equations (GEE) approach was suggested by Liang and Zeger (1986) and Zeger and Liang (1986). This method is discussed in depth in Section 7.9. Here we apply this method to a specific problem for the estimation of probit regression with a random intercept. An advantage of applying GEE to the probit model with normally distributed random intercepts is that the marginal mean admits a closed-form solution.

To compute the variance and covariance of the contaminated probit model, we use the following formulas, frequently mentioned in the framework of random effects models.

Let Y be a random variable (RV) as a function of another random variable u (Y may depend on other RVs, too). For example, Y might be an estimator that depends on the parameter θ, and u is an estimator for θ. Apparently, an estimator for θ would be $Y(u)$. We are concerned with the marginal variance of Y expressed in terms of u. The following general formula provides that variance,

$$\text{var}(Y) = \text{var}\left[E(Y|u)\right] + E\text{var}(Y|u). \tag{7.96}$$

We make several remarks. First, $E(Y|u)$ is a conditional expectation (a function of u), so var in the first term is the variance of this function over the distribution of u. In the second term, the conditional variance $\text{var}(Y|u)$ is the variance of Y when u is fixed. Thus, $\text{var}(Y|u)$ is also a function of u and the second term is the expectation of this function. Second, formula (7.96) may be viewed as the variance-decomposition formula. Indeed, in linear regression $Y = a + bX + \varepsilon$, where x and ε are independent random variables. Applying this formula, one obtains the familiar variance decomposition $\text{var}(Y) = \sigma^2 + \text{var}(\widehat{Y})$, where $\sigma^2 = \text{var}(\varepsilon)$ and $\widehat{Y} = a + bX$. In the following example, we apply formula (7.96) to a less trivial situation.

Example 1. Calculate the variance of the binary RV Y as a function of $u \sim \mathcal{N}(0, \sigma^2)$ defined by the conditional probability, $\Pr(Y = 1|u) = \Phi(s + u)$, where s is a fixed number.

Since for binary RV, probability = mean, we have $E(Y|u) = \Phi(s + u)$. From (7.15) we know that $E(Y) = E(E(Y|u)) = \Phi(s/\sqrt{1+\sigma^2})$, so

$$\text{var}\left[E(Y|u)\right] = E\left[E^2(Y|u)\right] - E^2[E(Y|u)] = E_u\Phi^2(s+u) - \Phi^2(s/\sqrt{1+\sigma^2}).$$

For binary RV, $\text{var}(Y|u) = \Phi(s+u)[1 - \Phi(s+u)]$, and finally,

$$
\begin{aligned}
&\text{var}(Y)\\
&= E_u\Phi^2(s+u) - \Phi^2(s/\sqrt{1+\sigma^2}) + \Phi(s/\sqrt{1+\sigma^2}) - E_u E_u\Phi^2(s+u)\\
&= \Phi(s/\sqrt{1+\sigma^2})[1 - \Phi(s/\sqrt{1+\sigma^2})].
\end{aligned}
$$

This formula is not surprising because for the marginal probability, $\Pr(Y = 1) = \Phi(s/\sqrt{1+\sigma^2})$.

∎

There is a vector generalization of formula (7.96). Let $\mathbf{Y}$ be a vector RV dependent on scalar RV u. Then

$$\text{cov}(\mathbf{Y}) = \text{cov}\left[E(\mathbf{Y}|u)\right] + E\text{cov}(\mathbf{Y}|u). \tag{7.97}$$

Example 2. Calculate the covariance between two binary RVs, Y_1 and Y_2, as functions of $u \sim \mathcal{N}(0, \sigma^2)$, defined by conditional probabilities, $\Pr(Y_j = 1|u) = \Phi(s_j + u)$, assuming that Y_1 and Y_2 are conditionally independent ($j = 1, 2$). For the first term of (7.97), we have

$$\text{cov}[\Phi(s_1 + u), \Phi(s_2 + u)] = E[\Phi(s_1 + u)\Phi(s_2 + u)]$$
$$-\Phi(s_1/\sqrt{1+\sigma^2})\Phi(s_2/\sqrt{1+\sigma^2}). \tag{7.98}$$

For the second term of (7.97), since Y_1 and Y_2 are conditionally independent, $E\text{cov}(\mathbf{Y}|u) = \mathbf{0}$, so the covariance between Y_1 and Y_2 is given by (7.98). Unfortunately, we do not know whether the first term can be written in closed form.

∎

Now using these examples, we approximate the $n_i \times n_i$ marginal covariance matrix, $\mathbf{V}_i$ of $\mathbf{y}_i = (y_{i1}, ..., y_{in_i})'$, as

$$(\mathbf{V}_i)_{jk} = \left\{ \begin{array}{l} \Phi(s_{ik}/\sqrt{1+\sigma^2})[1 - \Phi(s_{ik}/\sqrt{1+\sigma^2})] \text{ if } j = k \\ A_{ijk} - \Phi(s_{ij}/\sqrt{1+\sigma^2})\Phi(s_{ik}/\sqrt{1+\sigma^2}) \text{ if } j \neq k \end{array} \right.$$

where $s_{ik} = \boldsymbol{\beta}'\mathbf{x}_{ik}$ and $A_{ijk} = E[\Phi(s_{ik} + u)\Phi(s_{ij} + u)]$ or its approximate value ($j, k = 1, ..., n_i$). Two approximations can be suggested. First, letting $\Phi(s_{ij} + u) \simeq \Phi(s_{ij})$, we obtain, up to the first order, $A_{ijk} \simeq 0.5[\Phi(s_{ik}/\sqrt{1+\sigma^2}) \times \Phi(s_{ij}) + \Phi(s_{ik})\Phi(s_{ij}/\sqrt{1+\sigma^2})]$. Second, assuming without generality that $s_{ij} \leq s_{ik}$, we approximate $A_{ijk} \simeq \Phi(s_{ij}/\sqrt{1+\sigma^2}) - \Phi(s_{ij}) + \Phi(s_{ij})\Phi(s_{ik})$. Then the estimating equation for $\boldsymbol{\beta}$ is

$$\sum_{i=1}^{N} \mathbf{X}_i'\boldsymbol{\phi}_i\mathbf{V}_i^{-1}(\mathbf{y}_i - \boldsymbol{\Phi}_i) = \mathbf{0}, \tag{7.99}$$

where $\boldsymbol{\Phi}_i$ is an $n_i \times 1$ vector $(\Phi(s_{i1}/\sqrt{1+\sigma^2}), ..., \Phi(s_{in_i}/\sqrt{1+\sigma^2}))'$ and $\boldsymbol{\phi}_i$ is an $n_i \times n_i$ diagonal matrix with $\phi(\boldsymbol{\beta}'\mathbf{x}_{ij})$ on the diagonal. System (7.99) can be solved by the FS/IRLS algorithm as

$$\boldsymbol{\beta}_{s+1} = \boldsymbol{\beta}_s + \left(\sum_{i=1}^{N} \mathbf{X}_i'\boldsymbol{\phi}_i\mathbf{V}_i^{-1}\boldsymbol{\phi}_i\mathbf{X}_i\right)^{-1} \sum_{i=1}^{N} \mathbf{X}_i'\boldsymbol{\phi}_i\mathbf{V}_i^{-1}(\mathbf{y}_i - \boldsymbol{\Phi}_i). \tag{7.100}$$

An attractive feature of (7.99) is that it is robust to matrix $\mathbf{V}_i$ approximation because it does not change the unbiasedness of the estimating equation. The parameter σ^2 may be estimated from the variance least squares. More detail on the GEE approach are given in Section 7.9.

7.4.5   Implementation in R

As mentioned above, `glmmPQL` estimates the probit regression with random intercept using the option `family=binomilal(link=probit)`. The reader can easilily modify the codes for logistic regression to estimate the probit regression with random intercepts including `log FS` and `logFSL`. However, a conditional regression approach cannot be implemented for probit regression.

Problems for Section 7.4

1*. Develop the MLE algorithm for log-likelihood function (7.93), similar to that presented in Section 7.3.1. Write an R function and test it via simulations. Compare the performance with the `glmmPQL` algorithm.

2*. Write R functions that implement VARLINK and Heckman methods and test them with simulations. Compare the performance with the `glmmPQL` algorithm.

3. The compound symmetry correlation structure for mixed model with random intercepts is typically suggested as the working correlation structure in the GEE approach (see Section 7.9 for a discussion). Is it true that the correlation between binary observations within the same cluster is constant, assuming the probit model with a random intercept?

4*. Write an R function that implements the GEE for the probit model with random intercepts using iterations (7.100) and test it via simulations. Compare the performance with the `glmmPQL` algorithm.

5*. Apply the FSL algorithm described in Section 7.3.2 to the probit model. Write an R program and test it via simulations. Compare its performance with `glmmPQL`.

7.5   Poisson model with random intercept

In this section we discuss a clustered Poisson regression model following the line of discussion for logistic regression. We review the standard Poisson regression model briefly and then turn our attention to panel/clustered count data. A characteristic property of the Poisson distribution is that mean equals variance. In many applications, though, the count data do not exactly follow the Poisson distribution. For example, there might be omitted variables, counts might be measured with error, etc. There is no problem for linear regression if the error has zero mean and constant variance, but it does present a problem for logistic and Poisson regression, or any generalized linear model with a nonidentity link. Specifically, the convoluted count data implies *overdispersion* for Poisson regression when the variance is greater that the mean. This happens particularly for clustered data when intercepts are cluster-specific.

When the number of clusters is small and the number of observations per cluster is relatively large, the model with fixed intercepts may be reasonable, and we provide an efficient algorithm for the maximum likelihood estimation that eliminates nuisance intercepts. Otherwise, the model with random intercepts should be used. For this model, maximum likelihood leads to a one-dimensional integration. Several methods may be suggested to avoid integration, such as replacing the Poisson distribution with negative binomial, Laplace approximation, penalized quasi-likelihood, or VARLINK. These methods are straightforward generalizations of the logistic and probit regression models considered above.

Several methods for Poisson regression with random intercept are compared in asymptotic setting by Demidenko (2007a). Not surprisingly, MLE is the most efficient. Next to MLE stands the GEE approach with exact covariance matrix, called Exact GEE—we refer the reader to that paper for more detail.

7.5.1   Poisson regression for count data

In this section we model count/discrete data. Let random variable Y take nonnegative integer value k with probability $p_k \geq 0$, $k = 0, 1, 2, 3, ...$, so that $\sum_{k=1}^{\infty} p_k = 1$. Y may be the number of visits to a doctor, photon counts in optical imaging, telephone calls within a specific time interval, etc. A flexible way to specify probabilities p_k is via the Poisson distribution, where probabilities are defined as

$$\Pr(Y = k) = \frac{1}{k!} e^{-\lambda} \lambda^k, \quad k = 0, 1, ..., \tag{7.101}$$

parameterized by a positive λ. The Poisson distribution arises in many, mostly engineering applications, and the interested reader is referred to classical books such as Feller (1966) or Ross (1993). See also a book by Cameron and Trivedi (1998), which covers the Poisson regression in depth. A peculiar property of the Poisson distribution is that the expectation and the variance are the same and are equal to λ. Actually, one may view this property as a restriction because real count data often exhibit overdispersion. In most cases, one can expect that the variance is greater than the mean. We shall see that this is always true for clustered data.

The Poisson distribution is closely related to the binomial distribution. Namely, the limit of the binomial probability, when the number of trials (n) goes to infinity and the probability (p) goes to zero keeping $np = \lambda =$const is given by (7.101); see Rice (1995, p. 41). One may say that the Poisson distribution has the same importance for count data as the normal (Gaussian) distribution has for continuous data.

Poisson regression emerges when the mean is expressed as a linear combination of explanatory variables. Since parameter λ is positive it is convenient to express this parameter via an exponential function, $E(y_i) = \lambda_i = e^{\boldsymbol{\beta}' \mathbf{x}_i}$, where $\boldsymbol{\beta}$ is an $m \times 1$ vector of regression parameters and $\mathbf{x}_i$ is an $m \times 1$ vector of explanatory variables/covariates, $i = 1, 2, ..., n$. In the framework of generalized linear models, we say that Poisson regression has a log link because $\ln E(y_i) = \boldsymbol{\beta}' \mathbf{x}_i$. Usually, we assume that the first component of $\mathbf{x}_i$ is 1, so that β_1 is the intercept. For example, if y_i denotes the number of doctor visits per year, x_{i2} may be gender, x_{i3} age, and so on. Then e^{β_1} is the average number of annual doctor visits adjusted for gender and age.

To avoid degeneration, it is assumed that (7.1) holds. The log-likelihood function for the Poisson regression model, up to a constant term, takes the form

$$l(\boldsymbol{\beta}) = \sum_{i=1}^{n} \left(y_i \boldsymbol{\beta}' \mathbf{x}_i - e^{\boldsymbol{\beta}' \mathbf{x}_i} \right) = \boldsymbol{\beta}' \mathbf{r} - \sum_{i=1}^{n} e^{\boldsymbol{\beta}' \mathbf{x}_i}, \tag{7.102}$$

where vector $\mathbf{r} = \sum_{i=1}^{n} y_i \mathbf{x}_i$ is fixed. It is easy to prove that function (7.102) is concave since the negative matrix of the second derivatives (the Hessian), $\sum_{i=1}^{n} \mathbf{x}_i \mathbf{x}_i' e^{\boldsymbol{\beta}' \mathbf{x}_i}$, is positive definite. This implies that l has a unique maximum on R^m if the supremum is attained, similar to the logistic regression of Section 7.1.4. The MLE is the solution to the score vector equation, $\mathbf{r} - \sum_{i=1}^{n} \mathbf{x}_i e^{\boldsymbol{\beta}'\mathbf{x}_i} = \mathbf{0}$, or in an equivalent and compact form,

$$\mathbf{X}'(\mathbf{y} - \mathbf{e}) = \mathbf{0}, \tag{7.103}$$

where $\mathbf{y} = (y_1, ..., y_n)'$, $\mathbf{e} = \exp(\mathbf{X}\boldsymbol{\beta})$, and $\mathbf{X}$ is an $n \times m$ matrix with the ith row $\mathbf{x}_i'$. The FS algorithm for (7.102) takes the form

$$\boldsymbol{\beta}_{s+1} = \boldsymbol{\beta}_s + \left(\sum_{i=1}^{n} \mathbf{x}_i \mathbf{x}_i' e^{\boldsymbol{\beta}_s'\mathbf{x}_i} \right)^{-1} \left(\mathbf{r} - \sum_{i=1}^{n} \mathbf{x}_i e^{\boldsymbol{\beta}_s'\mathbf{x}_i} \right), \tag{7.104}$$

where s is the iteration index. A good starting point can be obtained by linear regression of $\ln y_i$ on $\{\mathbf{x}_i\}$, excluding zero observations.

7.5.2   Clustered count data

Now we turn our attention to clustered data with counts in a tabular/panel form, $\{y_{ij}, i = 1, ..., N, j = 1, ..., n_i\}$. Here i indicates the ith cluster/subject and j indicates the jth observation within subject i. For example, y_{ij} may count the annual number of doctor visits of person j in county i.

If we assume that the coefficients at $\mathbf{x}_{ij}$ do not change from cluster to cluster but intercepts do, we come to the subject (or cluster)-specific intercept Poisson regression model,

$$\Pr(y_{ij} = k | u_i) = \frac{1}{k!} \exp \left(k(u_i + \boldsymbol{\beta}'\mathbf{x}_{ij}) - e^{u_i + \boldsymbol{\beta}'\mathbf{x}_{ij}} \right). \tag{7.105}$$

Similarly to logistic regression, we make one of two assumptions on the intercepts: they are fixed or random. If the first component of $\mathbf{x}_{ij}$ is 1, u_i is interpreted as the *deviation* of the subject-specific intercept from the population-averaged intercept. If the $\{u_i\}$ are random, we shall assume that they are iid, and therefore we need to specify their common distribution for completeness.

A peculiar feature of the Poisson regression with random intercepts is that the ordinary Poisson regression (applied to the entire data set, ignoring clustering) yields consistent and asymptotically normally distributed estimates of *slope* coefficients. Indeed, if the first component of vector $\mathbf{x}_{ij}$ is 1, we write $\boldsymbol{\beta}'\mathbf{x}_{ij} = \beta_1 + \boldsymbol{\beta}_2'\mathbf{h}_{ij}$, where $\mathbf{h}_{ij}$ is the vector of covariates. Then, if the $\{u_i\}$ have common distribution F, we find that the marginal mean differs from the conditional mean by a factor

$$E(y_{ij}) = E_{u \sim F}[E(y_{ij}|u)] = (E_{u \sim F} e^u) e^{\boldsymbol{\beta}'\mathbf{x}_{ij}} = C e^{\boldsymbol{\beta}'\mathbf{x}_{ij}} = e^{\beta_{*1} + \boldsymbol{\beta}_2'\mathbf{h}_{ij}}, \tag{7.106}$$

where $\beta_{*1} = \ln C + \beta_1$ and $C = E_{u \sim F} e^u$. This means that clustering has little effect on the slope coefficients for Poisson regression, unlike the logistic and probit regressions. The Poisson clustered model somewhat resembles the linear mixed model, where ordinary least squares also produces consistent but less efficient estimates. Similarly, the ordinary Poisson regression does not yield efficient estimators of slopes unless the data are balanced. Again, we draw a parallel to the linear model where OLS is efficient for balanced data, Section 2.3. The aim of this section is to

discuss more efficient methods, including maximum likelihood and its approximations, which account for the intracluster correlation. Although the ordinary Poisson
regression for clustered data leaves the slopes consistent, their variances will be attenuated due to overdispersion. Providing the corrected variances for the slopes is
perhaps the major purpose of the clustered Poisson regression.

A unique property of the Poisson regression with random intercepts is that the
covariance matrix of $\mathbf{y}_i$ can be derived in closed form. We shall employ this property
to estimate the slopes by the GEE approach.

7.5.3   Fixed intercepts

When the number of clusters (N) is small and the number of observations per
cluster (n_i) is relatively large, say $\min n_i > N$, one may assume that the intercept
$a_i = \beta_1 + u_i$ is fixed and unknown $(i = 1, ..., N)$, as for logistic regression in Section
7.2.2. The advantage of this assumption for the Poisson regression model is that
intercepts can then be eliminated easily.

The Poisson model with fixed intercepts is written as

$$\Pr(y_{ij} = k) = \frac{1}{k!} \exp\left(k(a_i + \boldsymbol{\beta}'\mathbf{x}_{ij}) - e^{a_i + \boldsymbol{\beta}'\mathbf{x}_{ij}}\right), \quad k = 0, 1, 2, ..., \quad (7.107)$$

where it is assumed that $\mathbf{x}_{ij}$ does not have the unit component because a_i represents
the intercept. Observations $\{y_{ij}\}$ are independent within and between clusters. The
log-likelihood takes the form

$$l(a_1, ..., a_N, \boldsymbol{\beta}) = \boldsymbol{\beta}'\mathbf{r} + \sum_{i=1}^{N} a_i k_i - \sum_{i=1}^{N} e^{a_i} \sum_{j=1}^{n_i} e^{\boldsymbol{\beta}'\mathbf{x}_{ij}},$$

where $k_i = \sum_{j=1}^{n_i} y_{ij}$ and $\mathbf{r} = \sum_{i=1}^{N} \sum_{j=1}^{n_i} y_{ij}\mathbf{x}_{ij}$. The estimating equation for the
ith intercept is $\partial l / \partial a_i = k_i - e^{a_i} \sum_{j=1}^{n_i} e^{\boldsymbol{\beta}'\mathbf{x}_{ij}} = 0$, which yields the closed-form
solution

$$a_i = \ln k_i - \ln \sum_{j=1}^{n_i} e^{\boldsymbol{\beta}'\mathbf{x}_{ij}}. \quad (7.108)$$

Letting $e_{ij} = e^{\boldsymbol{\beta}'\mathbf{x}_{ij}}$ for convenience of notation, the estimating equation for $\boldsymbol{\beta}$ with
eliminated intercepts becomes

$$\mathbf{r} - \sum_{i=1}^{N} \frac{\sum_{j=1}^{n_i} \mathbf{x}_{ij} e_{ij}}{\sum_{j=1}^{n_i} e_{ij}} k_i = \mathbf{0}. \quad (7.109)$$

The Newton–Raphson algorithm leads to the iterations

$$\boldsymbol{\beta}_{s+1} = \boldsymbol{\beta}_s + \left(\sum_{i=1}^{N} \left[\frac{\sum_{j=1}^{n_i} \mathbf{x}_{ij}\mathbf{x}_{ij}' e_{ij}}{\sum_{j=1}^{n_i} e_{ij}} - \frac{\sum_{j=1}^{n_i} \mathbf{x}_{ij} e_{ij} \sum_{j=1}^{n_i} \mathbf{x}_{ij}' e_{ij}}{(\sum_{j=1}^{n_i} e_{ij})^2}\right] k_i\right)^{-1}$$

$$\times \left(\mathbf{r} - \sum_{i=1}^{N} \frac{\sum_{j=1}^{n_i} \mathbf{x}_{ij} e_{ij}}{\sum_{j=1}^{n_i} e_{ij}} k_i\right). \quad (7.110)$$

Following the line of proof of Lemma 34, one can show that the inverse matrix is positive definite. Iterations (7.110) are an economical version of maximum likelihood because intercepts are eliminated. Although standard Poisson regression software might be applied to maximize l, the update formula (7.110) reduces the original $(m + N)$-dimensional optimization problem to an m-dimensional problem. The inverse matrix at the final iteration is the covariance matrix of $\widehat{\boldsymbol{\beta}}_{ML}$.

7.5.4 Conditional Poisson regression

In this section we assume, for simplicity, that the intercepts $\{a_i\}$ are fixed and vary across clusters, as in the previous section. Conditional Poisson regression is a straightforward generalization of the conditional logistic regression of Section 7.2.3. We shall show that similar to logistic regression, conditional Poisson likelihood eliminates intercepts. The cluster index i will be omitted for awhile to shorten the notation.

Our plan is to derive the conditional likelihood of independent $y_1, ..., y_n$ conditioning on $\sum_{j=1}^{n} y_j = k$, a sufficient statistic for a. Let $z_1, z_2, ..., z_n$ be a sequence of nonnegative integers such that $\sum_{j=1}^{n} z_j = k$ is fixed. Then, in a way similar to (7.60), we obtain

$$\Pr(y_1 = z_1, ..., y_n = z_n) = \prod_{j=1}^{n} \frac{1}{z_j!} e^{-e^{a+\boldsymbol{\beta}'\mathbf{x}_j}} e^{(a+\boldsymbol{\beta}'\mathbf{x}_j)z_j}$$

$$= e^{ak - \sum_{j=1}^{n} e^{a+\boldsymbol{\beta}'\mathbf{x}_j}} \prod_{j=1}^{n} \frac{1}{z_j!} e^{\boldsymbol{\beta}'\mathbf{x}_j z_j}.$$

The probability to get $\sum_{j=1}^{n} y_j = k$ is

$$\frac{e^{ak - \sum_{j=1}^{n} e^{a+\boldsymbol{\beta}'\mathbf{x}_j}} \prod_{j=1}^{n} \frac{1}{y_j!} e^{\boldsymbol{\beta}'\mathbf{x}_j y_j}}{\sum_{\mathbf{z} \in \mathbf{Z}_k^n} e^{ak - \sum_{j=1}^{n} e^{a+\boldsymbol{\beta}'\mathbf{x}_j}} \prod_{j=1}^{n} \frac{1}{z_j!} e^{\boldsymbol{\beta}'\mathbf{x}_j z_j}} = \frac{\prod_{j=1}^{n} \frac{1}{y_j!} e^{\boldsymbol{\beta}'\mathbf{x}_j y_j}}{\sum_{\mathbf{z} \in \mathbf{Z}_k^n} \prod_{j=1}^{n} \frac{1}{z_j!} e^{\boldsymbol{\beta}'\mathbf{x}_j z_j}},$$

where $\mathbf{z} = (z_1, ..., z_n)$ and $\mathbf{Z}_k^n$ denotes the set of all vectors of $\mathbf{z}$ with the sum of nonnegative integer elements $k = \sum y_j$. Restoring the cluster index i, we arrive at the joint conditional log-likelihood function, up to a constant term,

$$l_c(\boldsymbol{\beta}) = \boldsymbol{\beta}'r - \sum_{i=1}^{N} \ln \left(\sum_{\mathbf{z} \in \mathbf{Z}_k^{n_i}} e^{\boldsymbol{\beta}' \sum_{j=1}^{n_i} \mathbf{x}_{ij} z_j - \ln p(\mathbf{z})} \right), \qquad (7.111)$$

where $p(\mathbf{z}) = \sum_{j=1}^{n_i} \max(1, z_j)$. Index sets $\{\mathbf{Z}_k^{n_i}\}$ and vectors $\{\sum_{j=1}^{n_i} \mathbf{x}_{ij} z_j\}$ do not change during the maximization procedure and can be computed beforehand. As follows from Andersen's theory, the conditional ML estimator is consistent and normally distributed for large N and bounded n_i under mild conditions. The gradient and the Hessian matrix for (7.111) are easy to obtain, similar to Section 7.2.3.

From Lemma 34, it follows that l_c is a concave function (the negative Hessian matrix is nonnegative definite). The inverse negative Hessian is an estimator for the covariance matrix of the $\boldsymbol{\beta}$ estimates.

Clearly, conditional Poisson regression may be used with random intercepts as well. Remarkably, we are not required to specify the distribution.

7.5.5 Negative binomial regression

Typically, the marginal mean of the dependent variable in nonlinear mixed models involves an integral. However, in some special cases, like the probit model with normally distributed intercepts, one can obtain a marginal mean of y_{ij} without integration. Then, pretending that the $\{y_{ij}\}$ are independent, the maximum likelihood with the marginal mean still yields consistent estimates when N goes to infinity and the $\{n_i\}$ are bounded because the estimating equation is unbiased. The Poisson regression model with intercepts distributed as log-Gamma also yields the marginal distribution of the $\{y_{ij}\}$ in closed form. This leads to a negative-binomial (NB) regression. Below we apply the NB regression to clustered count data taking into account overdispersion but assuming that the observations within each cluster are independent.

The gamma distribution is defined by two positive parameters, α and θ, and has the density $f(u; \alpha, \theta) = u^{\alpha-1}e^{-u/\theta}/(\theta^\alpha \Gamma(\alpha))$ for $u > 0$. For a positive integer α, we have $\Gamma(\alpha) = (\alpha - 1)!$ The following fact is central to negative binomial regression: if Y takes discrete values with the conditional Poisson distribution $\Pr(Y = k|\lambda) = e^{-\lambda}\lambda^k/k!$, where $\lambda > 0$ has a gamma distribution, the marginal distribution of Y is negative binomial. Indeed, the marginal probability, $\Pr(Y = k)$, is obtained by integrating out λ :

$$
\begin{aligned}
\int_0^\infty \Pr(Y &= k|\lambda)f(\lambda; a, \theta)d\lambda = \int_0^\infty \frac{1}{k!}e^{-\lambda}\lambda^k \frac{1}{\theta^\alpha \Gamma(\alpha)}\lambda^{\alpha-1}e^{-\lambda/\theta}d\lambda \\
&= \frac{1}{\theta^\alpha \Gamma(\alpha)k!}\int_0^\infty e^{-\lambda(1+1/\theta)}\lambda^{k+\alpha-1}d\lambda = \frac{\Gamma(\alpha+k)}{\Gamma(\alpha)k!}\frac{\theta^k}{(1+\theta)^{k+\theta}} \\
&= \binom{k+\alpha-1}{k}\left(\frac{\theta}{1+\theta}\right)^k \left(\frac{1}{1+\theta}\right)^\alpha,
\end{aligned}
\tag{7.112}
$$

where the binomial coefficient is computed as

$$
\binom{k+\alpha-1}{k} = \frac{(k+\alpha-1)(k+\alpha-2)...\alpha}{k!} = \frac{(k+\alpha-1)!}{k!(\alpha-1)!}.
$$

The distribution at the right-hand side of (7.112) is called a negative binomial. Symbolically,

$$
\text{Poisson + gamma = negative binomial.}
$$

For the negative binomial distribution, $E(Y) = \alpha\theta$ and $\text{var}(Y) = \alpha\theta(1+\theta)$. For Poisson distribution the mean and variance are equal, but for the NB distribution the variance is greater than the mean by $\alpha\theta^2$. Also, the Poisson distribution is specified by one parameter, but the NB distribution is specified by two parameters. After some calculus one can show that the Poisson distribution is a special case of the NB distribution when $\alpha \to \infty$ and $\theta \to 0$ such that the product, $\alpha\theta = \lambda$, is kept constant. The parameter $a = 1/\alpha$ is associated with the "extra-Poisson" variation because $\text{var}(Y) = \lambda + a\lambda^2$. This interpretation justifies a (λ, a)-parameterization of the NB distribution as

$$\Pr(Y = k; \lambda, a) = \binom{k + 1/a - 1}{k} \left(\frac{a\lambda}{1 + a\lambda}\right)^k \left(\frac{1}{1 + a\lambda}\right)^{1/a}. \tag{7.113}$$

Then $E(Y) = \lambda$ and $\text{var}(Y) = \lambda + a\lambda^2$, and $a = 0$ leads to the Poisson distribution. This parameterization is convenient for specifying the NB regression and for testing overdispersion as $H_0 : a = 0$ (Lawless, 1987).

Now we apply the NB distribution to clustered data assuming that $\exp(u_i)$ in model (7.105) has a gamma distribution. Then we say that u_i has the log-gamma distribution. Starting from this section, we assume that the first component of $\mathbf{x}_{ij}$ is 1, so that the first component of $\boldsymbol{\beta}$ represents the population-averaged intercept. Since for Poisson regression $\lambda_{ij} = e^{\boldsymbol{\beta}'\mathbf{x}_{ij}}$, applying (7.113) and assuming that the $\{y_{ij}\}$ are all independent, we obtain the log-likelihood function, up to a constant term,

$$l(\boldsymbol{\beta}, a) = \boldsymbol{\beta}'\mathbf{r} + \sum_{i=1}^{N} \sum_{j=1}^{n_i} \left[\sum_{k=0}^{y_{ij}-1} \ln(1 + ak) - (y_{ij} + 1/a)\ln(1 + ae^{\boldsymbol{\beta}'\mathbf{x}_{ij}})\right]. \tag{7.114}$$

When $a = 0$, we set the second term in brackets to be $e^{\boldsymbol{\beta}'\mathbf{x}_{ij}}$ because, by L'Hospital's rule,

$$\lim_{a \to 0} (y_{ij} + 1/a)\ln(1 + aB) = \lim_{a \to 0} \frac{\ln(1 + aB)}{a} = B,$$

where $B = e^{\boldsymbol{\beta}'\mathbf{x}_{ij}}$. When $y_{ij} = 0$, we let the first term of l be zero. The first derivatives of l are

$$\frac{\partial l}{\partial \boldsymbol{\beta}} = \mathbf{r} - \sum_{i=1}^{N} \sum_{j=1}^{n_i} \frac{(ay_{ij} + 1)e^{\boldsymbol{\beta}'\mathbf{x}_{ij}}}{1 + ae^{\boldsymbol{\beta}'\mathbf{x}_{ij}}}\mathbf{x}_{ij} = \sum_{i=1}^{N} \sum_{j=1}^{n_i} \frac{y_{ij} - e^{\boldsymbol{\beta}'\mathbf{x}_{ij}}}{1 + ae^{\boldsymbol{\beta}'\mathbf{x}_{ij}}}\mathbf{x}_{ij},$$

$$\frac{\partial l}{\partial a} = \sum_{i=1}^{N} \sum_{j=1}^{n_i} \left[\sum_{k=0}^{y_{ij}-1} \frac{k}{1 + ak} + a^2\ln(1 + ae^{\boldsymbol{\beta}'\mathbf{x}_{ij}}) - \frac{(y_{ij} + 1/a)}{1 + ae^{\boldsymbol{\beta}'\mathbf{x}_{ij}}}e^{\boldsymbol{\beta}'\mathbf{x}_{ij}}\right].$$

The estimates turn the first derivatives to zero. Following Lawless (1987), the information matrix blocks are

$$\mathcal{I}_{\boldsymbol{\beta}} = \sum_{i,j} \frac{e^{\boldsymbol{\beta}'\mathbf{x}_{ij}}}{1 + ae^{\boldsymbol{\beta}'\mathbf{x}_{ij}}}\mathbf{x}_{ij}\mathbf{x}_{ij}',$$

$$\mathcal{I}_a = a^{-4}\sum_{i,j} \left[\sum_{k=0}^{\infty}(1/a + k)^{-2}\Pr(Y_{ij} \geq k) - \frac{ae^{\boldsymbol{\beta}'\mathbf{x}_{ij}}}{1/a + e^{\boldsymbol{\beta}'\mathbf{x}_{ij}}}\right].$$

Taking the derivative of $\partial l/\partial \boldsymbol{\beta}$ with respect to a we see that the cross-derivative is zero, $\mathcal{I}_{\boldsymbol{\beta}a} = \mathbf{0}$. Remember that the same situation happens in the framework of the linear mixed effects model and nonlinear mixed model with a fixed matrix of random effects, Section 6.1. There are two consequences of the fact that the expected cross-derivative is zero, numerical and statistical: (a) function l can be maximized separately over $\boldsymbol{\beta}$ and a, and (b) any consistent estimator of a in the score equation $\partial l/\partial \boldsymbol{\beta} = \mathbf{0}$ leads to an efficient (asymptotically equivalent to the ML) estimation. However, the reader should be aware that the latter statement is true when the $\{y_{ij}\}$ are independent and follow the NB distribution. For our original clustered Poisson data, one loses the efficiency because the intracluster correlation is not taken into account.

Several comments on numerical issues of l maximization: The separate application of the FS for $\boldsymbol{\beta}$ and a is straightforward. Computation of $\Pr(Y_{ij} \geq k)$ may be time expensive, so we seek an approximation by the normal distribution. Using the fact that $E(Y_{ij}) = e^{\boldsymbol{\beta}'\mathbf{x}_{ij}}$ and $\text{var}(Y_{ij}) = e^{\boldsymbol{\beta}'\mathbf{x}_{ij}} + ae^{2\boldsymbol{\beta}'\mathbf{x}_{ij}}$, one obtains $\Pr(Y_{ij} \geq k) \simeq \Phi[(e^{\boldsymbol{\beta}'\mathbf{x}_{ij}} - k)/\sqrt{e^{\boldsymbol{\beta}'\mathbf{x}_{ij}} + ae^{2\boldsymbol{\beta}'\mathbf{x}_{ij}}}]$.

As was mentioned above, any consistent estimate of a would yield an efficient estimate of $\boldsymbol{\beta}$ for the NB regression. Advantages to using a consistent estimator of a, rather than the MLE, are that it is easier to compute and it may be robust to distribution misspecification. Specifically, Breslow (1984) suggested using a method of moments estimator for a, similar to our variance least squares of Section 3.12. His rather heuristic reasoning is as follows. Let us consider a linear model with heteroscedastic errors, $y_j = \boldsymbol{\beta}'\mathbf{x}_j + \varepsilon_j$, where $\varepsilon_j \sim \mathcal{N}(0, r_j^2)$ and r_j^2 are known. Let $\widehat{\boldsymbol{\beta}}$ be the $m \times 1$ weighted least squares estimator, then the expected value of the weighted sum of squares $\sum_{j=1}^{n}(y_j - \widehat{\lambda}_j)^2/r_j^2$ is $n - m$, where $\widehat{\lambda}_j = \boldsymbol{\beta}'\mathbf{x}_j$. Pretending that the Poisson model is linear and that $r_i^2 = \widehat{\lambda}_j(1 + a\widehat{\lambda}_j)$ and $\widehat{\lambda}_j = e^{\boldsymbol{\beta}'\mathbf{x}_j}$ are known, he finds a from the equation $\sum_{j=1}^{n}(y_j - \widehat{\lambda}_j)^2/r_j^2 = n - m$. Adapting this method to the clustered Poisson regression, we solve the system

$$\sum_{i=1}^{N}\sum_{j=1}^{n_i} \frac{y_{ij} - e^{\boldsymbol{\beta}'\mathbf{x}_{ij}}}{1 + ae^{\boldsymbol{\beta}'\mathbf{x}_{ij}}}\mathbf{x}_{ij} = \mathbf{0}, \tag{7.115}$$

$$\sum_{i=1}^{N}\sum_{j=1}^{n_i} \frac{(y_{ij} - e^{\boldsymbol{\beta}'\mathbf{x}_{ij}})^2}{e^{\boldsymbol{\beta}'\mathbf{x}_{ij}}(1 + ae^{\boldsymbol{\beta}'\mathbf{x}_{ij}})} = \sum_{i=1}^{N} n_i - m \tag{7.116}$$

for $\boldsymbol{\beta}$ and a. A good start is from the standard Poisson regression on the $\{y_{ij}\}$. First, we solve the second equation for a using Newton's algorithm. If the left-hand side of the second equation at $a = 0$ is less than the right-hand side, we let $\widehat{a} = 0$ meaning that no overdispersion is detected. After a is determined, we solve the first equation by the FS algorithm. As we mentioned above, this procedure generates estimates for $\boldsymbol{\beta}$ and a that are consistent for a large number of clusters and a finite number of observations per cluster. Also, one may iterate between $\boldsymbol{\beta}$ and a computation.

Exact GEE: accounting for correlation

The previous estimating equation (7.115) leads to consistent estimates because the estimating equation is unbiased, but we may gain some efficiency if the intracluster correlation were taken into account as we did for the probit model in Section 7.4.4. Thus, in this subsection we generalize (7.115) by applying the generalized estimating equations approach to clustered count data. For this we need to have the covariance matrix of $\mathbf{y}_i = (y_{i1}, ..., y_{i,n_i})'$. Fortunately, the log-Gamma distribution makes computation of the covariance matrix easy. Using the previous notation, one can show that

$$\mathbf{V}_i = \mathbf{E}_i + a\mathbf{e}_i\mathbf{e}_i', \tag{7.117}$$

where $\mathbf{e}_i = e^{\mathbf{X}_i\boldsymbol{\beta}} = E(\mathbf{y}_i)$ is an $n_i \times 1$ vector and $\mathbf{E}_i = \mathrm{diag}(\mathbf{e}_i)$ is an $n_i \times n_i$ matrix. The estimating equation for $\boldsymbol{\beta}$ is

$$\sum_{i=1}^N \mathbf{X}_i'\mathbf{E}_i\mathbf{V}_i^{-1}(\mathbf{y}_i - \mathbf{e}_i) = \mathbf{0}. \tag{7.118}$$

We call this approach exact GEE because the exact covariance matrix is used. The term *exact* is used to distinguish this from the traditional GEE where an approximate covariance matrix, based on the working correlation matrix, is used (see Section 7.9 for details).

Following the line of the Breslow argumentation, similar to (7.116), we come to the estimating equation for a:

$$\sum \mathbf{r}_i'\mathbf{V}_i^{-1}\mathbf{r}_i = \sum n_i - m, \tag{7.119}$$

where $\mathbf{r}_i = \mathbf{y}_i - \mathbf{e}_i$ is an $n_i \times 1$ residual vector. Holding a, we solve the first equation iteratively,

$$\boldsymbol{\beta}_{s+1} = \boldsymbol{\beta}_s + \left(\sum \mathbf{X}_i'\mathbf{E}_i\mathbf{V}_i^{-1}\mathbf{E}_i\mathbf{X}_i\right)^{-1}\sum \mathbf{X}_i'\mathbf{E}_i\mathbf{V}_i^{-1}\mathbf{r}_i. \tag{7.120}$$

When $\boldsymbol{\beta}$ is held fixed constant, equation (7.119) may be solved by Newton's algorithm with the derivative computed as $d(\mathbf{r}_i'\mathbf{V}_i^{-1}\mathbf{r}_i)/da = -(\mathbf{r}_i'\mathbf{V}_i^{-1}\mathbf{e}_i)^2$.

Another option is to estimate parameter a by variance least squares (VLS), Sections 3.12 and 6.1.4. When $\boldsymbol{\beta}$ is held, we find a, which minimizes $\sum_{i=1}^N \mathrm{tr}(\mathbf{r}_i\mathbf{r}_i' - \mathbf{E} - a\mathbf{e}_i\mathbf{e}_i')^2$, with the solution

$$\widehat{a}_{VLS} = \frac{\sum_{i=1}^N (\mathbf{r}_i'\mathbf{e}_i)^2 - \sum_{i=1}^N \sum_{j=1}^{n_i} e_{ij}^3}{\sum_{i=1}^N \|\mathbf{e}_i\|^4}. \tag{7.121}$$

One can alternate between solutions to (7.118) and (7.121) until convergence. The covariance matrix of the GEE estimate is given by

$$\mathrm{cov}(\widehat{\boldsymbol{\beta}}_{GEE}) = \left(\sum_{i=1}^N \mathbf{X}_i'\mathbf{E}_i\mathbf{V}_i^{-1}\mathbf{E}_i\mathbf{X}_i\right)^{-1}. \tag{7.122}$$

More discussion is given in Section 7.5.7, where exactly the same GEE approach is applied to a general, unspecified distribution.

7.5.6 Normally distributed intercepts

In this subsection we assume that random intercepts are iid and normally distributed, $u_i \sim \mathcal{N}(0, \sigma^2)$. The log-likelihood function takes generic form (7.64), where following the notation of Section 7.3.1 for the Poisson model,

$$h_i(\boldsymbol{\beta};u) = k_i u - u^2/(2\sigma^2) - e^u \sum_{j=1}^{n_i} e^{\boldsymbol{\beta}'\mathbf{x}_{ij}} \tag{7.123}$$

and $k_i = \sum_{j=1}^{n_i} y_{ij}$. The score equations and derivatives have the same form as (7.66), where for Poisson regression,

$$\mathbf{I}_{i3} = J_i \sum_{j=1}^{n_i} e^{\boldsymbol{\beta}'\mathbf{x}_{ij}} \mathbf{x}_{ij}, \quad \mathbf{I}_{i4} = J_i \sum_{j=1}^{n_i} e^{\boldsymbol{\beta}'\mathbf{x}_{ij}} \mathbf{x}_{ij}\mathbf{x}_{ij}', \tag{7.124}$$

and $J_i = \int_{-\infty}^{\infty} e^{h_i(\boldsymbol{\beta};\mathbf{u})+u} du$. We notice that the integrals are similar to logistic regression, except that u is presented in the exponential function. The MLE may be found by either method discussed in Section 7.3.1. The EFS algorithm is easier to implement because it requires only first derivatives.

To evaluate the integrals, one needs to replace an improper integral with a proper one finding the lower and upper limits such that the integrals differ by a small predefined number $\varepsilon > 0$. We can again use Lemma 35 for this purpose. For example, to compute the limits of integration for J_i, we use the inequalities $e^u \geq 1 + u + u^2/2$ for $u \geq 0$ and $e^u \geq 1 + u$ for $u < 0$. To compute $\int_{-\infty}^{\infty} u^2 e^{h_i(\boldsymbol{\beta};\mathbf{u})+u} du$, we use the inequality $\ln|u| \leq |u| - 1$ for the positive and negative parts.

PQL

The penalized quasi-likelihood approach, (7.84), can readily be applied to Poisson regression with normally distributed intercepts, resulting in the function to be maximized, assuming that σ^2 is fixed,

$$l_{PQL}(\boldsymbol{\beta},u_1,...,u_N) = \boldsymbol{\beta}'\mathbf{r} + \sum_{i=1}^{N} \left(u_i k_i - e^{u_i} \sum_{j=1}^{n_i} e^{\boldsymbol{\beta}'\mathbf{x}_{ij}} \right) - \frac{1}{2\sigma^2} \sum_{i=1}^{N} u_i^2. \tag{7.125}$$

This function may be viewed as the log-likelihood function with the fixed subject-specific intercepts penalized by the term $\sum u_i^2/(2\sigma^2)$. To find the maximum over $\boldsymbol{\beta}$ and u_i, we can use Newton's algorithm; see Section 7.4.1. Specifically, let $\boldsymbol{\beta}$ be held. Letting $B_i = \sum_{j=1}^{n_i} e^{\boldsymbol{\beta}'\mathbf{x}_{ij}}$, we want to solve the equation $\Psi(u_i) = k_i$, where $\Psi(u_i) = B_i e^{u_i} + u_i/\sigma^2$. This equation has a unique solution u_{*i} for each $i = 1, ..., N$. Then the Newton iterations yield the update formula

$$u_{s+1,i} = u_{s,i} - \frac{B_i e^{u_{s,i}} + u_{s,i}/\sigma^2 - k_i}{B_i e^{u_{s,i}} + 1/\sigma^2}, \quad s = 0, 1, 2, ...,$$

starting from $u_{0,i} = (k_i - B_i)(B_i + 1/\sigma^2)^{-1}$. One can prove that these iterations converge monotonically to the solution, see Section 7.2.2. When the $\{u_i\}$ are held, the maximization over $\boldsymbol{\beta}$ can be accomplished by the standard FS algorithm treating u_{*i} as an offset parameter. The Laplace approximation for the variance yields update formula (7.94). Since in the previous notation, $H_i = B_i e^{u_{*i}}$, this update formula simplifies to

$$\widehat{\sigma}_{s+1}^2 = \frac{1}{N} \sum_{i=1}^{N} \left(u_{*i}^2 + \frac{1}{\widehat{\sigma}_s^{-2} + B_i e^{u_{*i}}} \right). \tag{7.126}$$

As in the case of logistic regression, we start with $\widehat{\sigma}_0 = \infty$. Then, alternating iterations involve maximization of l_{PQL} and update formula (7.126).

Exact GEE: accounting for correlation

The beauty of the Poisson model with a normally distributed random intercept is that the marginal mean is easy to obtain using the fact that $Ee^{u+\beta} = e^{\beta + \sigma^2/2}$, where $u \sim \mathcal{N}(0, \sigma^2)$. This means that if the first component of $\mathbf{x}_{ij}$ is 1, only the intercept term is affected, namely, it increases by $\sigma^2/2$. Precisely for model (7.105) with normally distributed u_i, using (7.96) and (7.97), we obtain $E(\mathbf{y}_i) = \mathbf{e}_i$ and $\mathbf{V}_i = \mathbf{E}_i + a\mathbf{e}_i\mathbf{e}_i'$, where $a = e^{\sigma^2}(e^{\sigma^2} - 1)$. Therefore, we come to the same first moments for intercepts with a log-Gamma distribution. In the next section, we develop the exact GEE approach for a general, unspecified intercept distribution.

7.5.7 Exact GEE for any distribution

Two distributions for the intercepts were considered above—the log-Gamma and normal distributions—and it was found that they lead to the same estimating equations approach. In this section we summarize the findings merely assuming that $u_i \sim F$. From derivation (7.106) it follows that the marginal link is again the log-link with a modified population-averaged intercept. Furthermore, applying formula (7.97), we obtain the marginal covariance matrix,

$$\mathbf{V}_i = \mathrm{cov}(\mathbf{y}_i) = \mathbf{E}_i + \mathrm{var}(e^u)\mathbf{e}_i\mathbf{e}_i' = \mathbf{E}_i + a\mathbf{e}_i\mathbf{e}_i', \tag{7.127}$$

where $\mathbf{e}_i = \exp(\mathbf{X}_i\boldsymbol{\beta})$ and a is the overdispersion parameter. Thus, we infer that regardless of the distribution of the intercept, the exact covariance matrix of the Poisson clustered data $\{\mathbf{y}_i\}$ is given by (7.127). The exact GEE for $\boldsymbol{\beta}$ is the same, (7.118). We call it exact because the covariance matrix is exact.

Parameter a reflects the presence of the random intercept and there is a one-to-one relationship between the variance of the F distribution and a. For example, if $F = \mathcal{N}$, we have $a = 1 - e^{-\sigma^2}$. If $a = 0$ all intercepts are the same (no random effect); if $a > 0$ the intercepts vary from cluster to cluster. The overdispersion parameter, a may be estimated either from equation (7.119) or by VLS (7.121). Conversely, given a, regression estimates are obtained from iterations (7.120).

Assuming that a is known, one can estimate the covariance matrix of $\widehat{\boldsymbol{\beta}}_{GEE}$ from the sandwich formula, which produces the asymptotic covariance matrix (7.122).

Applying the dimension-reduction formula and noticing that $\mathbf{E}_i^{-1}\mathbf{e}_i = \mathbf{1}_i$, $\mathbf{E}_i\mathbf{1}_i = \mathbf{e}_i$, we simplify:

$$\mathbf{V}_i^{-1} = \mathbf{E}_i^{-1} - \frac{a}{1 + a\mathbf{e}_i'\mathbf{1}_i}\mathbf{1}_i\mathbf{1}_i',$$

where $\mathbf{1}_i$ is the $n_i \times 1$ vector of 1s. Hence, the asymptotic covariance matrix can be rewritten as

$$\mathrm{cov}(\widehat{\boldsymbol{\beta}}_{GEE}) = \left[\sum_{i=1}^N \left(\mathbf{X}_i'\mathbf{E}_i\mathbf{X}_i - \frac{a}{1 + a\mathbf{c}_i'\mathbf{1}_i}(\mathbf{X}_i'\mathbf{e}_i)(\mathbf{X}_i'\mathbf{e}_i)'\right)\right]^{-1}. \tag{7.128}$$

Below we consider the special case of balanced data, $n_i = n$ and $\mathbf{X}_i = \mathbf{X}$.

7.5.8 Exact GEE for balanced count data

We know from Subsections 2.4.1 and 2.4.2 that in a linear model with random intercepts and balanced data, neither the slopes nor their variances are affected by the random effect. The aim of this section is to prove that the same holds for the Poisson model with balanced count data if exact GEE is used. As before, we say that the data are balanced if $n_i = n$ and $\mathbf{X}_i = \mathbf{X}$.

First, we prove that the covariance matrix of slopes does not depend on a, the overdispersion parameter. To prove this, it suffices to demonstrate that the $(m-1) \times (m-1)$ submatrix of matrix (7.128) does not depend on a. Following the notation of Section 2.4.1, we represent $\mathbf{X} = [\mathbf{1}, \mathbf{U}]$. For balanced data we have

$$\text{cov}(\widehat{\boldsymbol{\beta}}_{GEE}) = \frac{1}{N}\left[\left(\mathbf{X'EX} - \frac{a}{1+a\mathbf{e'1}}(\mathbf{X'e})(\mathbf{X'e})'\right)\right]^{-1}.$$

Let the matrix to the inverse be partitioned as

$$\mathbf{X'EX} - \frac{a}{1+a\mathbf{e'1}}(\mathbf{X'e})(\mathbf{X'e})' = \begin{bmatrix} m_{11} & \mathbf{m}'_{21} \\ \mathbf{m}_{21} & \mathbf{M}_{22} \end{bmatrix}.$$

The matrix blocks can be found after some algebra:

$$[\mathbf{1}, \mathbf{U}]'\mathbf{E}[\mathbf{1}, \mathbf{U}] - \frac{a}{1+a\mathbf{e'1}}\begin{bmatrix}\mathbf{1'e} \\ \mathbf{U'e}\end{bmatrix}\begin{bmatrix}\mathbf{1'e} \\ \mathbf{U'e}\end{bmatrix}'$$

$$= \begin{bmatrix} \frac{\mathbf{1'e}}{1+a\mathbf{e'1}} & \frac{\mathbf{e'U}}{1+a\mathbf{e'1}} \\ \frac{\mathbf{U'e}}{1+a\mathbf{e'1}} & \mathbf{U'}\left(\mathbf{E} - \frac{a}{1+a\mathbf{e'1}}\mathbf{ee'}\right)\mathbf{U} \end{bmatrix}.$$

Thus, we have

$$m_{11} = \frac{\mathbf{1'e}}{1+a\mathbf{e'1}}, \quad \mathbf{m}_{21} = \frac{\mathbf{U'e}}{1+a\mathbf{e'1}}, \quad \mathbf{M}_{22} = \mathbf{U'}\left(\mathbf{E} - \frac{a}{1+a\mathbf{e'1}}\mathbf{ee'}\right)\mathbf{U}.$$

Using the well known formula, we find that the $(m-1) \times (m-1)$ inverted matrix is $(\mathbf{M}_{22} - \mathbf{m}_{21}\mathbf{m}'_{21}/m_{11})^{-1}$. But

$$\mathbf{M}_{22} - \frac{1}{m_{11}}\mathbf{m}_{21}\mathbf{m}'_{21} = \mathbf{U'}\left(\mathbf{E} - \frac{a}{1+a\mathbf{e'1}}\mathbf{ee'}\right)\mathbf{U} - \frac{1}{\mathbf{e'1}(1+a\mathbf{e'1})}\mathbf{U'ee'U}$$

$$= \mathbf{U'EU} - \frac{1}{\mathbf{e'1}}\mathbf{U'ee'U}.$$

This means that an $(m-1) \times (m-1)$ matrix of $\text{cov}(\widehat{\boldsymbol{\beta}}_{GEE})$, the covariance matrix of slopes, does not depend on a.

Second, we prove that the exact GEE estimates of slopes also do not depend on the overdispersion parameter. Precisely, we shall show that estimating equation (7.118) for balanced data collapses to standard Poisson regression. For balanced data, (7.118) simplifies to $\mathbf{X'EV}^{-1}(\overline{\mathbf{y}} - \mathbf{e}) = \mathbf{0}$, where $\overline{\mathbf{y}} = \sum_{i=1}^{N}\mathbf{y}_i/N$. Further, we have

$$
\begin{aligned}
\mathbf{X'EV}^{-1} &= \mathbf{X'E}\left(\mathbf{E}^{-1} - \frac{a}{1+a\mathbf{e'1}}\mathbf{11'}\right) = \mathbf{X'} - \frac{a}{1+a\mathbf{e'1}}\mathbf{X'E11'} \\
&= \mathbf{X'} - \frac{a}{1+a\mathbf{e'1}}\mathbf{X'e1'} = [\mathbf{1,U}]' - \frac{a}{1+a\mathbf{e'1}}[\mathbf{1,U}]'\mathbf{e1'} \\
&= \begin{bmatrix} \left[1 - \frac{a(\mathbf{e'1})}{1+a\mathbf{e'1}}\right]\mathbf{1'} \\ \mathbf{U'}\left[\mathbf{I} - \frac{a}{1+a\mathbf{e'1}}\mathbf{e1'}\right] \end{bmatrix} = \begin{bmatrix} \frac{1}{1+a\mathbf{e'1}}\mathbf{1'} \\ \mathbf{U'}\left[\mathbf{I} - \frac{a}{1+a\mathbf{e'1}}\mathbf{e1'}\right] \end{bmatrix},
\end{aligned}
$$

so the estimating equations simplify to $\mathbf{1'}(\overline{\mathbf{y}} - \mathbf{e}) = 0$ and $\mathbf{U'}(\overline{\mathbf{y}} - \mathbf{e}) = \mathbf{0}$, or combining,

$$
\mathbf{X'}(\overline{\mathbf{y}} - \mathbf{e}) = \mathbf{0}. \tag{7.129}
$$

But this is the score equation of the standard Poisson regression (7.103) applied to averaged data.

In summary, neither the slopes nor their variances depend on the overdispersion parameter if count data are balanced. The optimal method of estimation is the standard Poisson regression.

7.5.9   Heckman method for the Poisson model

Since standard Poisson regression gives consistent estimates of slopes and the intercept augmented by $\sigma^2/2$, we can estimate $\sum_{j=1}^{n_i} e^{\boldsymbol{\beta}'\mathbf{x}_{ij}}$ as $e^{-\sigma^2/2}B_i$, where $B_i = \sum_{j=1}^{n_i} e^{\widehat{\boldsymbol{\beta}}_0'\mathbf{x}_{ij}}$. Then, plugging this into the function (7.123), the original multivariate maximization problem will be reduced to a univariate one as we did for the probit model of Section 7.4.3. This reduction leads to the profile log-likelihood function,

$$
l(\sigma^2) = -\frac{N}{2}\ln 2\pi\sigma^2 - \frac{k}{2}\sigma^2 + \sum \ln I_i(\sigma^2),
$$

where $k = \sum_{i=1}^{N} k_i$ and $I_i(\sigma^2) = \int_{-\infty}^{\infty} e^{h_i(u;\sigma^2)}du$ with $h_i(u;\sigma^2) = k_i u - u^2/(2\sigma^2) - e^{u-\sigma^2/2}B_i$. One can find the maximum of this function by standard univariate optimization methods, as mentioned in Section 7.4.3.

Here we suggest a fixed-point approach. Taking the derivative of l with respect to σ^2, the score equation becomes

$$
-\frac{1}{2N\sigma^2} - \frac{k}{2} + \frac{1}{2\sigma^4}\sum\frac{K_i}{I_i} + \frac{1}{2}e^{-\sigma^2/2}\sum\frac{M_iB_i}{I_i} = 0,
$$

where

$$
K_i = \int_{-\infty}^{\infty} u^2 e^{h_i(u;\sigma^2)}du, \quad M_i = \int_{-\infty}^{\infty} e^{h_i(u;\sigma^2)+u}du.
$$

Solving the equation above for σ^2, we come to the recursive formula,

$$
\sigma^2_{s+1} = \frac{1 - \sqrt{1 - 4A(\sigma_s^2)C(\sigma_s^2)}}{2A(\sigma_s^2)}, \tag{7.130}
$$

where functions A and C are defined as follows:

$$
A = \frac{e^{-\sigma^2/2}}{N}\sum\frac{M_iB_i}{I_i} - \frac{k}{N}, \quad C = \frac{1}{N}\sum\frac{K_i}{I_i}.
$$

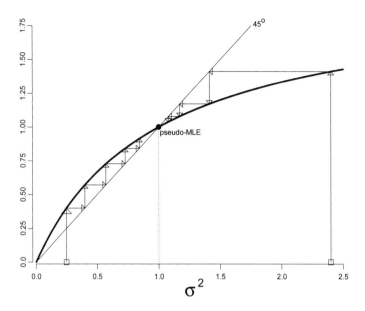

FIGURE 7.8. Fixed-point iterations (7.130) for Poisson regression with random intercepts using the Heckman method. Initial (starting) values for σ^2 are shown as empty squares. If the initial value is to the left of the fixed-point, iterations produce an increasing sequence; otherwise, the sequence is decreasing.

The right-hand side of (7.130) as a function of σ^2 takes zero at zero and approaches a constant when $\sigma^2 \to \infty$. Indeed, dividing, we see that $K_i(\sigma^2) \to 0$ and $I_i(\sigma^2) \to e^{B_i}$ when $\sigma^2 \to 0$. When $\sigma^2 \to \infty$, the term $u/(2\sigma^2)$ vanishes and therefore we have

$$\lim_{\sigma^2 \to \infty} \frac{K_i(\sigma^2)}{I_i(\sigma^2)} = \frac{\int_{-\infty}^{\infty} u^2 e^{k_i u - e^u B_i} du}{\int_{-\infty}^{\infty} e^{k_i u - e^u B_i} du},$$

and analogously for M_i/I_i. Further, applying the standard limit techniques we find that the right-hand side of (7.130) approaches a constant when $\sigma^2 \to \infty$. Importantly, since the limit at infinity exists, a large starting value, σ_0^2, may be used to start the fixed-point iterations (it is a bad idea to start with $\sigma_0^2 = 0$ because 0 is the fixed point). A typical function $F = F(\sigma^2)$, as the right-hand side of (7.130), is shown in Figure 7.8. The pseudo-MLE for σ^2 is derived from the intersection of $F(\sigma^2)$ with the 45° line. Initial values either to the left or to the right of the solution yield fixed-point convergence.

After $\widehat{\sigma}^2$ is determined, we can estimate the true intercept as $\widehat{\beta}_0 - \widehat{\sigma}^2/2$ and the co-variance matrix $\text{cov}(\widehat{\boldsymbol{\beta}}) \simeq (\sum \mathbf{X}_i' \mathbf{V}_i^{-1} \mathbf{X}_i)^{-1}$, where $\mathbf{V}_i = \text{diag}(\mathbf{e}_i) + e^{\widehat{\sigma}^2}(e^{\widehat{\sigma}^2} - 1)\mathbf{e}_i \mathbf{e}_i'$. Some additional details on the Fixed-Point algorithm are provided in Appendix 13.3.4.

7.5.10 Tests for overdispersion

It is straightforward to generalize the homogeneity tests developed in Section 7.3.7 to the Poisson regression with random intercepts. The F-test has the same form, (7.88).

An advantage of the Poisson model is that since the subject-specific intercepts admit a closed-form solution, (7.108), after some simplifications we get

$$l_{\min} = \widehat{\boldsymbol{\beta}}' \mathbf{r} + \sum \left(\ln k_i - \ln \sum_{j=1}^{n_i} e^{\widehat{\boldsymbol{\beta}}' \mathbf{x}_{ij}} - 1 \right) k_i,$$

where $\widehat{\boldsymbol{\beta}}$ is the limiting point of iterations (7.110).

Now we obtain the score test for $H_0 : \sigma^2 = 0$ in the Poisson model with normally distributed intercepts. Following the line of argumentation of Section 7.3.7, we obtain $l_i' = u \sum (y_{ij} - e^{\sigma u} e^{\boldsymbol{\beta}' \mathbf{x}_{ij}})$ and $l_i'' = -u^2 e^{\sigma u} e^{\boldsymbol{\beta}' \mathbf{x}_{ij}}$, so that the derivative at $\sigma = 0$ is proportional to the statistic

$$S = \sum_{i=1}^{N} \left(\sum_{j=1}^{n_i} (y_{ij} - e^{\widehat{\boldsymbol{\beta}}' \mathbf{x}_{ij}}) \right)^2 - \sum_{i=1}^{N} \sum_{j=1}^{n_i} e^{\widehat{\boldsymbol{\beta}}' \mathbf{x}_{ij}},$$

where $\widehat{\boldsymbol{\beta}}$ is the standard MLE. Applying Lemma 36, we find that the variance of statistic S is

$$v = \sum_{i=1}^{N} \left[\sum_{j=1}^{n_i} e^{\widehat{\boldsymbol{\beta}}' \mathbf{x}_{ij}} + 2 \left(\sum_{j=1}^{n_i} e^{\widehat{\boldsymbol{\beta}}' \mathbf{x}_{ij}} \right)^2 \right].$$

Finally, we reject overdispersion if $S > Z_{1-\alpha} \sqrt{v}$.

7.5.11   Implementation in R

Most algorithms discussed in this section are implemented as R functions. Poisson regression with random intercepts can be estimated by the PQL method using the previously discussed function `glmmPQL` with the option `family=poisson`. The following R functions can be downloaded from `"c:\\MixedModels\\Chapter07\\"`: `poissfix`, `poissGEE1`, `poissGEE`, `poissHeck`, and `poissMLE`. The calls to these functions are similar to the logistic and probit regression functions discussed earlier. The reader is welcome to modify and improve these functions.

Problems for Section 7.5

1. Write an R function for estimation of the Poisson regression using iterations (7.104) with an offset, $\ln E(y_i) = f_i + \boldsymbol{\beta}' \mathbf{x}_i$, where f_i is given offset. Prove that the Hessian of the log-likelihood is a positive definite matrix if the $\{\mathbf{x}_i\}$ have at least $m < n$ linearly independent vectors.

2*. Write an R function to implement the conditional Poisson regression model. Modify the `logric` function for this purpose. Test the function via simulations. Devise a method to estimate the variance of the random intercepts.

3. Demonstrate by simulations that the slope estimates in the Poisson model with random intercepts converge to the standard Poisson regression if the data become more balanced. Use $\text{var}(n_i)$ to characterize the balance.

4*. Conduct a simulation study for comparison of the methods for Poisson regression with random intercepts. What method would you recommend based on these simulations? Take into account the number of simulations when the algorithm did not converge.

5*. Evaluate the accuracy of the overdispersion test via simulations. Compute and plot the power function.

6*. The file `psdat.r` contains data on 9866 colon cancer patients; use `source("c:\\MixedModels\\Chapter07\\psdat.r")`. This dataframe has eight variables: `hrr`, `visitin`, `visitout`, `visittot`, `black`, `age10`, `female`, `daysfu`, where `visittot` is the number of visits to see a doctor after surgery and `hrr` codes the HRR hospital area. It is possible that hospital regions have geographic differences that lead to a Poisson model with a random intercept. The call

```
glmmPQL(fixed=visittot~black+female+I(age10-8)+I((age10-8)^2),
random=~1|hrr,data=psdat,family=poisson)
```

estimates the number of visits as a function of race, gender, and age using the PQL approach (this function requires `library(MASS)`). Plot the estimates of random intercepts. Use the test for overdispersion to conclude that the geographic differences are statistically significant.

7.6   Random intercept model: overview

The random intercept model is the simplest mixed model to use to address cluster heterogeneity and intracluster correlation. When the number of observations per cluster (n_i) is small (sparse data), conditional likelihood offers an efficient way to avoid integration in logistic or Poisson regression. This approach may be used when intercepts are fixed or random with little efficiency loss. An advantage of the conditional likelihood approach is that it does not require specification of the intercept distribution. Unfortunately, the conditional likelihood does not work for the probit model. Also, it is prohibitive when n_i is large; say, $n_i > 20$.

If n_i is relatively large, say $n_i > N$, the model with fixed subject-specific intercepts may be adequate. For the Poisson model, the intercepts may be eliminated with a closed-form formula.

The random intercept model takes a somewhat intermediate position and should be used when N and $\{n_i\}$ are relatively large. As follows from standard theory, maximum likelihood produces asymptotically unbiased (consistent) and efficient estimates when the number of clusters goes to infinity and the number of observations per cluster is bounded. Although the integrals involved are one-dimensional, the integration problem should not be underestimated, especially in the presence of outliers.

There are a variety of methods for approximate estimation of random effects models, as alternatives to ML. For example, if the marginal expectation were known, one could obtain consistent estimates simply by assuming that observations are independent. However, we gain efficiency if the within-cluster correlation structure is taken into account. There is no closed-form solution for the marginal expectation in logistic regression, but normally distributed intercepts do not change the link of probit or Poisson regression. These facts are the basis for the exact generalized estimating equations approach which avoids integration. Moreover, if the count data are balanced—the $\{y_{ij}\}$ have tabular form with no missing values—standard Poisson regression is efficient for slope coefficients.

The variance of the random intercept, σ^2, has different effects in different models: For the probit model, σ^2 attenuates all regression coefficients. For the Poisson model, it affects only the population-averaged intercept. Generally, introduction of the random effect has a different impact for different members of the generalized linear models family. In the model with fixed intercepts, they are treated as nuisance parameters. When intercepts are random, we can generalize the approach for the linear mixed effects model of Section 3.7 based on minimization (3.54). Since the counterpart of the first term is $-2l$, we estimate random effects $\{u_i\}$ that maximize function (7.84), assuming that σ^2 is known. Thus, the penalized quasi-likelihood function is a natural extension of the LME model to estimate random effect. Alternatively, one can use the original Laplace approximation log-likelihood (7.78). The difference between (7.78) and the PQL approach is that the last term is dropped. Principally, the same methods for $\{u_i\}$ estimation can be used for probit and Poisson models.

7.7   Mixed models with multiple random effects

The model with random intercepts can easily be generalized to a mixed model with multiple linear random effects. For example, the binary model with multiple linear random effects takes the form $\Pr(y_{ij} = 1|\mathbf{b}_i) = \mu(\boldsymbol{\beta}'\mathbf{x}_{ij} + \mathbf{b}_i'\mathbf{z}_{ij})$, where the $\{\mathbf{z}_{ij}\}$ are $k \times 1$ fixed vectors and $\mathbf{b}_i$ is the k-dimensional random effect. In this section we assume that the random effects are iid normally distributed, $\mathbf{b}_i \sim \mathcal{N}(\mathbf{0}, \mathbf{D}_*)$, where the covariance matrix $\mathbf{D}_*$ is subject to estimation along with the beta coefficients. In this book the subscript $*$ indicates that the covariance matrix is not scaled, $\mathbf{D}_* = \sigma^2\mathbf{D}$, where $\mathbf{D}$ is the *scaled* covariance matrix, following the line of our previous notation. The advantage of the normally distributed random effects is that $\mathbf{b}_i'\mathbf{z}_{ij}$ is also normally distributed as $\mathcal{N}(\mathbf{0}, \mathbf{z}_{ij}'\mathbf{D}_*\mathbf{z}_{ij})$. The maximum likelihood leads to a k-dimensional integral. Although a mixed model rarely has a large number of random effects (typically, $k = 2$ or 3), multidimensionality may substantially increase computation time, in addition to being a generally difficult problem of numerical quadrature for an improper integral; we refer the reader to the discussion at the end of Section 7.3.1. On the other hand, in image analysis we face estimation of GLMM with 255 random effects, Section 12.6.

Four types of algorithms and methods for the generalized linear mixed model (GLMM) are discussed: (a) maximum likelihood with numerical quadrature, (b) penalized quasi-likelihood (PQL), (c) specific methods in conjunction with Laplace approximation or the GEE approach, and (d) Monte Carlo methods for integral or log-likelihood approximation. We pay particular attention to special methods because they use specific properties of the link function, as in the case of probit or Poisson regression. We present a small simulation study to investigate the numerical and statistical properties of the algorithms discussed.

7.7.1   Multivariate Laplace approximation

To avoid integration, we approximate the multidimensional integral at the maximum point of the integrand, as in the one-dimensional case of Section 7.1.2. Omitting trivial algebra, we obtain a multivariate version of the Laplace approximation,

$$\int_{R^k} e^{h(\mathbf{x})} d\mathbf{x} \simeq (2\pi)^{k/2} e^{h_{\max}} \left| -\frac{\partial^2 h}{\partial \mathbf{x}^2} \right|_{\mathbf{x}=\mathbf{x}_{\max}}^{-1/2}. \qquad (7.131)$$

The right-hand side involves computation of function $h = h(\mathbf{x})$ and its Hessian matrix (determinant) at the maximum point, $\mathbf{x} = \mathbf{x}_{\max}$. Since the Hessian is evaluated at the maximum, it is at least nonnegative definite. Moreover, it is assumed that it is positive definite for the right-hand-side expression to exist. An implicit assumption is that function $h(\mathbf{x})$ is unimodal; it has one local minimum. Otherwise, approximation (7.131) may be imprecise.

We shall use a multivariate version of (7.31),

$$\frac{\int_{R^k} \mathbf{x}\mathbf{x}' e^{h(\mathbf{x})} d\mathbf{x}}{\int_{R^k} e^{h(\mathbf{x})} d\mathbf{x}} \simeq \mathbf{x}_{\max}\mathbf{x}'_{\max} + \left(-\frac{\partial^2 h}{\partial \mathbf{x}^2} \Big|_{\mathbf{x}=\mathbf{x}_{\max}} \right)^{-1}. \qquad (7.132)$$

This formula will be used to update the covariance matrix of random effects when the likelihood is approximated based on (7.131).

7.7.2   Logistic regression

We consider three methods for parameter estimation in logistic regression with normally distributed random effects. Maximum likelihood requires k-dimensional integration. If the integration is exact, the estimates are consistent and asymptotically unbiased when the number of clusters (N) increases to infinity, even if the number of observations per cluster is bounded. The other two methods avoid integration but are approximations to the likelihood. Therefore, one may expect a systematic bias, especially when the variances of the random effects are large. Penalized quasi-likelihood is a straightforward generalization of the random intercept. Two-probit approximation uses the facts that (a) the logit probability function may be uniformly approximated by a linear combination of probits with the absolute error 0.000526, and (b) the marginal mean of a probit with normally distributed random effects is again a probit.

Maximum likelihood

Estimation by maximum likelihood follows the line of logistic regression with random intercepts, Section 7.3.1. With multivariate random effects, it is more convenient to use the precision matrix parameterization. Recall that we used this parameterization for a linear mixed effects model in Section 2.2.4.

We want to express the log-likelihood function in terms of the precision matrix, $\mathbf{D}_- = \mathbf{D}_*^{-1}$. The log-likelihood function takes the form

$$l(\boldsymbol{\beta}, \mathbf{D}_-) = -\frac{Nk}{2}\ln(2\pi) + \frac{N}{2}\ln|\mathbf{D}_-| + \boldsymbol{\beta}'\mathbf{r} + \sum_{i=1}^{N} \ln \int_{R^k} e^{h_i(\boldsymbol{\beta};\mathbf{u})} d\mathbf{u}, \qquad (7.133)$$

where

$$h_i(\boldsymbol{\beta}; \mathbf{u}) = \mathbf{k}_i'\mathbf{u} - 0.5\mathbf{u}'\mathbf{D}_-\mathbf{u} - \sum_{j=1}^{n_i} \ln(1 + e^{\boldsymbol{\beta}'\mathbf{x}_{ij} + \mathbf{u}'\mathbf{z}_{ij}})$$

and $\mathbf{k}_i = \sum_{j=1}^{n_i} y_{ij}\mathbf{z}_{ij}$ is a $k \times 1$ vector. The first-order derivatives are:

$$\frac{\partial l}{\partial \boldsymbol{\beta}} = \mathbf{r} - \sum_{i=1}^{N} \frac{\mathbf{I}_{i3}}{I_{i1}}, \quad \frac{\partial l}{\partial \mathbf{D}_-} = \frac{1}{2}\left(N\mathbf{D}_-^{-1} - \sum_{i=1}^{N}\frac{\mathbf{I}_{i2}}{I_{i1}}\right), \tag{7.134}$$

where

$$I_{i1} = \int_{R^k} e^{h_i(\boldsymbol{\beta};\mathbf{u})}d\mathbf{u}, \quad \mathbf{I}_{i2} = \int_{R^k} \mathbf{u}\mathbf{u}'e^{h_i(\boldsymbol{\beta};\mathbf{u})}d\mathbf{u},$$

$$\mathbf{I}_{i3} = \int_{R^k} \left[\sum_{j=1}^{n_i} \mathbf{x}_{ij}\frac{e^{\boldsymbol{\beta}'\mathbf{x}_{ij}+\mathbf{u}'\mathbf{z}_{ij}}}{1 + e^{\boldsymbol{\beta}'\mathbf{x}_{ij}+\mathbf{u}'\mathbf{z}_{ij}}}e^{h_i(\boldsymbol{\beta};\mathbf{u})}\right]d\mathbf{u}.$$

The MLE for $\boldsymbol{\beta}$ and $\mathbf{D}_-$ is the solution to the score equations, $\partial l/\partial\boldsymbol{\beta} = \mathbf{0}$ and $\partial l/\partial\mathbf{D}_- = \mathbf{0}$. Now the reader appreciates the precision matrix parameterization because the derivative $\partial l/\partial\mathbf{D}_-$ is easy to compute. The score equations may be solved iteratively by the EFS algorithm. Alternatively, one can apply the Fixed-Point algorithm for the precision matrix, $\mathbf{D}_- = N(\sum \mathbf{I}_{i2}I_{i1}^{-1})^{-1}$. An advantage of the latter algorithm is that matrix $\mathbf{D}_-$ is always positive definite. The ML requires evaluation of $1 + m + k(k+1)/2$ k-dimensional integrals at each iteration.

Laplace approximation and penalized quasi-likelihood

To avoid integration, one can apply the Laplace approximation (7.131) and treat the new function as a new likelihood function. Thus, assuming that $\boldsymbol{\beta}$ and $\mathbf{D}_-$ are held, we find N estimates of the random effects as the maximizers of the individual penalized log-likelihood functions

$$l_i(\boldsymbol{\beta}, \mathbf{u}_i) - \frac{1}{2}\mathbf{u}_i'\mathbf{D}_-\mathbf{u}_i \Rightarrow \max_{\mathbf{u}_i}, \tag{7.135}$$

where the individual log-likelihood function is given by

$$l_i(\boldsymbol{\beta}, \mathbf{u}_i) = \sum_{y_{ij}=1} \ln\frac{e^{\boldsymbol{\beta}'\mathbf{x}_{ij}+\mathbf{u}_i'\mathbf{z}_{ij}}}{1 + e^{\boldsymbol{\beta}'\mathbf{x}_{ij}+\mathbf{u}_i'\mathbf{z}_{ij}}} + \sum_{y_{ij}=0} \ln\frac{1}{1 + e^{\boldsymbol{\beta}'\mathbf{x}_{ij}+\mathbf{u}_i'\mathbf{z}_{ij}}}$$

$$= \mathbf{r}_i'\boldsymbol{\beta} + \mathbf{u}_i'\mathbf{k}_i - \sum_{j=1}^{n_i}\ln(1 + e^{\boldsymbol{\beta}'\mathbf{x}_{ij}+\mathbf{u}_i'\mathbf{z}_{ij}}). \tag{7.136}$$

$\mathbf{r}_i = \sum_{j=1}^{n_i}\mathbf{x}_{ij}y_{ij}$ and $\mathbf{k}_i = \sum_{j=1}^{n_i}\mathbf{z}_{ij}y_{ij}$ are fixed $m \times 1$ and $k \times 1$ vectors. Let the solution to (7.135) be $\mathbf{u}_{*i}$, $i = 1, ..., N$. Then, applying the multivariate Laplace approximation, we obtain

$$l_{LA}(\boldsymbol{\beta}, \mathbf{D}_-) = \mathbf{r}'\boldsymbol{\beta} - \sum_{i=1}^{N} \left[\sum_{j=1}^{n_i} \ln(1 + e^{\boldsymbol{\beta}'\mathbf{x}_{ij} + \mathbf{u}'_{*i}\mathbf{z}_{ij}}) + 0.5\mathbf{u}'_{*i}\mathbf{D}_-\mathbf{u}_{*i} \right]$$

$$+ \frac{N}{2}\ln|\mathbf{D}_-| - \frac{1}{2}\sum_{i=1}^{N}\ln \left| \mathbf{D}_- + \sum_{j=1}^{n_i} \frac{e^{\boldsymbol{\beta}'\mathbf{x}_{ij} + \mathbf{u}'_{*i}\mathbf{z}_{ij}}}{(1 + e^{\boldsymbol{\beta}'\mathbf{x}_{ij} + \mathbf{u}'_{*i}\mathbf{z}_{ij}})^2} \mathbf{z}_{ij}\mathbf{z}'_{ij} \right|, \qquad (7.137)$$

where $\mathbf{r} = \sum_{i=1}^{N} \mathbf{r}_i$. Clearly, this is an obvious generalization of the univariate case (7.78). We make several comments on how to maximize this function over $\boldsymbol{\beta}$ and $\mathbf{D}_-$. Let us start with $\mathbf{D}_-$, assuming that $\boldsymbol{\beta}$ is fixed. Denoting

$$\mathbf{G}_i = \sum_{j=1}^{n_i} \frac{e^{\boldsymbol{\beta}'\mathbf{x}_{ij} + \mathbf{u}'_{*i}\mathbf{z}_{ij}}}{(1 + e^{\boldsymbol{\beta}'\mathbf{x}_{ij} + \mathbf{u}'_{*i}\mathbf{z}_{ij}})^2} \mathbf{z}_{ij}\mathbf{z}'_{ij}, \qquad (7.138)$$

we come to a minimization of $\sum(\mathbf{u}'_{*i}\mathbf{D}_-\mathbf{u}_{*i} + \ln|\mathbf{D}_- + \mathbf{G}_i|) - N\ln|\mathbf{D}_-|$ with the estimating equation

$$\mathbf{D}_-^{-1} - N^{-1}\sum(\mathbf{D}_- + \mathbf{G}_i)^{-1} = \overline{\mathbf{U}}, \qquad (7.139)$$

where $\overline{\mathbf{U}} = N^{-1}\sum \mathbf{u}_{*i}\mathbf{u}'_{*i}$. Several algorithms can be suggested to solve matrix equation (7.139). First, we can solve it using the FP iterations in conjunction with (7.132), which yields the recursive relation

$$\mathbf{D}_- = \left[\overline{\mathbf{U}} + \frac{1}{N}\sum_{i=1}^{N}(\mathbf{D}_- + \mathbf{H}_i)^{-1} \right]^{-1}. \qquad (7.140)$$

Second, we can solve (7.139) by the Newton–Raphson algorithm, applying the perturbation formula (2.106). Then, if $\Delta\mathbf{D}_-$ is the adjustment for $\mathbf{D}_-$, the inverse to the current matrix can be approximated as $\mathbf{D}_-^{-1} - \mathbf{D}_-^{-1}(\Delta\mathbf{D}_-)\mathbf{D}_-^{-1}$ and thus $(\mathbf{D}_- + \mathbf{H}_i)^{-1} - (\mathbf{D}_- + \mathbf{G}_i)^{-1}(\Delta\mathbf{D}_-)(\mathbf{D}_- + \mathbf{G}_i)^{-1}$. Plugging this approximation back into (7.139), we come to a linear matrix equation for $\Delta\mathbf{D}_-$ with the solution

$$\Delta\mathbf{D}_- = \left[N^{-1}\sum(\mathbf{D}_- + \mathbf{H}_i)^{-1} \otimes (\mathbf{D}_- + \mathbf{H}_i)^{-1} - \mathbf{D}_-^{-1} \otimes \mathbf{D}_-^{-1} \right]^{-1}$$

$$\times \text{vec}\left(\overline{\mathbf{U}} - \mathbf{D}_-^{-1} + N^{-1}\sum(\mathbf{D}_- + \mathbf{H}_i)^{-1} \right). \qquad (7.141)$$

The maximization of l_{LA} over $\boldsymbol{\beta}$ requires computation of the first and second derivatives.

The multivariate penalized quasi-likelihood is a straightforward generalization of (7.84) and (7.85):

$$l_{PQL}(\boldsymbol{\beta}, \mathbf{u}_1, ..., u_N) = \sum_{i=1}^{N} l_i(\boldsymbol{\beta}, \mathbf{u}_i) - \frac{1}{2}\sum_{i=1}^{N}\mathbf{u}'_i\mathbf{D}_-\mathbf{u}_i, \qquad (7.142)$$

where l_i is the individual log-likelihood function (7.136). To obtain an update for $\mathbf{D}_-$ we use the fixed-point algorithm where $\{\mathbf{u}_{*i}\}$ and $\boldsymbol{\beta}$ are derived from the maximization of (7.142). Now we discuss how to maximize l_{PQL} when $\mathbf{D}_-$ is fixed. One could maximize this function simultaneously over $m + Nk$ arguments but the inverse matrix will be large. Thus, we suggest alternating between $\boldsymbol{\beta}$ and $\{\mathbf{u}_i\}$ maximization. When $\boldsymbol{\beta}$ is fixed, we augment $\mathbf{u}_i$ by

$$
\left(\mathbf{D}_- + \sum_{j=1}^{n_i} \frac{e_{ij}}{(1 + e_{ij})^2} \mathbf{z}_{ij} \mathbf{z}'_{ij} \right)^{-1} \left(\mathbf{k}_i - \mathbf{D}_- \mathbf{u}_i - \sum_{j=1}^{n_i} \frac{e_{ij}}{1 + e_{ij}} \mathbf{z}_{ij} \right). \tag{7.143}
$$

When the $\{\mathbf{u}_i\}$ are fixed, we augment $\boldsymbol{\beta}$ by

$$
\left(\sum_{i=1}^{N} \sum_{j=1}^{n_i} \frac{e_{ij}}{(1 + e_{ij})^2} \mathbf{x}_{ij} \mathbf{x}'_{ij} \right)^{-1} \left(\mathbf{r} - \sum_{i=1}^{N} \sum_{j=1}^{n_i} \frac{e_{ij}}{1 + e_{ij}} \mathbf{x}_{ij} \right), \tag{7.144}
$$

where we denote $e_{ij} = \exp(\boldsymbol{\beta}' \mathbf{x}_{ij} + \mathbf{u}'_i \mathbf{z}_{ij})$ to shorten the notation. While iterations for $\{\mathbf{u}_i\}$ should be carried out until convergence, it usually suffices to make one iteration for $\boldsymbol{\beta}$ at each cycle.

Combining the steps, the PQL algorithm is as follows:

1. Compute standard logistic regression estimate $\widehat{\boldsymbol{\beta}}_0$ regressing $\{y_{ij}\}$ on $\{\mathbf{x}_{ij}\}$, $s = 0$. Choose a starting point $\mathbf{D}_0$ and compute $\mathbf{D}_- = \mathbf{D}_0^{-1}$.

2. Holding $\boldsymbol{\beta} = \widehat{\boldsymbol{\beta}}_s$ constant, compute $\mathbf{u}_{*i}$ using iterations (7.143) for each $i = 1, ..., N$.

3. Update $\mathbf{D}_-$ by formula (7.140).

4. Make one step (7.144) to obtain the next approximation, $\widehat{\boldsymbol{\beta}}_{s+1}$, and return to step 2 $(s = s + 1)$ if $\left\| \widehat{\boldsymbol{\beta}}_{s+1} - \widehat{\boldsymbol{\beta}}_s \right\| > \varepsilon$. Otherwise, stop.

At least two starting values for $\mathbf{D}_0$ should be tried to ensure that the iteration process converges to the same value. Possible initial values are $\mathbf{D}_0 = \mathbf{0}$ and $\mathbf{D}_0 = d\mathbf{I}$, where d is a large positive number.

Two-probit approximation

We can apply the two probit approximation to the logit probability function (7.17), as we did for the logistic-normal integral. Then we use the fact that the expectation of the probit probability with a normally distributed random effect is an attenuated probit probability. Letting $\nu = 0.4353$, $\tau_1 = 2.2967^2$, and $\tau_2 = 1.3017^2$, we obtain

$$
E_{\mathbf{u} \sim \mathcal{N}(\mathbf{0}, \mathbf{D}_*)} \frac{\exp(\boldsymbol{\beta}' \mathbf{x}_{ij} + \mathbf{u}' \mathbf{z}_{ij})}{1 + \exp(\boldsymbol{\beta}' \mathbf{x}_{ij} + \mathbf{u}' \mathbf{z}_{ij})}
$$

$$
\simeq \mu_{ij}(\boldsymbol{\beta}) = \nu \Phi \left(\frac{\boldsymbol{\beta}' \mathbf{x}_{ij}}{\sqrt{\tau_1 + \mathbf{z}'_{ij} \mathbf{D}_* \mathbf{z}_{ij}}} \right) + (1 - \nu) \Phi \left(\frac{\boldsymbol{\beta}' \mathbf{x}_{ij}}{\sqrt{\tau_2 + \mathbf{z}'_{ij} \mathbf{D}_* \mathbf{z}_{ij}}} \right).
$$

Denoting $\mathbf{s}_{1ij} = \mathbf{x}_{ij} / \sqrt{\tau_1 + \mathbf{z}'_{ij} \mathbf{D}_* \mathbf{z}_{ij}}$ and $\mathbf{s}_{2ij} = \mathbf{x}_{ij} / \sqrt{\tau_2 + \mathbf{z}'_{ij} \mathbf{D}_* \mathbf{z}_{ij}}$, we come to the approximate log-likelihood,

$$
l(\boldsymbol{\beta}) = \sum_{i=1}^{N} \sum_{j=1}^{n_i} \left[y_{ij} \ln \mu_{ij}(\boldsymbol{\beta}) + (1 - y_{ij}) \ln(1 - \mu_{ij}(\boldsymbol{\beta})) \right].
$$

Thus, instead of iterations (7.144), we make the FS steps $\widehat{\boldsymbol{\beta}}_{new} = \widehat{\boldsymbol{\beta}}_{old} + \mathbf{H}^{-1}\frac{\partial l}{\partial \boldsymbol{\beta}}$, where

$$
\frac{\partial l}{\partial \boldsymbol{\beta}} = \sum_{i=1}^{N}\sum_{j=1}^{n_i}\frac{h_{ij}(y_{ij} - \mu_{ij}(\boldsymbol{\beta}))}{\mu_{ij}(1 - \mu_{ij})}\mathbf{x}_{ij},
$$

$$
h_{ij} = \nu\frac{\phi(\boldsymbol{\beta}'\mathbf{s}_{1ij})}{\sqrt{\tau_1 + \mathbf{z}_{ij}'\mathbf{D}_*\mathbf{z}_{ij}}} + (1 - \nu)\frac{\phi(\boldsymbol{\beta}'\mathbf{s}_{2ij})}{\sqrt{\tau_2 + \mathbf{z}_{ij}'\mathbf{D}_*\mathbf{z}_{ij}}},
$$

$$
\mathbf{H} = \sum_{i=1}^{N}\sum_{j=1}^{n_i}\frac{h_{ij}^2}{\mu_{ij}(1 - \mu_{ij})}\mathbf{x}_{ij}\mathbf{x}_{ij}'.
$$

The inverse to matrix $\mathbf{H}$ may serve as an estimate of the covariance matrix for $\widehat{\boldsymbol{\beta}}$.

7.7.3 Probit regression

It is straightforward to generalize maximum likelihood estimation and likelihood approximations developed earlier for the random intercept model to the multivariate random effects probit model. Here, we discuss in more detail a combination of PQL and Laplace approximation for matrix $\mathbf{D}$ in conjunction with the fact that for the probit model with normally distributed random effects,

$$
\Pr(y_{ij} = 1) = \Phi\left(\frac{\boldsymbol{\beta}'\mathbf{x}_{ij}}{\sqrt{1 + \mathbf{z}_{ij}'\mathbf{D}_*\mathbf{z}_{ij}}}\right). \tag{7.145}
$$

The following algorithm is somewhat similar to the preceding one.

1. Estimate the ordinary probit model; let $\widehat{\boldsymbol{\beta}} = \widehat{\boldsymbol{\beta}}_0$. Choose a starting point, a positive definite matrix $\mathbf{D}_0$, and compute $\mathbf{D}_- = \mathbf{D}_0^{-1}$.

2. Maximize N penalized log-likelihoods by the FS algorithm to obtain an estimate $\mathbf{u}_{*i}$:

$$
l_{PQL,i}(\mathbf{u}) = l_i(\mathbf{u}) - \frac{1}{2}\mathbf{u}'\mathbf{D}_-\mathbf{u}, \tag{7.146}
$$

where

$$
l_i(\mathbf{u}) = \sum_{j=1}^{n_i}[y_{ij}\ln\Phi(g_{ij} + \mathbf{u}'\mathbf{z}_{ij}) + (1 - y_{ij})\ln(1 - \Phi(g_{ij} + \mathbf{u}'\mathbf{z}_{ij}))],
$$

treating $g_{ij} = \widehat{\boldsymbol{\beta}}'\mathbf{x}_{ij}$ as fixed offsets.

3. Update the precision matrix as

$$
\mathbf{D}_- = \left\{\frac{1}{N}\sum_{i=1}^{N}\left(\mathbf{u}_{*i}\mathbf{u}_{*i}' + \left[\mathbf{D}_- + \sum_{j=1}^{n_i}h_{ij}\mathbf{z}_{ij}\mathbf{z}_{ij}'\right]^{-1}\right)\right\}^{-1},
$$

where

$$
h_{ij} = \frac{\phi^2(g_{ij} + \mathbf{u}_{*i}'\mathbf{z}_{ij})}{\Phi(g_{ij} + \mathbf{u}_{*i}'\mathbf{z}_{ij})[1 - \Phi(g_{ij} + \mathbf{u}_{*i}'\mathbf{z}_{ij})]}.
$$

4. Compute $\mathbf{D}_* = \mathbf{D}_-^{-1}$ and run the ordinary probit regression with probability function $\Phi(\boldsymbol{\beta}'\mathbf{q}_{ij})$, where $\mathbf{q}_{ij} = \mathbf{x}_{ij}/\sqrt{1 + \mathbf{z}'_{ij}\mathbf{D}_*\mathbf{z}_{ij}}$, to obtain the next $\widehat{\boldsymbol{\beta}}$ approximation. Return to step 2 if the convergence criteria are not met.

As earlier, we recommend starting from several $\mathbf{D}_0$ to ensure that iterations converge to the same value. One of the choices is $d\mathbf{I}$, where d is a large positive number.

7.7.4 Poisson regression

Poisson regression with linear random effects is defined via conditional probability,

$$\Pr(y_{ij} = h|\mathbf{b}_i) = \frac{1}{h!} \exp\left[(\boldsymbol{\beta}'\mathbf{x}_{ij} + \mathbf{b}'_i\mathbf{z}_{ij})h - e^{\boldsymbol{\beta}'\mathbf{x}_{ij} + \mathbf{b}'_i\mathbf{z}_{ij}}\right], \quad h = 0, 1, 2, \ldots$$

In a special case when the number of random effects $k = 1$ and $z_{ij} = 1$, this model collapses to the random intercept model (7.105). Counts $\{y_{ij}, j = 1, \ldots, n_i, i = 1, \ldots, N\}$ are independent between clusters and conditionally independent within a cluster.

Maximum likelihood estimation is a slight modification of logistic regression. The log-likelihood function has the same form (7.133), but now

$$h_i(\boldsymbol{\beta}; \mathbf{u}) = \mathbf{k}'_i\mathbf{u} - 0.5\mathbf{u}'\mathbf{D}_-\mathbf{u} - \sum_{j=1}^{n_i} e^{\boldsymbol{\beta}'\mathbf{x}_{ij} + \mathbf{u}'\mathbf{z}_{ij}}.$$

The score equations are (7.134), with $\mathbf{I}_{i3}$ and $\mathbf{I}_{i4}$ defined by (7.124), where for Poisson regression, $J_i = \int_{R^k} e^{h_i(\boldsymbol{\beta};\mathbf{u}) + \mathbf{u}'\mathbf{D}_-\mathbf{u}} d\mathbf{u}$. The EFS or fixed-point algorithm can be applied to maximize l.

Exact GEE

We again take advantage of the fact that for the Poisson regression with normally distributed random effects, the first two moments can be computed exactly. This allows us to apply exact GEE. Indeed, if $\mathbf{z}_{ij} \sim \mathcal{N}(0, \mathbf{D}_*)$, the marginal mean is given by

$$E(y_{ij}) = e^{\boldsymbol{\beta}'\mathbf{x}_{ij} + 0.5\mathbf{z}'_{ij}\mathbf{D}_*\mathbf{z}_{ij}}. \tag{7.147}$$

Letting

$$\begin{aligned} v_{ijl} &= e^{\boldsymbol{\beta}'\mathbf{x}_{ij}} + e^{\boldsymbol{\beta}'(\mathbf{x}_{ij} + \mathbf{x}_{il}) + (\mathbf{z}_{ij} + \mathbf{z}_{il})'\mathbf{D}_*(\mathbf{z}_{ij} + \mathbf{z}_{il})/2} \\ &\quad - e^{\boldsymbol{\beta}'(\mathbf{x}_{ij} + \mathbf{x}_{il}) + \mathbf{z}'_{ij}\mathbf{D}_*\mathbf{z}_{ij}/2 + \mathbf{z}'_{il}\mathbf{D}_*\mathbf{z}_{il}/2}, \end{aligned}$$

for $j, l = 1, 2, \ldots, n_i$, the marginal covariance is given by

$$V_{ijl} = \text{cov}(y_{ij}, y_{il}) = \begin{cases} e^{\boldsymbol{\beta}'\mathbf{x}_{ij}} + v_{ijj} & \text{if } j = l \\ v_{ijl} & \text{if } j \neq l \end{cases}. \tag{7.148}$$

For the random intercept model, standard Poisson regression yields consistent estimates of slope coefficients. Generally, this does not hold for the Poisson model with multiple random effects. Thus, estimation of matrix $\mathbf{D}_*$ becomes essential.

Estimation by exact GEE alternates between solving estimating equation (7.118) for $\boldsymbol{\beta}$ and estimating matrix $\mathbf{D}_*$, where elements of vector $\mathbf{e}_i$ are defined by (7.147) and $\mathbf{V}_i$ is the $n_i \times n_i$ matrix, with the (j,l)th element defined by (7.148). Note that now we use the original intercept, not augmented by $\sigma^2/2$. One may obtain some consistent estimates of $\boldsymbol{\beta}$ and $\mathbf{D}$ by ordinary Poisson regression using (7.147) and expressing $\mathbf{z}_{ij}' \mathbf{D}_* \mathbf{z}_{ij}$ as a linear function of $\mathbf{D}_*$. Indeed, rewriting $\mathbf{z}_{ij}' \mathbf{D}_* \mathbf{z}_{ij} = \sum_{p,q} D_{*pq} z_{ijp} z_{ijq}$ and augmenting $\{\mathbf{x}_{ij}\}$ by $\{\mathbf{z}_{ijp} \mathbf{z}_{ijq}\}$ after possible term rearrangement, one arrives at ordinary Poisson regression, as suggested by Grömping (1996).

Example. In a univariate Poisson regression, let only the slope be random. Then $z_{ij} = x_{ij}$ and $E(y_{ij}) = \exp(\beta_1 + \beta_2 x_{ij} + 0.5 x_{ij}^2 D_*)$, so that the variance of the slope may be estimated consistently from ordinary Poisson regression.

Estimation by variance least squares

To estimate matrix $\mathbf{D}_*$, when $\boldsymbol{\beta}$ is held fixed, we employ Variance Least Squares (VLS). This general method was introduced for the linear mixed model in Section 3.12 and was then applied to the nonlinear marginal mixed model. The VLS method may be viewed as a multivariate version of the method of moments frequently used in the framework of the GEE approach; see Section 7.9. Let $\widehat{\boldsymbol{\beta}}$ be an estimate and $\widehat{\mathbf{e}}_i$ the $n_i \times 1$ residual vector from the ith cluster. For the Poisson model, we have $\widehat{\mathbf{e}}_i = \mathbf{y}_i - e^{\widehat{\boldsymbol{\beta}}' \mathbf{x}_{ij}}$. At each VLS iteration, we treat $\widehat{\mathbf{e}}_i$ as the observation vector so that the empirical covariance matrix $\widehat{\mathbf{e}}_i \widehat{\mathbf{e}}_i'$ would have mean $\mathbf{V}_i$ if $\widehat{\boldsymbol{\beta}}$ were the true vector. VLS finds $\mathbf{D}_*$ such that the sum of the squares of the differences between the empirical and theoretical quantity is the minimum, or mathematically,

$$S(\mathbf{D}_*) = \sum_{i=1}^N \mathrm{tr}\left(\widehat{\mathbf{e}}_i \widehat{\mathbf{e}}_i' - \mathbf{V}_i(\mathbf{D}_*)\right)^2 \Rightarrow \min_{\mathbf{D}_*}. \tag{7.149}$$

After elementary algebra, we can represent the sum as a function of $\mathbf{v}_i = \mathbf{v}_i(\mathbf{d}_*)$ $=\mathrm{vec}(\mathbf{V}_i(\mathbf{d}_*))$ as follows

$$S(\mathbf{d}_*) = \sum_{i=1}^N \|\widehat{\mathbf{e}}_i\|^2 - \sum_{i=1}^N \left[2(\mathbf{e}_i \otimes \mathbf{e}_i)' \mathbf{v}_i - \|\mathbf{v}_i\|^2\right],$$

where $\mathbf{d}_* = \mathrm{vech}(\mathbf{D}_*)$ is a $k(k+1)/2 \times 1$ vector of distinct elements of matrix $\mathbf{D}_*$. Denote $\mathbf{K}_i = \partial \mathbf{v}_i / \partial \mathbf{d}_* = \mathrm{vec}\{\partial V_{ijl}/\partial \mathbf{d}_*, j,l = 1,...,n_i\}$, the $n_i^2 \times k(k+1)/2$ matrix, then $\partial S/\partial \mathbf{d}_* = -2 \sum \mathbf{K}_i'[(\mathbf{e}_i \otimes \mathbf{e}_i) - \mathbf{v}_i]$ and

$$\frac{\partial V_{ijl}}{\partial \mathbf{d}_*} = \frac{1}{2} \mathcal{D}_+ e^{\boldsymbol{\beta}'(\mathbf{x}_{ij}+\mathbf{x}_{il}) + (\mathbf{z}_{ij}+\mathbf{z}_{il})'\mathbf{D}_*(\mathbf{z}_{ij}+\mathbf{z}_{il})/2}(\mathbf{z}_{ij} + \mathbf{z}_{il}) \otimes (\mathbf{z}_{ij} + \mathbf{z}_{il})$$

$$- \frac{1}{2} \mathcal{D}_+ e^{\boldsymbol{\beta}'(\mathbf{x}_{ij}+\mathbf{x}_{il}) + \mathbf{z}_{ij}'\mathbf{D}_*\mathbf{z}_{ij}/2 + \mathbf{z}_{il}'\mathbf{D}_*\mathbf{z}_{il}/2}[\mathbf{z}_{ij} \otimes \mathbf{z}_{ij} - \mathbf{z}_{il} \otimes \mathbf{z}_{il}],$$

where $\mathcal{D}_+$ is a duplication matrix, $\mathrm{vech}(\mathbf{D}_*) = \mathcal{D}_+ \mathrm{vec}(\mathbf{D}_*)$. The Gauss–Newton (GN) iterations are

$$\mathbf{d}_{*,s+1} = \mathbf{d}_{*s} + \left(\sum \mathbf{K}_i' \mathbf{K}_i\right)^{-1} \sum \mathbf{K}_i'[(\mathbf{e}_i \otimes \mathbf{e}_i) - \mathbf{v}_i]. \tag{7.150}$$

This update does not guarantee that the covariance matrix $\mathbf{D}_*$ will be positive definite at each iteration. To make it nonnegative definite, one can apply the projection operator as for the linear mixed effects model in Section 2.15.2. We let $\mathbf{D}_* = \mathbf{P}\mathbf{\Lambda}_+\mathbf{P}'$, where $\mathbf{P}$ is the $k \times k$ matrix of eigenvectors and $\mathbf{\Lambda}_+$ is the diagonal matrix of eigenvalues with the negative values replaced by zero. The estimation procedure involves alternation between estimating equation (7.118) and iterations (7.150).

Total GEE

Since for Poisson regression with normally distributed random effects, the marginal mean and covariance can be computed exactly we may use total GEE, Section 6.4. We notice that the Poisson model with normally distributed effects is a type III nonlinear marginal model (6.37), where $\boldsymbol{\theta}$ is the $(m + k(k+1)/2)$-dimensional parameter, which includes the beta coefficients and unique elements of matrix $\mathbf{D}_*$. In total GEE, beta coefficients and matrix $\mathbf{D}$ are found simultaneously. Since observations between clusters are independent, the estimating equation for $\boldsymbol{\theta} = (\boldsymbol{\beta}, \mathrm{vec}(\mathbf{D}_*))$ takes the form (6.50). Here, in the previous notation,

$$\mathbf{F}_i = \left[\begin{array}{cc} \frac{\partial \mathbf{f}_i}{\partial \boldsymbol{\beta}} & \frac{\partial \mathbf{f}_i}{\partial \mathbf{d}_*} \end{array} \right], \quad \mathbf{G}_i = \left[\begin{array}{cc} \frac{\partial \mathbf{v}_i}{\partial \boldsymbol{\beta}} & \mathbf{K}_i \end{array} \right]$$

are the $n_i \times (m+k^2)$ and $n_i^2 \times (m+k^2)$ matrices, where $\mathbf{f}_i = \{e^{\boldsymbol{\beta}'\mathbf{x}_{ij}+v_{ijj}}, j = 1, ..., n_i\}$ is the marginal mean, an $n_i \times 1$ vector. It is easy to find that

$$\frac{\partial \mathbf{f}_i}{\partial \boldsymbol{\beta}} = \mathbf{X}_i\mathbf{f}_i, \quad \frac{\partial f_{ij}}{\partial \mathbf{d}_*} = \frac{1}{2}f_{ij}(\mathbf{z}'_{ij} \otimes \mathbf{z}'_{ij}), \quad \frac{\partial V_{ijk}}{\partial \boldsymbol{\beta}} = (\mathbf{x}_{ij} + \mathbf{x}_{ik})V_{ijk}.$$

The solution to total GEE is found iteratively in (6.49), where matrices $\mathbf{P}$ and $\mathbf{Q}$ are defined by (6.51).

7.7.5   Homogeneity tests

The homogeneity tests developed earlier for models with random intercepts can easily be generalized to mixed models with multivariate random effects. The F-test (3.42) for $H_0 : \mathbf{D} = \mathbf{0}$, after replacing sum of squares S by $-2l$, transforms into

$$\frac{(l_{\max} - l_0)/(r - m)}{l_{\max}/(N_T - r)} \simeq F(r - m, N_T - r),$$

where r is the rank of matrix (2.34), l_0 is the maximum of the standard log-likelihood, and $l_{\max}$ is the maximum of the log-likelihood, treating $\mathbf{b}_{ij}$ as fixed parameters. For example, if $m = k$ and $\mathbf{x}_{ij} = \mathbf{z}_{ij}$, we have $r = Nm$. Theoretically, one may apply this test to an individual random effect $H_0 : D_{ll} = 0$ with the linear predictor $\mathbf{x}'_{ij}\boldsymbol{\beta}+b_{il}z_{ijl}$, but this would not imply positive definiteness of matrix $\mathbf{D}$ in the multivariate random effect model. Bonferroni adjustment can be used to account for multiple comparisons.

Alternatively, we can apply the score test. Particularly useful is its application to individual test $D_{ll} = 0$. The respective generalization of the random intercept model is straightforward. For example, for logistic regression, we have

$$S = \sum_{i=1}^{N} \left[\left(\sum_{j=1}^{n} z_{ij} \left(y_{ij} - \widehat{p}_{ij} \right) \right)^2 - \sum_{j=1}^{n_i} \widehat{p}_{ij} (1 - \widehat{p}_{ij}) z_{ij}^2 \right]$$

with the asymptotic variance

$$\sum_{i=1}^{N} \left[2 \left(\sum_{j=1}^{n} z_{ij}^2 \widehat{p}_{ij} (1 - \widehat{p}_{ij}) \right)^2 + \sum_{j=1}^{n} z_{ij}^4 (\widehat{p}_{ij} - 6\widehat{p}_{ij}^2 + 12\widehat{p}_{ij}^3 - 6\widehat{p}_{ij}^4) \right].$$

It is straightforward to generalize this test to probit or Poisson regression.

Problems for Section 7.7

1. Derive approximation (7.131) using the fact that $\int_{R^k} \exp(-\mathbf{x}'\mathbf{A}\mathbf{x})d\mathbf{x} = (2\pi)^{k/2}$ $\times \sqrt{|\mathbf{A}|}$, where $\mathbf{A}$ is a $k \times k$ positive definite matrix.

2. Derive approximation (7.132).

3. Prove that integrals and matrices of integrals, $I_{i1}, \mathbf{I}_{i2}$, and $\mathbf{I}_{i3}$ from Section 7.7.2 exist.

4*. Prove that matrix $\sum \mathbf{I}_{i2} I_{i1}^{-1}$ is positive definite, so that matrix $\mathbf{D}_-$ is positive definite. Develop a matrix FP algorithm, $\mathbf{D}_- = N(\sum \mathbf{I}_{i2} I_{i1}^{-1})^{-1}$ for logistic regression. Consult Section 13.3.4.

5. Prove that matrix $\mathbf{G}_i$ given by formula (7.138) is nonnegative definite. Prove that $\mathbf{G}_i$ is positive definite if matrix $\mathbf{Z}_i$ has full rank.

6*. Analyze convergency properties of the FP algorithm (7.140): Prove that iterations converge for $k = 1$ and provide some evidence that they converge for $k > 1$ (consult Section 13.3.4).

7*. Write an R function that implements the penalized quasi-likelihood algorithm for logistic regression with multiple random effects by means of iterations (7.143) and (7.144). Compare its performance with that of `glmmPQL`.

8*. Write an R function that implements the two-probit approximation for logistic regression with multiple random effects and compare it with `glmmPQL`.

9*. Use simulations to test whether D_* can be estimated consistently by the standard Poisson regression if only the slope is random as in the example in Section 7.7.4. Compute the MSE with increasing N. Generalize this idea when both intercept and slope are random.

10*. Write an R function to estimate the Poisson model with multiple random effects using a GEE approach with exact covariance matrix (exact GEE). Test this code via simulations.

11*. Generalize the score homogeneity test for probit and Poisson GLMMs with multiple random effects. Estimate the power of the test via simulations.

12*. Approximate the power of the homogeneity test from Section 7.7.5 based on the noncentral chi-square distribution.

7.8   GLMM and simulation methods

In this section we introduce the generalized linear mixed model (GLMM) via the exponential family distribution, as authors typically do. Although such a description unifies the logistic and Poisson models under one umbrella, the specificity of the models is lost. As we have demonstrated in this chapter, dealing with these models separately allows us to construct more efficient algorithms for statistical estimation and inference. Also, some important models, such as probit, are not members of the exponential family and require separate treatment anyway.

In this section we focus on approximations to maximum likelihood by statistical simulations (Monte Carlo). First, we introduce the GLMM via the exponential family distribution. Second, we briefly overview familiar Monte Carlo methods. Third, a novel and simple fixed simulation approach is introduced.

7.8.1   General form of GLMM via the exponential family

The logistic and Poisson models discussed in this chapter, and many others, can be derived from an exponential family distribution of the form

$$f(y; \theta, \phi) = \exp\left[\frac{\theta y - b(\theta)}{\phi} - c(y, \phi)\right], \tag{7.151}$$

where θ and ϕ are parameters. McCullagh and Nelder (1989) use (7.151) to consistently treat different members of this distribution family and respective GLM. Bickel and Doksum (2001) use this distribution as a platform for general statistical inference. Distribution (7.151) is very flexible and can specify continuous, binary, or count data. The first derivative of function b is the mean, $b'(\theta) = \mu$, and the second derivative is the variance, $b''(\theta) =$ var. Parameter θ is called the linear predictor and ϕ the scale parameter. In most cases of the generalized linear model, the variance is a simple function of the mean. For example, for binary data, var$= \mu(1 - \mu)$ and for count Poisson data, var$= \mu$. For these models, $\phi = 1$ and distribution (7.151) simplifies to $f(y; \theta) = e^{\theta y - b(\theta) - c(y)}$. For example, for logistic regression, $\theta = \beta x$, $b(\theta) = \ln(1 + e^\theta)$, and $c = 0$. For Poisson regression, $\theta = \beta x$, $b(\theta) = e^\theta$, and $c = -\ln y!$. The GLM with independent $\{y_i\}$ is specified by (7.151) with $\theta_i = \boldsymbol{\beta}'\mathbf{x}_i$.

For cluster data $\{y_{ij}\}$, assuming that $y_{ij}|\mathbf{u}_i$ are independent and following the exponential family distribution with the unit scale, where $\mathbf{u}_i$ is a normally distributed k-dimensional random effect, $\mathbf{u}_i \sim \mathcal{N}(\mathbf{0}, \mathbf{D}_*)$, the log-likelihood for the GLMM takes the form

$$l(\boldsymbol{\beta}, \mathbf{D}_*) = -\frac{Nk}{2}\ln(2\pi) - \frac{N}{2}\ln|\mathbf{D}_*| + \sum_{i=1}^N \ln \int_{R^k} e^{l_i(\boldsymbol{\beta}, \mathbf{u}) - \frac{1}{2}\mathbf{u}'\mathbf{D}_*^{-1}\mathbf{u}} d\mathbf{u}, \tag{7.152}$$

where

$$l_i(\boldsymbol{\beta}, \mathbf{u}) = \sum_{j=1}^{n_i}\left[(\boldsymbol{\beta}'\mathbf{x}_{ij} + \mathbf{u}'\mathbf{z}_{ij})y_{ij} - b(\boldsymbol{\beta}'\mathbf{x}_{ij} + \mathbf{u}'\mathbf{z}_{ij})\right]$$

is the ith conditional log-likelihood (the term $c(y)$ is omitted because it does not affect the likelihood maximization). It follows from GLM theory that conditionally,

$E(\mathbf{y}_i|\mathbf{u}) = b'(\boldsymbol{\beta}'\mathbf{x}_{ij} + \mathbf{u}'\mathbf{z}_{ij})$ and $\mathrm{var}(\mathbf{y}_i|\mathbf{u}) = b''(\boldsymbol{\beta}'\mathbf{x}_{ij} + \mathbf{u}'\mathbf{z}_{ij})$. It is easy to see that (7.133) is a special case of (7.152) after the precision matrix reparameterization $\mathbf{D}_- = \mathbf{D}_*^{-1}$.

It is straightforward to derive maximum likelihood, Laplace, and penalized quasi-likelihood methods of estimation for (7.152). However, since the most popular types of models, such as logit, probit, and Poisson, have already been covered, we skip this exercise.

7.8.2 Monte Carlo for ML

Only maximum likelihood is consistent when the number of clusters, N, goes to infinity and the number of observations per cluster, n_i, is finite. Unfortunately, the majority of approximate methods, such as Laplace or quasi-likelihood, require that both N and n_i go to infinity. This amplifies the need for ML despite its required integration. Another important argument in favor of ML is that it generates an estimate of the complete (beta coefficients plus variance parameters) asymptotic covariance matrix as the inverse of the information matrix. Methods of numerical integration for ML were discussed previously in Section 7.3.1; here we just provide some references to a well-developed area of the likelihood approximation via statistical simulations. There is extensive literature on the application of Monte Carlo methods to GLMM estimation. Simulation methods can work in conjunction with any optimization algorithm, such as Newton–Raphson, Fisher scoring or Expectation-Maximization (EM), although the latter is more popular, McCulloch (1997). Concise introductions have been provided by Fahrmeir and Tutz (2001), Agresti (2002), and McCulloch and Searle (2001). Markov Chain Monte Carlo (MCMC) methods of statistical simulation have become especially popular (Robert and Casella, 1999). Below we suggest a simulation method in which the sample does not change over maximization.

7.8.3 Fixed sample likelihood approach

In this section we generalize the approach of maximum likelihood approximation developed in Section 7.3.2 for binary models with random intercepts to multivariate random effects. The Fixed Sample Likelihood (FSL) approach combines Monte Carlo simulation and numerical integration under one scheme. The idea is to replace the integral with a weighted sum at fixed sampled values of the random effects and then treat that sum as a new likelihood function. The basis for this approximation is the observation that (a) all algorithms of numerical integration and Monte Carlo simulation attempt approximating the integral via a sum of the integrand computed at certain values with certain weights, and (b) beta coefficients and variance parameters can be combined into one parameter vector. Several authors applied technique similar to Gauss–Hermite quadrature. For example, Pinheiro and Bates (1995) applied this approach to the general nonlinear mixed effects model and Hedeker (2003) applied it to multinomial logistic regression with random effects. The FSL approach combines Gauss–Hermite quadrature and Monte Carlo under one methodological umbrella. For traditional approximations in the framework of GLMM estimation, such as Laplace approximation or Gauss–Hermite quadrature, we refer the reader to books by Vonesh (1997, 2012), Pinhero and Bates (2000).

We start by reparameterizing the log-likelihood function (7.152) in a slightly different manner as

$$l(\boldsymbol{\beta}, \mathbf{D}_c) = \sum_{i=1}^{N} \ln \frac{1}{(2\pi)^{k/2}} \int_{R^k} e^{\sum_{j=1}^{n_i} l(\boldsymbol{\beta}'\mathbf{x}_{ij} + \mathbf{z}_{ij}'\mathbf{D}_c'\mathbf{u})} e^{-\frac{1}{2}\|\mathbf{u}\|^2} d\mathbf{u}, \qquad (7.153)$$

where $\mathbf{D}_c$ is the $k \times k$ upper-triangular Cholesky decomposition factor (all elements of $\mathbf{D}_c$ below diagonal are zero), such that $\mathbf{D}_c'\mathbf{D}_c = \mathbf{D}_*$ and $\mathbf{u} \sim \mathcal{N}(\mathbf{0}, \mathbf{I})$. (Some authors assume $\mathbf{D}_c$ to be a lower-triangular matrix, then $\mathbf{D}_c\mathbf{D}_c' = \mathbf{D}_*$.) The advantage of (7.153) is that $\mathbf{u}$ does not depend on $\mathbf{D}$ and has fixed distribution. Furthermore, we represent the quantity $\mathbf{z}_{ij}'\mathbf{D}_c'\mathbf{u} = \sum_{l' \geq l} D_{cll'} z_{ijl} u_{l'}$ in such a way that $D_{cll'}$ can be treated as a coefficient at variable $z_{ijl} u_{l'}$. Then the vector $\boldsymbol{\beta}$ and nonzero elements of matrix $\mathbf{D}_c$ can be combined into one parameter vector. Specifically, let $\boldsymbol{\delta}$ be the $k(k+1)/2 \times 1$ vector of nonzero elements of $\mathbf{D}_c$ and $\mathbf{t}_{ij}$ be the $k(k+1)/2 \times 1$ vector with components $\{z_{ijl} u_{l'}\}$. Then introducing a vector of parameters $\boldsymbol{\theta} = (\boldsymbol{\beta}', \boldsymbol{\delta}')'$ and variables $\mathbf{g}_{ij} = (\mathbf{x}_{ij}', \mathbf{t}_{ij}')'$, we express the fixed and random parts as a linear combination, $\boldsymbol{\beta}'\mathbf{x}_{ij} + (\mathbf{D}_c\mathbf{z}_{ij})'\mathbf{u} = \boldsymbol{\theta}'\mathbf{g}_{ij}$. Thus, (7.153) simplifies to

$$l(\boldsymbol{\theta}) = \sum_{i=1}^{N} \ln \frac{1}{(2\pi)^{k/2}} \int_{R^k} e^{\sum_{j=1}^{n_i} l(\boldsymbol{\theta}'\mathbf{g}_{ij})} e^{-\frac{1}{2}\|\mathbf{u}\|^2} d\mathbf{u}, \qquad (7.154)$$

where the $(m + k(k+1)/2)$-dimensional vector $\mathbf{g}_{ij}$ does not contain unknown parameters.

Now we obtain a discretized version of (7.154), assuming that there exists a representative sample $\{\mathbf{u}_1, \mathbf{u}_2, ..., \mathbf{u}_S\}$ with weights $\{w_1, w_2, ..., w_S\}$. For example, if a statistical simulation is used, $\mathbf{u}_s$ is drawn randomly from $\mathcal{N}(\mathbf{0}, \mathbf{I})$ and the weight is $w_s = 1/S$. After replacing the integral in (7.154) by the weighted sum, we arrive at the discretized version of the log-likelihood function,

$$l_{FSL}(\boldsymbol{\theta}) = \sum_{i=1}^{N} \ln \sum_{s=1}^{S} w_s e^{\sum_{j=1}^{n_i} l_{ijs}(\boldsymbol{\theta})}, \qquad (7.155)$$

where $\mathbf{g}_{ijs} = (\mathbf{x}_{ij}', \mathbf{t}_{ijs}')'$ and $\mathbf{t}_{ijs}$ is the $k(k+1)/2 \times 1$ vector with components $\{z_{ijl} u_{l's}, l' \geq l\}$. Importantly, values $\{u_{l's}\}$ do not change with i or during iterations, so vectors $\{\mathbf{g}_{ijs}\}$ remain fixed. We treat l_{FSL} as a log-likelihood function. The formulas for the first derivatives (7.74) and the negative Hessian (7.75) remain unchanged and the Newton–Raphson algorithm has the same form, (7.77). Empirical FS algorithm is readily applied—this algorithm was used by Hedeker (2003). During maximization, we do not impose any restrictions on matrix $\mathbf{D}_c$ and the respective vector $\boldsymbol{\theta}$. After iterations are done, we estimate the covariance matrix as $\widehat{\mathbf{D}}_* = \widehat{\mathbf{D}}_c'\widehat{\mathbf{D}}_c$, which is a nonnegative definite matrix. We can test the presence of the random effects via the hypothesis $H_0 : D_{cll} = 0$ by the one-sided Wald test.

Table 7.2. Simulation results for logistic regression with random intercepts

Method	%Bias $\beta_2 = -1$	%RMSE	%Bias $\sigma^2 = 1$	%RMSE	Computation time, seconds
ML	-0.09	0.083	-0.52	32.2	755
FSL MC500	-0.74	0.083	1.12	32.2	50
FSL GH11	-0.77	0.083	1.05	31.2	33

Now we discuss how to use the Gauss–Hermite (GH) abscissas and weights in the framework of the FSL approach. Let K be the number of abscissas chosen, say $K = 11$ (see Table 7.1 in Section 7.1.2). First, one needs to rescale the abscissas and weights, multiplying them by $\sqrt{2}$ and $\pi^{-1/2}$, respectively. Let $\{u_1, u_2, ..., u_K\}$ be the set of resulting abscissas. We construct k-dimensional vectors $\mathbf{u}_s = (u_{s_1}, u_{s_2}, ..., u_{s_k})'$ by choosing the number of all possible samples from the index set $\{1, 2, ..., K\}$. The associated weight is the product of weights, $w_s = \prod_{h=1}^{k} w_{s_h}$. Clearly, the number of all vectors $\mathbf{u}_s$ is $S = K^k$. For example, if the number of random effects is three, then $S = 11^3 = 1331$. Although S increases exponentially with the number of random effects, practically, the number of random effects rarely exceeds five, so that modern computers can handle the computations. One may suggest an economical version of multivariate GH procedure by eliminating points where w_s is greater than a small number. For example, S decreases from 1331 to 425 if we take points where $w_s > 10^{-6}$.

The FSL approach can be applied to any link function and even nonnormal errors. For example, a robust GLMM model can be estimated assuming that random effects follow a double-exponential distribution, see Section 4.4 and Section 5.1.5. We illustrate this feature by logistic regression with random intercepts. If u has density $e^{-|u|/\sqrt{2}}/\sqrt{2}$, then $E(u) = 0$ and $\text{var}(u) = 1$. Generating $\{u_s\}$ from this distribution and maximizing (7.155) would be equivalent to assuming that intercepts follow a double–exponential distribution that allows outliers (large intercepts).

We show simulation results in Table 7.2 and Figure 7.9, where FSL is compared to ML for logistic regression with random intercepts (number of experiments = 100). The true beta parameters were $\beta_1 = 1$ (population-averaged intercept) and $\beta_2 = -1$ (slope) with SD intercept $\sigma = 1$. The statistical model has the form $\text{logit}(\mathbf{y}_i|u_i) = (\beta_1 + u_i) + \beta_2 \mathbf{x}_i$ with the covariate vector $\mathbf{x}_i = (1, 2, ..., n_i)'$ and $b_i \sim \mathcal{N}(0, \sigma^2)$. The number of clusters is $N = 200$, with the number of observations per cluster, n_i, ranging from 5 to 15. Maximum likelihood (ML) used the R function integrate to evaluate integrals (7.67) with the machine epsilon precision based on the adaptive 15-point Gauss–Kronrod quadrature algorithm. To maximize the log-likelihood function, the empirical FS algorithm was used, Section 7.3.1. The FSL Monte Carlo used $S = 100$ and $S = 500$. In Table 7.2 three methods are compared in terms of the quality of slope and variance estimation. FSL GH11 uses Gauss–Hermite sample with 11 abscissas. All three algorithms gave close results, and estimates of β and σ^2 were practically unbiased. Root MSE assesses the standard error of estimates in 100 experiments. Notice that while the slope is estimated very well, the estimates of σ^2 vary substantially, but in terms of methods there is almost no difference. However, in terms of the time of computation, methods differ substantially. Not surprisingly, Gauss–Hermite requires less time because the

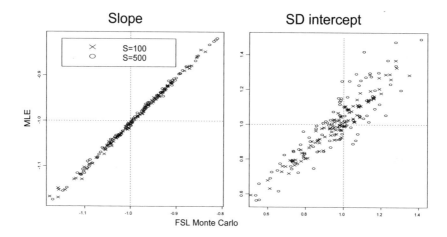

FIGURE 7.9. Scatter plot MLE versus FSL Monte Carlo ($S = 100$ and $S = 500$) for logistic regression with random intercepts.

sample size is 11 versus 500. Estimation by the straightforward ML is very slow because at each iteration it evaluates $200 \times 4 = 800$ integrals. It was more than 20 times slower than the FSL Gauss–Hermite algorithm. As the reader can see from the scatter plot, the correlation between FSL and ML is very high, especially for the slope.

The random effects can be estimated either after Laplace approximation from the penalized log-likelihood (7.135) or using the FSL/integration technique, see Section 8.15 for details. We shall apply the FSL approach to the general nonlinear mixed model in Section 8.14 as well.

Problems for Section 7.8

1. Derive log-likelihoods for the logistic and Poisson models with random intercepts as special cases using the general expression (7.153).

2. Estimate the log-likelihood function value (7.153) for a linear model by Monte Carlo methods by replacing the integral with the mean over simulated $\{\mathbf{u}_s, s = 1, ..., S\}$. Plot the result versus the number of simulations (S) and compare with the exact value (plot as a horizontal line). Can you see the convergence?

3*. Repeat the comparison as displayed in Figure 7.9 for the probit link (you have to use the FSL code in Problem 5 of Section 7.4).

7.9   GEE for clustered marginal GLM

There are two ways to model clustered data: conditional and marginal. The conditional approach based on random effects was discussed in great detail previously. To obtain the marginal mean, random effects should be integrated out. Here we discuss application of the marginal approach to model discrete (binary or count) data in the framework of the generalized linear model (GLM). In this approach, the GLM for clustered data is defined directly through its marginal mean, so no integration is required. Besides the mean, the within-cluster covariance structure should be specified (note that in the conditional approach, it is derived from the model). However, specification of the covariance structure for clustered data in the marginal approach is of secondary importance because it does not affect the unbiasedness of the estimating equation. Marginal models for continuous data were studied in the previous chapter; thus, some techniques and methods may be borrowed.

The centerpiece of the marginal GLM is the Generalized Estimating Equations (GEE) approach. Let us have clustered observations $\{y_{ij}, i = 1, ..., N, j = 1, ..., n_i\}$ with the first two moments defined as $E(y_{ij}) = \mu(\boldsymbol{\beta}'\mathbf{x}_{ij})$ and $\text{var}(y_{ij}) = v(\boldsymbol{\beta}'\mathbf{x}_{ij})$, where μ and ν are known functions. The marginal mean of y_{ij} is specified explicitly in the GEE approach. In many instances, repeated measurements (indexed by j) are associated with time—then we have longitudinal data. For a GLM, v is a function of μ. For example, for a binary model, $v = \mu(1 - \mu)$, and for a Poisson model, $v = \mu$. It is assumed that observations between clusters are independent, but within clusters are dependent, so one speaks of intracluster correlation. Indeed, we may ignore the intracluster correlation and still obtain consistent and asymptotically normally distributed estimates of $\boldsymbol{\beta}$ using the ordinary estimating equation

$$\sum_{i=1}^{N}\sum_{j=1}^{n_i}(y_{ij} - \mu_{ij})\frac{\mu_{ij}'}{v_{ij}}\mathbf{x}_{ij} = \mathbf{0} \tag{7.156}$$

as a straightforward generalization of (9.34). The consistency comes from the fact that $E(y_{ij} - \mu_{ij}) = 0$, and therefore (7.156) is an unbiased estimating equation, see Appendix 13.1.4. Here "asymptotic" means increasing N to infinity while $\{n_i\}$ may stay bounded.

However, to improve efficiency, one needs to account for intracluster correlation and therefore to specify the covariance matrix of $(y_{i1}, ..., y_{in_i})$ for each cluster $i = 1, ..., N$. Zeger and Liang (1986) and Liang and Zeger (1986) suggested specifying the covariance matrix via a *working* correlation matrix, the central concept of GEE for clustered data. Since then, this approach has gained much popularity, due to its convenience and algorithmic simplicity. If $\mathbf{R}_i$ is an $n_i \times n_i$ correlation matrix, $\mathbf{V}_i = \mathbf{D}_i^{1/2}\mathbf{R}_i\mathbf{D}_i^{1/2}$ is the covariance matrix for the $n_i \times 1$ vector $\mathbf{y}_i = (y_{i1}, ..., y_{in_i})'$, where $\mathbf{D}_i = \mathbf{D}_i(\boldsymbol{\beta})$ is a known function of $\boldsymbol{\beta}$, the diagonal matrix, $\text{diag}(v_{i1}, ..., v_{in_i})$. The elements of matrices $\mathbf{R}_i$ are usually connected through a low-dimension parameter vector, because otherwise, the number of unknown elements would be $\sum n_i(n_i - 1)/2$. More precisely, let us assume that the elements of $\mathbf{R}_i$ are known functions of a p-dimensional parameter $\boldsymbol{\gamma}$. For example, in a popular exchangeable (compound symmetry) correlation structure, all elements except the diagonal are $\gamma =$const. Finally, in vector notation, the clustered marginal GLM can be written as

$$E(\mathbf{y}_i) = \mu(\mathbf{X}_i\boldsymbol{\beta}), \quad \text{cov}(\mathbf{y}_i) \simeq \mathbf{V}_i = \mathbf{D}_i^{1/2}\mathbf{R}_i(\boldsymbol{\gamma})\mathbf{D}_i^{1/2}, \tag{7.157}$$

where $\mathbf{X}_i$ is an $n_i \times m$ matrix with a jth row $\mathbf{x}_{ij}$. We use "$\simeq$" to indicate that this is an approximation to the covariance matrix because $\mathbf{R}_i$ may not be the exact correlation matrix. Unlike the conditional/random effects model considered above, the distribution of $\mathbf{y}_i$ is unspecified. Moreover, the true covariance matrix of $\mathbf{y}_i$ may be different from what is assumed at the right-hand side of (7.157). An obvious modification of the estimating equation (7.156) to account for the intracluster correlation is

$$\sum_{i=1}^{N} \mathbf{X}'_i \dot{\boldsymbol{\mu}}_i \mathbf{V}_i^{-1}(\mathbf{y}_i - \boldsymbol{\mu}_i) = \mathbf{0}, \qquad (7.158)$$

where $\dot{\boldsymbol{\mu}}_i$ is an $n_i \times n_i$ diagonal matrix with $\dot{\mu}(\boldsymbol{\beta}'\mathbf{x}_{ij})$ on the diagonal. Clearly, (7.158) takes the form (7.156) under independence, $\mathbf{R}_i = \mathbf{I}_i$. In fact, we have used a special form of this estimating equation for the probit (7.99) and Poisson (7.118) mixed models. A distinctive feature of the GEE approach is that (a) no distribution is specified, and (b) the correlation matrix need not coincide with the true one. Therefore, sometimes (7.158) is viewed as a quasi-likelihood approach where a complete data distribution/statistical model is not specified. For a general discussion of the estimating equations approach, we refer the reader to Appendix 13.1.4.

According to our classification of nonlinear marginal models of Chapter 6, assuming that matrix $\mathbf{V}_i$ is a correct covariance matrix, model (7.157) is a type II nonlinear marginal model (6.36). As follows from Section 6.2.3, iteratively reweighted least squares (IRLS) leads to consistent and asymptotically normally distributed estimates. More precisely, from the sandwich formula, the GEE estimator from (7.158) is consistent and asymptotically normally distributed with the covariance matrix

$$\mathrm{cov}(\widehat{\boldsymbol{\beta}}_{GEE}) = \mathbf{M}^{-1} \left(\sum_{i=1}^{N} \mathbf{X}'_i \dot{\boldsymbol{\mu}}_i \mathbf{V}_i^{-1} \mathbf{V}_{Ti} \mathbf{V}_i^{-1} \dot{\boldsymbol{\mu}}_i \mathbf{X}_i \right) \mathbf{M}^{-1},$$

where $\mathbf{M} = \sum_{i=1}^{N} \mathbf{X}'_i \dot{\boldsymbol{\mu}}_i \mathbf{V}_i^{-1} \dot{\boldsymbol{\mu}}_i \mathbf{X}_i$ and $\mathbf{V}_{Ti} = \mathrm{cov}(\mathbf{y}_i)$ is the true covariance matrix. If $\mathbf{R}_i$ is guessed correctly, GEE produces asymptotically efficient estimates. In a robust or empirical version, the true covariance matrix is approximated by $\mathbf{V}_{Ti} \simeq (\mathbf{y}_i - \widehat{\boldsymbol{\mu}}_i)(\mathbf{y}_i - \widehat{\boldsymbol{\mu}}_i)'$. See Appendix 13.1.5 for a general discussion of the GEE approach.

The estimation algorithm alternates between $\boldsymbol{\beta}$ estimation from GEE (7.158) and $\boldsymbol{\gamma}$ estimation. When $\boldsymbol{\gamma}$ is held fixed, we iterate

$$\boldsymbol{\beta}_{s+1} = \boldsymbol{\beta}_s + \left(\sum_{i=1}^{N} \mathbf{X}'_i \dot{\boldsymbol{\mu}}_i \mathbf{V}_i^{-1} \dot{\boldsymbol{\mu}}_i \mathbf{X}_i \right)^{-1} \sum_{i=1}^{N} \mathbf{X}'_i \dot{\boldsymbol{\mu}}_i \mathbf{V}_i^{-1} (\mathbf{y}_i - \boldsymbol{\mu}_i). \qquad (7.159)$$

Methods of $\boldsymbol{\gamma}$ estimation when $\boldsymbol{\beta}$ is held fixed are discussed below. The criteria for convergence are discussed in Appendix 13.3.5.

7.9.1 Variance least squares

To estimate variance parameters $\boldsymbol{\gamma}$, we suggest using Variance Least Squares (VLS). This method was introduced in the framework of the linear mixed effects model in Section 3.12 and is used in this chapter to estimate the overdispersion parameter for clustered Poisson regression with random intercepts and for general random effects (7.149). Following the idea of VLS in model (7.157), at each iteration we compute the $n_i \times 1$ residual vector $\widehat{\mathbf{e}}_i = \mathbf{y}_i - \mu(\mathbf{X}_i \widehat{\boldsymbol{\beta}})$ and the $n_i \times n_i$ diagonal variance matrix $\mathbf{D}_i$. Then we minimize the total sum of squared differences between the empirical and theoretical matrices,

$$\sum_{i=1}^{N} \mathrm{tr} \left(\widehat{\mathbf{e}}_i \widehat{\mathbf{e}}'_i - \mathbf{D}_i^{1/2} \mathbf{R}_i(\boldsymbol{\gamma}) \mathbf{D}_i^{1/2} \right)^2. \qquad (7.160)$$

Denoting $\mathbf{r}_i = \text{vec}(\mathbf{R}_i)$, an $n_i^2 \times 1$ vector and $\mathbf{G}_i = \partial \mathbf{r}_i/\partial \boldsymbol{\gamma}$, an $n_i^2 \times p$ matrix, the estimating equation for $\boldsymbol{\gamma}$ in matrix form can be written as

$$\sum_{i=1}^{N} \mathbf{G}_i'(\boldsymbol{\gamma})(\mathbf{D}_i^{1/2} \otimes \mathbf{D}_i^{1/2})\text{vec}\left(\widehat{\mathbf{e}}_i\widehat{\mathbf{e}}_i' - \mathbf{D}_i^{1/2}\mathbf{R}_i(\boldsymbol{\gamma})\mathbf{D}_i^{1/2}\right) = \mathbf{0}, \qquad (7.161)$$

with the Gauss–Newton iterations

$$\boldsymbol{\gamma}_{s+1} = \boldsymbol{\gamma}_s + \left(\sum_{i=1}^{N} \mathbf{G}_{is}'(\mathbf{D}_i^{1/2} \otimes \mathbf{D}_i^{1/2})\mathbf{G}_{is}\right)^{-1} \qquad (7.162)$$

$$\times \sum_{i=1}^{N} \mathbf{G}_{is}'(\mathbf{D}_i^{1/2} \otimes \mathbf{D}_i^{1/2})\text{vec}\left(\widehat{\mathbf{e}}_i\widehat{\mathbf{e}}_i' - \mathbf{D}_i^{1/2}\mathbf{R}_{is}\mathbf{D}_i^{1/2}\right),$$

where $\mathbf{R}_{is} = \mathbf{R}_i(\boldsymbol{\gamma}_s)$ and $\mathbf{G}_{is} = \mathbf{G}_i(\boldsymbol{\gamma}_s)$. Obviously, if $\mathbf{R}_i$ is a linear function of $\boldsymbol{\gamma}$, iterations (7.162) converge at the first iteration. The advantage of VLS and iterative formula (7.162) is that they may be applied to any correlation structure $\mathbf{R}_i(\boldsymbol{\gamma})$ such as $MA(1)$ or $AR(1)$, see below and Section 4.3.4. We illustrate the VLS approach with some popular correlation structures.

There are alternative methods of $\boldsymbol{\gamma}$ estimation. For example, Chaganty (1997) used quasi-least squares; a detailed analysis of different methods of estimation is presented by Wang and Carey (2003). Although quasi-least squares is similar to variance least squares, it works with standardized residuals, $\mathbf{D}_i^{-1/2}\widehat{\mathbf{e}}_i$. We assert that such standardization may be a source of instability (see a more detailed explanation below).

Exchangeable correlation structure

For this structure, it is assumed that the correlation between observations of the same cluster is constant, ρ. Then the correlation matrix can be expressed as $\mathbf{R}_i = (1-\rho)\mathbf{I}_i + \rho\mathbf{1}_i\mathbf{1}_i'$, where $\mathbf{I}_i$ is the $n_i \times n_i$ identity matrix and $\mathbf{1}_i$ is the $n_i \times 1$ unit vector. Then letting $s_{ij} = \sqrt{D_{ijj}}$, the estimating equation (7.161) takes the form

$$\sum \text{tr}[(\widehat{\mathbf{e}}_i\widehat{\mathbf{e}}_i' - \mathbf{D}_i^{1/2}\mathbf{R}_i\mathbf{D}_i^{1/2})\mathbf{D}_i^{1/2}(\mathbf{1}_i\mathbf{1}_i' - \mathbf{I}_i)\mathbf{D}_i^{1/2}]$$

$$= \sum \left[\left(\sum \widehat{e}_{ij}s_{ij}\right)^2 - \sum \widehat{e}_{ij}^2 s_{ij}^2\right] - \rho\sum\left[\left(\sum s_{ij}^2\right)^2 - \sum s_{ij}^4\right],$$

which results in

$$\widehat{\rho} = \frac{\sum_{i=1}^{N}\left[\left(\sum_{j=1}^{n_i}\widehat{e}_{ij}s_{ij}\right)^2 - \sum_{j=1}^{n_i}\widehat{e}_{ij}^2 s_{ij}^2\right]}{\sum_{i=1}^{N}\left[\left(\sum_{j=1}^{n_i} s_{ij}^2\right)^2 - \sum_{j=1}^{n_i} s_{ij}^4\right]}. \qquad (7.163)$$

Alternatively, Liang and Zeger (1986) suggested a moment estimator,

$$\widehat{\rho} = \frac{\sum_{i=1}^{N}\sum_{j>l}^{n_i}(\widehat{e}_{ij}/s_{ij})(\widehat{e}_{il}/s_{il})}{0.5\sum_{i=1}^{N} n_i(n_i-1) - m}. \qquad (7.164)$$

These two estimators are closely related. First, the adjustment for the number of covariates, m, has little effect because typically, $0.5 \sum_{i=1}^{N} n_i(n_i - 1)$ is much greater than m. Second, since the numerator of (7.163) is $2 \sum_{i=1}^{N} \sum_{j>l}^{n_i} (e_{ij} s_{ij})(e_{il} s_{il})$, the two estimators differ by weights: In (7.163) the weights are $\{s_{ij}\}$, and in (7.164) the weights are $\{1/s_{ij}\}$, so the $\{\widehat{e}_{ij}/s_{ij}\}$ are standardized residuals. However, we assert that (7.163) is more robust to outliers. Indeed, if s_{ij} is very small but $\widehat{e}_{ij}$ is not that small estimator (7.164) produces an unstable estimate. For example, in logistic regression, this situation may occur when x_{ij} takes a large negative value and $\beta > 0$, so that $s_{ij} = e^{\beta_1/2 + \beta x_{ij}/2}/(1 + e^{\beta_1 + \beta x_{ij}})$ is small but $y_{ij} = 1$ and $\widehat{e}_{ij} \simeq 1$. In summary, standardized residuals may lead to unstable estimation of the correlation coefficient.

Linear correlation structure

In Section 4.3 we considered the covariance matrix as a linear combination of fixed symmetric matrices with constant unknown coefficients. Such structures are very flexible and may describe many correlation models. A particularly parsimonious covariance is generated based on the $MA(1)$ process using Toeplitz matrices of the form (4.115), $\mathbf{R}_i = \mathbf{I}_i + \rho_1 \mathbf{T}_{1i} + \rho_2 \mathbf{T}_{3i}$, where i indicates the dimension of the matrices. Obviously, $\rho_2 = 0$ gives an exchangeable correlation structure. One may derive estimates of ρ_1 and ρ_2 directly from minimization of the sum of squares (7.160), as we did for the exchangeable correlation structure, or using general formula (7.162); again it converges after the first iteration.

7.9.2   Limitations of the GEE approach

The core of the GEE approach (Liang and Zeger, 1986) is the concept of the working correlation matrix. The most frequently used correlation structure for binary clustered data is the exchangeable correlation structure (compound symmetry), which takes roots from the random intercepts model $y_{ij} = \boldsymbol{\beta}' \mathbf{x}_{ij} + \delta_i + \varepsilon_{ij}$, where δ_i is the deviation of the cluster-specific intercept from the population-averaged mean and ε_{ij} is the iid error term. Under normal assumptions, $\varepsilon_{ij} \sim \mathcal{N}(0, \sigma^2)$ and $\delta_i \sim \mathcal{N}(0, \sigma^2 d)$, so that the intracluster correlation coefficient $\rho = d/(1 + d) = \text{const}$. Use of GEE for a linear model with a continuous dependent random variable is difficult to justify because it may be studied more productively in the framework of linear mixed effects. So we concentrate on application of the GEE approach to discrete data and, specifically, to binary data modeled via logistic regression.

The aim of this section is to demonstrate that use of the Pearson correlation coefficient (ρ) for binary data is inadequate and troublesome. It is worthwhile to mention that originally, ρ was suggested to measure the association between continuous random variables. Moreover, major properties of the Pearson correlation coefficient, such as invariance to shifting and scaling, hold only for normally distributed random variables (Kendall and Stuart, 1961; Kagan et al., 1973). Perhaps, it is this property that makes the Pearson correlation coefficient so convenient and important. When the Pearson correlation coefficient is applied to nonnormal random variables, such as Bernoulli or Poisson distribution, it loses this principal property. As such, the entire idea of projecting the theory of multivariate normal distribution to discrete or binary variables through the working correlation matrix seems problematic.

Previous authors also reported limitations of the working correlation matrix approach. For example, Crowder (1995), Sutradhar and Das (1999), and Wang and Carey (2003) studied the impact of the wrong correlation matrix when the intracluster correlation is estimated by the method of moments. It was found that a wrong correlation structure may lead to breakdown of the estimation procedure and substantial loss of efficiency. In particular, if the true correlation structure is exchangeable but the working correlation matrix is $AR(1)$, the method of moments may produce a correlation coefficient estimate outside the interval $(-1, 1)$. In the next subsection we show that the Pearson correlation coefficient between two binary random variables satisfies intrinsic bounds and therefore cannot be modeled separate from the mean as in the GEE approach.

Admissible interval for the Pearson correlation coefficient

We emphasize that the Pearson correlation coefficient between two binary random variables cannot take an arbitrary number from $[-1, 1]$ but lies within certain admissible bounds that depend on the probabilities. Let y_1 and y_2 be two binary random variables and $\Pr(y_j = 1) = p_j$ for $j = 1, 2$. The Pearson correlation coefficient between y_1 and y_2 is given by $\rho = [\Pr(y_j = 1, y_k = 1) - p_j p_k]/\sqrt{p_1(1 - p_1)p_2(1 - p_2)}$. Using the fact that $0 \leq \Pr(y_j = 1, y_k = 1) \leq \min\{p_j, p_k\}$, it is easy to see that

$$-\sqrt{\frac{p_1 p_2}{(1 - p_1)(1 - p_2)}} \leq \rho \leq \min\left\{\sqrt{\frac{p_1(1 - p_2)}{p_2(1 - p_1)}}, \sqrt{\frac{p_2(1 - p_1)}{p_1(1 - p_2)}}\right\}. \tag{7.165}$$

Now we turn our attention to clustered binary data modeled via logistic regression with an exchangeable correlation structure. The response variable is binary $\{y_{ij}, i = 1, ..., N, j = 1, ..., n_i\}$, where i indexes the cluster and j the observation (subject) in cluster i, with the probability $\Pr(y_{ij} = 1) = \exp(\alpha + \boldsymbol{\beta}'\mathbf{x}_{ij})/(1 + \exp(\alpha + \boldsymbol{\beta}'\mathbf{x}_{ij}))$. Letting $p_1 = \exp(\alpha + \boldsymbol{\beta}'\mathbf{x}_{ij})/(1 + \exp(\alpha + \boldsymbol{\beta}'\mathbf{x}_{ij}))$ and $p_2 = \exp(\alpha + \boldsymbol{\beta}'\mathbf{x}_{ik})/(1 + \exp(\alpha + \boldsymbol{\beta}'\mathbf{x}_{ik}))$ from (7.165) and with the general restriction $\rho > -1/(n - 1)$, we obtain an admissible interval for ρ :

$$-\min\left\{\frac{1}{n - 1}, e^{\alpha + 0.5(\mathbf{x}_{ij} + \mathbf{x}_{ik})'\boldsymbol{\beta}}\right\} \leq \rho$$
$$\leq \min\left\{e^{0.5(\mathbf{x}_{ij} - \mathbf{x}_{ik})'\boldsymbol{\beta}}, e^{-0.5(\mathbf{x}_{ij} - \mathbf{x}_{ik})'\boldsymbol{\beta}}\right\}, \tag{7.166}$$

where the minimum is taken over $i = 1, ..., N$ and $j, k = 1, ..., n_i$. A similar but less precise upper bound for ρ is given by Oman and Zucker (2001).

An example of admissible values for the Pearson correlation coefficient as a function of β defined by inequalities (7.166) is shown in Figure 7.10, where $n_i = 10$ and $x_i \sim \mathcal{N}(0, 1)$ with zero intercept, $\alpha = 0$. We emphasize that the upper bound depends on β and x and therefore cannot be constant as in the exchangeable correlation structure. When the total number of observations increases to infinity, the admissible region shrinks to zero because $-1/(n - 1) \to 0$ and $\min e^{\pm 0.5(x_j - x_k)} \to 0$. Consequently, for large cluster size, the only valid exchangeable correlation structure is independent ($\rho = 0$).

Pros and cons of GEE

Positive features of GEE: (a) GEE applies to any GLM, and more generally, any regression model; (b) GEE is robust to specification of the correlation matrix and always produces consistent and asymptotically normally distributed estimates even if the number of observations per cluster is finite; (c) there exists a rich choice of correlation matrices, e.g., to reflect random intercepts or autocorrelation statistical phenomena; (d) the sandwich formula consistently estimates the variances of GEE estimates; and (e) estimation is simple and carried out by IRLS.

Negative features of GEE: (a) this is an estimation method for an unknown statistical model; in particular, there is a problem of generating binary data with specified parameters, covariates and correlation matrix; (b) there is no guarantee that there exists a statistical model that exactly obeys a given specification, and consequently, the correlation matrix can never be guessed correctly.

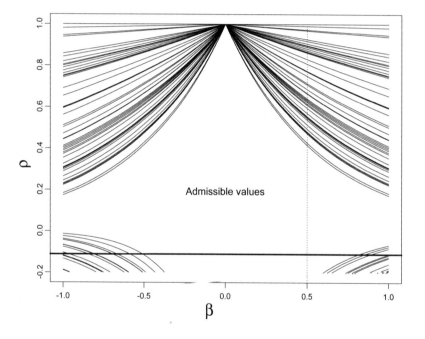

FIGURE 7.10. Admissible values for the Pearson correlation coefficient, ρ, assuming an exchangeable correlation structure with $n = 10$, as defined by inequalities (7.166). The bold horizontal line shows the lower limit $-1/(n-1)$. It is assumed that $x_i \sim \mathcal{N}(\alpha, 1)$, and each curve is defined by $\exp(0.5\beta(x_i - x_j))$ and $\exp(0.5\beta(x_j - x_i))$ for $i, j = 1, ..., n$. For example, if $\beta = 0.5$, ρ lies roughly in the interval $(-1/9, 0.4)$. Importantly, ρ cannot be constant, as it is a function of β.

7.9.3 Marginal or conditional model?

Marginal or conditional model? It is impossible to determine analytically which statistical model is more appropriate. Here, we summarize the properties of the two types of models and draw comparisons from a statistical point of view.

The marginal approach specifies the model in general form as

$$data = model + error. \tag{7.167}$$

On the other hand, the conditional model is defined as

$$data = model(error). \tag{7.168}$$

Model (7.167) has obvious roots from the linear/nonlinear regression model, while (7.168) is somewhat new to traditional regression analysis. If the *model* is linear, then $model(error) = model + error$, so the marginal and conditional approaches coincide. Otherwise, the two approaches are not equivalent. Although the marginal model is more familiar and and easier to handle, it is inadequate for modeling binary or discrete data. Indeed, if data are binary and the error distribution is modeled separately from the mean, the sum cannot produce 0 and 1 for any parameter value as the data dictate. In the conditional approach, error is intrinsic and usually requires integration to estimate parameters consistently. The marginal model is integration–free, and estimation is carried out by GEE.

Table 7.3. Relationship between marginal and conditional parameters for different GLM models with subject-specific intercepts

GLM	Relationship
Linear	$\beta_{\mathrm{marginal}} = \beta_{\mathrm{conditional}}$
Logistic	$\beta_{\mathrm{marginal}} \simeq \dfrac{1}{\sqrt{1+\sigma^2/1.7^2}} \beta_{\mathrm{conditional}}$
Probit	$\beta_{\mathrm{marginal}} = \dfrac{1}{\sqrt{1+\sigma^2}} \beta_{\mathrm{conditional}}$
Poisson/slope	$\beta_{\mathrm{marginal}} = \beta_{\mathrm{conditional}}$

In Table 7.3 we show the asymptotic relationship between (population-averaged) parameters of the two models. Precisely, a GLM with normally distributed random intercepts is assumed and β is the slope. Marginal and conditional approaches coincide for linear and Poisson models. GEE for logistic or probit regression produces attenuated population-averaged slopes—a larger variance of intercepts yields more attenuation. This attenuation cannot be compensated by the correlation matrix.

7.9.4   Implementation in R

Package **gee** contains a function **gee** that estimates the clustered marginal model with various assumptions as to the working correlation structure. For example, using the data on the number of visits to a doctor as a function of race, gender, and age from Problem 6 of Section 7.5, the call is

```
gee(visittot~black+female+I(age10-8)+I((age10-8)^2),id=hrr,
    data=psdat,family=poisson,corstr="exchangeable")
```

We use the option "exchangeable" for the correlation structure, as implied by the random intercept in the case of normally distributed data.

Problems for Section 7.9

1. Can iterations (7.159) be reduced to GLM estimation ($\mathtt{glm}$ call)?

2. Find a parallel between (7.160) and VLS for LME model as presented in Section 3.12.

3. Check if solution (7.163) can be derived from iterations (7.162) starting from any ρ_0.

4. Derive the closed-form expression for ρ in matrix $\mathbf{R}_i = \mathbf{R}_i(\rho)$, which is an identity matrix except that all elements on the main subdiagonal are ρ (only the neighboring elements of the residual vector correlate).

5. Find the VLS estimators of ρ_1 and ρ_2 when $\mathbf{R}_i = \mathbf{I}_i + \rho_1 \mathbf{T}_{1i} + \rho_2 \mathbf{T}_{3i}$.

6. Write an R program that reproduces Figure 7.10. Run this program with a larger n to demonstrate that the admissible area shrinks to zero.

7*. Explain why the working correlation matrix $\mathbf{R}_i$ can never be "guessed right" for GLM, so that GEE can never be efficient. Start with an LME model. Describe an LME model for which $\mathbf{R}_i$ can be "guessed right."

8. Explain rigorously the relationship in Table 7.3. Can the relationship between marginal and conditional approaches for the logistic regression model be expressed in a closed form exactly as in other cases?

7.10   Criteria for MLE existence for a binary model

There is quite a popular point of view that one does not need criteria for MLE existence. Let the algorithm for the log-likelihood function maximization run; if it finds the solution, MLE exists; if it fails, MLE does not exist. Such a pragmatic approach relies completely on the efficiency of the algorithm. However, what if the algorithm fails due to multicollinearity or the presence of an outlier and the inability to compute μ, e.g., Φ or $1 - \Phi$ in the probit model? Vice versa, what if the algorithm returns a maximum log-likelihood value close to zero (absolute maximum at infinity)? Does the final iteration give the true MLE, or does it indicate that MLE, in fact, simply does not exist? In any event, the success or failure of an algorithm cannot substitute for a criterion for MLE existence. Moreover, most software fails to recognize MLE nonexistence (Agresti, 2002, p. 195).

Weddenburn (1976) and Haberman (1979) formulated the condition for MLE existence for the probit and logistic models in terms of a separation plane. Silvapulle (1981) and Albert and Anderson (1984) did it for the logistic, and Lesaffre and Kaufmann (1992) for the probit model. That necessary and sufficient criterion is formulated in terms of separation of the data points in covariate space. However, a question remains: Does the separation plane exist? The goal of this section is to provide *constructive* criteria for MLE existence in a binary model with function μ, which satisfies properties 1 through 4 of Section 7.1. More general criteria for the existence of MLE are discussed by Demidenko (1981, 1989, 2000), and Nakamura and Lee (1993).

In this section we study the existence of the MLE with the log-likelihood function specified by equation (7.45). It is assumed that vectors $\{\mathbf{x}_i, i = 1, ..., n\}$ are not zero and have full rank.

Necessary and sufficient criteria for MLE existence in a binary model. The MLE for the binary model exists if and only if there is no $\boldsymbol{\beta}$ such that

$$\boldsymbol{\beta}'\mathbf{x}_i > 0 \quad \text{for all } i : y_i = 0 \quad \text{and} \quad \boldsymbol{\beta}'\mathbf{x}_i < 0 \text{ for all } i : y_i = 1. \tag{7.169}$$

This condition is referred to as the *separation condition*. Shortly, the separation condition may be rewritten as

$$(1 - 2y_i)\boldsymbol{\beta}'\mathbf{x}_i > 0, \quad i = 1, ..., n. \tag{7.170}$$

If there exists a nonzero vector $\boldsymbol{\beta}$ such that (7.170) is true, the MLE does not exist—there is perfect discrimination. Geometrically, the separation condition is illustrated in Figure 7.11.

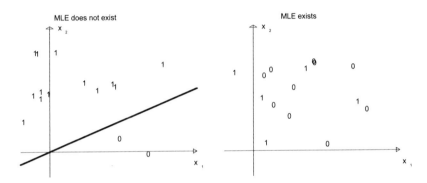

FIGURE 7.11. At the left, the separation line (bold) exists and divides observations in the covariate space (x_{i1}, x_{i2}) into two groups. The first group corresponds to $y_i = 1$, and the second group corresponds to $y_i = 0$; the MLE does not exist. At the right, there is no line that separates observations, and therefore the MLE exists.

To prove that (7.170) implies nonexistence, let us assume that it holds for $\boldsymbol{\beta}_*$ (clearly, $\boldsymbol{\beta}_* \neq \mathbf{0}$). Then letting $\boldsymbol{\beta} = \lambda\boldsymbol{\beta}_*$ and $\lambda \to -\infty$, we obtain

$$\lim_{\lambda \to -\infty} \mu(\lambda\boldsymbol{\beta}_*'\mathbf{x}_i) = \left\{ \begin{array}{l} 1 \text{ if } y_i = 1 \\ 0 \text{ if } y_i = 0 \end{array} \right. .$$

Clearly, it implies that $l(\lambda\boldsymbol{\beta}_*) \to 0$, where l is given by (7.45), and therefore the absolute upper bound of the log-likelihood function goes to infinity. Thus, the MLE does not exist.

Geometrically, the MLE does not exist if and only if there is a plane that separates points $\{\mathbf{x}_i, i = 1, ..., n\}$ into two groups according to the occurrence/nonoccurrence event y. Following Albert and Anderson (1984), points $\{\mathbf{x}_i, i = 1, ..., n\}$ are called *overlapped* if there is no separation plane. If (7.169) is not true for any $\boldsymbol{\beta}$, then $l(\boldsymbol{\beta}) \to -\infty$ if $\| \boldsymbol{\beta} \| \to \infty$. Otherwise, $\lim_{\lambda \to +\infty} l(\lambda\boldsymbol{\beta}_0'\mathbf{x}_i) = 0$, where $\boldsymbol{\beta}_0 \in R^k$ is such that $\boldsymbol{\beta}_0'\mathbf{x}_i > 0$ for $i \in S_0$ and $\boldsymbol{\beta}_0'\mathbf{x}_i < 0$ for $i \in S_1$, $\boldsymbol{\beta} \neq \mathbf{0}$.

We illustrate the separation condition by a one-covariate binary model: $\Pr(y_i = 1) = \mu(\beta_1 + \beta_2 x_i)$, see Figure 7.12. For this regression $m = 2$ and $\mathbf{x}_i = (1, x_i)' \in R^2$.

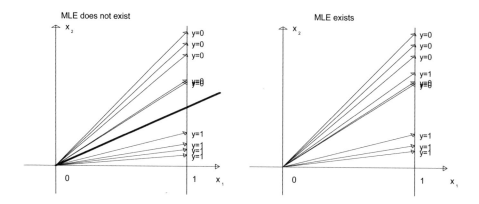

FIGURE 7.12. Due to the presence of the intercept term, all vectors $\mathbf{x}$ lie on the vertical line $x_1 = 1$. The separation condition may be expressed in terms of x_{i2}. At the left, the MLE does not exist because $\min_{y_i=0} x_{i2} > \max_{y_i=1} x_{i2}$. At the right, neither $m_0 < m_1 < M_0$ nor $m_0 < M_1 < M_0$ holds, and therefore the MLE exists.

We introduce the following quantities:

$$M_0 = \max_{y_i=0} x_i, \quad m_0 = \min_{y_i=0} x_i, \quad M_1 = \max_{y_i=1} x_i, \quad m_1 = \min_{y_i=1} x_i.$$

Vectors $\{\mathbf{x}_i, i = 1, ..., n\}$ can be separated by a line if and only if the intervals (m_0, M_0) and (m_1, M_1) do not overlap, which occurs when $M_0 \leq m_1$ or $M_1 \leq m_0$. Therefore, the MLE exists if and only if

$$m_0 < m_1 < M_0 \text{ or } m_0 < M_1 < M_0. \tag{7.171}$$

In particular, there should be at least one data point with $y = 0$ or $y = 1$ for the MLE to exist. The MLE does not exist if all $y_i = 0$ (or $y_i = 1$), $i = 1, ..., n$.

The condition of separation is difficult to verify for a higher dimension ($m > 2$). We aim to construct sufficient criteria for the MLE existence for an arbitrary parameter dimension. We introduce the following index sets:

$$S_0 = \{i : y_i = 0\}, \quad S_1 = \{i : y_i = 1\}.$$

Clearly, the union of S_0 and S_1 is $\{1, ..., n\}$ and the intersection is empty. Our criteria are expressed in terms of the vectors

$$\mathbf{v}_i = (1 - 2y_i)\mathbf{x}_i = \begin{cases} \mathbf{x}_i & \text{if } i \in S_0 \\ -\mathbf{x}_i & \text{if } i \in S_1 \end{cases}, \quad i = 1, ..., n. \tag{7.172}$$

The statements of the following theorem can be viewed as reformulations of the separation condition (7.169). Equivalently, they can be expressed in terms of the existence of the solution of a system of homogeneous inequalities. The last statement is the well known Gordan theorem (1873). See also Cottle et al. (1992) for a modern formulation and further detail.

Theorem 37 *The following statements are equivalent:*
(i) The MLE for a binary model exists.
(ii) There are no $\boldsymbol{\beta} \neq \mathbf{0}$ such that $\boldsymbol{\beta}'\mathbf{v}_i \geq 0$ for all $i = 1, ..., n$.
(iii) For any $\boldsymbol{\beta} \neq \mathbf{0}$ there is vector $\mathbf{v}_j$ from $\{\mathbf{v}_i, \ i = 1, ..., n\}$ such that $\boldsymbol{\beta}'\mathbf{v}_j < 0$.
(iv) The system of homogeneous linear inequalities $\boldsymbol{\beta}'\mathbf{v}_i > 0$ for $\boldsymbol{\beta}$ has no solution.
(v) There exist $\gamma_1 \geq 0, ..., \gamma_n \geq 0$ not all equal to zero such that $\sum_{i=1}^n \gamma_i \mathbf{v}_i = \mathbf{0}$.

Consequently, if a vector $\mathbf{v}_j$ is a linear combination of other vectors $\{\mathbf{v}_i\}$ with nonnegative coefficients, it can be removed from MLE existence consideration because it does not affect the existence of a solution to a system of homogeneous inequalities.

A simple sufficient criterion is formulated below. Before formulating the criterion, let us make some comments on the geometry of the Euclidean space R^m. We define an axis-vector as a vector with zero elements except one that may be either 1 or -1. Then the space can be divided into 2^m octants. An open octant can be defined as an open cone spanned by m neighboring axis vectors. We call m axis vectors neighboring if none of the remaining axis vectors can be expressed as a positive linear combination of them. Note that components of two vectors from the same open octant have the same sign, particularly if their scalar product is positive.

Theorem 38 *(Sufficient Criterion I). The MLE for binary model exists if every open octant of R^m contains a vector from $\{\mathbf{v}_i, \ i = 1, ..., n\}$.*

Proof. We prove that for any vector $\boldsymbol{\beta} \neq \mathbf{0}$, there exists a vector $\mathbf{v}_j$ from $\{\mathbf{v}_i, \ i = 1, ..., n\}$ such that $\boldsymbol{\beta}'\mathbf{v}_j > 0$, using (iii) of Theorem 37. Indeed, let $\boldsymbol{\beta} \neq \mathbf{0}$ be given and belong to an octant O of R^m. By the condition of the Theorem we can find a vector $\mathbf{v}_j$ from system $\{\mathbf{v}_i\}$ in the same octant O. Then the scalar product $\boldsymbol{\beta}'\mathbf{v}_j$ is positive. ∎

This criterion is simple but quite restrictive. For instance, for a one-covariate model with the intercept term, it works only if x takes positive values for $y = 0$ and negative values for $y = 1$. Notice that it does not work for data in the right-hand graph of Figure 7.12 because none of the vectors $\{\mathbf{v}_i\}$ belongs to the second octant. A better sufficient criterion is formulated below. To simplify the notation, the vectors $\mathbf{x}_i$ are supplied with the superindex 0 or 1. Thus, $\mathbf{x}_i^0$ corresponds to the covariate vector with $y_i = 0$, and $\mathbf{x}_j^1$ corresponds to $y_j = 1$. Also, $\mathbf{x}^0$ are supplied with the subindex i, and $\mathbf{x}^1$ are supplied with the subindex j. As follows from (7.169), the MLE does not exist if and only if sets $\{\mathbf{x}_i^0\}$ and $\{\mathbf{x}_j^1\}$ can be separated by a plane. With certain ambiguity, by *positive linear combination* we understand linear combination with positive coefficients.

Theorem 39 *(Sufficient Criterion II). The MLE exists if there exists $\mathbf{x}_p^0$ which can be represented as a positive linear combination of vectors $\{\mathbf{x}_j^1\}$ or there exists $\mathbf{x}_p^1$, which can be represented as a positive linear combination of vectors $\{\mathbf{x}_j^0\}$.*

Proof. Let vector $\mathbf{x}_p^0$ be represented as a positive linear combination, $\sum \lambda_j \mathbf{x}_j^1$, where $\lambda_j > 0$. We use (iv) of Theorem 37 to prove that the MLE exists. On the contrary, if $\boldsymbol{\beta}$ exists such that $\boldsymbol{\beta}'\mathbf{x}_j^1 > 0$ and $\boldsymbol{\beta}'\mathbf{x}_i^0 < 0$, then for vector $\mathbf{x}_p^0$ we have

$$\boldsymbol{\beta}'\mathbf{x}_p^0 = \boldsymbol{\beta}' \sum \lambda_j \mathbf{x}_j^1 = \sum \lambda_j \boldsymbol{\beta}'\mathbf{x}_j^1 > 0,$$

a contradiction. Analogously, we prove the MLE existence if $\mathbf{x}_p^1$ can be expressed as a positive linear combination of vectors $\mathbf{x}_i^0$.

∎

By this criterion the MLE for the right-hand graph of Figure 7.12 exists because the vector corresponding to $y = 1$ can be represented as a positive linear combination of two extreme vectors with $y = 0$ (loosely speaking, we may say that one observation with $y = 1$ is between observations with $y = 0$). The following algorithm, based on this theorem, determines if the MLE exists.

Algorithm 1 (sufficient)

1. Pick a vector $\mathbf{x}_p^0$ from $\{\mathbf{x}_i^0\}$.

2. Pick m linearly independent vectors from $\{\mathbf{x}_j^1\}$.

3. Express $\mathbf{x}_i^0$ as a linear combination of m vectors from step 2 solving the according system of linear equations. If all coefficients of the solution are positive, the MLE exists, and quit. Otherwise, return to step 2 until all m linearly independent vectors from $\{\mathbf{x}_j^1\}$ are exhausted.

4. Return to step 1 to pick another vector.

The necessary and sufficient criterion for the MLE existence is formulated next.

Theorem 40 *(Necessary and Sufficient Criterion). The MLE does not exist if and only if there are $m - 1$ vectors $\mathbf{w}_1, \mathbf{w}_2, ..., \mathbf{w}_{m-1}$ among $\{\mathbf{v}_i, i = 1, ..., n\}$ for which all n determinants,*

$$D_i = \det \begin{bmatrix} v_{i1} & v_{i2} & \cdots & v_{im} \\ w_{11} & w_{12} & \cdots & w_{1m} \\ \cdots & & & \\ w_{m-1,1} & w_{m-1,2} & \cdots & w_{m-1,m} \end{bmatrix}, \quad i = 1, 2, ..., n \quad (7.173)$$

have the same sign.

Proof. Let the MLE not exist. Then there exists $\boldsymbol{\beta} \neq \mathbf{0}$ as the solution to n homogeneous inequalities $\boldsymbol{\beta}'\mathbf{v}_i \geq 0$, $i = 1, ..., n$. It is well known that the solutions to the system of homogeneous inequalities is a polyhedral cone C^+ conjugate to the cone C spanned by the vectors $\{\mathbf{v}_i, i = 1, ..., n\}$, see, for example, Hoffman (1999). Each edge of C^+ is orthogonal to at least $m - 1$ vectors of $\{\mathbf{v}_i, i = 1, ..., n\}$. Hence, it is possible to pick a $\boldsymbol{\beta}_* \neq \mathbf{0}$ and $m-1$ vectors $\mathbf{w}_1, ..., \mathbf{w}_{m-1}$ among $\{\mathbf{v}_i\}$ such that $\boldsymbol{\beta}_*'\mathbf{v}_i \geq 0$ for all $i = 1, ..., n$ and $\boldsymbol{\beta}_*'\mathbf{w}_j = 0$ for $j = 1, ..., m - 1$. Thus, in searching for a plane that separates $\{\mathbf{x}_i^0\}$ and $\{\mathbf{x}_j^1\}$, without loss of generality, we can restrict ourselves to planes which go through $m - 1$ points from $\{\mathbf{v}_i\}$. Further, it is well known that the position of vector $\mathbf{v} = (v_1, ..., v_m)'$ about the plane defined by m points $(\mathbf{0}, \mathbf{w}_1, ..., \mathbf{w}_{m-1})$ is determined by the sign of (7.173). Therefore, the MLE does not exist if and only if all D_i have the same sign for all $\mathbf{v}_i$ and certain group of $m - 1$ vectors from $\{\mathbf{v}_i\}$.

∎

The following algorithm verifies whether the MLE exists.

Algorithm 2 (necessary and sufficient)

1. Pick any $m - 1$ different vectors $\mathbf{w}_1, ..., \mathbf{w}_{m-1}$ from $\{\mathbf{v}_i, i = 1, ..., n\}$. There are $\binom{n}{m-1}$ ways to pick $m - 1$ different vectors $\mathbf{w}_1, ..., \mathbf{w}_{m-1}$.

2. Compute n determinants (7.173), skipping when $\mathbf{v}_i$ coincides with one of $\mathbf{w}_1, ..., \mathbf{w}_{m-1}$. If all determinants have the same sign, the MLE does not exist, and quit. Otherwise, go to step 1 and pick another group of $m - 1$ vectors.

This algorithm may be time consuming because it has an exhaustive nature.

Problems for Section 7.10

1^*. Is it true that when MLE does not exist, the maximum of the log-likelihood is zero? Does the reverse statement hold?

2^*. Write an R program that implements Algorithm 2. Select (y_i, x_i) such that the MLE does not exist using (7.171). Verify that your program confirms that MLE does not exist, and finally, run glm. Explain the result.

3^*. Derive sufficient criteria for the existence of the MLE with the Poisson regression model. Extend these results to the Poisson model with random intercepts.

4^*. Generalize the results of this section to the GEE approach.

5^*. Generalize the results of this section to the binary mixed model with random intercept.

7.11 Summary points

- Typically, the study of generalized linear mixed models is carried out in a deductive fashion under the umbrella of the exponential distribution family. We argue that the inductive approach, when logistic, probit, and Poisson models are studied separately, is more effective. Practically, only these three models are used. Theoretically, each model allows a specific approach that simplifies statistical inference significantly. For example, binomial data with a beta distribution for probability leads to the beta-binomial model; probit regression with normally distributed random effects lead again to a probit regression; Poisson regression with normally distributed random effects is again a Poisson regression.

- Several probability functions/links can be used to model binary outcomes. The logit link (logistic regression) is popular in epidemiology because the coefficients have a clear interpretation via the odds ratio. Probit regression is widely used in econometrics and dose-response studies, where only thresholds of a normally distributed latent variable are observable. The complementary log-log link function is adequate when the original count Poisson data are reduced to binary.

- There exists a close relationship between logit and probit probability functions. The logit function can be approximated by one- or two-probit functions with increasing precision. For example, the probit function with argument divided by 1.7 approximates the logit probability function with the absolute error less than 0.01. A linear combination of two probits approximates the logit probability function with the absolute error 0.0005. These approximations are useful for estimating logistic regression with normally distributed random effects.

- The logistic-normal integral is often encountered in the framework of the measurement error problem. This integral also emerges in logistic regression with normally distributed random effects. There are several methods to approximate this integral using one- or two-probit approximations, link approximation, first and second approximation, and Laplace approximation. The link and two-probit approximations are most robust and are fairly precise.

- Laplace approximation assumes that there exists a unique maximum of the integrand. Otherwise, the approximation may be poor. We introduce an improved Laplace approximation expressed in terms of two standard normal cumulative distribution functions.

- Numerical integration/quadrature can evaluate integrals with any given precision. However, a proper solution to the quadrature problem would involve an assessment of the error of approximation, usually a step missing in maximum likelihood estimation. First, we need to replace an improper integral with the proper one, and find the lower and the upper limits of integration such that the difference between two integrals is sufficiently small. Second, an appropriate number of nodes should be chosen to provide the needed accuracy. Sometimes simpler methods, such as summation with a sufficient number of terms, outperform complicated methods of integral approximation in terms of time of computation.

- There is no exact integral evaluation unless the integral can be expressed in a closed-form. Thus, one needs to think in terms of the integral approximation and the error of approximation. A proper error analysis would involve an analytical investigation of the integrand and its high-order derivatives in the entire range of the parameters involved. Often, such an analysis is absent, so we do not know the error of approximation. Therefore, strictly speaking, maximum likelihood can be viewed as just another approximate method of estimation. Due to the error uncertainty, use of at least two different starting points is recommended to ensure that iterations converge to the same parameter value and are not affected by, for example, the number of nodes.

- Although the log-likelihood function for the generalized linear model without random effects is concave, it does not guarantee the existence of the MLE. For example, the maximum likelihood estimate for a binary model approaches infinity if there is a plane that separates observations with $y = 0$ and $y = 1$. Several algorithms are available to detect whether such a separation plane exists. Unfortunately, commercial software does not check the existence of the MLE and may report an estimate where the solution, in fact, does not exist.

- The most important model for clustered data is a model with cluster/subject-specific intercepts. When the number of clusters (N) is small and the number of observations per cluster (n_i) is large, say $n_i > N$, the model with fixed random intercepts is adequate. When n_i is small, conditional likelihood for logit and Poisson models is almost as efficient as maximum likelihood but does not require distribution specification. Otherwise, the random effects model should be used.

- Ignoring random effects attenuates the coefficients of the logit and probit models but does not change the slope coefficients of the Poisson model. In this respect, the Poisson model resembles the linear mixed effects model, where ignoring random effect leaves the estimates unbiased. Different members of GLM react differently to introduction of the random effect.

- Only maximum likelihood is consistent when N goes to infinity and the $\{n_i\}$ are bounded for binary data; all approximate methods of estimation require n_i to be large as well. Two general approximate methods of GLMM estimation are Laplace and penalized quasi-likelihood. These methods differ by a term that vanishes when $n_i \to \infty$. There are several specific approximate methods for members of the GLM family that can outperform general methods.

- The Poisson model with normally distributed random effects is the easiest among GLMM because the first two moments admit a closed-form solution. This is the only GLM model for which the PA and SS slope coefficients coincide. The ordinary Poisson regression for balanced data with random intercepts yields an efficient estimate of slopes. Exact or Total GEE produces highly efficient estimates for the Poisson model with multiple random effects.

- An important part of GLMM analysis is the homogeneity test that random effects are zero. Two tests are available: the F-test, as a generalization of LME test, and the score test. These tests can be applied to simultaneous or individual random effects. In the former case, Bonferroni adjustment for the significance level may be used.

- The generalized estimating equation (GEE) approach estimates parameters of an unknown statistical model. In particular, there is a problem of generating data that comply with the GEE specification. If the covariate is normally distributed, the only valid GEE model with logit link is the model with zero intracluster correlation when N goes to infinity. The concept of a "working correlation matrix," based on the Pearson correlation coefficient, is appropriate for continuous but not binary data.

- The generalized linear model for cluster/longitudinal data may be studied in a conditional or marginal setting. The conditional setting assumes random effects that describe subject-specific intercepts or coefficients. In the marginal setting, the cluster nature of data is addressed through the correlation matrix. Although GEE is straightforward, the statistical validity of a marginal model for binary or discrete data may be questionable. A conditional/mixed model is a valid statistical model, but it may be computationally intensive.

- We prefer the conditional model with random effects because it implies a valid statistical model. The drawback usually mentioned, which is associated with difficulties of estimation and numerical integration, can be facilitated by the Fixed Sample Likelihood (FSL) approach, which combines Monte Carlo and Gauss–Hermite schema in a general framework. In the FSL approach the likelihood integral is approximated by a sum and treated as a new likelihood with combined beta and variance parameters. Our practice showed that this approach outperforms many approximate estimation techniques and produces estimates very close to MLE and about 10 times faster. Unlike many approximate methods it provides the joint covariance matrix for population-averaged coefficients and variance parameters. It is quite rare that GLMM has more than five random effects, so modern computers can handle the FSL computation.

8

Nonlinear Mixed Effects Model

8.1 Introduction

The nonlinear mixed effects (NLME) model is a further generalization of the marginal mixed effects model considered in Chapter 6 and the generalized linear mixed model of Chapter 7. As in Chapter 6, we shall assume that we deal with continuous data. Modeling of binary and count data was discussed in the previous chapter. Unlike the marginal model, the likelihood function for the general NLME model does not admit a closed-form solution because the random effects enter the model in a nonlinear fashion. Consequently, to obtain the marginal distribution of the dependent variable, a formidable integration problem emerges, especially when the number of random effects is large. A special nonlinear mixed effects model, the generalized linear mixed model (GLMM), was considered in Chapter 7. As we learned from Section 7.3.1, even one random effect may create challenges to the quadrature problem when the maximum likelihood (ML) applies.

Early authors attempted to avoid integration by using simplified, approximate solutions. For instance, Pockock et al. (1981) and Berkey and Laird (1986) suggested an intuitively appealing two-stage estimator when all parameters of the growth curve are random (subject-specific). Another approach, based on a first-order approximation around the population-averaged mean, extracting the random effects from the nonlinear regression function, was proposed by Sheiner and Beal (1980) and developed further by Vonesh and Carter (1992). An alternative method, which uses the first-order approximation, was suggested by Lindstrom and Bates (1990); however, they approximate the nonlinear function around the subject-specific means. Later it was found that their original algorithm can be derived through the Laplace approximation to the likelihood function (Wolfinger, 1993; Pinheiro and Bates, 1995; Vonesh, 1996; Vonesh et al., 2002). Many approximation methods aim to reduce the NLME model to the marginal mixed model studied in Chapter 6. Therefore, the techniques developed in that chapter can be very useful, particularly GEE and total GEE. However, it is worthwhile to remember that unlike in Chapter 6, the marginal models obtained in this chapter are approximations to the original nonlinear mixed effects models. Therefore, the maximum likelihood estimation may be inadequate because it is sensitive to distribution misspecification.

After introducing the NLME model in general terms, an example of modeling the height of girls and boys is considered. Four methods of estimation are discussed in this chapter: maximum likelihood, two-stage, first-order approximation, and Laplace approximation. In fact, these methods were applied to generalized linear mixed models in Chapter 7, so in this chapter we extend them to the general nonlinear mixed effects model. The asymptotic properties of the estimators are illustrated by a simple one-parameter exponential model, where the estimate admits a closed-form solution and allows exact calculation of the asymptotic bias. The result, the asymptotic equivalence of three estimators, is presented in Section 8.10. The bias-corrected version of the two-stage estimator is suggested in Section 8.11. The effect of distribution misspecification is discussed in Section 8.12. Finally, we discuss the integration problem and the FSL approach as a generalization of that for the generalized linear mixed models.

8.2   The model

The NLME model is a straightforward generalization of the marginal mixed effects model and is written in two stages (Sheiner and Beal, 1985; Lindstrom and Bates, 1990; Davidian and Giltinan, 1995; Vonesh and Chinchilli, 1997). The first stage of the NLME model consists of N nonlinear regression models with some random (subject-specific) parameters,

$$\mathbf{y}_i = \mathbf{f}_i(\boldsymbol{\gamma}, \mathbf{a}_i) + \boldsymbol{\epsilon}_i, \quad i = 1, ..., N, \tag{8.1}$$

where $\mathbf{y}_i$ is an $n_i \times 1$ vector of the dependent variable; $\mathbf{f}_i$ is a nonlinear $n_i \times 1$ vector function,

$$\mathbf{f}_i(\boldsymbol{\gamma}, \mathbf{a}_i) = (f(\boldsymbol{\gamma}, \mathbf{a}_i; \mathbf{x}_{i1}), f(\boldsymbol{\gamma}, \mathbf{a}_i; \mathbf{x}_{i2}), ..., f(\boldsymbol{\gamma}, \mathbf{a}_i; \mathbf{x}_{i,n_i}))';$$

$\mathbf{x}_{ij}$ is a vector of covariates; $\boldsymbol{\gamma}$ is a $q \times 1$ vector of unknown (deterministic) parameters; $\boldsymbol{\epsilon}_i$ is an $n_i \times 1$ error vector with $E(\boldsymbol{\epsilon}_i) = \mathbf{0}$ and $\text{cov}(\boldsymbol{\epsilon}_i) = \sigma^2 \mathbf{I}$; and $\mathbf{a}_i$ is a $k \times 1$ vector of unobservable subject-specific random parameters with the unknown $k \times k$ covariance matrix

$$\text{cov}(\mathbf{a}_i) = \mathbf{D}_* = \sigma^2 \mathbf{D}.$$

Following the line of our notation, we call $\mathbf{D}$ the *scaled* covariance matrix. Sometimes σ^2 is called the within-subject variance. Sometimes, to shorten the notation, we combine the variance parameters into a $(k(k+1)/2+1)$-dimensional vector $\boldsymbol{\theta}$, as we did for the linear mixed effects model. Index i refers to the ith subject (cluster/individual/experimental unit), and n_i denotes the number of observations for the ith subject. The total number of observations is $N_T = \sum_{i=1}^{N} n_i$. Although the assumption that the components of the error vector are independent seems restrictive, conceptually little changes if one, for example, assumes that $\sigma^2(\mathbf{I} + \boldsymbol{\Omega}_i(\boldsymbol{\tau}))$, where $\boldsymbol{\Omega}_i$ is an $n_i \times n_i$ matrix dependent on unknown parameter $\boldsymbol{\tau}$. See Section

4.3.4, where $\mathbf{\Omega}_i$ accounts for autocorrelation. To be exact, equation (8.1) should be written in conditional form $\mathbf{y}_i|\mathbf{a}_i$ since $\mathbf{a}_i$ is random.

The second stage of the NLME model is the same as for the linear growth curve model (Section 4.1) and has the form

$$\mathbf{a}_i = \mathbf{A}_i\boldsymbol{\beta} + \mathbf{b}_i, \tag{8.2}$$

where $\mathbf{A}_i$ is a $k \times m$ design matrix, $\boldsymbol{\beta}$ is an $m \times 1$ vector of population-averaged parameters, and $\mathbf{b}_i$ is a $k \times 1$ vector of random effects, $E(\mathbf{b}_i) = \mathbf{0}$, $\text{cov}(\mathbf{b}_i) = \sigma^2\mathbf{D}$. Random effects $\mathbf{b}_i$ and error terms $\boldsymbol{\epsilon}_i$ are assumed mutually independent and independent across subjects. Also, it is assumed that matrix $\sum \mathbf{A}_i'\mathbf{A}_i$ has full rank, $\sigma^2 > 0$ and matrix $\mathbf{D}$ is nonnegative definite. The combined vector $\boldsymbol{\theta} = (\sigma^2, \text{vech}'(\mathbf{D}))'$ is called the *variance parameter*. Sometimes the mixed model is called the repeated measurements model, where the repeated measurements are indexed by $j = 1, ..., n_i$. Often, the repeated measurements/data are longitudinal, as in the example in Section 8.3.

In a special case when the vector parameter $\boldsymbol{\gamma}$ is absent, the NLME model (8.1) is a nonlinear generalization of the growth curve model considered in Chapter 4. Such a model will be called a *nonlinear growth curve model*. It is specified by the following pair of equations:

$$\mathbf{y}_i = \mathbf{f}_i(\mathbf{a}_i) + \boldsymbol{\epsilon}_i, \quad \mathbf{a}_i = \mathbf{A}_i\boldsymbol{\beta} + \mathbf{b}_i. \tag{8.3}$$

In this model all growth curve parameters are subject-specific. This nonlinear growth curve model is somewhat simpler than (8.1) because, for example, we can *separately* estimate each $\mathbf{a}_i$ by nonlinear least squares and then apply a weighting procedure to estimate $\boldsymbol{\beta}$ (see the two-stage method of estimation, Section 8.5).

The NLME model, specified by equations (8.1) and (8.2), can be rewritten as $\mathbf{y}_i = \mathbf{f}_i(\boldsymbol{\gamma}, \mathbf{A}_i\boldsymbol{\beta} + \mathbf{b}_i) + \boldsymbol{\varepsilon}_i$ so that parameters $\boldsymbol{\gamma}$ and $\boldsymbol{\beta}$ can be combined into one population-averaged parameter $\boldsymbol{\chi} = (\boldsymbol{\gamma}', \boldsymbol{\beta}')'$. We prefer the current specification, however, because it indicates that $\boldsymbol{\gamma}$ is fixed and that random effects $\mathbf{b}_i$ are associated with $\boldsymbol{\beta}$.

Naturally, one may ask an essential question: Why do we need random effects? Why is it adequate to assume that parameters of the growth curve are random? In Chapter 1 we explained why random effects are useful for repeated or cluster measurements. Now we illustrate the point in the framework of a nonlinear model of male height, see Figure 8.1. Let i index the person and j index the year his height is measured, so that y_{ij} is the height of person i at time t_j. The logistic growth curve (or its generalization) is an appropriate model for the height (we consider the modeling of children's height at length in the next section). The standard nonlinear regression model (zero random effects) assumes that all individuals have the same parameters, including adult height. Moreover, since there is only one source of error, the generated time series data may not be increasing, which is unacceptable. If the growth curve with random parameters is used (nonzero random effects) it would assume that everyone has his/her own growth curves parameters, including adult height. It is less likely that the random effects model produces a nonmonotonic time series. Consequently, the growth curve with random parameters is better for growth data.

The NLME model is different from the marginal mixed model because random parameters, $\mathbf{a}_i$, are "inside" a nonlinear function. This means that generally the

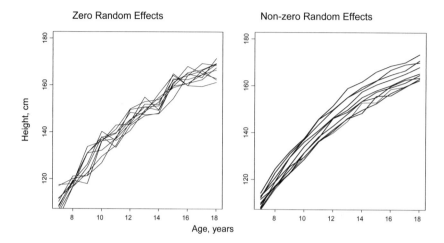

FIGURE 8.1. Simulated male height using a logistic growth curve. At the left it is assumed that there are no random effects. That is, parameters of the growth curve are the same for everyone and the only source of variation is the error term. We notice that height, generated by this model, may go up and down; that is absolutely unacceptable. At the right it is assumed that each person has his own parameter of growth, including adult height (the asymptote). There are two sources of variation: one is modeled via the usual error term and another via random effects, as the deviation of the subject-specific from population-averaged parameters. The nonzero random effects model is more accurate.

marginal expectation of the dependent variable cannot be expressed in terms of population-averaged parameters in closed terms: namely,

$$E(\mathbf{y}_i) = E_{\mathbf{b}_i} \{\mathbf{f}_i(\boldsymbol{\gamma}, \mathbf{A}_i\boldsymbol{\beta} + \mathbf{b}_i)\} \neq \mathbf{f}_i(\boldsymbol{\gamma}, \mathbf{A}_i\boldsymbol{\beta}).$$

This is a characteristic property of the NLME model. Consequently, it is very difficult to establish statistical properties of estimators in the NLME model in finite samples even when the variance parameters are known, a common difficulty with all nonlinear statistical models. Therefore, asymptotic consideration (when the number of observations goes to infinity/large sample) is useful.

In a repeated measurements model, the following three asymptotic situations may be considered:

1. The number of subjects, N, goes to infinity, but the number of observations per subject n_i remains finite (uniformly bounded).

2. The number of subjects, N, is fixed, but the number of observations per subject n_i goes to infinity.

3. The number of subjects, N, goes to infinity along with the minimum number of observations per subject, $\min n_i$.

For linear mixed effects models, the first condition is sufficient to guarantee consistency, asymptotic normality, and efficiency. As we shall learn later, for the NLME model this is true only for maximum likelihood estimation, and all approximate methods require both N and n_i to go to infinity. The asymptotic properties of the NLME model in these three situations are considered in Sections 8.9 and 8.10.

Problems for Section 8.2

1^*. Is it correct to say that the NLME model is a nonlinear regression model with random parameters? Prove that the latter model, $y_i = f_i(a_i) + \varepsilon_i$, where $a_i = \beta + b_i$, with normally and independently distributed errors is not identifiable $(i = 1, 2, ..., N)$. What makes the NLME model identifiable?

2. Describe the three asymptotic situations using the stochastic scheme from Section 3.6.2; use the representation $\mathbf{f}_i = \mathbf{f}(x_i)$.

8.3   Example: height of girls and boys

Before advancing to estimation methods, we consider the following motivational example of the NLME model.

The data are from the Longitudinal Studies of Child Health Development, initiated in 1929 at the Harvard School of Public Health (the full description of the project is given by Stuart and Reed, 1929) and consist of the heights of 67 girls and 67 boys aged from 7 to 18, see Figure 8.2. The growth curve analysis for the preschool children was carried out previously by Berkey and Laird (1986); thus, we focus on the modeling of school-aged children.

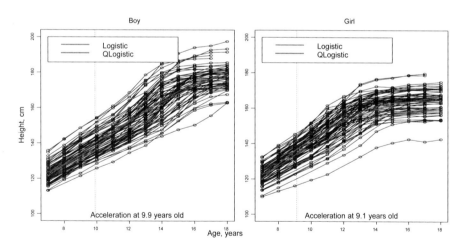

FIGURE 8.2. Height of 67 girls and 67 boys. Nonlinear growth is evident, particularly as the height approaches an asymptote.

The data, as an R object/dataframe, is downloaded to the R session as source ("c:\\MixedModels\\Chapter08\\height.dat"). It has 1404 observations with sex=1 corresponding to girl and sex=0 corresponding to boy.

Clearly, the linear growth model is not appropriate for these data because the growth has an evident asymptote, and therefore some type of nonlinear growth would be appropriate. The choice of a suitable nonlinear model is critical to regression analysis, and to the mixed model especially, due to its complexity. The wrong model may lead to computational difficulties, such as lack of convergence, negative variances of random effects, computer program overflow, etc. A good start is to compute the mean height, which eliminates the variation among children, see Figure 8.2. The mean height data facilitate the choice of the model. As follows from this figure, until age 12, girls and boys grow at a closely similar rate; however, after 12, boys continue growing while girls slow down. We may expect the mean adult height for males to be a little less than 180 cm and the adult height for females to be about 160 cm.

Table 8.1. Nonlinear regression fit of height with two logistic growth curves

	a_1	a_2	a_3	a_4	$\widehat{\sigma}$	Accel.
		Girls				
Logistic	171.0	0.904	0.251		6.97	
(SE)	(1.24)	(0.093)	(0.014)			
QLogistic	164.7	-2.15	-0.425	0.0386	6.79	9.1
(SE)	(0.32)	(0.043)	(0.009)	(0.006)		
		Boys				
Logistic	213.7	0.626	0.128		7.65	
(SE)	(6.73)	(0.026)	(0.010)			
QLogistic	182.3	-1.001	-0.161	0.0177	7.53	9.9
(SE)	(1.917)	(0.331)	(0.067)	(0.0037)		

There is plenty of literature on growth curve models. All growth curves can be derived as the solution to the respective differential equation, the interested reader is referred to Banks (1994) and to a chapter in Seber and Wild (1989). The most popular growth curve with an asymptote is the three-parameter *logistic* curve,

$$f_t(a_1, a_2, a_3) = \frac{a_1}{1 + e^{a_2 - a_3 t}}, \quad t = 1, ..., n. \tag{8.4}$$

As the reader can verify, the logistic curve, (8.4), satisfies the differential equation $df/dt = a_3 f(a_1 - f)$. Parameter a_1 is the asymptote, and a_3 is the rate at which f approaches a_1. However, it is well documented that teenagers grow very rapidly between 9 and 11, and the transition time to adult height is much shorter than can be modeled using a logistic curve (8.4). Hence, to describe a faster/accelerated growth, we suggest a quadratic-logistic growth curve (QLogistic):

$$f_t(a_1, a_2, a_3, a_4) = \frac{a_1}{1 + e^{a_2 - a_3 t - a_4 t^2}}, \quad t = 1, ..., n. \tag{8.5}$$

Parameter a_4 may be interpreted as the acceleration parameter. Results of fitting to the growth data using the `nls` function are presented in Table 8.1. It is elementary to show that the fastest growth occurs at the time when the second derivative of f_t with respect to t vanishes, which yields $t_{\text{accel}} = (\sqrt{2a_4} - a_3)/(2a_4)$ displayed in the last column of the table. The R function `heightlog`, which produces Figure 8.2 and estimates the logistic growth with `nls`, can be downloaded as `source("c:\\MixedModels\\Chapter08\\heightlog.r")`. Remember that the data frame `height.dat` should be downloaded first in order to run `heightlog`.

As follows from Table 8.1, the quadratic-logistic growth curve gives better results then the standard logistic regression: (a) the regression SD ($\widehat{\sigma}$) is smaller; (b) the adult height for males is more realistic; (c) standard errors for most parameters are smaller; (d) the quadratic term is statistically significant; (e) girls accelerate with twofold speed; and (f) as follows from this model, girls accelerate at about 9 and boys accelerate at about 10. As follows from QLogistic fit, the height of adult males is about 182 cm and adult females 165 cm, on average. Notice that the estimate of the adult male is overestimated using the standard Logistic curve–this is a drawback of using the average data—we obtain a more reliable estimate using the nonlinear mixed effects approach in Section 8.16. To apply the quadratic logistic growth curve model (8.5) to individual data, we assume that some parameters are subject-specific. In mixed modeling a large part of the decision has to do with what parameters are random (subject-specific) and what parameters are common to all subjects (population-averaged). The asymptote (adult height, a_1) should be subject-specific. Also, the initial height (the height at age 7) is probably also subject-specific, leading us to the assumption that a_2 is subject-specific as well. The decision on the randomness of a_3 and a_4 can be checked empirically by fitting the NLME model and examining the covariance matrix of the random effects. For example, for girls, assuming that all four parameters are subject-specific, the NLME model is

$$y_{ij} = \frac{a_1 + b_{1i}}{1 + e^{(a_2 + b_{i2}) - (a_3 + b_{i3})t_{ij} - (a_4 + b_{i4})t_{ij}^2}} + \varepsilon_{ij}, \tag{8.6}$$

where $i = 1, ..., 67, j = 1, ..., n_i$, and $\varepsilon_{ij} \sim \mathcal{N}(0, \sigma^2)$, $\mathbf{b}_i = (b_{i1}, b_{i2}, b_{i3}, b_{i4})' \sim \mathcal{N}(0, \sigma^2 \mathbf{D})$. It is interesting to determine what growth parameters are gender specific, leading to the question of whether the data on boys and girls can be combined under one model. Notice that if only the adult height is subject-specific, the model becomes marginal, see Section 6.2.4.

Problems for Section 8.3

1*. Modify `heightlog` code to fit Logistic and QLogistic curves to the mean data (average height for each age=7,8,...,18). Compare the results with Table 8.1. Why are the results different? When would be the results the same? What fit is more efficient?

2. Derive the formula for the acceleration time for the quadratic-logistic model. Does acceleration time exist for the standard logistic model?

3. Explain why the sign of a_3 is different for Logistic and QLogistic models.

8.4   Maximum likelihood estimation

If the random terms ϵ_i and $\mathbf{b}_i$ are normally distributed, the NLME model can be rewritten compactly as

$$\mathbf{y}_i \mid \mathbf{a}_i \sim \mathcal{N}\left(\mathbf{f}_i(\boldsymbol{\gamma}, \mathbf{a}_i), \sigma^2 \mathbf{I}\right), \tag{8.7}$$

$$\mathbf{a}_i \sim \mathcal{N}\left(\mathbf{A}_i \boldsymbol{\beta}, \sigma^2 \mathbf{D}\right) \tag{8.8}$$

with the log-likelihood function, up to a constant term $-(N_T + Nk)\ln\sqrt{2\pi}$,

$$l(\gamma, \beta, \theta) \tag{8.9}$$

$$= -\frac{1}{2}\left[N\ln|\mathbf{D}| + \sum_{i=1}^{N}(n_i + k)\ln(\sigma^2) + \sum_{i=1}^{N}\ln\int_{R^k} g_i(\gamma, \mathbf{a}, \beta, \theta)d\mathbf{a}\right]$$

where

$$g_i(\gamma, \mathbf{a}, \beta, \theta) = \exp\left\{-\frac{1}{2\sigma^2}\left[\|\mathbf{y}_i - \mathbf{f}_i(\gamma, \mathbf{a})\|^2 + (\mathbf{a} - \mathbf{A}_i\beta)'\mathbf{D}^{-1}(\mathbf{a} - \mathbf{A}_i\beta)\right]\right\}.$$

It is elementary to show that (8.9) gives (4.14) if the NLME model is linear, $\mathbf{f}_i = \mathbf{Z}_i\mathbf{a}$. In this case (8.7) and (8.8) can be written compactly as (4.5). As the reader can see, the likelihood function involves an improper integral, which does not have a closed-form solution unless the model is linear. The presence of the integral is the major issue in NLME model estimation. The integral in (8.9) makes the maximum likelihood procedure cumbersome, especially for multidimensional random effects. Several estimators of β are considered in detail in subsequent sections. They all coincide for a linear mixed effects model when the variance parameters are known. However, they all are different and have quite different statistical properties for the general NLME model.

As follows from the maximum likelihood theory, the MLE is consistent, asymptotically normally distributed, and efficient when N goes to infinity and and $\{n_i\}$ are bounded, see Section 8.2. The asymptotic variance based on the information matrix is crucial for efficiency comparisons. However, calculation of the information matrix for the NLME model again leads to an integration problem. Below we derive an absolute lower bound for the covariance matrix of beta coefficients.

We use the following lemma, which provides an upper bound for the information matrix in a model with two random vector variables $\mathbf{Y}$ and $\mathbf{A}$, where $\mathbf{A}$ is unobservable. It is well known that the information based on $\mathbf{Y}$ is less than the information based on $\mathbf{A}$ if $\mathbf{Y}$ is a function of $\mathbf{A}$ (Schervish, 1995). We generalize this result to the case when $\mathbf{Y}$ depends on $\mathbf{A}$ stochastically.

Lemma 41 *Let* $\mathbf{Y}$ *and* $\mathbf{A}$ *be two random vector variables,* $\mathbf{A}$ *is unobservable with marginal density* $f_2(\mathbf{a}; \tau)$, *where* τ *is the parameter vector. Variable* $\mathbf{Y}$ *is observable, the conditional density of* $\mathbf{Y} \mid \mathbf{A}$ *is* $f_1(\mathbf{y}, \mathbf{a})$, *and the marginal density* $f(\mathbf{y}; \tau)$ $= \int f_1(\mathbf{y}, \mathbf{a})f_2(\mathbf{a}; \tau)d\mathbf{a}$. *Then*

$$\mathcal{I}_{\mathbf{Y}} \leq \mathcal{I}_{\mathbf{A}}; \tag{8.10}$$

that is, matrix $\mathcal{I}_{\mathbf{A}} - \mathcal{I}_{\mathbf{Y}}$ *is nonnegative definite, where* $\mathcal{I}_{\mathbf{Y}}$ *is the Fisher information about* τ *from* $\mathbf{Y}$ *and* $\mathcal{I}_{\mathbf{A}}$ *is the information from* $\mathbf{A}$.

Proof. We use the following vector analog of the Cauchy inequality (Rao, 1973): if $d\mu(\mathbf{x})$ is a measure, $\mathbf{u}(\mathbf{x})$ is an integrable vector, and $f(\mathbf{x})$ is an integrable scalar function, then

$$\left(\int \mathbf{u}(\mathbf{x})f(\mathbf{x})d\mu(\mathbf{x})\right)\left(\int \mathbf{u}(\mathbf{x})f(\mathbf{x})d\mu(\mathbf{x})\right)'$$

$$\leq \left(\int f^2(\mathbf{x})d\mu(\mathbf{x})\right)\left(\int \mathbf{u}(\mathbf{x})\mathbf{u}'(\mathbf{x})d\mu(\mathbf{x})\right). \tag{8.11}$$

Omitting, for simplicity of notation, arguments of functions, we obtain

$$\frac{\partial \ln f}{\partial \tau} = \left(\int f_1 f_2 d\mathbf{a} \right)^{-1} \left(\int f_1 \frac{\partial f_2}{\partial \tau} d\mathbf{a} \right),$$

so that the marginal information matrix becomes

$$\mathcal{I}_\mathbf{Y} = \int \left\{ \left(\int f_1 \frac{\partial f_2}{\partial \tau} d\mathbf{a} \right) \left(\int f_1 \frac{\partial f_2}{\partial \tau} d\mathbf{a} \right)' \left(\int f_1 f_2 d\mathbf{a} \right)^{-1} \right\} d\mathbf{y}. \qquad (8.12)$$

But by inequality (8.11),

$$\left(\int f_1 \frac{\partial f_2}{\partial \tau} d\mathbf{a} \right) \left(\int f_1 \frac{\partial f_2}{\partial \tau} d\mathbf{a} \right)'$$

$$= \left[\int \left(\sqrt{\frac{f_1}{f_2}} \frac{\partial f_2}{\partial \tau} \right) \left(\sqrt{f_1 f_2} \right) d\mathbf{a} \right] \left[\int \left(\sqrt{\frac{f_1}{f_2}} \frac{\partial f_2}{\partial \tau} \right) \left(\sqrt{f_1 f_2} \right) d\mathbf{a} \right]'$$

$$\leq \left[\int \left(\frac{\partial f_2}{\partial \tau} \right) \left(\frac{\partial f_2}{\partial \tau} \right)' \frac{f_1}{f_2} d\mathbf{a} \right] \left(\int f_1 f_2 d\mathbf{a} \right). \qquad (8.13)$$

Substituting this into (8.12), we come to the desired inequality

$$\mathcal{I}_\mathbf{Y} \leq \int \left[\int \left(\frac{\partial f_2}{\partial \tau} \right) \left(\frac{\partial f_2}{\partial \tau} \right)' \frac{f_1}{f_2} d\mathbf{a} \right] d\mathbf{y}$$

$$= \int \left[\frac{1}{f_2} \left(\frac{\partial f_2}{\partial \tau} \right) \left(\frac{\partial f_2}{\partial \tau} \right)' \left(\int f_1 d\mathbf{y} \right) \right] d\mathbf{a} = \mathcal{I}_\mathbf{A},$$

because $\int f_1 d\mathbf{y} = 1$ for any $\mathbf{a}$.

∎

Now we apply this lemma to the model defined by (8.7) and (8.8). Information $\mathcal{I}_\mathbf{Y}$ is determined from the marginal distribution, and information $\mathcal{I}_\mathbf{A}$ is determined from the second-stage model (8.8). From the properties of the multivariate normal distribution, it follows that $\mathcal{I}_\mathbf{A} = \sum_{i=1}^{N} \mathbf{A}_i'(\sigma^2 \mathbf{D})^{-1} \mathbf{A}_i$. Thus, the absolute lower bound for the covariance matrix for the NLME model is given by

$$\text{cov}(\widehat{\boldsymbol{\beta}}_{ML}) \geq \sigma^2 \left(\sum_{i=1}^{N} \mathbf{A}_i' \mathbf{D}^{-1} \mathbf{A}_i \right)^{-1}. \qquad (8.14)$$

We notice that this inequality is true whether or not $\boldsymbol{\gamma}$ and $\boldsymbol{\theta}$ are known. This inequality may be viewed as the Cramér–Rao bound for the NLME model assuming normal distribution of $\mathbf{a}_i$. Interestingly, the lower bound depends neither on the first-stage model nor on the number of observations per subject, n_i. As follows from Section 8.10, if $\boldsymbol{\gamma}$ is not presented, this inequality turns into an equality when $N \to \infty$ and $\min n_i \to \infty$. In a special random parameters case, $\mathbf{A}_i = \mathbf{I}$, the lower covariance bound is $\mathbf{D}_*/N$.

Inequality (8.14) has an interesting interpretation: it turns into equality under a hypothetical situation when the $\{\mathbf{a}_i\}$ are observable. Indeed, in that case the best estimator, as follows from (8.8), would be the generalized least squares estimator with the covariance matrix coinciding with the right-hand side of (8.14). In fact, the condition $\min n_i \to \infty$ means that $\mathbf{a}_i$ can be estimated with infinite precision.

Problems for Section 8.4

1. Prove that the log-likelihood function (8.9) reduces to (4.14) if $\mathbf{f}_i$ are linear functions as for the LME model.

2. Justify the consistency and asymptotic normality of MLE for the NLME model using a stochastic scheme (Section 3.6.2). Use representation $\mathbf{f}_i = \mathbf{f}(\mathbf{x}_i)$ and think of n_i as a random sample from a meta-distribution.

3. Prove Lemma 41 for the case when $\mathbf{Y}$ is a function of $\mathbf{A}$ (the Schervish result).

4*. Derive inequality (8.14) for the LME model directly using the results of Chapter 4. Does inequality (8.14) turn into an equality for the LME model? Under what conditions does this inequality become an equality?

8.5   Two-stage estimator

This estimation method was one of the first suggested in the literature and seems natural in the framework of the nonlinear growth curve model (8.3); see Swamy (1971), Pocock et al. (1981), Beal and Sheiner (1982), Steimer et al. (1984), and Berkey and Laird (1986). Importantly, it is assumed that subjects do not share fixed parameters (no $\boldsymbol{\gamma}$). Thus, such a model can be called an all-random parameter model. Although we generalize the two-stage (TS) estimator to the model with fixed shared parameters as well (see the end of this section), it becomes less attractive due to the increased computational burden.

The idea is to use the subject-specific (individual) nonlinear least squares estimates of the regression parameters in the second-stage model applying the Generalized Least Squares (GLS) method. This two-stage method of estimation is a straightforward generalization of its analog for linear models discussed in Section 4.1. Indeed, after individual estimates are obtained, estimation procedures for the second-stage model become very similar. More precisely, the two-stage procedure to estimate the vector of population parameters $\boldsymbol{\beta}$ in model (8.3) is as follows:

1. Estimate $\mathbf{a}_i$, along with its covariance matrix, individually by nonlinear least squares.

2. Substitute the estimates of $\mathbf{a}_i$ into the second-stage model (8.2) and apply GLS using the estimate of the covariance matrix of individual parameters from the first step.

At the first step, N individual nonlinear regression problems are solved using standard techniques, such as Gauss–Newton or Levenberg–Marquardt, as described by Bard (1974), Nash and Walker-Smith (1987), Bates and Watts (1988), Seber and Wild (1989), and Demidenko (1989),

$$\| \mathbf{y}_i - \mathbf{f}_i(\boldsymbol{\alpha}_i) \|^2 \Longrightarrow \min_{\boldsymbol{\alpha}_i}, \qquad i = 1, ..., N \tag{8.15}$$

to obtain $\mathbf{a}_i^o$. We refer the reader to Section 6.1.3 for the computational detail and to Appendix 13.3 for a general discussion of optimization techniques. The conditional (asymptotic, when $n_i \to \infty$) covariance matrix of $\mathbf{a}_i^o$, as follows from the standard theory of nonlinear regression, is

$$\text{cov}(\mathbf{a}_i^o \,|\mathbf{b}_i|) \simeq \mathbf{T}_i = \widehat{\sigma}^2 (\mathbf{R}_i' \mathbf{R}_i)^{-1}, \tag{8.16}$$

where $\mathbf{R}_i$ is the $n_i \times k$ derivative matrix of $\mathbf{f}_i$ at $\mathbf{a}_i^o$. Analogously to the LME model, the estimator of σ^2 is the pooled variance, namely,

$$\widehat{\sigma}^2 = \frac{1}{\sum(n_i - k)} \sum_{i=1}^{N} \parallel \mathbf{y}_i - \mathbf{f}_i(\mathbf{a}_i^o) \parallel^2 . \tag{8.17}$$

Again, as in the linear model, the following variance/covariance decomposition holds (see also Section 7.4.4):

$$\text{cov}(\mathbf{a}_i^o) = \text{cov}(\mathbf{a}_i^o | \mathbf{b}_i) + \text{cov}(\mathbf{b}_i) \simeq \mathbf{T}_i + \mathbf{D}_*. \tag{8.18}$$

There are two options in proceeding toward $\boldsymbol{\beta}$ estimation given individual estimates $\mathbf{a}_i^o$ and matrices $\mathbf{T}_i$. First, similar to the linear growth curve model of Section 4.1, we can apply the maximum likelihood procedure to the second-stage model, assuming that the $\{\mathbf{a}_i^o\}$ have a normal distribution; see Davidian and Giltinan (1995), Stukel and Demidenko (1997b). Second, we can estimate matrix $\mathbf{D}$ by the method of moments and then apply GLS.

The R function `heightlog2S` below plots and estimates individual growth data using the `nls` function.

```
heightlog2S=function(sex=0)
{
dump("heightlog2S","c:\\MixedModels\\Chapter08\\heightlog2S.r")
gender=c("Boy","Girl")
if(sex==1) a0=c(165,-2.2,-0.42,0.039) else a0=c(182,-1,-0.16,0.018)
                    #start
da=height.dat[height.dat$sex==sex,] #extract gender set
nkids=nrow(da)
id=da$id
xx=seq(from=7,to=18,by=.1) #values to plot the curve
uid=unique(id);nud=length(uid)
par4cov=matrix(nrow=nud,ncol=4+4^2) #matrix of all fits
par(mfrow=c(7,10),mar=c(2,2,1,1))
Scov=matrix(0,4,4)
Sa=rep(0,4)
SSres=0;dfpool=0
```

```
 for(i in 1:nud)
{
x=da$year[id==uid[i]];y=da$height[id==uid[i]]
y=y[order(x)];x=x[order(x)] # order to make lines
plot(x,y,type="o",xlab="",ylab="",main=paste(gender[sex+1],uid[i]))
oi=try(nls(y~a1/(1+exp(a2-a3*x-a4*x^2)),start=
              list(a1=a0[1],a2=a0[2],a3=a0[3],a4=a0[4])
              ,nls.control(maxiter=200))) # prevent from stop
if(attr(oi,"class")!="try-error")
{
a=coef(oi)
par4cov[i,1:4]=a
yp=a[1]/(1+exp(a[2]-a[3]*xx-a[4]*xx^2))
lines(xx,yp,col=2,lwd=3)
covpar=summary(oi)$cov.unscaled # cov matrix/sigma2i
par4cov[i,5:20]=as.vector(covpar)
SSres=SSres+sum((y-predict(oi))^2)
dfpool=dfpool+length(y)-4
i.covpar=solve(covpar)
Sa=Sa+i.covpar%*%a
Scov=Scov+i.covpar
}
}
s2pool=SSres/dfpool # pooled variance
print(gender[sex+1])
meanpar=as.data.frame(matrix(ncol=2,nrow=4))
names(meanpar)=c("Mean","Weighted Mean")
row.names(meanpar)=c("a1","a2","a3","a4")
for(i in 1:4) meanpar[i,1]=mean(par4cov[,i],na.rm=T)
meanpar[,2]=solve(Scov)%*%Sa #weighted mean
print(meanpar)
par4cov[,5:20]=par4cov[,5:20]*s2pool # matrices Ti
# par4cov.height0=heightlog2S(sex=0)
return(par4cov) # return all ind fits for further analysis
}
```

We make several comments regarding this code: (1) the argument sex specifies
which growth data to analyze; by default, boys' growth is analyzed; (2) array a0 is
used as the start values for nls; these values are taken from Table 8.1; (3) array
par4cov contains four parameters and their covariance matrix for each person, this
information will be used for computation of the weighted mean, an example of saving
this matrix is shown at the end of the code; (4) the 4×4 matrix Scov is the sum

of inversed covariance matrices and the 4×1 array `Sa` is the weighted parameter vector; (5) the command `try` prevents the code from stopping when iterations do not converge; the maximum number of iterations is controlled by `nls.control`; we increase it to 200 because the default number 50 may not be sufficient; (6) the first four columns of matrix `par4cov` are the `nls` parameters themselves and the remaining 16 columns contain the covariance matrix divided by $\widehat{\sigma}_i^2$ and stored as a vector; (7) the dataframe `meanpar` contains parameter averages as the first column and the vector of the weighted mean as the second column, the weighted mean is computed as

$$\widetilde{\mathbf{a}} = \left(\sum_{i=1}^{N} \mathbf{P}_i^{-1} \right)^{-1} \left(\sum_{i=1}^{N} \mathbf{P}_i^{-1} \widehat{\mathbf{a}}_i \right),$$

where $\widehat{\mathbf{a}}_i$ is the NLS estimate and $\mathbf{P}_i = (\mathbf{R}_i' \mathbf{R}_i)^{-1}$ is the 'unscaled' covariance matrix. A more efficient way to compute the weighted parameter mean is discussed below.

8.5.1 Maximum likelihood estimation

Based on (8.18), it is reasonable to approximate

$$\mathbf{a}_i^o \simeq \mathcal{N}(\mathbf{A}_i \boldsymbol{\beta}, \mathbf{T}_i + \mathbf{D}_*), \qquad i = 1, ..., N, \tag{8.19}$$

treating $\mathbf{a}_i^o$, $\mathbf{T}_i$, and $\widehat{\sigma}^2$ as given but parameters $\boldsymbol{\beta}$ and $\mathbf{D}_*$ as subject to estimation. Then the Two-Stage Maximum Likelihood (TSML) estimator maximizes the log-likelihood function,

$$l_2(\boldsymbol{\beta}, \mathbf{D}_*) = -\frac{1}{2} \sum_{i=1}^{N} \{ \ln | \mathbf{T}_i + \mathbf{D}_* | + (\mathbf{a}_i^o - \mathbf{A}_i \boldsymbol{\beta})' (\mathbf{T}_i + \mathbf{D}_*)^{-1} (\mathbf{a}_i^o - \mathbf{A}_i \boldsymbol{\beta}) \}.$$

In the restricted version of MLE, the function to maximize takes the form

$$\begin{aligned}
l_{2R}(\boldsymbol{\beta}, \mathbf{D}_*) = \; & -\frac{1}{2} \sum_{i=1}^{N} \{ \ln | \mathbf{T}_i + \mathbf{D}_* | + \ln | \mathbf{A}_i' (\mathbf{T}_i + \mathbf{D}_*)^{-1} \mathbf{A}_i | \\
& + (\mathbf{a}_i^o - \mathbf{A}_i \boldsymbol{\beta})' (\mathbf{T}_i + \mathbf{D}_*)^{-1} (\mathbf{a}_i^o - \mathbf{A}_i \boldsymbol{\beta}) \}.
\end{aligned}$$

These two functions are the same as for the linear mixed effects model considered in Chapter 4, so the reader is referred to that chapter. The maximization can be accomplished by either of three algorithms: (1) Newton–Raphson, (2) Fisher scoring, or (3) EM (fixed-point). Davidian and Giltiman (1995) called this method the "global TS" estimation method.

8.5.2 Method of moments

An alternative way is to estimate matrix $\mathbf{D}_*$ by the Method of Moments (MM), analogously to the linear growth curve model, and then apply GLS to model (8.19). Therefore, based on decomposition (8.18), assuming that $\mathbf{T}_i$ is fixed, we estimate

$\widehat{\mathbf{D}}_* = (\sum \mathbf{d}_i \mathbf{d}_i' - \mathbf{T}_i)/N$, where $\mathbf{d}_i$ is the OLS residual vector of the second-stage model,

$$\mathbf{d}_i = \mathbf{a}_i^o - \mathbf{A}_i \left(\sum_{j=1}^N \mathbf{A}_j' \mathbf{A}_j \right)^{-1} \sum_{j=1}^N \mathbf{A}_j' \mathbf{a}_j^o. \tag{8.20}$$

Sometimes matrix $\widehat{\mathbf{D}}_*$ may not be nonnegative definite; then we modify the estimate as

$$\widehat{\mathbf{D}}_* = \frac{1}{N} \sum \mathbf{d}_i \mathbf{d}_i' - \lambda \frac{1}{N} \sum \mathbf{T}_i, \tag{8.21}$$

where λ is the minimum eigenvalue of matrix $(\mathbf{T}')^{-1/2} \sum \mathbf{d}_i \mathbf{d}_i' \mathbf{T}^{-1/2}$. It is elementary to prove that (8.21) is then a nonnegative definite matrix. A similar procedure was suggested by Vonesh and Carter (1992). The GLS estimator applied to (8.19) yields the Two-Stage MM (TSMM) estimator,

$$\widehat{\boldsymbol{\beta}}_{TS} = \left[\sum \mathbf{A}_i' (\mathbf{T}_i + \widehat{\mathbf{D}}_s)^{-1} \mathbf{A}_i \right]^{-1} \left[\sum \mathbf{A}_i' (\mathbf{T}_i + \widehat{\mathbf{D}}_s)^{-1} \mathbf{a}_i^o \right]. \tag{8.22}$$

The TSML and TSMM estimators have the same form as the GLS estimator and differ only by the choice of the estimator for matrix $\mathbf{D}_*$. The covariance matrix for the two estimators is given by

$$\left[\sum \mathbf{A}_i' (\mathbf{T}_i + \widehat{\mathbf{D}}_*)^{-1} \mathbf{A}_i \right]^{-1}, \tag{8.23}$$

where for TSML, $\widehat{\mathbf{D}}_*$ is the MLE from l_2 or l_{2R}, and for TSMM it is (8.21).

8.5.3 Disadvantage of two-stage estimation

The disadvantage of TS estimation is that individual estimation may fail, especially when the number of observations per subject, n_i, is small. Thus, the condition that the number of observations per subject/cluster is large is not only a theoretical but a practical requirement. Perhaps the simplest way to treat failed cases is just not to include them in the second stage. See Section 8.9, where we study the properties of the TS estimator for a simple exponential model. There is another pitfall of TS estimation: Since the decision on nonconvergence is always nonformal, the inclusion of a poor individual estimate in the second-stage model may lead to severe bias in the final beta estimator. To make the TS estimate more robust, Davidian and Giltinan (1995) suggest using absolute rather than squared residuals when minimizing l_2 or l_{2R}. Fortunately, the individual outliers are often accompanied by large covariance matrices $\mathbf{T}_i$, reducing the effect of poor estimation at the second stage. Clearly, the number of successful individual regressions must be large enough to allow inversion of the matrix in (8.22) or to find the maximum of the log-likelihood function. We refer the reader to a paper by Yeap and Davidian (2001), where the robust TS method for nonlinear mixed models is explored further.

8.5.4 Further discussion

Now let us discuss the case when the second-stage model is the rectangular growth curve model of Section 4.1.5. Then all components of the subject-specific parameters have the same set of explanatory variables, $\mathbf{A}_i = \mathbf{I} \otimes \mathbf{q}_i'$, where $\mathbf{I}$ is the $k \times k$ identity matrix and $\mathbf{q}_i$ is a $p \times 1$ vector of common explanatory variables (vector $\boldsymbol{\beta}$ has dimension $m = pk$). If, in addition, the first-stage model is balanced, the growth curve is called double balanced and the GLS collapses to the OLS estimator (we again refer the reader to Section 4.1.5). This does not remain true for the nonlinear growth curve model. Specifically, if in model (8.3) we have $\mathbf{f}_i = \mathbf{f}$, $n_i = n$, and $\mathbf{A}_i = \mathbf{I} \otimes \mathbf{q}_i'$, GLS and OLS produce different estimates. This stems from the fact that in the nonlinear model, $\mathbf{R}_i \neq$ const since derivatives are evaluated at different points $\mathbf{a}_i^o$, and consequently, $\mathbf{T}_i$ are not the same, unlike the double-balanced linear growth curve model.

As shown in Chapter 4, the two-stage estimator for the linear mixed effects model is consistent, asymptotically normally distributed, and efficient when $N \to \infty$ and $\{n_i\}$ are fixed. Later in the chapter it will be shown that the TS estimator is consistent for a nonlinear mixed model when *both* the number of subjects and the number of observations per subject increase to infinity. One can see from (8.16) that when n_i goes to infinity, $\mathbf{R}_i' \mathbf{R}_i = O(n_i)$ and matrix $\mathbf{T}_i$ vanishes. This means that as follows from (8.23), the covariance matrix approaches $(\sum \mathbf{A}_i' \mathbf{D}^{-1} \mathbf{A}_i^{-1})^{-1}$, where $\mathbf{D}$ is the scaled covariance matrix. But as follows from (8.14), this matrix coincides with the absolute lower bound for $\boldsymbol{\beta}$, meaning that when $N \to \infty$ and n_i are large, the TS estimator is efficient.

8.5.5 Two-stage method in the presence of a common parameter

Ordinarily, the two-stage method of estimation assumes that there is no common parameter $\boldsymbol{\gamma}$. However, one may generalize the TS to model (8.1) by minimization of the total sum of squares,

$$\sum_{i=1}^{N} \| \mathbf{y}_i - \mathbf{f}_i(\boldsymbol{\gamma}, \boldsymbol{\alpha}_i) \|^2 . \tag{8.24}$$

Obviously, in the absence of $\boldsymbol{\gamma}$, this minimization collapses to N separate nonlinear least squares. In the presence of $\boldsymbol{\gamma}$, problem (8.24) does not collapse into separate minimizations. To facilitate the computational burden, one may apply a modification of the Gauss–Newton algorithm described in Section 8.7.3. From (8.24) we obtain estimates $\mathbf{a}_i^o$ and its covariance matrix and proceed to estimation of the second-stage model.

Problems for Section 8.4

1. The code `heightlog2S` computes the weighted mean using matrices $\mathbf{P}_i = (\mathbf{R}_i' \mathbf{R}_i)^{-1}$. Show that the estimate $\widetilde{\mathbf{a}}$ does not change if $\mathbf{P}_i$ is replaced by the covariance matrix of $\widehat{\mathbf{a}}_i$: namely, $\mathbf{T}_i = \widehat{\sigma}^2 \mathbf{P}_i$.

2. Run `heightlog2S` for girls and boys and compare the results with Table 8.1. What estimate is more reliable based on the prediction of the adult height?

3*. Derive the Newton-Raphson algorithm for maximization of $l_2(\boldsymbol{\beta}, \mathbf{D}_*)$ and $l_{2R}(\boldsymbol{\beta}, \mathbf{D}_*)$ following the line of derivation in Section 2.10. Use the matrix derivative $\partial \ln | \mathbf{T}_i + \mathbf{D}_* | / \partial \mathbf{D}_* = (\mathbf{T}_i + \mathbf{D}_*)^{-1}$ and inverse matrix approximation $(\mathbf{T}_i + \mathbf{D}_{**})^{-1} \simeq \mathbf{R}_i^{-1} - \mathbf{R}_i^{-1} \boldsymbol{\Delta} \mathbf{R}_i^{-1}$ where $\mathbf{R}_i = \mathbf{T}_i + \mathbf{D}_*$ and $\boldsymbol{\Delta} = \mathbf{D}_{**} - \mathbf{D}_*$. Obtain the score equation for $\mathbf{D}_*$ and solve it using the vec operator. Derive the MLE for $\boldsymbol{\beta}$ and $\mathbf{D}_*$ when the data are balanced, $\mathbf{T}_i = \mathbf{T}$. Write an R function that implements this algorithm. Test whether your function converges to the analytic solution in the case of balanced data. Apply this algorithm for the height data.

4. Simplify the MM for the all-random parameter model as coded in the function **heightlog2S**. Derive a simple expression for (8.20) and compute (8.21) and (8.22) for the height of boys and girls.

5. Compare (8.23) with (8.14) derived previously inequality. Does the former comply with the latter? When does (8.14) turn into an equality, or better stated, when is the left-hand side close to the right-hand side?

6. Write an R program that models the height data with the QLogist model assuming that only adult height (a_1) varies from person to person. Reduce the estimation problem to **nls** alternating between an estimation of 67 individual a_{1i} and fixed a_2, a_3, and a_4.

8.6   First-order approximation

To circumvent the integration problem, several authors have suggested replacing the original nonlinear regression function with its linear analog using the first-order approximation (FOA), see Sheiner and Beal (1980), Beal and Sheiner (1982, 1992), and Vonesh and Carter (1992). The advantage of this approach is that in the linearized model the random effects become linear and therefore we arrive at the *marginal* mixed model, studied in Chapter 6.

Thus, replacing $\mathbf{f}_i(\boldsymbol{\gamma}, \mathbf{A}_i\boldsymbol{\beta} + \mathbf{b}_i)$ with its linear counterpart around $E(\mathbf{a}_i) = \mathbf{A}_i\boldsymbol{\beta}$, one obtains a pseudo-model

$$\mathbf{y}_i = \mathbf{f}_i(\boldsymbol{\gamma}, \mathbf{A}_i\boldsymbol{\beta}) + \mathbf{Z}_i(\boldsymbol{\beta})\mathbf{b}_i + \boldsymbol{\epsilon}_i, \tag{8.25}$$

where $\mathbf{Z}_i = \partial \mathbf{f}_i / \partial \mathbf{a}_i$ and $\mathbf{b}_i \sim \mathcal{N}(\mathbf{0}, \sigma^2 \mathbf{D})$. We use the term *pseudo* to emphasize that the model (8.25) is not the same as the original model. It is worthwhile to remember that this approximation is done around the population-averaged mean; later, we consider an approximation around the subject-specific mean. The key to the first-order approximation is that it turns the original model into a marginal model with the varied matrix of random effects (6.17) of Section 6.2. The reader should remember that the original and pseudo-models are not equivalent. To estimate (8.25), one could simply follow the recipes of Section 6.2. For completeness, we review several schemes to estimate the pseudo-model (8.25).

8.6.1   GEE and MLE

As mentioned earlier in Section 6.2, the marginal model with a varied matrix of random effects may be estimated by either MLE or GEE using iteratively reweighted least squares (IRLS) to update $\boldsymbol{\beta}$ and $\boldsymbol{\gamma}$, see Section 6.2.3 for details. Under the normal assumption, the former method is more efficient, but it is not robust to distribution and model specification. Since (8.25) is an approximate model, estimating by GEE is well justified. Following the line of Sections 6.1 and 6.2, $\boldsymbol{\gamma}$, $\boldsymbol{\beta}$, and the variance parameters, σ^2 and $\mathbf{D}$, may be estimated by the ML with the log-likelihood function

$$l(\boldsymbol{\gamma},\boldsymbol{\beta},\sigma^2,\mathbf{D}) = -\frac{1}{2}\left\{N_T \ln\sigma^2 + \sum[\ln|\mathbf{V}_i| + \sigma^{-2}(\mathbf{y}_i - \mathbf{f}_i)'\mathbf{V}_i^{-1}(\mathbf{y}_i - \mathbf{f}_i)]\right\} \quad (8.26)$$

where

$$\mathbf{f}_i = \mathbf{f}_i(\boldsymbol{\gamma},\mathbf{A}_i\boldsymbol{\beta}), \quad \mathbf{V}_i = \mathbf{V}_i(\mathbf{D}) = \mathbf{I} + \mathbf{Z}_i\mathbf{D}\mathbf{Z}_i'. \quad (8.27)$$

Notice that we deliberately indicate in (8.27) that matrices $\mathbf{V}_i$ and $\mathbf{Z}_i$ are not functions of $\boldsymbol{\gamma}$ and $\boldsymbol{\beta}$ but functions of $\mathbf{D}$ only, so that the estimating equation for $\boldsymbol{\chi} = (\boldsymbol{\gamma}',\boldsymbol{\beta}')'$ is $\sum\mathbf{R}_i\mathbf{V}_i^{-1}(\mathbf{y} - \mathbf{f}_i) = \mathbf{0}$ where $\mathbf{R}_i = \partial\mathbf{f}_i/\partial\boldsymbol{\chi}$. After the maximum of l is found, we update $\mathbf{Z}_i$ and $\mathbf{V}_i$ and restart the maximization process, iterating in such a manner until convergence. We can eliminate σ^2 and obtain a profile log-likelihood such as (6.6). Below we consider another method to estimate the variance parameters.

8.6.2   Method of moments and VLS

Instead of the likelihood-based variance parameters estimation, one can use a Method of Moments (MM) estimator as in the two-stage method discussed above or as discussed in Section 6.1.4. In particular, in the case when $\mathbf{A}_i$ has the form $(\mathbf{I} \otimes \mathbf{q}_i')$, Vonesh and Carter (1992) proposed a MM estimator for the covariance matrix of random effects,

$$\widehat{\mathbf{D}}_* = \frac{1}{N-m}\sum_i \mathbf{d}_i\mathbf{d}_i' - \lambda\frac{1}{N-m}\sum_i\left[1 - \mathbf{q}_i'\left(\sum\mathbf{q}_j\mathbf{q}_j'\right)^{-1}\mathbf{q}_i\right]\mathbf{T}_i \quad (8.28)$$

where $\mathbf{T}_i$ and $\mathbf{d}_i$ are as defined in (8.16) and (8.20). Scalar λ provides the nonnegative definiteness of matrix $\widehat{\mathbf{D}}_*$ and can be chosen as for the TS estimator described above. In the general case, we use the MM estimator (8.21). Vonesh and Carter proved that for pseudo-model (8.25), the FOA estimator is asymptotically equivalent to the MLE when both $N \to \infty$ and $\min n_i \to \infty$. However, it is important to note that model (8.25) does not coincide with the original model (8.1, 8.2), and consequently, the properties of this estimator do not necessarily remain true for the original model. Moreover, as shown in Section 8.9, the FOA estimator is not consistent for model (8.1) in either of two asymptotic situations.

By analogy with a linear mixed effects model, variance parameters σ^2 and $\mathbf{D}$ can be estimated based on residuals $\mathbf{e}_i = \mathbf{y}_i - \mathbf{f}_i(\widehat{\boldsymbol{\gamma}},\mathbf{A}_i\widehat{\boldsymbol{\beta}}_0)$ and matrix $\mathbf{R}_i$ using the Variance Least Squares (VLS) estimator, see Section 3.12 and Section 6.1.4.

Problems for Section 8.6

1. Describe the NLME model for which the pseudo-model (8.25) is equivalent to the original model. Provide an example.

2. Following the nomenclature of Section 6.3, to what type of nonlinear marginal model does the pseudo-model (8.25) belong.

3. Obtain a closed-form solution of MLE for $\mathbf{D}$ given $\boldsymbol{\beta}$ using function (8.26) when $\mathbf{Z}_i = \mathbf{Z}$.

4*. Consider the exponential model with random intercept, $y_{ij} = \exp(\alpha + \beta x_{ij} + b_i) + \varepsilon_{ij}$, where b_j is the random effect ($\alpha + b_i$ is the random intercept) and the error term are independent and normally distributed with zero mean and variances σ_b^2 and σ^2 respectively, $j = 1, 2, ..., n; i = 1, 2, ..., N$. Find a consistent estimator of the slope using standard nonlinear least squares assuming that $nN \to \infty$. Estimate β using maximization of the log-likelihood function (8.26); make necessary simplifications. Write an R program to investigate the small-sample properties of the two estimators as a function of n and N (assume that $x_{ij} = i$). Is the FOA estimator consistent when $N \to \infty$ and n is fixed, say, $n = 2$. Support your analytical derivation with simulations.

5. The conditions are same as Problem 4 but the slope is also random, $y_{ij} = \exp(\alpha + (\beta + \delta_i)x_{ij} + b_i) + \varepsilon_{ij}$.

8.7   Lindstrom–Bates estimator

Lindstrom and Bates (1990) suggested approximating the nonlinear function $\mathbf{f}_i$ not around the population means $E(\mathbf{a}_i) = \mathbf{A}_i\boldsymbol{\beta}$, as in the first-order approximation method, but around the subject-specific means $E(\mathbf{a}_i) + \widehat{\mathbf{b}}_i$, where $\widehat{\mathbf{b}}_i$ is an "estimate" of $\mathbf{b}_i$. The iterative procedure consists of two steps (originally, there were no $\boldsymbol{\gamma}$):

1. Penalized nonlinear least squares (PLS). When $\mathbf{D}$ is being held, the following minimization problem is solved:

$$\sum_{i=1}^{N} \left[\| \mathbf{y}_i - \mathbf{f}_i(\boldsymbol{\gamma}, \mathbf{A}_i\boldsymbol{\beta} + \boldsymbol{\tau}_i) \|^2 + \boldsymbol{\tau}_i' \mathbf{D}^{-1} \boldsymbol{\tau}_i \right] \Longrightarrow \min_{\boldsymbol{\gamma}, \boldsymbol{\beta}, \boldsymbol{\tau}_1, ..., \boldsymbol{\tau}_N}. \qquad (8.29)$$

The solution to (8.29) is denoted as $\widehat{\boldsymbol{\gamma}}$, $\widehat{\boldsymbol{\beta}}$, and $\{\widehat{\boldsymbol{\tau}}_1, \widehat{\boldsymbol{\tau}}_2, ..., \widehat{\boldsymbol{\tau}}_N\}$.

2. Linear mixed effects (LME). Given estimates of the random effects $\widehat{\boldsymbol{\tau}}_i$ and population-averaged parameters $\widehat{\boldsymbol{\gamma}}$ and $\widehat{\boldsymbol{\beta}}$ from step 1, apply the linear mixed effects maximum likelihood estimation procedure based on the model

$$\mathbf{w}_i \sim N\left(\mathbf{R}_i\mathbf{A}_i\boldsymbol{\beta}, \sigma^2(\mathbf{I} + \mathbf{R}_i\mathbf{D}\mathbf{R}_i')\right) \qquad (8.30)$$

with the pseudo-observation $\mathbf{w}_i$:

$$\mathbf{w}_i = \mathbf{y}_i - \mathbf{f}_i(\widehat{\boldsymbol{\gamma}}, \mathbf{A}_i\widehat{\boldsymbol{\beta}} + \widehat{\boldsymbol{\tau}}_i) + \mathbf{R}_i(\widehat{\boldsymbol{\tau}}_i + \mathbf{A}_i\widehat{\boldsymbol{\beta}}), \quad \mathbf{R}_i = \left. \frac{\partial \mathbf{f}_i}{\partial \mathbf{a}_i} \right|_{\mathbf{a}_i = \mathbf{A}_i\widehat{\boldsymbol{\beta}} + \widehat{\boldsymbol{\tau}}_i}.$$

Next find estimates for $\widehat{\boldsymbol{\beta}}$, $\widehat{\sigma}^2$, and $\widehat{\mathbf{D}}$ (the regular or restricted ML estimation procedure can be applied) and return to step 1, iterating until convergence. The resulting estimator is called the LB estimator.

It is instructive to see what the LB estimator turns into for a linear growth curve model, $\mathbf{y}_i = \mathbf{Z}_i\mathbf{a}_i + \boldsymbol{\varepsilon}_i$, where $\mathbf{a}_i = \mathbf{A}_i\boldsymbol{\beta} + \mathbf{b}_i$, see Section 4.1. Then $\mathbf{f}_i(\boldsymbol{\gamma}, \mathbf{a}) = \mathbf{Z}_i\mathbf{a}$ and $\mathbf{R}_i = \mathbf{Z}_i$. The pseudo-observation takes the form

$$\mathbf{w}_i = \mathbf{y}_i - \mathbf{Z}_i(\mathbf{A}_i\widehat{\boldsymbol{\beta}} + \widehat{\boldsymbol{\tau}}_i) - \mathbf{Z}_i(\widehat{\boldsymbol{\tau}}_i + \mathbf{A}_i\widehat{\boldsymbol{\beta}}) = \mathbf{y}_i,$$

so that model (8.30) turns into linear growth curve model (4.5), and consequently, LB = ML. For this model, PLS is not required.

A question arises as to the numerical consistency of the two steps arises because parameter $\boldsymbol{\beta}$ is estimated on different grounds: in PLS, it is the solution to (8.29), and in LME, it is the estimate of fixed effects. We show that these two estimates coincide at convergence (both procedures produce the same $\boldsymbol{\beta}$-estimate). To prove this, it suffices to show that if $\boldsymbol{\beta}_1$ minimizes

$$\sum_{i=1}^{N} \left[\| \, \mathbf{y}_i - \mathbf{f}_i(\boldsymbol{\gamma}, \mathbf{A}_i\boldsymbol{\beta} + \boldsymbol{\tau}_i) \, \|^2 + \boldsymbol{\tau}_i' \mathbf{D}^{-1} \boldsymbol{\tau}_i \right] \tag{8.31}$$

and $\boldsymbol{\beta}_2$ minimizes

$$\sum \left[(\mathbf{w}_i - \mathbf{R}_i\mathbf{A}_i\boldsymbol{\beta})'(\mathbf{I} + \mathbf{R}_i\mathbf{D}\mathbf{R}_i')^{-1}(\mathbf{w}_i - \mathbf{R}_i\mathbf{A}_i\boldsymbol{\beta}) \right], \tag{8.32}$$

assuming that $\boldsymbol{\gamma}$ and $\mathbf{D}$ are fixed, where

$$\mathbf{w}_i = \mathbf{y}_i - \mathbf{f}_i(\boldsymbol{\gamma}, \mathbf{A}_i\boldsymbol{\beta}_1 + \boldsymbol{\tau}_i) + \mathbf{R}_i\boldsymbol{\tau}_i + \mathbf{R}_i\mathbf{A}_i\boldsymbol{\beta}_1, \quad \mathbf{R}_i = \left. \frac{\partial \mathbf{f}_i}{\partial \mathbf{a}_i} \right|_{\mathbf{a}_i = \mathbf{A}_i\boldsymbol{\beta}_1 + \boldsymbol{\tau}_i},$$

then $\boldsymbol{\beta}_1 = \boldsymbol{\beta}_2$. Indeed, the first-order conditions for $\boldsymbol{\beta}$ and $\boldsymbol{\tau}_i$ from (8.31) can be written, respectively, as

$$\sum \mathbf{A}_i'\mathbf{R}_i'\mathbf{e}_i = \mathbf{0}, \qquad \mathbf{D}\mathbf{R}_i'\mathbf{e}_i + \boldsymbol{\tau}_i = \mathbf{0}, \tag{8.33}$$

where $\mathbf{e}_i = \mathbf{y}_i - \mathbf{f}_i(\boldsymbol{\gamma}, \mathbf{A}_i\boldsymbol{\beta} + \boldsymbol{\tau}_i)$. The first-order condition for $\boldsymbol{\beta}$ from the linear mixed effects problem is written as

$$\sum \mathbf{A}_i'\mathbf{R}_i'(\mathbf{I} + \mathbf{R}_i\mathbf{D}\mathbf{R}_i')^{-1}(\mathbf{w}_i - \mathbf{R}_i\mathbf{A}_i\boldsymbol{\beta}_2) = \mathbf{0}. \tag{8.34}$$

We aim to show that (8.33) and (8.34) imply that $\boldsymbol{\beta}_1 = \boldsymbol{\beta}_2$. Indeed, applying the dimension-reduction formula (2.21), we rewrite (8.34) as

$$\begin{aligned}
\mathbf{0} = &\sum \mathbf{A}_i'\mathbf{R}_i'(\mathbf{I} + \mathbf{R}_i\mathbf{D}\mathbf{R}_i')^{-1}\mathbf{R}_i'\left(\mathbf{e}_i + \mathbf{R}_i\boldsymbol{\tau}_i\right) \\
&+ \left(\sum \mathbf{A}_i'\mathbf{R}_i'(\mathbf{I} + \mathbf{R}_i\mathbf{D}\mathbf{R}_i')^{-1}\mathbf{R}_i\mathbf{A}_i\right)(\boldsymbol{\beta}_1 - \boldsymbol{\beta}_2).
\end{aligned} \tag{8.35}$$

But for the first term, using (8.33), we obtain after some algebra

$$\sum \mathbf{A}_i'\mathbf{R}_i'(\mathbf{I} + \mathbf{R}_i\mathbf{D}\mathbf{R}_i')^{-1}\mathbf{R}_i'(\mathbf{I} - \mathbf{D}\mathbf{R}_i'\mathbf{R}_i)\mathbf{e}_i = \mathbf{0},$$

so that the first term in (8.35) vanishes, implying that $\boldsymbol{\beta}_1 = \boldsymbol{\beta}_2$. ∎

One can use this fact to simplify the computations in the LB procedure. First, we can take $\boldsymbol{\beta}$ from the PLS. Thus, let $\boldsymbol{\gamma} = \widehat{\boldsymbol{\gamma}}$ and $\boldsymbol{\beta} = \widehat{\boldsymbol{\beta}}$ in (8.29) be held fixed, so that $\widehat{\mathbf{a}}_i = \mathbf{A}_i\widehat{\boldsymbol{\beta}}$ is fixed. Then the optimization problem (8.29) collapses into N separate optimization problems,

$$\| \, \mathbf{y}_i - \mathbf{f}_i(\widehat{\mathbf{a}}_i + \boldsymbol{\tau}) \, \|^2 + \boldsymbol{\tau}'\mathbf{D}^{-1}\boldsymbol{\tau} \Longrightarrow \min_{\boldsymbol{\tau}}, \ i = 1, ..., N.$$

They can be solved by the Gauss–Newton algorithm,

$$\boldsymbol{\tau}_{s+1} = \boldsymbol{\tau}_s + \lambda_s(\mathbf{R}_i'\mathbf{R}_i + \mathbf{D}^{-1})^{-1}\mathbf{R}_i'(\mathbf{y}_i - \mathbf{f}_i(\widehat{\boldsymbol{\gamma}}, \widehat{\mathbf{a}}_i + \boldsymbol{\tau}_s)),$$

where $\mathbf{R}_i$ is the derivative of $\mathbf{f}_i$ calculated at $\widehat{\mathbf{a}}_i + \boldsymbol{\tau}_s$ and $0 < \lambda_s \leq 1$ is the step length to guarantee the drop in the sum of squares at each iteration $s = 0, 1, ...$

The second way to simplify the LB procedure is to solve (8.29) for $\boldsymbol{\gamma}, \boldsymbol{\beta}, \boldsymbol{\tau}_1, ..., \boldsymbol{\tau}_N$ but to use the linear mixed effects model without fixed effects to obtain estimates for the variance parameters, namely,

$$\mathbf{y}_i - \mathbf{f}_i(\widehat{\boldsymbol{\gamma}}, \mathbf{A}_i\widehat{\boldsymbol{\beta}} + \widehat{\boldsymbol{\tau}}_i) + \mathbf{R}_i\widehat{\boldsymbol{\tau}}_i \sim N\left(\mathbf{0}, \sigma^2(\mathbf{I} + \mathbf{R}_i\mathbf{D}\mathbf{R}'_i)\right).$$

Computational aspects of simultaneous minimization over all parameters in PLS are discussed below in the Section 8.7.3.

The relationship between the LB method and Laplace approximation is studied in Section 8.8.2. We shall show that LB is equivalent to the penalized quasi-likelihood method.

8.7.1   What if matrix $\mathbf{D}$ is not positive definite?

An implicit assumption of penalized nonlinear least squares is that during iterations, matrix $\mathbf{D}$ remains positive definite. Although we can assume that $\mathbf{D}$ is nonnegative definite, because it is the outcome of the ML solution, it is possible to get $\det(\mathbf{D}) = 0$ at some iteration. A naive solution to take a generalized inverse of matrix $\mathbf{D}$ in (8.29) is unsatisfactory. To illustrate this comment, let us assume that there are two uncorrelated random effects: matrix $\mathbf{D}$ is 2×2 and $D_{12} = D_{21} = 0$. Let $D_{22} = 0$ and let the first diagonal element be positive. The generalized inverse of $\mathbf{D} = \mathrm{diag}(D_{11}, 0)$ is $\mathrm{diag}(1/D_{11}, 0)$. This implies that the second component of vector $\boldsymbol{\tau}_i$ becomes unrestricted in the penalized least squares. To the contrary, since $\mathrm{var}(\tau_{i2}) = 0$, this component must be zero.

An appropriate way to cope with situations in which $\mathbf{D}$ becomes singular is as follows. For singular $\mathbf{D}$, using eigenvalue decomposition, we represent

$$\mathbf{D} = [\mathbf{P}_1, \mathbf{P}_2] \begin{bmatrix} \mathbf{0} & \mathbf{0} \\ \mathbf{0} & \boldsymbol{\Lambda} \end{bmatrix} \begin{bmatrix} \mathbf{P}'_1 \\ \mathbf{P}'_2 \end{bmatrix}, \tag{8.36}$$

where $\boldsymbol{\Lambda}$ is the diagonal matrix of nonzero eigenvalues. Let $\mathbf{D}^+ = \mathbf{P}_2\boldsymbol{\Lambda}^{-1}\mathbf{P}_2$ be the generalized inverse of matrix $\mathbf{D}$. Then the penalized nonlinear least squares takes the form

$$\sum_{i=1}^{N} \left[\| \mathbf{y}_i - \mathbf{f}_i(\boldsymbol{\gamma}, \mathbf{A}_i\boldsymbol{\beta} + \boldsymbol{\tau}_i) \|^2 + \boldsymbol{\tau}'_i\mathbf{D}^+\boldsymbol{\tau}_i\right] \Rightarrow \min_{\boldsymbol{\beta}, \mathbf{P}'_1\boldsymbol{\tau}_i = \mathbf{0}}.$$

In other words, we replace the original PLS by the restricted PLS, $\mathbf{P}'_1\boldsymbol{\tau}_i = \mathbf{0}$, $i = 1, 2, ..., N$.

8.7.2   Relation to the two-stage estimator

The TS and LB estimates are closely related. Let δ be any positive scalar and let $\widehat{\boldsymbol{\beta}}(\delta)$ be the solution to the PLS

$$\sum_{i=1}^{N} \left[\| \mathbf{y}_i - \mathbf{f}_i(\boldsymbol{\gamma}, \mathbf{A}_i\boldsymbol{\beta} + \boldsymbol{\tau}_i) \|^2 + \delta\boldsymbol{\tau}'_i\mathbf{D}^{-1}\boldsymbol{\tau}_i\right]. \tag{8.37}$$

Clearly, (8.37) is equivalent to (8.29) for $\delta = 1$. We aim to show that when δ approaches zero, the LB estimate converges to the TS estimate, namely,

$$\lim_{\delta \to 0} \widehat{\boldsymbol{\beta}}(\delta) = \widehat{\boldsymbol{\beta}}, \tag{8.38}$$

where $\widehat{\boldsymbol{\beta}}$ is the TS estimate, defined as

$$\widehat{\boldsymbol{\beta}} = \left(\sum_{i=1}^{N} \mathbf{A}_i' \mathbf{D}^{-1} \mathbf{A}_i \right)^{-1} \left(\sum_{i=1}^{N} \mathbf{A}_i' \mathbf{D}^{-1} \mathbf{a}_i^o \right), \tag{8.39}$$

where the $\{\mathbf{a}_i^o\}$ minimize the total sum of squares (8.24). To prove this, we denote $\boldsymbol{\alpha}_i = \mathbf{A}_i \boldsymbol{\beta} + \boldsymbol{\tau}_i$ and rewrite (8.37) as

$$\sum \left[\| \mathbf{y}_i - \mathbf{f}_i(\boldsymbol{\gamma}, \boldsymbol{\alpha}_i) \|^2 + \delta(\boldsymbol{\alpha}_i - \mathbf{A}_i \boldsymbol{\beta})' \mathbf{D}^{-1}(\boldsymbol{\alpha}_i - \mathbf{A}_i \boldsymbol{\beta}) \right]. \tag{8.40}$$

The first-order conditions for minimization for $\boldsymbol{\alpha}_i$ are

$$\frac{\partial \mathbf{f}_i}{\partial \boldsymbol{\alpha}_i}(\mathbf{y}_i - \mathbf{f}_i(\boldsymbol{\gamma}, \boldsymbol{\alpha}_i)) + \delta \mathbf{D}^{-1}(\boldsymbol{\alpha}_i - \mathbf{A}_i \boldsymbol{\beta}) = \mathbf{0}, \quad i = 1, ..., N \tag{8.41}$$

and the first-order condition for $\boldsymbol{\beta}$ is

$$\mathbf{A}_i' \mathbf{D}^{-1}(\boldsymbol{\alpha}_i - \mathbf{A}_i \boldsymbol{\beta}) = \mathbf{0}. \tag{8.42}$$

Since $\delta \to 0$, equations (8.41) become equivalent to $\frac{\partial \mathbf{f}_i}{\partial \boldsymbol{\alpha}_i}(\mathbf{y}_i - \mathbf{f}_i(\boldsymbol{\alpha}_i)) = \mathbf{0}$, leading to the individual least squares solution, $\boldsymbol{\alpha}_i = \mathbf{a}_i^o$. Substituting them into (8.42), we come to (8.39)—the limit (8.38) is proved. In fact, (8.37) may define a new family of estimators as a function of $\delta \in (0, 1]$. When $\delta = 1$, we obtain the LB estimator; when $\delta \to 0$, we come to the TS estimator.

The close relationship between the two methods of estimation explains their statistical equivalence when $\min n_i \to \infty$, see details in Section 8.10. Referring to (8.40), the LB estimator can be viewed as an adjusted version of the TS estimator. The penalty term, $(\boldsymbol{\alpha}_i - \mathbf{A}_i \boldsymbol{\beta})' \mathbf{D}^{-1}(\boldsymbol{\alpha}_i - \mathbf{A}_i \boldsymbol{\beta})$, can be interpreted as a tentative restriction on the dispersion of individual estimates. Several authors have pointed out the connection between the LB estimator and MLE via the Laplace approximation to the log-likelihood function. The relevant discussion is given in Section 8.8.

8.7.3 Computational aspects of penalized least squares

Simultaneous minimization of the criterion function (8.29) involves a large number of parameters, $q + Nk + m$. Consequently, a straightforward application of the Gauss–Newton algorithm or any of its modifications would require a $(q + Nk + m) \times (q + Nk + m)$ matrix inverse. As already mentioned, a characteristic feature of (8.29) is that holding $\boldsymbol{\beta}$, one comes to N separate optimization problems. This kind of problem was called a "loosely coupled" nonlinear least squares problem by Soo and Bates (1992). They made use of this peculiar property and proposed a special algorithm avoiding the large matrix inverse based on orthogonal-triangular matrix decomposition. Here we suggest an alternative way to solve (8.29) in the framework of the Gauss–Newton algorithm and provide an explicit solution for the parameter increments.

Let $\boldsymbol{\gamma}_{new} = \boldsymbol{\gamma} + \boldsymbol{\Delta\gamma}$, $\boldsymbol{\beta}_{new} = \boldsymbol{\beta} + \boldsymbol{\Delta\beta}$, and $\boldsymbol{\tau}_{i,new} = \boldsymbol{\tau}_i + \boldsymbol{\Delta\tau}_i$ where $\boldsymbol{\gamma}, \boldsymbol{\beta}$, and $\boldsymbol{\tau}_i$ are values from the previous iteration. The idea is to find the increments $\boldsymbol{\Delta\gamma}$, $\boldsymbol{\Delta\beta}$ and $\boldsymbol{\Delta\tau}_i$ by linearization of the nonlinear regression functions in (8.29). Denoting the residuals from the previous iteration as $\mathbf{e}_i = \mathbf{y}_i - \mathbf{f}_i(\boldsymbol{\gamma}, \mathbf{A}_i\boldsymbol{\beta} + \boldsymbol{\tau}_i)$, the criterion function can be approximated by a quadratic function as follows:

$$\sum_{i=1}^{N} \left[\| \mathbf{e}_i - \mathbf{E}_i\boldsymbol{\Delta\nu} - \mathbf{R}_i\boldsymbol{\Delta\tau}_i) \|^2 + (\boldsymbol{\tau}_i + \boldsymbol{\Delta\tau}_i)'\mathbf{D}^{-1}(\boldsymbol{\tau}_i + \boldsymbol{\Delta\tau}_i) \right], \qquad (8.43)$$

where $\boldsymbol{\nu}$ is the combined parameter vector,

$$\boldsymbol{\nu} = \left[\begin{array}{c} \boldsymbol{\gamma} \\ \boldsymbol{\beta} \end{array} \right], \quad \mathbf{E}_i = \left[\begin{array}{c} \partial\mathbf{f}_i/\boldsymbol{\gamma} \\ \mathbf{R}_i\mathbf{A}_i \end{array} \right].$$

If $\boldsymbol{\Delta\beta}$ is held, the minimization of (8.43) falls into N separate quadratic problems for $\boldsymbol{\Delta\tau}_i$ with the solution

$$\boldsymbol{\Delta\tau}_i = (\mathbf{R}_i'\mathbf{R}_i + \mathbf{D}^{-1})^{-1}(\mathbf{R}_i'\mathbf{e}_i - \mathbf{D}^{-1}\boldsymbol{\tau}_i - \mathbf{R}_i'\mathbf{E}_i\boldsymbol{\Delta\nu}), \quad i = 1, ..., N.$$

Substituting $\boldsymbol{\Delta\tau}_i$ back into (8.43), the profile criterion function takes the form of a regular sum of squares, $\sum \| \mathbf{v}_i - \mathbf{Q}_i\boldsymbol{\Delta\nu} \|^2$, where

$$\begin{array}{rcl} \mathbf{v}_i & = & \mathbf{e}_i - \mathbf{R}_i(\mathbf{R}_i'\mathbf{R}_i + \mathbf{D}^{-1})^{-1}(\mathbf{R}_i'\mathbf{e}_i - \mathbf{D}^{-1}\boldsymbol{\tau}_i), \\ \mathbf{Q}_i & = & \mathbf{E}_i - \mathbf{R}_i(\mathbf{R}_i'\mathbf{R}_i + \mathbf{D}^{-1})^{-1}\mathbf{R}_i'\mathbf{E}_i, \end{array}$$

with the solution $\boldsymbol{\Delta\nu} = \left(\sum \mathbf{Q}_i'\mathbf{Q}_i \right)^{-1} \left(\sum \mathbf{Q}_i'\mathbf{v}_i \right)$. Finally, the Gauss–Newton iterations have the form

$$\boldsymbol{\nu}_{new} = \boldsymbol{\nu} + \lambda\boldsymbol{\Delta\nu}, \quad \boldsymbol{\tau}_{i,new} = \boldsymbol{\tau}_i + \lambda\boldsymbol{\Delta\tau}_i$$

where $0 < \lambda \leq 1$ is the step length, to ensure a decrease in the original criterion function at each iteration.

If there is no common parameter $\boldsymbol{\gamma}$ in the nonlinear growth curve model, we can apply N separate penalized nonlinear least squares to find $\boldsymbol{\tau}_i$, and we can find $\boldsymbol{\beta}$ from LME (8.30).

8.7.4   Implementation in R: the function nlme

The Lindstrom-Bates estimation procedure is implemented in the function nlme from the library of the same name; we have used this function before in Section 6.4.6. Three components should be specified in the nlme call: (1) the nonlinear function $\mathbf{f}_i$ as a function of fixed and random parameters (the syntax is the same as in the nls function); (2) fixed effects parameters; and (3) random effects parameters. When specifying random effects, we use the same syntax as in lme. Also as in lme we can specify the structure of the covariance matrix of random effects, $\text{cov}(\mathbf{b}_i) = \mathbf{D}_*$. Recall that random=pdDiag(alpha+beta~1) in function phototum means that parameters alpha and beta are random and do not correlate, i.e. matrix $\mathbf{D}_*$ is diagonal; `random=alpha+beta~1` would mean that there is no restriction on matrix $\mathbf{D}_*$, i.e. the off-diagonal is not zero and subject to estimation. As in the case of `nls`, the user should specify the starting values for the fixed parameters; they can be obtained from the `nls` fit. Function $\mathbf{f}_i$ can be specified as a formula in the `nlme` call or can exist as a stand-alone function in the `R` session (it cannot be specified locally).

We illustrate the `nlme` function with the `QLogist` model applied to the height data. The function `QLogist` must exist in the `R` session:

```
QLogist=function(a1,a2,a3,a4,x)
{
dene=a2-a3*x-a4*x^2
y=a1/(1+exp(dene))
return(y)
}
```

The function `heightlog.nlme` contains several `nlme` calls; one of them is as follows:

```
outnlme<-nlme(height~QLogist(a1,a2,a3,a4,x=year),
        fixed=a1+a2+a3+a4~1,random=a1+a2+a4~1,groups=~id,
        data=da,start=c(a1=a0[1],a2=a0[2],a3=a0[3],a4=a0[4]))
```

Alternatively, one can call

```
outnlme<-nlme(height~a1/(1+exp(a2-a3*year-a4*year^2)),
        fixed=a1+a2+a3+a4~1,random=a1+a2+a4~1,groups=~id,
        data=da,start=c(a1=a0[1],a2=a0[2],a3=a0[3],a4=a0[4]))
```

The latter call is efficient when the model is given by a short formula; otherwise it should be defined as a stand-alone function, such as `QLogist`. In the calls above, parameters $a_1, a_2,$ and a_4 are assumed random with unstructured covariance matrix. The function `heightlog.nlme` plots the individual height data together with the modeled growth assuming that only adult height (parameter a_1) is random and subject-specific. The function `nlme` is quite flexible and allows autocorrelation within the cluster and nonconstant variance. However, it may fail to converge when the matrix $\mathbf{D}$ tends not to be positive definite during iteration, as happens with the function `lme` (see details in Section 2.16).

Problems for Section 8.7

1. Relate (8.29) with the results of Section 3.7, particularly equation (3.54). Provide an interpretation of the PLS.

2. What is the difference between (8.30) and the FAO approach? Is there a difference if $\mathbf{f}_i$ is a linear function?

3. Using spectral matrix decomposition (8.36) prove that $\mathbf{D}^+ = \mathbf{P}_2\boldsymbol{\Lambda}^{-1}\mathbf{P}_2$ is the generalized matrix inverse. See sections 2.2.3 and 13.2.2 for examples. Use function `ginverse.sym` to verify this formula by a numerical example.

4. Show that the LB estimate converges to the TS estimate for linear model when $\delta \to 0$ directly using closed-form formulas.

5. Apply the algorithm from Section 8.7.3 to a linear model, and verify that it needs one iteration to converge.

8.8   Likelihood approximations

Laplace approximation to the likelihood is the major approximation in the framework of nonlinear mixed models. We used this approximation extensively for GLMM in the previous chapter. Several authors, including Wolfinger (1993), Pinheiro and Bates (1995), and Vonesh (1996), pointed out a close relationship between the Laplace approximation, penalized quasi-likelihood, and the Lindstrom–Bates estimator. In this section we overview the relevant results; we refer the reader to Sections 7.7.1 and 7.7.2.

Let $l(\mathbf{y}_i|\mathbf{b}_i; \boldsymbol{\gamma}, \boldsymbol{\beta}, \sigma^2)$ be the conditional log-likelihood function or the log-likelihood function of the first-stage model (8.1),

$$
\begin{aligned}
& l(\mathbf{y}_i|\mathbf{b}_i; \boldsymbol{\gamma}, \boldsymbol{\beta}, \sigma^2) \\
= {} & -0.5 \left\{ n_i \ln(2\pi) + n_i \ln \sigma^2 + \sigma^{-2} \parallel \mathbf{y}_i - \mathbf{f}_i(\boldsymbol{\gamma}, \mathbf{A}_i\boldsymbol{\beta} + \mathbf{b}_i) \parallel^2 \right\}.
\end{aligned}
\tag{8.44}
$$

The marginal log-likelihood function for $\mathbf{y}_i$ is obtained after integrating out the random effects,

$$
l(\mathbf{y}_i; \boldsymbol{\gamma}, \boldsymbol{\beta}, \sigma^2) = \ln \int e^{l(\mathbf{y}_i|\mathbf{b}; \boldsymbol{\gamma}, \boldsymbol{\beta}, \sigma^2)} \phi(\mathbf{b}; \mathbf{D}) d\mathbf{b},
\tag{8.45}
$$

where ϕ is the density of the normally distributed random effects $\mathbf{b}^{k \times 1}$,

$$
\phi(\mathbf{b}; \mathbf{D}) = (2\pi)^{-k/2} (\sigma^2)^{-k/2} |\mathbf{D}|^{-1/2} \exp\left(-\frac{1}{2\sigma^2} \mathbf{b}'\mathbf{D}^{-1}\mathbf{b} \right).
\tag{8.46}
$$

As the reader can see, log (8.45) is just (8.9) with $\mathbf{b}$ as the integration variable instead of $\mathbf{a}_i$. Integral (8.45) generally does not admit a closed-form solution, so an approximation is sought.

8.8.1   Linear approximation of the likelihood at zero

It is instructive to start with the first-order approximation of function $\mathbf{f}_i$ in (8.44) to derive an approximation of the likelihood. We show that the FOA model, derived in Section 8.6, can be obtained as an approximation of the log-likelihood, Wolfinger and Lin (1997).

Since $E(\mathbf{b}_i) = \mathbf{0}$, function $\mathbf{f}_i(\boldsymbol{\gamma}, \mathbf{A}_i\boldsymbol{\beta} + \mathbf{b}_i)$ may be approximated at zero by a linear function as

$$
\mathbf{f}_i(\boldsymbol{\gamma}, \mathbf{A}_i\boldsymbol{\beta} + \mathbf{b}_i) \simeq \mathbf{f}_i(\boldsymbol{\gamma}, \mathbf{A}_i\boldsymbol{\beta}) + \mathbf{R}_i\mathbf{b}_i,
\tag{8.47}
$$

where

$$
\mathbf{R}_i = \left. \frac{\partial \mathbf{f}_i(\boldsymbol{\gamma}, \mathbf{A}_i\boldsymbol{\beta} + \mathbf{b})}{\partial \mathbf{b}} \right|_{\mathbf{b}=\mathbf{0}}
\tag{8.48}
$$

is the $n_i \times k$ matrix of derivatives calculated at $\mathbf{b}_i = \mathbf{0}$. Having (8.47), we approximate the log-likelihood function (8.44) by

$$-0.5 \left[n_i \ln(2\pi) + n_i \ln \sigma^2 + \sigma^{-2} \parallel \mathbf{e}_i - \mathbf{R}_i \mathbf{b}_i \parallel^2 \right], \tag{8.49}$$

where $\mathbf{e}_i = \mathbf{y}_i - \mathbf{f}_i(\boldsymbol{\gamma}, \mathbf{A}_i \boldsymbol{\beta})$ is the $n_i \times 1$ residual vector. As a result of this approximation, the exponent in (8.45) becomes a quadratic function of $\mathbf{b}$, and therefore the integral admits a closed-form solution. However, instead of doing a straightforward multivariate integral calculation we interpret (8.49) as the log-likelihood function of the model $\mathbf{e}_i | \mathbf{b}_i \sim \mathcal{N}(\mathbf{R}_i \mathbf{b}_i, \sigma^2 \mathbf{I})$ and couple this with the model for random effects, $\mathbf{b}_i \sim \mathcal{N}(\mathbf{0}, \sigma^2 \mathbf{D})$. Then integration (8.45) gives the marginal model for $\mathbf{e}_i$, namely, $\mathbf{e}_i \sim \mathcal{N}(\mathbf{0}, \sigma^2(\mathbf{I} + \mathbf{R}_i \mathbf{D} \mathbf{R}_i))$. Finally, in terms of $\mathbf{y}_i$, the likelihood approximation (8.47) yields the approximate model

$$\mathbf{y}_i \sim \mathcal{N}\left(\mathbf{f}_i(\boldsymbol{\gamma}, \mathbf{A}_i \boldsymbol{\beta}), \sigma^2(\mathbf{I} + \mathbf{R}_i(\boldsymbol{\beta})\mathbf{D}\mathbf{R}_i'(\boldsymbol{\beta}))\right), \tag{8.50}$$

which yields a previously derived first-order approximation (8.25) with the joint log-likelihood function (8.26). Thus, approximation of the mean function of Section 8.6 and the likelihood approximation leads to a nonlinear marginal model with a varied matrix of random effects (6.17) or the pseudo-model (8.25) previously studied in Section 6.2.

8.8.2   Laplace and PQL approximations

The aim of the log-likelihood approximation is to eliminate the integral. According to the Laplace approximation, one approximates the integral where the integrand (8.45), as a function of $\mathbf{b}$, takes maximum value, see Subsections 7.1.2, 7.3.4 and 7.7.1. Let $\boldsymbol{\gamma}, \boldsymbol{\beta}$, and $\mathbf{D}$ be fixed; then maximization leads to N penalized nonlinear least squares,

$$\parallel \mathbf{y}_i - \mathbf{f}_i(\boldsymbol{\gamma}, \mathbf{A}_i \boldsymbol{\beta} + \mathbf{b}_i) \parallel^2 + \mathbf{b}_i' \mathbf{D}^{-1} \mathbf{b}_i \Rightarrow \min_{\mathbf{b}_i}. \tag{8.51}$$

Denote the solutions/maximizers $\{\mathbf{b}_{*i}, i = 1, ..., N\}$. Assuming that $\mathbf{b}_{*i}$ are being held fixed, the multivariate Laplace approximation (7.131) gives the following approximation to the joint log-likelihood, up to a constant,

$$l_{LA}(\boldsymbol{\chi}, \sigma^2, \mathbf{D}) = -0.5[N_T \ln(2\pi\sigma^2) + N \ln |\mathbf{D}| \tag{8.52}$$

$$+ \sum_{i=1}^{N} \ln \left| \mathbf{D}^{-1} + \mathbf{R}_{*i}' \mathbf{R}_{*i} + \mathbf{H}_{*i} \right| + \sigma^{-2} \sum_{i=1}^{N} (\parallel \mathbf{y}_i - \mathbf{f}_{*i}(\boldsymbol{\chi}) \parallel^2 + \mathbf{b}_{*i}' \mathbf{D}^{-1} \mathbf{b}_{*i})],$$

where $\mathbf{f}_{*i}(\boldsymbol{\chi}) = \mathbf{f}_i(\boldsymbol{\gamma}, \mathbf{A}_i \boldsymbol{\beta} + \mathbf{b}_{*i})$ is an $n_i \times 1$ vector of the mean/regression functions, $\mathbf{R}_{*i}$ is an $n_i \times m$ matrix of the first derivatives of $\mathbf{f}_i$ and

$$\mathbf{H}_{*i} = \sum_{j=1}^{n_i} (y_{ij} - f_{*ij}) \frac{\partial^2 f_{ij}}{\partial \mathbf{b}_i^2} \tag{8.53}$$

is the $m \times m$ matrix evaluated at $\boldsymbol{\gamma}, \mathbf{A}_i \boldsymbol{\beta} + \mathbf{b}_{*i}$. Notice that we use the notation $\boldsymbol{\chi} = (\boldsymbol{\gamma}', \boldsymbol{\beta}')'$ for the entire vector of population-averaged parameters. The reader can see an obvious parallel to the LA method (7.137) for logistic regression with random effects. Both LA and FOA use linear approximation, but in the latter we approximate around zero and in the former we approximate around an estimate of the random effect as the solution to (8.51).

The estimation process based on (8.51) and (8.52) consists of two alternating steps: (a) solving N penalized least squares (8.51) assuming that τ and $\mathbf{D}$ are being held fixed, (b) maximizing function (8.52) over parameters τ, σ^2, and $\mathbf{D}$ assuming that $\{\mathbf{b}_{*i}\}$ are being held. Numerical details are discussed in the next subsection.

In penalized quasi-likelihood, the term with second derivatives, $\mathbf{H}_{*i}$, is ignored, see Chapter 7. One can justify this by observing that $E(\mathbf{H}_{*i}) \simeq \mathbf{0}$ because $E(y_{ij} - f_{*ij}) \simeq 0$. Thus, we have

$$l_{PQL}(\chi, \sigma^2, \mathbf{D}) = -0.5[N_T \ln(2\pi\sigma^2) + N \ln|\mathbf{D}| \tag{8.54}$$
$$+ \sigma^{-2} \sum (\| \mathbf{y}_i - \mathbf{f}_{*i}(\chi) \|^2 + \mathbf{b}'_{*i}\mathbf{D}^{-1}\mathbf{b}_{*i}) + \sum \ln \left| \mathbf{D}^{-1} + \mathbf{R}'_{*i}\mathbf{R}_{*i} \right|)],$$

as derived by Vonesh (1996). The difference between LA and PQL approximations should be small when n_i is large. Wolfinger and Lin (1997) showed that PQL = LB, or in other words, penalized quasi-likelihood is equivalent to the Lindstrom–Bates method. It suffices to show that

$$\|\mathbf{e}_{*i}\|^2 + \mathbf{b}'_{*i}\mathbf{D}^{-1}\mathbf{b}_{*i} + \ln\left|\mathbf{I} + \mathbf{D}\mathbf{R}'_{*i}\mathbf{R}_{*i}\right| \tag{8.55}$$
$$= (\mathbf{e}_{*i} + \mathbf{R}_{*i}\mathbf{b}_{*i})'\mathbf{V}_i^{-1}(\mathbf{e}_{*i} + \mathbf{R}_{*i}\mathbf{b}_{*i}) + \ln|\mathbf{V}_i|,$$

where $\mathbf{V}_i = \mathbf{I} + \mathbf{R}_{*i}\mathbf{D}\mathbf{R}'_{*i}$ and $\mathbf{b}_{*i}$ comprise the solution to PLS; they satisfy the equation $\mathbf{R}'_{*i}\mathbf{e}_{*i} = \mathbf{D}^{-1}\mathbf{b}_{*i}$. Using the dimension-reduction formula (2.22), we see that the log determinant at the left- and right-hand sides are equal. Next, substituting $\mathbf{b}_{*i} = \mathbf{D}\mathbf{R}'_{*i}\mathbf{e}_{*i}$ into the left-hand sides of (8.55), we obtain $\mathbf{e}'_{*i}\mathbf{V}_i\mathbf{e}_{*i}$. Substituting the same at the right-hand side, we obtain $\mathbf{e}'_{*i}\mathbf{V}_i\mathbf{V}_i^{-1}\mathbf{V}_i\mathbf{e}_{*i} = \mathbf{e}'_{*i}\mathbf{V}_i\mathbf{e}_{*i}$, and equality (8.55) is established.

It is instructive to show that for the LME and the nonlinear marginal model with a fixed (6.1) or varied (6.17) matrix of random effects, LA (8.52) and PQL (8.54) yield the ordinary log-likelihood function (6.18). Apparently, since for these models, random effects are linear, $\mathbf{H}_{*i} = \mathbf{0}$ and $l_{LA} = l_{PQL}$. Further, as follows from Section 3.7, the solution to PLS (8.51) is $\widehat{\mathbf{b}}_i = \mathbf{D}\mathbf{Z}'_i(\mathbf{I} + \mathbf{P}_i)^{-1}\mathbf{e}_i$, where $\mathbf{e}_i = \mathbf{y}_i - \mathbf{f}_i$ and $\mathbf{P}_i = \mathbf{Z}_i\mathbf{D}\mathbf{Z}'_i$. The minimum is a quadratic form of $\mathbf{e}_i$ with the matrix

$$[\mathbf{I} - \mathbf{P}_i(\mathbf{I} + \mathbf{P}_i)^{-1}][(\mathbf{I} - (\mathbf{I} + \mathbf{P}_i)^{-1}\mathbf{P}_i] + (\mathbf{I} + \mathbf{P}_i)^{-1}\mathbf{P}_i(\mathbf{I} + \mathbf{P}_i)^{-1}. \tag{8.56}$$

It is elementary to show that (8.56) simplifies to $\mathbf{V}_i^{-1} = (\mathbf{I} + \mathbf{P}_i)^{-1}$. Also, for a mixed model with linear random effects, $\mathbf{R}_i = \mathbf{Z}_i$ and $\mathbf{H}_i = \mathbf{0}$. Hence, using formula (2.22), we finally infer that l_{LA} coincides with (6.18).

Problems for Section 8.8

1. Derive the marginal log-likelihood function (8.45) for problem 4 of Section 8.7. Derive the linear approximation of the likelihood at zero.

2*. Write an R function that estimates the exponential model from Problem 4 of Section 8.7 by maximum likelihood. Use `integrate` to compute (8.45) and other integrals needed for function maximization that emerge in the score equation. Use the Empirical Fisher scoring algorithm for iterations, see Section 7.3.1 and Appendix 13.3.4.

3. Show how estimation of model (8.50) can be reduced to alternation between the weighted nonlinear least squares and LME.

4*. Derive an iterative algorithm for maximization of function (8.54) alternating between `nls` and `lme`. Write an `R` function that implements it; compare with `nlme` on simulated data using problem 4 of Section 8.7.

8.9 One-parameter exponential model

In this section a simple example of a nonlinear mixed effect model is considered, a one-random parameter exponential model. The simplicity of this model allows us to find a closed-form solution to estimate the population-averaged parameter and to calculate the bias directly, or at least to find a good approximation to the bias for all four estimators considered in the previous section. Remarkably, this model reflects all features of more complicated real-life nonlinear mixed effects models, such as bias or possible nonexistence of nonlinear least squares estimates sometimes experienced in practice (Demidenko, 1989, 1996). Based on this model, we show that all estimators considered above, except the MLE, are inconsistent when $\{n_i\}$ are finite and $N \to \infty$. In the next section this model is used to illustrate the asymptotic mean square error (MSE) calculation and efficiency comparison.

The following one-parameter balanced exponential model is considered to illustrate estimation methods,

$$y_{ij} = e^{a_i} + \epsilon_{ij}, \quad \epsilon_{ij} \sim \mathcal{N}(0, \sigma^2), \quad i = 1, ..., N, \, j = 1, ..., n \tag{8.57}$$

with the second-stage model

$$a_i = \beta + b_i, \quad b_i \sim N(0, \sigma^2 \omega^2), \tag{8.58}$$

where the ϵ_{ij} and b_i are independent. This is a balanced model because the number of observations in each cluster is the same, n. The assumptions imply that $\bar{y}_i = \sum y_{ij}/n$, $i = 1, ..., N$, are independent and identically distributed (iid). To simplify, only β, the parameter of interest, is assumed to be unknown in this section, i.e., the parameters $\sigma^2 > 0$ and $\omega^2 > 0$ are known. Sometimes, ω is referred to as the relative SD of the random effect. In this section we determine the asymptotic bias, as a function of n, for three estimators when $N \to \infty$. It should be noted that for finite n, some estimators may not exist with a nonzero probability even for infinitely large N. Therefore, we have to take this into account when comparing estimators.

8.9.1 Maximum likelihood estimator

The likelihood function for the ith subject/cluster, as follows from the model defined by the pair of equations (8.57) and (8.58), is given by

$$l_i(\beta; y_{i1}, ..., y_{in}) = C(2\pi\sigma^2)^{-n/2} \int_{-\infty}^{+\infty} e^{-\frac{1}{2\sigma^2}\sum_{j=1}^n (y_{ij}-e^a)^2} e^{-\frac{1}{2\omega^2\sigma^2}(a-\beta)^2} da,$$

where $C = (2\pi\sigma^2\omega^2)^{-1/2}$. The Fisher information (scalar) for the ith cluster is

$$
\begin{aligned}
\mathcal{I}_\beta &= \int_{R^n} \frac{(dl/d\beta)^2}{l} dy_1 \cdots dy_n \\
&= \frac{C}{\sigma^4\omega^4}(2\pi\sigma^2)^{-n/2} \int_{R^n} \frac{g_1^2(\sum_1^n y_j)}{g_2(\sum_1^n y_j)} e^{-\frac{1}{2\sigma^2}\sum_1^n y_j^2} dy_1 \cdots dy_n \\
&= \frac{C}{\sigma^4\omega^4} E_{\overline{y}}\left(\frac{g_1^2(\overline{y})}{g_2(\overline{y})}\right) = \frac{\sqrt{n}}{(2\pi)^{3/2}\sigma^7\omega^6} \int_{-\infty}^{\infty} \frac{g_1^2(s)}{g_2(s)} \exp\left(-\frac{ns^2}{2\sigma^2}\right) ds, (8.59)
\end{aligned}
$$

where the functions g_1, g_2 and p are defined as

$$
\begin{aligned}
g_1(s) &= \int_{-\infty}^{+\infty} (a-\beta)p(a,s)da, \quad g_2(s) = \int_{-\infty}^{+\infty} p(a,s)da \\
p(a,s) &= \exp\left(n\frac{2e^a s - e^{2a}}{2\sigma^2} - \frac{(a-\beta)^2}{2\omega^2\sigma^2}\right).
\end{aligned}
$$

The asymptotic variance $\mathrm{var}_{as}(\sqrt{N}\widehat{\beta}_{ML}) = \mathcal{I}_\beta^{-1} \geq \sigma^2\omega^2$, as follows from (8.14). There is no closed-form solution to the MLE, even for this simple model. From maximum likelihood theory it follows that $\widehat{\beta}_{ML}$ is consistent and asymptotically normally distributed when $N \to \infty$ and n is fixed. As will be shown later, the asymptotic variance of the MLE approaches its absolute lower bound $\sigma^2\omega^2$ when $n \to \infty$. We shall use the formula for $\mathcal{I}_\beta$ in Section 8.10 when comparing the MSE of different estimates.

8.9.2 First-order approximation

Following the idea of the first-order approximation (FOA), we replace the original model, defined by equations (8.57) and (8.58), with the marginal model, the so-called pseudo-model,

$$
y_{ij} = e^\beta + \eta_{ij}, \tag{8.60}
$$

where $\eta_{ij} = e^\beta b_i + \epsilon_{ij}$. Letting $\boldsymbol{\eta}_i = (\eta_{i1}, \eta_{i2}, ..., \eta_{in})'$ and $\mathbf{1} = (1,1,...,1)'$, the covariance matrix for the random vector term $\boldsymbol{\eta}_i$ can be written as $\mathrm{cov}(\boldsymbol{\eta}_i) = \sigma^2\mathbf{V}(\beta)$, where $\mathbf{V} = \mathbf{V}(\beta) = \mathbf{I} + e^{2\beta}\omega^2\mathbf{11}'$. Let an initial estimate of β be given, β_*. Then the FOA estimator is the solution to the following nonlinear regression problem with the weight matrix $\mathbf{V}_* = \mathbf{V}(\beta_*)$:

$$
\sum_{i=1}^{N} (\mathbf{y}_i - e^\beta\mathbf{1})' \mathbf{V}_*^{-1} (\mathbf{y}_i - e^\beta\mathbf{1}) \Rightarrow \min_\beta.
$$

Clearly, the solution is

$$
\widehat{\beta}_{FOA} = \ln\left(\frac{\sum_i \mathbf{1}'\mathbf{V}_*^{-1}\mathbf{y}_i}{N\mathbf{1}'\mathbf{V}_*^{-1}\mathbf{1}}\right). \tag{8.61}
$$

The special structure of $\mathbf{V}_*$ allows us to find the explicit form for its inverse,

$$
\mathbf{V}_*^{-1} = \mathbf{I} - \frac{e^{2\beta_*}\omega^2}{1 + e^{2\beta_*}\omega^2 n}\mathbf{11}'. \tag{8.62}
$$

Then substituting (8.62) back into (8.61), we obtain

$$
\begin{aligned}
\mathbf{1}'\mathbf{V}_*^{-1}\mathbf{1} &= n - \frac{e^{2\beta_*}\omega^2}{1 + e^{2\beta_*}\omega^2 n}n^2 = \frac{n}{1 + e^{2\beta_*}\omega^2 n}, \\
\mathbf{1}'\mathbf{V}_*^{-1}\mathbf{y}_i &= \left(1 - \frac{e^{2\beta_*}\omega^2 n}{1 + e^{2\beta_*}\omega^2 n}\right)\sum_{j=1}^{n} y_{ij} = \frac{1}{1 + e^{2\beta_*}\omega^2 n}\sum_{j=1}^{n} y_{ij}.
\end{aligned}
$$

Hence, the FOA estimator simplifies to

$$
\widehat{\beta}_{FOA} = \ln\left(\frac{1}{Nn}\sum_{i,j} y_{ij}\right). \tag{8.63}
$$

It is interesting to notice that for this model the FOA estimator does not depend on the initial estimate β_*, or even matrix $\mathbf{V}$. We encountered a similar situation before: for the double-balanced LME model GLS = OLS, Section 4.1.5.

Now we calculate the asymptotic limit of (8.63). We have

$$
\begin{aligned}
\frac{1}{Nn}\sum y_{ij} &= \frac{1}{N}\sum_i \left(\frac{1}{n}\sum_j \left(e^{\beta+b_i} + \epsilon_{ij}\right)\right) \\
&= \frac{1}{N}\sum_i \left(e^{\beta+b_i} + \frac{1}{n}\sum_j \epsilon_{ij}\right) = \frac{1}{N}\sum_i e^{\beta+b_i} + \frac{1}{Nn}\sum_{i,j}\epsilon_{ij}.
\end{aligned}
$$

But $e^{\beta+b_i}$ has the lognormal distribution, which implies that $E(e^{\beta+b_i}) = e^{\beta+\sigma^2\omega^2/2}$, Rao (1973). Thus, $E(y_{ij}) = E\left(e^{\beta+b_i} + \epsilon_{ij}\right) = e^{\beta+\sigma^2\omega^2/2}$, and by the law of large numbers,

$$
\lim_{N\to\infty}\frac{1}{N}\sum_i e^{\beta+b_i} = e^{\beta+\sigma^2\omega^2/2}, \quad \lim_{N\to\infty}\frac{1}{Nn}\sum_{i,j}\epsilon_{ij} = 0
$$

for any n. Combining these two limits, we finally obtain

$$
\lim_{N\to\infty}\widehat{\beta}_{FOA} = \ln e^{\beta+\sigma^2\omega^2/2} = \beta + \frac{1}{2}\sigma^2\omega^2. \tag{8.64}
$$

Thus, we conclude that the FOA estimator is inconsistent and has a systematic positive bias even if n goes to infinity along with N.

Also, the FOA estimator may not exist for finite N and n because $\sum y_{ij}$ can be nonpositive. However, the probability that the FOA estimator exists goes to 1 when $N \to \infty$, regardless of n, because $\sum y_{ij}/Nn$ converges to $e^{\beta+\sigma^2\omega^2/2} > 0$ with probability 1.

8.9.3   Two-stage estimator

The individual least squares estimation of (8.57) leads to the subject-specific estimator, $\widehat{a}_i = \ln \bar{y}_i$. Given an estimate of a_i, one can apply GLS and obtain the

TS estimator, which in our balanced model collapses to a simple average of the individual estimates,

$$\widehat{\beta}_{TS} = \frac{1}{N}\sum_{i=1}^{N}\ln\overline{y}_i. \tag{8.65}$$

Now we study its asymptotic properties when $N \to \infty$. Again, by the law of large numbers

$$\lim_{N\to\infty}\widehat{\beta}_{TS} = E\ln\left(\overline{y}_1\right) = E\ln\left(e^{\beta+b_1} + \overline{\epsilon}_1\right), \tag{8.66}$$

with probability 1, where $\overline{\epsilon}_1 = n^{-1}\sum_{j=1}^{n}\epsilon_{1j} \sim N\left(0, \sigma^2/n\right)$ and $b_1 \sim N(0, \sigma^2\omega^2)$; b_1 and $\overline{\epsilon}_1$ are independent.

The TS estimator has a systematic negative bias for fixed n even for infinitely large N. This follows from the elementary inequality $\ln(a + x) < \ln(a) + x/a$ for $x \neq 0, a > 0, a + x > 0$, and the fact that b_1 and ϵ_1 are independent. Specifically,

$$\begin{aligned}\lim_{N\to\infty}\widehat{\beta}_{TS} &= E\ln\left(e^{\beta+b_1} + \overline{\epsilon}_1\right) < E\left(\ln e^{\beta+b_1} + \overline{\epsilon}_1 e^{-(\beta+b_1)}\right)\\ &= \beta + E\left(\overline{\epsilon}_1 e^{-(\beta+b_1)}\right) = \beta + E(\overline{\epsilon}_1)Ee^{-(\beta+b_1)} = \beta.\end{aligned}$$

Expectation (8.66) can be calculated exactly as a two-dimensional integral or approximated as

$$Er(u,v) \simeq r(0,0) + \frac{1}{2}\mathrm{var}(u)\left.\frac{\partial^2 r}{\partial u^2}\right|_{u=0,v=0} + \frac{1}{2}\mathrm{var}(v)\left.\frac{\partial^2 r}{\partial v^2}\right|_{u=0,v=0}, \tag{8.67}$$

where $r = r(u, v)$ is any function of independent random variables u and v with zero means. To apply (8.67) to (8.66), we let $u = b_1$, $v = \overline{\epsilon}_1$, and $r(u, v) = e^{\beta+u} + v$. Remarkably, the second derivative with respect to the random effect is zero; that is, the second term in the approximation disappears (as we shall learn later, this is true for any NLME model, see Section 8.11). Since $\mathrm{var}(b_1) = \sigma^2\omega^2$ and $\mathrm{var}(\overline{\epsilon}_1) = \sigma^2/n$, the asymptotic bias for fixed n can be approximated as

$$\lim_{N\to\infty}\widehat{\beta}_{TS} - \beta \simeq -\frac{\sigma^2}{2n}e^{-2\beta}. \tag{8.68}$$

As we see, the bias is negative and has the order of $1/n$. Also, the bias does not depend on the variance of the random effect, ω^2. Consequently, if σ^2 is close to zero, one can expect unbiased estimation by the two-stage method. This statement applies to general NLME models: the two-stage estimation will work well if the within-subject variance (σ^2) is relatively small and the individual fits are good.

In Section 8.5 we mentioned a serious drawback of the TS estimator: it may not exist when n is small (in practice one faces a failure to estimate by nonlinear least squares). We illustrate this phenomenon by model (8.57). Indeed, for this exponential model, formula (8.65) fails when $\overline{y}_i \leq 0$. Since $\overline{y}_i$ is a continuous variable with the range $(-\infty, \infty)$ and all $\{\overline{y}_i\}$ are iid, $\Pr(\overline{y}_i > 0) = \Pr(\overline{y}_1 > 0) = q_n < 1$, so that

$$\Pr(\widehat{\beta}_{TS} \text{ does not exist}) = 1 - q_n^N \to 1, \qquad N \to \infty,$$

because q_n is constant for fixed n. Therefore, the TS estimator does not exist with probability 1 for fixed n and $N \to \infty$. In fact, it may not exist even if $n \to \infty$. To obtain the existence with probability 1, the following must hold: $N \ln q_n \to 0$. Since $q_n \to 0$ when $n \to \infty$ it means that n must be large enough to satisfy the condition above.

However, there is a remedy: if $\bar{y}_i \leq 0$, we simply do not include the corresponding term in sum (8.65). Then the corrected TS estimator becomes

$$\tilde{\beta}_{TS} = \frac{\sum_{\bar{y}_i > 0} \ln \bar{y}_i}{\#(y_i > 0, i = 1, ..., N)} \simeq \frac{\sum_{\bar{y}_i > 0} \ln \bar{y}_i}{N q_n},$$

which exists now with probability 1. The approximate formula for the bias (8.68) works for $\tilde{\beta}_{TS}$ as well. Now we can prove the consistency of the corrected TS estimator when $n \to \infty$:

$$\lim_{N \to \infty} \lim_{n \to \infty} \tilde{\beta}_{TS} = \lim_{N \to \infty} \frac{1}{Nq} \sum_{\bar{y}_i > 0} \ln \left(\lim_{n \to \infty} (\bar{y}_i \mid \bar{y}_i > 0) \right)$$

$$= \lim_{N \to \infty} \frac{1}{Nq} \sum_{i=1}^{N} q \ln \left(e^{\beta + b_i} + \lim_{n \to \infty} \frac{1}{n} \sum_{j=1}^{n} \varepsilon_{ij} \mid e^{\beta + b_i} + \frac{1}{n} \sum_{j=1}^{n} \varepsilon_{ij} > 0 \right)$$

$$= \lim_{N \to \infty} \frac{1}{N} \sum_{i=1}^{N} (\beta + b_i) = \beta + \lim \frac{1}{N} \sum_{i=1}^{N} b_i = \beta,$$

where $\mid \bar{y}_i > 0$ means "under condition $\bar{y}_i > 0$."

As follows from (8.66), the asymptotic bias for the corrected TS estimator when $N \to \infty$ can be calculated exactly through two two-dimensional integrals

$$E(\tilde{\beta}_{TS}) - \beta = \frac{G_n}{q_n} - \beta, \tag{8.69}$$

where

$$G_n = \frac{\sqrt{n}}{2\pi\omega\sigma^2} \int \int_{e^{\beta + x} + y > 0} \ln(e^{\beta + x} + y) \exp\left(-\frac{1}{2\sigma^2\omega^2} x^2 - \frac{n}{2\sigma^2} y^2\right) dx dy, \tag{8.70}$$

and

$$q_n = \frac{\sqrt{n}}{2\pi\omega\sigma^2} \int \int_{e^{\beta + x} + y > 0} \exp\left(-\frac{1}{2\sigma^2\omega^2} x^2 - \frac{n}{2\sigma^2} y^2\right) dx dy$$

is the probability of the existence of the corrected TS estimator.

Summing up, the two-stage estimate may not exist for some i. However, if we omit those, the TS estimator remains valid.

8.9.4   Lindstrom–Bates estimator

Since σ^2 and ω^2 are known, we implement only the penalized nonlinear least squares step. The Lindstrom–Bates (LB) estimator, $\tilde{\beta}_{LB}$, is the solution to the following $(N + 1)$-dimensional optimization problem:

$$\frac{1}{N} \sum_{i=1}^{N} \left(\frac{1}{n} \sum_{j=1}^{n} (y_{ij} - e^{\beta + \tau_i})^2 + \frac{1}{n\omega^2} \tau_i^2 \right) \Rightarrow \min_{\beta, \tau_1, ..., \tau_N}.$$

The estimating equations for the nuisance parameters, $\widehat{\tau}_1, ..., \widehat{\tau}_N$ (which can be interpreted as estimates of the random effects), and $\widehat{\beta}_{LB}$ are

$$e^{2(\beta+\tau_i)} - e^{\beta+\tau_i}\overline{y}_i + \frac{1}{n\omega^2}\tau_i = 0, \quad i = 1, ..., N, \tag{8.71}$$

$$\frac{1}{N}\sum_{i=1}^{N}\left(e^{2(\beta+\tau_i)} - e^{\beta+\tau_i}\overline{y}_i\right) = 0. \tag{8.72}$$

Summing equations (8.71) over i and substituting the result into (8.72) leads to the estimating equation for the LB estimator:

$$\frac{1}{N}\sum_{i=1}^{N}\widehat{\tau}(\beta,\overline{y}_i) = 0, \tag{8.73}$$

where $\widehat{\tau}_i = \widehat{\tau}(\beta,\overline{y}_i)$ is the solution to (8.71) as a function of β and $\overline{y}_i$.

The LB estimator is inconsistent when n =const and $N \to \infty$. To determine the systematic bias, the following fact will be used. Let $u_1, u_2, ..., u_N$ be iid random variables with a distribution dependent on parameter β; the true parameter is denoted by β_0. Let the estimating equation for $\widehat{\beta}_N$ be $N^{-1}\sum_{i=1}^{N}S(u_i;\beta) = 0$. Then $\lim_{N\to\infty}\widehat{\beta}_N = \beta_*$ with probability 1, where β_* is the unique solution to the equation $\overline{S}(\beta,\beta_0) = E_{\beta_0}S(u_1;\beta) = 0$, see Appendix 13.1.4.

Based on this fact, to compute the bias for $\widehat{\beta}_{LB}$ we introduce the function $\overline{S}(\beta,\beta_0) = E_{\beta_0}\widehat{\tau}(\beta,\overline{y})$, where $\widehat{\tau}(\beta,\overline{y})$ is the solution to the nonlinear equation

$$e^{2(\beta+\tau)} - e^{\beta+\tau}\overline{y} + \tau/(n\omega^2) = 0. \tag{8.74}$$

This equation can be solved by Newton's iterations

$$\tau_{s+1} = \tau_s - \frac{e^{2(\beta+\tau_s)} - e^{\beta+\tau_s}\overline{y} + \tau_s/(n\omega^2)}{2e^{2(\beta+\tau)} - e^{\beta+\tau}\overline{y} + 1/(n\omega^2)}$$

starting from $\tau_0 = \ln\overline{y} - \beta$.

The asymptotic limit of $\widehat{\beta}_{LB}$ when $N \to \infty$ and n is fixed is the root of the equation $\overline{S}(\beta,\beta_0) = 0$, where the function $\overline{S}$ is computed as a two-dimensional integral:

$$\overline{S}(\beta,\beta_0) = \int_{-\infty}^{\infty}\int_{-\infty}^{\infty}\widehat{\tau}(\beta,e^{\beta_0+x}+y)\exp\left(-\frac{x^2}{2\sigma^2\omega^2} - \frac{ny^2}{2\sigma^2}\right)dxdy,$$

where $\widehat{\tau}$ is the root of the nonlinear equation (8.74). To find the root of this equation, we again use Newton's algorithm,

$$\beta_{s+1} = \beta_s - \frac{\overline{S}(\beta_k,\beta_0)}{\overline{S}'(\beta_k,\beta_0)},$$

where $\overline{S}'(\beta_k,\beta_0)$ is the derivative of $\overline{S}$ with respect to β. The derivative of $\widehat{\tau}$, as the root of equation (8.74), with respect to β is found from differentiation of equation (8.74),

$$2(1+\tau')e^{2(\beta+\tau)} - (1+\tau')e^{\beta+\tau}\overline{y} + \tau'/(n\omega^2) = 0,$$

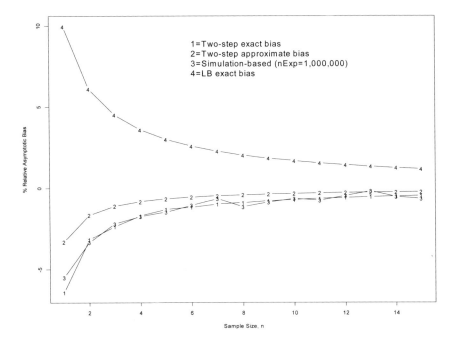

FIGURE 8.3. Relative asymptotic bias of two estimators for the one-parameter balanced exponential model ($\beta = 0.5$, $\sigma = 0.3$, $\omega = 2$) for $N = \infty$ and different n. The percent relative bias of FOA estimator is 40% (not shown).

which yields

$$\tau' = \frac{e^{\beta+\tau} - 2e^{2(\beta+\tau)}}{2e^{2(\beta+\tau)} - e^{\beta+\tau} + (n\omega^2)^{-1}}.$$

The functions S and $\overline{S}'$ are computed via the GH quadrature after expressing

$$\overline{S}(\beta, \beta_0) = \frac{2\sigma^2\omega}{\sqrt{n}} \int_{-\infty}^{\infty} \int_{-\infty}^{\infty} \widehat{\tau}(\beta, e^{\beta_0 + \sqrt{2}\sigma\omega x} + \sqrt{2/n}\sigma y)e^{-x^2-y^2} dxdy.$$

These computations coded in the R function INT.ch08 are depicted in Figure 8.3, where we compare the relative asymptotic bias $(\widehat{\beta} - \beta_0)/\beta_0 \cdot 100\%$ of two estimators with $\sigma = 0.3$, $\omega = 2$, $\beta_0 = 0.5$ when $N \to \infty$ and n is fixed. The FOA estimator is not shown since its bias, $0.5\sigma^2\omega^2 = 0.28$, does not depend on n (the relative bias is 40%). As we can see, the approximation formula for the TS estimator bias (8.68) works fairly well. The probability of the nonexistence of the TS estimator is low: for $n = 1$ we have $1 - q = 0.0182$, which drops to 0.0003 for $n = 15$. It is interesting to observe that the bias of the LB estimator for this model is positive and larger in absolute value than that of the TS estimator.

We compare the MSE in the next section.

Problems for Section 8.9

1*. The function onexpML located at c:\\MixedModels\\Chapter08\\ computes the log-likelihood $\sum_{i=1}^{N} \ln l_i(\beta)$, where l_i is defined through the integral in Section

(8.9.1), and its maximum is on the grid of beta values. Modify this function to investigate the sample properties of $\widehat{\beta}_{ML}$ assuming that σ^2 and ω^2 are known. Compute the derivative $d(\ln l_i)/d\beta\,\widehat{\beta}_{ML}$ as an integral and use Empirical FS to find $\widehat{\beta}_{ML}$ via iterations. Plot the MSE as a function of N with fixed n to demonstrate the MLE consistency. Store the $\widehat{\beta}_{ML}$ values and use `density` to demonstrate the asymptotic normality for large N.

2*. Using the Central Limit Theorem, estimate the probability that $\widehat{\beta}_{FOA}$ given by formula (8.63) does not exists . Use simulations to verify your analytical result. Estimate $E(\widehat{\beta}_{FOA})$ via simulations and plot it against increasing N. Confirm that it approaches the right-hand side of (8.64).

3. Compute the probability that $\widehat{\beta}_{TS}$ does not exist by evaluating $1-q_n = \Pr(\overline{y}_1 \leq 0)$ using the GH quadrature discussed in Section 7.1.3. Plot this probability as a function of n for different σ^2. Use `INT.ch08` for reference.

4*. Compute the bias of $\widetilde{\beta}_{TS}$ given by formula (8.69) through integration of G_n and g_n, see Section 7.1.3. Reduce the double integral to integration of the normal cdf Φ.

5. The function `onexpSIM` does the following: (1) simulates y_{ij} for given n, N, σ, ω, and β; (2) estimates β by `nlme` (σ and ω are estimated as well), and (3) returns the mean of all $\widehat{\beta}$ when `nlme` converged. Modify this function to see how the bias is affected by N and n when all other parameters are fixed.

6*. Compare three methods of estimation via simulations: FOA, TS, and LB (`nlme`) using MSE as a figure of merit for different n, N, σ, and ω.

8.10   Asymptotic equivalence of the TS and LB estimators

The FOA estimator is dropped from consideration because it is not consistent even when $\min n_i \rightarrow \infty$, as shown in the previous section. The aim of this section is to show that the Two-Stage (TS) and Lindstrom–Bates (LB) estimators are asymptotically equivalent. Basically, this result comes from the observation that the contribution of the penalty term $\delta = O(1/n_i)$ in PLS vanishes when $n_i \rightarrow \infty$, see Section 8.7.2; see also Vonesh et al. (2002).

Theorem 42 *Under mild asymptotic conditions, the maximum likelihood, two-stage and Lindstrom–Bates estimators have the same limiting normal distribution with the covariance matrix*

$$\sigma^2(\sum \mathbf{A}_i'\mathbf{D}^{-1}\mathbf{A}_i)^{-1} \tag{8.75}$$

when the number of subjects and the number of observations per subject go to infinity. That is, these estimators are asymptotically equivalent when $N \rightarrow \infty$ and $\min n_i \rightarrow \infty$.

These mild conditions and the proof are given in Section 8.18. As follows from the proof, all three estimators ML, LB, and TS are equivalent to the following simplified

TS estimator

$$\widehat{\boldsymbol{\beta}} = \left(\sum_{i=1}^{N} \mathbf{A}_i' \widehat{\mathbf{D}}_1^{-1} \mathbf{A}_i \right)^{-1} \left(\sum_{i=1}^{N} \mathbf{A}_i' \widehat{\mathbf{D}}_1^{-1} \mathbf{a}_i^o \right), \tag{8.76}$$

where $\widehat{\mathbf{D}}_1$ is defined by (8.21). This estimator follows directly from (8.22) because $\mathbf{T}_i \rightarrow \mathbf{0}$ and $\widehat{\mathbf{D}}_2 \rightarrow \mathbf{0}$ with probability 1 when $\min n_i \rightarrow \infty$. As follows from this theorem, when the number of observations per subject goes to infinity, the covariances matrix of the estimators achieve their absolute lower bound (8.14).

To assess the quality of the ML and TS estimators for fixed $n_i = n$, we compute the asymptotic MSE for the univariate balanced exponential model (8.57), (8.58). The LB estimator is dropped from the analysis because it is equivalent to the TS estimator. Note that the absolute lower bound for the MSE is $\sigma^2 \omega^2$. The asymptotic MSE for the TS estimator is calculated as a two-dimensional integral,

$$MSE_{TS} = \frac{1}{q_n} \frac{\sqrt{n}}{2\pi\omega\sigma^2} \int \int_{e^{\beta+x}+y>0} G(x,y)dxdy, \tag{8.77}$$

where

$$G(x,y) = \left(\beta - \ln(e^{\beta+x} + y) \right)^2 \exp \left(-\frac{1}{2\sigma^2\omega^2} x^2 - \frac{n}{2\sigma^2} y^2 \right)$$

and q_n is as given in Section 8.9.3. The MSE for the MLE is equal to $\mathcal{I}_\beta^{-1}$, where $\mathcal{I}_\beta$ is defined by (8.59).

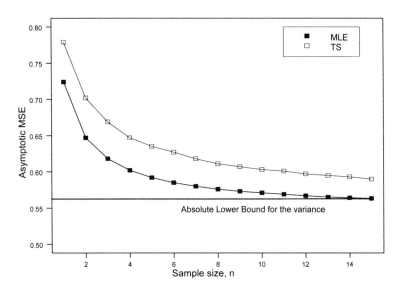

FIGURE 8.4. Asymptotic MSE of the MLE and two-stage estimators for the one-parameter balanced exponential model when $N \rightarrow \infty$ and n is fixed. The Absolute Lower Bound (bold horizontal line) for the asymptotic variance of any estimator is $\sigma^2 \omega^2 = 0.56$.

In Figure 8.4, the asymptotic MSE is shown for different values of n and parameters defined as in Figure 8.3. The MSE of the MLE is less than that of the TS estimator, as one could expect from the maximum likelihood theory. When $n \rightarrow \infty$, the MSEs of both estimators approach the absolute lower bound derived in Section 8.9.1.

Problems for Section 8.10

1. Demonstrate Theorem 42 by simulations using the one-exponential model (8.57). Modify the code `onexpSIM` for this purpose: run simulations and compute MSE with increasing N and n. Show that the MSEs for both methods converge to (8.75).

2. Reconstruct the MSEs in Figure 8.4. Compute TS MSE by formula (8.77) and ML MSE by formula (8.59) using the GH quadrature discussed in Section 7.1.3.

3*. Study the small-sample properties of TS, FOA, and LB estimators via simulations using the exponential model from Problem 4 of Section 8.7. Use `nlme` to compute the LB estimator.

8.11   Bias-corrected two-stage estimator

As follows from the proof of Theorem 42, the bias of the TS estimator is due to the fact that individual least squares (LS) estimates $\{\mathbf{a}_i^o, i = 1, ..., N\}$ are biased for finite n_i. Therefore, to find a bias correction to the TS estimator (8.22), we have to evaluate the bias in $\mathbf{a}_i^o$, conditional on random effects. This is the objective of this section.

Omitting i, the normal equation for the individual LS estimator in the nonlinear regression $\mathbf{y} = \mathbf{f}(\boldsymbol{\alpha}) + \boldsymbol{\varepsilon}$ can be written as $\mathbf{R}(\boldsymbol{\alpha})(\mathbf{y} - \mathbf{f}(\boldsymbol{\alpha})) = \mathbf{0}$, or in terms of $\boldsymbol{\varepsilon}$ and $\mathbf{b}$ as

$$\mathbf{R}(\boldsymbol{\alpha}) \left(\mathbf{f}(\mathbf{A}\boldsymbol{\beta} + \mathbf{b}) + \boldsymbol{\varepsilon} - \mathbf{f}(\boldsymbol{\alpha}) \right) = \mathbf{0}. \tag{8.78}$$

The solution to (8.78), $\mathbf{a}_i^o$, is an implicit function of $\boldsymbol{\varepsilon}$ and $\mathbf{b}$. We aim to evaluate the bias using the second-order approximation to $\mathbf{a}_i^o$ in the neighborhood of $\boldsymbol{\varepsilon} = \mathbf{0}$ and $\mathbf{b} = \mathbf{0}$, as an implicit function of $\mathbf{b}$ and $\boldsymbol{\varepsilon}$. One can expect that such an approximation would work well for small σ^2 and $\mathbf{D}$. The approximation can be viewed as a generalization of (8.68). Since $\boldsymbol{\varepsilon}$ and $\mathbf{b}$ are independent, the cross-derivative term vanishes in the second-order approximation, so we only need to find

$$\left. \frac{\partial^2 \mathbf{a}_i^o}{\partial \boldsymbol{\varepsilon}^2} \right|_{\boldsymbol{\varepsilon}=\mathbf{0},\mathbf{b}=\mathbf{0}} \quad \text{and} \quad \left. \frac{\partial^2 \mathbf{a}_i^o}{\partial \mathbf{b}^2} \right|_{\boldsymbol{\varepsilon}=\mathbf{0},\mathbf{b}=\mathbf{0}}. \tag{8.79}$$

Notice that for $\boldsymbol{\varepsilon} = \mathbf{0}$ and $\mathbf{b} = \mathbf{0}$, we have $\mathbf{a}_i^o = \mathbf{A}\boldsymbol{\beta}$.

As we learned from the exponential model of Section 8.9, the second derivative of the TS estimator with respect to the random effect is zero. We shall show that this holds for any nonlinear model. First, let us consider the univariate case when α and b are scalars. Then (8.78) can be rewritten as

$$\left(\mathbf{f}(\gamma + b) + \boldsymbol{\varepsilon} - \mathbf{f}(\alpha) \right)' \dot{\mathbf{f}}(\alpha) = 0, \tag{8.80}$$

where $\gamma = \mathbf{A}\boldsymbol{\beta}$ and $\dot{\mathbf{f}}$ is an $n \times 1$ vector of the first derivatives. Differentiating (8.80) with respect to b, we obtain

$$\left(\dot{\mathbf{f}}(\gamma + b) - \dot{\mathbf{f}}(\alpha) \frac{\partial \alpha}{\partial b} \right)' \dot{\mathbf{f}}(\alpha) + \left(\mathbf{f}(\gamma + b) + \boldsymbol{\varepsilon} - \mathbf{f}(\alpha) \right)' \ddot{\mathbf{f}}(\alpha) \frac{\partial \alpha}{\partial b} = 0. \tag{8.81}$$

At $\varepsilon = \mathbf{0}$ and $b = 0$, we find that

$$\left. \frac{\partial a_i^o}{\partial b} \right|_{\varepsilon=\mathbf{0},b=0} = 1. \tag{8.82}$$

To find the second derivatives at $\varepsilon = \mathbf{0}$ and $b = 0$, we observe that we do not need to differentiate the second factors of the two terms in (8.81) because the first factors vanish at $\varepsilon = \mathbf{0}$ and $b = 0$. Therefore, differentiating the first factors in (8.81) with respect to b, one obtains

$$\left(\ddot{\mathbf{f}}(\gamma + b) - \ddot{\mathbf{f}}(\alpha) \left(\frac{\partial \alpha}{\partial b} \right)^2 - \dot{\mathbf{f}}(\alpha) \frac{\partial^2 \alpha}{\partial b^2} \right)' \dot{\mathbf{f}}(\alpha)$$

$$+ \left(\dot{\mathbf{f}}(\gamma + b) - \dot{\mathbf{f}}(\alpha) \frac{\partial \alpha}{\partial b} \right)' \ddot{\mathbf{f}}(\alpha) \frac{\partial \alpha}{\partial b} = 0$$

at $\varepsilon = \mathbf{0}$ and $b = 0$. Calculating the last expression at $\varepsilon = \mathbf{0}$ and $b = 0$, we obtain

$$\left(\ddot{\mathbf{f}}(\gamma) - \ddot{\mathbf{f}}(\gamma) \left(\frac{\partial \alpha}{\partial b} \right)^2 - \dot{\mathbf{f}}(\gamma) \frac{\partial^2 \alpha}{\partial b^2} \right)' \dot{\mathbf{f}}(\gamma) = 0.$$

Finally, using (8.82), we obtain that the second derivative is zero,

$$\left. \frac{\partial^2 a_i^o}{\partial b^2} \right|_{\varepsilon=\mathbf{0},b=0} = 0.$$

In the multivariate case, we repeat the steps above for every component of vectors $\mathbf{b}$ and $\boldsymbol{\alpha}$. Thus, we conclude that the individual LS estimate depends linearly on the random effects in the neighborhood of zero, and consequently, $E(\mathbf{a}_i^o | \mathbf{b}_i) \simeq \mathbf{0}$.

To find the bias of $\mathbf{a}_i^o$ due to ε_i, we adopt the theory on the bias in nonlinear estimation based on the second-order approximation developed by Box (1971). Box's formula for the bias is

$$\mathbf{a}_i^o - E\mathbf{a}_i^o \simeq -\frac{\sigma^2}{2} (\mathbf{R}'\mathbf{R})^{-1} \mathbf{R}' \mathbf{d}, \tag{8.83}$$

where $\mathbf{d}$ is an $n \times 1$ vector with the jth element,

$$d_j = \mathrm{tr}\left((\mathbf{R}'\mathbf{R})^{-1} \mathbf{H}_j \right), \quad \text{where} \quad \mathbf{H}_j = \frac{\partial^2 f_j}{\partial \boldsymbol{\alpha}^2}, \quad j = 1, ..., n.$$

Since $E(\mathbf{a}_i^o | \mathbf{b}_i) \simeq \mathbf{0}$, the only bias is (8.83), so that finally the bias-corrected version of the TS estimator (8.22) has the form

$$\widehat{\boldsymbol{\beta}}_{TS}^c = \widehat{\boldsymbol{\beta}}_{TS} + \left[\sum \mathbf{A}_i' (\mathbf{T}_i + \widehat{\mathbf{D}})^{-1} \mathbf{A}_i \right]^{-1} \sum \mathbf{A}_i' (\mathbf{T}_i + \widehat{\mathbf{D}})^{-1} \mathbf{c}_i, \tag{8.84}$$

where $\widehat{\boldsymbol{\beta}}_{TS}$ is the ordinary TS estimator and $\mathbf{c}_i = 0.5\widehat{\sigma}_i^2 (\mathbf{R}_i'\mathbf{R}_i)^{-1} \mathbf{R}_i' \mathbf{d}$. Here $\mathbf{d}_i$ is an $n_i \times 1$ vector with the jth element $\mathrm{tr}\left((\mathbf{R}_i'\mathbf{R}_i)^{-1} \mathbf{H}_{ij} \right)$, where $\mathbf{H}_{ij} = \partial^2 f_{ij}/\partial \boldsymbol{\alpha}^2$ is the matrix of second derivatives and $\widehat{\sigma}_i^2$ is the residual variance.

Problems for Section 8.11

1. Apply Box's formula for the bias (8.83) to nonlinear regression $y_i = e^\alpha + \varepsilon_i$, where $\varepsilon_i \sim \mathcal{N}(0, \sigma^2)$. Use simulations to assess how precise the bias is. Take care of simulations when the NLS estimate does not exist. Does the bias correction improve MSE?

2. Apply the formula for the bias (8.83) to model (8.57).

8.12   Distribution misspecification

The assumption of a normal distribution of random variables in the NLME model is practically unverifiable. What is the implication of a distribution misspecification? What happens if the distribution, in fact, is not normal but we use maximum likelihood for parameter estimation? To illustrate, we start with ordinary nonlinear regression.

Example: *Distribution misspecification in nonlinear regression.* Ordinary nonlinear regression has the form $y_i = f(\mathbf{x}_i; \boldsymbol{\beta}) + \sigma \varepsilon_i$, where $\mathbf{x}_i$ is the design (fixed) vector and $\{\varepsilon_i,\ i = 1, ..., N\}$ are iid random variables with zero mean and unit variance. To simplify, the variance σ^2 is assumed known. Denote the density of ε_i as $p(\cdot)$, so that

$$E(\varepsilon_i) = \int t p(t) dt = 0, \quad \text{var}(\varepsilon_i) = \int t^2 p(t) dt = 1. \tag{8.85}$$

It is assumed that the limit

$$\lim_{N \to \infty} \frac{1}{N} \sum_{i=1}^{N} \left(\frac{\partial f(\mathbf{x}_i; \boldsymbol{\beta})}{\partial \boldsymbol{\beta}} \right) \left(\frac{\partial f(\mathbf{x}_i; \boldsymbol{\beta})}{\partial \boldsymbol{\beta}} \right)' = \mathbf{Q} \tag{8.86}$$

exists and that $\mathbf{Q} = \mathbf{Q}(\boldsymbol{\beta})$ is a nonsingular matrix for all $\boldsymbol{\beta}$. Also, it is assumed that all other standard conditions required for consistency and asymptotic normality of the least squares (LS) estimator and the MLE hold (Jennrich, 1969; Wu, 1981). In the absence of misspecification LS = ML. Otherwise, we obtain an LS estimator $\widehat{\boldsymbol{\beta}}_{LS}$ that differs from $\widehat{\boldsymbol{\beta}}_{ML}$. Despite the distribution misspecification, the LS estimator is consistent and asymptotically normally distributed as

$$\sqrt{N}(\widehat{\boldsymbol{\beta}}_{LS} - \boldsymbol{\beta}) \simeq \mathcal{N}(\mathbf{0}, \sigma^2 \mathbf{Q}^{-1}), \qquad N \to \infty.$$

The MLE, $\widehat{\boldsymbol{\beta}}_{ML}$, as the solution to the score equation

$$\frac{1}{N} \sum_{i=1}^{N} \left(\frac{d \ln p(t)}{dt} \bigg|_{t=(y_i - \mathbf{x}_i'\boldsymbol{\beta})/\sigma} \right) \mathbf{x}_i = \mathbf{0},$$

is also consistent and asymptotically normally distributed as

$$\sqrt{N}(\widehat{\boldsymbol{\beta}}_{ML} - \boldsymbol{\beta}) \simeq \mathcal{N}\left(\mathbf{0}, \frac{\sigma^2}{\gamma^2} \mathbf{Q}^{-1} \right), \tag{8.87}$$

where

$$\gamma^2 = E\left(\frac{d\ln p(t)}{dt}\right)^2 = \int \left(\frac{d\ln p(t)}{dt}\right)^2 p(t)dt.$$

We prove that $\gamma^2 \geq 1$. Indeed, from integration by parts

$$E\left(t\frac{d\ln p(t)}{dt}\right) = \int t\frac{dp(t)}{dt}dt = \int p(t)dt = 1$$

and by the Cauchy inequality,

$$1 = E^2\left(t\frac{d\ln p(t)}{dt}\right) \leq E(t^2)E\left(\frac{d\ln p(t)}{dt}\right)^2 = \gamma^2$$

because from (8.85) we have $E(t^2) = 1$. ∎

From (8.87) it follows that the asymptotic variance of the MLE is less than or equal to the variance of the LS estimator. Also, from Cauchy inequality, it follows that the LS estimator does not lose efficiency if and only if $d\ln p(t)/dt$ is proportional to t, which holds only for normal distribution. For example, if ε_i had heavier tails, as for the Laplace (double-exponential) distribution $p(t) = (2\lambda)^{-1}e^{-|t|/\lambda}$, the assumption of the normal distribution would lead to the least squares estimator while the true MLE would lead to the median estimator. It is easy to compute the efficiency loss when the true distribution is, in fact, exponential: $\gamma = 2$, the standard deviation of the LS estimator would be two times larger than that for the median. Note that we could derive the variance of the estimators under a misspecified distribution using the sandwich formula of Appendix 13.1.4.

Summing up, when the distribution in a nonlinear regression model is misspecified, we still obtain consistent but less efficient estimates. However, as follows from the example below, the implication of the misspecification in the random effects for the NLME model is much more severe—one loses consistency!

To assess the asymptotic bias for infinitely large N and fixed n under distribution misspecification in the NLME model, we again consider the one-random parameter exponential model (8.57, 8.58). The true distribution of the random effect is assumed to be Laplace/double-exponential with parameter $\lambda = 2\sigma^2\omega^2$, meaning that $\text{var}(b) = \sigma^2\omega^2$ but ε_{ij} remains normally distributed. Parameter β is estimated based on the incorrect assumption that $b \sim \mathcal{N}(0, \sigma^2\omega^2)$. The asymptotic bias, when $N \to \infty$ and n is fixed, is calculated from the two-dimensional integral. The method of the bias calculation is the same as in Section 8.9.4. The reader is also referred to Appendix 13.1.4. The expected value of the estimating equation is given by the two-dimensional integral

$$\overline{S}_n(\beta, \beta_0)$$
$$= \int \int \left\{ \frac{\int (a-\beta)Q_n(a,x,y;\beta,\beta_0)da}{\int Q_n(a,x,y;\beta,\beta_0)da} \exp\left(-\frac{|x|}{2\sigma^2\omega^2} - \frac{ny}{2\sigma^2}\right) dxdy \right\}$$

where

$$Q_n(a,x,y;\beta,\beta_0) = \exp\left[\frac{ne^a\left(2(e^{\beta_0+x}+y) - e^a\right)}{2\sigma^2} - \frac{(a-\beta)^2}{2\sigma^2\omega^2} - c\right]$$

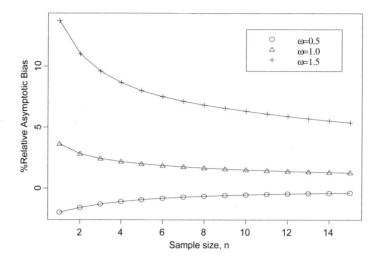

FIGURE 8.5. Relative asymptotic bias under misspecification of the distribution of the random effect in the one-parameter exponential model ($\beta_0=0.7$, $\sigma=0.5$) for infinitely large N and relative SD of the random effect, ω. The true distribution of the random effect b is double exponential; however, β is estimated by ML assuming normal distribution.

and $c = 2\sigma^{-2}n(e^{\beta_0+x}+y)^2$, the normalizing constant (integration is over the entire space R^2). Given β_0, the true value, the misspecified estimator converges to the root of the equation $\overline{S}_n(\beta, \beta_0) = 0$. We find the root by Newton's algorithm,

$$\beta_{s+1} = \beta_s - \frac{\overline{S}_n(\beta_s, \beta_0)}{\overline{S}'_n(\beta_s, \beta_0)}, \quad s = 0, 1, ...,$$

where $\overline{S}'_n(\beta_s, \beta_0)$ is the derivative of $\overline{S}_n(\beta, \beta_0)$ with respect to β. The relative asymptotic bias for different relative SDs of the random effects (ω) is shown in Figure 8.5. As we see, the absolute bias decreases with n; however, it is negative for $w = 0.5$ and positive for $w = 1$ and $w = 1.5$.

In summary, misspecification of the distribution of random effects is disastrous to maximum likelihood estimation: the MLE becomes systematically biased even for an infinitely large number of subjects. However, the bias vanishes when the number of observations per subject increases along with the number of subjects. Interestingly, misspecification of the distribution of ε_{ij} is not so harmful because it leaves the estimator consistent but with some loss of efficiency. An analysis of misspecified assumptions based on a simulation study was conducted by Hartford and Davidian (2000). It was found that the LA method of estimation is more precise than FOA in case of the normality misspecification but has a slower convergence rate.

Problems for Section 8.12

1*. Develop the asymptotic efficiency comparison for the median against the mean when the data have heavy tails but the mean is used to estimate the center of the distribution. More specifically, assume that $y_i = \beta + \sigma\varepsilon_i$, where iid ε_i have Laplace distribution with the density $\frac{1}{\sqrt{2}}e^{-\sqrt{2}|t|}$. Prove that the MLE of β in this model is the median. Use simulations to generate the data from Laplace distribution and estimate β using the mean (LS). Use inverse cdf to generate random numbers from Laplace distribution. Plot the ratio of two empirical MSE for the mean and the median as a function of increasing N and display the theoretical ratio as a horizontal line.

2*. Reproduce Figure 8.5. Use the GH quadrature for double integration to compute function $\overline{S}_n(\beta, \beta_0)$, see Section 7.1.3. Then use Newton's iterations to compute β for given n. Use the function INT.ch08.

8.13   Partially nonlinear marginal mixed model

In many applications a nonlinear statistical model has only a few intrinsically nonlinear parameters, while other parameters are linear. Such a model is called *partial nonlinear regression*. For example, in the log-Gompertz curve of Section 6.1.7, defined by the equation $\beta_1 - \beta_2 e^{-\beta_3 t}$, there is only one intrinsically nonlinear parameter, β_3, and parameters β_1 and β_2 are linear. Estimation of nonlinear regression with partially linear parameters is well studied in the literature (sometimes it is related to separable nonlinear least squares). The idea is to reduce the parameter space by eliminating linear parameters, Golub and Pereyra (1973). A recent review of the topic, with a large number of applications in different fields, is given by Golub and Pereyra (2003). For example, if nonlinear regression with linear parameters has the form $\mathbf{y} = \mathbf{X}(\boldsymbol{\beta})\boldsymbol{\gamma} + \boldsymbol{\varepsilon}$, where $\mathbf{X}$ is an $n \times m$ matrix function of a $p \times 1$ parameter vector $\boldsymbol{\beta}$ and $\boldsymbol{\gamma}$ is an $m \times 1$ linear parameter vector, we can eliminate $\boldsymbol{\gamma}$ using least squares as $\widehat{\boldsymbol{\gamma}} = (\mathbf{X}'(\boldsymbol{\beta})\mathbf{X}(\boldsymbol{\beta}))^{-1}\mathbf{X}'(\boldsymbol{\beta})\mathbf{y}$. Then, plugging it in back into the original regression we reduce the dimension from $p + m$ to p parameters, $\mathbf{y} = \mathbf{K}(\boldsymbol{\beta})\mathbf{y} + \boldsymbol{\varepsilon}$, where $\mathbf{K}(\boldsymbol{\beta}) = (\mathbf{X}'(\boldsymbol{\beta})\mathbf{X}(\boldsymbol{\beta}))^{-1}\mathbf{X}'(\boldsymbol{\beta})$ is an idempotent matrix. It is easy to show that the least squares for the new regression is equivalent to maximization of $\mathbf{y}'\mathbf{K}(\boldsymbol{\beta})\mathbf{y}$. This reduction is especially effective when p is small (say, 1 or 2) and m is large. Also, it was found that this reduction improves statistical inference on $\boldsymbol{\beta}$, such as confidence intervals (Macaskill, 1993).

It is straightforward to generalize the partial nonlinear regression model to a mixed model with random parameters,

$$\mathbf{y}_i = \mathbf{X}_i(\mathbf{b}_i)\mathbf{g}_i + \boldsymbol{\varepsilon}_i, \quad i = 1, ..., N, \ j = 1, ..., n_i, \tag{8.88}$$

where $\mathbf{y}_i$ is the $n_i \times 1$ vector of the dependent variable, $\mathbf{X}_i$ is the $n_i \times m$ matrix function of the p-dimensional random intrinsically nonlinear parameter $\mathbf{b}_i$, $\mathbf{g}_i$ is the m-dimensional linear vector parameter and $\boldsymbol{\varepsilon}_i$ is the $n_i \times 1$ vector of iid errors. We assume that $\mathbf{b}_i, \mathbf{g}_i$, and $\boldsymbol{\varepsilon}_i$ are normally distributed and that $\boldsymbol{\varepsilon}_i \sim \mathcal{N}(\mathbf{0}, \sigma^2\mathbf{I})$ is independent of $(\mathbf{b}_i, \mathbf{g}_i)$. Instead of specifying the joint normal distribution of random parameters, we specify $\mathbf{b}_i \sim \mathcal{N}(\boldsymbol{\beta}, \mathbf{D}_1)$ and the conditional normal distribution $\mathbf{g}_i|\mathbf{b}_i \sim \mathcal{N}(\boldsymbol{\gamma} + \boldsymbol{\Gamma}\mathbf{b}_i, \mathbf{D}_2)$, where $\boldsymbol{\gamma}$ is an $m \times 1$ vector and $\boldsymbol{\Gamma}$ is an $m \times p$ matrix. Then model (8.88) can be written as

$$\mathbf{y}_i|\mathbf{b}_i \sim \mathcal{N}\left(\mathbf{X}_i(\mathbf{b}_i)(\boldsymbol{\gamma} + \boldsymbol{\Gamma}\mathbf{b}_i), \mathbf{I} + \mathbf{X}_i(\mathbf{b}_i)\mathbf{D}_2\mathbf{X}_i'(\mathbf{b}_i)\right). \tag{8.89}$$

Thus, the original mixed model with $m + p$ random parameters is reduced to p random parameters. Again, this reduction is especially effective when p is small and m is large. Although we do not eliminate linear parameters, as in nonlinear regression, the dimension of the integral is reduced. The joint log-likelihood is

$$l(\boldsymbol{\beta}, \boldsymbol{\gamma}, \boldsymbol{\Gamma}, \mathbf{D}_1, \mathbf{D}_2) = \sum_{i=1}^{N} \int_{R^p} e^{\frac{1}{2} l_i (\mathbf{b}; \boldsymbol{\beta}, \boldsymbol{\gamma}, \boldsymbol{\Gamma}, \mathbf{D}_1, \mathbf{D}_2)} d\mathbf{b},$$

where l_i is the twice-negative log-likelihood function of the ith subject defined as

$$\ln |\mathbf{I} + \mathbf{X}_i(\mathbf{b}_i) \mathbf{D}_2 \mathbf{X}'_i(\mathbf{b}_i)| + \ln |\mathbf{D}_1|$$
$$+ \mathbf{e}'_i [\mathbf{I} + \mathbf{X}_i(\mathbf{b}_i) \mathbf{D}_2 \mathbf{X}'_i(\mathbf{b}_i)]^{-1} \mathbf{e}_i + (\mathbf{b}_i - \boldsymbol{\beta})' \mathbf{D}_1^{-1} (\mathbf{b}_i - \boldsymbol{\beta}),$$

where $\mathbf{e}_i = \mathbf{y}_i - \mathbf{X}_i(\mathbf{b}_i)(\boldsymbol{\gamma} + \boldsymbol{\Gamma} \mathbf{b}_i)$.

To illustrate, we again consider the log-Gompertz growth curve (6.16) but now assuming that all three parameters are random, $\mathbf{y}_i | (b_{i1}, b_{i2}, b_{i3}) = (\beta_1 + b_{i1}) - (\beta_2 + b_{i2}) e^{-(\beta_3 + b_{i3}) \mathbf{t}_i} + \boldsymbol{\varepsilon}_i$, where $\mathbf{t}_i$ is an $n_i \times 1$ vector. In the previous notation, $p = 1$ and $m = 2$, so that D_1 is a scalar, with $\mathbf{X}_i(b) = [\mathbf{1}, -e^{-bt_i}]$. Thus, the original three-dimensional integral is reduced to a one-dimensional integral.

Problems for Section 8.13

1. Reduce the estimation of a three-random-parameter log-Gompertz model to a one-random parameter model. Write an R function that estimates this NLME model using the GH quadrature for integral approximation. Apply this function for estimation of the growth of spheroids with the data in the file TUMspher.txt (see Section 6.1.7). Compare your results with nlme.

8.14   Fixed sample likelihood approach

We can easily generalize the Fixed Sample Likelihood (FSL) approach of Section 7.8.3 to the NLME model. As mentioned earlier, the FSL approach combines the Gauss-Hermite quadrature with Monte Carlo integral approximation. The difference between those is how the integration nodes are computed: the former uses predefined formulas (the gauher function in R) and in the latter the nodes are sample values from the normal distribution. The interested reader can learn more about application of the GH quadrature to generalized linear and nonlinear mixed models from Liu and Pierce (1994), Pinheiro and Bates (1995), Pinheiro and Bates (2000, pp. 319-322), and Vonesh (2012, pp. 276-279). An attractive idea for using the FSL approach is that the covariance matrix for random effects (actually its Cholesky factor) can be combined with the fixed effects coefficients and therefore treated under one scheme of estimation.

Let $\mathbf{D}_{*c}$ be the Cholesky factor of matrix $\mathbf{D}_* = \sigma^2 \mathbf{D}$. Then the model (8.7), (8.8) can be parameterized as

$$\mathbf{y}_i | \mathbf{u}_i \sim \mathcal{N}(\mathbf{f}_i(\boldsymbol{\gamma}, \mathbf{A}_i \boldsymbol{\beta} + \mathbf{D}'_{*c} \mathbf{u}_i), \sigma^2 \mathbf{I})$$

with the log-likelihood

$$l = -\frac{N_T \ln \sigma^2}{2} + \sum_{i=1}^{N} \ln \int e^{-\frac{1}{2\sigma^2} \left\| \mathbf{y}_i - \mathbf{f}_i (\boldsymbol{\gamma}, \mathbf{A}_i \boldsymbol{\beta} + \sqrt{2} \mathbf{D}'_{*c} \mathbf{u}) \right\|^2} e^{-\|\mathbf{u}\|^2} d\mathbf{u} + c,$$

where $c = N \ln \sqrt{2} - N_T \ln \sqrt{2\pi}$, a constant. The presence of the constant is required to compare different likelihood approximations. Note that in the parametrization the integration kernel is $e^{-\|\mathbf{u}\|^2}$ for convenience of the Gauss-Hermite quadrature, see Section 7.1.3. If $\{\mathbf{u}_s\}$ and weights $\{w_s\}$ are derived using the `gauher` function, the discrete version of the log-likelihood function takes the form of a sum,

$$l_{FSL}(\boldsymbol{\gamma}, \boldsymbol{\beta}, \sigma^2, \boldsymbol{\delta}) = -\frac{N_T \ln \sigma^2}{2} + \sum_{i=1}^{N} \ln \sum_{s=1}^{S} w_s e^{-\frac{1}{2\sigma^2} \|\mathbf{y}_i - \mathbf{f}_i(\boldsymbol{\gamma}, \mathbf{A}_i \boldsymbol{\beta} + \mathbf{U}_s \boldsymbol{\delta})\|^2} + c,$$

where $\mathbf{U}_s$ is a $k \times (k(k+1)/2)$ matrix and $\boldsymbol{\delta}$ is a $(k(k+1)/2) \times 1$ vector of nonzero elements of matrix $\mathbf{D}_{*c}$. Specifically, let $\mathbf{U}_s = \sqrt{2}(\mathbf{u}_s' \otimes \mathbf{I}_k)\mathcal{D}_k$, where $\mathcal{D}_k$ is the $k^2 \times (k(k+1)/2)$ duplication matrix. Then as follows from the representation

$$\begin{aligned} \mathbf{D}_{*c}' \mathbf{u}_s &= \text{vec}(\mathbf{D}_{*c}' \mathbf{u}_s) = \text{vec}(\mathbf{I}_k \mathbf{D}_{*c}' \mathbf{u}_s) = (\mathbf{u}_s' \otimes \mathbf{I}_k)\text{vec}(\mathbf{D}_{*c}') \\ &= (\mathbf{u}_s' \otimes \mathbf{I}_k)\mathcal{D}_k \text{vech}(\mathbf{D}_{*c}') = (\mathbf{u}_s' \otimes \mathbf{I}_k)\mathcal{D}_k \boldsymbol{\delta}. \end{aligned}$$

Introducing an $n_i \times 1$ nonlinear function, $\mathbf{h}_{is}(\boldsymbol{\tau}) = \mathbf{f}_i(\boldsymbol{\gamma}, \mathbf{A}_i \boldsymbol{\beta} + \mathbf{U}_s \boldsymbol{\delta})$, where $\boldsymbol{\tau}$ is the combined parameter vector $\boldsymbol{\gamma}, \boldsymbol{\beta}$, and $\boldsymbol{\delta}$, we come to the function maximization over $\boldsymbol{\tau}$,

$$l_{FSL}(\boldsymbol{\tau}) = -\frac{N_T \ln \sigma^2}{2} + \sum_{i=1}^{N} \ln \sum_{s=1}^{S} w_s e^{-\frac{1}{2\sigma^2} \|\mathbf{y}_i - \mathbf{h}_{is}(\boldsymbol{\tau})\|^2} + c. \tag{8.90}$$

Several algorithms can be suggested, perhaps the simplest of which is Empirical Fisher scoring (EFS), see Section 7.3.1 and Appendix 13.3.4. The required derivatives are

$$\frac{\partial l_{FSL}}{\partial \sigma^2} = -\frac{N_T}{2\sigma^2} + \frac{1}{2\sigma^4} \sum_{i=1}^{N} \frac{\sum_{s=1}^{S} w_s e_{is} \|\mathbf{y}_i - \mathbf{h}_{is}(\boldsymbol{\tau})\|^2}{\sum_{s=1}^{S} w_s e_{is}},$$

$$\frac{\partial l_{FSL}}{\partial \boldsymbol{\tau}} = \frac{1}{\sigma^2} \sum_{i=1}^{N} \frac{\sum_{s=1}^{S} w_s e_{is} \mathbf{H}_{is}'(\mathbf{y}_i - \mathbf{h}_{is}(\boldsymbol{\tau}))}{\sum_{s=1}^{S} w_s e_{is}},$$

where $e_{is} = e^{-\frac{1}{2\sigma^2}\|\mathbf{y}_i - \mathbf{h}_{is}(\boldsymbol{\tau})\|^2}$ and $\mathbf{H}_{is} = \partial \mathbf{h}_{is}/\partial \boldsymbol{\tau}$. Thus, letting

$$\mathbf{d}_i = \begin{bmatrix} -\frac{n_i}{2\sigma^2} + \frac{1}{2\sigma^4} \left(\sum_{s=1}^{S} w_s e_{is}\right)^{-1} \left(\sum_{s=1}^{S} w_s e_{is} \|\mathbf{y}_i - \mathbf{h}_{is}(\boldsymbol{\tau})\|^2\right) \\ \frac{1}{\sigma^2} \left(\sum_{s=1}^{S} w_s e_{is}\right)^{-1} \left(\sum_{s=1}^{S} w_s e_{is} \mathbf{H}_{is}'(\mathbf{y}_i - \mathbf{h}_{is}(\boldsymbol{\tau}))\right) \end{bmatrix}$$

by the EFS algorithm, we iterate as $\boldsymbol{\tau}_{new} = \boldsymbol{\tau} + \lambda(\sum \mathbf{d}_i \mathbf{d}_i')^{-1} \sum \mathbf{d}_i$, where λ is a positive step length to ensure that l_{FSL} increases (usually $\lambda = 1$).

Use `source("c:\\MixedModels\\Chapter08\\callnlmeFSL.r")` to download a version of FSL (`nlmeFSL`) applied to the `Qlogist` function with `heightlog.dat` data.

8.14.1   Example: one-parameter exponential model

We use the one-parameter exponential model specified by equations (8.57) and (8.58) to illustrate the FSL approach. The log-likelihood function after slight simplification takes the form

$$l_{FSL}(\beta,\sigma^2,\omega^2) = -\frac{Nn\ln\sigma^2}{2} + \sum_{i=1}^{N}\ln\sum_{k=1}^{K}w_k e^{-\frac{1}{2\sigma^2}\left(s_i^2+n(\overline{y}_i-e^{\beta+U_k\omega})^2\right)} + c,$$

where $s_i^2 = \|\mathbf{y}_i\|^2$, $U_k = \sqrt{2}x_k$, and x_k and w_k are the abscissa and the weight of the Gauss-Hermite quadrature (the output of **gauher** function). Denote $\boldsymbol{\tau}^{2\times 1} = (\beta,\omega)'$ and $\mathbf{h}_k^{n\times 1} = \mathbf{1}h_k(\boldsymbol{\tau})$, where $h_k(\boldsymbol{\tau}) = e^{\beta+U_k\omega} = e^{\mathbf{g}_k'\boldsymbol{\tau}}$ and $\mathbf{g}_k^{2\times 1} = (1,U_k)'$. Then the log-likelihood function takes the form (8.90) with derivatives

$$\frac{\partial l_{FSL}}{\partial \sigma^2} = -\frac{Nn}{2\sigma^2} + \frac{1}{2\sigma^4}\sum_{i=1}^{N}\frac{\sum_{k=1}^{K}w_k e_{ik}\left(s_i^2+n(\overline{y}_i-e^{\beta+U_k\omega})^2\right)}{\sum_{k=1}^{K}w_k e_{ik}},$$

$$\frac{\partial l_{FSL}}{\partial \beta} = \frac{n}{\sigma^2}\sum_{i=1}^{N}\frac{\sum_{k=1}^{K}w_k e_{ik}h_k(\overline{y}_i-e^{\beta+U_k\omega})}{\sum_{k=1}^{K}w_k e_{ik}},$$

$$\frac{\partial l_{FSL}}{\partial \omega} = \frac{n}{\sigma^2}\sum_{i=1}^{N}\frac{\sum_{k=1}^{K}w_k e_{ik}h_k(\overline{y}_i-e^{\beta+U_k\omega})U_k}{\sum_{k=1}^{K}w_k e_{ik}}$$

where $e_{ik} = e^{-\frac{1}{2\sigma^2}\left(s_i^2+n(\overline{y}_i-e^{\beta+U_k\omega})^2\right)}$.

This method is programmed in function **onexpFSL**. Two versions for the choice of U_k are available: if **method="gauher"** x_k and w_k are chosen as in Gauss-Hermite quadrature; otherwise, $w_k = 1/K$ and x_k is a sample from a normal distribution with zero mean and SD=$\sqrt{2}$. The function **onexpSIM** does simulations and computes MSE for **nlme** and **onexpFSL**. Both functions are downloaded into the R session as **source("c:\\MixedModels\\Chapter08\\onexpSIMFSL.r")**.

Problems for Section 8.14

1. Write an R function that estimates the height of girls using the **Qlogist** function with only adult height being random (parameter a_1), see Section 8.3. Modify the function **onexpSIM**. Compare the results of estimation with **nlme**.

2*. Write an R function that estimates the height of girls using **Qlogist** function with all four parameters being random. Compare the results of estimation with **nlme**.

8.15 Estimation of random effects and hypothesis testing

8.15.1 Estimation of the random effects

There are two approaches to estimating the random effects, $\mathbf{b}_i$, after estimates for all parameters $\boldsymbol{\gamma}, \boldsymbol{\beta}, \sigma^2$, and $\mathbf{D}$ are available: approximate and exact. In the approximate approach, after applying Laplace approximation, we come to N penalized least squares (PLS),

$$\| \mathbf{y}_i - \mathbf{f}_i(\widehat{\boldsymbol{\gamma}}, \mathbf{A}_i\widehat{\boldsymbol{\beta}} + \boldsymbol{\tau}_i) \|^2 + \boldsymbol{\tau}_i'\widehat{\mathbf{D}}^{-1}\boldsymbol{\tau}_i, \tag{8.91}$$

which mimics the PLS for the linear mixed model (3.54). Since $\widehat{\boldsymbol{\gamma}}, \widehat{\boldsymbol{\beta}}$, and $\widehat{\mathbf{D}}$ are fixed, the total PLS (8.29) collapses to N separate PLSs (8.91). Then the estimate of the random effect $\mathbf{b}_i$ is the minimizer $\widehat{\boldsymbol{\tau}}_i$. Hence, if the NLME model is estimated by LB or LA, the estimate of the random effect is obtained as a by-product of the estimation procedure.

In the exact approach, we recall that for the LME model the PLS is equivalent to the posterior/conditional mean of the random effect, see Section 3.7. This gives rise to exact estimation of the random effect as the conditional mean in NLME model. To find the conditional mean of $\mathbf{b}$ given data $\mathbf{y}$, we express the posterior distribution of the random effect as $f(\mathbf{b}|\mathbf{y}) = f(\mathbf{y}|\mathbf{b})f(\mathbf{b})/f(\mathbf{y})$. Thus, using the notation of Section 8.8, we obtain

$$\widehat{\mathbf{b}}_i = \frac{\int \mathbf{b} e^{l(\mathbf{y}_i|\mathbf{b};\widehat{\boldsymbol{\gamma}},\widehat{\boldsymbol{\beta}},\widehat{\sigma}^2)} \phi(\mathbf{b};\widehat{\mathbf{D}}) d\mathbf{b}}{\int e^{l(\mathbf{y}_i|\mathbf{b};\widehat{\boldsymbol{\gamma}},\widehat{\boldsymbol{\beta}},\widehat{\sigma}^2)} \phi(\mathbf{b};\widehat{\mathbf{D}}) d\mathbf{b}}, \tag{8.92}$$

where $l(\mathbf{y}_i|\mathbf{b};\widehat{\boldsymbol{\gamma}},\widehat{\boldsymbol{\beta}},\widehat{\sigma}^2)$ is the conditional log density of $\mathbf{y}_i$ defined by equation (8.44). Moreover, one may find the posterior/conditional covariance matrix of the random effects by computing (8.92), where instead of $\mathbf{b}$ one has the matrix $(\mathbf{b}-\widehat{\mathbf{b}}_i)(\mathbf{b}-\widehat{\mathbf{b}}_i)'$. The exact approach requires integral evaluation and therefore is convenient when ML or FSL is used. Obviously, for a linear model the approximate and exact approaches are the same, $\widehat{\boldsymbol{\tau}}_i = \widehat{\mathbf{b}}_i$.

8.15.2   Hypothesis testing for the NLME model

Two kinds of hypothesis testing can be distinguished in the framework of a nonlinear mixed effects model: hypothesis testing regarding (a) population-averaged parameters $\boldsymbol{\gamma}$ and $\boldsymbol{\beta}$, and (b) the variance parameters of random effects (elements of matrix $\mathbf{D}$). To test (a), such as the significance of a component of $\boldsymbol{\gamma}$ or $\boldsymbol{\beta}$, the Wald test may be applied based on the covariance matrix of the population-averaged parameters. The likelihood ratio test also can be applied, but it requires double estimation, under the null hypothesis (restricted) and unrestricted estimation. For nonlinear models profile-likelihood confidence intervals may be better than standard Wald confidence intervals, see Section 3.4.

To test the presence of the random effects, $H_0 : \mathbf{D} = \mathbf{0}$, neither the Wald nor the likelihood ratio test is valid because the null hypothesis belongs to the boundary of the parameter set. We have developed an exact F-test for the LME model in Section 3.5 and generalized it to the nonlinear marginal mixed model in Section 6.1.5. Now we further generalize it to the NLME model. The idea is to compare two sums of squares: First, assume that there are no random effects ($\mathbf{b}_i = \mathbf{0}$); and second, give the random effects complete freedom, i.e., assume that $\mathbf{b}_i$ are fixed unknown parameters. The two SSs are

$$S_{OLS} = \min_{\boldsymbol{\gamma},\boldsymbol{\beta}} \sum \|\mathbf{y}_i - \mathbf{f}_i(\boldsymbol{\gamma}, \mathbf{A}_i\boldsymbol{\beta})\|^2, \quad S_{\min} = \min_{\boldsymbol{\gamma},\mathbf{b}_1,\ldots,\mathbf{b}_N} \sum \|\mathbf{y}_i - \mathbf{f}_i(\boldsymbol{\gamma}, \mathbf{b}_i)\|^2. \tag{8.93}$$

Note that in the second minimization, we ignore the term $\mathbf{A}_i\boldsymbol{\beta}$ because it is consumed by $\mathbf{b}_i$. Letting $r = m + Nk$, we compute the statistic (3.42) and proceed as in the F-test. When $\mathbf{f}_i$ is linear, this test gives the exact type I error.

As a final comment, various types of testing require a joint covariance matrix of fixed and random effects. For the LME model, this matrix has a block diagonal form, and therefore one can ignore the precision of the variance parameters. This does not hold for the general NLME model, and therefore the entire covariance matrix is needed to carry out an asymptotically valid statistical testing. Unfortunately, the approximate methods do not produce the entire covariance matrix; only the maximum likelihood (or FSL) does. This is a strong point in favor of maximum likelihood estimation because statistical inference usually does not end with estimation and requires covariance matrix assessment as well. Alternatively, AIC or HAIC can be used for the model selection, see Section 1.6.

Apparently, there is no satisfactory test for variance-covariance matrix $\mathbf{D}$ and much work has to be done, especially when the number of clusters is small.

Problems for Section 8.15

1*. Write down the equation for estimation of the random effect (8.91) for the one-parameter exponential model (8.57). Derive the Newton's algorithm to iteratively solve N equations for b_i starting from zero. Generate data and run `nlme` to obtain estimates for β and random effects, b_i. Then use your algorithm to compute $\widehat{b}_i$. Compare the results.

2*. Let matrix $\mathbf{D}$ be known. Derive estimates for γ, β, and τ_i as minimizers of $\sum_{i=1}^{N} \left(\parallel \mathbf{y}_i - \mathbf{f}_i(\gamma, \mathbf{A}_i\beta + \tau_i) \parallel^2 + \tau_i' \mathbf{D}^{-1} \tau_i \right)$. To what method of NLME model estimation does it relate? Compare with the LME model. Develop a method for minimization and apply it to the one-parameter exponential model. Use simulations to study its sample properties.

3*. Develop the Wald and likelihood ratio tests for the one-parameter exponential model, see Section 8.9. Use simulations to compare the power functions for testing $H_0 : \beta = 0.5$. Do the two tests yield the specified type I error ($\alpha = 0.05$)? Modify the function `onexpSIM` to write the simulation program.

4*. Use the Wald, likelihood ratio, and F-test based on computation of sum of squares (8.93) to test that the variance of the random effect is zero. Use simulations to compare the power functions for testing $H_0 : \omega = 0$. What test do you prefer? Is there an overall champion?

8.16   Example (continued)

In this section we illustrate the methods of NLME model estimation with the height example of Section 8.3 assuming model (8.6). Thus, all parameters are random. This data set may be a rather nontrivial example to compare approximation methods; as we shall see later, different methods give quite different estimation results, and some of them fail. Having four random effects creates challenges for maximum likelihood estimation as well.

The parameter estimates obtained for average data may serve as good starting points for more complicated procedures. Since all parameters are assumed random, one can obtain individual estimates for each girl or boy. The densities of the individual estimates are displayed in Figure 8.6. As the reader can see, some individual

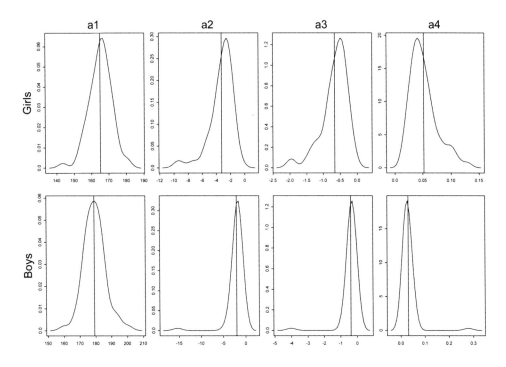

FIGURE 8.6. Densities of individual nonlinear least squares estimates for girls' and boys' heights. The vertical line indicates the TS estimate. Notice the long tails of the estimate densities. This means that some individual estimates have large values or possibly diverge.

estimates are not stable, which is reflected in the long density tails—a common situation with small sample sizes.

The results of estimation with different methods are presented in Table 8.2. Function `callnlmeFSL`, located in the directory `c:\\MixedModels\\Chapter08\\`, estimates the model using the FSL approach. Two options for choosing $\mathbf{U}_s$ and w_s are available: (1) `method="gauher"` produces abscissas and weights as suggested by the GH quadrature (function `gauher`), (2) otherwise, a random sample from a four-dimensional normal distribution is used with weights=1/`SS` where `SS` is the sample size. This function is not optimized in terms of computation and requires a long time (perhaps overnight).

Notice that all methods indicate a relatively small standard error for all parameters, the acceleration year is shown in the last column. As noted earlier, girls accelerate a year earlier and approach their adult height before boys do.

The corrected and uncorrected two-stage methods for girls yield the same result; however, for boys the correction is significant. Interestingly, after the correction, the Two-Stage and First-Order approximation methods become closer.

As a general comment, since boys keep growing after 18, it would be desirable to have data on height for at least three more years. The absence of these data makes the estimation results somewhat unstable with an overestimated male adult height.

Table 8.2. Fitting the height with the QLogistic growth curve
(all four parameters are subject-specific)

	a_1	a_2	a_3	a_4	Acc.
		Girls			
TS	165.2 (.799)	-3.17 (.254)	-.646 (.057)	.0502 (.0032)	9.6
TSC	165.2 (.799)	-3.17 (.254)	-.646 (.057)	.0502 (.0032)	9.6
FOA	173.2 (.672)	-1.21 (.078)	-.193 (.017)	.0214 (.0014)	9.3
FSL (1000)	165.5 (.20)	-2.92 (.16)	-.601 (.034)	.048 (.0018)	9.5
FSL (GH:11)	167.2 (.093)	-2.18 (.126)	-.567 (.029)	.0452 (.0016)	9.6
`nlme`	165.2 (.079)	-2.40 (.109)	-.471 (.023)	.040 (.0014)	9.3
		Boys			
TS	179.2 (.838)	-2.03 (.244)	-.038 (.062)	.0301 (.0041)	10.4
TSC	178.9 (.838)	-1.36 (.244)	-.263 (.062)	.0234 (.0041)	10.3
FOA	183.5 (.710)	-.887 (.077)	-.126 (.016)	.0154 (.0017)	9.8
FSL (1000)	185.4 (.609)	-1.144(.112)	-.197 (.023)	.0188 (.0012)	11.2
FSL (GH:11)	184.2 (.474)	-1.276 (.102)	-.230 (.021)	.0210 (.0011)	10.4
`nlme`	185.5 (1.03)	-.855 (.082)	-.131 (.016)	.0155 (.0009)	9.9

TS=Two-Stage, TSC=Two-Stage Corrected, FOA=First-Order Approximation, FSL=Fixed Sample Likelihood (`callnlmeFSL`); the number in the parentheses for FSLindicates the sample size

Problems for Section 8.16

1*. Reproduce the results of Table 8.2: write your own R functions (for this purpose, modify functions `heightlog.nlme`, `callnlmeFSL`, and `nlmeFSL`). Create a similar table with matrix **D** estimates.

2*. Test the hypothesis that the only the adult height is subject-specific (random). Use three tests: Wald, likelihood ratio, and F. Do they concur?

3. Optimize function `nlmeFSL` by replacing the loop over SS with matrix multiplication.

8.17   Practical recommendations

Estimation of nonlinear statistical modes, with random effects particularly, may be a complex business. Indeed, even estimation of a LME model can be problematic when the covariance matrix of random effects becomes deficient during the log-likelihood maximization.

In estimating nonlinear models, we urge the reader to follow the principle *from simple to complex*. Start by estimating the model without random effects using standard nonlinear regression techniques. To see whether the model is adequate, fitting the average data may help, as we did in Section 8.3. Choice of the model is more important than choice of the estimation method, so the effort should be spent accordingly. A good nonlinear model should have a sound justification, requiring a detailed understanding of the modeling subject. Examples of choosing the right nonlinear model for tumor regrowth after cancer treatment may be found in Chapter

10. In fact, we spent more time on the model than on its estimation. Computation of the post-estimation model characteristics, such as maximum growth or inflection point (where the rate of growth is maximum), may be insightful.

Add one random effect at a time. It is a bad practice to start with the assumption that all parameters are subject-specific (random), even if you are using commercial software and fitting seems easy. Pay attention to the standard errors (SEs) of the estimated parameters and the magnitude of the variances of the random effects. If the random effect becomes irrelevant, the quality of the statistical models drops or the estimation procedure just fails. For statistical testing of the presence of the random effects, the results of Section 8.15 may be used.

For sound statistical inference, besides the estimate itself, one needs to have a satisfactory standard error. A major drawback of approximate methods of estimation, such as LB or LA, is that they usually underestimate the SE. For example, if the SE comes from the LME step, (8.30), it implicitly assumes that the random effects $\{\widehat{\boldsymbol{\tau}}_i\}$ are perfectly estimated and that the population-averaged and variance parameters are uncorrelated. To the contrary, FSL provides consistent SE assessment because it takes this correlation into account by inverting the joint Fisher information matrix.

8.18   Appendix: Proof of theorem on equivalence

The plan of the proof is as follows ($N \to \infty$ is assumed):

1. The LB and TS estimators are equivalent when $\min n_i \to \infty$ and σ^2 and $\mathbf{D}$ are fixed.

2. The TS estimator is consistent and normally distributed with the covariance matrix equal to the lower bound (8.14).

3. The LB and TS estimators produce consistent estimators of σ^2 and $\mathbf{D}$.

4. The TS estimator is equivalent to the MLE when $\min n_i \to \infty$ and $\mathbf{D}$ is substituted for by a consistent estimator.

The "mild" asymptotic conditions are: (a) the probability that the individual LS estimator for (8.15) exists is positive and bounded from below; (b) elements of matrices $\{\mathbf{A}_i\}$ are bounded and the limit matrix,

$$\lim_{N \to \infty} N^{-1} \sum_{i=1}^{N} \mathbf{A}_i' \mathbf{D}^{-1} \mathbf{A}_i = \mathbf{M},$$

is nonsingular, and (c) standard asymptotic assumptions for the ith nonlinear regression of (8.1), conditionally on $\mathbf{a}_i$, are fulfilled (e.g., Gallant, 1989 or Wu, 1981). The latter implies that the individual nonlinear least squares estimators $\mathbf{a}_i^o$ are consistent for $\mathbf{a}_i$, are asymptotically normally distributed, and are efficient when $n_i \to \infty$.

1. The asymptotic equivalence between LB and TS estimators follows from Section 8.7.2. Based on this result, we prove that the LB estimator is asymptotically equivalent to (8.76) with probability 1. Since $\mathbf{D}$ is fixed in the LB procedure, we have to consider only the penalized nonlinear least squares step:

$$\sum_{i=1}^{N} \left[n_i^{-1} \parallel \mathbf{y}_i - \mathbf{f}_i(\mathbf{A}_i \boldsymbol{\beta} + \mathbf{b}_i) \parallel^2 + \frac{1}{n_i} \mathbf{b}_i' \mathbf{D}^{-1} \mathbf{b}_i \right] \Rightarrow \min_{\boldsymbol{\beta}, \mathbf{b}_1, \ldots, \mathbf{b}_N}.$$

To apply (8.38), we show that there exists a constant A such that, with probability 1,

$$n_i^{-1} \parallel \mathbf{y}_i - \mathbf{f}_i(\mathbf{A}_i\boldsymbol{\beta} + \mathbf{b}_i) \parallel^2 \geq A > 0, \quad i = 1, ..., N \to \infty \qquad (8.94)$$

when $\min n_i \to \infty$. In fact, letting $\mathbf{p}_i = \mathbf{A}_i\boldsymbol{\beta} + \mathbf{b}_i$, conditionally on the random variables $\mathbf{a}_i$, we have

$$\lim_{n_i \to \infty} n_i^{-1} \parallel \mathbf{y}_i - \mathbf{f}_i(\mathbf{p}_i) \parallel^2 = \lim_{n_i \to \infty} n_i^{-1} \parallel \mathbf{y}_i - \mathbf{f}_i(\mathbf{a}_i) \parallel^2$$
$$+2 \lim_{n_i \to \infty} n_i^{-1} (\mathbf{y}_i - \mathbf{f}_i(\mathbf{a}_i))'(\mathbf{f}_i(\mathbf{a}_i) - \mathbf{f}_i(\mathbf{p})) + \lim_{n_i \to \infty} n_i^{-1} \parallel \mathbf{f}_i(\mathbf{a}_i) - \mathbf{f}_i(\mathbf{p}_i) \parallel^2 .$$

However, by standard arguments of nonlinear regression theory, conditionally on $\mathbf{a}_i$, with probability 1 uniformly for $i = 1, ..., N$, we have

$$\lim_{n_i \to \infty} n_i^{-1} \parallel \mathbf{y}_i - \mathbf{f}_i(\mathbf{a}_i) \parallel^2 = \sigma^2, \quad \lim_{n_i \to \infty} n_i^{-1}(\mathbf{y}_i - \mathbf{f}_i(\mathbf{a}_i)'(\mathbf{f}_i(\mathbf{a}_i) - \mathbf{f}_i(\mathbf{p}_i)) = 0,$$
$$\lim_{n_i \to \infty} n_i^{-1} \parallel \mathbf{f}_i(\mathbf{a}_i) - \mathbf{f}_i(\mathbf{p}_i) \parallel^2 \geq 0.$$

Therefore, in (8.94) we can set $A = \sigma^2$. Denoting $\delta = 1/n_i$ and applying (8.38), we prove that the LB estimator is asymptotically equivalent to (8.76) when $\min n_i \to \infty$.

Now we show that the TS estimator (8.22) is equivalent to (8.76). As mentioned above, from the standard theory of nonlinear regression, conditionally on $\mathbf{a}_i$, we have

$$\lim_{n_i \to \infty} \mathbf{a}_i^o = \mathbf{a}_i, \quad \sqrt{n_i}(\mathbf{a}_i^o - \mathbf{a}_i) \simeq \mathcal{N}(\mathbf{0}, \sigma^2 \mathbf{T}_i^{-1}), \qquad (8.95)$$

where

$$\mathbf{T}_i = \mathbf{E}_{\mathbf{x}_i} \left[\mathbf{R}_i(\mathbf{x}_i; \mathbf{a}_i) \mathbf{R}_i'(\mathbf{x}_i; \mathbf{a}_i) \big| \mathbf{a}_i \right], \quad \mathbf{R}_i(\mathbf{x}_i; \mathbf{a}_i) = \frac{\partial f(\mathbf{a}_i; \mathbf{x}_i)}{\partial \boldsymbol{\alpha}_i} \bigg|_{\boldsymbol{\alpha}_i = \mathbf{a}_i} .$$

Thus, $\mathbf{T}_i = O(n_i^{-1})$ and $\widehat{\mathbf{D}}_2 \to \mathbf{0}$, so for given σ^2 and $\mathbf{D}$, the TS estimator (8.22) is asymptotically equivalent to (8.76).

2. Starting from this point, we can deal only with the second-stage model (8.2), assuming that instead of observations $\mathbf{a}_i$ we have $\mathbf{a}_i^o$ with properties (8.95). Letting $\boldsymbol{\delta}_i = \mathbf{a}_i - \mathbf{a}_i^o$, we have $\sqrt{N}(\widehat{\boldsymbol{\beta}} - \boldsymbol{\beta}) = \mathbf{s}_N + \mathbf{u}_N$, where

$$\mathbf{s}_N = \left(N^{-1} \sum \mathbf{A}_i' \mathbf{D}^{-1} \mathbf{A}_i \right)^{-1} \left(N^{-1/2} \sum \mathbf{A}_i' \mathbf{D}^{-1} \mathbf{b}_i \right),$$
$$\mathbf{u}_N = \left(N^{-1} \sum \mathbf{A}_i' \mathbf{D}^{-1} \mathbf{A}_i \right)^{-1} \left(N^{-1/2} \sum \mathbf{A}_i' \mathbf{D}^{-1} \boldsymbol{\delta}_i \right).$$

Obviously, $\mathbf{s}_N \simeq \mathcal{N}(\mathbf{0}, \sigma^2 \mathbf{M}^{-1})$. Also, since $\text{cov}(\boldsymbol{\delta}_i) = O(1/n_i)$, we have $\mathbf{u}_N \to \mathbf{0}$ with probability 1. That proves that the estimator (8.76) is asymptotically normally distributed as $\sqrt{N}(\widehat{\boldsymbol{\beta}} - \boldsymbol{\beta}) \simeq \mathcal{N}(\mathbf{0}, \sigma^2 \mathbf{M}^{-1})$.

3. First, we prove that in (8.21) $\widehat{\mathbf{D}} \to \mathbf{D}$. It follows from part **1** that $\widehat{\mathbf{D}}_2 \to \mathbf{0}$, so we have to show that $\widehat{\mathbf{D}}_1 \to \mathbf{D}$. We decompose the matrix estimator into four parts:

$$\widehat{\mathbf{D}}_1 = \widehat{\mathbf{D}}_{11} + \widehat{\mathbf{D}}_{12} + \widehat{\mathbf{D}}_{12}' + \widehat{\mathbf{D}}_{22}, \qquad (8.96)$$

where

$$\widehat{\mathbf{D}}_{11} = N^{-1} \sum_i (\mathbf{a}_i^o - \mathbf{A}_i \boldsymbol{\beta}) (\mathbf{a}_i^o - \mathbf{A}_i \boldsymbol{\beta})',$$

$$\widehat{\mathbf{D}}_{12} = N^{-1} \sum_i (\mathbf{a}_i^o - \mathbf{A}_i \boldsymbol{\beta}) \left(\boldsymbol{\beta} - (\sum_j \mathbf{Z}_j' \mathbf{A}_j)^{-1} (\sum_j \mathbf{Z}_j' \widehat{\boldsymbol{\alpha}}_j^{LS}) \right)' \mathbf{A}_i',$$

$$\widehat{\mathbf{D}}_{22} = N^{-1} \sum_i \mathbf{A}_i \left(\boldsymbol{\beta} - (\sum_j \mathbf{Z}_j' \mathbf{A}_j)^{-1} (\sum_j \mathbf{Z}_j' \widehat{\boldsymbol{\alpha}}_j^{LS}) \right)$$
$$\times \left(\boldsymbol{\beta} - (\sum_j \mathbf{Z}_j' \mathbf{A}_j)^{-1} (\sum_j \mathbf{Z}_j' \widehat{\boldsymbol{\alpha}}_j^{LS}) \right)' \mathbf{A}_i'$$

and $i, j = 1, ..., N$. As follows from (8.95), when calculating the asymptotic limits of these matrices, we can replace $\mathbf{a}_i^o$ with $\mathbf{a}_i$, which implies immediately that $p \lim \widehat{\mathbf{D}}_{11} = \mathbf{D}$. Now we show that the other three components in (8.96) converge to zero in probability. Indeed, $\widehat{\mathbf{D}}_{12}$ is equivalent to

$$-N^{-1} \sum_i \mathbf{b}_i \mathbf{b}_i' \mathbf{Z}_i (\sum_j \mathbf{Z}_j' \mathbf{A}_j)^{-1} \mathbf{A}_i' - N^{-1} \sum_i \mathbf{b}_i (\sum_{j \neq i} \mathbf{b}_j' \mathbf{Z}_j) (\sum_j \mathbf{Z}_j' \mathbf{A}_j)^{-1} \mathbf{A}_i'. \quad (8.97)$$

But

$$E \left(N^{-1} \sum_i \mathbf{b}_i \mathbf{b}_i' \mathbf{Z}_i (\sum_j \mathbf{Z}_j' \mathbf{A}_j)^{-1} \mathbf{A}_i' \right) = N^{-1} \mathbf{D} \sum_i \mathbf{Z}_i (\sum_j \mathbf{Z}_j' \mathbf{A}_j)^{-1} \mathbf{A}_i' \to \mathbf{0}$$

because

$$\mathrm{tr} \left(\sum_i \mathbf{Z}_i (\sum_j \mathbf{Z}_j' \mathbf{A}_j)^{-1} \mathbf{A}_i' \right) = \sum_i \mathrm{tr} \left(\mathbf{Z}_i (\sum_j \mathbf{Z}_j' \mathbf{A}_j)^{-1} \mathbf{A}_i' \right)$$
$$= \mathrm{tr} \left(\sum_j (\mathbf{Z}_j' \mathbf{A}_j)^{-1} \sum_i (\mathbf{Z}_i' \mathbf{A}_i) \right) = m. \quad (8.98)$$

The second term in (8.97) has zero expectation because $\mathbf{b}_i$ and $\mathbf{b}_j$ are independent for $i \neq j$. Let $\mathbf{c}$ be any unit vector $\mathbf{c}'\mathbf{c} = 1$. We will prove that

$$\mathrm{var} \left(\frac{1}{N} \mathbf{c}' \sum_i \mathbf{b}_i \mathbf{b}_i' \mathbf{Z}_i (\sum_j \mathbf{Z}_j' \mathbf{A}_j)^{-1} \mathbf{A}_i' \mathbf{c} \right) \to \mathbf{0}. \quad (8.99)$$

Since $\mathrm{var}(\mathbf{u}'\mathbf{A}\mathbf{u}) = 2\mathrm{tr}(\mathbf{A}\mathbf{D})^2$ for $\mathbf{u} \sim \mathcal{N}(\mathbf{0}, \mathbf{D})$ we find that the left-hand side of (8.99) is bounded from above,

$$\frac{2\sigma^4}{N^2} \sum_i \left(\mathbf{c}' \mathbf{D} \mathbf{Z}_i (\sum_j \mathbf{Z}_j' \mathbf{A}_j)^{-1} \mathbf{A}_i' \mathbf{c} \right)^2 \leq \frac{2\sigma^4}{N^2} \left(\mathbf{c}' \mathbf{D} \sum_i \mathbf{Z}_i (\sum_j \mathbf{Z}_j' \mathbf{A}_j)^{-1} \mathbf{A}_i' \mathbf{c} \right)^2,$$

which approaches null when $N \to \infty$, as follows from (8.98). This implies that the second term in (8.97) vanishes when $\min n_i \to \infty$. Similarly, we prove that $p \lim \widehat{\mathbf{D}}_{22} = \mathbf{0}$. This all proves that $\widehat{\mathbf{D}}$ is a consistent estimator of $\mathbf{D}$ when $\min n_i \to \infty$.

Now we shall show that the Lindstrom and Bates procedure, based on linear mixed effects, provides a consistent estimator of $\mathbf{D}$, too. As follows from part **1**,

$\mathbf{A}_i\widehat{\boldsymbol{\beta}} + \widehat{\mathbf{b}}_i \sim \mathbf{a}_i^o \sim \mathbf{a}_i$, where $\sim$ indicates asymptotic equivalence with probability 1. To prove that the linear mixed effects model provides a consistent estimator for σ^2 and $\mathbf{D}$ based on (8.30), it suffices to show that $E(\mathbf{w}_i) = \mathbf{R}_i\mathbf{A}_i\boldsymbol{\beta}$ and $\mathrm{cov}(\mathbf{w}_i) = \sigma^2(\mathbf{I} + \mathbf{R}_i\mathbf{D}\mathbf{R}_i')$ when $\mathbf{A}_i\widehat{\boldsymbol{\beta}} + \widehat{\mathbf{b}}_i = \mathbf{a}_i$ and $\widehat{\boldsymbol{\beta}} = \boldsymbol{\beta}$. Indeed, for a linear mixed effects model, $\mathbf{w}_i = \mathbf{y}_i - \mathbf{f}_i(\mathbf{a}_i) + \mathbf{R}_i(\mathbf{a}_i - \mathbf{A}_i\boldsymbol{\beta}_i) + \mathbf{R}_i\mathbf{A}_i\boldsymbol{\beta}$, and we have

$$E(\mathbf{w}_i) = E\left(E(\mathbf{y}_i - \mathbf{f}_i(\mathbf{a}_i) + \mathbf{R}_i(\mathbf{a}_i - \mathbf{A}_i\boldsymbol{\beta}_i) + \mathbf{R}_i\mathbf{A}_i\boldsymbol{\beta}|\mathbf{a}_i)\right) = \mathbf{R}_i\mathbf{A}_i\boldsymbol{\beta},$$

$$\mathrm{cov}(\mathbf{w}_i) = E\mathrm{cov}(\mathbf{w}_i|\mathbf{a}_i) + \mathrm{cov}(E(\mathbf{w}_i|\mathbf{a}_i)) = E\mathrm{cov}(\mathbf{w}_i|\mathbf{a}_i) = \sigma^2(\mathbf{I} + \mathbf{R}_i\mathbf{D}\mathbf{R}_i'),$$

as we set out to prove.

4. As follows from parts **1** to **3**, when $N \to \infty$ and $\min n_i \to \infty$, the NLME model is asymptotically equivalent to the linear model, $\mathbf{a}_i \sim \mathcal{N}(\mathbf{A}_i\boldsymbol{\beta}, \sigma^2\mathbf{D})$. But in the linear model, the information matrix for $\boldsymbol{\beta}$ and $(\sigma^2, \mathbf{D})$ is block diagonal; consequently, pseudo MLE is equivalent to the full MLE, Section 2.11 and Appendix 13.1.3. In other words, one obtains an asymptotically efficient estimator for $\boldsymbol{\beta}$ by substituting a consistent estimator for $\mathbf{D}$ in the generalized least squares estimator. This implies that the LB and TS estimators are equivalent to (8.76) when $\mathbf{D}$ is replaced with its consistent estimator, or more precisely,

$$\sqrt{N}(\widehat{\boldsymbol{\beta}}^{LB} - \boldsymbol{\beta}) \sim \mathcal{N}\left(\mathbf{0}, \sigma^2\mathbf{M}^{-1}\right), \quad \sqrt{N}(\widehat{\boldsymbol{\beta}}^{TS} - \boldsymbol{\beta}) \sim \mathcal{N}\left(\mathbf{0}, \sigma^2\mathbf{M}^{-1}\right).$$

Finally, this means that the covariances of the LB and TS estimators attain the lower bound (8.14). Therefore, all the estimators are asymptotically equivalent, and the theorem is proved.

8.19   Summary points

- The nonlinear mixed effects (NLME) model is a straightforward generalization of LME and the linear growth curve model and is written in a hierarchical fashion. The first-stage model consists of a set of individual or subject-specific nonlinear regressions with random parameters. The second-stage model is a linear model with population parameters to estimate. The difference between the NLME and the marginal mixed model is that in the former model the expected value of the dependent variable is not a closed-form function of population-averaged parameters, so an integration problem emerges. The NLME model can be viewed as a generalization of GLMM since the latter can be expressed in generic form as $f_i(\boldsymbol{\beta}) = \mu(\boldsymbol{\beta}'\mathbf{x}_i)$, where μ is an inverse link function.

- Maximum likelihood estimation of the NLME model involves, generally, a multidimensional integral because the subject-specific parameters are unobservable and therefore must be integrated out. To avoid the integration problem several approximation methods for the NLME model estimation have been proposed.

- The approximation methods for estimation of the NLME model can be divided into two groups. In the Two-Stage (TS) methods, subject-specific parameters are estimated by nonlinear least squares individually from the first-stage model and are then treated as observations for the second-stage model. The TS estimator works well when the within-cluster variance (σ^2) is relatively small and the number of observations per cluster is large enough to fit the individual models well. The TS method allows bias correction using the nonlinear regression technique suggested by Box (1971). This bias correction requires second-order derivatives of the nonlinear regression model.

- In the second group, the NLME function is approximated by a linear function, so the model is reduced to a nonlinear marginal mixed model. If the function is approximated at zero random effects, we obtain the FOA, which can be treated further as the nonlinear marginal mixed model with varied matrix of random effects, Section 6.2. According to Laplace, a better approximation can be derived if the function is approximated at an estimate of the random effects from the PLS.

- Penalized least squares naturally emerges to estimate population-averaged and subject-specific (random effects) parameters via an approximation to the likelihood, assuming that the variance parameters are known. The penalty term is the reciprocal of the scaled covariance matrix of the random effect: if the random effects have large variances, the penalty is small; otherwise, it is large. Thus, a satisfactory estimation of variance parameters is crucial.

- Laplace approximation of the integral involves second derivatives. Since the expectation of the term with the second derivatives is zero, one can ignore it and we come to the penalized quasi-likelihood, as we did for GLMM. It turns out that LB = PQL, so the Lindstrom–Bates and penalized quasi-likelihood approaches are equivalent.

- When the number of clusters (N) and the number of observations per cluster (n_i) goes to infinity, the TS, LB/PQL and ML methods of NLME model estimation become equivalent. Namely, they converge to the same normal distribution with the covariance matrix as the lower limit. Indeed, as n_i increases, the contribution of the penalty term in PLS vanishes, so PLS collapses to individual nonlinear least squares. FOA has a systematic bias even when $n_i \to \infty$.

- Unfortunately, there is a price for approximate methods of estimation: to yield consistent estimates, they require not only a large number of subjects/clusters but also a large number of observations per cluster. Maximum Likelihood (ML) requires only a large number of clusters; consistent estimates can be derived even with a small number of observations per cluster.

- The MLE loses it consistency if the distribution of the random effect is misspecified. However, it regains its asymptotic properties when the number of observations per cluster goes to infinity along with the number of clusters.

- The difficulties with maximum likelihood estimation are sometimes overstated. In practice, it is quite rare to need more than five random effects (producing a five-dimensional integral). The advantages of ML are that (a) it does not require a large number of observations per cluster to obtain consistent estimates, and (b) it produces a joint covariance matrix of population-averaged and variance parameters, and consequently the correct standard error for all estimates.

- The Fixed Simulated Likelihood (FSL) approach is a convenient way to combine Gauss–Hermite quadrature and Monte Carlo under one umbrella. One need only provide sample values and the weights to replace the multidimensional integral by a weighted sum. Several samples may be tried to ensure that the resulting estimates are close.

9

Diagnostics and Influence Analysis

9.1 Introduction

Influence analysis and influential observations diagnostics is a necessary part of comprehensive statistical analysis. The statistical analyst must be sure that there are no influential observations, irrelevant to the study, that affect the major statistical inference. Many articles and books address the problem of influential observations and outliers. The interested reader is referred to books by Belsley et al. (1980), Cook and Weisberg (1982), and Neter et al. (1990), and to seminal papers by Pregibon (1981), Chatterjee and Hadi (1986), and Cook (1977, 1986). Two principal types of influence analyses for linear models are developed. In the first, the calculation of leverage and standardized residuals plays a central role. The second is based on the influence of case deletion and is called *case deletion diagnostics*.

In this book influence is understood to be the sensitivity of a statistic to a small (infinitesimal) perturbation of data or model, so that influence analysis might equivalently be called sensitivity analysis. In fact, we make use of an old definition of influence formulated by Cook and Weisberg (1982, p. 101): "The basic idea in influence analysis is quite simple. We introduce a small perturbation in the problem formulation, and monitor how the perturbation changes the outcome of the analysis." To distinguish this type of influence analysis, we call it infinitesimal (infinitely small), after Pregibon (1981), who introduced this influence analysis. Since we are interested in infinitesimal change, the *derivative* naturally emerges as the measure of influence. The idea of measuring the sensitivity of a statistic by its derivative is not new. Hodges and Moore (1972) were probably the first to suggest measuring the impact of a small change in the individual observation of the explanatory variable on the Ordinary Least Squares (OLS) estimate via derivative (following our definition, this is an example of infinitesimal data influence). The main advantage of infinitesimal influence analysis is that it is easily applied to complex statistical models such as nonlinear regression and linear and nonlinear mixed effects models. It only requires taking a derivative.

Two types of infinitesimal influence analysis can be considered: (a) the influence of small change in individual observations, and (b) the influence of model assumptions. The first analysis is referred to as infinitesimal *data* influence, and the second analysis is referred to as infinitesimal *model* influence. Hampel (1974) developed the concept of *influence function* and demonstrated its application to robust statistics. Cook (1986) applied this concept to measure the model sensitivity as the maximum curvature of log-likelihood displacement, and called it *local influence.* (In our definition, this is an infinitesimal model influence.) In this chapter we combine the two approaches under one umbrella of infinitesimal influence and show how this approach works for many statistical characteristics in a variety of settings. For instance, as shown later, the Cook and Hodges–Moore approaches are equivalent to the linear regression model. In fact, Cook's local influence is a special case of our approach because we can take the likelihood displacement as the characteristic of the infinitesimal analysis.

Infinitesimal influence analysis has several advantages:

- It has an intuitively appealing interpretation—the partial derivative indicates what is affected by what and with what magnitude.

- It is easy to compute; the analysis is based on the current estimate and does not involve additional computation rather than taking a derivative.

- It allows broad graphical support which is very helpful for observation diagnostics.

- It is a general tool and can be applied to any statistic as the influence of data or model assumption perturbation.

The goal of this chapter is to introduce infinitesimal influence analysis and illustrate it by several examples of linear, nonlinear, and logistic regression models. We start with influence analysis for the linear regression model and its relationship on local influence. Then we consider influence analysis for nonlinear regression and binary models (we study particularly the sensitivity of misclassification in logistic regression). Next, we apply the idea of model influence to correlated data and measurement error in the binary model. At the end of the chapter, infinitesimal influence analysis is applied to mixed models.

9.2   Influence analysis for linear regression

Traditional influence analysis for the linear regression model is concentrated around two major concepts:

- Leverage, as the diagonal element of the hat matrix, and standardized residuals.

- Case deletion diagnostics and Cook's distance.

Now we provide a quick overview of these concepts. Comprehensive coverage of the topic may be found in books by Belsley et al. (1980), Cook and Weisberg (1982), and Chatterjee and Hadi (1986).

The ordinary linear regression model is written in the form

$$y_i = \boldsymbol{\beta}'\mathbf{x}_i + \varepsilon_i, \qquad i = 1, ..., n, \tag{9.1}$$

where $\mathbf{x}_i$ is the $m \times 1$ vector of explanatory or independent variables (covariates) and $\boldsymbol{\beta}$ is the $m \times 1$ parameter of interest. It is assumed that $\varepsilon_1, ..., \varepsilon_n$ are independent and identically distributed (iid) with zero mean and constant variance σ^2. The Ordinary Least Squares (OLS) estimator of $\boldsymbol{\beta}$ is

$$\widehat{\boldsymbol{\beta}} = (\mathbf{X}'\mathbf{X})^{-1}\mathbf{X}'\mathbf{y} = \left(\sum_{i=1}^{n}\mathbf{x}_i\mathbf{x}_i'\right)^{-1}\left(\sum_{i=1}^{n}\mathbf{x}_i y_i\right), \tag{9.2}$$

where the ith row of matrix $\mathbf{X}$ is $\mathbf{x}_i'$, and it is assumed that $\mathbf{X}$ has full rank (matrix $\mathbf{X}'\mathbf{X}$ is nonsingular). The goal of influence analysis is to detect influential observation(s). Such an observation might be an outlier, an incorrectly recorded result, or just an observation irrelevant to the study. In any event, an influential observation deserves a close look in terms of its correctness and adequateness in light of the model postulated. The core of influence analysis is the measure/characteristic of influence. Usually, it is not difficult to detect an influential observation(s) *after* a definition or measure of influence is given. Importantly, traditional influence analysis detects influential *cases,* which consist of observations of the dependent and explanatory variables, $(y_i, \mathbf{x}_i')$. Later, we shall learn how to distinguish the influence with respect to dependent and explanatory variables by the means of infinitesimal influence analysis.

The first step in finding an influential case is to compute the OLS residuals, $r_i = y_i - \widehat{y}_i$, where $\widehat{y}_i$ is the OLS predicted value, $\widehat{y}_i = \widehat{\boldsymbol{\beta}}'\mathbf{x}_i$. However, a large residual does not always point to an influential case. The traditional characteristic of influence is *leverage,* the diagonal element of the hat matrix $\mathbf{H} = \mathbf{X}(\mathbf{X}'\mathbf{X})^{-1}\mathbf{X}'$. The ith diagonal element of this matrix is $p_i = \mathbf{x}_i'(\mathbf{X}'\mathbf{X})^{-1}\mathbf{x}_i$. It is easy to prove that $0 \leq p_i < 1$ and $\sum_{i=1}^{n} p_i = m$. Indeed, $p_i \geq 0$ because matrix $(\mathbf{X}'\mathbf{X})^{-1}$ is positive definite. The latter identity follows from elementary matrix algebra,

$$\sum_{i=1}^{n}p_i = \sum_{i=1}^{n}\mathbf{x}_i'(\mathbf{X}'\mathbf{X})^{-1}\mathbf{x}_i = \sum_{i=1}^{n}\text{tr}\left[\mathbf{x}_i'(\mathbf{X}'\mathbf{X})^{-1}\mathbf{x}_i\right] = \sum_{i=1}^{n}\text{tr}\left[(\mathbf{X}'\mathbf{X})^{-1}\mathbf{x}_i\mathbf{x}_i'\right]$$

$$= \text{tr}\sum_{i=1}^{n}\left[(\mathbf{X}'\mathbf{X})^{-1}\mathbf{x}_i\mathbf{x}_i'\right] = \text{tr}\left[(\mathbf{X}'\mathbf{X})^{-1}\sum_{i=1}^{n}\mathbf{x}_i\mathbf{x}_i'\right] = \text{tr}\left[(\mathbf{X}'\mathbf{X})^{-1}(\mathbf{X}'\mathbf{X})\right]$$

$$= \text{tr}(\mathbf{I}) = m.$$

Cases with high leverage are called influential. Characteristically, in the traditional approach there are no further details as to *what* is influential. We shall learn later that the infinitesimal approach provides such an interpretation; leverage reflects how the predicted value is influential in the observation of the dependent variable (Rao and Toutenburg, 1999).

A better indicator of influential cases, in terms of their departure from the fitted model, is the standardized residual, $r_i/(s\sqrt{1-p_i})$, where $s^2 = \sum r_i^2/(n-m)$ is the estimated variance.

Another measure of influence comes from the idea of case deletion. A case is called influential if the OLS estimate changes significantly after deleting this case from the data. Fortunately, it is not necessary to recalculate the regression after case deletion. Beckman and Trussel (1974) and Miller (1974) proved that if $\widehat{\boldsymbol{\beta}}_{(i)}$ denotes the OLS estimate after the ith case was deleted (leave-one-out), it may be derived as

$$\widehat{\boldsymbol{\beta}}_{(i)} = \widehat{\boldsymbol{\beta}} - \frac{r_i}{1-p_i}(\mathbf{X}'\mathbf{X})^{-1}\mathbf{x}_i. \tag{9.3}$$

Proof. The following matrix formula is used:

$$(\mathbf{A} - \mathbf{bb}')^{-1} = \mathbf{A}^{-1} + \frac{\mathbf{A}^{-1}\mathbf{bb}'\mathbf{A}^{-1}}{1 - \mathbf{b}'\mathbf{A}^{-1}\mathbf{b}},$$

where $\mathbf{A}$ is a positive definite matrix and $\mathbf{b}$ is a vector column of appropriate length. If $\mathbf{X}_{(i)}$ denotes a matrix $\mathbf{X}$ with the ith row deleted, applying this formula, one obtains

$$
\begin{aligned}
(\mathbf{X}'_{(i)}\mathbf{X}_{(i)})^{-1}\mathbf{x}_i &= (\mathbf{X}'\mathbf{X} - \mathbf{x}_i\mathbf{x}_i')^{-1}\mathbf{x}_i \\
&= (\mathbf{X}'\mathbf{X})^{-1}\mathbf{x}_i + (\mathbf{X}'\mathbf{X})^{-1}\frac{\mathbf{x}_i\mathbf{x}_i'}{1 - \mathbf{x}_i'(\mathbf{X}'\mathbf{X})^{-1}\mathbf{x}_i}(\mathbf{X}'\mathbf{X})^{-1}\mathbf{x}_i \\
&= \left(1 + \frac{\mathbf{x}_i'(\mathbf{X}'\mathbf{X})^{-1}\mathbf{x}_i}{1 - \mathbf{x}_i'(\mathbf{X}'\mathbf{X})^{-1}\mathbf{x}_i}\right)(\mathbf{X}'\mathbf{X})^{-1}\mathbf{x}_i = \frac{1}{1-p_i}(\mathbf{X}'\mathbf{X})^{-1}\mathbf{x}_i.
\end{aligned}
\tag{9.4}
$$

Therefore, using formulas (9.3) and (9.4), we obtain

$$
\begin{aligned}
\widehat{\boldsymbol{\beta}}_{(i)} &= (\mathbf{X}'_{(i)}\mathbf{X}_{(i)})^{-1}\mathbf{X}'_{(i)}\mathbf{y}_{(i)} = (\mathbf{X}'_{(i)}\mathbf{X}_{(i)})^{-1}(\mathbf{X}'\mathbf{y} - \mathbf{x}_iy_i) \\
&= (\mathbf{X}'_{(i)}\mathbf{X}_{(i)})^{-1}\mathbf{X}'\mathbf{y} - (\mathbf{X}'_{(i)}\mathbf{X}_{(i)})^{-1}\mathbf{x}_iy_i \\
&= \widehat{\boldsymbol{\beta}} + (\mathbf{X}'\mathbf{X})^{-1}\frac{\mathbf{x}_i\mathbf{x}_i'}{1 - \mathbf{x}_i'(\mathbf{X}'\mathbf{X})^{-1}\mathbf{x}_i}\widehat{\boldsymbol{\beta}} - \frac{1}{1-p_i}(\mathbf{X}'\mathbf{X})^{-1}\mathbf{x}_iy_i \\
&= \widehat{\boldsymbol{\beta}} - \frac{y_i - \mathbf{x}_i'\widehat{\boldsymbol{\beta}}}{1-p_i}(\mathbf{X}'\mathbf{X})^{-1}\mathbf{x}_i = \widehat{\boldsymbol{\beta}} - \frac{r_i}{1-p_i}(\mathbf{X}'\mathbf{X})^{-1}\mathbf{x}.
\end{aligned}
$$

∎

An alternative way to assess the influence of the ith case is to calculate the difference in the predicted values after case deletion. As follows from linear regression theory, the $(1-\alpha)$th confidence ellipsoid is defined as

$$E = \{\boldsymbol{\beta} : (\boldsymbol{\beta}-\widehat{\boldsymbol{\beta}})'\mathbf{X}'\mathbf{X}(\boldsymbol{\beta}-\widehat{\boldsymbol{\beta}}) \le ms^2 F_{1-\alpha}\}, \tag{9.5}$$

where $F_{1-\alpha}$ is the $(1-\alpha)$th quantile of the F-distribution with $(m, n-m)$ degrees of freedom. Thus, according to Cook (1977), the ith case is influential if

$$D_i = \frac{1}{ms^2}(\widehat{\boldsymbol{\beta}}_{(i)}-\widehat{\boldsymbol{\beta}})'\mathbf{X}'\mathbf{X}(\widehat{\boldsymbol{\beta}}_{(i)}-\widehat{\boldsymbol{\beta}}) > F_{1-\alpha}. \tag{9.6}$$

The quantity D_i is called Cook's distance. Equivalently, it may be represented via the $n \times 1$ predicted vector $\widehat{\mathbf{y}}_{(i)}$ after the ith case was deleted, $D_i = \| \widehat{\mathbf{y}} - \widehat{\mathbf{y}}_{(i)} \|^2 / (ms^2)$. With the implication of formula (4.97), it is possible to express D_i via complete data:

$$D_i = \frac{r_i^2}{ms^2} \frac{p_i}{(1 - p_i)^2}. \tag{9.7}$$

This influence measure is computed in the statistical package SAS (procedure dfbeta). There are some other measures of influence for linear regression. The interested reader is referred to the literature cited above; a concise discussion of the topic appears in the books by Rao and Toutenburg (1999).

Problems for Section 9.2

1. Derive formula $\widehat{\beta}_{(i)}$ for a simple average model, $y_i = \beta + \varepsilon_i$. Express the leave-one-out analysis in terms of $y_{\min}$ and $y_{\max}$.

2. Is it true that the average of $\widehat{\beta}_{(i)}$ is the OLS estimate? When is it true?

3. Derive Cook's distance formula (9.7).

4*. Investigate the ability of Cook's distance measure to identify an outlier via simulations. Simulate n observations using the linear regression model $y_i = \alpha + \beta x_i + \varepsilon_i$. Then simulate an outlier as the $(n + 1)$th observation using the model $y_{n+1} = \alpha + \beta_* x_{n+1} + \varepsilon_{n+1}$, where $\beta_* \neq \beta$, and add it to the sample. Count the proportion of cases when $\max D_i$ corresponds to the last observation. Display the results as a function of $|\beta - \beta_*|$. Another way to simulate an outlier is to use $\text{var}(\varepsilon_{n+1}) > \sigma^2$.

9.3   The idea of infinitesimal influence

As mentioned in the Introduction, we distinguish two types of influences: the influence of an individual observation (data influence) and the influence of the underlying assumptions (model influence). This distinction is quite ambiguous, and sometimes we treat model perturbation via data influence, e.g., misclassification of the binary data. See Sections 9.4.3 and 9.6.4 for details.

The aim of this section is to show how the idea of using the derivative as the measure of infinitesimal influence works for many statistics in many statistical models and settings. At the end of this chapter we apply this analysis to linear and nonlinear mixed effects models. For brevity, infinitesimal influence is referred to as I-influence.

9.3.1   Data influence

Let $\mathbf{D}$ be a data vector comprised of individual observations of dependent and independent variables and $\mathbf{t} = \mathbf{t}(\mathbf{D})$ be any statistic or characteristic of interest. For instance, $\mathbf{t}$ might be an estimate itself, the vector of predicted values, a test statistic, etc. I-influence analysis suggests a measure of how a slight perturbation in an observation affects the statistic. Thus, if D_i is the ith element of the data, the change ΔD leads to a change in the statistic, $\mathbf{t}(\mathbf{D} + \Delta D \mathbf{e}_i) - \mathbf{t}(\mathbf{D})$, where $\mathbf{e}_i$ is the Kronecker vector, consisting of zeros except for the ith element, which is 1. Then the *infinitesimal* change in statistic $\mathbf{t}$ due to the data perturbation can be defined as

$$\lim_{\Delta D \to 0} \frac{\mathbf{t}(\mathbf{D} + \Delta D \mathbf{e}_i) - \mathbf{t}(\mathbf{D})}{\Delta D}. \tag{9.8}$$

Observations with high values of limit (9.8) are called *influential*. The reader has probably already realized that the quantity (9.8) is just the partial derivative of $\mathbf{t}$ with respect to D_i, namely,

$$\frac{\partial \mathbf{t}(\mathbf{D})}{\partial D_i}. \tag{9.9}$$

The influence analysis based on the derivative (9.9) is referred to as *infinitesimal data influence analysis*. The kth element of vector (9.9) indicates how a small perturbation in the ith element of data affects the kth element of the statistic $\mathbf{t}$. When statistic $\mathbf{t}$ does not admit a closed-form solution, (9.9) is computed as the derivative of the implicit function. Importantly, the partial derivative is evaluated at the current data, so no reestimation is required.

9.3.2   Model influence

Let $l(\boldsymbol{\theta})$ be the log-likelihood of the postulated model subject to influence analysis. We nest this model into a more general model that is dependent on an additional parameter $\boldsymbol{\omega}$; we shall call it the *parent model*. The log-likelihood of the parent model is denoted as $l(\boldsymbol{\theta} \mid \boldsymbol{\omega})$. Mathematically, the nesting property, without loss of generality, can be written as $l(\boldsymbol{\theta} \mid \boldsymbol{\omega} = \mathbf{0}) = l(\boldsymbol{\theta})$, which means that the postulated model is just a specific case of the parent model at $\boldsymbol{\omega} = \mathbf{0}$. Let $\mathbf{t}(\boldsymbol{\omega})$ be any statistic or characteristic of interest as a function of $\boldsymbol{\omega}$, e.g., the Maximum Likelihood Estimate (MLE), which maximizes the log-likelihood $l(\boldsymbol{\theta} \mid \boldsymbol{\omega})$ assuming that $\boldsymbol{\omega}$ is known. Then the influence of $\mathbf{t}$ with respect to a possible departure from the postulated model is measured as

$$\left. \frac{\partial \mathbf{t}}{\partial \boldsymbol{\omega}} \right|_{\boldsymbol{\omega}=0}. \tag{9.10}$$

Influence analysis based on the derivative (9.10) is called *infinitesimal model influence analysis*. It is worth mentioning that analogously to data influence, we do not need to re-estimate the postulated model; all calculations of (9.10) are carried out at the current estimate.

The difference between this and Cook's local influence is that he took the likelihood displacement, the difference of the log-likelihood function, as the measure of the model departure. In contrast, in our approach the model departure is expressed in terms of the characteristic of interest, $\mathbf{t}$. Consequently, (9.10) has a clearer interpretation. The two analyses are closely related. For instance, as we show in Section 9.4.2, the influence of an individual observation of the explanatory variable on the OLS coefficient in a linear model based on Cook's local influence approach is equivalent to the I-influence based on the partial derivative as obtained by Hodges and Moore (1972). Model influence can be viewed as the analysis of model misspecification.

We make a few comments on how to calculate (9.9) or (9.10) when $\mathbf{t}$ does not admit a closed-form solution. For example, we illustrate how to calculate (9.10) when $\mathbf{t}$ is the MLE. By definition, $\mathbf{t}$ is the solution to the score equation $\partial l(\boldsymbol{\theta} \mid \boldsymbol{\omega})/\partial\boldsymbol{\theta} = \mathbf{0}$

and the needed derivative, as follows from the formula for the derivative of an implicit function, is given as

$$
\frac{\partial \mathbf{t}}{\partial \boldsymbol{\omega}}\bigg|_{\boldsymbol{\omega}=0} = \left(-\frac{\partial^2 l(\mathbf{t} \mid \boldsymbol{\omega})}{\partial \mathbf{t}^2}\bigg|_{\boldsymbol{\omega}=0} \right)^{-1} \left(\frac{\partial^2 l(\mathbf{t} \mid \boldsymbol{\omega})}{\partial \mathbf{t} \partial \boldsymbol{\omega}}\bigg|_{\boldsymbol{\omega}=0} \right). \tag{9.11}
$$

It is interesting to note that the inverse matrix is the asymptotic covariance of the MLE, so that (9.11) can be rewritten as

$$
\frac{\partial \mathbf{t}}{\partial \boldsymbol{\omega}}\bigg|_{\boldsymbol{\omega}=0} = \mathrm{cov}(\mathbf{t}) \left(\frac{\partial^2 l(\mathbf{t} \mid \boldsymbol{\omega})}{\partial \mathbf{t} \partial \boldsymbol{\omega}}\bigg|_{\boldsymbol{\omega}=0} \right).
$$

As a general result, we find that a poorly estimated parameter vector is more likely to be sensitive to the model perturbation because then the covariance matrix is large.

Obviously, if in I-influence analysis we take $\mathbf{t}$ to be the likelihood displacement, we come to Cook's local influence approach. Therefore, the I-influence is a more general approach and covers local influence as a special case.

Problems for Section 9.3

1^*. The effect of the quadratic term in linear regression is investigated via the model influence. Using the expression for $\partial \mathbf{t}/\partial \boldsymbol{\omega}$, investigate the dependence of the OLS estimate of the slope coefficient β on the quadratic term coefficient γ in the linear regression $y_i = \alpha + \beta x_i + \gamma x_i^2 + \varepsilon_i$.

9.4   Linear regression model

I-influence analysis for linear regression model (9.1) is well developed, although it has not been considered on a systematic basis. The aim of this section is to review relevant formulas and illustrate the approach graphically for several examples. Infinitesimal influence analyses for nonlinear regression and binary data are developed in Section 9.5 and Section 9.6.

In this section, an ordinary linear regression model in the form (9.1) is considered. To be specific, index i is referred to as the ith individual. Since $\widehat{\mathbf{y}} = \mathbf{Hy}$ and $\partial \widehat{y}_i/\partial y_i = p_i$, we infer that from the I-influence point of view, leverage measures the influence of observation y_i on the predicted value, $\widehat{y}_i$. Although leverage is an important characteristic of influence analysis, one should remember that it measures the influence of the individual observation of the dependent variable on the predicted value for the same individual. However, we argue that the estimate itself is of interest, not the predicted value, unless the only purpose of the model is to predict the ith individual. Therefore, the question we pose is: How is the OLS estimate affected by an individual observation of the dependent or explanatory variable? Thus, unlike traditional influence analysis, we distinguish the influence of the dependent and independent variables. The influence with respect to the *dependent* variable is called the *Y-influence*, and the influence with respect to the *explanatory* variable is called the *X-influence*. These types of influence reveal the cause of the influence—the dependent or independent variable—and which independent variable

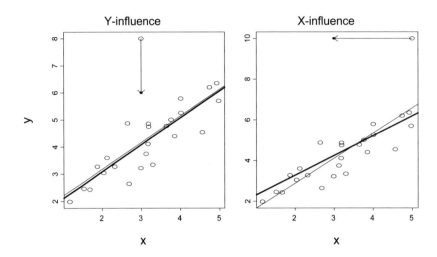

FIGURE 9.1. Y- and X-influences. Original (solid) and perturbed regression line (bold) after an individual observation changed (circle on the top). Left: Y-influence, the *dependent* variable changes. Right: X-influence, the *explanatory* variable changes. The same magnitude of perturbation in y and x leads to different changes in the regression slope. Apparently, for this example the slope is more influenced by a change in the explanatory variable.

is most influential. The difference between these two types of influences is illustrated in Figure 9.1. For the Y-influence we change an observation of the dependent variable and seek how the regression line changes (the empty circle moves to a filled one). In particular, for this example the slope does not change much and the major change is in the intercept term. On the contrary, for X-influence we seek how a change of an explanatory observation changes the regression line. For this example we conclude that the Y-influence is less significant than the X-influence because in the latter case the slope changes more significantly.

9.4.1 Influence of the dependent variable

The I-influence of the ith observation of the dependent variable on the OLS estimate is measured as the m-dimensional derivative vector,

$$\frac{\partial \widehat{\boldsymbol{\beta}}}{\partial y_i} = (\mathbf{X}'\mathbf{X})^{-1}\mathbf{x}_i, \qquad i = 1, ..., n. \tag{9.12}$$

The kth element of vector (9.12) is interpreted as the rate of change in the estimate of the kth regression coefficient due to a small change in y_i. High absolute values of the derivative are associated with influential observations of y. We shall learn later that vector $(\mathbf{X}'\mathbf{X})^{-1}\mathbf{x}_i$ is an important quantity of the influence analysis. It may be large when two conditions hold: (a) the length of $\mathbf{x}_i$ is relatively large, i.e., $\mathbf{x}_i$ lies outside the bulk of data $\{\mathbf{x}_i\}$; (b) $\mathbf{x}_i$ lies in the direction where the scatter plot is squeezed rather than stretched out. Thus, (9.12) reflects outstanding observations $\mathbf{x}_i$ and multicollinearity as well (Cook and Weisberg, 1982, p. 13).

9.4.2 Influence of the continuous explanatory variable

We revive the idea of measuring the influence of individual observations of explanatory variable x_{ik} on the OLS estimate via a derivative, as suggested by Hodges and Moore (1972). Thus, the question we pose is: How is the OLS estimate affected by a small perturbation in the ith observation of the kth covariate, x_{ik}? To make the infinitesimal approach work, we assume here that x_{ik} is continuous (in the next subsection, an approach is developed for the binary explanatory variable). Following the line of the I-influence, the sensitivity of $\widehat{\boldsymbol{\beta}}$ to small change in x_{ik} is measured via a partial derivative:

$$\frac{\partial \widehat{\boldsymbol{\beta}}}{\partial x_{ik}}, \qquad 1 \le i \le n, \ 1 \le k \le m. \tag{9.13}$$

Thus, the jth element of this vector is interpreted as the rate of departure from the jth OLS coefficient under a small perturbation in the ith case of the kth covariate. To derive the expression for (9.13), we write

$$
\begin{aligned}
&\frac{\partial}{\partial x_{ik}} \left(\sum \mathbf{x}_i \mathbf{x}_i' \right)^{-1} \left(\sum \mathbf{x}_i y_i \right) \\
&= -(\mathbf{X}'\mathbf{X})^{-1} \left(\frac{\partial}{\partial x_{ik}} \sum \mathbf{x}_i \mathbf{x}_i' \right) \widehat{\boldsymbol{\beta}} + (\mathbf{X}'\mathbf{X})^{-1} \left(\frac{\partial}{\partial x_{ik}} \sum \mathbf{x}_i y_i \right) \\
&= -(\mathbf{X}'\mathbf{X})^{-1} \left(\mathbf{x}_i \mathbf{e}_k' + \mathbf{e}_k \mathbf{x}_i' \right) \widehat{\boldsymbol{\beta}} + (\mathbf{X}'\mathbf{X})^{-1} \mathbf{e}_k y_i \\
&= (\mathbf{X}'\mathbf{X})^{-1} \left(\mathbf{e}_k (y_i - \mathbf{x}_i' \widehat{\boldsymbol{\beta}}) - \mathbf{x}_i (\mathbf{e}_k' \widehat{\boldsymbol{\beta}}) \right) = (\mathbf{X}'\mathbf{X})^{-1} (\mathbf{e}_k r_i - \mathbf{x}_i \widehat{\beta}_k),
\end{aligned}
\tag{9.14}
$$

where r_i is the ith OLS residual, $y_i - \widehat{\boldsymbol{\beta}}' \mathbf{x}_i$, $\widehat{\beta}_k$ is the kth OLS coefficient, and $\mathbf{e}_k$ is the $m \times 1$ Kronecker vector. Thus, the influence of observation x_{ik} on the OLS estimate can be measured as (Hodges and Moore, 1972)

$$\frac{\partial \widehat{\boldsymbol{\beta}}}{\partial x_{ik}} = (\mathbf{X}'\mathbf{X})^{-1} (\mathbf{e}_k r_i - \mathbf{x}_i \widehat{\beta}_k), \qquad 1 \le i \le n, \ 1 \le k \le m. \tag{9.15}$$

This influence measure is easy to interpret: one unit change of x_{ik} leads to the $\widehat{\boldsymbol{\beta}}$ change specified by (9.15). Certainly, the influence analysis based on this formula does not make sense for certain explanatory variables, e.g., gender or intercept term. As we see, perturbation in the kth covariate implies changes in other coefficients unless covariates are orthogonal. The influence of x_{ik} on the estimate, as follows from (9.15), has two components. The first component, $r_i (\mathbf{X}'\mathbf{X})^{-1} \mathbf{e}_k$, is associated with a large residual, and the second component, $\widehat{\beta}_k (\mathbf{X}'\mathbf{X})^{-1} \mathbf{x}_i$, is the coefficient times the vector of the Y-influence.

It is interesting to note that (9.15) is equivalent to that derived by Cook (1986) using his approach of local influence, assuming that the distribution of ε is normal. He suggested measuring the influence of x_{ik} on $\widehat{\beta}_k$ as $r_i - \widehat{\beta}_k q_i$, where q_i is the ith residual in regression of x_k on the remainder of the explanatory variables.

Now we will show that $r_i - \widehat{\beta}_k q_i$ is proportional to the kth component of vector (9.15), meaning that the I-influence and the local influence are equivalent. Without loss of generality we can assume that $k = 1$. Let $\mathbf{X}$ be partitioned as $[\mathbf{x}_1; \mathbf{X}_2]$, so that

$$(\mathbf{X}'\mathbf{X})^{-1} = \begin{bmatrix} a & \mathbf{b}' \\ \mathbf{b} & \mathbf{A} \end{bmatrix},$$

where a is a scalar, $\mathbf{b}$ is a $(m-1) \times 1$ vector, and $\mathbf{A}$ is a $(m-1) \times (m-1)$ symmetric matrix. As follows from the formula for the inverse of a partitioned matrix,

$$a = \frac{1}{\mathbf{x}_1'\mathbf{x}_1} + \frac{1}{(\mathbf{x}_1'\mathbf{x}_1)^2}\mathbf{x}_1'\mathbf{M}\mathbf{x}_1, \qquad \mathbf{X}_2\mathbf{b} = -\frac{1}{\mathbf{x}_1'\mathbf{x}_1}\mathbf{M}\mathbf{x}_1,$$

where

$$\mathbf{M} = \mathbf{H} + \frac{1}{\mathbf{x}_1'\mathbf{x}_1 - \mathbf{x}_1'\mathbf{H}\mathbf{x}_1}\mathbf{H}\mathbf{x}_1\mathbf{x}_1'\mathbf{H},$$

and $\mathbf{H} = \mathbf{X}_2(\mathbf{X}_2'\mathbf{X}_2)^{-1}\mathbf{X}_2'$ is an $n \times n$ projection matrix. After some algebra one obtains $a = (\mathbf{x}_1'\mathbf{x}_1 - \mathbf{x}_1'\mathbf{H}\mathbf{x}_1)^{-1}$. Next we find that

$$
\begin{aligned}
\mathbf{x}_1'\mathbf{M}\mathbf{x}_1 &= \mathbf{x}_1'\left(\mathbf{H} + \frac{1}{\mathbf{x}_1'\mathbf{x}_1 - \mathbf{x}_1'\mathbf{H}\mathbf{x}_1}\mathbf{H}\mathbf{x}_1\mathbf{x}_1'\mathbf{H}\right)\mathbf{x}_1 \\
&= \mathbf{x}_1'\mathbf{H}\mathbf{x}_1 + \frac{(\mathbf{x}_1'\mathbf{H}\mathbf{x}_1)^2}{\mathbf{x}_1'\mathbf{x}_1 - \mathbf{x}_1'\mathbf{H}\mathbf{x}_1} = \frac{\mathbf{x}_1'\mathbf{x}_1 \cdot \mathbf{x}_1'\mathbf{H}\mathbf{x}_1}{\mathbf{x}_1'\mathbf{x}_1 - \mathbf{x}_1'\mathbf{H}\mathbf{x}_1}
\end{aligned}
$$

and

$$
\begin{aligned}
\mathbf{M}\mathbf{x}_1 &= \left(\mathbf{H} + \frac{1}{\mathbf{x}_1'\mathbf{x}_1 - \mathbf{x}_1'\mathbf{H}\mathbf{x}_1}\mathbf{H}\mathbf{x}_1\mathbf{x}_1'\mathbf{H}\right)\mathbf{x}_1 \\
&= \mathbf{H}\mathbf{x} + \frac{\mathbf{x}_1'\mathbf{H}\mathbf{x}_1}{\mathbf{x}_1'\mathbf{x}_1 - \mathbf{x}_1'\mathbf{H}\mathbf{x}_1}\mathbf{H}\mathbf{x}_1 = \left(\frac{\mathbf{x}_1'\mathbf{x}_1}{\mathbf{x}_1'\mathbf{x}_1 - \mathbf{x}_1'\mathbf{H}\mathbf{x}_1}\right)\mathbf{H}\mathbf{x}_1.
\end{aligned}
$$

Then, the first column of matrix $\mathbf{X}(\mathbf{X}'\mathbf{X})^{-1}$ can be represented as

$$
\begin{aligned}
&a\mathbf{x}_1 + \mathbf{X}_2\mathbf{b} \\
&= \left(\frac{1}{\mathbf{x}_1'\mathbf{x}_1}\mathbf{I} + \frac{1}{(\mathbf{x}_1'\mathbf{x}_1)^2} \cdot \frac{\mathbf{x}_1'\mathbf{x}_1 \cdot \mathbf{x}_1'\mathbf{H}\mathbf{x}_1}{\mathbf{x}_1'\mathbf{x}_1 - \mathbf{x}_1'\mathbf{H}\mathbf{x}_1}\mathbf{I} - \frac{1}{\mathbf{x}_1'\mathbf{x}_1}\frac{\mathbf{x}_1'\mathbf{x}_1}{\mathbf{x}_1'\mathbf{x}_1 - \mathbf{x}_1'\mathbf{H}\mathbf{x}_1}\mathbf{H}\right)\mathbf{x}_1 \\
&= \left(\frac{1}{\mathbf{x}_1'\mathbf{x}_1}\mathbf{I} + \frac{1}{\mathbf{x}_1'\mathbf{x}_1} \cdot \frac{\mathbf{x}_1'\mathbf{H}\mathbf{x}_1}{\mathbf{x}_1'\mathbf{x}_1 - \mathbf{x}_1'\mathbf{H}\mathbf{x}_1}\mathbf{I} - \frac{1}{\mathbf{x}_1'\mathbf{x}_1 - \mathbf{x}_1'\mathbf{H}\mathbf{x}_1}\mathbf{H}\right)\mathbf{x}_1 \\
&= \left(\frac{1}{\mathbf{x}_1'\mathbf{x}_1 - \mathbf{x}_1'\mathbf{H}\mathbf{x}_1}\mathbf{I} - \frac{1}{\mathbf{x}_1'\mathbf{x}_1 - \mathbf{x}_1'\mathbf{H}\mathbf{x}_1}\mathbf{H}\right)\mathbf{x}_1 = \frac{1}{\mathbf{x}_1'\mathbf{x}_1 - \mathbf{x}_1'\mathbf{H}\mathbf{x}_1}(\mathbf{I} - \mathbf{H})\mathbf{x}_1 \\
&= a\mathbf{q},
\end{aligned}
$$

where $\mathbf{q} = (\mathbf{I} - \mathbf{H})\mathbf{x}_1$, the residual vector in regression $\mathbf{x}_1$ on $\mathbf{X}_2$. Finally, returning to formula (9.15) in vector form

$$\frac{\partial\widehat{\beta}_1}{\partial\mathbf{x}_1} = (\mathbf{X}'\mathbf{X})_{11}^{-1}\mathbf{r} - \widehat{\beta}_1\left(\mathbf{X}(\mathbf{X}'\mathbf{X})^{-1}\right)_{\cdot 1} = a(\mathbf{r} - \widehat{\beta}_1\mathbf{q}),$$

where $_{\cdot 1}$ indicates the first column. Hence, the $\{r_i - \widehat{\beta}_1 q_i\}$ are proportional to $\{\partial\widehat{\beta}_1/\partial x_{i1}\}$ with the factor $a = (\mathbf{X}'\mathbf{X})_{11}^{-1}$.

■

Formula (9.15) is even more general than the Cook's local influence formula because it is distribution-free and allows assessing the influence of the kth explanatory variable on the jth OLS coefficient when $k \neq j$.

9.4.3 Influence of the binary explanatory variable

In some cases the explanatory variable is not continuous; for example, it may take either the value 0 or 1 (dichotomous variable). We can still apply the I-influence, employing the idea of misclassification. Following our definition in Section 9.3, this is an example of infinitesimal model influence analysis. The idea of misclassification is developed further for the logistic regression model in Section 9.6.

If x_{ik} is binary and observed, we can interpret it as an outcome of a classification procedure; without loss of generality we can assume that $k = m$. The sensitivity of the OLS coefficient to the binary variable is understood as the sensitivity to the probability of misclassification. To set the model up with misclassification, we shall assume that the regression model is given as $E(y|z) = \alpha + \beta_m z$, where z is the true unobserved binary explanatory variable misclassified with the probability q and $\alpha = \beta_1 x_1 + \dots + \beta_{m-1} x_{m-1}$. However, we do not observe z but observe x_m such that $\Pr(z = 1|x_m = 0) = \Pr(z = 0|x_m = 1) = q$; a symmetric misclassification is assumed. Then, in terms of observed data, the regression conditioned on $x_m = 1$ can be rewritten as

$$
\begin{aligned}
E(y|x_m &= 1) = E(y|z = 1, x_m = 0)\Pr(z = 1|x_m = 1) \\
+E(y|z &= 0, x_m = 0)\Pr(z = 0|x_m = 1).
\end{aligned}
$$

Also, we shall assume that the misclassification does not depend on the regression, or more precisely, $\Pr(y|x_m, z) = \Pr(y|z)$. Hence, it is easy to see that $E(y|x_m) = \alpha + \beta_m(x_m + (1 - 2x_m)q)$. Therefore, assuming that x_{im} is binary, in the notations of (9.15), the impact of misclassification on the OLS estimate can be measured as

$$
\left.\frac{\partial\widehat{\boldsymbol{\beta}}}{\partial q_i}\right|_{q_i=0} = (1 - 2x_{im})(\mathbf{X}'\mathbf{X})^{-1}(\mathbf{e}_k r_i - \mathbf{x}_i\widehat{\beta}_k). \tag{9.16}
$$

Interestingly, the misclassification becomes asymptotically negligible when x_{im} takes zero and 1 with equal probability because then $E(1 - 2x_{im}) = 1 - 2\Pr(x_{im} = 1) = 0$. As we see, this formula very closely resembles (9.15), and they have the same absolute value.

9.4.4 Influence on the predicted value

As mentioned in Section 9.4, the diagonal element of the hat matrix measures the influence of the dependent variable on its predicted value. Of no less importance is how the predicted value is affected by the explanatory variable. Omitting fairly simple algebra and using (9.15), one obtains

$$
\frac{\partial\widehat{y}_i}{\partial x_{ik}} = \widehat{\beta}_k(1 - p_i) + \mathbf{x}_i'(\mathbf{X}'\mathbf{X})^{-1}\mathbf{e}_k r_i \qquad 1 \le i \le n,\ 1 \le k \le m, \tag{9.17}
$$

where p_i is the leverage.

We make a few comments on how to calculate derivatives when there are replicates, the regression is curvilinear, or the explanatory variables are functionally related. In the case of replicates—when several observations of the dependent variable y_i are available for the same value of x_{ik}—formula (9.15) is written as

$$\frac{\partial \widehat{\beta}}{\partial x_{ik}} = (\mathbf{X}'\mathbf{X})^{-1}(\mathbf{e}_k \sum_{x=x_{ik}} r_i - \mathbf{x}_i \widehat{\beta}_k).$$

In the case of curvilinear regression—when $\mathbf{x}_i$ enters the regression model as $\widetilde{\mathbf{x}}_i = g(\mathbf{x}_i)$, where $g(\cdot)$ is a known function—formula (9.15) is written as

$$\frac{\partial \widehat{\beta}}{\partial x_{ik}} = (\widetilde{\mathbf{X}}'\widetilde{\mathbf{X}})^{-1}(\mathbf{e}_k r_i g'(x_{ik}) - \widetilde{\mathbf{x}}_i \widehat{\beta}_k), \tag{9.18}$$

where g' denotes the derivative of g; see Section 9.4.9, where $g(s) = \ln(s + 1)$. Also, it is easy to obtain the expression for the derivative in the case when some explanatory variables are functionally related, as in quadratic regression.

9.4.5   Case or group deletion

The theory of case deletion, particularly infinitesimal deletion based on weights, has been developed by Belsley et al. (1980), Pregibon (1981), and Cook and Weisberg (1982). We briefly review the theory for further extension to nonlinear and logistic regressions.

We introduce weight w_i for case i and assume that all other cases have weight 1. Then, the weighted normal equation for the least squares estimate is written as

$$\sum_{j \neq i}(y_j - \beta'\mathbf{x}_j)\mathbf{x}_j + w_i(y_i - \beta'\mathbf{x}_i)\mathbf{x}_i = \mathbf{0}. \tag{9.19}$$

The solution to this equation is the weighted LS estimate, $\widehat{\beta}=\widehat{\beta}(w_i)$. In the infinitesimal deletion approach, one assesses how a small departure w_i from affects the regression estimate. The rate of this change is measured as the derivative of the estimate with respect to w_i. Two types of infinitesimal deletion may be distinguished according to the point at which the derivative is evaluated. When the derivative is evaluated at $w_i = 1$, we call it the *I-influence of deletion at inclusion*. If the derivative is evaluated at $w_i = 0$ we call it the *I-influence of deletion at exclusion*. The formula for the derivative at inclusion has been derived by Belsley et al. (1980):

$$\left.\frac{\partial \widehat{\beta}}{\partial w_i}\right|_{w_i=1} = r_i(\mathbf{X}'\mathbf{X})^{-1}\mathbf{x}_i, \tag{9.20}$$

where, as before, r_i is the OLS residual. This formula can be derived from (9.19) by differentiating with respect to w_i. As mentioned above, another option is to calculate the derivative at the point where the ith case is excluded ($w_i = 0$). We will prove that

$$\left.\frac{\partial \widehat{\beta}}{\partial w_i}\right|_{w_i=0} = \frac{r_i}{(1 - p_i)^2}(\mathbf{X}'\mathbf{X})^{-1}\mathbf{x}_i. \tag{9.21}$$

Proof. Indeed, using (9.3), one obtains

$$
\left.\frac{\partial \widehat{\boldsymbol{\beta}}}{\partial w_i}\right|_{w_i=0} = \left.\frac{\partial}{\partial w_i}(\mathbf{X}'\mathbf{X}-w_i\mathbf{x}_i\mathbf{x}_i')^{-1}(\mathbf{X}'\mathbf{y}-w_i\mathbf{x}_iy_i)\right|_{w_i=0}
$$

$$
= (\mathbf{X}_{(i)}'\mathbf{X}_{(i)})^{-1}\mathbf{x}_i\mathbf{x}_i'(\mathbf{X}_{(i)}'\mathbf{X}_{(i)})^{-1}\mathbf{X}_{(i)}'\mathbf{y}_{(i)} - (\mathbf{X}_{(i)}'\mathbf{X}_{(i)})^{-1}\mathbf{x}_iy_i
$$

$$
= \frac{1}{(1-p_i)^2}(\mathbf{X}'\mathbf{X})^{-1}\mathbf{x}_i\mathbf{x}_i'(\mathbf{X}'\mathbf{X})^{-1}(\mathbf{X}'\mathbf{y} - \mathbf{x}_iy_i) - \frac{1}{1-p_i}(\mathbf{X}'\mathbf{X})^{-1}\mathbf{x}_iy_i
$$

$$
= \left(\frac{p_iy_i - \widehat{y}_i}{(1-p_i)^2} + \frac{y_i}{1-p_i}\right)(\mathbf{X}'\mathbf{X})^{-1}\mathbf{x}_i = \frac{r_i}{(1-p_i)^2}(\mathbf{X}'\mathbf{X})^{-1}\mathbf{x}_i.
$$

Formula (9.21) is proved.

■

All three measures (9.3), (9.20), and (9.21) look alike. Moreover, we want to show that the former is approximately the average of the latter two. Indeed, half of the sum of (9.20) and (9.21), assuming that $p_i^2 \simeq 0$, is

$$
\frac{1}{2}r_i\left(1 + \frac{1}{(1-p_i)^2}\right)(\mathbf{X}'\mathbf{X})^{-1}\mathbf{x}_i \tag{9.22}
$$

$$
= \frac{1}{2}r_i\left(\frac{2}{1-p_i} + \frac{p_i^2}{(1-p_i)^2}\right)(\mathbf{X}'\mathbf{X})^{-1}\mathbf{x}_i \simeq \frac{r_i}{1-p_i}(\mathbf{X}'\mathbf{X})^{-1}\mathbf{x}_i.
$$

There is an important feature of the influence measure (9.20): it can be used to study the influence of the *group deletion*. Indeed, this follows from the fact that the derivative of a sum is the sum of the derivatives. Let a group of cases $\mathcal{I}$ (suspected of being influential) be chosen, and we want to find how the deletion of this entire group affects the OLS estimate. Introducing weights $w = w_i, i \in \mathcal{I}$, we come to an estimating equation similar to (9.19):

$$
\sum_{i\notin\mathcal{I}}(y_i - \boldsymbol{\beta}'\mathbf{x}_i)\mathbf{x}_i + w\sum_{i\in\mathcal{I}}(y_i - \boldsymbol{\beta}'\mathbf{x}_i)\mathbf{x}_i = \mathbf{0}.
$$

Then the influence of the entire group $\mathcal{I}$ deletion on the OLS estimate is measured as $(\mathbf{X}'\mathbf{X})^{-1}\sum_{i\in\mathcal{I}} r_i\mathbf{x}_i$, which is the sum of individual deletion measures. In other words, by identifying a group of observations with large values from (9.20), we actually identify a *group* of influential cases. It is worthwhile to note that this property does not hold for the standard case deletion diagnostic.

Derivatives (9.20) and (9.21) can be used to predict the effect of case deletion on the OLS estimates. Indeed, using the classic calculus formula $f(x) - f(x_0) \simeq f'(x_0)(x - x_0)$, we can approximate the OLS estimate upon deletion at inclusion as

$$
\widehat{\boldsymbol{\beta}} - \widehat{\boldsymbol{\beta}}_{(i)} \simeq (1 - 0) \times \left.\frac{\partial \widehat{\boldsymbol{\beta}}(w_i)}{\partial w_i}\right|_{w_i=1} = r_i(\mathbf{X}'\mathbf{X})^{-1}\mathbf{x}_i.
$$

Similarly, deletion at exclusion yields

$$
\widehat{\boldsymbol{\beta}}_{(i)} - \widehat{\boldsymbol{\beta}} \simeq (0 - 1) \times \left.\frac{\partial \widehat{\boldsymbol{\beta}}(w_i)}{\partial w_i}\right|_{w_i=0} = -\frac{r_i}{(1-p_i)^2}(\mathbf{X}'\mathbf{X})^{-1}\mathbf{x}_i.
$$

Note that the exact difference between $\widehat{\beta}_{(i)}$ and $\widehat{\beta}$ is given by (9.3). These approximations are computed in Section 9.4.8. We benefit from the I-influence of case deletion, especially in nonlinear models where no closed-form solution exists for the estimate upon case deletion.

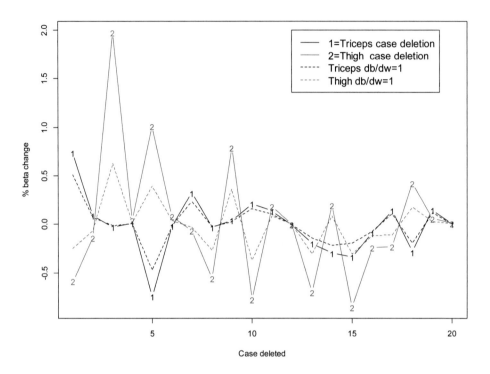

FIGURE 9.2. Women's body fat influence analysis. This plot is created by the R function call `wbf()`. The solid line depicts the % coefficient change upon case deletion and the dashed line depicts the approximation using the I-influence computed by formula (9.20).

9.4.6 R code

Below we provide a sample of an R code that computes two beta coefficients for each case deletion and compares that with the I-influence of deletion at exclusion using formula (9.20). The data and other relevant influence analyses are discussed in Section 9.4.8. We make a few comments on the code below. The `dump` command saves the code as a text file (the code is restored using the `source` command). The option `weights` is used to delete the ith case from the data when computing the OLS estimate by `lm`. First, we compute the OLS beta coefficients, residuals, and quantities (9.20) for the entire data set, and then we compute the beta coefficients with the case deleted. `iXtX%*%t(ri*X)` is a compact way to compute (9.20). Note that `ri*X` is an equivalent but economical version for `diag(ri,n,n)%*%X`. The result of this code is displayed in Figure 9.2. As can be seen from this plot, approximation (9.20) is a fair assessment of case deletion, especially for the coefficient at thigh, although the percent change is small in large samples. This I-influence analysis would be especially useful for large data sets when the case-by-case deletion is time consuming.

```
wbf=function()
{
    dump("wbf","c:\\MixedModels\\Chapter09\\wbf.r") # save the code
    #Influence analysis for Chapter 9
    #Example 1: Women's body fat, data in WomenBF.dat
    dat=read.table("c:\\MixedModels\\Chapter09\\WomenBF.dat")
    n=nrow(dat)
    outlm=lm(Fat~Triceps+Thigh,data=dat)
    betaALL=coef(outlm)[2:3]
    ri=outlm$residuals
    betai=matrix(nrow=n,ncol=2)
    dbdw1=dbdw0=matrix(nrow=n,ncol=2)
    X=as.matrix(cbind(rep(1,n),dat[,2:3]))
    iXtX=solve(t(X)%*%X)
    dbdw1=iXtX%*%t(ri*X)
    for(i in 1:n)
    {
        w=rep(1,n); w[i]=0
        outi=lm(Fat~Triceps+Thigh,data=dat,weights=w)
        betai[i,]=(coef(outi)[2:3]-betaALL)/betaALL*100
    }
    matplot(1:n,betai,lty=1,type="b",xlab="Case deleted",
            ylab="% beta change")
    lines(1:n,-100*dbdw1[2,],lty=2)
    lines(1:n,-100*dbdw1[3,],lty=2,col=2)
    legend(12,2,c("1=Triceps case deletion","2=Thigh case deletion",
            "Triceps db/dw=1","Thigh db/dw=1"),
            lty=c(1,1,2,2),col=c(1,2,1,2))
}
```

9.4.7 Influence on regression characteristics

Sometimes, besides regression coefficients themselves, we are interested in regression characteristics as a part of influence analysis. For instance, in investigating the effect of a new treatment, the key characteristic might be the t-statistic of the OLS estimate at the treatment effect variable (1 = new treatment, 0 = old treatment), where y is the treatment outcome and the set of other covariates may include age, gender, etc. No influence analysis is available for regression characteristics, such as the t-statistic or the coefficient of determination in traditional regression diagnostics. As mentioned above, one of the advantages of the I-influence approach is that it can be applied to any statistic as a function of data. In this section we illustrate this feature by the I-influence analysis for the coefficient of determination and t-statistic. Following the line of the previous discussion, we distinguish two types of influences: the influence of the dependent (Y-influence) and independent (X-influence) variables.

Y-influence

Coefficient of determination. We start the analysis with the Residual Sum of Squares (RSS). The influence of the observation of the dependent variable y_i on the RSS is measured as the partial derivative of the RSS with respect to y_i. Then, if r_i denotes the ith OLS residual, the Y-influence of the RSS is measured as

$$\frac{\partial RSS}{\partial y_i} = \frac{\partial}{\partial y_i} \sum_{j=1}^{n} (y_j - \mathbf{x}_j'\widehat{\boldsymbol{\beta}})^2 = 2r_i - 2\sum_{j=1}^{n} r_j \mathbf{x}_j'(\mathbf{X}'\mathbf{X})^{-1}\mathbf{x}_i = 2r_i, \qquad (9.23)$$

since $\sum r_j \mathbf{x}_j = 0$. Thus, the rate of change of RSS with respect to a small change in the dependent variable, y_i, is proportional to the OLS residual. Omitting some algebra, we obtain the formula for the Y-influence of the coefficient of determination, R^2:

$$\frac{\partial R^2}{\partial y_i} = \frac{2}{\sum (y_j - \overline{y})^2} \left[(1 - R^2)(y_i - \overline{y}) - r_i \right]. \qquad (9.24)$$

As follows from equation (9.24), the Y-influence for the coefficient of determination consists of two parts: the first part is associated with the y-residual about the mean, and the second part is associated with the OLS residual.

t-statistic. Let $\mathbf{D} = \text{diag}((\mathbf{X}'\mathbf{X})^{-1})$ denote an $m \times m$ diagonal matrix of the inverse to $\mathbf{X}'\mathbf{X}$; then the vector of t-statistics can be written as $\mathbf{t} = s^{-1}\mathbf{D}^{-1/2}\widehat{\boldsymbol{\beta}}$, where $s^2 = RSS/(n - m)$. Omitting some algebra and using previously derived formulas (9.15) and (9.23), one obtains

$$\frac{\partial \mathbf{t}}{\partial y_i} = \frac{1}{s}\mathbf{D}^{-1/2}(\mathbf{X}'\mathbf{X})^{-1}\mathbf{x}_i - \frac{u_i}{RSS}. \qquad (9.25)$$

Hence, plotting these derivatives against i, one can identify influential observations of the dependent variable in terms of the sensitivity of t-statistics to small changes in observation of the dependent variable. (See the next section for an example.)

X-influence

The influence of an independent variable on the RSS is trivial. It easy to show that the derivative of RSS and R^2 with respect to x_{ik} is proportional to the OLS residual. The X-influence of the t-statistic is measured as the partial derivative,

$$\frac{\partial \mathbf{t}}{\partial x_{ik}} = \frac{\widehat{\beta}_k u_i}{RSS}\mathbf{t} + \frac{1}{s}\mathbf{D}^{-1/2}(\mathbf{X}'\mathbf{X})^{-1}(\mathbf{e}_k u_i - \mathbf{x}_i\widehat{\beta}_k) + \frac{1}{s}\mathbf{p}, \qquad (9.26)$$

where $\mathbf{p}$ is the $m \times 1$ vector with the jth component,

$$p_j = ((X'X)_{jj}^{-1})^{-3/2}(X'X)_{jk}^{-1}\sum_{l=1}^{m}(X'X)_{jl}^{-1}x_{il}\widehat{\beta}_j.$$

This influence analysis will be especially useful for correlated explanatory variables; then it can identify influential observations that cause low t-statistics values.

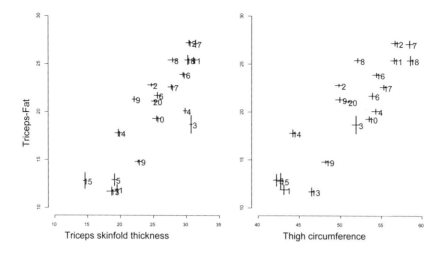

FIGURE 9.3. Cross-influence plot for the women's body fat example. The length of the vertical bar of the cross is proportional to the influence of the respective body fat observation on the predicted value, leverage. The length of the horizontal bar is proportional to the influence of the respective independent variable on the predicted value of fat. For example, observation 3 has little X-influence but a large Y-influence.

9.4.8 Example 1: Women's body fat

To illustrate the I-influence approach, we consider the regression of Body Fat (y_i) on Triceps skinfold thickness (x_{i1}) and Thigh circumference (x_{i2}) for 20 women from Neter et al. (1990). The estimated multivariate regression is $\widehat{y}_i = 0.2224x_1 + 0.6594x_2 - 19.174$. R code with case deletion analysis is presented in Section 9.4.6 and depicted in Figure 9.2. Here we continue the influence analysis using other measures.

The standard technique in visualizing influential cases is to use a proportional influence plot, a scatter plot where the ith observation point is represented by a circle of radius proportional to the leverage, p_i. Larger circles in the plot identify more influential cases. Such a plot is implemented in the statistical package STATA. However, we can make this graph more informative, displaying the influence of both the dependent and independent variables, where the latter is calculated by formula (9.17). Such a graph is called a *cross influence plot*. Since our example has two continuous variables, it is relevant to study the influence of an individual observation of triceps and thigh on the predicted value of body fat, see Figure 9.3. Each case is represented by a cross. The length of the vertical bar is proportional to the leverage, p_i, and is equal to the diameter of the circle in the standard proportional influence graph. The length of the horizontal bar is proportional to (9.17). As we see, the longest vertical bar corresponds to case 3. On the other hand, the horizontal bar for this case is relatively small, especially for triceps-influence. It means that the predicted value for case 3 is sensitive to perturbation of the dependent variable and not sensitive to perturbation in the explanatory variables.

The *star influence plot* shows the influence of individual observations on the OLS coefficient, see Figure 9.4. To compare the magnitude of the influence, the percent

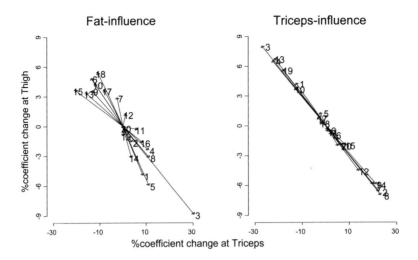

FIGURE 9.4. Star influence plot for women's body fat example based on formula (9.15). As follows from the fat-influence analysis, an increase of the third observation of fat by one unit leads an approximate 35% in increase the intercept and an 8% decrease in the second slope. The arrows in the right graph lie closely to a line because of multicollinearity.

change in beta coefficient is displayed. Coefficient $\widehat{\beta}_1 = 0.2224$ is more sensitive to perturbation and its rate lies in the range -20 to 35%. Our interpretation is as follows: if the third observation of fat increases by 1 then the first OLS, the $\widehat{\beta}_1$ coefficient would increase by 35% and would become $0.2224 + 0.35 \times 0.2224 = 0.3$. At the same time, the second coefficient would become $0.6594 - 0.08 \times 0.6594 = 0.6067$. Similarly, we can compute the effect of a perturbation of triceps on the second OLS slope, $\widehat{\beta}_2$.

A *bar influence plot* is shown in Figure 9.5 and displays relative changes in the beta coefficients in a different manner.

This graph should be read from right to left. In the right-hand graph, one can identify maximum influence located at the end-points. By projecting the bars on the left graph it is easy to locate the influential cases. Bar influence plots are useful for detecting groups of influential observations and for the comparison of influence for different regression coefficients. As we see, $\widehat{\beta}_1$ is slightly more sensitive to perturbation in both dependent and independent variables. For the dependent variable it ranges from -20 to 30%, whereas $\widehat{\beta}_2$ only ranges from -10 to 7%.

The influence of case deletion is illustrated in Figure 9.6, where relative changes in beta coefficients are shown. Three bars, according to formulas (9.20), (4.97), and (9.21) for three regression coefficients, are displayed. As noted in Section 9.4.5, the influence of deletion is equal to approximately half the sum of the two others. The most influential case is 3; deletion of this case would lead to an increase of 100% in the OLS coefficient. Looking at Figure 9.5, we see that this is due to the observations of body fat and triceps. Bar influence in combination with deletion influence plots can help identify which individual observation of what variable is influential. Notice that the standard deletion diagnostics do not allow one to identify which variable makes the case influential.

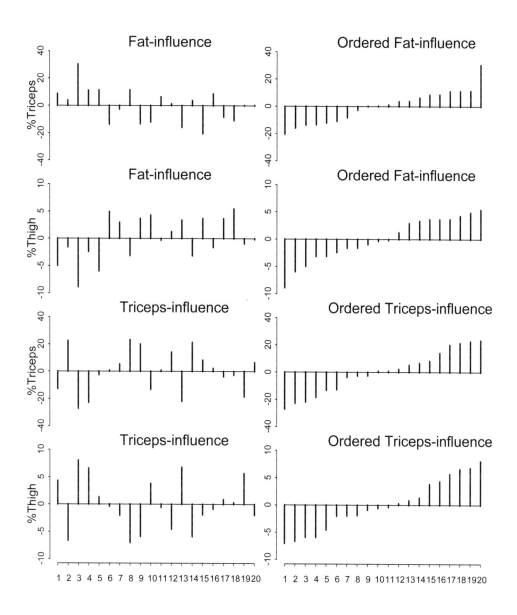

FIGURE 9.5. Bar influence plot for the women's body fat example. In the graphs at the right, the influence is ordered so that influential observations are located at the left and right. The influential case number can be found on the left-hand graph by projecting the influence bar from right to left. This type of graph is convenient for group influence detection. For instance, we can identify four observations of triceps that are influential on $\widehat{\beta}_1$ — they are located at the right side.

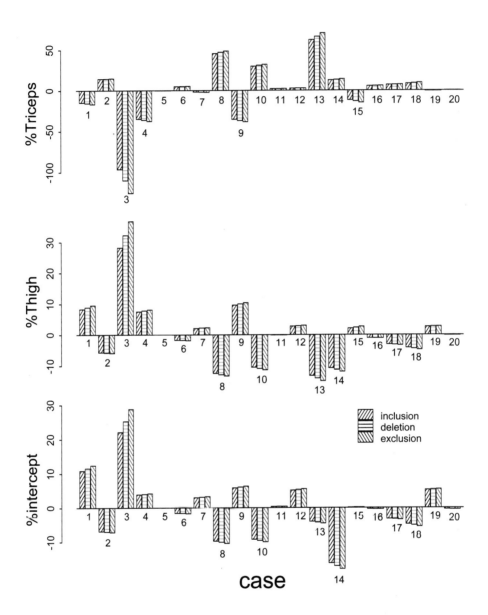

FIGURE 9.6. Case deletion influence plot for the women's body fat example as a percentage of change in the OLS estimate. For each case the left bar corresponds to infinitesimal deletion at inclusion, the middle bar corresponds to full case deletion, and the third bar corresponds to deletion at exclusion. The length of the influence bar is proportional to the change in the beta coefficient after the ith case is deleted. Obviously, the three measures of influence are highly correlated. Moreover, 'deletion' is the half-sum of 'inclusion' and 'exclusion', see expression (9.22).

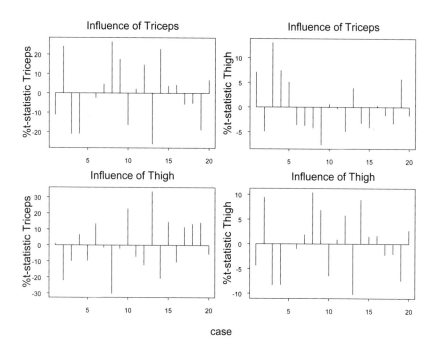

FIGURE 9.7. I-influence on t-statistics. The bottom graph on the left reveals that an increase by 1 in the 13th observation of the thigh variable would increase the t-statistic by 30%.

In Figure 9.7 we show how t-statistics depend on an infinitesimal change in the independent variables triceps and thigh computed by formula (9.26). For example, a unit increase in the thigh variable in the eight observation would lead to a drop of 30% in the t-statistic.

9.4.9   Example 2: gypsy moth study

In this section we illustrate how I-influence analysis can be applied to curvilinear regression (linear in parameters but nonlinear in covariates). We use burlap data from a gypsy moth study (Buonaccorsi, 1994) to illustrate the I-influence in curvilinear regression. The objective, as formulated by Buonaccorsi, was "to see how well counts of gypsy moth egg mass found under burlap bands on trees can be used to predict the egg mass density for a large area." The data consist of 51 measurements of egg mass, denoted as *megg*, in the area and egg mass under burlap, denoted as *mburlap*. Due to the objective of prediction, we look for relationship of megg on mburlap, the left-hand plot in Figure 9.8.

As we see from that graph, there is a cluster of observations in the neighborhood of zero with small values. Unlike Bounaccorsi, who studied the relationship of mburlap on megg, we suggest: (1) using the reverse relationship, i.e., megg on mburlap, and (2) taking logarithms of variables plus 1. There is an interesting property of this transformation: for large mburlap and megg, we obtain a power relationship, and

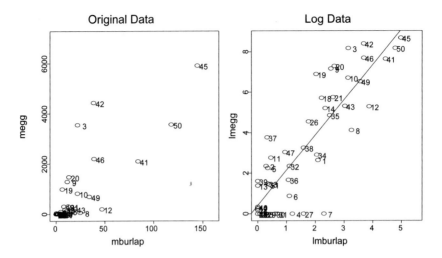

FIGURE 9.8. Gypsy moth study, burlap data. The left-hand graph: scatter plot of original data. The right-hand graph: scatter plot of log plus 1 megg (lmegg) with the regression line. The transformation makes the scatter plot more informative.

for small values of mburlap it is linear. In fact, if $\ln(y+1) = a + b\ln(x+1)$, then $y = c(x+1)^b - 1$, where $c = \exp(a)$, and we have $\lim y/x^b \simeq c$ for large x. If $x \simeq 0$, we can approximate $(x+1)^b \simeq 1 + bx$ and then $y \simeq (c-1) + (cb)x$. Therefore, the regression model we suggest is curvilinear,

$$\text{lmegg}_i = a + b \cdot \text{lmburlap}_i + \varepsilon_i,$$

where $\text{lmegg}_i = \ln(\text{megg}_i + 1)$ and $\text{lmburlap}_i = \ln(\text{mburlap}_i + 1)$. The transformation makes the scatter plot more informative; compare the two graphs in Figure 9.8.

We show only the star influence plot for this example. It shows how a small perturbation in megg and mburlap affects the OLS estimate for the intercept and slope, Figure 9.9. The derivatives are calculated similar to formula (9.18), where $g(s) = \ln(s+1)$. The left-hand plot shows the impact of small changes in megg, and the right-hand plot shows the impact of mburlap. The star influence plot helps us to view directions of data influence in the parameter space. Clearly, case 7 is influential. However, the seventh observation of megg is not influential on the slope and has a positive outstanding influence on the intercept. The seventh observation of mburlap is influential on both slope and intercept. Therefore, one can infer that the 7th case is influential because of an incorrect measurement of mburlap, not megg. We notice that we could not detect the impact of mburlap using standard techniques based on leverage or case deletion diagnostics because the influence would then be associated with the case as a whole.

Problems for Section 9.4

1. Derive the influence measure (9.12) explicitly for a simple linear regression $y_i = \alpha + \beta x_i + \varepsilon_i$. Is it correct to say that this quantity measures how far x_i is from the bulk of x-data?

2. Derive the influence measure (9.15) explicitly for a simple linear regression, as in the previous problem.

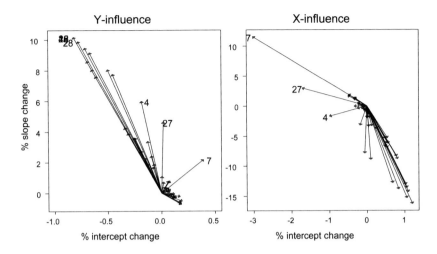

FIGURE 9.9. Star influence plot, burlap data. Case 7 is influential. An increase of mburlap by 1 would increase the slope by 10%.

3. Consider the linear regression on the log scale: $y_i = \alpha + \beta \ln z_i, + \varepsilon_i$, meaning that $x_i = \ln z_i$. Is it correct to say that (9.15) measures the relative change of the beta estimate?

4. Develop the I-influence of continuous explanatory variable on the coefficient of determination.

5. Adopt the R code from Section 9.4.6 to the leave-one-out analysis for the gypsy moth data in file `GypsyM.dat`.

6*. Conduct a simulation study to investigate how satisfactory the I-influence of deletion measures (9.20) and (9.21) identify influential cases (outliers). Use a linear regression with two independent variables $y_i = \alpha + \beta_1 x_{i1} + \beta_2 x_{i2} + \varepsilon_i$ to generate the data for $i = 1, 2, ..., n$. Use $y_{n+1} = \alpha^* + \beta_1^* x_{n+1,1} + \beta_2^* x_{n+1,2} + \varepsilon_{n+1}$ to generate the $(n + 1)$th observation/outlier. Compute the proportion of simulations that produce extreme values for (9.20) and (9.21) which indicate that the last observation is influential for a grid of values β_1^* (and/or β_2^*) starting from the true value β_1. You can use your own values for x_1 and x_2 or let $x_1 = 1, 2, ..., n$ and $x_2 = x_1^2$ as in quadratic regression.

7*. Develop the I-influence of case deletion on the t-statistic. Test your analytical derivations via simulations as in the previous problem, adopt the R code from Section 9.4.6.

8*. The data `coloncancer.dat` contains Medicare reimbursements for 10,109 colon cancer patients over a 10 period of times (t1,t2,t3,...,t10); the total number of observations is 101,090 (use `read.table` to read the file, see also problem 3 of Section 9.9). Other covariates include gender (female=1, male=0), stage2, stage3, and Charlson (morbidity) index. As was suggested by Demidenko and Stukel (2005), one of the model to describe the total cost for colon cancer treatment (y) takes the form of a linear regression $\ln(y + 100) = \alpha + \beta_1 \times female + \beta_2 \times stage2 + \beta_2 \times stage3 + \beta_4 \times Charlson + \beta_5 \times t1 + \varepsilon$. Compute and display the I-influence measures (9.20) and (9.21). Compute and display I-influence of y on t-statistics (9.25).

9.5   Nonlinear regression model

I-influence analysis is especially useful in complex statistical models such as nonlinear regression, where case deletion diagnostics would lead to time expensive regression recalculations. The nonlinear regression model is written as $y_i = f_i(\boldsymbol{\beta}; \mathbf{x}_i) + \epsilon_i$, where $\mathbf{x}_i$ is the vector of explanatory variables subject to influence analysis. The Least Squares (LS) estimate, $\widehat{\boldsymbol{\beta}}$, satisfies the vector normal equation

$$\sum_{i=1}^{n}(y_i - f_i(\boldsymbol{\beta}; \mathbf{x}_i))\frac{\partial f_i(\boldsymbol{\beta}; \mathbf{x}_i)}{\partial \boldsymbol{\beta}} = \mathbf{0}. \tag{9.27}$$

Apparently, $\widehat{\boldsymbol{\beta}}$ can be viewed as a function of y_i and $\mathbf{x}_i$. How is $\widehat{\boldsymbol{\beta}}$ affected by an individual observation of the dependent or explanatory variable? Following the approach of *I*-influence analysis, this influence is measured as $\partial\widehat{\boldsymbol{\beta}}/\partial y_i$ and $\partial\widehat{\boldsymbol{\beta}}/\partial x_{ik}$, respectively. There is no closed-form solution to the LS estimate (LSE) in nonlinear regression, so we need to find the derivatives above by treating $\widehat{\boldsymbol{\beta}}$ as an implicit function of y_i and $\mathbf{x}_i$.

9.5.1   Influence of the dependent variable on the LSE

The necessary derivative can be found either by direct differentiation of (9.27) or by applying the formula for the derivative of an implicit function that leads to

$$\frac{\partial\widehat{\boldsymbol{\beta}}}{\partial y_i} = \mathbf{H}^{-1}\frac{\partial f_i}{\partial \boldsymbol{\beta}}, \tag{9.28}$$

where

$$\mathbf{H} = \sum_{j=1}^{n}\left[\left(\frac{\partial f_j}{\partial \boldsymbol{\beta}}\right)\left(\frac{\partial f_j}{\partial \boldsymbol{\beta}}\right)' - (y_j - f_j)\frac{\partial^2 f_j}{\partial \boldsymbol{\beta}^2}\right]$$

is the half-Hessian of the sum of squares and all derivatives are calculated at $\boldsymbol{\beta} = \widehat{\boldsymbol{\beta}}$. Following Bates and Watts (1988), the matrix $\mathbf{H}$ may be approximated by $\mathbf{G}'\mathbf{G}$, where $\mathbf{G} = \partial\mathbf{f}/\partial\boldsymbol{\beta}$ is the $n \times m$ matrix of first derivatives of $\{f_i\}$.

9.5.2   Influence of the explanatory variable on the LSE

Again, to find $\partial\widehat{\boldsymbol{\beta}}/\partial x_{ik}$, we can either differentiate the normal equation (9.27) or apply the formula for the derivative of an implicit function,

$$\frac{\partial\widehat{\boldsymbol{\beta}}}{\partial x_{ik}} = \mathbf{H}^{-1}\left[r_i\frac{\partial^2 f_i}{\partial \boldsymbol{\beta}\partial x_{ik}} - \frac{\partial f_i}{\partial x_{ik}}\frac{\partial f_i}{\partial \boldsymbol{\beta}}\right]. \tag{9.29}$$

It is not difficult to obtain the formula for influence in the case when the explanatory variable is binary by employing the idea of misclassification as was done for the linear model in Section 9.4.3.

9.5.3 Influence on the predicted value

Following the I-influence approach, we measure the influence of an individual obser-
vation y_i on $\mathbf{f}(\widehat{\boldsymbol{\beta}}) = (f_1(\boldsymbol{\beta}; \mathbf{x}_1), ..., f_n(\boldsymbol{\beta}; \mathbf{x}_n))'$ as $\partial \mathbf{f}(\widehat{\boldsymbol{\beta}})/\partial y_i$. The use of this derivative for influence analysis in nonlinear regression was suggested by Emerson et al.
(1984) and later generalized by Laurent and Cook (1992, 1993). To find $\partial \mathbf{f}(\widehat{\boldsymbol{\beta}})/\partial y_i$,
we use formula (9.28) and apply the chain rule:

$$\frac{\partial \mathbf{f}(\widehat{\boldsymbol{\beta}})}{\partial y_i} = \frac{\partial \mathbf{f}(\widehat{\boldsymbol{\beta}})}{\partial \widehat{\boldsymbol{\beta}}} \frac{\partial \widehat{\boldsymbol{\beta}}}{\partial y_i} = \mathbf{G} \frac{\partial \widehat{\boldsymbol{\beta}}}{\partial y_i} = \mathbf{G} \mathbf{H}^{-1} \frac{\partial f_i}{\partial \boldsymbol{\beta}}. \tag{9.30}$$

Laurent and Cook called the matrix consisting of vectors (9.30) the *Jacobian leverage*. For a linear regression model, the ith component of vector (9.30) is the usual
leverage, p_i.

9.5.4 Influence of case deletion

The influence of case deletion on parameter estimates in nonlinear regression has
been studied by Cook and Weisberg (1982) and by Ross (1987). A straightforward
implementation of case deletion would lead to regression reestimation. To avoid this,
one can use a one-step approximation, as suggested by Pregibon (1981) and Preisser
and Qaqish (1996) for the generalized linear model. Analogously to the linear model,
two kinds of I-influence of case deletion can be considered: the influence at inclusion
and exclusion. In the first type of influence the derivative is evaluated at $w_i = 1$,
and in the second, at $w_i = 0$. Omitting a fairly simple algebra, the influence at
inclusion and at exclusion is

$$\left. \frac{\partial \widehat{\boldsymbol{\beta}}}{\partial w_i} \right|_{w_i=1} = r_i \mathbf{H}^{-1} \frac{\partial f_i}{\partial \boldsymbol{\beta}}, \qquad \left. \frac{\partial \widehat{\boldsymbol{\beta}}}{\partial w_i} \right|_{w_i=0} \simeq \frac{r_i}{(1-p_i)^2} (\mathbf{G}'\mathbf{G})^{-1} \frac{\partial f_i}{\partial \boldsymbol{\beta}}, \tag{9.31}$$

respectively, where r_i is the ith LS residual and

$$p_i = \left(\frac{\partial f_i}{\partial \boldsymbol{\beta}} \right)' (\mathbf{G}'\mathbf{G})^{-1} \left(\frac{\partial f_i}{\partial \boldsymbol{\beta}} \right)$$

is an analog of the leverage (it is easy to see that p_i is the standard leverage if f_i
is a linear function). These influence measures are called *exclusion 1*. We can use
another definition of leverage based on (9.30):

$$\left. \frac{\partial \widehat{\boldsymbol{\beta}}}{\partial w_i} \right|_{w_i=0} \simeq \frac{r_i}{(1-p_i^*)^2} \mathbf{H}^{-1} \frac{\partial f_i}{\partial \boldsymbol{\beta}}, \tag{9.32}$$

where

$$p_i^* = \left(\frac{\partial f_i}{\partial \boldsymbol{\beta}} \right)' \mathbf{H}^{-1} \left(\frac{\partial f_i}{\partial \boldsymbol{\beta}} \right).$$

This measure is called *exclusion 2*. Notice that all derivatives are evaluated at the
LS estimate, so we do not need to reestimate the regression. The three measures
are compared in the following example.

9.5.5   Example 3: logistic growth curve model

We take an example that Laurent and Cook (1993) borrowed from Bates and Watts (1988). The dependent variable y, radioactivity counts in rat heart tissue, is related to molar concentration of nifedipene (NIF), $x = \log_{10}(\text{concentration NIF})$ via a logistic growth curve model

$$f(\boldsymbol{\theta}; x_i) = \theta_1 + \frac{\theta_2}{1 + e^{\theta_4(x_i - \theta_3)}}, \quad i = 1, ..., 16. \tag{9.33}$$

The R code that computes the theta parameters upon case deletion is shown below.

```
nlsnif=function()
{
    dump("nlsnif","c:\\MixedModels\\Chapter09\\nlsnif.r")
    dat=read.table("c:\\MixedModels\\Chapter09\\NLSNIF.dat")
    n=nrow(dat)
    thetaDEL=matrix(ncol=4,nrow=n)
    outnls=nls(y~theta1+theta2/(1+exp(theta4*(x-theta3))),
    start=c(theta1=2000,theta2=3200,theta3=-8.3,theta4=1.3)
        ,data=dat)
    thetaALL=coef(outnls)
    for(i in 1:n)
    {
        w=rep(1,n);w[i]=0
        outnlsi=nls(y~theta1+theta2/(1+exp(theta4*(x-theta3))),
            weights=w,start=list(theta1=thetaALL[1],
            theta2=thetaALL[2],theta3=thetaALL[3],
            theta4=thetaALL[4]),data=dat,
            control=list(maxiter=500))
        thetaDEL[i,]=coef(outnlsi)
    }
    return(thetaDEL)
}
```

To compute theta parameters with the ith case deleted, we use the same method as in the case of linear regression by setting the `weights` vector component to 0 for the deleted case and 1 for other components. The default maximum number of iterations in `nls` is 50; we have to increase it to 500 to get convergence for all deleted cases.

An interesting feature of these data is that for the first two observations ($i = 1, 2$), the concentration is zero, formally $x = -\infty$ and $f(\boldsymbol{\theta}; x_1) = f(\boldsymbol{\theta}; x_2) = \theta_1 + \theta_2$. The observation points with the fitted curve are shown in Figure 9.10. Apparently, the real concentration should be positive, so that one might admit that the measurement tool is just not precise enough to detect a tiny concentration. Therefore, as a part of influence analysis, it is of interest to assess the influence of these points. Also, since the sample size is fairly small, one can expect that each case is influential to a certain degree. To display points we arbitrarily set $x_1 = x_2 = -27$, as Laurent and Cook did. The nonlinear least squares estimates with t-statistics in the parentheses are: $\widehat{\theta}_1 = 1923.52\,(5.2)$, $\widehat{\theta}_2 = 3194.92\,(6.7)$, $\widehat{\theta}_3 = -8.3214\,(21)$, and $\widehat{\theta}_4 = 1.269\,(2.2)$.

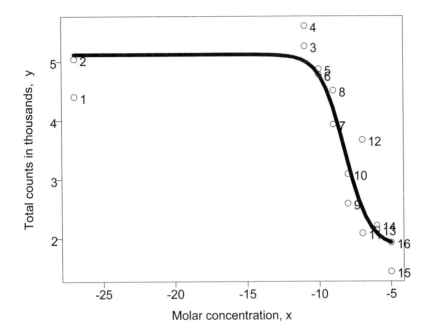

FIGURE 9.10. Observation points and the fitted curve for the logistic nonlinear regression model. For each molar concentration, there is a pair of total counts. We set the x-value of the first pair of observations ($x = -\infty$) to -27 as the original authors did.

We begin our influence analysis by assessing how a small perturbation in an individual observation of the dependent or independent variable affects the LS estimate using formulas (9.28) and (9.29); see Figure 9.11 (influence plots for the second and third theta parameters are not shown).

Since x is controllable in this example, the influence analysis with respect to x may answer the question of how well the experiment is designed and what should be done to improve it. First, we observe that $\widehat{\theta}_1$ is more sensitive than $\widehat{\theta}_4$; probably because $\widehat{\theta}_1$ is less significant, the fact is likely to be general. Second, parameters are much more sensitive to y-observations than to x-observations. This fact could not be revealed using standard case deletion diagnostics because the influence of the dependent and independent variables are not separated. As we also see, the two left-hand endpoints have little effect on parameters. On the other hand, the right-hand endpoints have maximum influence on the first and fourth parameters. A close look at Figure 9.11 clarifies the reason for this: Parameter θ_4 corresponds to the rate of y change with respect to x, and the two right-hand x-observations bring substantial information for the estimation parameter θ_4. Hence, in order to

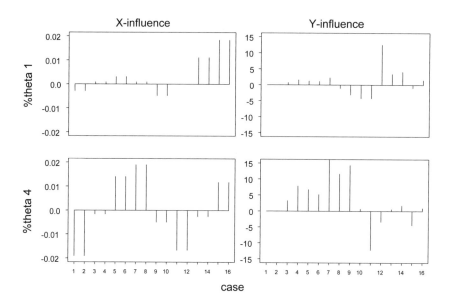

FIGURE 9.11. Bar influence plot for logistic growth curve model (9.33). The twelveth observation of total counts affects $\widehat{\theta}_1$ (the increase in y_{12} by 1000 increases $\widehat{\theta}_1$ by approximately 12%, top-right graph). To the contrary, y_{12} does not affect $\widehat{\theta}_4$. On the other hand, $\widehat{\theta}_4$ is affected by the seventh observation of counts—see the bottom-right graph.

get more precise estimates of the rate parameter, the researcher should add design points with $x > -5$.

Now, let us consider the influence of case deletion on parameter estimation, Figure 9.12 (first and fourth parameters).Five measures of case deletion are computed as the relative changes to the LS estimate. The first three measures are calculated by formulas (9.31, 9.32); the fourth measure, deletion, corresponds to precise case deletion and regression recalculation. As we see, the influence of case deletion in a certain way accumulates the influences driven by the dependent and independent variables considered above. Case 15 is influential for all parameters, this part of influence inference coincides with the conclusion of Laurent and Cook (1993) based on the Jacobian leverage (9.30). However, in contrast to their analysis, case 16 is not influential, which can be verified by looking at Figure 9.11. For this example, all five measures behave quite differently for some cases; however, generally, they are correlated.

Problems for Section 9.5

1. Derive the influence at inclusion and exclusion measures computed by formula (9.31) for linear regression, $f_i(\boldsymbol{\beta}) = \mathbf{x}'_i\boldsymbol{\beta}$. Find the respective counterpart formulas in the previous section. Are the influences at exclusion measures given by (9.31) and (9.32) different for linear regression?

2. Reproduce Figure 9.12 by adopting the R code.

3*. Write an R code to compare the influence measures (9.31) and (9.32) with the exact leave-one-out computations for model (9.33) by adopting the R code.

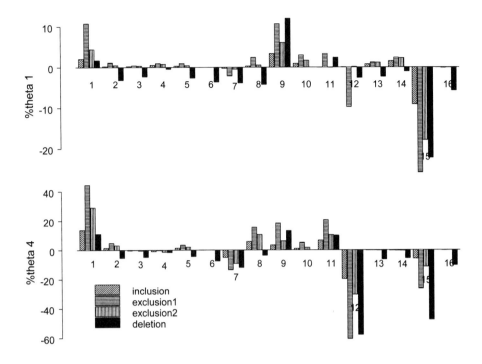

FIGURE 9.12. Case deletion diagnostics for a logistic nonlinear regression model (9.33). Four measures correlate, although the brute-force deletion is closest to the inclusion formula (9.31).

Plot measures (9.31) and (9.32) together with $\widehat{\boldsymbol{\theta}} - \widehat{\boldsymbol{\theta}}_{(i)}$ for $i = 1, 2, ..., n$ for all four parameters. Which parameter is most sensitive to case deletion? For each parameter, identify which case deletion is most influential.

9.6 Logistic regression for binary outcome

In this section we deal with the binary dependent variable. Thus, let y_i code the occurrence of a certain event: $y_i = 1$ means that the event took place, $y_i = 0$ means that it did not. For instance, $y_i = 1$ may mean that individual i has the disease, and $y_i = 0$ means individual i is disease-free. As before, the $m \times 1$ vector $\mathbf{x}_i$ denotes the correspondent vector of explanatory variables (covariates), such as age, weight, and smoking status. In logistic regression, the occurrence of the event y_i given $\mathbf{x}_i$ is modeled via probability, defined as

$$\Pr(y_i = 1) = \frac{e^{\boldsymbol{\beta}' \mathbf{x}_i}}{1 + e^{\boldsymbol{\beta}' \mathbf{x}_i}}, \qquad i = 1, ..., n, \tag{9.34}$$

where the $m \times 1$ vector $\boldsymbol{\beta}$ is the parameter of interest. Commonly, logistic regression (9.34) is estimated by maximum likelihood. The log-likelihood function for data $(y_i, \mathbf{x}_i)$ has the form $\boldsymbol{\beta}' \sum_{y_i=1} \mathbf{x}_i - \sum_{i=1}^{n} \ln(1 + e^{\boldsymbol{\beta}' \mathbf{x}_i})$, and the MLE $\widehat{\boldsymbol{\beta}}$ is determined from the score (estimating) equation,

$$\sum_{i=1}^{n} \frac{1}{1+e^{\beta' \mathbf{x}_i}} \mathbf{x}_i - \sum_{y_i=0} \mathbf{x}_i = \mathbf{0}. \tag{9.35}$$

We refer the reader to Section 7.1 for detail. The aim of this section is to describe techniques of detecting an influential observation in logistic regression. In other words, we answer the question of how an individual observation, y_i or $\mathbf{x}_i$, affects the MLE or another statistic, such as predicted probability. In a pioneering paper, Pregibon (1981) introduced the infinitesimal influence analysis and applied it to case deletion diagnostics for logistic regression. Here we extend his approach to the influence analysis of individual observations and misclassification of the dependent variable. Following our approach, we measure the infinitesimal influence via the derivative of $\widehat{\boldsymbol{\beta}}$ with respect to individual observation of either the dependent or the independent variable.

9.6.1   Influence of the covariate on the MLE

The influence of an individual observation x_{ik} on the MLE is measured as $\partial \widehat{\boldsymbol{\beta}}/\partial x_{ik}$. We find the derivative differentiating (9.35) with respect to x_{ik},

$$\frac{\partial \widehat{\boldsymbol{\beta}}}{\partial x_{ik}} = \mathbf{H}^{-1} \left(\mathbf{e}_k r_i - \frac{e^{\widehat{\boldsymbol{\beta}}' \mathbf{x}_i}}{(1+e^{\widehat{\boldsymbol{\beta}}' \mathbf{x}_i})^2} \mathbf{x}_i \widehat{\beta}_k \right), \tag{9.36}$$

where $r_i = y_i - e^{\widehat{\boldsymbol{\beta}}' \mathbf{x}_i}/(1+e^{\widehat{\boldsymbol{\beta}}' \mathbf{x}_i})$ is the ith residual of the logistic regression and the negative Hessian (information) matrix is defined as

$$\mathbf{H} = \sum_{i=1}^{n} \frac{e^{\widehat{\boldsymbol{\beta}}' \mathbf{x}_i}}{(1+e^{\widehat{\boldsymbol{\beta}}' \mathbf{x}_i})^2} \mathbf{x}_i \mathbf{x}_i'. \tag{9.37}$$

As the reader can see, formula (9.36) resembles its linear analog (9.15). Formula (9.36) has a simple interpretation: increasing x_{ik} by 1 would change the MLE by the value (9.36).

9.6.2   Influence on the predicted probability

In some instances we may be interested in the predicted probabilities, Johnson (1985). Then the characteristic of interest is $\widehat{p}_i = e^{\widehat{\boldsymbol{\beta}}' \mathbf{x}_i}/(1+e^{\widehat{\boldsymbol{\beta}}' \mathbf{x}_i})$, which may be analyzed with respect to the influence of misclassification of the binary variable, individual observation of covariate, or case deletion. We find the derivative of $\widehat{p}_i$ based on the derivative of the MLE by applying the chain rule. We start by calculating the influence of $\widehat{p}_i$ with respect to x_{ik} based on formula (9.36). Hence, applying the chain rule, we obtain

$$\frac{\partial \widehat{p}_i}{\partial x_{ik}} = \left(\frac{\partial \widehat{p}_i}{\partial \widehat{\boldsymbol{\beta}}} \right)' \left(\frac{\partial \widehat{\boldsymbol{\beta}}}{\partial x_{ik}} \right) = \frac{e^{\widehat{\boldsymbol{\beta}}' \mathbf{x}_i}}{(1+e^{\widehat{\boldsymbol{\beta}}' \mathbf{x}_i})^2} \mathbf{x}_i' \mathbf{H}^{-1} \left(r_i \mathbf{e}_k - \frac{e^{\widehat{\boldsymbol{\beta}}' \mathbf{x}_i}}{(1+e^{\widehat{\boldsymbol{\beta}}' \mathbf{x}_i})^2} \mathbf{x}_i \widehat{\beta}_k \right).$$

Now we find how $\widehat{p}_i$ is sensitive to misclassification q_i. Again, using the chain rule, one obtains

$$\frac{\partial \widehat{p}_i}{\partial q_i} = \left(\frac{\partial \widehat{p}_i}{\partial \widehat{\boldsymbol{\beta}}}\right)' \left(\frac{\partial \widehat{\boldsymbol{\beta}}}{\partial q_i}\right) = \frac{e^{\widehat{\boldsymbol{\beta}}'\mathbf{x}_i}(e^{\widehat{\boldsymbol{\beta}}'\mathbf{x}_i} - 1)}{(1 + e^{\widehat{\boldsymbol{\beta}}'\mathbf{x}_i})^3} \mathbf{x}_i' \mathbf{H}^{-1} \mathbf{x}_i. \tag{9.38}$$

Recall that in the linear model, the influence of the dependent variable on the predicted value is measured via the diagonal element of the hat matrix, the leverage. Therefore, (9.38) can be viewed as a generalization of the leverage for logistic regression. It is interesting to note that the quadratic form $\mathbf{x}_i'\mathbf{H}^{-1}\mathbf{x}_i$ is similar to the linear model; however, the scalar factor in (9.38) is specific to the logistic regression and reflects the binary nature of the dependent variable. This influence is minimal when y_i is equally likely to take the value zero or 1 (the numerator is zero).

9.6.3 Influence of the case deletion on the MLE

The theory of I-influence for the case deletion in logistic regression was developed by Pregibon (1981). Following Pregibon, let i be fixed and w_i be the weight of the ith case (other cases do not change). Then the MLE becomes a function of w_i and we aim to find $\partial\widehat{\boldsymbol{\beta}}/\partial w_i$. If $y_i = 1$, the score equation takes the form

$$\sum_{j \neq i} \frac{1}{1 + e^{\boldsymbol{\beta}'\mathbf{x}_i}}\mathbf{x}_i + \frac{w_i}{1 + e^{\boldsymbol{\beta}'\mathbf{x}_i}}\mathbf{x}_i - \sum_{y_i = 0} \mathbf{x}_i = \mathbf{0}.$$

It is easy to write a similar score equation if $y_i = 0$. Differentiation with respect to w_i leads to two formulas, corresponding to deletion at inclusion and exclusion,

$$\left.\frac{\partial\widehat{\boldsymbol{\beta}}}{\partial w_i}\right|_{w_i=1} = r_i \mathbf{H}^{-1}\mathbf{x}_i, \qquad \left.\frac{\partial\widehat{\boldsymbol{\beta}}}{\partial w_i}\right|_{w_i=0} \simeq \frac{r_i}{(1 - p_i)^2}\mathbf{H}^{-1}\mathbf{x}_i,$$

where r_i is the ith residual defined above. It is easy to calculate the derivative for the predicted probability based on the chain rule. For example, as follows from the first formula, if $\widehat{\boldsymbol{\beta}}$ is the MLE for all data, the estimate after the ith case is deleted would be $\widehat{\boldsymbol{\beta}} + r_i\mathbf{H}^{-1}\mathbf{x}_i$. The influence of the case deletion by omitting the ith case and recomputing the regression has been discussed by Fay (2002).

9.6.4 Sensitivity to misclassification

In some applications the assignment 0/1 to the response variable may be under question and not trivial. Consequently, one may ask how sensitive our statistical inference is to flipping 0/1 in an observation of the dependent variable. Since y_i takes values 0 and 1, a straightforward solution would be to recalculate the logistic regression replacing $y_i = 1$ with $y_i = 0$, and vice versa, which would involve a number of reestimations equal to the number of observations. However, it is possible to avoid such massive calculation, employing the idea of misclassification, similar to what we did in Section 9.4.3.

Indeed, let us fix i and assume that the observed event y_i is *symmetrically misclassified* with probability q_i, assuming that other observations are well classified

($q_j = 0$ for $j \neq i$). It is assumed that the true, "well-classified" binary event z_i is not observable with probability modeled via logistic regression as $\Pr(z_i = 1) = e^{\boldsymbol{\beta}'\mathbf{x}_i}/(1 + e^{\boldsymbol{\beta}'\mathbf{x}_i})$. The condition on misclassification can be written as

$$\Pr(y_i = 1 | z_i = 0) = \Pr(y_i = 0 | z_i = 1) = q_i, \qquad (9.39)$$

where q_i is assumed known. Then, using standard formulas of the theory of probability, we find the marginal probability of the observed event $y_i = 1$ as

$$
\begin{aligned}
\Pr(y_i &= 1) \\
&= \Pr(y_i = 1, z_i = 1) + \Pr(y_i = 1, z_i = 0) \\
&= \Pr(y_i = 1 | z_i = 1) \Pr(z_i = 1) + \Pr(y_i = 1 | z_i = 0) \Pr(z_i = 0) \\
&= (1 - q_i)\frac{e^{\boldsymbol{\beta}'\mathbf{x}_i}}{1 + e^{\boldsymbol{\beta}'\mathbf{x}_i}} + q_i\frac{1}{1 + e^{\boldsymbol{\beta}'\mathbf{x}_i}} = \frac{(1 - q_i)e^{\boldsymbol{\beta}'\mathbf{x}_i} + q_i}{1 + e^{\boldsymbol{\beta}'\mathbf{x}_i}}. \qquad (9.40)
\end{aligned}
$$

We notice that in special cases, when misclassification is absent ($q_i = 0$), probability (9.40) collapses to (9.34). Conversely, $q_i = 1$ corresponds to the reverse coding. The idea of introducing a misclassification parameter into the logistic regression model belongs to Copas (1988). However, he assumed that $q_i = q$ and all observations were misclassified. We, in contrast, are looking for the influence of *individual* observations, and therefore, $q_j = 0$ for $j \neq i$. Also unlike Copas, we do not compute the MLE under misclassification but characterize the influence by the rate at which the MLE changes upon a small misclassification of y_i.

Now we assess how sensitive the MLE is to a low probability of misclassification q_i using formula (9.40). For convenience of notation, we use vector probabilities $\{q_j, j = 1, ..., n\}$, where $q_j = 0$ if $j \neq i$ and $q_i > 0$. Then, the log-likelihood function of the logistic regression under misclassification (9.40) is given as

$$l(\boldsymbol{\beta}) = \sum_{j=1}^{n} \left[y_j \ln \frac{(1 - q_j)e^{\boldsymbol{\beta}'\mathbf{x}_j} + q_j}{1 + e^{\boldsymbol{\beta}'\mathbf{x}_j}} + (1 - y_j) \ln \frac{q_j e^{\boldsymbol{\beta}'\mathbf{x}_j} + (1 - q_j)}{1 + e^{\boldsymbol{\beta}'\mathbf{x}_j}} \right]. \qquad (9.41)$$

We notice that the MLE $\widehat{\boldsymbol{\beta}} = \widehat{\boldsymbol{\beta}}(q_i)$, as the solution to the score equation

$$\sum_{j=1}^{n} \left(\frac{y_j(1 - q_j)e^{\boldsymbol{\beta}'\mathbf{x}_j}}{(1 - q_j)e^{\boldsymbol{\beta}'\mathbf{x}_j} + q_j} + \frac{(1 - y_j)q_j e^{\boldsymbol{\beta}'\mathbf{x}_j}}{q_j e^{\boldsymbol{\beta}'\mathbf{x}_j} + (1 - q_j)} - \frac{e^{\boldsymbol{\beta}'\mathbf{x}_j}}{1 + e^{\boldsymbol{\beta}'\mathbf{x}_j}} \right) \mathbf{x}_j = \mathbf{0} \qquad (9.42)$$

is a function of q_i. Therefore, the derivative $\partial\widehat{\boldsymbol{\beta}}/\partial q_i$ calculated at $q_i = 0$ can be interpreted as an influence measure of y_i on the MLE. Differentiating the score equation (9.42) with respect to q_i, after some algebra we come to the derivative desired,

$$\left. \frac{\partial\widehat{\boldsymbol{\beta}}}{\partial q_i} \right|_{q_i = 0} = (1 - 2y_i)e^{(1 - 2y_i)\widehat{\boldsymbol{\beta}}'\mathbf{x}_i}\mathbf{H}^{-1}\mathbf{x}_i, \qquad (9.43)$$

where $\mathbf{H}$ is the information matrix defined by (9.37). As follows from (9.43), the coefficient at $\mathbf{H}^{-1}\mathbf{x}_i$ is $\exp(\widehat{\boldsymbol{\beta}}'\mathbf{x}_i)$ if $y_i = 0$, and $-\exp(-\widehat{\boldsymbol{\beta}}'\mathbf{x}_i)$ if $y_i = 1$. We interpret (9.43) as by how much the MLE changes upon flipping 0/1 in the ith observation.

The reader is referred to the top-left graph in Figure 9.13 as an example, where the MLE under misclassification, as the solution to the score equation (9.42), is plotted against the probability of misclassification for the fourth observation of the response variable, q_4 (Finney data; see the example below). The straight line has a slope equal to the derivative of the MLE at zero calculated by formula (9.43).

In applications to clinical studies, where the response variable codes the occurrence of a disease, the misclassification may not be symmetric. For example, if y denotes the presence of cancer, the doctor usually does not make a mistake when there is no cancer: namely, $\Pr(y = 1|z = 0) = 0$. On the other hand, the doctor may overlook the cancer, which translates mathematically into $\Pr(y = 0|z = 1) = q > 0$. This leads to an asymmetrical misclassification

$$\Pr(y_i = 1|z_i = 0) = 0, \quad \Pr(y_i = 0|z_i = 1) = q_i,$$

with the marginal probability $\Pr(y_i = 1) = (1 - q_i)e^{\beta' x_i}/(1 + e^{\beta' x_i})$. It is quite straightforward to apply the influence analysis above to this asymmetrical misclassification.

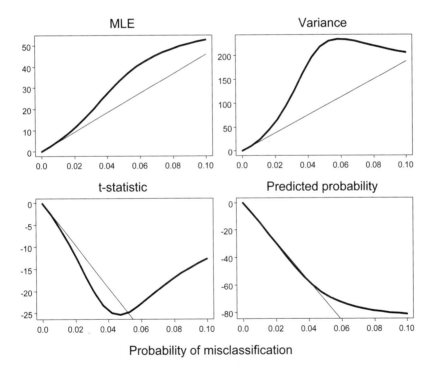

FIGURE 9.13. Percent change of the MLE of β_2 and other quantities under misclassification of the fourth observation in the response variable (Finney data). Bold: %MLE change as the solution to the score equation for different probabilities of misclassification, q_i. The slope of the straight line is the derivative evaluated at zero ($q_i = 0$). A nonlinear relationship of the characteristics as a function of q_i is evident, especially for larger probability values.

Sensitivity of the variance and significance testing

Often, we are interested not only in the odds ratio (exponent of the beta coefficient, see the detail in Section 7.1) *per se*, but also in significance testing. Does the new drug statistically significantly decrease the post-treatment disease recurrence? Does the exposure or a risk factor have a statistically significant effect on the incidence rate? Clearly, misclassification may jeopardize our statistical testing. The aim of this section is to provide a sensitivity analysis of the MLE variance and t-statistic to misclassification, as a generalization of Section 9.4.7.

We start with the sensitivity of the MLE variance to misclassification described by model (9.40). The MLE variance of the kth logistic regression coefficient, σ_k^2, under misclassification is calculated as the (k, k)th diagonal element of the inverse information matrix, defined as the negative derivative of the score equation (9.42). Therefore, differentiating (9.42) with respect to β, the MLE variance of the kth beta regression coefficient is the (k, k)th element of the matrix inverse to

$$\mathbf{G} = \sum_{j=1}^{n} \left[\frac{\widehat{e}_j}{(1 + \widehat{e}_j)^2} - y_j \frac{q_j(1 - q_j)\widehat{e}_j}{((1 - q_j)\widehat{e}_j + q_j)^2} - (1 - y_j) \frac{q_j(1 - q_j)\widehat{e}_j}{(q_j\widehat{e}_j + (1 - q_j))^2} \mathbf{x}_j \mathbf{x}_j' \right],$$

where $\widehat{e}_j = \exp(\widehat{\boldsymbol{\beta}}' \mathbf{x}_j)$, and $\widehat{\boldsymbol{\beta}}$ is the MLE under misclassification of the ith response variable with probability q_i. Then the MLE variance of the kth regression coefficient is $\mathbf{e}_k' \mathbf{G}^{-1} \mathbf{e}_k$, where $\mathbf{e}_k$ is the Kronecker vector. Therefore, the sensitivity of the MLE variance to misclassification is given by

$$\left. \frac{\partial \sigma_k^2}{\partial q_i} \right|_{q_i=0} = -\mathbf{e}_k' \mathbf{H}^{-1} \left(\left. \frac{\partial \mathbf{G}}{\partial q_i} \right|_{q_i=0} \right) \mathbf{H}^{-1} \mathbf{e}_k, \tag{9.44}$$

where

$$\left. \frac{\partial \mathbf{G}}{\partial q_i} \right|_{q_i=0} = \sum_{j=1}^{N} \left[\frac{\widehat{e}_j(1 - \widehat{e}_j)}{(1 + \widehat{e}_j)^3} \mathbf{x}_j \mathbf{x}_j' \mathbf{x}_j' \left(\left. \frac{\partial \widehat{\boldsymbol{\beta}}}{\partial q_i} \right|_{q_i=0} \right) \right] - (y_i \widehat{e}_i^{-1} + (1 - y_i)\widehat{e}_i) \mathbf{x}_i \mathbf{x}_i'. \tag{9.45}$$

The derivative $\partial \boldsymbol{\beta} / \partial q_i$ is defined by (9.43), and the matrix $\mathbf{H}$ is defined by (9.37).

Now we define a measure of sensitivity for the t-statistic. Following the line of our approach, we measure this sensitivity as the derivative of the t-statistic to the probability of misclassification at zero. Since the t-statistic is the ratio of the MLE to the square root of the variance, the desired derivative is

$$\frac{\partial t_k}{\partial q_i} = \left(\widehat{\beta}_k^{-1} \frac{\partial \widehat{\beta}_k}{\partial q_i} - \frac{1}{2\sigma_k^2} \frac{\partial \sigma_k^2}{\partial q_i} \right) t_k, \tag{9.46}$$

where the derivative of the MLE is defined by (9.43), and the derivative of the variance σ_k^2 is defined by (9.44). Note that all quantities are computed at $q_i = 0$, and σ_k^2 and t_k are the MLE variance and t-statistic of the standard logistic regression. The reader is referred to Figure 9.13 (the top-right and bottom-left graphs), where the variance and the t-statistic are plotted against the probability of misclassification with the derivative at zero calculated by formulas (9.44) and (9.46), respectively. Plotting these derivatives against i can identify influential observations of the response variable in terms of the sensitivity of the variance or the t-statistic to a small misclassification of the response variable.

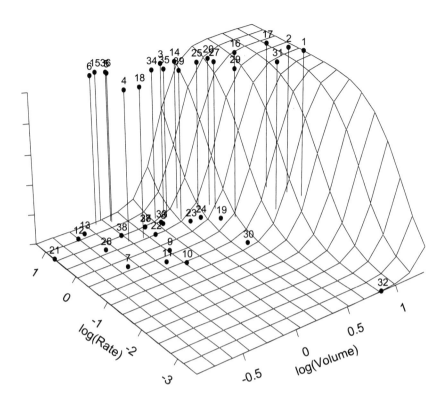

FIGURE 9.14. 3D plot of logistic regression model (Finney data). Observations are shown by the filled circles. Notice that case 32 stands apart from the bulk of the data.

Sensitivity to the predicted probability

Sometimes we are interested in the prediction of probabilities (Johnson, 1985). Then the characteristic of interest is $\widehat{p}_i = e^{\widehat{\beta}'\mathbf{x}_i}/(1 + e^{\widehat{\beta}'\mathbf{x}_i})$, which may also be analyzed in terms of its sensitivity to the misclassification. Following our approach, we measure the sensitivity as the derivative of $\widehat{p}_i$ with respect to misclassification probability, q_i, calculated at $q_i = 0$. Applying the chain rule and formula (9.43), we find that

$$\left.\frac{\partial \widehat{p}_i}{\partial q_i}\right|_{q_i=0} = \left(\left.\frac{\partial \widehat{p}_i}{\partial \widehat{\beta}}\right|_{q_i=0}\right)' \left(\left.\frac{\partial \widehat{\beta}}{\partial q_i}\right|_{q_i=0}\right) = (1-2y_i)\frac{e^{2(1-y_i)\widehat{\beta}'\mathbf{x}_i}}{(1+e^{\widehat{\beta}'\mathbf{x}})^2}\mathbf{x}_i'\mathbf{H}^{-1}\mathbf{x}_i. \quad (9.47)$$

Measure (9.47) may be considered as a generalization of leverage in linear regression. Recall that for the linear regression model, the leverage is the derivative of the predicted value $\widehat{y}_i$ with respect to the value of the response variable,

$$\frac{\partial \widehat{y}_i}{\partial y_i} = \mathbf{x}_i'\mathbf{H}^{-1}\mathbf{x}_i. \quad (9.48)$$

Our formula (9.47) is similar to (9.48), with the scalar factor pertinent to logistic regression, where, instead of y_i, it is the probability of misclassification under consideration. Thus, derivative (9.47) can be called the *logistic regression lever-age*. Derivative (9.47) has a clear interpretation: flipping 0/1 in the ith observation would lead to a change in the predicted probability by amount (9.47). The reader is referred to Figure 9.13 (right-bottom graph), where the predicted probability is plotted against the probability of misclassification, with the derivative at zero calculated by formula (9.47).

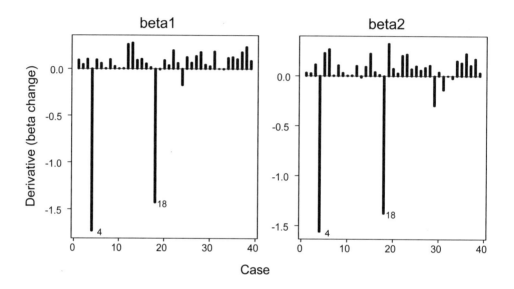

FIGURE 9.15. Pregibon's coefficient sensitivity to case deletion. Cases 4 and 18 are influential because their deletion from the data changes the regression coefficients substantially (downwards).

9.6.5   *Example: Finney data*

To illustrate influence analysis for logistic regression, we take an example from Pregibon (1981) based on Finney data. The dependent variable y indicates the occurrence (1) or nonoccurrence (0) of vasoconstriction in the skin of the digits; x_1 and x_2 are the logs of the Volume and Rate of air inspired on a transient vasoconstriction; number of cases $n = 40$. The logistic regression has the form $\text{logit}(y) = \beta_1 \ln(\text{Volume}) + \beta_2 \ln(\text{Rate}) + \beta_3$ with the MLE $\widehat{\beta}_1 = 5.18$ and $\widehat{\beta}_2 = 4.56$; the 3D plot is depicted in Figure 9.14.

The analysis of case deletion and infinitesimal deletion was conducted by Pregibon. As shown in Figure 9.15, cases 4 and 18 are influential because their deletion significantly affects the MLE (the derivatives were computed by formulas from Section 9.6.3).

Below we show the R code to compute the logistic regression and to run the leave-one-out analysis. The I-influence measures depicted in Figure 9.15 should correlated with the exact deletion results (Problem 1).

```
finney=function()
{
dump("finney","c:\\MixedModels\\Chapter09\\finney.r")
dat=read.table("c:\\MixedModels\\Chapter09\\Finney.dat")
n=nrow(dat)
lnv=log(dat$Volume)
lnr=log(dat$Rate)
dat=cbind(dat,lnv,lnr)
outL=glm(y~lnv+lnr,data=dat,family=binomial)
beta1OUT=matrix(nrow=n,ncol=2)
for(i in 1:n)
{
    w=rep(1,n);w[i]=0
    outLi=glm(y~lnv+lnr,weights=w,data=dat,family=binomial)
    beta1OUT[i,]=coef(outLi)[2:3]
}
beta1OUT
}
```

Now we concentrate on the I-influence of misclassification and individual observations of Volume and Rate based on formulas (9.36) and (9.43). Notice that the former formula should be modified because the covariates enter regression in logarithms. The influence of Volume and Rate on the MLE is depicted in Figure 9.16, where $(\partial \widehat{\beta}_j / dx)/\widehat{\beta}_j \times 100\%$ is displayed for each beta coefficient ($j = 1, 2$). As one can see, both estimates are very sensitive to observation change; a 1 unit change in the 4th or 18th observation of Volume would lead to a decrease in $\widehat{\beta}_1$ to approximately -150% (the top-left graph). Interestingly, these observations of Volume do not affect $\widehat{\beta}_2$ as much. Now we investigate the effect of misclassification using formula (9.43). Both $\widehat{\beta}_1$ and $\widehat{\beta}_2$ are highly sensitive to misclassification of the 4th and 18th observations of y. This finding is confirmed by the 3D plot in Figure 9.14: observations 4 and 18 are surrounded by observations with $y = 0$ and seem to appear in the "wrong" place; therefore, replacing $y_4 = 1$ and $y_{18} = 1$ with $y_4 = 0$ and $y_{18} = 0$ would change the MLE coefficients dramatically. Possible misclassification of the response variable in cases 4 and 18 also has a considerable effect on t-statistics.

Summing up, sensitivity to misclassification may explain further why deletion of a specific case is influential.

Problems for Section 9.6

1. Adopt the R code above to show the exact values of the beta-coefficient change and their infinitesimal change on the same plot, as in Figure 9.15.

2. Write an R code to reproduce Figure 9.13.

3*. Develop I-influence measures for probit regression.

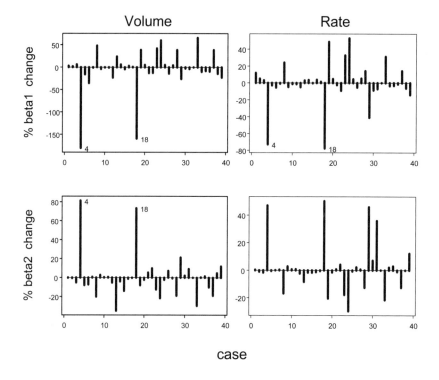

FIGURE 9.16. Bar influence plot for logistic regression (Finney data). Individual change in obervation of Volume and/or Rate may significantly affect the MLEs.

9.7 Influence of correlation structure

One assumption of ordinary regression is that the errors are uncorrelated. What is the influence of this assumption on the OLS estimate? What are the consequences of a possibly missing correlation structure? In particular, this question might be reasonable when regression analysis is applied to time series data as follows.

We write the standard linear regression model as $y_t = \boldsymbol{\beta}'\mathbf{x}_t + \varepsilon_t$, where $t = 1, ..., T$ denotes the time index. Let us assume that the correlation structure is induced by the first-order autoregression, $\varepsilon_t = \rho\varepsilon_t + \eta_t$, where η_t are iid random variables with zero mean and variance σ^2. The (i, j)th element of the $T \times T$ correlation matrix $\boldsymbol{\Omega} = \boldsymbol{\Omega}(\rho)$ for $\epsilon_1, ..., \epsilon_T$ is equal to $\rho^{|i-j|}$, and the weighted least squares estimator has the form

$$\widehat{\boldsymbol{\beta}}(\rho) = (\mathbf{X}'\boldsymbol{\Omega}^{-1}(\rho)\mathbf{X})^{-1}\mathbf{X}'\boldsymbol{\Omega}^{-1}(\rho)\mathbf{y},$$

where $\boldsymbol{\Omega}(0) = \mathbf{I}$. Clearly, a small departure of ρ from zero changes the estimate at the rate

$$\left. \frac{d\widehat{\boldsymbol{\beta}}(\rho)}{d\rho} \right|_{\rho=0} = -(\mathbf{X}'\mathbf{X})^{-1}\mathbf{X}'\mathbf{u}, \tag{9.49}$$

where $\mathbf{u}' = (r_2, r_1 + r_3, ..., r_{T-1})$ and r_t is the tth OLS residual. A similar formula can be obtained for nonlinear regression. Thus, one can assess the influence of a possible missing correlation structure on the beta coefficients by examining the components of vector (9.49) prior to ρ estimation, as a part of preliminary data analysis.

Problems for Section 9.7

1. Prove that the correlation coefficient between y_i and y_j is $\rho^{|i-j|}$.
2. Find the expected value of the rate vector (9.49). Find $\mathbf{X}$ for which this expected value is zero (use the fact that $\mathbf{X}'\mathbf{r} = \mathbf{0}$).

9.8   Influence of measurement error

Covariates often contain measurement errors. There is a well-established theory of errors-in-variables (Fuller, 1987; Carroll et al., 1995). Generally, if there is measurement error in a covariate (independent or explanatory variable), parameters of the model are not identifiable unless additional information is provided. In particular, the MLE exists if the variance of measurement error, σ^2, is known. In practice, a calibration or validation study might be undertaken to obtain an estimate of that variance (Spiegelman et al., 2000). However, since such studies are usually expensive, it might be very useful to assess the effect of measurement error on parameter estimates *prior* to the validation study. It is well known that in simple linear regression with errors-in-variables, the OLS slope is attenuated (bias toward null). In multivariate linear regression, due to correlation among covariates, the effect of measurement error may not be mitigated so easily. The effect of measurement error becomes more complicated in nonlinear models, such as generalized linear models or nonlinear regressions. The aim of this section is to show how to assess the effect of measurement error on the MLE via the I-influence approach without knowing σ^2. Our plan is as follows:

- Set up the model with a known error variance σ^2.

- Calculate $d\widehat{\boldsymbol{\beta}}(\sigma^2 = 0)/d\sigma^2$, where $\widehat{\boldsymbol{\beta}}$ is the MLE, as a function of σ^2.

Then the derivative vector would indicate how the MLE is sensitive to small measurement error. In fact, by computing this derivative, we obtain the first-order approximation to the MLE in the neighborhood of small variance: $\widehat{\boldsymbol{\beta}} \simeq \widehat{\boldsymbol{\beta}}_0 + \sigma^2 d\widehat{\boldsymbol{\beta}}(\sigma^2 = 0)/d\sigma^2$, where $\widehat{\boldsymbol{\beta}}_0$ is the MLE assuming no measurement error (naive estimate). This method provides (a) information on what coefficients are most sensitive to measurement error, (b) the direction of change in the naive ML estimate, and (c) the crude coefficient estimate given the value of the error variance. Following the line of I-influence approach, we do not require estimation of σ^2 because the derivative is evaluated at the naive MLE.

Let the set of covariates consist of a fixed vector $\mathbf{u}_i$ measured without error and an unobserved scalar covariate x_i measured with an error/surrogate. To simplify, we shall assume the Berkson measurement error model (Berkson, 1950; Fuller, 1987): $x_i = z_i + \sigma s_i$ where z_i is the design variable and s_i is the standardized measurement error with zero mean and unit variance. Thus, the variance of the measurement error is σ^2. We do not specify the distribution of the measurement error, so our analysis is distribution-free. The true regression model is expressed in terms of x_i

and to derive the log-likelihood function for available observations (y_i, z_i), we have to integrate out the measurement error s.

The binary model is defined via conditional probability: $\Pr(y_i = 1 \mid x_i) = H(\boldsymbol{\gamma}'\mathbf{u}_i + \tau x_i)$, where H is the probability function and $\boldsymbol{\beta} = (\boldsymbol{\gamma}', \tau)'$ is the vector of the model coefficients. If $H = \exp/(1+\exp)$, we come to logistic regression; if $H = \Phi$, where $\Phi(\cdot)$ is the normal distribution function, we come to probit regression (see Section 7.1). The *observed* model can be written as

$$\Pr(y_i = 1 \mid z_i) = E_s H(\boldsymbol{\gamma}'\mathbf{u}_i + \tau z_i + \sigma \tau s)), \tag{9.50}$$

where E_s means expectation over s; for a special case, $s \sim \mathcal{N}(0, 1)$. As shown in Section 9.10, the derivative of the MLE with respect to the variance of the measurement error, in a large sample, can be approximated as

$$\left. \frac{d\widehat{\boldsymbol{\beta}}}{d\sigma^2} \right|_{\sigma^2 = 0} \simeq -\frac{1}{2}\tau^2 \mathbf{H}^{-1} \left(\sum_{i=1}^{n} \frac{H_i'' H_i'}{H_i(1 - H_i)} \begin{bmatrix} \mathbf{u}_i \\ z_i \end{bmatrix} \right), \tag{9.51}$$

where H_i and its derivatives (H_i'' and H_i') are evaluated at $\widehat{\boldsymbol{\gamma}}'\mathbf{u}_i + \widehat{\tau} z_i$. The MLE $\widehat{\boldsymbol{\gamma}}$ and $\widehat{\tau}$ are naive estimates (no measurement error), and the information matrix $\mathbf{H}$ is defined as

$$\mathbf{H} = \sum_{i=1}^{n} \frac{H_i'^2}{H_i(1 - H_i)} \begin{bmatrix} \mathbf{u}_i \\ z_i \end{bmatrix} \begin{bmatrix} \mathbf{u}_i \\ z_i \end{bmatrix}'. \tag{9.52}$$

We illustrate measure (9.51) by the probit model ($H = \Phi$) with a normally distributed measurement error. This choice means that the *observed* model (9.50) is again probit; see the discussion around formula (7.15). More precisely, in our notation,

$$\Pr(y_i = 1 \mid z_i) = \Phi\left(\frac{\boldsymbol{\gamma}'\mathbf{u}_i + \tau z_i}{\sqrt{1 + \sigma^2 \tau^2}} \right),$$

meaning that the (naive) MLE ignoring measurement error will be attenuated by the factor $(1 + \sigma^2 \tau^2)^{-1/2}$. This implies that the MLE as a function of σ^2 in large samples can be expressed via the naive MLE as

$$\widehat{\gamma}_{ML} = \frac{\widehat{\gamma}_0}{\sqrt{1 - \sigma^2 \widehat{\tau}_0^2}}, \qquad \widehat{\tau}_{ML} = \frac{\widehat{\tau}_0}{\sqrt{1 - \sigma^2 \widehat{\tau}_0^2}}, \tag{9.53}$$

where $\widehat{\gamma}_0$ and $\widehat{\tau}_0$ are the MLE at zero variance, i.e., based on the model $\Phi(\boldsymbol{\gamma}'\mathbf{u}_i + \tau z_i)$. In particular, sensitivity of the MLE τ to the variance of measurement error can be assessed as

$$\left. \frac{d\widehat{\tau}_{ML}}{d\sigma^2} \right|_{\sigma^2 = 0} = \frac{1}{2}\widehat{\tau}_0^3, \tag{9.54}$$

the derivative of $\widehat{\tau}_{ML}$ with respect to σ^2 evaluated at zero, as is easy to see from (9.53). It is instructive to verify that our approximation formula (9.51) gives the

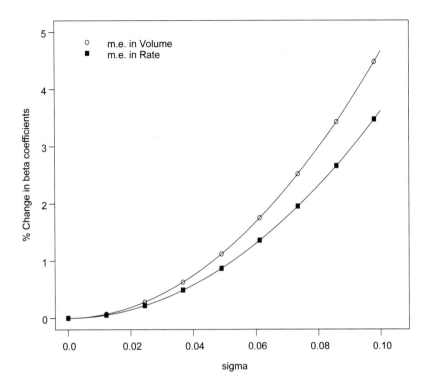

FIGURE 9.17. Impact of a small measurement error (m.e.) in ln(Volume) and ln(Rate) on the MLE for a logistic regression model, Finney data. The MLE is more sensitive to measurement error in Volume. Approximately 10% m.e. in Volume would lead to a 5% increase in beta coefficients.

same result for the probit model $H_i = \Phi_i' = \phi_i$ and $H_i'' = -(\boldsymbol{\gamma}'\mathbf{u}_i + \tau z_i)\phi_i$, so that

$$\mathbf{H}^{-1}\left(\sum_{i=1}^n \frac{H_i'' H_i'}{H_i(1-H_i)}\begin{bmatrix} \mathbf{u}_i \\ z_i \end{bmatrix}\right) = -\left(\sum_{i=1}^n \frac{\phi_i^2}{\Phi_i(1-\Phi_i)}\begin{bmatrix} \mathbf{u}_i \\ z_i \end{bmatrix}\begin{bmatrix} \mathbf{u}_i \\ z_i \end{bmatrix}'\right)^{-1}$$

$$\times \left(\frac{\phi_i^2}{\Phi_i(1-\Phi_i)}\begin{bmatrix} \mathbf{u}_i \\ z_i \end{bmatrix}\begin{bmatrix} \mathbf{u}_i \\ z_i \end{bmatrix}'\begin{bmatrix} \boldsymbol{\gamma} \\ \tau \end{bmatrix}\right) = -\begin{bmatrix} \boldsymbol{\gamma} \\ \tau \end{bmatrix},$$

which leads to the exact derivative using the relationship (9.53).

For logistic regression, we have

$$\left.\frac{d\widehat{\boldsymbol{\beta}}}{d\sigma^2}\right|_{\sigma^2=0} = -\frac{1}{2}\tau^2 \mathbf{H}^{-1}\sum_{i=1}^n \frac{e_i(1-e_i)}{(1+e_i)^3}\begin{bmatrix} \mathbf{u}_i \\ z_i \end{bmatrix}, \tag{9.55}$$

where $\mathbf{H}$ is the information matrix for the naive MLE defined by (9.37), and $e_i = \exp(\widehat{\boldsymbol{\gamma}}'\mathbf{u}_i + \widehat{\tau}z_i)$. Interestingly, measurement error will have little effect for symmetric data, $e_i \simeq 1$, or equivalently, $\widehat{\boldsymbol{\gamma}}'\mathbf{u}_i + \widehat{\tau}z_i \simeq 0$.

We illustrate the sensitivity analysis for the logistic regression model to measurement error (m.e.) by Pregibon's example of Section 9.6.5. Multiplicative error is assumed (additive error on the log scale). Figure 9.17 shows that the relative bias is close to a quadratic function of σ. Interestingly, the MLE is more sensitive to m.e. in Volume; a 10% m.e. would lead to a 4.5% increase in the MLE.

There is an indication that the approximation based on (9.51) is fairly good for other real-life data. We refer the reader to the graphs on pp. 91 and 93 in the book by Carroll et al. (1995), where the ML estimates of a logistic regression model are displayed as functions of the variance of measurement error (Framingham Heart Study data). Those functions look quite linear in the neighborhood of zero, and therefore a linear approximation based on (9.51) should be pretty accurate. Again, formula (9.51) does not require recalculation, knowledge of the variance of measurement error, or simulations.

Problems for Section 9.8

1. Set up the Berkson measurement error scheme for a linear model, $\boldsymbol{\gamma}'\mathbf{u}_i + \tau z_i$. Does the OLS estimator imply bias for $\boldsymbol{\gamma}$ and τ? Do the results hold for a quadratic regression $\boldsymbol{\gamma}'\mathbf{u}_i + \tau z_i + \varphi z_i^2$?

2. Find/approximate the expected sensitivity (9.55).

3*. The data `alckid.dat` contains information on underage alcohol drinking for 5,469 U.S. teenagers. The variables are: yn=1 if ever drunk (0=never), agen=age-10, sensn=1 if a sensation seeker (0 otherwise), frn=number of friends who drinks, alcmov= exposure to alcohol scenes in movies on the log scale. The R code below reads the data and runs the logistic regression model. To get started:

```
alckid=function()
{
  dump("alckid","c:\\MixedModels\\Chapter09\\alckid.r")
  dat=read.csv("c:\\MixedModels\\Chapter09\\alckid.dat")
  outL=glm(yn~agen+sensn+frn+alcmov,family=binomial,data=dat)
  summary(outL)
}
```

An interested reader can get more insights on the association between adolescent drinking and movie watching from recent papers by Sargent et al. (2012) and Demidenko et al. (2012). The information on drinking was self-recorded and understandably subject to underreporting ('misclassification,' in our language). Use results of Section 9.6.4 to study the influence of misclassification.

4*. Write an R code to test (9.55) through simulations. Compute the average ML as a function of σ^2, as in Figure 9.17, and plot the tangent line with the expected slope (9.55). Use Finney data in the file `Finney.dat` on the log scale for `Volume` and `Rate` (use `read.table` to read the file). Use probit regression and the relationship between probit and logit for the approximation (9.55).

9.9   Influence analysis for the LME model

In this section we develop I-influence analysis for the Linear Mixed Effects (LME) model in formulation (2.5). The influence analysis for the LME model based on the local influence approach has been discussed extensively in two books by Verbeke and Molenberghs (2000) and Pan and Fang (2002). The application of local influence analysis to a nonlinear mixed effects model has been discussed recently by Lee and Xu (2003); Turkan and Toktamis (2012) discuss the local influence approach to the linear mixed model. The discussion below follows a paper by Demidenko and Stukel (2005).

Recall that the local influence approach measures the sensitivity by the maximum curvature of the log-likelihood function. The flexibility of the I-influence is that it allows examination of the impact in a small change of a single observation or individual (cluster) on any statistic or parameter of interest, regardless of the distribution. For example, one can consider the I-influence of the dependent/independent variable or case deletion on the MLE, variance estimate, predicted value, estimates of random effects, etc. The attractive feature of the I-influence is that it specifies what influences what and with what magnitude. To be concrete, we assume model (2.14) with parameters estimated by maximum likelihood. Since the information matrix for $\boldsymbol{\beta}$ and the variance parameters $(\sigma^2, \mathbf{D})$ is block diagonal, we may treat variance parameters as fixed when examining the influence of the MLE.

We start by constructing an analog of leverage for the LME model. As mentioned earlier, the leverage in a standard linear model can be viewed as an infinitesimal influence of a small change in the observation of the dependent variable on the predicted value, or symbolically, $p_i = \partial \widehat{y}_i / \partial y_i$. Analogously for the LME model, we define the leverage *matrix* as

$$\mathbf{P}_i = \frac{\partial \widehat{\mathbf{y}}_i}{\partial \mathbf{y}_i},$$

where $\widehat{\mathbf{y}}_i = \mathbf{X}_i \widehat{\boldsymbol{\beta}}$ is the predicted value, and

$$\widehat{\boldsymbol{\beta}} = \mathbf{H}^{-1}\mathbf{s}$$

is the MLE, where

$$\mathbf{H} = \sum_{i=1}^{N} \mathbf{X}_i' \mathbf{V}_i^{-1} \mathbf{X}_i^{-1}, \quad \mathbf{s} = \sum_{i=1}^{N} \mathbf{X}_i' \mathbf{V}_i^{-1} \mathbf{y}_i, \quad \mathbf{V}_i = \mathbf{I} + \mathbf{Z}_i \widehat{\mathbf{D}} \mathbf{Z}_i'.$$

Then, as is easy to see, the leverage matrix is

$$\mathbf{P}_i = \mathbf{X}_i \mathbf{H}^{-1} \mathbf{X}_i' \mathbf{V}_i^{-1}, \quad i = 1, ..., N. \tag{9.56}$$

The sum of the traces of the leverage matrices is equal to the dimension of vector $\boldsymbol{\beta}$,

$$
\begin{aligned}
\mathrm{tr}\left(\sum_{i=1}^{N} \mathbf{P}_i\right) &= \sum_{i=1}^{N} \mathrm{tr}\mathbf{P}_i = \sum_{i=1}^{N} \mathrm{tr}\left(\mathbf{H}^{-1}\mathbf{X}_i'\mathbf{V}_i^{-1}\mathbf{X}_i\right) \\
&= \mathrm{tr}\left(\mathbf{H}^{-1}\sum_{i=1}^{N}\mathbf{X}_i'\mathbf{V}_i^{-1}\mathbf{X}_i\right) = \mathrm{tr}\mathbf{I}_m = m.
\end{aligned}
$$

Thus, the average value of $\{\mathrm{tr}\mathbf{P}_i\}$ is m/N, and a value of $\mathrm{tr}\mathbf{P}_i$ much higher than the average points to an influential cluster.

Now we determine how the beta coefficients are sensitive to small changes in the dependent or independent variable. The I-influence of $\mathbf{y}_i$ and $\mathbf{X}_i$ on the MLE is defined by

$$\frac{\partial \widehat{\boldsymbol{\beta}}}{\partial \mathbf{y}_i} = \mathbf{H}^{-1} \mathbf{X}_i' \mathbf{V}_i^{-1}, \tag{9.57}$$

and similar to the derivation of (9.14),

$$
\begin{aligned}
\frac{\partial \widehat{\boldsymbol{\beta}}}{\partial x_{ijk}} &= -\mathbf{H}^{-1} \left(\frac{\partial \mathbf{H}}{\partial x_{ijk}} \right) \mathbf{H}^{-1} \mathbf{s} + \mathbf{H}^{-1} \frac{\partial \mathbf{s}}{\partial x_{ijk}} \\
&= \mathbf{H}^{-1} \left(\mathbf{E}_{ijk}' \mathbf{V}_i^{-1} \mathbf{y}_i - [\mathbf{E}_{ijk}' \mathbf{V}_i^{-1} \mathbf{X}_i + \mathbf{X}_i' \mathbf{V}_i^{-1} \mathbf{E}_{ijk}] \widehat{\boldsymbol{\beta}} \right) \\
&= \mathbf{H}^{-1} \left(\mathbf{E}_{ijk}' \mathbf{V}_i^{-1} \mathbf{r}_i - \mathbf{X}_i' \mathbf{V}_i^{-1} \mathbf{E}_{ijk} \widehat{\boldsymbol{\beta}} \right),
\end{aligned} \tag{9.58}
$$

where $\mathbf{E}_{ijk}$ is the $n_i \times m$ matrix of zeros except the (j,k)th element, which is 1, and $\mathbf{r}_i = \mathbf{y}_i - \mathbf{X}_i \widehat{\boldsymbol{\beta}}$ is an $n_i \times 1$ residual vector, $j = 1, ..., n_i, k = 1, ..., m$.

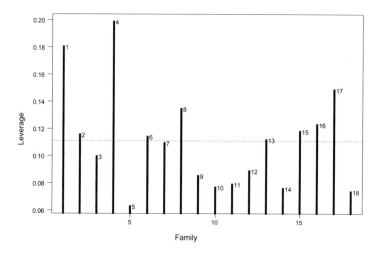

FIGURE 9.18. Leverage $\{tr\mathbf{P}_i\}$ versus family number. The dotted horizontal line represents the average leverage, $2/N$. Families 1 and 4 seem influential.

Now we develop cluster deletion diagnostics analogously to case deletion in the standard linear model. Thus, after picking cluster i, we want to know how deletion of this cluster affects $\widehat{\boldsymbol{\beta}}$. A straightforward and time-consuming solution would be recalculating $\widehat{\boldsymbol{\beta}}$ after cluster deletion. However, it is possible to derive an update formula similar to (9.3) that avoids massive reestimation. Following the line of previous notation, we denote $\widehat{\boldsymbol{\beta}}_{(i)}$ as the MLE with the ith cluster deleted, namely,

$$\widehat{\boldsymbol{\beta}}_{(i)} = [\mathbf{H} - \mathbf{X}_i' \mathbf{V}_i^{-1} \mathbf{X}_i]^{-1} [\mathbf{s} - \mathbf{X}_i' \mathbf{V}_i^{-1} \mathbf{y}_i], \quad i = 1, ..., N. \tag{9.59}$$

Using the matrix formula

$$(\mathbf{H} - \mathbf{X}_i' \mathbf{V}_i^{-1} \mathbf{X}_i)^{-1} = \mathbf{H}^{-1} + \mathbf{H}^{-1} \mathbf{X}_i' (\mathbf{V}_i - \mathbf{X}_i \mathbf{H}^{-1} \mathbf{X}_i')^{-1} \mathbf{X}_i \mathbf{H}^{-1},$$

we obtain

$$[\mathbf{H} - \mathbf{X}_i'\mathbf{V}_i^{-1}\mathbf{X}_i]^{-1}\mathbf{X}_i'\mathbf{V}_i^{-1}$$
$$= \left[\mathbf{H}^{-1} + \mathbf{H}^{-1}\mathbf{X}_i'(\mathbf{V}_i - \mathbf{X}_i\mathbf{H}^{-1}\mathbf{X}_i')^{-1}\mathbf{X}_i\mathbf{H}^{-1}\right]\mathbf{X}_i'\mathbf{V}_i^{-1}$$
$$= \mathbf{H}^{-1}\mathbf{X}_i'\mathbf{V}_i^{-1} + \mathbf{H}^{-1}\mathbf{X}_i'(\mathbf{V}_i - \mathbf{X}_i\mathbf{H}^{-1}\mathbf{X}_i')^{-1}\mathbf{X}_i\mathbf{H}^{-1}\mathbf{X}_i'\mathbf{V}_i^{-1}$$
$$= \mathbf{H}^{-1}\mathbf{X}_i'(\mathbf{V}_i - \mathbf{X}_i\mathbf{H}^{-1}\mathbf{X}_i')^{-1}[(\mathbf{V}_i - \mathbf{X}_i\mathbf{H}^{-1}\mathbf{X}_i')\mathbf{V}_i^{-1} + \mathbf{X}_i\mathbf{H}^{-1}\mathbf{X}_i'\mathbf{V}_i^{-1}]$$
$$= \mathbf{H}^{-1}\mathbf{X}_i'(\mathbf{V}_i - \mathbf{X}_i\mathbf{H}^{-1}\mathbf{X}_i')^{-1}.$$

Applying this formula to (9.59), yields

$$\widehat{\boldsymbol{\beta}}_{(i)}$$
$$= \boldsymbol{\beta} + \mathbf{H}^{-1}\mathbf{X}_i'(\mathbf{V}_i - \mathbf{X}_i\mathbf{H}^{-1}\mathbf{X}_i')^{-1}\mathbf{X}_i\boldsymbol{\beta} - \mathbf{H}^{-1}\mathbf{X}_i'(\mathbf{V}_i - \mathbf{X}_i\mathbf{H}^{-1}\mathbf{X}_i')^{-1}\mathbf{y}_i$$
$$= \boldsymbol{\beta} - \mathbf{H}^{-1}\mathbf{X}_i'\mathbf{V}_i^{-1}(\mathbf{I} - \mathbf{X}_i\mathbf{H}^{-1}\mathbf{X}_i'\mathbf{V}_i^{-1})^{-1}\mathbf{r}_i$$
$$= \boldsymbol{\beta} - \mathbf{H}^{-1}\mathbf{X}_i'\mathbf{V}_i^{-1}(\mathbf{I} - \mathbf{P}_i)^{-1}\mathbf{r}_i,$$

where $\mathbf{P}_i$ is the leverage matrix given by (9.56). Thus, the analog of (9.3) for the LME model is

$$\widehat{\boldsymbol{\beta}} - \widehat{\boldsymbol{\beta}}_{(i)} = \mathbf{H}^{-1}\mathbf{X}_i'\mathbf{V}_i^{-1}(\mathbf{I} - \mathbf{P}_i)^{-1}\mathbf{r}_i. \tag{9.60}$$

Ignoring the fact that we used an estimate of $\mathbf{D}$, the $(1-\alpha)100\%$ ellipsoid for beta coefficients is defined as

$$\{\boldsymbol{\beta} \in R^m \colon (\boldsymbol{\beta} - \widehat{\boldsymbol{\beta}})'\mathbf{H}(\boldsymbol{\beta} - \widehat{\boldsymbol{\beta}}) \le m\widehat{\sigma}^2 F_{1-\alpha}\},$$

where $\widehat{\sigma}^2$ is the MLE of σ^2 and $F_{1-\alpha}$ is the $(1-\alpha)100\%$ quantile of the F-distribution with $(m, \sum n_i - m)$ degrees of freedom. Thus, if

$$D_i = \frac{1}{m\widehat{\sigma}^2}\mathbf{r}_i'(\mathbf{I} - \mathbf{P}_i)^{-1}\mathbf{V}_i^{-1}\mathbf{X}_i\mathbf{H}^{-1}\mathbf{X}_i'\mathbf{V}_i^{-1}(\mathbf{I} - \mathbf{P}_i)^{-1}\mathbf{r}_i > F_{1-\alpha}, \tag{9.61}$$

we say that cluster i is influential because its deletion changes the MLE significantly. The reader can notice an obvious similarity between the left-hand side of the inequality (9.61) and Cook's distance (9.6). Formula (9.60) was derived previously by Banerjee and Frees (1997). Practically, it is more informative to report and/or plot the p-values associated with D_i. See the next example.

To apply the I-analysis to case deletion, we consider the MLE as a function of the weight for the ith cluster,

$$\widehat{\boldsymbol{\beta}}_{(i)}(w) = [\mathbf{H} - w\mathbf{X}_i'\mathbf{V}_i^{-1}\mathbf{X}_i]^{-1}[\mathbf{s} - w\mathbf{X}_i'\mathbf{V}_i^{-1}\mathbf{y}_i], \tag{9.62}$$

where w is the weight. Current MLE means that $w = 0$, and $w = 1$ corresponds to deletion of the ith cluster. In I-influence analysis, we determine how a small departure of w from zero affects the estimate by computing the rate of change,

$$\left.\frac{d\widehat{\boldsymbol{\beta}}_{(i)}(w)}{dw}\right|_{w=0} = \mathbf{H}^{-1}\mathbf{X}_i'\mathbf{V}_i^{-1}\mathbf{X}_i\mathbf{H}^{-1}\mathbf{s} - \mathbf{H}^{-1}\mathbf{X}_i'\mathbf{V}_i^{-1}\mathbf{y}_i$$
$$= -\mathbf{H}^{-1}\mathbf{X}_i'\mathbf{V}_i^{-1}\mathbf{r}_i. \tag{9.63}$$

This formula differs from the change $\widehat{\boldsymbol{\beta}}_{(i)}(0) - \widehat{\boldsymbol{\beta}}_{(i)}(1)$, determined by (9.60), by matrix factor $(\mathbf{I} - \mathbf{P}_i)^{-1}$ because (9.60) determines the exact, and (9.63) an approximate, change upon cluster deletion. These measures of influence are illustrated in the following example.

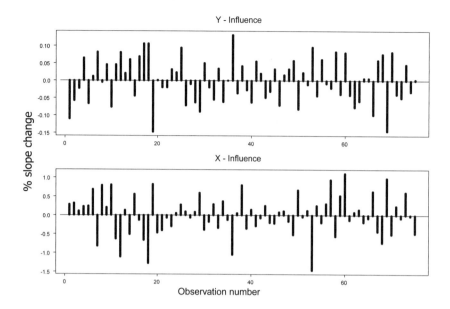

FIGURE 9.19. Influence on the slope of a small change in Weight (Y-influence) and Height (X-influence) individual observations. No apparent influential observations are seen.

9.9.1 Example: Weight versus height

In this section we illustrate the measures of influence for the linear mixed effects model by familial data, Weight versus Height, see the motivating example in Section 2.1. We start with the leverage matrix (9.56) and plot $\{\mathrm{tr}\mathbf{P}_i, i = 1, ..., 19\}$ versus family number, Figure 9.18. According to this plot, the leverage values of families 1 and 4 are obviously above the average, $2/19$. The influence of individual observations of Weight and Height on the slope using formulas (9.57) and (9.58) is displayed in Figure 9.19. It shows that the slope is not sensitive to small individual changes in either Weight or Height. Figure 9.20 displays the effect of cluster deletion. In the upper plot, the probability of (9.61) is plotted against family number, and in the bottom plot we plot the percent slope change upon deletion of the ith family using formulas (9.62) and (9.63). As follows from the D_i probability plot, families 4 and 15 are influential; their deletion from the data would affect the MLE. Interestingly, family 1 is not as influential to the MLE but is influential in terms of the predicted value as follows from previous analysis. Instead, family 15 comes into play; indeed, one member of this family seems to be an outlier. The bottom plot reveals that exclusion of the 15th family would decrease the estimate of slope by 10%. Interestingly, the membership test, developed in Section 3.8.1, pointed to the same family.

Problems for Section 9.9

1*. Develop an infinitesimal cluster deletion diagnostic for t-statistics.

2*. Apply the dimension-reduction formulas from Section 2.2.3 to (9.60) and (9.61).

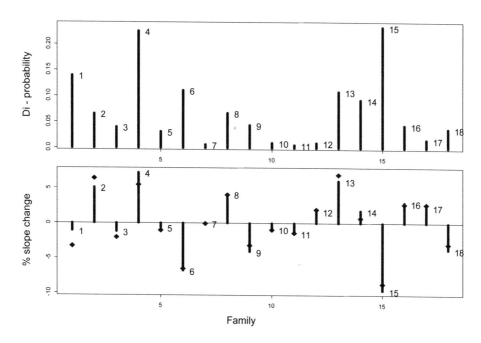

FIGURE 9.20. Family (cluster) deletion diagnostic for the LME model (bars are computed using the infinitesimal deletion diagnostic formula, and points are computed using the exact formula). Families 4 and 15 are fairly influential as can be seen from the D_i probabilities plot. Removal of the 4th family from the data would increase the slope by 5%, and removal of the 15th family would decrease the slope by 10%. The length of the bar in the bottom plot is proportional to infinitesimal deletion, and the symbol on the bar indicates true deletion.

3*. Compute a cluster deletion diagnostic measures (9.60) and (9.61) for a linear mixed model using Medicare data `coloncancer.dat` also used in Problem 8 of Section 9.4. The R code below reads the data and runs the `lme` function (the cluster is the individual):

```
coloncancer=function()
{
library(nlme)
dump("coloncancer","c:\\MixedModels\\Chapter09\\coloncancer.r")
dat=read.table("c:\\MixedModels\\Chapter09\\coloncancer.dat")
out.lme=lme(LNtotexpplus1~female+black+age+stage2+stage3+xchrlson
      +t1,random=~1|id,data=dat)
summary(out.lme)
}
```

The reader can use other covariates, such as t2, t3, etc., but it is important to know that most expenses are made in the first six months after cancer diagnosis (t1). A multilevel/nested model also can be used with the cluster `hrr` (hospital region); see Demidenko and Stukel (2005).

9.10   Appendix: MLE derivative with respect to σ^2

Here we derive formula (9.51). The score equation for the MLE under fixed σ is

$$\frac{\partial L(\boldsymbol{\beta};\sigma)}{\partial \boldsymbol{\beta}} = \sum_{y_i=1} \frac{\mathbf{v}_i}{H_i} - \sum_{y_i=0} \frac{\mathbf{v}_i}{1-H_i} = \mathbf{0}, \tag{9.64}$$

where

$$\mathbf{v}_i = \left[\begin{array}{c} \mathbf{u}_i E_s H_i' \\ E_s((z_i + \sigma s)H_i') \end{array} \right],$$

and $H_i = H(\boldsymbol{\gamma}'\mathbf{u}_i + \tau(z_i + \sigma s))$, where $'$ denotes the derivative of H. We aim to find the derivative of $\widehat{\boldsymbol{\beta}}$ with respect to σ^2, as the solution to the score equation (9.64), and evaluate the derivative at $\sigma^2 = 0$. We first calculate

$$\frac{\partial^2 L(\boldsymbol{\beta};\sigma)}{\partial \boldsymbol{\beta} \partial \sigma} = \sum_{y_i=1} \left(\frac{1}{H_i} \mathbf{w}_i - \frac{\tau E_s s H_i'}{H_i^2} \mathbf{v}_i \right) - \sum_{y_i=0} \left(\frac{1}{1-H_i} \mathbf{w}_i + \frac{\tau E_s s H_i'}{(1-H_i)^2} \mathbf{v}_i \right), \tag{9.65}$$

where

$$\mathbf{w}_i = \left[\begin{array}{c} \tau \mathbf{u}_i E_s s H_i'' \\ E_s(\tau s(z_i + \sigma s)H_i'' + s H_i') \end{array} \right].$$

Then, as is easy to see,

$$\frac{\partial^2 L(\boldsymbol{\beta};\sigma)}{\partial \boldsymbol{\beta} \partial (\sigma^2)} = \frac{1}{2} \frac{\partial^3 L(\boldsymbol{\beta};\sigma)}{\partial \boldsymbol{\beta} \partial \sigma \partial \sigma},$$

so again we need to differentiate (9.65) with respect to σ. First, let us consider cases with $y_i = 1$. We have

$$\frac{\partial}{\partial \sigma} \left(\frac{1}{H_i} \mathbf{w}_i - \frac{\tau E_s s H_i'}{H_i^2} \mathbf{v}_i \right) = \frac{\partial \mathbf{w}_i}{\partial \sigma} \frac{1}{H_i} - \frac{1}{H_i^2} \frac{\partial H_i}{\partial \sigma} \mathbf{w}_i - \frac{\tau^2 E_s s^2 H_i''}{H_i^2} \mathbf{v}_i$$
$$+ 2 \frac{\tau E_s s H_i'}{H_i^3} \frac{\partial H_i}{\partial \sigma} \mathbf{v}_i - \frac{\tau E_s s H_i'}{H_i^2} \frac{\partial \mathbf{v}_i}{\partial \sigma}.$$

Then we evaluate the derivative at zero,

$$\begin{aligned} \frac{\partial H_i}{\partial \sigma}\Big|_{\sigma=0} &= \tau \, E_s s H'(\boldsymbol{\gamma}'\mathbf{u}_i + \tau(z_i + \sigma s))|_{\sigma=0} = \tau E_s s H'(\boldsymbol{\gamma}'\mathbf{u}_i + \tau z_i) \\ &= \tau H'(\boldsymbol{\gamma}'\mathbf{u}_i + \tau z_i) E(s) = 0 \end{aligned}$$

because $E(s) = 0$. Further, because $E(s^2) = 1$, we have

$$\begin{aligned} \frac{\partial \mathbf{w}_i}{\partial \sigma}\Big|_{\sigma=0} &= E_s \left[\begin{array}{c} \tau^2 \mathbf{u}_i s^2 H_i''' \\ \tau s^2 H_i'' + \tau^2 s^2(z_i + \sigma s)H_i''' + \tau s^2 H_i'' \end{array} \right]\Big|_{\sigma=0} \\ &= \left[\begin{array}{c} \tau^2 \mathbf{u}_i H_i''' \\ 2\tau H_i'' + \tau^2 z_i H_i''' \end{array} \right]. \end{aligned}$$

Moreover,

$$\frac{\partial \mathbf{v}_i}{\partial \sigma}\bigg|_{\sigma=0} = E_s \left[\begin{array}{c} \tau \mathbf{u}_i s H_i'' \\ s H_i' + \tau s(z_i + \sigma s) H_i'' \end{array} \right]\bigg|_{\sigma=0} = \mathbf{0}.$$

Combining the results, we obtain

$$\begin{aligned} \mathbf{p}_{1i} &= \frac{\partial}{\partial \sigma}\left(\frac{1}{H_i}\mathbf{w}_i - \frac{\tau E_s s H_i'}{H_i^2}\mathbf{v}_i \right)\bigg|_{\sigma=0} \\ &= \frac{1}{H_i}\left[\begin{array}{c} \tau^2 \mathbf{u}_i H_i''' \\ 2\tau H_i'' + \tau^2 z_i H_i''' \end{array} \right] - \frac{\tau^2 H_i'' H_i'}{H_i^2}\left[\begin{array}{c} \mathbf{u}_i \\ z_i \end{array} \right]. \end{aligned}$$

Analogously,

$$\begin{aligned} \mathbf{p}_{0i} &= \frac{\partial}{\partial \sigma}\left(\frac{1}{1-H_i}\mathbf{w}_i - \frac{\tau E_s s H_i'}{(1-H_i)^2}\mathbf{v}_i \right)\bigg|_{\sigma=0} \\ &= \frac{1}{1-H_i}\left[\begin{array}{c} \tau^2 \mathbf{u}_i H_i''' \\ 2\tau H_i'' + \tau^2 z_i H_i''' \end{array} \right] + \frac{\tau^2 H_i'' H_i'}{(1-H_i)^2}\left[\begin{array}{c} \mathbf{u}_i \\ z_i \end{array} \right]. \end{aligned}$$

Finally, using the formula for the derivative of an implicit function we obtain

$$\frac{d\widehat{\boldsymbol{\beta}}}{d\sigma^2}\bigg|_{\sigma^2=0} = \frac{1}{2}\left(-\frac{\partial^2 L}{\partial \boldsymbol{\beta}^2} \right)^{-1}\left(\sum_{y_i=1}\mathbf{p}_{1i} - \sum_{y_i=0}\mathbf{p}_{0i} \right),$$

where

$$\begin{aligned} \frac{\partial^2 L}{\partial \boldsymbol{\beta}^2} &= \sum_{y_i=1}\frac{H_i H_i'' - H_i'^2}{H_i^2}\left[\begin{array}{c} \mathbf{u}_i \\ z_i \end{array} \right]\left[\begin{array}{c} \mathbf{u}_i \\ z_i \end{array} \right]' \\ &\quad - \sum_{y_i=0}\frac{(1-H_i)H_i'' + H_i'^2}{(1-H_i)^2}\left[\begin{array}{c} \mathbf{u}_i \\ z_i \end{array} \right]\left[\begin{array}{c} \mathbf{u}_i \\ z_i \end{array} \right]'. \end{aligned}$$

When n is large, $-n^{-1}\partial^2 L/\partial \boldsymbol{\beta}^2 \simeq \mathbf{H}$ where matrix $\mathbf{H}$ is defined in (9.52). Also, when $n \to \infty$, by the Law of Large Numbers,

$$\begin{aligned} \frac{1}{n}\left(\sum_{y_i=1}\mathbf{p}_{1i} - \sum_{y_i=0}\mathbf{p}_{0i} \right) &\simeq -\sum_{i=1}^{n}(H_i\mathbf{p}_{1i} - (1-H_i)\mathbf{p}_{0i}) \\ &= -\tau^2\sum_{i=1}^{n}\left(\frac{H_i'' H_i'}{H_i} + \frac{H_i'' H_i'}{1-H_i} \right)\left[\begin{array}{c} \mathbf{u}_i \\ z_i \end{array} \right], \end{aligned}$$

which finally gives (9.51).

9.11   Summary points

- An important part of statistical analysis and parameter estimation is the analysis of influential observations, or more broadly, the influence on postulated model assumptions. We make use of infinitesimal (infinitely small) influence analysis that measures the sensitivity of an estimate, or any other statistic, to a small perturbation in data or model via the partial derivative, Pregibon (1981). For instance, the I-influence on the OLS estimate of a small change in continuous individual observation of the explanatory variable is measured by a partial derivative of the estimate with respect to that observation. The I-influence approach is especially useful for complex statistical models such as nonlinear or logistic regression.

- The I-influence approach may be used to measure the *sensitivity* to data or model assumptions following the line of the local influence approach proposed by Cook (1986). I-influence analysis has a clear interpretation because it measures the influence *directly* on the parameter of interest, unlike local influence, where the measure of influence is the log-likelihood displacement. An advantage of I-influence analysis is that it does not require a distribution assumption.

- Two types of data influence may be distinguished: the influence of the dependent variable and the influence of the explanatory variable (standard influence analysis based mostly on case-deletion diagnostics does not distinguish these types of influence). We prove that Cooks's local influence of the explanatory variable in linear regression can be viewed as a special case of I-influence.

- I-influence analysis is graphically supported. Several types of influence graphs are introduced: Y-and X-influences, and star and bar I-influence plots. Each has a clear interpretation: For example, the influence of an observation of the independent variable, measured as a partial derivative, indicates change in the LS estimate by a 1-unit change of the variable.

- An influence analysis based on the idea of misclassification is proposed for a binary explanatory variable and dependent variable in the logistic regression model. Examples demonstrate that misclassification analysis may provide more detail on why a specific case is influential.

- The concept of I influence is generalized to the nonlinear regression model. Several measures of influence can be considered: influence of the dependent or independent variable on the least squares estimate or predicted value, influence of infinitesimal case deletion on regression parameters, etc. In particular, the I-influence of the dependent variable on the predicted value can be viewed as a generalization of leverage.

- I-influence analysis may be applied to study how an estimate is sensitive to model assumptions. We demonstrated this technique by the influence of residual correlation and the influence of measurement error in the covariate of the binary model. Again, the advantage of this analysis is that it does not require parameter re-estimation because the derivative is evaluated at the postulated model. This analysis is a fairly easy to accomplish and is especially useful at the stage of model formulation.

- I-influence analysis can be generalized to the linear mixed effects model. We may study the influence of an individual observation or an entire cluster.

Cook's distance is generalized to the LME model; one may use either infinitesimal or exact deletion diagnostics.

- Since I-influence analysis requires merely derivative computation, it may easily be extended to nonlinear mixed effects models. When the characteristic of interest does not admit a closed-form expression, the chain rule or an implicit differentiation can be carried out.

10
Tumor Regrowth Curves

Growth curve theory is a well-established topic and has a long history in biomathematics and biostatistics. A fairly complete account of available growth curves and their statistical estimation by nonlinear least squares is given in the book by Seber and Wild (1989). Banks (1994) describes many examples of growth curves and their applications from differential equation theory. However, while growth curves are helpful for modeling an untreated tumor, they cannot be applied to a *treated* tumor since the tumor may shrink and regrow after such treatment as radiation. In this chapter we develop a new theory of nonmonotonic growth as a function of time and dose, such as radiation dose, and apply the mixed model approach to longitudinal data to estimate parameters of the regrowth curve. In particular, our methodology enables us:

- To assess a radiosensitivity parameter *in vivo,* a milestone characteristic of the radiation treatment.

- To assess the fraction of surviving/killed cells at the time of treatment using longitudinal measurements of tumor volume.

- To evaluate the *synergistic* (supra-additive) effect, whether a *combination* of treatments is more effective than both treatments applied separately.

Statistical modeling of tumor response to treatment can be used in many ways and its potential application is well recognized (Steel, 1977; Wheldon, 1988; Heitjan, 1991; Norton and Day, 1991; Heitjan et al., 1993; Bajzer and Vuk-Pavlovic, 1997). First, a statistical model can be the basis for comparisons of different radiotherapy outcomes, such as doubling time and tumor growth delay. Second, mathematical modeling may provide objective evidence for nonconventional choices of radiotherapy regimens to optimize such treatment outcomes as tumor growth delay or damage to normal tissue. Third, regrowth curves may define a better model for tumor control probability in fractionated radiotherapy because they adequately describe tumor regrowth between irradiations. Fourth, they create an opportunity for a better prediction of tumor response to treatment by accounting for individual characteristics, such as age or tumor stage, that are critical in clinical oncology.

Modeling of treated tumors is a long-standing problem in mathematical biology and biostatistics. There are a few attempts to model post-irradiated tumor regrowth. For example, Looney et al. (1975) used a linear combination of two exponential curves. Norton and Simon (1977) proposed a complicated version of the Gompertz curve. Durrleman and Simon (1989) used polynomial splines for nonparametric smoothing. However, those models, perhaps useful for data interpolation, have no biological interpretation and cannot predict tumor response given the radiation dose. Heitjan (1991) suggested a model for prostate tumor reaction to androgen withdrawal by castration, but this model assumes that the tumor vanishes after treatment. Rygaardt and Spang-Thomsen (1997) used exponential and Gompertz curves after the tumor starts regrowing, with the time to regrowth determined subjectively. To the best of our knowledge, there are no tumor regrowth *statistical* models/curves that describe tumor shrinkage and regrowth that depends explicitly on radiation dose.

On the other hand, there is an extensive literature on the use of mathematical modeling to describe post-irradiated tumor growth and regrowth quantitatively based on a *cell kinetics* approach. Several theoretical settings for optimal radiation treatment have been developed based on this theory and many of them emerged in the late 1970s (Aherne et al., 1977; Steel, 1977; Eisen, 1979; Goldie and Coldman, 1979; Day, 1986a, 1986b; Knolle, 1988; Wheldon, 1988; Martin and Teo, 1994). Attempts have been made to use these models to establish optimal fractionation dose and time schedules through clinical trials and studies (Tubiana et al., 1990; Perez and Brady, 1992). Several studies used mathematical approaches designed to find the optimal schedule for fractionated radiation based on the theory of optimization (Sachs et al., 1996; Shahine et al., 1997; Yakovlev et al., 1997). A number of other authors tried to resolve the dilemma between the repair of normal tissue and tumor regrowth using stochastic models (Yakovlev and Zorin, 1988; Yakovlev and Tsodikov, 1995; Afenya, 1996). There are several obstacles in applying those models to post-irradiated tumor regrowth data: all those models require, as specific input, values for radiobiological parameters and other information, such as the proportion of cells actively cycling, cell-cycle time, and the alpha/beta ratio in the survival curve, to name a few. In many instances these values are taken arbitrarily or based on sparse radiobiological experiment (Martin and Teo, 1994; Mao and Wheldon, 1996). No statistical testing of those models has been performed to determine their adequacy and validity to describe actual experimental data. Generally, the parameters of stochastic models for cell population growth could not be estimated properly due to the large number of cell kinetics parameters involved.

Thus, there is a striking gap between theoretical cell kinetics modeling and statistical models of post-irradiated tumor regrowth based on serial experimental measurements of such tumor growth characteristics as tumor volume. Probably, this gap is responsible for the failure of many theoretical models to fit existing cancer data and their failure to apply in clinical settings (Norton and Day, 1991). A new approach to the modeling of growth dynamics is needed to describe *parsimoniously* how tumors respond to treatment. We combine the following existing theories to create new biologically based statistical models of treated tumor:

1. Classical growth curve models, such as exponential or Gompertz curves used to describe unperturbed tumor growth.

2. Cell kinetics modeling that describes major biological processes of growth on the cellular level in terms of differential equations.

3. Survival curve theory that describes the proportion of cells surviving treatment/irradiation.

Our regrowth curve theory is a product of combining two existing theories: traditional growth curve theory and survival curve theory. To model the dynamics of tumor after treatment, we use the traditional growth curve to describe the further growth of surviving cells, and we use the survival curve to model the proportion of cells killed by the treatment. So, symbolically, our regrowth curve has the form

$$\text{Regrowth curve} = \text{Growth curve} \times \text{Survival curve.} \tag{10.1}$$

Thus, one may use any combination of growth and survival curves to create a new parsimonious regrowth curve that describes the post-treatment dynamics of the tumor.

We pay special attention to a proper estimation of our regrowth curves using the mixed effects approach. Statistical analysis of animal and human data is complicated by a broad (sometimes wild) range of response to treatment. Tumor and cell heterogeneity is well recognized in modern cancer research and several recent papers address this phenomenon. See for example, Heitjan et al. (1993) and Hill and Skarsgard (1999). The mixed effects methodology is well suited to address heterogeneity, and in several papers it was proven to be an adequate statistical model for tumor growth and regrowth, e.g., O'Hara et al. (2001), Pogue et al. (2003), Sundaram et al. (2003). We demonstrated the application of the mixed model technique in Section 6.1.7, where cellular spheroid volume was modeled via the log-Gompertz curve with random parameters. Following this approach, some parameters of the regrowth curve are allowed to be subject/human-specific, reflecting differences in microenvironment and treatment/drug delivery. On the contrary, cell-specific parameters, such as rate of growth, are less likely to be subject-specific and may be addressed via statistical hypothesis testing. Determining what parameters of growth or regrowth are fixed/genetically driven and what parameters are environmentally dependent is a fundamental biological question. Several recent papers of mine deal with tumor regrowth theory and estimation via mixed model (Demidenko, 2006a, 2010).

10.1   Survival curves

The Survival Curve (SC), a major component of the tumor regrowth model, is fundamental to radiobiology and it understood as an idealized relationship between the fraction of cells surviving radiation against the dose given (Casarett, 1968;

Elkind, 1988; Tubiana et al., 1990; Hall, 2000). Several papers address the problem of survival curve parameter estimation (Thames et al., 1986; Roberts and Hendry, 1993, 1998). The survival curve may be viewed as a dose-response relationship in a cellular context. Estimation of dose-response relationships has a long history in biostatistics with a vast literature. In our approach we estimate the parameters of the survival curve indirectly using longitudinal tumor volume data. Mathematically, SC can be represented as a decreasing function of dose, $S = S(D)$, where D is the radiation dose and S is the fraction of tumor cells surviving the radiation. Following this relationship, if there is no irradiation ($D = 0$), the tumor remains unchanged; for a large amount of radiation, the tumor is killed completely (at least hypothetically). Mathematically, this can be written as $S(0) = 1$ and $S(\infty) = 0$.

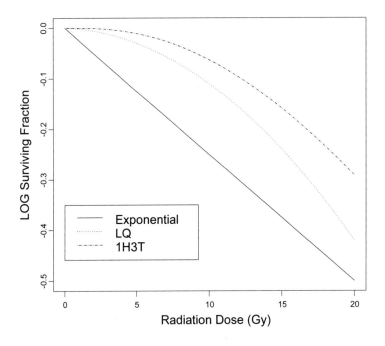

FIGURE 10.1. Three survival curves on a semilogarithmic scale (LQ = linear quadratic, 1H3T = one-hit-three-target). LQ and 1H3T curves have a characteristic shoulder for small radiation doses. It is expected that these curves are better suited for modeling *in vivo* data.

Several mathematical models have been suggested for cell survival. The simplest is of exponential type, has been confirmed empirically for viruses, bacteria, and haploid yeasts, and has the form $S = e^{-\alpha D}$, where $\alpha > 0$ is the *radiosensitivity* parameter, the rate at which cells are killed by radiation. Often, SC is displayed on a semilogarithmic scale, see Figure 10.1. However, it was discovered that survival curves for most mammalian cells differ from those of most bacterial cells by having a "shoulder" in the low-dose region (DeVita et al., 1995). The shoulder indicates a reduced efficiency of cell killing which may be explained by a resistance to low doses and repair, or to the inability to deliver ionization electrons to the tumor site due to dispersion. The simplest SC that accounts for this effect is called Linear-Quadratic

(LQ), $S(D) = e^{-\alpha D - \beta D^2}$, and is widely used in clinical oncology (DeVita et al., 1995). A special case of the LQ survival curve is $e^{-\beta D^2}$, and we shall find that this SC sometimes gives a better fit. Several models for survival curves with shoulders in the low-dose region have been developed based on the *target theory*. The central assumption of this theory is that to kill a cell, several hits or cell targets may be required, due to cell repair, Casarett (1968), Hall (2000), Hanin et al. (1993). For instance, if the lethal event happens in a one-hit-multi-target (1HMT) model, the SC has the form $S = 1 - (1 - e^{-\gamma D})^n$, where n is the number of targets needed to achieve the lethal event of the cell. To derive this SC, we assume that to kill a cell, one needs to hit n targets, each with probability $1 - e^{-\gamma D}$, where $e^{-\gamma D}$ is the probability of missing (target survival). Second, we assume that probabilities are independent. Third, it is assumed that the cell is killed if all n targets are hit. Then the probability of hitting all n targets is $(1 - e^{-\gamma D})^n$ and the probability of survival is $1 - (1 - e^{-\gamma D})^n$. It is expected that LQ and target theory SC are better suited to modeling *in vivo* data.

It is worth noting that existing approaches of experimental biology to estimate parameters of survival curves are based on *in vitro* data, with direct counts of surviving/killed cells using histology methods. Incorporating SC into the regrowth curve facilitates the recovery of *in vivo* parameters having only fairly simply derived longitudinal observations of tumor volume.

Problems for Section 10.1

1. Is the 1HMT survival curve concave (the second derivative is negative) for any n?

2. Does the survival curve $S(D) = \left(1 - (1 - e^{-\gamma D})^n\right)^m$ meet your expectation of being a multi-hit-multi-target dose-response relationship? Does the probability of surviving decrease with m? Plot several SC curves for different n and m.

3. Many dose-response relationships are defined on the log scale of dose, such as $\Phi(\beta \ln D)$ or $\exp(\beta \ln D)/(1 + \exp(\beta \ln D))$. Redefine survival curves introduced in this section, as functions of $\ln D$, and interpret the parameters as a percent decrease in survival per a 1% increase in D.

10.2   Double-exponential regrowth curve

Now we derive our first regrowth curve in a series of models to describe the dynamics of post-irradiated tumors based on the two-compartment model for cell proliferation. This regrowth curve may adequately describe the regrowth of radiosensitive *fast-growing* tumors because after some time, the tumor regains exponential growth.

Since proliferating cells are the most sensitive to radiation, we distinguish two population compartments: proliferating (clonogenic), P, and quiescent (nonproliferating or resting), Q. Two fundamental and opposite processes occur in any living organism: birth and death. Three hypotheses generate the two-compartment model: (i) proliferating cells divide at a constant rate, ν, (ii) quiescent cells die at a constant rate, ϕ (cell loss), and (iii) a portion of proliferating cells become quiescent at rate τ (Eisen, 1979; Baserga, 1981). The first hypothesis leads to a simple differential equation $dP/dt = \nu P$, implying exponential growth of proliferating cells. The

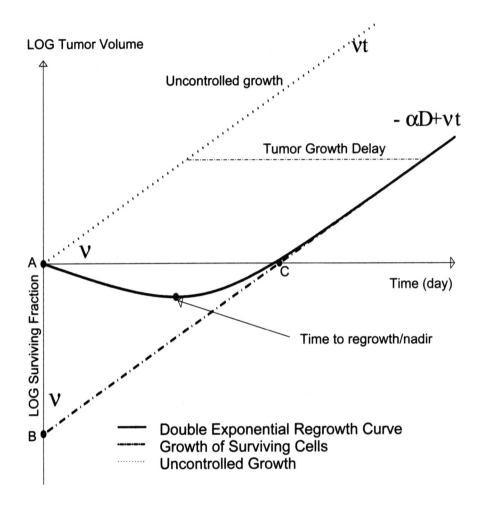

FIGURE 10.2. Double-Exponential (DE) regrowth curve on a logarithmic scale. Uncontrolled cell growth has rate ν, and on a log scale it is a straight (dotted) line because the growth is exponential. After treatment (e.g., radiation) the proportion of surviving cells is θ, so the length of the segment $AB = -$ LOG Surviving Fraction $= -\log\theta = \alpha D$. It is assumed that after treatment the surviving cells proliferate at the same rate ν (dashed bold line with slope ν). The double–exponential regrowth curve is the sum of surviving cells and doomed (quiescent) cells that leave the tumor following a decay law. The DE curve decreases from the initial tumor volume to time to regrowth/nadir, due to delayed death and washout of cells affected by the treatment. It may take several cell cycles before damaged cells leave the tumor. According to the DE regrowth curve, after a period of time, the tumor regrows at the same rate ν and the DE curve approaches the dashed line $-\alpha D + \nu t$. The relationship Tumor Growth Delay $= -$LOG Surviving Fraction$/\nu$ follows from triangle ABC with slope ν.

second and third hypotheses lead to the differential equation $dQ/dt = \tau P - \phi Q$. Combining these equations leads to the following simple yet fundamental pair of differential equations (Codington and Levinson, 1955; Knolle, 1988; Wheldon, 1988):

$$\frac{dP}{dt} = \nu P, \qquad \frac{dQ}{dt} = \tau P - \phi Q. \tag{10.2}$$

This simple system of differential equations represents the main features of tumor growth as the sum of proliferating and quiescent cells. This system will be generalized later for a more adequate tumor regrowth model for slow growing tumors. From the first equation, we deduce that proliferating (clonogenic, malignant) cells grow exponentially according to $P(t) = P_0 e^{\nu t}$, where ν is the rate of growth and P_0 reprsents the number of proliferating cells at the initial time $(t = 0)$. Substituting this solution into the second equation, we find that the total number of cells at time t is the sum $N(t) = P(t) + Q(t)$ with the closed-form solution,

$$N(t) = N_0 \left(\theta e^{\nu t} + (1 - \theta) e^{-\phi t} \right), \qquad t \geq 0, \tag{10.3}$$

where θ is the proportion of proliferating cells. Formula (10.3) can model nonincreasing growth when the initial number of proliferating cells is small so that during a certain period of time the total number of cells will decrease due to dying quiescent cells. However, with time, the number of proliferating cells will increase and the total number of cells will, eventually, grow exponentially. This model has been used by Looney et al. (1975), but we suggest a special interpretation for parameter θ as a fraction of surviving cells modeled via the survival curve, as described below.

To introduce radiation dose as a factor of regrowth, we employ the notion of the survival curve, which describes the proportion of cells surviving the radiation. Since in our model θ is the proportion of surviving cells, it is natural to set $\theta = S(D)$, where S is a survival curve as a function of dose D, as described in the previous subsection. This leads to a regrowth curve,

$$N(t) = N_0 \left(S(D) e^{\nu t} + (1 - S(D)) e^{-\phi t} \right). \tag{10.4}$$

The fraction of cells killed by dose D is $1 - S(D)$. In particular, taking the simplest exponential survival curve, we arrive at the *Double-Exponential* (DE) regrowth curve:

$$N(t) = N_0 \left(e^{-\alpha D + \nu t} + (1 - e^{-\alpha D}) e^{-\phi t} \right). \tag{10.5}$$

This model describes two cell compartments, see Figure 10.2 for a geometrical illustration. The first compartment is defined by equation $N_0 e^{-\alpha D} e^{\nu t}$ and represents cells not affected by radiation—it continues growing exponentially after treatment. The second compartment, $N_0(1 - e^{-\alpha D}) e^{-\phi t}$, represents cells affected by radiation (doomed cells) and decreases following a decay law with the rate ϕ. When there is no irradiation ($D = 0$), the tumor continues growing exponentially because the second term in (10.5) vanishes. It is worth mentioning that model (10.4) is suitable for fast-growing tumors when the treatment effect occurs immediately after $t = 0$. Later, we generalize regrowth curve to allow the tumor to grow after treatment and then to shrink and regrow.

As follows from Figure 10.2, three fundamental radiobiological concepts are related through

$$\text{Tumor Growth Delay} = \frac{\ln(\text{Surviving Fraction})}{\text{Rate of Growth } (\nu)}. \tag{10.6}$$

Remarkably, in texts on radiobiology such as Kallman (1987), Tubiana et al. (1990) and Hall (2000) one cannot find relationship (10.6). Moreover, in such fundamental papers as that of Rofstadt (1981), the three quantities have been analyzed separately.

Assuming that the total number of tumor cells (N) is proportional to tumor volume (V), we can estimate such tumor growth parameters as the rate of death (ϕ) and the radiosensitivity parameter (α) from post-irradiated *in vivo* tumor-volume data. A statistical model is formulated below, and we shall see how the assumption on the proportion of total number of cells and tumor volume may be eased. However, before addressing estimation issues, we show how several important radiobiological treatment outcomes (e.g., Begg, 1983) may be expressed in terms of the DE regrowth model. The following treatment end-points admit a closed-form solution for the DE regrowth curve. For more complicated curves an iterative solution must be applied.

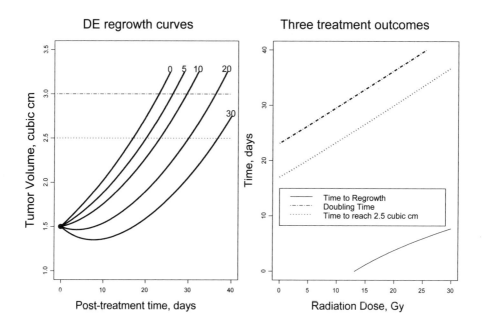

FIGURE 10.3. Double exponential regrowth curves with three radiotherapy treatment outcomes as functions of a single radiation dose. Left: tumor volume as a function of time with initial volume 1.5 cm^3. Right: Time to regrowth, Doubling time, and Time to reach 2.5 cm^3 as functions of radiation dose. As we see, the tumor shrinks when the dose exceeds 13 Gy. Doubling time and Time to reach 2.5 cm^3 as functions of D are close to straight lines.

10.2.1   Time to regrowth, T_R

The advantage of the DE regrowth curve is that such an important radiobiological treatment outcome as time to regrowth can be expressed explicitly in terms of the regrowth curve parameters. See Figure 10.3 for an illustration. Indeed, to find the minimum of the DE curve, we differentiate (10.3) with respect to t and equate the derivative to zero, leading to the formula for the time to regrowth (or nadir):

$$T_R = \frac{1}{\nu + \phi} \ln \left(\frac{1 - \theta}{\theta} \frac{\phi}{\nu} \right). \tag{10.7}$$

As follows from this formula, the tumor shrinks ($T_R > 0$) when the proportion of surviving cells is less than $\phi/(\nu + \phi)$. For a simple exponential survival curve, $\theta = e^{-\alpha D}$, we can easily find the minimum radiation dose to achieve tumor shrinkage, $D_0 = \alpha^{-1} \ln[\phi^{-1}(\nu + \phi)]$. For a dose greater than D_0, the tumor shrinks; for a dose less than D_0, the tumor growth slows down but does not shrink.

10.2.2   Time to reach specific tumor volume, T_*

When comparing the outcomes of different treatment groups, researchers may be interested in the time T_* to reach a specific tumor volume N_*, assuming that $N_* > N_0$. To compute this time using the DE regrowth curve, we need to solve the following equation for $t = T_*$:

$$N_0 \left(\theta e^{\nu t} + (1 - \theta)e^{-\phi t} \right) = N_*. \tag{10.8}$$

This is a transcendental equation, so we solve it iteratively applying Newton's algorithm (here it is assumed that $0 < \theta < 1$ and $\nu > 0, \phi > 0$). We show that iterations

$$t_{s+1} = t_s - \frac{\theta e^{\nu t_s} + (1 - \theta)e^{-\phi t_s} - (N_*/N_0)}{\nu \theta e^{\nu t_s} - \phi(1 - \theta)e^{-\phi t_s}}, \quad s = 0, 1, ..., \tag{10.9}$$

starting from $t_0 = \nu^{-1} \ln[N_*(\theta N_0)^{-1}]$, converge to the solution of (10.8). Moreover, the sequence is descending, $t_{s+1} < t_s$. To see this, we notice that the function $\theta e^{\nu t} + (1 - \theta)e^{-\phi t}$ is a convex and increasing function of t for $t > T_*$. To justify the starting point t_0, we notice that $\theta e^{\nu t} + (1 - \theta)e^{-\phi t} > \theta e^{\nu t}$, and therefore the equation $\theta e^{\nu t} = N_*/N_0$ leads to $t_0 > T_*$.

10.2.3   Doubling time, T_D

Tumor volume doubling time is a popular measure to characterize treatment outcome in experimental biology. It may be viewed as a special case of (10.8) for $N_* = 2N_0$. Thus, we are interested in the time required to double the initial volume. Doubling time is somewhat more objective because it eliminates N_0 and therefore may be useful when comparing treatment outcomes for animals with different initial tumor volumes. By the definition, tumor volume doubling time, $t = T_D$, is the solution to the equation $\theta e^{\nu t} + (1 - \theta)e^{-\phi t} = 2$, and therefore procedure (10.9) is valid with $N_*/N_0 = 2$. In radiobiology, potential doubling time, $T_{pot} = \ln 2/\nu$, means the time to double the initial tumor volume of un untreated tumor. Thus, to describe the effect of treatment, the ratio T_D/T_{pot} may be of interest and it may be plotted against dose D (Steel, 1977).

The R function that follows solves the equation $e^{A+\nu t} + e^{B-\lambda t} = 1$ for t using Newton's algorithm (10.9). Besides the solution itself, it computes its variance (it is assumed that both A and B are negative). This variance is computed via the delta-method based on the 4×4 covariance matrix of the parameter estimates obtained from `nlme`.

```
decE <- function(A, nu, B, la, Cmat, maxiter=10, eps=10^-8)
  {
  # Cmat is the 4x4 covariance matrix for A, nu, B, la
      t0 <- - A/nu
      for(iter in 1:maxiter) {
          exp1 <- exp(A + nu * t0)
          exp2 <- exp(B - la * t0)
          t1 <- t0 - (exp1 + exp2 - 1)/(nu * exp1 - la * exp2)
          if(abs(exp1 + exp2 - 1) < eps) break
          t0 <- t1
      }
      dFdA <- exp1
      dFdB <- exp2
      dFdnu <- t1 * exp1
      dFdla <- exp2 * t1
      dFdt <- nu * exp1 - exp2 * la
      h <- - c(dFdA, dFdnu, dFdB, dFdla)/dFdt #derivative vector
      var1 <- as.numeric(t(h) %*% Cmat %*% h) # delta-method
      return(c(t1, var1))
  }
}
```

For example, to compute the time to regrowth as the solution to (10.8) we set $A = \ln N_0 + \ln \theta - \ln N_*$ and $B = \ln N_0 + \ln(1 - \theta) - \ln N_*$. For the doubling time $A = \ln 2 + \ln \theta$ and $B = \ln 2 + \ln(1 - \theta)$.

10.2.4 Statistical model for regrowth

In this section we describe how the Double–exponential regrowth curve is estimated using mixed effects methodology when longitudinal tumor measurement data are available for different subjects/animals. To simplify, we assume that the data comprise serial measurements of individual tumor volumes from one treatment group. More specifically, let there be N mice treated at day 0. Let Y_{ij} denote the tumor volume of animal i at time t_{ij} and $y_{ij} = \ln Y_{ij}$, $i = 1, 2, ..., N$, and $j = 1, 2, ..., n_i$. If the parameters of the DE regrowth curve do not change across animals (no heterogeneity), assuming multiplicative error as in Section 6.1.7, we come to a nonlinear regression model,

$$y_{ij} = y_0 + \ln \left[\theta e^{\nu t_{ij}} + (1 - \theta)e^{-\phi t_{ij}} \right] + \varepsilon_{ij}, \qquad (10.10)$$

where y_0 denotes the logarithm of the initial tumor volume. In this model ε_{ij} is the independent error term with zero mean and constant variance. We can estimate nonlinear regression (10.10), combining data into one pool (numerical issues are discussed later). Notice that model (10.10) assumes that tumor volume is proportional to the total number of cells, a common simplifying assumption. However, we may ease this assumption by assuming that Y_{ij} is related to the total number of cells through a power function, $Y_{ij} = \tau N_{ij}^{\gamma}$ that would lead to relationship (10.10) with an additional coefficient γ. It is well known in radiobiology that the relationship between the number of tumor cells and tumor volume may be quite complex (e.g., tumor volume may involve a tumor bed), so accommodating the power relationship into (10.10) may be adequate (Kallman, 1987).

Having estimates for the parameters from nonlinear regression model (10.10), one can explore the possibility of incorporating random effects by assuming that some parameters of the regrowth are random (see earlier chapters). The simplest random effects model would account for a mouse-specific initial tumor volume, $y_{0i} = y_0 + \delta_i$:

$$y_{ij} = y_0 + \ln\left[\theta e^{\nu t_{ij}} + (1-\theta)e^{-\phi t_{ij}}\right] + \delta_i + \varepsilon_{ij}, \qquad (10.11)$$

where $E(\delta_j) = 0$ and $\mathrm{var}(\delta_i) = \sigma^2 d$. Clearly, model (10.11) is a nonlinear marginal model with a fixed matrix of random effects, Section 6.1. As follows from this model, animals do not correlate, but longitudinal observations within the same animal have a constant correlation $d/(1+d)$. One may further complicate this model by allowing other parameters to be animal-specific (random), but then we arrive at the nonlinear mixed effects model of Chapter 8. Following the line of arguments of Section 6.1.7, we may assume that parameters ν and ϕ reflect tumor cell type and are constant across animals. If it is believed that treatment alters the regrowth curve parameters, one should estimate the parameters of the DE regrowth curve separately for each group. See our example on chemotherapy in Section 10.2.7.

If parameter θ is related to the survival curve via dose D we can simultaneously estimate regrowth curve parameters using data from all treatment groups. Thus, if $l = 1, 2, ..., L$ counts, the number of treatment groups irradiated with dose D_l, assuming that $\theta = e^{-\alpha D_l}$, we come to the three-level cluster mixed model:

$$y_{ijl} = y_0 + \ln\left[e^{\nu t_{ijl} - \alpha D_l} + (1 - e^{-\alpha D_l})e^{-\phi t_{ijl}}\right] + \delta_i + \eta_l + \varepsilon_{ijl}.$$

Clearly, this model assumes that parameters y_0, ν and ϕ are constant across treatment groups. There are many variants to ease this assumption by incorporating random effects. For example, one may assume that the radiosensitivity parameter is treatment-specific, $\alpha_l = \alpha + \omega_l$, where ω_l is the random effect.

10.2.5 Variance estimation for tumor regrowth outcomes

In order to use the regrowth curve characteristics T_R (time to regrowth), T_* (time to reach a specific tumor volume), and T_D (doubling time) for statistical inference, one needs to assess their variances. We use the delta-method, which provides an estimate of the variance based on the linear approximation around its mean (Rao, 1973; Bickel and Doksum, 2001). According to this method, if a random variable Y is a nonlinear function f of p random variables $\mathbf{X} = (X_1, ..., X_p)'$ with a known covariance matrix, then

$$\mathrm{var}(Y) \simeq \left(\frac{\partial f}{\partial \mathbf{X}}\right)' \mathrm{cov}(\mathbf{X}) \left(\frac{\partial f}{\partial \mathbf{X}}\right). \qquad (10.12)$$

Since all these characteristics are functions of regrowth curve parameters with the covariance matrix derived from an estimation procedure, it suffices to obtain partial derivatives with respect to the parameters. To illustrate, we start with the time to regrowth (10.7), where the proportion of surviving cells is modeled via simple exponential SC, as in (10.5). Thus, if $\mathbf{p} = (\widehat{\alpha}, \widehat{\nu}, \widehat{\phi})'$ is the vector of estimates from model (10.10) or (10.11), an estimate of the time to regrowth is

$$\widehat{T}_R = \frac{\ln(e^{\widehat{\alpha}D} - 1) + \ln\widehat{\phi} - \ln\widehat{\nu}}{\widehat{\nu} + \widehat{\phi}}.$$

From this estimate the variance is computed by formula (10.12), where $\partial f / \partial \mathbf{X}$ is the vector of partial derivatives of $\widehat{T}_R$ with respect to $\mathbf{p}$ and $\text{cov}(\mathbf{X})$ is the covariance matrix of $\mathbf{p}$ (the calculation of partial derivatives for T_R is straightforward). To use the delta-method for doubling time, we use the formula for the derivative of an implicit function. Indeed, since T_D is the solution to equation (10.8), we have

$$\frac{\partial \widehat{T}_D}{\partial \theta} = -\frac{\partial \left(\theta e^{\nu t} + (1-\theta)e^{-\phi t}\right)/\partial \theta}{\partial \left(\theta e^{\nu t} + (1-\theta)e^{-\phi t}\right)/\partial t}\Bigg|_{t=\widehat{T}_D} = -\frac{e^{\nu \widehat{T}_D} - e^{-\phi \widehat{T}_D}}{\theta \nu e^{\nu \widehat{T}_D} - (1-\theta)\phi e^{-\phi \widehat{T}_D}}.$$

Similarly, one finds partial derivatives with respect to other parameters. We emonstrate these calculations in a chemotherapy example in Section 10.2.7.

10.2.6 Starting values

The choice of starting values for parameters is crucial for nonlinear estimation because poor initial values often lead to a poor fit. Here we suggest a procedure to obtain rough estimates for parameters y_0, ν, ϕ, and θ of the DE regrowth curve (10.10):

1. Obtain an estimate for the rate of untreated tumor growth ν and initial ln(Tumor Volume), y_0. Since the DE curve assumes that the untreated tumor grows exponentially, we apply linear regression $y = \gamma_1 + \gamma_2 t + \varepsilon$, where y is the ln(Tumor Volume), to combined data for control group and other groups before treatment. Then we set $\widehat{\nu}_0 = \widehat{\gamma}_2$ and $\widehat{y}_0 = \widehat{\gamma}_1$.

2. Obtain an estimate of the cell loss rate ϕ by regressing y on t for treatment group data *before* the tumor regrows, $y = \eta_1 + \eta_2 t + \varepsilon$, and set $\widehat{\phi} = \widehat{\eta}_2$ (another option is to set $\eta_1 = \widehat{y}_0$ and to estimate a one-parameter regression).

3. Obtain an estimate for the radiosensitivity parameter α. There are at least two ways. The first way is to rewrite (10.10), provided estimates $\widehat{\nu}$ and $\widehat{\phi}$, as

$$e^{y_{ij} - \widehat{y}_0} - e^{-\widehat{\phi} t_{ij}} = e^{-\alpha D_j}\left(e^{\widehat{\nu} t_{ij}} - e^{-\widehat{\phi} t_{ij}}\right)$$

and apply LS (least squares) to a one-parameter linear regression, $z = \gamma D + \varepsilon$, where

$$z = \ln \frac{e^{y_{ij} - \widehat{y}_0} - e^{-\widehat{\phi} t}}{e^{\widehat{\nu} t} - e^{-\widehat{\phi} t}},$$

and then set $\widehat{\alpha} = -\widehat{\gamma}$. Another way is to use the fact that after regrowth cells proliferate with the rate ν and, for post-treatment tumor, $y_{ij} = -\alpha D_j + \widehat{\nu} t_{ij}$, as illustrated in Figure 10.2.

Clearly, all estimates must be positive, and negative values would indicate a failure of the procedure.

10.2.7 Example: chemotherapy treatment comparison

We consider an example of the DE regrowth curve estimation and its application to compare tumor treatment outcomes. We illustrate how the data can be analyzed by different mixed models and show how treatment outcomes can be compared by three cancer treatment end-points.

The data comprise longitudinal measurements of tumor volume Y_{ij} in four groups of mice, $i = 1, 2, 3, 4 = N$ (Table 10.1). The first group is untreated (control group), and the other three groups are treated with the chemotherapeutic drug *cisplatin*. See Figure 10.4. In groups 2 and 3, the tumor was treated with 10 mg/kg, and in group 4 with 25 mg/kg cisplatin. Two methods of drug delivery are compared: intratumor (ITu, groups 3 and 4) and intravenous (IV, group 2). In the former method, cisplatin was injected directly into tumor, and in the latter it was injected into the tail of the mouse. In all groups cisplatin slowed tumor growth. The question is whether the treatment effect is statistically significantly different. First, we notice that the tumor grows fairly rapidly and the treatment effect occurs as early as the next day after drug delivery. This means that the DE regrowth curve may be adequate to model tumor shrinkage and regrowth. Since the mechanisms of venous and tumor drug delivery are quite different, we may expect that the parameters of the regrowth curve will not be the same in different treatment groups. Therefore, we apply the DE regrowth curve to each group separately. As mentioned above, the aim of the study is to compare treatment groups using three cancer treatment end-points: time to regrowth/nadir (T_T), time to reach 1 cm^3 (T_1), and doubling time (T_D). In Figure 10.4, T_1 is the time when the tumor regrowth curve intersects the zero horizontal line.

Table 10.1. Results of the DE regrowth curve estimation in four groups of mice

	Group 1 Exponential[1]	Group 2	Group 3 Double–exponential Regrowth Curve[2]	Group 4
β_1	-1.47 (0.0545)	-8.105 (0.36)	-5.48 (0.44)	-6.72 (0.34)
β_2	0.325 (0.0085)	0.323 (0.015)	0.244 (0.018)	0.241 (0.011)
β_3		-0.839 (0.094)	-0.688 (0.076)	-0.813 (0.051)
β_4		0.2033 (0.012)	0.122 (0.013)	0.111 (0.007)
σ_δ		0.79	0.9	0.71
σ_η		0.37	0.32	0.22
ρ		0.83	0.38	-0.69
σ		0.34	0.26	0.24
%SF	100	0.12 (0.038)	1.02 (0.45)	0.35 (0.12)
T_R		11.8 (0.34)	10.3 (0.7)	13.8 (0.67)
T_1	3.5 (0.20)	23.1 (0.60)	20.8 (0.98)	26.0 (0.9)
T_D	2.1 (0.06)	23.8 (2.9)	21.3 (4.4)	26.9 (3.5)

[1]Reduced to a random intercept LME model (Section 2.4).

[2]Estimated by the Lindstrom–Bates method using the R function `nlme` (Section 8.7).

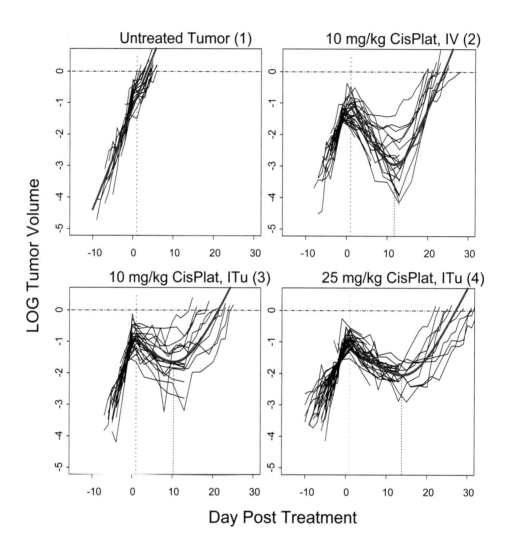

FIGURE 10.4. Chemotherapeutic treatment in three groups of mice (groups 2 to 4). In the control group (1) tumor was not treated, and its volume increases rapidly with time following the linear model for LOG Tumor volume. In the other three groups, the tumor was treated at day 0 with the chemotherapeutic drug cisplatin. Tumor volume drops the next day, comes to its minimum, and then regrows. We fit the data with a DE regrowth curve (bold) in each group separately. One of the characteristics of treatment is the time to reach 1 cm^3, which corresponds to the point where the regrowth curve hits the zero line (dashed). The vertical dotted line shows the estimated time to regrowth.

Control group. Assuming multiplicative error, the statistical model for exponential growth is $Y_{ij} = e^{\beta_1 + \beta_2 t_{ij} + \varepsilon_{ij}}$. This model is equivalent to the linear model $y_{ij} = \beta_1 + \beta_2 t_{ij} + \varepsilon_{ij}$, where i indicates the mouse and y_{ij} indicates ln(tumor volume) measured at time t_{ij}. Clearly, β_1 estimates ln(initial volume) at time zero, and β_2 estimates the rate of uncontrolled growth (in previous notation, ν). One may address animal heterogeneity by assuming that β_1 and/or β_2 are random (mouse-specific). Here we assume that the intercept is mouse-specific but the rate β_2 is the same across mice, leading to a linear mixed effects model with random intercepts, Section 2.4. The doubling time for exponential growth is denoted by T_{pot}, and it is determined from the equation $e^{\beta_1 + \beta_2 t} = 2e^{\beta_1}$, which yields $T_{pot} = \ln 2/\beta_2$. The variance of T_{pot} is estimated by the delta-method, $\operatorname{var}(T_{pot}) \simeq \operatorname{var}(\widehat{\beta}_2)(\ln 2)^2/\widehat{\beta}_2^4$. The time to reach 1 cm^3 is found from the equation $\beta_1 + \beta_2 t = 0$ which gives $T_1 = -\beta_1/\beta_2$. Again using the delta-method (10.12), we obtain

$$\operatorname{var}(T_1) \simeq \operatorname{var}(\widehat{\beta}_1)/\widehat{\beta}_2^2 - 2\widehat{\beta}_1 \operatorname{cov}(\widehat{\beta}_1, \widehat{\beta}_2)/\widehat{\beta}_2^3 + \widehat{\beta}_1^2 \operatorname{var}(\widehat{\beta}_2)/\widehat{\beta}_2^4.$$

In the R code below we show how to read/plot the data for untreated mice and compute Doubling Time (T_D) with its standard error (file untrlme.r).

```
library(nlme) # see Figure 10.5
dat = read.table("c:\\MixedModels\\Chapter10\\DEregrowth.dat",
                   stringsAsFactor=F)
names(dat)=c("TreatmentGroup","MiceID","TumorVolume","Day")
utrgr=unique(dat[,1])
plot(1,1,xlim=c(-10,30),ylim=c(-5,1),main=utrgr[1],type="n")
xd=seq(from=-10,to=30,by=.1)
daUNTR=dat[dat$TreatmentGroup==utrgr[1] | dat$Day<=0,]
y=log(daUNTR$TumorVolume); day=daUNTR$Day
id=daUNTR$MiceID; uid=unique(id); nid=length(uid)
for(j in 1:nid) {
    yi=y[id==uid[j]];xi=day[id==uid[j]]
    lines(xi,yi);points(xi,yi,pch=16)
}
o=lme(fixed=y~day,random=~1|id); print(summary(o))
aUNTR=as.vector(o$coefficients$fixed)
lines(xd,aUNTR[1]+aUNTR[2]*xd,col=2,lwd=3)
segments(0,-6,0,2,col=3)
covpar <- o$varFix
DT <- log(2)/aUNTR[2]
lines(c(-12,DT,DT),c(aUNTR[1]+log(2),aUNTR[1]+log(2),-6),col=3)
SE.TD <- DT/aUNTR[2] * sqrt(covpar[2, 2])
text(10,-4,paste("Doubling Time =", round(DT,1), "\nSE =",
         round(SE.TD,2)),adj=0,cex=1.25)
```

We make several remarks on the code: (1) the data for all four treatment groups are in the file DEregrowth.dat; the data on untreated mice are composed of a control group plus the data from three other groups prior to treatment (Day<=0); (2) since the multiplicative error scheme is assumed the exponential growth for untreated mice reduces to a linear function estimated by lme; (3) the standard error for the doubling time is estimated using the delta-method (matrix o$varFix contains the variance-covariance of the fixed effects parameters, intercept and slope); and (4) the difference in SE for T_D in Table 10.1 and Figure 10.5 is because the R code uses data for all untreated mice, but in Table 10.1 only Control/Group 1 data are used.

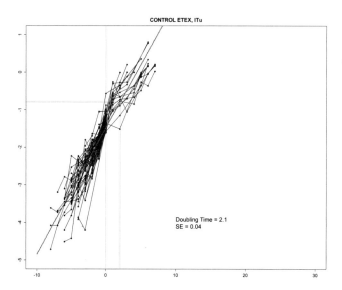

FIGURE 10.5. Tumor volume on the log scale for untreated mice estimated with lme.

Treatment groups. Using the DE regrowth curve with multiplicative error, we first fit the data in each treatment group using a statistical model,

$$y_{ij} = \ln(e^{\beta_1 + \beta_2 t_{ij}} + e^{\beta_3 - \beta_4 t_{ij}}) + \varepsilon_{ij},$$

assuming that mice have the same parameters, $\varepsilon_{ij} \sim \mathcal{N}(0, \sigma^2)$. Since parameters are fixed, this model reduces to nonlinear regression (starting values are derived as outlined in Section 10.2.6).

There are several ways to address heterogeneity of response to treatment. First, one can assume that parameters β_1 and β_3 are random but that β_2 and β_4 are fixed, leading to the following nonlinear mixed effects model:

$$Y_{ij} = (e^{\beta_1 + \beta_2 t_{ij} + \delta_i} + e^{\beta_3 - \beta_4 t_{ij} + \eta_i})e^{\varepsilon_{ij}}, \tag{10.13}$$

where random terms are normally distributed as $\delta_i \sim \mathcal{N}(0, \sigma_\delta^2)$ and $\eta_i \sim \mathcal{N}(0, \sigma_\eta^2)$ with correlation coefficient ρ. Several methods may be used to estimate the mixed model (10.13). After taking the natural log, one arrives at the nonlinear mixed effects model,

$$y_{ij} = \ln\left(e^{\beta_1 + \beta_2 t_{ij} + \delta_i} + e^{\beta_3 - \beta_4 t_{ij} + \eta_i}\right) + \varepsilon_{ij}, \tag{10.14}$$

studied in the previous chapter. In particular, model (10.14) may be estimated using such standard software as statistical packages nlme (R) or proc mixed (SAS). Second, one can use the fact that Y_{ij} has a lognormal distribution with the first moment $E(Y_{ij}) = e^{\tau_1 + \beta_2 t_{ij}} + e^{\tau_2 - \beta_4 t_{ij}}$, where $\tau_1 = \beta_1 + (\sigma^2 + \sigma_\delta^2)/2$ and $\tau_2 = \beta_3 + (\sigma^2 + \sigma_\eta^2)/2$. Further, one can find the exact covariance matrix and apply the IRLS or total GEE approach, as we did for the log-Gompertz curve of Section 6.4.5.

The R code below reads and plots the data for the three groups of treated mice shown in Figure 10.4 and estimates the response to treatment using the DE regrowth curve according to model (10.14) via the nlme function (Lindtsrom and Bates method). Use source("c:\\MixedModels\\Chapter10\\trnlme.r") to download the R function. Only data starting on day 1 after treatment are used. Days to regrowth is TR, and the standard error (SETR) is estimated via the delta method, where the 4×4 covariance matrix is extracted from the output of nlme as o$varFix.

```
dat = read.table("c:\\kluwer\\DEregrowth.dat",stringsAsFactor=F)
names(dat)=c("TreatmentGroup","MiceID","TumorVolume","Day")
xd=seq(from=1,to=30,by=.1)
utrgr=unique(dat[,1])
par(mfrow=c(1,3))
for(ig in 2:4)
{
    print(utrgr[ig])
    plot(1,1,xlim=c(0,30),ylim=c(-5,1),main=utrgr[ig],type="n",
            xlab="",ylab="")
    daUNTR=dat[dat$TreatmentGroup==utrgr[ig] & dat$Day>0,]
    y=log(daUNTR$TumorVolume); day=daUNTR$Day
    id=daUNTR$MiceID; uid=unique(id); nid=length(uid)
    for(j in 1:nid)
    {
        yi=y[id==uid[j]];xi=day[id==uid[j]]
        lines(xi,yi);points(xi,yi,pch=16)
    }
    o <- nlme(model=y~log(exp(a1+a2*day)+exp(a3-a4*day)),
        fixed=list(a1~1,a2~1,a3~1,a4~1), random=a1+a3~1|id,
        start=c(-7.,0.2,-0.8,0.2))
    print(summary(o))
    a <- as.vector(o$coefficients[[1]])
    yfit=log(exp(a[1]+a[2]*xd)+exp(a[3]-a[4]*xd))
    lines(xd,yfit,col=2,lwd=3)
    TR <- (log(a[4]/a[2])-a[1]+a[3])/(a[4]+a[2])
    ytr <-log(exp(a[1]+a[2]*TR)+exp(a[3]-a[4]*TR))
```

```
    segments(-1, 0, 30, 0, col=3,lty=2)
    segments(TR, ytr, TR, -7, col=3)
    d1 <- -1/(a[2] + a[4]); d2 <- - d1; al <- log(a[4]/a[2])
    d3 <- (-a[2]*al+a[2]*(a[1]-a[3])-a[2]-a[4])/(a[2]+a[4])^2/a[2]
    d4 <- (-a[4]*al+a[4]*(a[1]-a[3])+a[2]+a[4])/(a[2]+a[4])^2/a[4]
    dd <- c(d1, d3, d2, d4)
    SETR <- sqrt(t(dd) %*% o$varFix %*% dd)
    text(20,-4,paste("TR=",round(TR,1),"\nSE=",round(SETR,1)
        ,sep=""),adj=0,cex=2)
  }
mtext(side=1,"Days Post Treatment",outer=T,cex=1.5,line=-1.5)
mtext(side=2,"LOG Tumor Volume",outer=T,cex=1.5,line=-1.5)
```

There is a slight difference of time to regrowth estimates compared to the Table 10.1 values, due to difference in the data sets. We do not provide code for computation of other treatment outcome parameters since it is fairly straightforward. The computation of time to reach 1 cm^3 (T_1) and doubling time (T_D) requires the function decE shown above.

Table 10.2. p-values for group comparisons.

Group Comparison	T_R	T_1	T_D
2 versus 3	0.064	0.027	0.648
2 versus 4	0.0065	0.0016	0.536
3 versus 4	0.0003	<0.0001	0.348

The results of estimation by the Lindstrom–Bates method (Section 8.7) are shown in Table 10.1. All estimates have a small standard error and are statistically significant. This is a very rapidly growing tumor; for the control group, it takes only 2.1 days to double the tumor volume. Clearly, treatment has a profound effect–the doubling time increases from 2 days in the control group to more than 20 days in the treatment groups. Based on model (10.14), we can assess the Surviving Fraction (SF) as $e^{\beta_1}/(e^{\beta_1} + e^{\beta_3})$, the proportion of clonogenic cells at $t = 0$. The estimation results reveal different treatment effects in the three groups. In Group 2 the surviving fraction is the smallest, however, the kill effect has the shortest duration since the rate of the post-treatment growth is the highest, 32.3% a day, just slightly less than that of untreated tumor. In Group 3 the same dose of cisplatin is used, but the effect of treatment is prolonged, with a rate of growth of 24.4% a day. Group 4 has a slightly lower rate of post-treatment growth than that of the previous group and a smaller surviving fraction. This analysis suggests that an equivalent concentration of intratumor cisplatin injection leads to slower tumor regrowth: the 2.5-fold increase in cisplatin concentration (Group 4) has almost the same rate of regrowth but is much more toxic. This conclusion is confirmed by the tumor growth delay characteristics, such as time to regrowth (T_R), time to reach 1 cm^3 (T_1), and doubling time (T_D). In Table 10.2, p-values are shown for group comparison. Interestingly, treatment affects doubling time less, so the time to reach 1 cm^3 contrasts the groups better than does the time to regrowth.

Problems for Section 10.2

1. Check that equation (10.3) satisfies the system (10.2).
2. Solve the ODE $dQ/dt = \tau C e^{\nu t} - \phi Q(t)$, where C is a positive constant.
3. Prove that the DE as a function of D is convex (the second derivative is positive).
4. Derive the time to regrowth formula (10.7).
5. Prove that iterations (10.9) produce a descending sequence.
6. Using the derivation of implicit function, prove that doubling time is a decreasing function of ν and an increasing function of ϕ.
7. Adopt the code on page 548 to compute T_1 and T_D with SE for each treatment group.
8*. Derive a formula for maximum tumor volume reduction as the expected tumor volume at T_R and its standard error using the delta-method. Write an R code for computation and apply it to DEregrowth.dat data set. Append Table 10.2 to compare the tumor volume reduction across the groups.

10.3   Exponential growth with fixed regrowth time

Sometimes, nonlinear estimation fails and one needs simpler, more reliable statistical models. Here we suggest a simplified approach that reduces to a linear model after making the following assumptions on regrowth: (a) growth of untreated and treated tumors, after a certain time T_*, is exponential with the same rate, and (b) the regrowth time T_* is known. In particular, this approach was used in a recent paper by Demidenko (2010).

The idea of fixed regrowth time is illustrated in Figure 10.2: the uncontrolled growth (untreated/control group) and the growth of the treated group, after time $T_* = C$, is exponential with the rate ν. The key point of this approach is that on the log scale the intercept (say, h) measures the logarithm surviving fraction, which can be used to contrast treatments. When several treatment groups are studied and the post-treatment growth rate is the same, which often is the case, we can combine the data and estimate intercepts/SF simultaneously using a linear mixed effects model. Then the question of the relative efficacy of the treatments translates into a linear statistical hypothesis. A convenient way to pool group data is to use the method of dummy variables/intercepts (Draper and Smith, 1998). To be specific, let us assume that in two treatment groups (A and B) at day t_* after treatment at day $t = 0$, tumor regains its exponential growth rate ν. Let the surviving fraction in treatment groups A and B be h_1 and h_2, respectively. We combine observations from the three groups (the first group is a control) by introducing two dummy binary variables d_{i1} and d_{i2}, such that $d_{i1} = 1$ if and only if the ith animal belongs to treatment group A and zero otherwise. Analogously, $d_{i2} = 1$ codes treatment group B. Then the unified model for the three groups takes the form

$$y_{ijt} = h_0 + h_1 d_{i1} + h_2 d_{i2} + \nu t_{ij} + \varepsilon_{ijt}, \tag{10.15}$$

where y_{ijt} is the tumor volume logarithm of the ith animal at time t_{ij} from group $j = 1, 2, 3$ (if measurements are taken at the same time, we have a balanced model). We include all observations from the control group, but for the treatment groups, we take only those for which $t \geq T_*$. Note that if relative volume is used, $h_0 = 0$. As follows from this model, if animal i belongs to the control group, $y_{i2t} = h_0 + \nu t_{i1} + \varepsilon_{i1t}$, where h_0 is the ln(tumor volume) of the control group. For animals from treatment group A, the equation is $y_{i2t} = h_0 + h_1 + \nu t_{i2} + \varepsilon_{i2t}$, where h_1 is the ln volume of surviving cells in group A. Then the logarithm surviving fraction is equal to $h_1 - h_0$ for group A and $h_2 - h_0$ for group B. Model (10.15) is the multivariate regression model because all observations are independent and have the same variance. A more adequate assumption is that the intercepts are animal- and treatment group-specific, leading us to a two-level linear mixed effects model:

$$y_{ijt} = h_0 + h_1 d_{i1} + h_2 d_{i2} + \nu t_{ij} + \delta_i + \tau_j + \varepsilon_{ijt}, \tag{10.16}$$

where $\delta_i \sim \mathcal{N}(0, \sigma_\delta^2)$, $\tau_j \sim \mathcal{N}(0, \sigma_\tau^2)$, and $\varepsilon_{ijt} \sim \mathcal{N}(0, \sigma_\varepsilon^2)$ are independent. Further, this model can be reduced to the LME model studied in Chapters 2 and 3, and one can incorporate serial autocorrelation using methods described in Section 4.3.4.

10.3.1 Statistical hypothesis testing

After tumor regrowth models (10.15) or (10.16) are estimated, we can compute several treatment end-points as functions of the model parameters and test various statistical hypotheses. For example, to answer the question of whether group A is statistically significantly different from the control, we test the linear hypothesis $H_0 : h_1 = 0$. To test whether groups A and B are different, we test $H_0 : h_1 = h_2$. The doubling time for group A is estimated as $(\ln 2 - h_1)/\nu$ and for group B as $(\ln 2 - h_2)/\nu$. To contrast treatment groups by T_D, we take the difference $(h_2 - h_1)/\nu$.

10.3.2 Synergistic or supra-additive effect

Often, new cancer treatments are sought as a combination of existing treatments. A major problem is to prove that a combination of treatments leads to a greater therapeutic effect than treatments applied separately. If there exists such a special effect, we call it a *synergistic* or *supra-additive* effect. Below we provide a definition of the synergistic effect in terms of the surviving fraction and show how to test it using linear hypotheses in the framework of models (10.15) or (10.16).

Let A and B be two treatments aimed at killing cancer cells. After treatment A, let the fraction of surviving cells be SF_1, and after treatment B, let the fraction be SF_2, assuming that they are applied alone. Now if treatment B is applied after A, we expect the fraction of surviving cells to be the product $SF_1 \times SF_2$ because treatment B only affects cells surviving treatment A. We obtain the same answer when treatment B comes first because $SF_1 \times SF_2 = SF_2 \times SF_1$.

Definition 43 *We say that two treatments in combination have a synergistic effect if the surviving fraction of the combined treatment is less than the product of the surviving fractions when the treatments are applied alone.*

We emphasize that we take the product of the surviving fractions, which translates into the sum on the log scale.

Now let C be the treatment group with combined treatments A and B, and let all three groups be described by a model similar to (10.15) or (10.16) with three intercepts, $h_j, j = 1, 2, 3$, where the third group is C. Since the logarithm of the SF of the third group is h_3, we see that there is a synergistic effect if $h_3 < h_1 + h_2$. If there is no supra-additive effect, then $h_3 = h_1 + h_2$. Hence, the presence of the synergistic effect may be tested by the linear hypothesis $H_0 : h_3 = h_1 + h_2$. One can define the Relative Synergistic Effect (RSE) as

$$\text{RSE} = \frac{\text{SF}_1\text{SF}_2 - \text{SF}_3}{\text{SF}_1\text{SF}_2} 100\%, \tag{10.17}$$

where SF_1, SF_2, and SF_3 are surviving fractions in groups A, B, and C. RSAE is close to 100% when the combined treatment kills the tumor almost completely ($\text{SF}_3 = 1$). Vice versa, RSE=0% when the combined treatment plan has the same effect as if treatments were applied separately. If RSE is negative, the combined treatment is worse than separate.

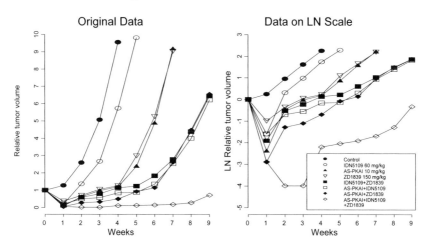

FIGURE 10.6. GEO tumor colon cancer xenograft growth delay data (Tortora et al., 2001) shown on two scales (mean values). Although the original scale helps to judge the relative tumor volume *value*, the logarithmic scale is more informative for analysis of the tumor *growth rate* in different treatment groups. In fact, it is possible to show the original scale at the right, see the next figure. Particularly, as follows from the right-hand graph (a) post-treatment tumors regain exponential growth at week 2 after treatment, and (b) all treatments introduce a tumor growth delay, but after week 2, tumors grow at the rate of the control group (the lines are parallel).

10.3.3   Example: combination of treatments

Tortora et al. (2001) describe a study designed to verify that combined oral administration of three novel agents that block multiple cancer cells signaling pathways reduces tumor growth significantly in nude mice bearing GEO colon cancer xenografts. Although a combination of new drugs seemed to affect the tumor growth in seven treatment groups, no statistical analysis was presented by the authors. We apply our approach to contrast treatment groups via traditional tumor growth time delay and doubling time using the exponential tumor regrowth model assuming that the time after which tumors regain exponential growth is defined. Our particular interest is in assessing the percent cancer cell kill in each treatment group and testing the significance of the synergistic effect.

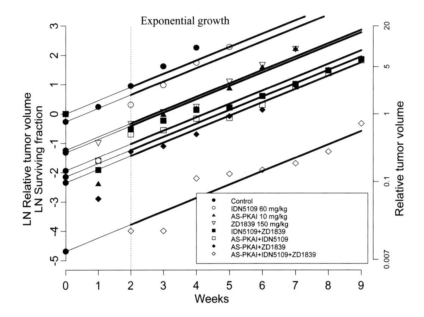

FIGURE 10.7. Linear mixed effects model fit to Tortora et al. (2001) data on the logarithmic scale. It is assumed that after week 2, tumors in all treatment groups regain exponential growth of the control group (46% volume increase per week). Since the data are ln(relative tumor volume), the control group starts from zero. The intercept, ln(Surviving Fraction), is determined by back projection of the treatment group line onto the y-axis. SF is a minimum for the last group when all three treatments are combined.

Seven treatment groups are considered, with approximately eight mice in each group. Groups received three types of inhibitors targeting the respective kinases as different doses in mg/kg, alone and in combination. The mean group data are shown on two scales in Figure 10.6. At the left the relative mean tumor volume is plotted against time in the way that it was presented in the original work. Although it is easy to judge the *value* of the relative volume when the data are plotted on the original scale, the logarithmic scale reveals two important features of the data: (a) after a period of time, i.e., after week 2, tumors regain exponential growth (the growth curves are almost straight lines) (b) the rate of growth of the post-treatment tumors is the same as that in the control (sham-treated) group of mice. These two observations give rise to the following assumption: After week 2 the natural logarithm of the relative volume in each mouse group is a linear function of time with a common slope ν but a different intercept pertinent to the treatment group. Generating seven dummy variables $d_{i1}, d_{i2}, ..., d_{i7}$, where i codes mouse so that $d_{ij} = 1$ if mouse i belongs to the jth treatment group and zero otherwise, we come to a linear mixed effects model,

$$
\begin{aligned}
y_{ijt} = {} & h_1 d_{i1} + h_2 d_{i2} + h_3 d_{i3} + h_4 d_{i4} + h_5 d_{i5} + h_6 d_{i6} + h_7 d_{i7} \\
& + \nu t_{ij} + \delta_i + \tau_j + \varepsilon_{ijt},
\end{aligned}
$$

with eight coefficients to estimate; y_{ijt} is the natural logarithm of the relative tumor volume after week 2, ν is the common growth rate, ε_{ijt} is the error term, and τ_j and δ_i are treatment- and mouse-specific random effects (there is no common intercept term because data are in relative volume format). As follows from this model, the relative tumor volume in the control group grows exponentially as $e^{\nu t}$; the tumor volume in the group IDN5109 60 mg/kg grows according to $e^{h_1 + \nu t}$; in the group AS-PKAI 10 mg/kg, tumors grow according to $e^{h_2 + \nu t}$; and so on.

The results of the estimation are illustrated in Figure 10.7 and presented in Table 10.3. The exponential growth rate, $\nu = 0.456$, means that the volume of the untreated tumors and post-treatment tumors after week 2 increases by 45.6% each week. Since data are presented as the natural logarithm of the relative tumor volume, the intercept for the control group is zero. Doubling time (DT) for the control group is calculated as $T_{pot} = \ln 2/\nu = 1.5$ weeks, with SE $= \ln 2/\nu^2 \times SE_\nu$. Tumor growth delay (TGD) is calculated as the difference between DT and T_{pot}. All treatment outcomes are statistically significant.

Treatment group comparison

We can compare treatment groups by two end-points, cell kill/surviving fraction and doubling time. However, since tumors in all treatment groups grow with the same rate one may expect that the results will be similar. As follows from Table 10.4 only groups (3,4), (5,6), and (6,7) failed to show contrast; the other pairs differ significantly in terms of surviving fraction and doubling time.

Table 10.3. Estimation results with three treatment end-points (common growth rate $\nu = 0.456$)

Treat. Group	Intercept, ln SF, h_j (SE)	Surviving Fraction $100e^{h_j}$	Cell Kill	Doubling Time (SE) weeks	Tumor Growth Delay
1	0	100%	0%	1.50 (0.06)	0
2	-0.26 (0.16)	76.8%	23.2%	2.10 (0.40)	0.60 (0.34)
3	-1.32 (0.15)	26.7%	73.3%	4.42 (0.45)	2.90 (0.27)
4	-1.24 (0.15)	29.0%	71.0%	4.23 (0.45)	2.71 (0.27)
2+3	-1.94 (0.15)	14.4%	86.6%	5.77 (0.52)	4.25 (0.23)
2+4	-2.15 (0.15)	11.7%	88.3%	6.23 (0.54)	4.71 (0.23)
3+4	-2.34 (0.15)	9.6%	90.4%	6.66 (0.55)	5.13 (0.23)
2+3+4	-4.69 (0.15)	0.9%	99.1%	11.80 (0.75)	10.28 (0.20)

Treatment groups: 1–Control, 2. IDN5109 60 mg/kg, 3. AS-PKAI 10 mg/kg, 4. ZD1839 150 mg/kg.

Table 10.4. Treatment group pairwise comparison (difference) for logarithm
surviving fraction and doubling time

Group	3	4	5	6	7	8
2 lnSF	1.06*	0.97*	1.67*	1.89*	2.08*	4.42*
DT	-2.32*	-2.13*	-3.67*	-4.13*	-4.56*	-9.70*
3 lnSF		-0.08	0.61*	0.82*	1.02*	3.36*
DT		0.19	-1.35*	-1.81*	-2.24*	-7.38*
4 lnSF			0.70*	0.91*	1.10*	3.45*
DT			-1.53*	-1.99*	-2.42*	-7.56*
5 lnSF				0.21	0.41*	2.75*
DT				-0.46	-0.89*	-6.03*
6 lnSF					0.19	2.54*
DT					-0.43	-5.58*
7 lnSF						2.34*
DT						-5.14*

Note. The asterisk indicates that the p-value is less than or equal to 0.01.

Testing the synergistic effect

The results of statistical testing of the synergistic effect are presented in Table 10.5. The goal of this testing is to determine whether the combination of drugs leads to a greater cell kill than that of the individual drugs. As follows from the preceding section, the synergistic hypothesis is reduced to conventional statistical hypothesis testing on the intercepts in the linear model. As follows from Table 10.5, the combinations of inhibitors IDN5109 with AS-PKAI and AS-PKAI with ZD1839 do not have much of an effect compared to the case when administered separately. However, the combinations of IDN5109 with ZD1839 and all three inhibitors have a dramatic synergistic effect. For example, the percent surviving fraction when IDN5109 and ZD1839 used separately, would be 92% higher than when these drugs are used in combination. Interestingly, this combination of drugs has a greater relative effect than when the three drugs are combined (85%).

Table 10.5. Statistical testing of the synergistic effect of combined treatments

Treatm. group	Separate effect	Combined Effect	Difference SAE (SE)	$p-$ Value	RSE %
2+3	$h_1 + h_2 = -1.58$	$h_4 = -1.94$	0.36 (0.22)	0.118	30
2+4	$h_1 + h_3 = -1.50$	$h_5 = -2.15$	0.65 (0.22)	0.005	48
3+4	$h_2 + h_3 = -2.56$	$h_6 = -2.34$	-0.22 (0.21)	0.302	-24
2+3 +4	$h_1 + h_2 + h_3$ $= -2.82$	$h_7 = -4.69$	1.87 (0.28)	<0.001	85

Problems for Section 10.3

1. Use the delta method to derive formulas for SE for estimates of T_1 and T_D from a linear mixed model.

2. Use the delta method to compute the SE for RSE.

3*. Use the fixed regrowth time to estimate T_1 and T_D with their SE for the data set DEregrowth.dat.

4*. The file \\MixedModels\\Chapetr10\\tumdat.csv contains another data on tumor regrowth in four groups of mice with 0 (control), 3, 5, and 10 Gy of radiation. The R code is in the file R.growth.r and a detailed description of the data with the output is in file Regrowth.pdf. Use the DE regrowth model estimated with nlme for treated groups and compare the result with the fixed regrowth time approach implemented in the function R.growth. Compare the results. Which approach is better? Justify.

10.4 General regrowth curve

We can generalize the DE regrowth curve taking any growth curve G and survival curve S by the rule

$$R(t) = S(D) \times G(t) + G(0) \times (1 - S(D))e^{-\phi t}, \quad t \geq 0, \qquad (10.18)$$

where $R(t)$ is a regrowth curve, $S(D)$ is a survival curve with treatment dose D and $G(t)$ is a growth curve. Here $G(0)$ is the value of the growth curve at time 0 and it is assumed that doomed cells wash out from the tumor with exponential rate $\phi > 0$. It is easy to see that DE curve (10.5) is a special case of (10.18) when $G(t) = e^{\ln N_0 + \nu t}$ and $S(D) = e^{-\alpha D}$. Combining the Gompertz growth curve with exponential SC, we arrive at the Gompertz regrowth curve, which can be written as

$$R(t) = A \left[e^{-\alpha D - e^{-\nu t}} + (1 - e^{-\alpha D})e^{-\phi t} \right].$$

Here $A = R(0)$ is the initial tumor volume and $Ae^{-\alpha D}$ is the maximum tumor volume after treatment with dose D. As follows from formula (10.18),

$$R(0) = S(D)G(0) + G(0)(1 - S(D)) = G(0).$$

That is, the regrowth curve is a continuous function of time for any dose D. It is worthwhile to note that the regrowth curve (10.18) can model tumor dynamics only if the tumor shrinks immediately after treatment in a way that can be expressed mathematically as

$$R'(0) = S(D) \times G'(0) - \phi G(0) \times (1 - S(D)) < G'(0).$$

In other words, (10.18) is not a smooth function at $t = 0$. This kind of model can be used for very responsive tumors. To describe the dynamics of smoothly regrowing tumors (less responsive), a more complicated model is required. This is our aim in the next section.

Problems for Section 10.4

1*. Apply the Gompertz regrowth curve to the data set DEregrowth.dat. Do you see any advantage of this curve compared with the DE regrowth curve?

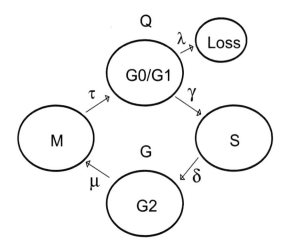

FIGURE 10.8. Smooth regrowth curves are built to model less responsive tumors. They originate from the cell-cycle model, well accepted in tumor biology. Four cell-cycle phases, corresponding to four model compartments, are distinguished: Phases G_0 and G_1 are combined to constitute the first compartment, Q. Cells from this compartment either move to the DNA synthetic phase S at rate γ or die at rate λ. Cells from compartment S move to the next compartment, G at rate δ, and from G to mitotic compartment M at rate μ. After mitosis, cells enter compartment Q at rate τ. This scheme is represented mathematically via a system of four differential equations of the first order, (10.19).

10.5   Double-exponential transient regrowth curve

The aim of this section is to generalize the DE regrowth curve to account for possible (transient) growth immediately after treatment based on the textbook four-compartment cell cycle model, see Figure 10.8. It is well known that the cell cycle comprises four phases, e.g., Murray and Hunt (1993):

- The G_1 phase represents the DNA presynthetic phase.

- The S phase represents the phase during which the DNA synthesis happens; this phase is an intermediate step between the G_1 and G_2 phases.

- The G_2 phase represents cells between the S phase and mitosis or cell division (the post-synthetic phase).

- The M phase represents actual cell division where the mother cell divides into two daughter cells.

I addition to these four cell groups/phases there is another relatively large portion of quiescent cells that are not involved in the cell cycle but enter G_1 after receiving a signal for cell division. In particular, these cells play the role of recruiters after treatment/irradiation. The first compartment constitutes quiescent cells (G_0) and cells from phase G_1 denoted by Q. The second compartment constitutes cells from phase S, compartment G holds cells from phase G_2, and M denotes mitotic cells. We want to describe the dynamics of compartments and how cells from one compartment move to another compartment in time. To derive a parsimonious model, we have to describe the most important part of cell promotion in the manner of the simplest birth/death model (10.2). We start from the first compartment: the number of cells increases by newborn cells from compartment M at rate τ and decreases as cells die at rate λ. Further, it is assumed that cells from compartment Q move to compartment S at rate γ, cells from compartment S move on to compartment G at the rate δ, and finally to the mitotic compartment at the rate μ. In mathematical terms the interactions among the four compartments of the cell cycle may be written via a system of differential equations:

$$\frac{dQ}{dt} = \tau M - \lambda Q, \quad \frac{dS}{dt} = \gamma Q, \quad \frac{dG}{dt} = \delta S, \quad \frac{dM}{dt} = \mu G. \tag{10.19}$$

After subsequent differentiation and substitution, we can reduce this system to one Ordinary Differential Equation (ODE) of the fourth order,

$$\frac{d^4 Q}{dt^4} = \kappa Q - \lambda \frac{d^3 Q}{dt^3}, \tag{10.20}$$

where $\kappa = \delta\gamma\mu\tau$. To find a solution to this ODE, we must solve the characteristic (polynomial) equation $C(z) = \kappa$, where $C(z) = z^4 + \lambda z^3$ (Codington and Levinson, 1955; Bartlett and Hiorus, 1973). See Figure 10.9 for a geometrical illustration.

Proposition 44 *The fourth-order algebraic equation $z^4 + \lambda z^3 = \kappa$, where constants λ and κ are positive, has two real roots, one positive (ν) and one negative ($-\phi$), and a couple of conjugate complex roots with a negative real part, $-\zeta \pm \omega i$.*

Proof. First, we prove that the function $C(z) = z^4 + \lambda z^3$ is strictly increasing for positive z. This follows from the fact that the derivative is positive, $dC/dz = 4z^3 + 3\lambda z^2 > 0$ for $z > 0$. Since $C(0) = 0$, it follows that $C(z) = \kappa$ has a unique positive root. Second, we prove that the equation $C(z) = \kappa$ has a unique negative root. Indeed, the function $C(z)$ attains its minimum at $z_{\min} = -3\lambda/4$ which gives $C_{\min} = -3^3\lambda^4/4^4 < 0$. In the interval $(-\infty, z_{\min})$, the function $C(z)$ is decreasing and $C(-\infty) = +\infty$. This implies that $C(z) = \kappa$ has a unique negative root. It is known that the equation $z^4 + \lambda z^3 = \kappa$ has four roots in the complex domain; since it has only two real roots, it must have two conjugate complex roots, $-\zeta \pm \omega i$. ∎

As follows from ODE theory, the solution to (10.20) can be written as

$$Q(t) = C_1 e^{\nu t} + C_2 \left(e^{-\phi t} + T(t) \right), \tag{10.21}$$

where $T(t)$, called the *transient* function, is defined as $T(t) = Ce^{-\zeta t}\sin(\omega t)$. Constants C_1 and C_2 specify the number of surviving and damaged cells, respectively, at time zero. Interestingly, equation (10.21) contains an oscillation part associated with period $2\pi/\omega$. The oscillation of the surviving cells is a well-documented phenomenon

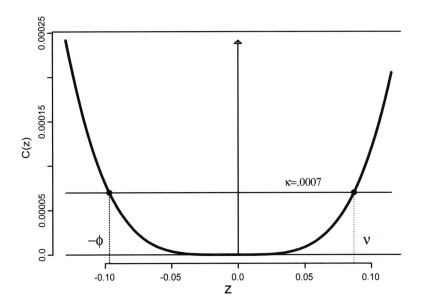

FIGURE 10.9. Characteristic equation $C(z) = \kappa$ with $\kappa = 0.0007$ and $\lambda = 0.02$ where $C(z) = z^4 + \lambda z^3$. This algebraic equation of the fourth order has four roots: two real roots (one of each is positive and another is negative, dots) and a couple of conjugate complex roots. The positive root (ν) is the rate of growth rate of clonogenic/cancer cells, the negative root $(-\phi)$ is that rate at which doomed cells leave the tumor. Complex roots correspond to an oscillating pattern of doomed tumor cells.

in vitro and *in vivo* (Brown, 1975; Chignola et al., 1999). It is easy to show that the total number of cells in the four compartments, $N(t) = Q(t) + S(t) + G(t) + M(t)$, follows an equation similar to (10.21):

$$N(t) = C_1 e^{\nu t} + C_2 \left(e^{-\phi t} + T(t) \right). \tag{10.22}$$

This growth curve contains three parts. The first part, $C_1 e^{\nu t}$ describes the exponential growth of proliferating cells; $C_2 e^{-\phi t}$ describes the fraction of doomed cells that leave the tumor with constant rate ϕ; and the third part corresponds to the transient function, $T(t)$ which reflects mitotic death.

Now we apply this growth curve to model tumor dynamics after a single dose D. If N_0 is the total number of cells at the time of treatment $(t = 0)$, then, as follows from equation (10.22), C_1/N_0 represents the fraction of surviving cells and C_2/N_0 represents the fraction of killed cells washing out from the tumor according to exponential law at a negative rate. Following the line of our general approach, the surviving fraction is modeled via survival curve $S = S(D)$, and therefore equation (10.22) takes the form $(t \geq 0)$

$$N(t) = N_0 \left[S(D) e^{\nu t} + (1 - S(D)) \left(e^{-\phi t} + C e^{-\zeta t} \sin(\omega t) \right) \right]. \tag{10.23}$$

Note that if $D = 0$, no treatment, cells continue growing exponentially, $N(t) - N_0 e^{\nu t}$. At the time of treatment

$$N(0) = N_0 \left[S(D) + (1 - S(D)) (1 + C \sin(0)) \right] = N_0,$$

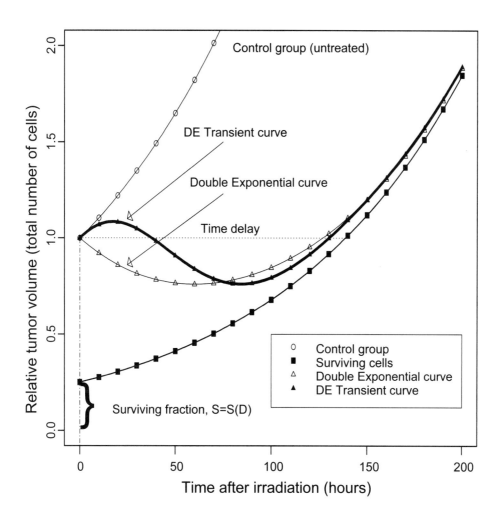

FIGURE 10.10. Principal idea of the Double-Exponential Transient regrowth curve. The fraction of surviving cells is modeled via a survival (dose-response) relationship, $S = S(D)$. It is assumed that the unaffected fraction of cells continues growing at the rate of the control group (filled squares). Cells immediately affected by the irradiation wash out from the tumor (group B). According to the DE regrowth curve the total number of cells drops right after the time of radiation (empty triangles). A more comprehensive DET regrowth curve (bold) has a smooth character: it is assumed that cells may go through a few cell cycles before dying and eventually washing out from the tumor (apoptosis). A characteristic property of a transient curve is that it has a local maximum and a minimum and that the rate of growth at time zero is a continuous function of time.

so that $N(t)$ is a continuous function, assuming that for $t < 0$, cells grew according to $N_0 e^{\nu t}$. To make the function (10.23) smooth at $t = 0$, we equate the rate of exponential growth for $t < 0$ to the rate at $t = 0$,

$$\left. \frac{d\left(N_0 e^{\nu t}\right)}{dt} \right|_{t=0} = \left. \frac{d\left(N(t)\right)}{dt} \right|_{t=0} \tag{10.24}$$

for all doses D. This leads to the condition $\nu = -\phi + C\omega$. Expressing constant C in terms of rates ν and ϕ, we finally arrive at the regrowth curve for the total number of post-treatment tumor cells

$$N(t) = N_0 \left[S(D)e^{\nu t} + (1 - S(D))\left(e^{-\phi t} + \frac{\nu + \phi}{\omega}e^{-\zeta t}\sin(\omega t)\right)\right]. \tag{10.25}$$

This regrowth curve is smooth at $t = 0$ because the rate of growth at time zero is equal to the rate of uncontrolled exponential growth ($t \leq 0$), as follows from condition (10.24). This function is called the *General Double–Exponential Transient (GDET)* regrowth curve. Function (10.25) defines a family of regrowth curves dependent on the choice of survival curve S. For example, taking the simplest exponential survival curve $S(D) = e^{-\alpha D}$, we arrive at the *Double–Exponential Transient (DET)*,

$$N(t) = N_0 \left[e^{-\alpha D}e^{\nu t} + (1 - e^{-\alpha D})\left(e^{-\phi t} + \frac{\nu + \phi}{\omega}e^{-\zeta t}\sin(\omega t)\right)\right]. \tag{10.26}$$

The DET regrowth curve (10.26) comprises three groups corresponding to cells not affected by the irradiation (A), doomed cells (B) and lethally damaged/apoptotic cells (C); namely $N(t) = P(t) + K(t) + A(t)$. A geometrical illustration of the DET regrowth curve is presented in Figure 10.10. More precisely, the three groups are specified as follows:

A Cells not affected by irradiation retain the ability to proliferate exponentially with the rate ν. The number of cells at time t is $P(t) = N_0 e^{-\alpha D}e^{\nu t}$.

B Cells killed by irradiation wash out from the tumor almost immediately following a decay law, $K(t) = N_0(1 - e^{-\alpha D})e^{-\phi t}$.

C Apoptotic cells lethally damaged by irradiation may not die immediately. They may go through a few cell cycles before dying and washing out from the tumor, $A(t) = N_0(1 - e^{-\alpha D})e^{-\zeta t}\sin(\omega t)(\nu + \phi)/\omega$, a damped sine. This group contains cells with damaged DNA and apoptotic cells, Tubiana et al. (1990), Hall (2000). Several radiobiological studies have confirmed an oscillating pattern of apoptotic cells (Rockwell and Kallman, 1974; Higashikubo et al., 1996). Also, oscillation may be due to a profound tumor bed effect *in vivo* (Begg, 1983; Kallman, 1987).

The parameters of the DET curve have biological interpretations:

- α is the radiosensitivity parameter pertinent to the specified tumor cell type, and $e^{-\alpha D}$ is the surviving fraction after single dose D.

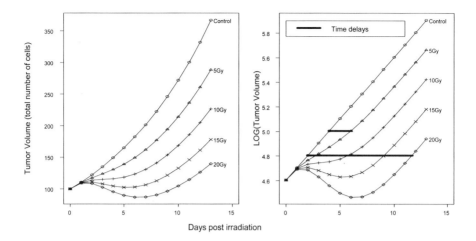

FIGURE 10.11. Double-Exponential Transient (DET) regrowth curve as a function of different radiation doses. The control group (untreated tumor) grows exponentially, treated tumors slow down after radiation and then regrow. A characteristic property of the DET curve is that it can model tumors that do not shrink immediately after irradiation but can grow awhile and then shrink. At the right, the same curves are displayed on a logarithmic scale. This scale illuminates the concept of tumor growth time delay. For example, a single dose of 5 Gy at day 0 leads to a 2-day delay, and 20 Gy leads to an 8.5-day delay. These regrowth curves closely resemble hand drawings of the desirable shape of regrowth curves as depicted in classical radiobiological texts, such as those of Kallman (1987), Tubiana et al. (1990), and Hall (2000).

- $(1 - e^{-\alpha D})$ is the fraction of cells lethally damaged by the treatment.

- ζ is the rate at which damaged cells wash out from the tumor, $\zeta < \phi$.

- ω is proportional to the frequency of damaged cell oscillation; namely, at $\pi/(2\omega)$ after irradiation, the population of lethally damaged cells reaches its maximum. It then goes down, reaching its minimum at $1.5\pi/\omega$. We may not see the oscillation pattern in tumor growth delay data because it damps at the rate ζ.

Figure 10.11 displays different patterns of post-irradiated tumor regrowth as a response to different radiation doses using our DET model (10.26), with the radiosensitivity parameter α corresponding to the RUC-2 malignant cell line (Tubiana et al., 1990). As follows from this graph, a bigger radiation dose kills more cells and delays tumor growth. For example, tumors treated with 15 and 20 Gy radiation doses begin shrinking and then regrow. When tumor receives a single 5 Gy radiation dose, the time delay is about 2 days, and the delay is about 8.5 days for 20 Gy. Remarkably, these graphs are similar to hand-drawings that illustrate tumor response to radiation in many radiobiological texts, such as those of Kallman (1987), Tubiana et al. (1990), and Hall (2000).

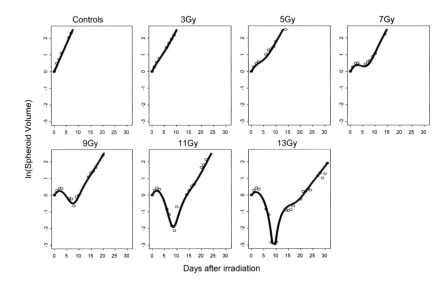

FIGURE 10.12. Double Exponential Transient (DET) regrowth curve (10.27) for Carlsson and Yuhas (1984) data (LAN-1 neuroblastoma spheroids) estimated by the **nlme** function of S-Plus. This type of malignant cell is very responsive to radiation, and therefore we use a quadratic SC. Notice the excellent fit in all groups.

10.5.1   Example: treatment of cellular spheroids

In this subsection, we fit the DET regrowth curve to the volume of human LAN-1 neuroblastoma spheroids treated with six graded radiation doses (cesium-137 gamma rays), as described by Carlsson and Yuhas (1984); see Figure 10.12. The cellular spheroid is an important 3D model in tumor biology because of its intermediate status between *in vitro* and *in vivo;* see Acker et al. (1984). In particular, spheroids suit our modeling well because volume/total number of cells is measured fairly precisely. As follows from Figure 10.12, some spheroids continue growing after irradiation and, therefore a DE regrowth curve of the form (10.25) seems adequate. We found that a normalizing factor should be included, reflecting the fact that the number of cells is not proportional to the tumor volume (nonuniform cell density). According to Carlsson and Yuhas, this type of cancer cell is responsive to radiation treatment. Mathematically, this means that the Linear-Quadratic (LQ) survival curve of Section 10.1 might be a good candidate. We found that coefficient α is close to zero, and therefore in (10.25), we use $S(D) = e^{-\beta D^2}$. The statistical model for the seven radiation dose groups takes the form

$$y_{ij} = (A + \delta_j)\ln[e^{-\alpha D_i^2 + \nu t_{ij}} \tag{10.27}$$
$$+ (1 - e^{-\alpha D_i^2})(e^{-\phi t_{ij}} + \frac{\nu + \phi}{\omega} e^{-\zeta t_{ij}} \sin(\omega t_{ij}))] + \varepsilon_{ij},$$

where t_{ij} represents the day when spheroid volume was measured; $j = 1, 2, ..., 7$ is the treatment group with a single radiation dose D: 0, 3, 5, 7, 9, 11, 13 Gy at day 0. As follows from model (10.27), all parameters but the normalizing factor are assumed fixed across treatment groups. This model was estimated by the **nlme** function, and the estimation results are presented in Table 10.6. Notice that all parameters are highly significant.

Table 10.6. Estimation of the DET regrowth curve for cellular spheroids (Carlsson and Yuhas, 1984).

Parameter	Estimate	SE	Z-statistic
Rate of uncontrolled growth, ν	0.216	0.022	9.61
Rate of loss, killed cells, ϕ	0.185	0.023	7.99
Rate of loss, damaged cells, ζ	0.126	0.023	5.46
Frequency of oscillation, ω	0.508	0.010	49.9
Radiosensitivity parameter, α	2.661	0.29	9.15
Normalizing factor, A	1.219	0.14	8.57

Using the estimate of the radiosensitivity parameter, one can predict that 20 Gy radiation would kill the tumor almost completely because $e^{-2.661 \times 20^2} \simeq 0$ (however, at least theoretically, it suffices to have one cell to develop a tumor). We notice that the damaged cells leave the tumor at a lower rate, 0.126, than that of killed cells, 0.185. The period of oscillation, according to this model, is $(2\pi)/0.508 = 12.4$ days. A small dose of radiation for this tumor has almost no effect because the derivative of S with respect to D is zero at $D = 0$.

Problems for Section 10.5

1. Plot several DET curves (10.26) as a function of time t for several ϕ, ζ, D, and ω, e.g. as shown in Figure 10.11. Plot three groups of cells, **A**, **B**, and **C**. Provide an explanation.

2. Using parameter values from Table 10.6, compute the nadir and minimum tumor volume for $D = 20$ Gy. Plot the curve and display your answer as the point on the curve.

3*. Develop the Newton algorithm for computation of the time delay, as shown in the right-hand plot of Figure 10.11. Write an R code.

10.6   Gompertz transient regrowth curve

Many studies demonstrate that the Gompertz curve is an adequate model for unperturbed tumor with limited growth. Statistical issues of Gompertz curve estimation are discussed in Section 6.1.7. We can easily modify our cell cycle model (10.19) to account for limited growth. Indeed, as a differential equation, the Gompertz curve is written as $dN/dt = \nu N(\ln N_\infty - \ln N)$, where N_∞ is the tumor size limit and $N = N(t)$ is the tumor size at time t. Thus, instead of the term τM, which implies exponential growth, we use $\nu M(\ln M_\infty - \ln M)$ to account for limited growth, where M_∞ is the maximum size of the mitotic compartment. Unfortunately, this system of differential equations will not have a closed-form solution, so that we use the simplified approach of modifying (10.26) directly. Since the Gompertz curve has the equivalent form $\exp(n_\infty - (n_\infty - n_0)e^{-\nu t})$, where $n_\infty = \ln N_\infty$ and $n_0 = \ln N_0$ are the logarithm maximum and initial tumor size/volume, respectively (Section 6.1.7), the *Gompertz Transient* (GT) regrowth curve takes the form ($t \geq 0$)

$$N(t) = e^{n_\infty - (n_\infty - n_0)e^{-\nu t} - \alpha D} + e^{n_0}(1 - e^{-\alpha D})$$
$$\times \left(e^{-\phi t} + \frac{\nu(n_\infty - n_0) + \phi}{\omega} e^{-\zeta t} \sin(\omega t) \right).$$

It is straightforward to show that this regrowth curve: (a) collapses to a traditional Gompertz growth curve when $D = 0$, (b) is continuous at $t = 0$, and (c) is smooth at $t = 0$ (continuous first derivative) for any dose D. The GT regrowth curve is adequate to model the behavior of large post-treated tumors. It is obvious how to modify the GT regrowth curve using more complicated survival curves, as in (10.25).

10.6.1 Example: tumor treated in mice

We apply the Gompertz Transient regrowth curve to *in vivo* data from Rygaardt and Spang-Thomsen (1997), with the kind permission of the authors. The experiment consisted of four groups of immune-deficient mice with human tumor xenografts implanted at day 14 prior to the irradiation. On day 0, three groups of mice received a single radiation dose of 3, 5, or 10 Gy, respectively. The authors used the Gompertz curve to fit the control group, and the regrowth data in radiation groups were fit by an exponential function with a subjectively chosen day of regrowth.

We start by fitting the logarithmic Gompertz curve to the control group and with mice from the other three radiation groups prior to radiation using a nonlinear mixed effects approach, assuming that maximum and initial tumor size is mouse-specific, namely,

$$y_{ij} = n_{j\infty} - (n_{j\infty} - n_{j0})e^{-\nu t_{ij}} + \varepsilon_{ij}, \qquad (10.28)$$

where $i = 1, ..., n_j$ is the number of longitudinal measurements of tumor volume, and $\varepsilon_{ij} \sim \mathcal{N}(0, \sigma_\varepsilon^2)$ (see section 6.1.7 for more detail on this Gompertz curve estimation). Since maximum and initial tumor size is mouse-specific, we may assume that

$$\begin{bmatrix} n_{j\infty} \\ n_{j0} \end{bmatrix} \sim \mathcal{N}\left(\begin{bmatrix} n_\infty \\ n_0 \end{bmatrix}, \begin{bmatrix} \sigma_\infty^2 & \sigma_{\infty 0} \\ \sigma_{\infty 0} & \sigma_0^2 \end{bmatrix} \right). \qquad (10.29)$$

Model (10.28) belongs to the type II nonlinear mixed models (varied matrix of random effects); Section 6.2. The estimated model is

$$\widehat{y}_{ij} = 9.29 - (9.29 - 4.89)\, e^{-0.027 t_{ij}}, \qquad (10.30)$$

with estimated covariance matrix

$$\begin{bmatrix} \sigma_\infty^2 & \sigma_{\infty 0} \\ \sigma_{\infty 0} & \sigma_0^2 \end{bmatrix} = \begin{bmatrix} 0.999^2 & 0.5 \times 0.838 \times 0.999 \\ 0.5 \times 0.838 \times 0.999 & 0.838^2 \end{bmatrix}.$$

As follows from (10.30), the untreated tumor may grow up to 9.29 mm^3. The rate at which the tumor approaches this limit is 2.7% a day.

Table 10.7. Estimation of the GT regrowth curve for tumor volume in mice,
Rygaardt and Spang-Thomsen (1997)

Parameter	Estimate	SE	Z-statistic
Rate of uncontrolled growth, ν	0.024	0.0025	9.6
Rate of loss, killed cells, ϕ	0.0507	0.0133	3.8
Rate of loss, damaged cells, ζ	0.0892	0.0294	3.1
Frequency of oscillation, ω	0.5306	0.028	18.6
Radiosensitivity parameter, α	0.203	0.0194	10.4
ln initial tumor volume, n_0	4.898	0.0819	59.8
ln maximum tumor volume, n_∞	10.38	0.387	26.7

Now we apply the GT regrowth curve with mouse-specific n_∞ and n_0 to the treated tumors,

$$
\begin{aligned}
y_{ij} = \ln \Big[& e^{n_\infty - (n_{j\infty} - n_{j0})e^{-\nu t} - \alpha D} + e^{n_{j0}}(1 - e^{-\alpha D}) \\
& \times \Big(e^{-\phi t} + \frac{\nu(n_{j\infty} - n_{j0}) + \phi}{\omega} e^{-\zeta t} \sin(\omega t) \Big) \Big] + \varepsilon_{ij},
\end{aligned}
\tag{10.31}
$$

where random $n_{j\infty}$ and n_{j0} have joint distribution (10.29). The estimation results are presented in Table 10.7 and the fit to individual growth data is presented in Figure 10.13. First, we notice that all parameters are well estimated and the GT curve goes close to all data points. Second, the radiosensitivity to 1 Gy is 0.23 Gy^{-1}, implying that 10 Gy kills $100(1 - e^{-2.3})\% \simeq 90\%$ of the cancer cells. Third, parameters $n_{j\infty}$ and n_{j0} are close to the control group. Fourth, the oscillation parameter is very close to what we obtained for spheroid data (period $= 2\pi/0.5 \simeq 12$ days). Whether or not this is a coincidence is a matter for future investigation.

A fragment of an R code is shown below (the code is incomplete due to the lack of space; the data may be found in the file Gompertz.dat). The mouse-specific regrowth curves plotted in Figure 10.13 use the matrix of ar coefficients (the number of rows equal to the number of mice, $N = 46$).

```
rstGT()
{
da=read.table("C:\\MixedModels\\Chapter10\\Gompertz.dat")
da0 <- da[da$day>=0, ] # only data after radiation are used
o<-nlme(LOGTV~log(exp(a1-a2*Dose-exp(-a3*day)*(a1-a4))+exp(a4)*
(1-exp(-a2*Dose))*(exp(-a5*day)+(a5+a3*(a1-a4))/a7*exp(-a6*
day)*sin(a7*day))),fixed=a1+a2+a3+a4+a5+a6+a7~1,
random=a1+a4~1|id,data=da0,start=c(11,0.19,0.02,5,0.06,0.09,0.55))
print(summary(o))
a <-as.vector(o$coefficients[[1]]) # fixed effects parameters
ar <-(o$coefficients[[2]])$id # mouse-specific parameters
}
```

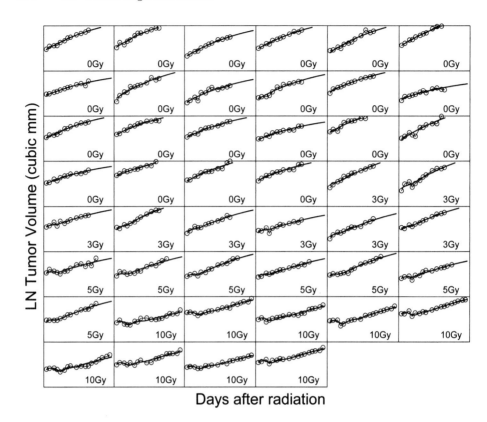

Days after radiation

FIGURE 10.13. Individual predictions of 46 tumor volumes in mice in four radiation groups from day 0 to day 43 by a GT regrowth curve, assuming that initial and maximum tumor volumes are mouse-specific (random).

Problems for Section 10.6

1. Why isn't the DE transient curve appropriate for `Gompertz.dat` data? Provide a justification.

2. Add lines nessesary to code in the function `rstGT` to reproduce Table 10.7 and Figure 10.13.

3*. Derive formulas for doubling time, time to reach a specific volume, and time to regrowth for GT curve along with SEs estimated by the delta method. Write the R code and compute these quantities using `Gompertz.dat` data.

4*. Explore more complicated structures for random effects in GT mixed model. Do mouse-specific ν, ϕ, and ω produce reasonable results?

10.7 Summary points

- Existing growth curve models, such as exponential, logistic, and Gompertz, cannot be used to model the post-treatment tumor volume dynamics because they are monotonic functions of time, but tumor growth delay data may not be monotonic. In particular, tumors after treatment may shrink in volume, reach nadir, and then regrow.

- Elaborated cell kinetics models cannot be used to model tumor growth delay data because they contain large numbers of unknown parameters impossible to estimate from limited longitudinal tumor regrowth data.

- We build our parsimonious tumor regrowth models combining classical growth curve models with a survival curve that models the proportion of surviving cells as a function of treatment dose, such as radiation. For example, the Double–exponential (DE) regrowth curve for radiotherapy data with fast-growing, responsive tumors is specified by three parameters: rate of growth of clonogenic cells, rate at which doomed cells wash out from the tumor, and radiosensitivity, which determines how cancer cells are affected by radiation. Fitting this curve to tumor growth delay data enables assessment of the radiosensitivity *in vivo*. Important endpoints of radiotherapy, such as time to regrowth/nadir and tumor growth delay, can be defined in the framework of the DE regrowth curve.

- Exponential and Gompertz transient curves are designed for less responsive tumors that respond to radiation not immediately but with some delay described by the transient function. We derive this curve from a system of differential equations that describe the cell cycle with four phases. We show that this system is equivalent to an ordinary differential equation of the fourth order and provide a closed-form solution that involves a sine component.

- Parameters of our regrowth curves have biological interpretations such as radiosensitivity, the growth rate of clonogenic cells, and frequency of oscillation of apoptotic cells. Direct assessment of these parameters is very expensive even *in vitro*, and almost impossible *in vivo*.

- There exists a simple relationship between three fundamental variables of cancer treatment: tumor growth delay is equal to the ratio of the logarithm of the surviving fraction to the rate of growth of clonogenic cells.

- Mixed model methodology is well suited to analyzing longitudinal tumor growth delay data. Parameters of regrowth curves may be population-based (genetically driven) or subject-specific.

- If, after a certain time T_*, treated tumors regain the exponential growth of untreated tumors, and T_* is known, the regrowth data may be analyzed by a linear model. Then the intercept measures the logarithm of the surviving fraction, and the question of treatment efficacy can be reduced to linear statistical hypothesis testing.

- Sometimes, new treatment drugs are combinations of old ones. A question arises as to whether the combined drug has a stronger killing effect than that of separate administration. We define this synergistic (supra-additive) effect in terms of a dose-response (survival) curve and show how it can be verified by statistical testing in the framework of the regrowth curve.

11

Statistical Analysis of Shape

11.1 Introduction

An impetus for the application of mixed models to the statistical analysis of shape is the fact that, on one hand, shapes come from the same population but, on the other hand, shapes vary and are subject-specific. Thus, the mixed model methodology may be useful in describing shape variation. In the language of a mixed model, mean shape is specified by population-averaged parameters (or fixed effects), and subject-specific variation is specified by random effects.

A characteristic property of a shape is that it is invariant in translation, rotation and size transformations. For example, we say that all equilateral triangles have the same shape because after size elimination, they become congruent. Eliminating irrelevant features associated with those transformations is the major issue in shape analysis.

Statistical shape analysis is widely employed in many fields and disciplines of science and engineering. We do not provide a complete coverage of the applications but just to name a few. For example, Lu (1965) analyzed human faces via a combination of Fourier series and ANOVA modeling. Wang et al. (2003) used a Procrustes shape model for gait recognition in surveillance systems. Shape analysis is used to characterize brain asymmetry and to detect schizophrenia or Alzheimer's disease (Wang et al., 2001). In geology, shape analysis is used to study particles and particularly sand grain variation (Bowman et al., 2001). In dentistry, shape analysis has been used to compare teeth (Ferrario et al., 1999). Shape analysis is widely used in biology to study specimen shapes that belong to the same population; this discipline is called *morphology*, see the review Rohlf (1990), and Lestrel (1997). For example, Horgan (2001) studied the shape of carrots of a specific type, Rohlf and Archie (1984) studied the wings of mosquitoes and Ferson et al. (1985) studied the shape of shells. A review on the topic and a methods comparison may be found in papers by McLellan, and Endler (1998) and Rohlf (2003).

Geometrical issues of shape, especially three-dimensional shape, are discussed comprehensively by Kendall et al. (1999). However, we consider only planar, or two-dimensional, shapes. The basis for statistical analysis is the fact that shapes can be *quantified* and therefore represented as a set of numbers. There are two ways to quantify shape; by landmarks and via digital image processing. An adequate set of landmarks determines the shape configuration, and digital image processing techniques specify the digital shape, the outline. For obvious reasons, earlier authors concentrated on the first approach. Technical aspects of extracting the shape from a digital image are discussed by Costa and Cesar (2001). Extracting a shape as an outline or outer contour of an image is not a difficult problem for modern photo-processing software such as PaintShop Pro (Jasc Software, Inc.). The two techniques imply different statistical analyses. In landmark analysis, the order of points is known, but the size and angle of rotation may be different. Several methods to deal with landmark data are available. First, one can use the raw data, the coordinates of the landmarks. If the orientation and variation in size are substantial a Procrustes model can be applied, Small (1996). Second, one can compute the relative distances between landmark points or angles (Bookstein, 1986, 1991; Kendall, 1989; Kendall et al., 1999; Lele and Richtsmeier, 2001). An obvious advantage of this approach is that the orientation of the shape, sometimes arbitrary, is eliminated. To analyze digital shapes, more complicated methods such as Fourier descriptor analysis are applied.

Several tasks are pursued in the statistical theory of shape:

- To estimate/reconstruct the true unknown shape μ, assuming that the shape samples are given up to rotation, translation, and scaling.

- To compare two samples of shape and test that they came from the same general population.

- To test whether the $(N+1)$th shape belongs to N given shapes, the membership test.

Specifically, we confine our consideration to two-dimensional shape, or more precisely to polygons. Since a polygon is defined by n points, the data take the form of $n \times 2$ matrices, $\mathbf{u}_1, \mathbf{u}_2, ..., \mathbf{u}_N$. We assume that the shapes are independent and identically distributed. The latter means that there exists an $n \times 2$ matrix (shape) μ such that after translation, rotation and scaling the mean of $\mathbf{u}_i$ is μ, which is called the *mean shape*.

We start the shape analysis with the simplest shape problem—triangular shapes or random triangles—and illustrate how the membership test can be used for human face identification. Next, we discuss how a linear mixed model can be applied to landmark analysis and how to model the correlation between neighboring landmarks via the Toeplitz covariance structure of Section 4.3.4. To eliminate shape orientation and size, a Procrustes model is used. First, we apply the Fourier descriptor analysis to round shapes and then to arbitrary shapes, where the random effects reflect the shape variation. The results of a balanced growth curve model apply. We illustrate the Fourier descriptor analysis by leaf analysis.

11.2   Statistical analysis of random triangles

We start with the simplest two-dimensional (planar) shape, the triangle. We deal with *random triangles,* so that the length of the side is a random variable. It is assumed that the triangles are independent and identically distributed (iid). Since the triangular shape is uniquely specified by the lengths of its sides, we reduce the statistical analysis to an analysis of n iid triples. The triples are independent and belong to the same general population. Statistical analysis of triangles is a relatively old shape problem and has been considered by a number of authors, Watson (1986), Mardia (1989), and Goodall and Lange (1989), to name a few. However, unlike previous studies, we assume that the triangles come just slightly rotated and scaled so that we know the order of the sides (shape reconstruction of planar figures that may be rigidly transformed is considered later). In fact, in many applied problems we know the tops and bases of the triangles, so the order of the sides is known. For instance, this assumption will hold later for our face identification problem.

In particular, we solve the following membership problem: given a sequence of N iid triangles, determine whether the $(N+1)$th triangle belongs to the same general population. We refer the reader to Section 3.8, where the membership problem is described in terms of a linear statistical model.

Thus, let us have N iid random triangles with the lengths of the sides specified by the *triangle model*

$$\mathbf{s}_i = \boldsymbol{\mu} + \boldsymbol{\varepsilon}_i, \quad i = 1, ..., N, \tag{11.1}$$

where $\mathbf{s}_i = (s_{i1}, s_{i2}, s_{i3})'$ denotes the vector of the lengths of the three sides and the vector $\boldsymbol{\mu} = (\mu_1, \mu_2, \mu_3)'$ is unknown. The error vector $\boldsymbol{\varepsilon}_i = (\varepsilon_{i1}, \varepsilon_{i2}, \varepsilon_{i3})' \sim \mathcal{N}(\mathbf{0}, \boldsymbol{\Omega})$, where $\boldsymbol{\Omega}$ is the 3×3 covariance matrix. The vector $\boldsymbol{\mu}$ specifies the mean triangular shape and the matrix $\boldsymbol{\Omega}$ specifies the covariance matrix of the error vector, both unknown and to be estimated (unstructured parameterization). The correlation between sides may reflect the fact that the sides were computed from random vertex coordinates. If the randomness of the length of the sides is due to measurement error, one may assume that all $\{\varepsilon_{ij}\}$ have the same variance, leading to a more compact parameterization, $\boldsymbol{\Omega} = \sigma^2 \mathbf{R}$, where the correlation matrix is given by

$$\mathbf{R} = \begin{bmatrix} 1 & \rho_{12} & \rho_{13} \\ \rho_{12} & 1 & \rho_{23} \\ \rho_{13} & \rho_{23} & 1 \end{bmatrix}. \tag{11.2}$$

An alternative (isotropic) parameterization would be to assume that all three sides correlate at the same magnitude, $\rho_{12} = \rho_{13} = \rho_{23} = \rho$. This model has a nice interpretation as a model to account for intra-cluster (intra-triangle) correlation. Indeed, let us assume that the length is subject to a pure measurement error but that the triangles differ in size. This can be captured by the model $s_{ij} = \mu_j + b_i + \varepsilon_{ij}$, where $\varepsilon_{ij} \sim \mathcal{N}(0, \tau^2)$ is associated with the measurement error and $b_i \sim \mathcal{N}(0, \tau^2 d)$ reflects the difference in size (d is the scaled variance). It is elementary to check that in the previous notation, $\sigma^2 = \tau^2(1 + d)$ and $\rho = d/(1 + d)$. The theory of linear mixed effects and the balanced growth curve model of Section 4.1 are particularly applicable.

A problem may emerge with the model (11.1) when the measurements are very imprecise because the sum of two sides may be less than the value of the other side. However, we ignore this possibility.

One hundred random triangles are shown in Figure 11.1. The question we pose is: Assuming that the first 99 triangles are iid and following the model (11.1), does the last triangle (bold) belong to the same general population? We will use the membership test from Section 3.8.1 to answer this question. A simplified version of the test based on the chi-squared distribution will be used.

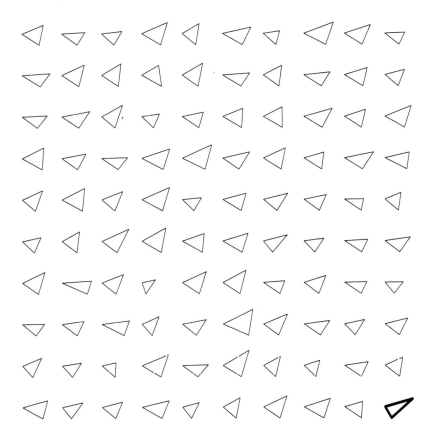

FIGURE 11.1. The first 99 independent triangles belong to the same general population. Does the 100th triangle (bold) belong to the same population?

We start by estimating of $\boldsymbol{\mu}$ and $\boldsymbol{\Omega}$ using the data given $\{\mathbf{s}_i, i = 1, ..., N\}$. The log-likelihood function for model (11.1) is

$$l(\boldsymbol{\mu}, \boldsymbol{\Omega}) = -\frac{1}{2}\left\{N \ln |\boldsymbol{\Omega}| + \sum_{i=1}^{N}(\mathbf{s}_i - \boldsymbol{\mu})'\boldsymbol{\Omega}^{-1}(\mathbf{s}_i - \boldsymbol{\mu})\right\}.$$

The maximum of this function admits a closed-form solution under unstructured parameterization because model (11.1) is balanced (no missing measurements),

$$\bar{\mathbf{s}} = \frac{1}{N}\sum_{i=1}^{N}\mathbf{s}_i, \quad \widehat{\boldsymbol{\Omega}}_{ML} = \frac{1}{N}\sum_{i=1}^{N}(\mathbf{s}_i - \bar{\mathbf{s}})(\mathbf{s}_i - \bar{\mathbf{s}})'.$$

Also, we can use an unbiased method of moments estimator for $\boldsymbol{\Omega}$,

$$\widehat{\boldsymbol{\Omega}}_{MM} = \frac{1}{N-1}\sum_{i=1}^{N}(\mathbf{s}_i - \bar{\mathbf{s}})(\mathbf{s}_i - \bar{\mathbf{s}})'. \tag{11.3}$$

When matrix $\boldsymbol{\Omega}$ is defined as $\sigma^2\mathbf{R}$, where matrix $\mathbf{R}$ is parameterized by three parameters (11.2), there is no closed-form solution to the MLE. However we can use the method of moments and estimate $\widehat{\rho}_{jk}$ as the correlation coefficient between s_{ij} and s_{ik}. Finally, $\widehat{\sigma}^2 = \sum(\mathbf{s}_i - \bar{\mathbf{s}})'\widehat{\mathbf{R}}^{-1}(\mathbf{s}_i - \bar{\mathbf{s}})/(3N)$.

Now we turn our attention to the membership problem: if an $M = N+1$ triangle (triple) is given, does that triangle belong to the same triangle population? We assume that $\mathbf{s}_{N+1} = \boldsymbol{\mu}_* + \boldsymbol{\varepsilon}_{N+1}$, where $\boldsymbol{\varepsilon}_{N+1} \sim \mathcal{N}(\mathbf{0}, \boldsymbol{\Omega})$. In other words, the sides of the triangle may be different but the covariance matrix is the same. We rephrase the membership problem in terms of statistical hypothesis testing $H_0 : \boldsymbol{\mu}_* = \boldsymbol{\mu}$ with the alternative that for at least one j we have $\mu_{*j} \neq \mu_j$ ($j = 1, 2, 3$). Under the null (the last triangle belongs to the population), $\bar{\mathbf{s}} - \mathbf{s}_{N+1} \sim \mathcal{N}\left(\mathbf{0}, \frac{N+1}{N}\boldsymbol{\Omega}\right)$, and replacing $\boldsymbol{\Omega}$ with $\widehat{\boldsymbol{\Omega}}$, we obtain, approximately,

$$S = \frac{N}{N+1}(\bar{\mathbf{s}} - \mathbf{s}_{N+1})'\widehat{\boldsymbol{\Omega}}^{-1}(\bar{\mathbf{s}} - \mathbf{s}_{N+1}) \sim \chi^2(3), \tag{11.4}$$

the chi-squared distribution with 3 degrees of freedom. Thus, if the test statistic S takes a value greater than $q_{1-\alpha}$, the $(1-\alpha)$th quantile of the chi-squared distribution, H_0 is rejected.

In Figure 11.1, the first 99 random triangles are generated with $\boldsymbol{\mu} = (2.5, 2.5, 3)'$ and $\Omega_{11} = 0.2$, $\Omega_{12} = 0.05$, $\Omega_{13} = 0.07$, $\Omega_{22} = \Omega_{33} = 0.1$, and $\Omega_{23} = 0.03$ and the 100th triangle was generated with $\boldsymbol{\mu}_* = (1.5, 2.0, 3.0)$, so it does not belong to the same population (all triangles are slightly rotated). The chi-squared test (11.4) rejects H_0 for the sample depicted in Figure 11.1 at $\alpha = 0.05$ with the p-value 0.036. The last triangle is different.

In the R code that follows, the function **randtr** generates 16 random polygons with m vertices (the default shape is triangle). The average distance from 0 is 1 with **roeps** as the deviation from 1 for each vertex. Two types of distributions can be used: unifrom and normal. The rotation is accomplished via the 2×2 matrix

$$\mathbf{P} = \begin{bmatrix} \cos\theta & -\sin\theta \\ \sin\theta & \cos\theta \end{bmatrix},$$

where θ is the (counterwise) random rotation angle uniformly distributed on $[0, 2\pi]$. This model is different from (11.1) and makes it possible to generate random polygons with an arbitrary number of vertices (this shape model is used later in Section 11.6).

```
randtr(roeps=.2,distr="run",m=3)
{
  par(mfrow=c(4,4),mar=c(1,1,1,1))
  ang=(2*pi)/m*(0:(m-1)) # angles for vertices
  Prot=matrix(ncol=2,nrow=2)
  for(itr in 1:16)
  {
      plot(c(-1.5,1.5),c(-1.5,1.5),type="n",xlab="",ylab="",axes=F)
      if(distr=="run") leng=runif(n=m,min=1-roeps,max=1+roeps)
      else leng=rnorm(n=m,mean=1,sd=roeps) #rotation distribution
      x=leng*cos(ang);y=leng*sin(ang)
      theta=runif(n=1,min=0,max=2*pi) #rotation angle
      Prot[1,1]=cos(theta);Prot[1,2]=-sin(theta) #rotation matrix
      Prot[2,1]=sin(theta);Prot[2,2]=cos(theta)
      xtr=Prot%*%t(cbind(x,y))
      xtr=cbind(xtr,xtr[,1]) # connectivity
      polygon(xtr[1,],xtr[2,],col=2)
      lines(xtr[1,],xtr[2,],lwd=4)
  }
}
```

Problems for Section 11.2

1*. Modify the function **randtr** to plot random triangles using model (11.1).

2. List advantages and disadvantages of the two random triangle models.

11.3   Face recognition

Face recognition and identification comprise a classic problem of pattern recognition. Much literature exists on the topic, and many scientific conferences and meetings are devoted to the subject, mostly in engineering and computer science circles. For a recent review, the interested reader is referred to a collection of papers of the Third International Conference on person authentication that includes face, speech, and fingerprint image processing and recognition (Bigun and Smeraldi, 2001). Surveys of methods on face recognition may be found in Samal and Iyengar (1992) and Chellappa et al. (1995). Numerous methods and algorithms have been suggested.

The basis for our approach is the observation that regardless of the facial expression, the distance between the eyes and the tip of the nose does not change; thus, our triangle model (11.1) can be applied. Particularly, we want to solve the following membership problem: given a sequence of photos of one person with possibly different facial expressions, is the next photo of the same person?

We use the Yale face database, which contains 165 gray images of 15 people at

http://cvc.yale.edu/projects/yalefaces/yalefaces.html

There are 11 facial expression per person. For illustrative purposes we consider only 11 photos of the first person and one photo of the second person, Figure 11.2. Since the lower part of the face moves with different facial expressions, we choose the following landmark triangle to quantify the image: right eye (left on the photo), left eye, and tip of the nose. This triangle is specified by the lengths of its sides. Thus, s_{11} is the distance between the eyes in the first photo in Figure 11.2; s_{12} is the distance between the left eye and the nose; and s_{13} is the distance between the nose and the right eye of the "centerlight" photo. The landmark points are identified manually and therefore are subject to measurement error. Below we show the mean distances for the first person ($i = 1, ..., 11$), the vector of distances of the second person ($i = 12$), standard errors of the mean, and the correlation matrix.

$$\widehat{\boldsymbol{\mu}}_{11} = \begin{bmatrix} 56.57 \\ 41.65 \\ 41.94 \end{bmatrix}, \quad \mathbf{s}_{12} = \begin{bmatrix} 53.08 \\ 42.80 \\ 45.00 \end{bmatrix},$$

$$SE(\widehat{\boldsymbol{\mu}}_{11}) = \begin{bmatrix} 0.43 \\ 0.43 \\ 0.71 \end{bmatrix}, \quad \text{cor}(\widehat{\boldsymbol{\mu}}_{11}) = \begin{bmatrix} 1 & 0.19 & 0.29 \\ 0.19 & 1 & -0.01 \\ 0.29 & -0.01 & 1 \end{bmatrix}.$$

We use an unbiased MM estimator (11.3) for matrix $\boldsymbol{\Omega}$ with $N = 11$. We decide that the last photo is of the same person if vector $\mathbf{s}_{12}$ is within the "normal" range of $\widehat{\boldsymbol{\mu}}_{11}$. More precisely, we compute statistic (11.4) and base our decision on its value. Since under the assumption that the last photo is of the same person, statistic S has the chi-squared distribution with 3 degrees of freedom, and the threshold value is 7.81 with significance level $\alpha = 0.05$ (the error of rejecting the face when it is really of the same person). Our data give $S = 10.1$, and therefore we reject the null hypothesis with the p-value 0.018.

Several modifications can be made to improve this face model. First, we can assume that the distance between the eyes and the nose is the same, $\mu_2 = \mu_3$. Second, we can use other facial features such as the width of the face. Third, we can use a structured model for the covariance matrix (11.2), especially useful when the number of landmark points is large.

11.4 Scale-irrelevant shape model

In this section we consider a generalization of the triangle model (11.1), where size does not matter. Thus, triangles follow the linear model (11.1) but may be of different sizes. We are still interested in whether the 100th triangle in Figure 11.1 belongs to the population of the previous 99 triangles. When size does not matter, instead of the side length we can consider the angle; the model (11.1) remains the same, but $\mathbf{s}_i$ is the two-element vector of angles (we ignore the third angle because the sum of the angles is π).

When the shape is defined by $n > 3$ numbers, the statistical model for a scale-irrelevant shape can be defined as

$$\mathbf{s}_i = c_i \boldsymbol{\mu} + \boldsymbol{\varepsilon}_i, \quad i = 1, ..., N, \tag{11.5}$$

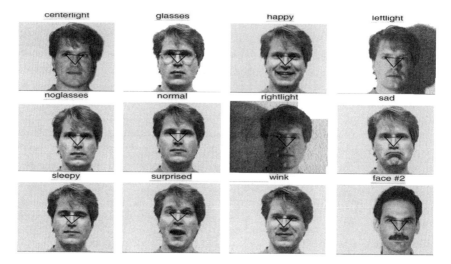

FIGURE 11.2. Twelve faces from the Yale face database. The first 11 photos are of the same person with different facial expressions. The last photo is of a different person. We apply the triangle membership test of Section 11.2 to show that the last photo is of a different person. This test seems adequate because facial expressions do not change the distance between the eyes and the tip of the nose.

where $s_i = (s_{i1}, ..., s_{in})'$ is the $n \times 1$ vector of shape observations, $\boldsymbol{\mu} = (\mu_1, ..., \mu_n)'$ defines the true unknown shape, c_i is a positive scale coefficient associated with size, and $\boldsymbol{\varepsilon}_i$ is the $n \times 1$ random error term. For example, a quadrangle (a polygon with four sides) can be defined by the length of four sides plus one diagonal, $n = 5$ (this representation is called *triangulation*, see Small 1996). Again, we assume that the order of sides is known. For clarity of presentation, we shall assume that the components of the error term are independent and normally distributed random variables with zero mean and variance σ^2. If $c_i = 1$ and $n = 3$, we come to the triangle model (11.1) with $\boldsymbol{\Omega} = \sigma^2 \mathbf{I}$. Regarding the scale coefficients $\{c_i\}$ we assume that they are fixed and unknown and we treat them as nuisance parameters (below we also consider a model where sizes are random). Since they are unknown, we have to restrict the length of the vector $\boldsymbol{\mu}$ because otherwise $\boldsymbol{\mu}$ would be nonidentifiable. Thus, it is assumed that $\|\boldsymbol{\mu}\| = 1$. The log-likelihood function for model (11.5) takes the form

$$l(\boldsymbol{\mu}, \sigma^2, c_1, ..., c_N) = -\frac{1}{2} \left\{ nN \ln \sigma^2 + \frac{1}{\sigma^2} \sum_{i=1}^{N} \|\mathbf{s}_i - c_i \boldsymbol{\mu}\|^2 \right\}. \qquad (11.6)$$

Maximization over c_i gives $\widehat{c}_i = s_i' \boldsymbol{\mu}$, and after some algebra, we express the sum of squares as

$$\sum \|\mathbf{s}_i - \widehat{c}_i \boldsymbol{\mu}\|^2 = \sum \|\mathbf{s}_i - \boldsymbol{\mu}\boldsymbol{\mu}' \mathbf{s}_i\|^2 = \text{tr} \left[(\mathbf{I} - \boldsymbol{\mu}\boldsymbol{\mu}')^2 \sum \mathbf{s}_i \mathbf{s}_i' \right]$$
$$= \text{tr} \left[(\mathbf{I} - \boldsymbol{\mu}\boldsymbol{\mu}')^2 \mathbf{M} \right] = \text{tr} \left[(\mathbf{I} - \boldsymbol{\mu}\boldsymbol{\mu}') \mathbf{M} \right] = \text{tr} \mathbf{M} - \boldsymbol{\mu}' \mathbf{M} \boldsymbol{\mu},$$

where $\mathbf{M} = \sum_{i=1}^{N} \mathbf{s}_i \mathbf{s}_i'$, a fixed matrix. Hence, the maximum likelihood estimate of the true shape, $\widehat{\boldsymbol{\mu}}_{ML}$, is the dominant eigenvector of matrix $\mathbf{M}$, and

$$\widehat{\sigma}^2_{ML} = (\text{tr}\mathbf{M} - \widehat{\boldsymbol{\mu}}'_{ML}\mathbf{M}\widehat{\boldsymbol{\mu}}_{ML})/(Nn).$$

This model can be used for further statistical inference. For example, the membership test to test whether the $(N + 1)$th shape belongs to the same size-irrelevant family of shapes.

Model (11.5) has a large number of nuisance parameters, $\{c_i\}$, which increases with the sample size (shapes). Consequently, we cannot use standard maximum likelihood theory because the $\{\mathbf{s}_i\}$ are not identically distributed. Also, parameter c_i cannot be estimated consistently when N goes to infinity with a fixed n. Since our primary interest is $\boldsymbol{\mu}$, a question arises as to whether the mean shape $\widehat{\boldsymbol{\mu}}_{ML}$ is consistent. The answer is positive. Indeed, let us assume that the $\{|c_i|\}$ are bounded and $\lim_{N\to\infty} N^{-1} \sum_{i=1}^{N} c_i^2 = A > 0$. Then with probability 1 from the law of large numbers, $N^{-1}\mathbf{M} \to \sigma^2\mathbf{I} + A\boldsymbol{\mu}\boldsymbol{\mu}'$. The dominant eigenvector of the latter matrix is unique and equal to $\boldsymbol{\mu}$ because $(\sigma^2\mathbf{I} + A\boldsymbol{\mu}\boldsymbol{\mu}')\boldsymbol{\mu} = (\sigma^2 + A)\boldsymbol{\mu}$. Since the unique dominant eigenvector is a continuous function of the matrix, we find that $\widehat{\boldsymbol{\mu}}_{ML} \to \boldsymbol{\mu}$ with probability 1. It is easy to show that $\widehat{\sigma}^2_{ML}$ is consistent as well.

The scale-irrelevant shape model may be modified to account for correlation between neighboring points, as in the triangle model. Thus, let us assume that $\text{cov}(\boldsymbol{\varepsilon}_i) = \boldsymbol{\Omega}$. Now, instead of $\boldsymbol{\mu}'\boldsymbol{\mu} = 1$, using a normalizing restriction $\boldsymbol{\mu}'\boldsymbol{\Omega}^{-1}\boldsymbol{\mu} = 1$, we obtain that $\widehat{\boldsymbol{\mu}}_{ML} = \boldsymbol{\Omega}^{1/2}\boldsymbol{\tau}$, where $\boldsymbol{\tau}$ is the dominant eigenvector vector of matrix $\boldsymbol{\Omega}^{-1/2}\mathbf{M}\boldsymbol{\Omega}^{-1/2}$. If all elements of matrix $\boldsymbol{\Omega}$ are unknown, a large number of shapes are required because the total number of unknown parameters is $N + n + n(n+1)/2$. For example, a parsimonious specification would be to assume that the correlation between neighboring points is the same. Later we discuss how to avoid estimating a large parameter further when considering the Procrustes shape model.

11.4.1   Random effects scale-irrelevant shape model

We argue that the scale coefficients c_i, under certain sample designs, may be meaningful and be a part of the population feature. For example, if in the face identification problem, the distance from the camera to the face is held fixed and faces are of adults, size c_i may represent the subject-specific size and one can talk about a distribution of face sizes. On the other hand, if the camera position varies or if the sample of faces contains faces of children, we cannot assume that the $\{c_i\}$ belong to the same population. If the shapes are drawn from the same population and the size is a part of the subject-specific shape variation, we may assume that the $\{c_i\}$ are random and iid so that they have the same mean. This leads to the *random effects scale-irrelevant shape* model. As with many random/mixed effects models, this model can be written in a hierarchical manner: The first-stage model has the conditional form $\mathbf{s}_i|c_i \sim \mathcal{N}(c_i\boldsymbol{\mu}, \sigma^2)$ and the second-level model is $c_i \sim \mathcal{N}(1, \sigma_c^2)$. Note that we assume that $E(c_i) = 1$ because otherwise the model becomes nonidentifiable since $\boldsymbol{\mu}$ is unknown. Denoting the scaled variance as $d = \sigma_c^2/\sigma^2$, we obtain the marginal model $\mathbf{s}_i = \boldsymbol{\mu} + \boldsymbol{\eta}_i$, where $\mathbf{s}_i \sim \mathcal{N}(\boldsymbol{\mu}, \sigma^2(\mathbf{I} + d\boldsymbol{\mu}\boldsymbol{\mu}'))$, $i = 1, 2, ..., N$. Clearly, if shapes are of the same size (no shape-specific size), we have $d = 0$. The latter model is not the LME model of the form (2.5) because the covariance matrix depends on $\boldsymbol{\mu}$. This is a peculiar case of the marginal mixed model considered in Chapter 6. Two approaches may be taken to estimate the true shape, $\boldsymbol{\mu}$ and the variance parameters, σ^2 and d: a distribution-free approach using Variance Least Squares (VLS) of Section 3.12 and maximum likelihood based on the normal assumption.

Since $E(\mathbf{s}_i) = \boldsymbol{\mu}$, we can unbiasedly estimate the true shape as $\widehat{\boldsymbol{\mu}} = \bar{\mathbf{s}} = N^{-1} \sum_{i=1}^{N} \mathbf{s}_i$. The VLS estimates for σ^2 and σ_c^2 are found such that the difference between the empirical and theoretical covariance matrices is a minimum,

$$\sum_{i=1}^{N} \mathrm{tr}\left(\widehat{\mathbf{e}}_i \widehat{\mathbf{e}}_i' - \sigma^2 \mathbf{I} - \sigma_c^2 \bar{\mathbf{s}} \bar{\mathbf{s}}'\right)^2 = \min,$$

where $\widehat{\mathbf{e}}_i = \mathbf{s}_i - \bar{\mathbf{s}}$. Differentiating with respect to σ^2 and σ_c^2, we come to a system of linear equations $\sigma^2 n + \sigma_c^2 \|\bar{\mathbf{s}}\|^2 = N^{-1} \sum \|\mathbf{s}_i - \bar{\mathbf{s}}\|^2$ and $\sigma^2 \|\bar{\mathbf{s}}\|^2 + \sigma_c^2 \|\bar{\mathbf{s}}\|^4 = N^{-1} \sum ((\mathbf{s}_i - \bar{\mathbf{s}})' \bar{\mathbf{s}})^2$.

Alternatively, we assume that the distribution is normal and apply the maximum likelihood approach. The twice-negative log-likelihood function takes the form

$$nN \ln \sigma^2 + N \ln |\mathbf{I} + d\boldsymbol{\mu}\boldsymbol{\mu}'| + \frac{1}{\sigma^2} \sum_{i=1}^{N} (\mathbf{s}_i - \boldsymbol{\mu})' \left(\mathbf{I} + d\boldsymbol{\mu}\boldsymbol{\mu}'\right)^{-1} (\mathbf{s}_i - \boldsymbol{\mu}).$$

Similar to the random intercepts model of Section 2.4, using the dimension-reduction formulas $|\mathbf{I} + d\boldsymbol{\mu}\boldsymbol{\mu}'| = 1 + d\|\boldsymbol{\mu}\|^2$ and $(\mathbf{I} + d\boldsymbol{\mu}\boldsymbol{\mu}')^{-1} = \mathbf{I} - d\boldsymbol{\mu}\boldsymbol{\mu}/(1 + d\|\boldsymbol{\mu}\|^2)$, the expression above can be simplified to

$$nN \ln \sigma^2 + N \ln(1 + d\|\boldsymbol{\mu}\|^2) + \frac{1}{\sigma^2} \sum_{i=1}^{N} \left[\|\mathbf{s}_i - \boldsymbol{\mu}\|^2 - d\frac{(\boldsymbol{\mu}'(\mathbf{s}_i - \boldsymbol{\mu}))^2}{1 + d\|\boldsymbol{\mu}\|^2}\right].$$

Differentiating with respect to $\boldsymbol{\mu}$, we obtain the MLE of the true shape, $\boldsymbol{\mu} = \lambda \bar{\mathbf{s}}$. Plugging this expression back into the log-likelihood, one can find λ and the variance parameters that maximize the log-likelihood function.

11.4.2   Scale-irrelevant shape model on the log scale

One may expect that the larger the shape, the larger the deviation from the true shape. This assumption leads to a multiplicative error model, $\mathbf{s}_i = c_i \boldsymbol{\mu} e^{\boldsymbol{\varepsilon}_i}$ (Rao and Suryawanshi, 1996). The advantage of this model is that after taking a logarithm, this model transforms into an additive scale-irrelevant model,

$$\mathbf{t}_i = \boldsymbol{\nu} + h_i + \boldsymbol{\eta}_i, \tag{11.7}$$

where $\mathbf{t}_i = \ln \mathbf{s}_i$, $\boldsymbol{\nu} = \ln \boldsymbol{\mu}$, $h_i = \ln c_i$, and $\boldsymbol{\eta}_i \sim \mathcal{N}(\mathbf{0}, \sigma^2 \mathbf{I})$. Clearly, this model assumes that the components of vector $\boldsymbol{\mu}$ are positive, such as when $\boldsymbol{\mu}$ is the distance between vertices of a polygon. Model (11.7) is a special case of the random intercepts model of Section 2.4. If the $\{h_i\}$ are treated as fixed, we can eliminate them by taking the differences, $\{t_{ij} - \bar{t}_i, i = 1, ..., N, j = 1, ..., n\}$. If the $\{h_i\}$ are treated as random, namely, $h_i \sim \mathcal{N}(0, \sigma^2 d)$, the results of Section 2.4 and Section 4.1.5 apply.

We can also account for correlation between components of vector $\mathbf{t}_i$ that would lead to a correlation matrix similar to (11.2) with $\rho_{12} = \rho_{23}$. A more general way to account for correlation is to model the covariance matrix via a Toeplitz matrix as $\mathrm{cov}(\boldsymbol{\eta}_i) = \sigma^2 \mathbf{V}$, where $\mathbf{V} = \mathbf{I} + \sum_{k=1}^{K} \theta_k \mathbf{T}_k$, see Section 4.3.4 for detail. Then the variance component θ_1 determines the correlation between points j and $j+1$; θ_2 determines the correlation between points j and $j+2$, etc. Assuming normal distribution, we come to a linear mixed effects (LME) model $\mathbf{t}_i \sim \mathcal{N}(\boldsymbol{\nu}, \sigma^2(\mathbf{1}\mathbf{1}' + \mathbf{V}))$. This is a balanced LME model, and as follows from the results of Section 2.3, the MLE estimate of the true shape is a simple arithmetic mean, $\bar{\mathbf{t}}$. Although a complex covariance structure does not affect computation of the true mean, it does affect the shape comparison and the membership test.

11.4.3   Fixed or random size?

The choice of how to treat size $\{c_i\}$ in shape analysis, random or fixed, is similar to the choice of random or fixed effects in a mixed model. Two issues should be taken into account. If size is a population feature, such as leaves from the same tree or skulls of the same type of adult animal, then $\{c_i\}$ can be assumed random with a well-interpreted mean. In particular, we may be interested in the variance of the size. Under a fixed-size design, the $\{c_i\}$ do not have an interpretation as a population feature. For example, we come to the fixed-size model when the shape is derived from digital pictures taken at different distances. However, it is worthwhile to remember that although the random size design seems more restrictive, it is statistically more attractive because it does not lead to a large number of nuisance parameters. Random size leads to a random effects model and is preferable. Consequently, if shapes are derived from digital images they should be taken at the same camera position. In summary, the choice of fixed or random size should be driven by the sampling design, not by the preference or expertise of the analyst.

Problems for Section 11.4

1. Prove that the ML estimator of $\boldsymbol{\mu}$ with the log-likelihood function (11.6) is the maximum (dominant) eigenvector of matrix $\mathbf{M}$.

2. Write an R function that generates a random quadrangle defined by five sides of two triangles.

3*. Modify the code from the previous problem to incorporate a correlation between sides. Visually compare quadrangles with independent and correlated sides.

4*. Find the ML estimator of λ in the random effect scale-irrelevant shape model.

11.5   Gorilla vertebrae analysis

We illustrate use of the random effects model to shape analysis by vertebrae data. The key is to distinguish two sources of variation: the variation within a shape and the variation between the shapes in each group. In a recent paper, Albert et al. (2003) analyzed the configuration of landmarks of the cervical vertebrae of 10 species of *Gorilla gorilla gorilla* (GGG) and seven species of *Gorilla gorilla berengei* (GGB), see Figure 11.3. In particular, the question is whether the data can distinguish between the two gorilla groups.

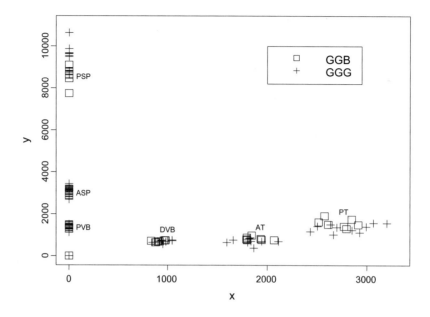

FIGURE 11.3. Landmarks of the vertebrae of 10 species of gorillas GGG and seven species of GGB. The names of the landmark veterbrae are indicated.

Table 11.1. Results of estimation of the LME model for the two gorilla groups (on a log scale)

Landmark	$\widehat{\mu}$ GGG	$\widehat{\mu}$ GGB	St. Diff.
PVBy	7.22	7.24	0.436
DVBx	6.86	6.83	0.717
DVBy	6.53	6.55	0.436
ASPy	8.04	8.02	0.479
PSPy	9.15	9.06	2.10
ATx	7.50	7.54	0.690
ATy	6.53	6.70	-3.81
PTx	7.93	7.91	0.573
PTy	7.18	7.34	-3.59
SD ε	0.088	0.064	
SD b	0.077	0.031	

Several linear mixed effects models for the landmark analysis can be suggested. We found that the multiplicative/relative error model works better (see detail in Section 11.4.2), so we take the logarithm of the nonzero coordinates. An indication that the relative error is better can be seen from Figure 11.3: the larger the absolute value of the landmark, the larger the variation. Thus, if z_{ij} represents the log of a nonzero coordinate of the ith gorilla of the jth landmark, then $z_{ij} = \mu_j + b_i + \varepsilon_{ij}$, where μ_j is the true coordinate, b_i is the random effect/size and ε_{ij} is the error term. Assuming that b_i and ε_{ij} are independent and normally distributed random variables, we come to the VARCOMP model. A variance of ε_{ij} represents the variation *within* vertebrae shape, and the variance of b_i represents the variation *between* vertebrae shapes. Estimations for two linear mixed models are presented in Table 11.1. Since the data are balanced (no missing values), the estimate of the landmark mean is the geometric mean. In the third column, we show the standardized difference, $(\widehat{\mu}_{GGG} - \widehat{\mu}_{GGB})/\sqrt{\text{var}(\widehat{\mu}_{GGG}) + \text{var}(\widehat{\mu}_{GGB})}$. The last two rows of the table are estimates of the standard deviations of the error term (variation within shape) and the standard error of the random effect (variation among shapes). Although the variation within shape is larger, the random effect is significant.

As follows from the last column, the vertebrae of the two gorilla groups differ in height, particularly for landmarks PSPy, ATy, and PTy. This can also be seen in Figure 11.3. Also, as follows from the last row of the table, the landmark variation for GGB is half that of GGG. A simple chi-squared test confirms that the two gorilla groups have significantly different cervical vertebrae (the authors of the original article came to the same conclusion using a more sophisticated statistical technique).

11.6   Procrustes estimation of the mean shape

Shapes may come in different sizes and be rotated arbitrarily. To eliminate these irrelevant shape features the Procrustes[1] model has been suggested; see Mardia and Dryden (1989), Goodall (1991), Dryden et al. (1997).

Let there be N shapes defined by n points, $\mathbf{u}_{ij} = (x_{ij}, y_{ij})' \in R^2$, where $i = 1, ..., N$ and $j = 1, ..., n$. Let $\boldsymbol{\mu}_j$ be the jth (x, y) coordinate of an unknown vector, which defines the true shape. We want to reconstruct an n-dimensional shape configuration using data on N shapes, $\{\mathbf{u}_{i1}, ..., \mathbf{u}_{in}\}$. Let $\mathbf{t}_i \in R^2$, $r_i > 0$ and θ_i be the unknown shape-specific translation vector, scale coefficient, and rotation angle. Then the Procrustes statistical model for shape is given by

$$(\mathbf{u}_{ij} - \mathbf{t}_i)r_i\mathbf{R}(\theta_i) = \boldsymbol{\mu}_j + \boldsymbol{\varepsilon}_{ij}, \tag{11.8}$$

where $\mathbf{R}$ is the 2×2 rotation matrix,

$$\mathbf{R}(\theta) = \begin{bmatrix} \cos\theta & -\sin\theta \\ \sin\theta & \cos\theta \end{bmatrix},$$

and $\boldsymbol{\varepsilon}_{ij}$ is the two-dimensional error vector with zero mean and constant variance. We do not restrict r_i to be positive, so reflection is allowed. Although it seems that the Procrustes model for $n = 3$ is equivalent to the triangle model (11.1), in fact, it is more general because we do not know the order of the triangle sides.

The Procrustes model (11.8) leads to a peculiar estimation problem because the number of nuisance parameters increases with the sample size, N. Additionally, one cannot assert optimal properties of the maximum likelihood theory because the $\{\mathbf{u}_{i1}, ..., \mathbf{u}_{in}\}$ are not iid. Moreover, as demonstrated by Neyman and Scott (1948), a statistical problem with an increasing number of unknown nuisance parameters may be inconsistent. We have encountered a problem with a large number of parameters

---

[1]Procrustes ("The Stretcher"), in Greek mythology a robber who tortured his victims by cutting them down to fit his bed (Procrustes' bed) if they were too tall, or hammering and stretching them, if they were too short, was captured by the Greek hero Theseus, who inflicted upon Procrustes the same kind of torture that he had imposed upon his victims.

in the general linear growth curve model of Section 4.2. As was shown by Lele (1993) and later by Kent and Mardia (1997), if the $\{\varepsilon_{ij}\}$ are normally distributed with an unstructured covariance matrix, $\widehat{\mu}_{ML}$ is inconsistent. However, if the $\{\varepsilon_{ij}\}$ are iid with $\Omega = \sigma^2 \mathbf{I}$, the MLE is consistent. A similar situation occurs in the errors-in-variables structural model (Kendall and Stuart, 1961). Therefore, we assume that the error term in (11.8) has uncorrelated components with the same variance, $\varepsilon_{ij} \sim \mathcal{N}(\mathbf{0}, \sigma^2 \mathbf{I}_2)$. In the shape literature, such errors are called *isotropic*.

Next we derive the maximum likelihood estimator of μ. Given $2nN$ observations, we want to estimate $4N + n + 1$ unknown parameters. The two-element vectors $\{\mu_j, j = 1, ..., n\}$ are the parameters of interest and the rest are treated as nuisance parameters. Since the size is unspecified, we have to restrict the length of μ to make statistical estimation identifiable, so we let $\|\mu\| = 1$.

First, we notice that since r_i and θ_i are unknown, we can define new parameters as $p_i = r_i \cos \theta_i$ and $q_i = r_i \sin \theta_i$ so that the elements of matrix $\mathbf{R}$ become linear functions. Second, we eliminate the translation parameter $\mathbf{t}_i$ by putting a linear restriction on vectors μ_j as $n^{-1} \sum_{j=1}^n \mu_j = \mathbf{0}$. To comply with this restriction, we centerize $\mathbf{u}_{ij}$ so that we set $\widehat{\mathbf{t}}_i = n^{-1} \sum_{j=1}^n \mathbf{u}_{ij}$. Third, we stack all observations into a $(2n) \times 1$ vector; the first n elements are x-coordinates and the last n elements are y-coordinates, $\mathbf{u}_i = (x_{i1}, x_{i2}, ..., x_{in}, y_{i1}, y_{i2}, ..., y_{in})'$. Also, we introduce a $(2n) \times 1$ vector $\mathbf{v}_i = (-y_{i1}, -y_{i2}, ..., -y_{in}, x_{i1}, x_{i2}, ..., x_{in},)'$. Then, the Procrustes model (11.8) can be rewritten compactly as

$$p_i \mathbf{u}_i + q_i \mathbf{v}_i = \mu + \varepsilon_i, \quad i = 1, ..., N, \tag{11.9}$$

where $\varepsilon \sim \mathcal{N}(\mathbf{0}, \sigma^2 \mathbf{I}_{2n})$, and p_i and q_i are unknown (nuisance) parameters. The log-likelihood function takes a familiar form,

$$l = -\frac{1}{2} \left\{ 2Nn \ln(2\pi\sigma^2) + \frac{1}{\sigma^2} \sum_{i=1}^N \|p_i \mathbf{u}_i + q_i \mathbf{v}_i - \mu\|^2 \right\}. \tag{11.10}$$

The maximum likelihood estimates for p_i and q_i when μ is being held are given by $\widehat{p}_i = \Delta_i^{-1}(b_i \mathbf{u}_i - c_i \mathbf{v}_i)'\mu$ and $\widehat{q}_i = \Delta_i^{-1}(a_i \mathbf{v}_i - c_i \mathbf{u}_i)'\mu$, where

$$a_i = \|\mathbf{u}_i\|^2, \ b_i = \|\mathbf{v}_i\|^2, \ c_i = \mathbf{u}_i'\mathbf{v}_i, \ \Delta_i = a_i b_i - c_i^2.$$

Substituting the estimates for p_i and q_i back into l, we reduce the likelihood maximization to minimization of the quadratic form $\sum_{i=1}^N \mu' \mathbf{Q}_i' \mathbf{Q}_i \mu$, where

$$\mathbf{Q}_i = \Delta_i^{-1} (b_i \mathbf{u}_i \mathbf{u}_i' - c_i \mathbf{u}_i \mathbf{v}_i' - c_i \mathbf{v}_i \mathbf{u}_i' + a_i \mathbf{v}_i \mathbf{v}_i') - \mathbf{I}, \tag{11.11}$$

the $(2n) \times (2n)$ matrix. Finally, the MLE of the true shape is the dominant eigenvector:

$$\widehat{\mu}_{ML} = \mu_{\max} \left(\sum_{i=1}^N \mathbf{Q}_i' \mathbf{Q}_i \right). \tag{11.12}$$

The MLE for the variance of the error term is $\widehat{\sigma}_{ML}^2 = \lambda_{\max}/(2Nn)$ and $l_{\max} = -Nn \ln(2\pi e \widehat{\sigma}_{ML}^2)$. This maximum may be used for statistical testing by the likelihood ratio test.

Now we derive the Procrustes solution under a different parameterization. Indeed, since the size of the true shape can be taken to be arbitrary, we suggest fixing the last component of vector $\boldsymbol{\mu}$. To obtain a closed-form solution for $\boldsymbol{\mu}$, we use the following simple fact: the minimum of $\boldsymbol{\nu}'\mathbf{A}\boldsymbol{\nu}$, where $\boldsymbol{\nu} = (\boldsymbol{\nu}'_1, c)'$ and c is a fixed number, is attained at $\boldsymbol{\nu}_1 = -c\mathbf{A}_{11}^{-1}\mathbf{a}_{n1}$, where $\mathbf{A}_{11}$ is the first $(n-1) \times (n-1)$ submatrix of matrix $\mathbf{A}$ and $\mathbf{a}_{n1}$ is the $(n-1) \times 1$ vector column at the nth position. Since the sum of the elements of vector $\boldsymbol{\mu}$ must be zero, we finally obtain the MLE of the true shape:

$$\widehat{\boldsymbol{\mu}}_{1,ML} = -\left(\sum_{i=1}^{N}\mathbf{Q}'_i\mathbf{Q}_i\right)_{11}^{-1}\left(\sum_{i=1}^{N}\mathbf{Q}'_i\mathbf{Q}_i\right)_{n1}, \quad \widehat{\boldsymbol{\mu}}_{2n,ML} = -\sum_{i=1}^{2n-1}\widehat{\boldsymbol{\mu}}_{1i,ML}. \quad (11.13)$$

The closed-form formula (11.13) is useful for studying statistical properties and gives the same shape as the dominant eigenvector solution (11.12).

The R function below plots the true regular hexagon and 15 random irregular hexagons with `sigma` as the parameter that controls the magnitude of the irregularity.

```
shapeh=function(sigma=.01, N=15)
{
dump("shapeh","c:\\MixedModels\\Chapter11\\shapeh.r")
angtrue=(2*pi)*(0:5)/6 # true shape
mutrue=cbind(cos(angtrue),sin(angtrue)) #regular hexagon
par(mfrow=c(4,4),mar=c(0,0,0,0))
plot(c(-1.25,1.25),c(-1.25,1.25),type="n",axes=F,xlab="",ylab="")
lines(c(mutrue[,1],mutrue[1,1]),c(mutrue[,2],mutrue[1,2]),lwd=4)
text(0,0,"True shape",cex=1.5)
u6=rep(1,6);R=matrix(ncol=2,nrow=2) # random rotation matrix
for(i in 1:15)
{
    mur=mutrue+matrix(sigma*rnorm(2*6),ncol=2,nrow=6)
    ti=rnorm(2,mean=0,sd=.1) #random shift
    ri=runif(1,min=.9,max=1.1) # random size
    theta=runif(1,min=0,max=2*pi) #random angle
    R[1,1]=cos(theta);R[1,2]=-sin(theta);
    R[2,1]=sin(theta);R[2,2]=cos(theta)
    ui=u6%*%t(ti)+mur%*%t(solve(R))/ri # get u[i,j] from eqn 11.8
    plot(c(-1.25,1.25),c(-1.25,1.25),type="n",axes=F,xlab="",ylab="")
    polygon(c(ui[,1],ui[1,1]),c(ui[,2],ui[1,2]),col=3)
    lines(c(ui[,1],ui[1,1]),c(ui[,2],ui[1,2]),lwd=4)
}
}
```

11.6.1   Polygon estimation

To illustrate the Procrustes model, we took six points on the plane as vertices of a (true) convex hexagon, see Figure 11.4. Then we added normal noise to the coordinates of the six vertices, and randomly rotated and resized the polygon to produce 28 random hexagons. Basically, the same function shape6 was used but with mutrue, which defines an irregular hexagon. The mean hexagon, as an estimate of the true hexagon, is computed by (11.13). As we see, the estimate is satisfactory (one needs visually to rotate the mean by roughly 60° clockwise to overlap with the true hexagon).

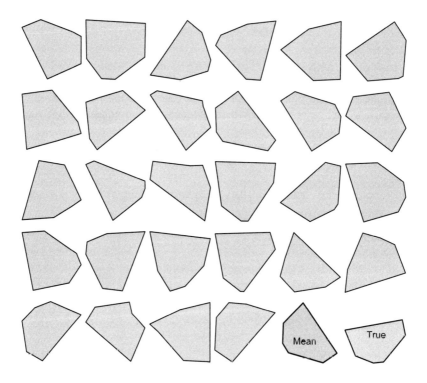

FIGURE 11.4. Mean shape estimation from 28 iid random hexagons. The last hexagon was randomly rotated, scaled, and shifted to produce 28 polygon shapes. The shape estimate/mean was computed by formulas (11.13).

11.6.2   Generalized Procrustes model

The Procrustes model, (11.8) or equivalently (11.9), is useful when the number of landmark points is not large and they are uncorrelated. When the shape is obtained as an outline of a digital image, the shape is fairly smooth, and therefore the neighboring points become highly correlated. It is straightforward to generalize the Procrustes model assuming that the $(2n) \times 1$ vectors ε_i in (11.9) are correlated, or more specifically, $\mathrm{cov}(\varepsilon_i) = \mathbf{W} = \mathbf{I}_2 \otimes \mathbf{\Omega}$, where $\mathbf{I}_2$ is the 2×2 identity matrix.

Then the log-likelihood function, up to the constant $-Nn \ln(2\pi)$, takes the form

$$l = -\frac{1}{2} \left\{ 2N \ln |\boldsymbol{\Omega}| + \boldsymbol{\mu}' \left(\sum_{i=1}^{N} \mathbf{Q}_i' \mathbf{W}^{-1} \mathbf{Q}_i \right) \boldsymbol{\mu} \right\},$$

where $\mathbf{W}^{-1} = \mathbf{I}_2 \otimes \boldsymbol{\Omega}^{-1}$. The $(2n) \times (2n)$ matrix $\mathbf{Q}_i$ is defined as previously, (11.11), where $a_i = \mathbf{u}_i' \mathbf{W}^{-1} \mathbf{u}_i$, $b_i = \mathbf{v}_i \mathbf{W}^{-1} \mathbf{v}_i$, and $c_i = \mathbf{u}_i' \mathbf{W}^{-1} \mathbf{v}_i$. Following the line of the isotropic case, we come to the Generalized Procrustes (GP) solution,

$$\widehat{\boldsymbol{\mu}}_{ML} = \boldsymbol{\mu}_{\max} \left(\sum_{i=1}^{N} \mathbf{Q}_i' \mathbf{W}^{-1} \mathbf{Q}_i \right), \tag{11.14}$$

assuming that matrix $\boldsymbol{\Omega}$ is being held fixed. Now we discuss how to parameterize matrix $\boldsymbol{\Omega}$. When the number of landmarks is large, the estimation of an unrestricted matrix $\boldsymbol{\Omega}$ leads to an ill-identified problem because it requires estimation of $n(n+1)/2$ elements. A parsimonious covariance parameterization would assume that: (a) all elements of $\boldsymbol{\varepsilon}_i$ have the same variance, and (b) the correlation between elements ε_{i1} and ε_{j1} is a function of $|i-j|$. Recall that we encountered the same covariance parameterization problem for the time series linear mixed effects model of Section 4.3.4. Therefore, we define matrix $\boldsymbol{\Omega}$ as a linear combination of elementary Toeplitz matrices with unknown coefficients, namely,

$$\boldsymbol{\Omega} = \sum_{k=0}^{K} \theta_k \mathbf{T}_k. \tag{11.15}$$

Here $\mathbf{T}_0$ is the identity matrix and $\mathbf{T}_k$ is a symmetric elementary Toeplitz matrix defined as $(\mathbf{T}_k)_{ij} = 1$ if $|i-j| = k$ and zero elsewhere. Examples of $\mathbf{T}$ matrices with $k = 1$ and 2 are given in (4.115). The number K determines the depth of the correlation of the components of the shape vector $\mathbf{u}_i$. To find the maximum of l, we alternate between (11.14) and maximization over $\{\theta_k\}$ until convergence.

11.6.3   Random effects shape model

The Procrustes model is very liberal and allows arbitrary rotation, size transformation, and translation. Although it makes the sampling design very flexible, the price is that the number of parameters grows with the number of shapes. In Section 11.4.1 we suggested modeling the shape size via the random effect—this can easily be generalized to the Procrustes model as follows. We rewrite the Procrustes model in a slightly different manner as

$$\mathbf{u}_{ij} = \begin{bmatrix} h_i & g_i \\ -g_i & h_i \end{bmatrix} \boldsymbol{\mu}_j + \mathbf{t}_i + \boldsymbol{\varepsilon}_{ij}, \tag{11.16}$$

where $\mathbf{u}_{ij}$ is the 2×1 vector of coordinates of the jth point on the ith shape, $\boldsymbol{\mu}_j$ is the 2×1 vector of the true unknown shape. and $h_i, g_i, \mathbf{t}_i = (t_{i1}, t_{i2})'$ are random variables (random effects). It is assumed that the shape observations are obtained as a random rotation, scale, and translation of an unknown shape $\boldsymbol{\mu}$. Assuming that the distribution is normal and the error term has zero mean and constant variance σ^2 (isotropic case), we finalize the random effects shape model (11.16) by writing

$$\begin{bmatrix} h_i \\ g_i \end{bmatrix} \sim \mathcal{N}\left(\begin{bmatrix} 1 \\ 0 \end{bmatrix}, \sigma^2 \begin{bmatrix} \sigma_h^2 & \sigma_{hg} \\ \sigma_{hg} & \sigma_g^2 \end{bmatrix}\right),$$

$$\mathbf{t}_i \sim \mathcal{N}\left(\begin{bmatrix} 0 \\ 0 \end{bmatrix}, \sigma^2 \begin{bmatrix} \tau_1^2 & \tau_{12} \\ \tau_{12} & \tau_2^2 \end{bmatrix}\right). \tag{11.17}$$

Note that $E(h_i) = 1$, which implies that the expectation of the observed shape coincides with the true shape. Model (11.16) allows between-shape variation, and the variance parameters reflect the strength of the heterogeneity. Introducing $(2n) \times 1$ vectors of observations $\mathbf{u}_i$ and the true shape $\boldsymbol{\mu}$ as at the beginning of this section, we rewrite model (11.16) in marginal form as $\mathbf{u}_i \sim \mathcal{N}(\boldsymbol{\mu}, \sigma^2 \mathbf{V}(\boldsymbol{\mu}))$. To express $\mathbf{V}$ as a function of $\boldsymbol{\mu}$, we introduce a 2×2 fixed matrix $\mathbf{L}$ with the elements $L_{11} = L_{22} = 0$ and $L_{21} = -L_{12} = 1$. Then the first term on the right-hand side of equation (11.16) can be rewritten as $(h_i \mathbf{I}_{2n} + g_i(\mathbf{L} \otimes \mathbf{I}_n))\boldsymbol{\mu}$, and hence

$$\begin{aligned} \mathbf{V}(\boldsymbol{\mu}) &= \mathbf{I}_{2n} + \mathbf{I}_n \otimes \mathbf{T} + \sigma_h^2 \boldsymbol{\mu}\boldsymbol{\mu}' + \sigma_{hg}[\boldsymbol{\mu}\boldsymbol{\mu}'(\mathbf{L}' \otimes \mathbf{I}_n) + (\mathbf{L} \otimes \mathbf{I}_n)\boldsymbol{\mu}\boldsymbol{\mu}'] \\ &\quad + \sigma_g^2(\mathbf{L} \otimes \mathbf{I}_n)\boldsymbol{\mu}\boldsymbol{\mu}'(\mathbf{L}' \otimes \mathbf{I}_n), \end{aligned}$$

where $\mathbf{T} = \sigma^{-2}\mathrm{cov}(\mathbf{t}_i)$. Similar to the random size model of Section 11.4.1, we can estimate model (11.17) by either VLS or ML. Since the model is balanced, GLS is equivalent to OLS, $\widehat{\boldsymbol{\mu}}_{GLS} = \widehat{\boldsymbol{\mu}}_{OLS} = \overline{\mathbf{u}}$. The variance parameters can be estimated by VLS. For the maximum likelihood approach, $\widehat{\boldsymbol{\mu}}_{ML} \neq \overline{\mathbf{u}}$, and it requires simultaneous maximization over $\boldsymbol{\mu}$ and seven variance parameters.

Sometimes, due to the sampling design, some transformation parameters are under control and can be assumed random but some are arbitrary, such as translation. A model similar to the general growth curve model of Section 4.2 may be applied with a combination of mixed and random effects to analyze such shapes.

11.6.4   Random or fixed (Procrustes) effects model?

Comparison of random- and fixed-size shape models applies to the more complex Procrustes and random effects shape models, (11.16). In the former model, the transform parameters are fixed, and in the latter model they are random. The choice between the two models should be dictated by the experimental design. If the size and orientation vary slightly and are part of the shape heterogeneity, as in landmark analysis, the random effects model is adequate. For example, the random effects shape model would not be adequate to describe the hexagon shapes in Figure 11.4. If shapes are arbitrarily rotated and obtained as an image outline taken at different (nonrandom) camera positions, the Procrustes model is preferred. For example, the Procrustes model would be needed for analyzing sand particles taken with different camera magnifications.

11.6.5   Maple leaf analysis

The R function that follows reads and plots the nine maple leaf shapes shown in Figure 1.6. The xy data are in the files `maple#.xy`, where # runs from 1 to 9. The point on the top may be viewed as the reference point.

```
maple=function()
{
dump("maple","c:\\MixedModels\\Chapter11\\maple.r")
par(mfrow = c(3, 3), mar = c(0, 0, 0, 0))
for(i in 1:9) {
 pf <- paste("c:\\MixedModels\\Chapter11\\maple", as.character(i),
     ".xy", sep = "")
 d <- matrix(scan(pf), ncol = 2)
 d <- d[!is.na(d[, 1]) & !is.na(d[, 2]), ]
 n <- nrow(d)
 dy <- min(d[, 2])
 im <- (1:n)[d[, 2] == dy]
 plot(d[, 1], - d[, 2], type = "l", xlab = "", ylab = "", axes = F)
 points(d[im, 1], - d[im, 2], pch = 1, cex = 1.5,col=2)
 polygon(x = d[, 1], y = - d[, 2], col = 3)
 lines(d[, 1], - d[, 2],lwd=4)
}
}
```

The Procrustes shape model (11.8) can be used to estimate the average shape using observed μ_i as the matrix of xy coordinates, with the top point as the reference. Since the shapes need to have the same number of points, some sort of downsampling (or interpolation) is required.

Problems for Section 11.6

1. Prove that the ML estimator of μ with the log-likelihood function (11.6) is the maximum (dominant) eigenvector of matrix $\mathbf{M}$.

2. Write an R function that generates a random quadrangle defined by five sides of two adjacent triangles.

3. Modify the **shapeh** function to plot random polygons with an arbitrary number of vertices.

4*. Write an R function which estimates the polygon shape by maximum likelihood with the log-likelihood function given by (11.10). Use two parameterizations of the true shape, with the unit norm and the fixed last component. Carry out simulations to test whether the estimation code reconstructs the true shape satisfactory.

5*. Generate random polygons using the generalized Procrustes model with representation (11.15) for the covariance matrix.

6*. Develop an algorithm for the maximum likelihood estimation of random shapes/polygons with random effects. Write an R function that implements this algorithm and tests it via simulations.

7*. Estimate the average maple leaf shape using the data in function **maple** by Procrustes model (11.8).

11.7   Fourier descriptor analysis

Landmark analysis is useful when the number of landmarks is relatively small. When the shape is derived as the outline of an image, other techniques to quantify and analyze the shape may be more appropriate. When shape is defined by a large number of points, it would be attractive to assume that the true mean shape is fairly smooth and therefore may be described by a relatively small number of parameters. In shape theory, such parameters are called shape descriptors or simply *descriptors*. Since the shape is intrinsically a periodic function, Fourier series or harmonic decomposition naturally emerges. Then the coefficients of Fourier decomposition are the shape descriptors. Two types of Fourier decomposition are discussed in this section. First, we apply the Fourier decomposition to the radius function of a relatively simple star or round (potato-like) shape (Lu, 1965; Ehrlich and Weinberg, 1970; Hobolth et al., 2003). The second type of shape is more general and requires two Fourier series to specify the shape (Zahn and Roskies, 1972). For an overview see the paper by Lestler (1997) and many other papers on biological applications listed in that book. Previous authors assumed that the Fourier coefficients are fixed. We argue that each individual shape has its own set of harmonic coefficients, but a common population mean. In the language of the mixed effects model, the coefficients are shape- or subject-specific. This leads to the *Random* Fourier Descriptor (RFD) model. We apply the theory of mixed effects models developed in Chapters 1 to 8 to estimate and study shapes with random Fourier coefficients. Although random descriptors were studied previously under a Bayesian approach (Grenander and Miller, 1994) mixed model methodology does not require complete specification of the prior distribution and therefore is more robust. RFD analysis is illustrated using a leaf example.

11.7.1   Analysis of a star shape

Sometimes, there is a point within the shape, called a *centroid*, which can be connected to any other point on the shape by a segment within the shape. We call such a shape a *star* shape. For example, if the shape is specified by a sequence of points $\{(x_i, y_i), i = 1, ..., n\}$, the centroid may be chosen as $(\overline{x}, \overline{y})$. A special case of a star shape is a convex shape. For a convex shape, *any* point within the shape may serve as a centroid. Let us assume that the centroid, (x_0, y_0) is known. Then, in polar coordinates any point (x, y) on the shape can be represented as $(r(\theta) \cos \theta + x_0, r(\theta) \sin \theta + y_0)$, where θ is the angle between the ray to (x_0, y_0) and the x-axis, see Figure 11.5. Usually, we specify θ by a sequence of equally spaced angles, for example, $\theta_j = 2\pi(j-1)/J, j = 1, 2, ..., J = 360$. Then the shape is determined completely by the radius function $r(\theta_j)$. The star shape guarantees that there is a unique intersection of the ray with the shape; if the ray does not intersect the shape, one may take either the closest point on the shape or a linear interpolation between points. After the shape is expressed in polar coordinates, one may plot r as a function of the angle, θ, on the interval $[0, 2\pi)$ and apply further statistical analysis.

Star shapes can be analyzed using two approaches. The first approach is called semiparametric and does not specify the model for the mean shape in the way that

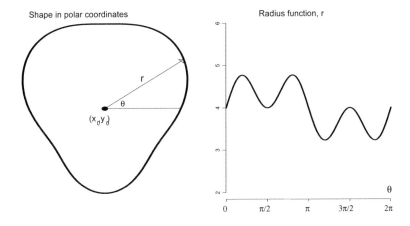

FIGURE 11.5. Star-shaped representation in polar coordinates. The radius function defines the shape.

we dealt with landmarks. Although this approach requires fewer assumptions, the number of shapes should be large. In a more complicated Fourier descriptor analysis, the radius function is modeled by a few harmonics.

Semiparametric model for the star shape

We merely assume that the mean shape is the average of the shapes after an appropriate size and orientation transformation. Let $\boldsymbol{\theta}$ be the $J \times 1$ vector of angles $(\theta_1, ..., \theta_J)'$ so that the radius data for the N shapes takes the form of a $J \times N$ matrix, $\mathbf{R} = \{\mathbf{r}_i(\boldsymbol{\theta}), i = 1, ..., N\}$. Similar to Section 11.4.2, we assume that the radius function is on the log scale, making the size additive:

$$\mathbf{r}_i(\boldsymbol{\theta} + \kappa_i \mathbf{1}) = h_i \mathbf{1} + \boldsymbol{\mu} + \boldsymbol{\varepsilon}_i, \quad i = 1, ..., N, \tag{11.18}$$

where h_i is the size and κ_i is the angle of rotation. In this section we assume that the angle of rotation is taken modulo 2π. The true radius function $\boldsymbol{\mu}$ is not specified and is subject to estimation. Two assumptions on h_i and κ_i lead to two different models, fixed or random effects.

In the *fixed effects* star-shaped model, h_i and κ_i are fixed and unknown. We get rid of the nuisance parameter h_i by centerizing the data, or more precisely by replacing $\mathbf{r}_i(\boldsymbol{\theta})$ with $\mathbf{r}_i(\boldsymbol{\theta}) - J^{-1} \sum_{j=1}^{J} (\mathbf{r}_i(\theta_j) - \overline{r})$ for each $i = 1, ..., N$. If the κ_i were known, the true radius function would be $\widehat{\boldsymbol{\mu}} = N^{-1} \sum_{i=1}^{N} \mathbf{r}_i(\boldsymbol{\theta} + \kappa_i \mathbf{1})$. Now we discuss how to estimate angle rotations $\kappa_1, ..., \kappa_N$. First, one needs to find satisfactory initial values. Let the true shape be the first shape. Then for every other shape $i = 2, ..., N$ we can find κ_i such that the ith sum of squares $S_i = \|\mathbf{r}_1(\boldsymbol{\theta}) - \mathbf{r}_i(\boldsymbol{\theta} + \kappa_i \mathbf{1})\|^2$ is minimum (obviously, $\kappa_1 = 0$). Then we try the second shape as the mean shape, etc. Among all the shapes, we find the mean shape and the initial vector $\{\widehat{\kappa}_i\}$ that gives an overall minimum $\sum_{i=1}^{N} S_i$. In fact, we can continue in this fashion computing $\widehat{\boldsymbol{\mu}} = N^{-1} \sum_{i=1}^{N} \mathbf{r}_i(\boldsymbol{\theta} + \widehat{\kappa}_i \mathbf{1})$ and finding the next approximation for the angle rotation that minimizes $\sum_{i=1}^{N} \|\widehat{\boldsymbol{\mu}} - \mathbf{r}_i(\boldsymbol{\theta} + \kappa_i \mathbf{1})\|^2$, iterating until convergence. Recall that $\boldsymbol{\theta} + \kappa_i \mathbf{1}$ is taken modulo 2π.

Also, we can estimate κ simultaneously by minimizing the sum of squares,

$$S(\kappa_1, ..., \kappa_N) = \sum_{i=1}^{N} \left\| \mathbf{r}_i(\boldsymbol{\theta} + \kappa_i \mathbf{1}) - N^{-1} \sum_{l=1}^{N} \mathbf{r}_l(\boldsymbol{\theta} + \kappa_l \mathbf{1}) \right\|^2 = \text{tr}(\mathbf{RJR}'), \qquad (11.19)$$

where $\mathbf{J} = \mathbf{I} - N^{-1}\mathbf{1}\mathbf{1}'$ is the $N \times N$ projection matrix. The function S can be minimized with the Gauss–Newton algorithm as $\boldsymbol{\kappa}_{s+1} = \boldsymbol{\kappa}_s - (\mathbf{G}'\mathbf{G})^{-1} \times \text{diag}(\mathbf{G}'\mathbf{RJ})$, where $\mathbf{G}$ is the $J \times N$ matrix of differences with the ith row $[\mathbf{r}_i(\boldsymbol{\theta} + (\kappa_i + d)\mathbf{1}) - \mathbf{r}_i(\boldsymbol{\theta} + \kappa_i \mathbf{1})]/d$ and d is an integer (step), say $d = 1$. Although the Gauss–Newton algorithm is faster, a separate rotation may be more precise. Alternatively, one can use the derivative-free method (DUD) described in Section 12.7.7.

Next we discuss briefly the *random effects* star-shaped model. The model is specified by the same equation (11.18), but now it is assumed that κ_i and h_i are random (again it is assumed that the radius function is on the log scale). This model is adequate when the shapes are from the same general population and are uniformly registered (e.g., as the top-right leaf). Then we assume that $h_i \sim \mathcal{N}(0, \sigma_h^2)$ and $\kappa_i \sim \mathcal{N}(0, \sigma_\kappa^2)$, so that model (11.18) becomes the nonlinear mixed effects model of Chapter 8.

Example: leaf analysis

Figure 11.6 shows 29 independent and identically deformed leaves. We want to find the mean star shape using the semiparametric fixed effects model (11.18). Two types of radius functions are shown in Figure 11.7. At the left, the radius functions are unadjusted (no rotation). At the right, the leaves were rotated to minimize the total residual sum of squares. The light line determines the mean shape shown in Figure 11.6. When shapes are widely rotated, as in this example, the arithmetic mean for the true shape may not be a satisfactory estimate (in our example it produces a circle, a constant radius function).

Random Fourier descriptor analysis for the star shape

The radius function is periodic on the interval $0 \leq \theta < 2\pi$, and therefore a *discrete* Fourier series representation of the form

$$r(\theta_j) = c_0 + \sum_{k=1}^{K} (a_k \cos k\theta_j + b_k \sin k\theta_j) + \varepsilon_j, \quad j = 1, ..., J \qquad (11.20)$$

can be used, where the error term ε_i has zero mean and constant variance σ^2. The kth harmonic is specified by the coefficients a_k and b_k. It is assumed that K is known—we discuss the choice of K later. It is also assumed that the number of unknown harmonic coefficients is less than the number of observations, $2K + 1 < J$. Coefficients with small k account for the global shape, and coefficients with high k account for fine detail. The Fourier representation (11.20) for vector $\mathbf{r} = (r(\theta_1), ..., r(\theta_J))'$ can be rewritten as a linear statistical model $\mathbf{r} = \mathbf{Z}\mathbf{a} + \boldsymbol{\varepsilon}$, where the $J \times (2K + 1)$ design matrix is given by

$$\mathbf{Z} = \sqrt{\frac{2}{n}} \left[\frac{1}{\sqrt{2}}, \cos(1 \times \boldsymbol{\theta}), \sin(1 \times \boldsymbol{\theta}), ..., \cos(K \times \boldsymbol{\theta}), \sin(K \times \boldsymbol{\theta}) \right], \qquad (11.21)$$

and $\mathbf{a} = (c_0, a_1, b_1, a_2, b_2, ..., a_K, b_K)'$ is the $(2K+1) \times 1$ total vector of coefficients. The matrix $\mathbf{Z}$ is orthogonal, $\mathbf{Z}'\mathbf{Z} = \mathbf{I}_{2K+1}$. This property drastically simplifies the Fourier coefficients estimation.

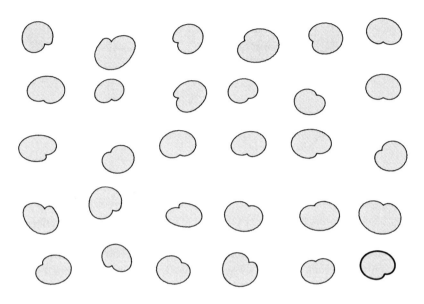

FIGURE 11.6. Twenty-nine independent identically deformed and rotated leaves. The last leaf (bold) is the estimated mean shape using a fixed effects semiparametric model.

Now we apply discrete Fourier decomposition to a sequence or a sample of shapes drawn independently from the same general population, $\{\mathbf{r}_i, i = 1, ..., N\}$. It is assumed that the shapes have different shape-specific coefficients with the same population mean, namely,

$$\mathbf{r}_i = \mathbf{Z}\mathbf{a}_i + \varepsilon_i, \quad \mathbf{a}_i = \boldsymbol{\beta} + \mathbf{b}_i, \quad i = 1, ..., N, \tag{11.22}$$

where $\boldsymbol{\beta}$ is the $(2K+1) \times 1$ population vector of coefficients and $\mathbf{a}_i$ is the ith shape-specific vector of coefficients ($\mathbf{b}_i$ is the deviation). It is assumed that the $\{\mathbf{b}_i\}$ are iid with zero mean and covariance matrix $\sigma^2 \mathbf{D}$. We call model (11.22) a *Random Fourier Descriptor* (RFD) model. To motivate the RFD model, we suggest Figure 11.8. The true shape is defined by the radius function as $r_j = r(\theta_j) = \sum_{k=1}^{K=11} [a_k \sin(k\theta_j) + b_k \cos(k\theta_j)]$, where $\theta_j = 2(j-1)\pi/360$. The traditional Fourier descriptor model involves one random error term, so the generated shape is $y_j = r_j + \varepsilon_j$, where $\varepsilon_j \sim \mathcal{N}(0, \sigma_\varepsilon^2)$. We show two generated shapes with $\sigma = 1/10$ and $\sigma = 2/10$ in the upper row. The RFD model assumes that the Fourier coefficients are random as well and the generated shape takes the form $y_j = \sum_{k=1}^{K=11} [(a_k + \zeta_k) \sin(k\theta_j) + (b_k + \delta_k) \cos(k\theta_j)] + \varepsilon_j$, where $\zeta_k, \delta_k, \varepsilon_j$ are normally distributed random variables. We show three RFD shapes with increasing shape variation in the lower row. Clearly, these shapes look more familiar, and therefore the RFD model is preferable.

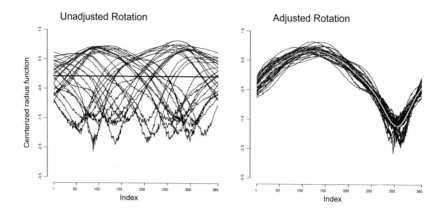

FIGURE 11.7. Radius functions for 29 leaves. At the left, the unadjusted/raw radius functions are shown (the horizontal line is the mean). At the right, the leaves are rotated properly to produce the mean shape (light line).

The key observation is that the RFD model (11.22) is a linear mixed effects model or more precisely, a balanced growth curve model of Section 2.3. Thus, the theory on mixed models developed in earlier chapters applies to the analysis in full!

Various hypotheses can be tested. For example, if the diagonal elements of matrix $\mathbf{D}$ are zero, the respective coefficient does not change from shape to shape. If the shape is symmetric along the y-axis, the sine coefficients are zero, $\alpha_k = 0$. If the shape is circular, all Fourier coefficients are zero. The membership test can be applied to determine whether a specific shape belongs to another group of shapes, Section 3.8.

Now we discuss issues of Fourier coefficient estimation. There are several important consequences of the fact that the RFD model (11.22) is a balanced random-coefficient model, as follows from Section 2.3. Estimation of Fourier coefficients of the true shape, $\boldsymbol{\beta}$ is reduced to an average, $\bar{\mathbf{r}} = N^{-1} \sum_{i=1}^{N} \mathbf{r}_i$. The optimal estimation of $\boldsymbol{\beta}$ is the ordinary least squares, regardless of the covariance matrix $\mathbf{D}$,

$$\widehat{\boldsymbol{\beta}} = \mathbf{Z}'\bar{\mathbf{r}}. \tag{11.23}$$

To estimate variances, we apply maximum likelihood. As follows from Theorem 2, the estimates admit a closed-form solution. In particular, as follows from (2.59), the unbiased estimator of the error term variance is given by

$$\widehat{\sigma}^2 = \frac{1}{N(J - 2K - 1)} \sum_{i=1}^{N} \left(\|\mathbf{r}_i\|^2 - \|\mathbf{Z}'\mathbf{r}_i\|^2 \right). \tag{11.24}$$

The estimated true radius vector is $\widehat{\mathbf{r}} = \mathbf{Z}\widehat{\boldsymbol{\beta}} = \mathbf{Z}\mathbf{Z}'\bar{\mathbf{r}}$. We compute the $(2K + 1) \times (2K + 1)$ shape-specific Fourier coefficients matrix variation as

$$\mathbf{A} = \frac{1}{N-1} \sum_{i=1}^{N} (\widehat{\mathbf{a}}_i - \widehat{\boldsymbol{\beta}})(\widehat{\mathbf{a}}_i - \widehat{\boldsymbol{\beta}})' = \frac{1}{N-1} \sum_{i=1}^{N} (\mathbf{Z}'\mathbf{r}_i - \widehat{\boldsymbol{\beta}})(\mathbf{Z}'\mathbf{r}_i - \widehat{\boldsymbol{\beta}})',$$

where $\widehat{\mathbf{a}}_i$ is the individual Fourier vector of coefficients. Then, as follows from formula (2.61), the unbiased estimator of the covariance matrix of Fourier coefficients is given by

$$\widehat{\mathbf{D}}_{RML} = \frac{1}{\widehat{\sigma}^2}\mathbf{A} - \mathbf{I}_{2K+1}. \tag{11.25}$$

Due to the dimension-reduction formula (2.25) the formula for the covariance matrix of Fourier coefficients simplifies to

$$\mathrm{cov}(\widehat{\boldsymbol{\beta}}) = \widehat{\sigma}^2\mathbf{A}^{-1}. \tag{11.26}$$

As follows from Section 3.52, an estimate of the Fourier coefficients of the ith radius shape is $\widehat{\mathbf{a}}_i = \widehat{\boldsymbol{\beta}} + \widehat{\mathbf{b}}_i$. Plugging estimates (11.24) and (11.25) into this expression, we yield the BLUP estimate for an individual shape, $\widetilde{\mathbf{a}}_i = \widehat{\mathbf{a}}_i + \widehat{\sigma}^2\mathbf{A}^{-1}(\widehat{\boldsymbol{\beta}} - \widehat{\mathbf{a}}_i)$. As the reader can see, the BLUP estimate is an adjusted ordinary individual estimate.

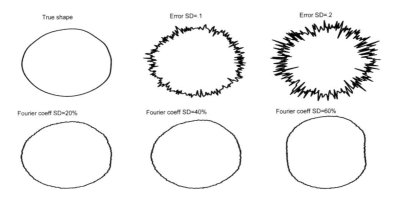

FIGURE 11.8. Two statistical models for a round shape analysis. The true shape is shown in the upper-left panel. Two shapes generated by a traditional model *shape+error* are shown in the upper row. Due to the independence of the error term, the generated shapes look ragged. In contrast, if the shape variation comes from Fourier coefficients the generated shapes look more familiar, as in the lower row.

Leaf analysis (continued)

We apply the RFD model to the analyzed previously leaf data, Figure 11.6. Several fitting characteristics may be used to chose the appropriate number of harmonics, K. First, one can rely on the Z-score of the Fourier coefficient (the ratio of the estimate to its standard error). Typically, after a certain K, the Z-score decreases. Second, one can use an F-test to identify at what K, the fit does not improve. Third, one can use numerous techniques of regression variable selection, including Akaiki information. The result of fitting with a different number of harmonics is shown in Figure 11.9. A detailed four-harmonic Fourier series fit is shown in Table 11.2. As the reader can see, four harmonics with nine parameters ($1 + 2 \times 4 = 9$) provide a good fit to the mean shape data. The contribution of the kth harmonic, $\sqrt{a_k^2 + b_k^2}$, in Fourier decomposition (11.20) decreases quite fast. Standard errors of the estimates are computed by formula (11.26). The Z-score of the estimate indicates that the Fourier coefficients are statistically significant up to the third harmonic. The

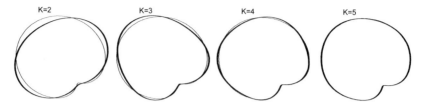

FIGURE 11.9. Random Fourier descriptor model for reconstruction of the mean leaf shape using several harmonics. The five-harmonic model fits the mean shape perfectly.

column SE RE shows the square root of the diagonal elements of matrix $\widehat{\sigma}^2 \widehat{\mathbf{D}}_{RML}$, the covariance matrix of the random effects/coefficients. The last column shows the relative leaf variability, SE RE/estimate $\times 100\%$. As follows from this analysis, maximum variability comes from the third sine harmonic.

11.7.2 Random Fourier descriptor analysis

Often, shapes are more complex and consequently cannot be quantified by a single radius function. An example of shapes where two Fourier series are needed is the nine-maple-leaf example from Chapter 1, shown in Figure 1.6. Several methods have been suggested to quantify a general shape with a large number of points (such as those derived from a digital image), Zahn and Roskies (1972). We focus on a method widely used in image processing (Gonzalez and Woods, 2002). To start the shape quantification, an origin point on the shape should be picked, say at the maximum x-coordinate. Let the origin point be (x_1, y_1). Then, traversing clockwise, we record consecutive coordinate pairs (x_j, y_j) so that the $(n+1)$th step should yield (x_0, y_0). Notice that x and y are periodic functions, and therefore we can represent them as functions on the interval $[0, 2\pi)$ using the mapping $\theta_j = 2\pi(j-1)/n$. Hence, similar to the star shape of Section 11.7.1, a general shape can be quantified by a pair of periodic functions $\{x(\theta_j), y(\theta_j), j = 1, ..., n\}$. A generalization of the shape analysis is now straightforward—instead of one periodic function, the radius function for the star shape, we have two periodic functions. Let N shapes be indexed by $i = 1, ..., N$ and let $\mathbf{z}_i$ denote the $n \times 2$ matrix of the ith shape's consecutive coordinates. Several statistical models may be suggested as generalizations of Section 11.4. For example, if shapes are of the same size and perfectly oriented, the model $\mathbf{z}_i = \mathbf{1}\mathbf{h}_i' + \boldsymbol{\mu} + \boldsymbol{\varepsilon}_i$ accounts for the translation, where $\mathbf{h}_i$ is the 2×1 translation vector and $\boldsymbol{\mu}$ is the $n \times 2$ true shape. An easy way to eliminate translation is to centerize the coordinates. If translation is random, we may assume that $\mathbf{h}_i \sim \mathcal{N}(\mathbf{0}, \boldsymbol{\Omega})$, leading to a linear mixed effects model, or more precisely, to the balanced growth curve model. One can use an isotropic model for the error term, assuming that there is no correlation between the x and y coordinates and equal variance, or generally, $\boldsymbol{\varepsilon}_{ij} \sim \mathcal{N}(\mathbf{0}, \boldsymbol{\Lambda})$, where $\boldsymbol{\Lambda}$ is the 2×2 unknown covariance matrix. If the shapes' orientation is arbitrary and translation is eliminated, model (11.18) takes the form $\mathbf{z}_i(\boldsymbol{\theta} + \kappa_i \mathbf{1}) = \boldsymbol{\mu} + \boldsymbol{\varepsilon}_i$, where κ_i is the nuisance rotation parameter. If estimates of $\{\kappa_i\}$ were known, the mean shape is the simple average, $\widehat{\boldsymbol{\mu}} = N^{-1} \sum_{i=1}^{N} \mathbf{z}_i(\boldsymbol{\theta} + \widehat{\kappa}_i \mathbf{1})$. The rotation parameters $\widehat{\kappa}_i$ may be chosen to minimize the total or weighted sum of squares, similar to (11.19).

Table 11.2. Estimation of the mean leaf shape with a RFD model using four harmonics (see Figures 11.6 and 11.9)

$\widehat{\beta}$	Estimate	$\sqrt{a_k^2 + b_k^2}$	SE $\widehat{\beta}$	Z-score	SE RE	RE-score, %
$\widehat{c}_0$	-3.05		0.024	-124.8	2.29	75.5
$\widehat{a}_1$	-7.78		0.49	-15.8	1.07	13.8
$\widehat{b}_1$	12.34	14.6	0.39	31.5	0.79	6.39
$\widehat{a}_2$	1.39		0.30	4.7	0.97	69.4
$\widehat{b}_2$	3.34	3.6	0.135	24.7	1.07	32.1
$\widehat{a}_3$	1.91		0.59	3.2	0.77	40.5
$\widehat{b}_3$	0.576	2.0	0.42	1.4	1.18	298.0
$\widehat{a}_4$	0.761		1.06	0.71	0.79	104.2
$\widehat{b}_4$	-0.595	0.97	0.772	-0.82	0.65	109.4

Estimation of the RFD model with two coordinate data is similar to (11.22): $\mathbf{x}_i = \mathbf{Z}_1(\boldsymbol{\beta}_1 + \mathbf{b}_{i1}) + \boldsymbol{\varepsilon}_{i1}$ and $\mathbf{y}_i = \mathbf{Z}_2(\boldsymbol{\beta}_2 + \mathbf{b}_{i2}) + \boldsymbol{\varepsilon}_{i2}$. Assuming that these mixed models do not share common parameters and that the error term is isotropic, the analysis is carried out separately and the previous formulas apply.

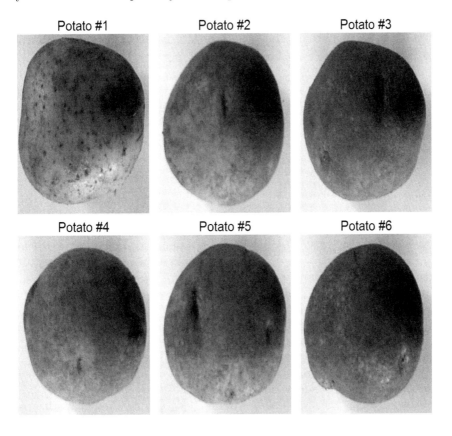

FIGURE 11.10. Siz real potato grayscale images plotted with the R function potato.

11.7.3 Potato project

In the function below we read and plot six data files that represent grayscale images of real potatoes in 8-bit format (see Figure 11.10). The intensity of each pixel is expressed via an integer on a scale of 0 (absolutely black) to 255 (absolutely white) according to the PGM format; see the next chapter for more information about images. The original pictures of potatoes were in JPG format and then saved in PGM (Portable GrayMap) format using PaintShop Pro software.

```
potato=function()
{
par(mfrow=c(2,3),mar=c(1,1,3,1))
for(i in 1:6)
{
potdat=scan(paste("c:\\MixedModels\\Chapter11\\pot",i,".pgm",
      sep=""),what="",quiet=T) # reading the image files
nr=as.numeric(potdat[3]);nc=as.numeric(potdat[2])
potdat=matrix(as.numeric(potdat[5:length(potdat)]),byrow=T,
      ncol=nc,nrow=nr) # the matrix image
image(1:nr,1:nc,potdat,xlab="",ylab="",axes=F,col=gray(0:255/255))
mtext(side=3, paste("Potato #",i,sep=""),cex=2,line=.5)
}
```

These images give rise to the shape analysis after the shape/boundary extraction and are used in one of the problems below.

Problems for Section 11.7

1. Plot 16 different shapes with the radius function $r(\theta) = 1 + [1 + 0.2\cos(2\theta) - 0.4\sin(3\theta)](1 + \cos^2(4\theta))$ using the model (11.18) with various μ, κ_i, and h_i. Use the same xlim and ylim.

2. As a continuation of the previous problem, estimate μ, κ_i, and h_i by minimizing the sum of squares (11.19).

3. As a modification of problem 1, plot 16 different shapes with the radius function $r(\theta + \eta_i)$, where r is as specified in Problem 1 and $\eta_i \sim \mathcal{N}(0, \pi^2)$, using model (11.18) with various ϕ_i, μ, κ_i, and h_i.

4*. Use simulations with the true shape from the previous problem to estimate the true shape from n realizations. Compute and plot a BLUP estimate of the shape. Repeat simulations with increased n. Is the ML shape estimator consistent?

5*. Based on the data from the function potato, extract the shape of potatoes and use fixed and/or random Fourier descriptor shape analysis to compute the mean shape. Develop the membership criterion to determine whether another potato belongs to this group of six potatoes. Generate a potato shape that does not belong to this group of shapes and verify whether the membership test rejects the null hypothesis. Do simulations to test the quality of the membership pest (compute the power function).

11.8   Summary points

- Shape analysis is widely used in science and engineering. For example, morphology is a part of systematic biology and examines the shapes of various biological subjects, vegetables, insects, animals, and humans. In engineering and computer science, shape analysis is typically used in the framework of computer vision, radar, and image recognition.

- There are two ways to obtain shape data; using landmarks or as an outline of a digital image. Landmarks are chosen manually to represent some distinguished or important points of the shape. Usually, the number of landmarks is fairly small (say, <30), but a digital shape may include thousands of points.

- A characteristic feature of shape analysis is the fact that shapes usually come in different sizes and are arbitrarily rotated, translated, or even reflected. These are irrelevant features and should be excluded from the shape analysis.

- Two assumptions may be made when analyzing the shape: that size, rotation, and translation are fixed and arbitrary for each shape, or that shapes are just slightly and randomly transformed. The first hypothesis leads to the Procrustes model, with the number of nuisance parameters increasing with the number of shapes. The second hypothesis leads to a random effects model.

- The choice of a fixed- or random-transformation model should be dictated by the sampling design. For example, if the shape of particles is analyzed, the rotation and translation may be out of the experimentalist's control, and therefore it is better to assume a fixed model. If skull landmarks or leaves of mature subjects of the same type are analyzed, the experimentalist may record the shapes just slightly rotated—then the random model would be appropriate.

- A mixed effects model is well suited for shape analysis to describe the shape variation across individuals within a common general population. The theory of mixed effects developed in earlier chapters becomes a powerful and unified model to analyze random iid shapes. For example, linear mixed effects, or more precisely, the balanced growth curve model can be applied to landmark analysis. A combination of a shape-specific transformation and a random effect such as size may be modeled by the general growth curve model of Section 4.2. Random rotation leads to a nonlinear mixed model.

- The Fourier descriptor model is adequate to study shape outlines obtained from digital images. A star shape is represented uniquely by one periodic radius function, and a general shape may be represented by two periodic functions. These functions can be described parsimoniously by a few harmonics of Fourier series with random coefficients (Random Fourier Descriptor = RFD). The balanced random-coefficient model of Section 2.3, as a special case of the LME model, applies. Estimation and analysis of the RFD model is drastically simplified because the design matrix is orthogonal.

12

Statistical Image Analysis

12.1 Introduction

We are witnessing a tremendous development in digital imaging. Ten years ago, one needed special equipment to take digital images and quantify them—today it is a routine task. *Image processing* is a well-established discipline with a number of textbooks on the subject: Starck et al. (1998), Petrou and Bosdogianni (1999), Seul et al. (2000), Gonzales and Woods (2002), and Petrou and Petrou (2010). Image processing is concerned with picture enhancement, restoration, and segmentation and is a part of *signal processing.* However, we are concerned with image analysis, particularly *statistical* analysis of a sample of images (we prefer the word *ensemble*). We refer the reader to a book by Barrett and Myers (2004) for a complete in-depth discussion of image science and image reconstruction.

Our primary assumption is that images are random. For example, if one is interested in the quality of paint finishing, one can assume that images of different parts of the painted object will differ up to a certain degree. One wants to know if the image variation is within established limits. Since images are random, the statistical approach becomes relevant. Typical questions of statistical analysis of images are: (a) are two images the same up to a random deviation, or in statistical language, do two images belong to the same general population? (b) are two ensembles of images the same, like a series of images taken before and after treatment? (c) can we generalize a t-test for images? and (d) can we compute a p-value for image comparison as we routinely do in statistics for sample comparison? *Pattern recognition,* as a part of signal processing, also deals with image comparison but in terms of image classification. Although the problems of statistical image comparison and classification are close, they are not the same and, in particular, the latter does not address image-specific variation.

We have to admit that today, statistical image analysis and comparison are unsatisfactory. Perhaps the most advanced image statistics application is functional MRI (fMRI), where time series image frames are analyzed to detect the signal around the brain activation area. But image analysis should go far beyond fMRI because image appeal becomes commonplace in scientific research. For example, a routine practice in cancer research showing two microscopic tissue images before and after treatment as proof of a method's validity is unacceptable. Images vary considerably across sections and animals (or humans). Proper analysis would involve the comparison of dozens or hundreds of images; in our terminology, an *ensemble* of images. This is where the human eye cannot judge and statistics come into play.

The idea of distinguishing two types of image variation, within image and between images, leads immediately to the mixed model as the workhorse of statistical image analysis. Thus, the theory developed in previous chapters becomes the key to the statistical analysis of digital images. For example, images of the same tissue taken at different locations or different time points can be viewed as repeated measurements and therefore may be analyzed by the relevant statistical methodology.

It is routine to use least squares as a criterion in image processing: for example, for image registration. Why least squares? Why not weighted least squares? Why sum of squares? We suggest an elaborative statistical model for images that implies a justified criterion enabling statistical image analysis and comparison.

The goal of this chapter is to lay out the foundation for statistical analysis of images using mixed effects modeling techniques for repeated measurements as described in Chapters 2 through 8. Depending on the level of complexity and sophistication, statistical image models can lead to either linear mixed effects, or the generalized linear or nonlinear mixed effects models. In no way can our description be considered as complete; it serves only as a start for future, more sophisticated statistical image modeling.

12.1.1   What is a digital image?

Mathematically, a digital image is a matrix. Consequently, matrix algebra is the major mathematical tool in image analysis. There are two kinds of image, grayscale and color. A grayscale (monochrome) image is a matrix with intensity represented as integer values from 0 (black) to 255 (white). A grayscale image has 256 levels (0 to 255) because the human eye can distinguish approximately this many levels, and because that number fits conveniently in one byte (a byte has 8 bits, $2^8 = 256$). A *binary* image is a special case of the grayscale format; it has intensity values of only 0 and 255, or pure black and pure white.

Each matrix element corresponds to a pixel on the image. If an image is represented as a $P \times Q$ matrix M, the value at each point on the image is rescaled as $255(M - M_{\min})/(M_{\max} - M_{\min})$ and rounded. In digital imaging, P and Q may be hundreds or even thousands, leading to very large files. For example, a file of a 121×74 gray image will be $121 \times 74 = 8954$ bytes, although the actual size of the image file depends on the format used. See Section 12.5 for a discussion of image compression.

Because the three primary colors (Red, Green and Blue) can be combined to produce other colors, a color image can be represented by three gray images—the

RGB format. Thus, a color image can be represented numerically by a triple of $P \times Q$ matrices with integer values from 0 to 255 as color saturation values. Although to the human eye, color and three gray images do not seem to be equivalent, they are mathematically. We take this approach in this book when dealing with color images. Thus, instead of displaying a color image, we display three gray images. The original color images may be viewed on the Internet.

Many formats are used to store images. Popular image formats include jpg, gif, and tiff. Gray images may be converted to a text file using the Portable Graymap (pgm) format, and color images may be converted to a text file using the Portable Pixelmap (ppm) format. Although the resulting text file will be much larger, the format gives the researcher full access to the image data for further processing. There are many photo-editing, image-processing, and file-conversion products; we use PaintShop Pro from Jasc Software, Inc.

In image analysis we often treat matrix elements as a function of the indices, so in this chapter we use the notation $M(p,q)$ to refer to the (p,q)th element. For example, we work with p and q as arguments for image alignment. Moreover, we shall deal with random p and q.

12.1.2   Image arithmetic

Like matrices, images can be added, subtracted, and even multiplied and divided. However, there is a substantial limitation to image arithmetic because images are generally not aligned. For example, if one is interested in finding the image difference between *before* and *after,* it is tempting to take image difference by subtracting pixel intensities. However, it will soon be realized that pixels on the first image do not exactly correspond to pixels on the second image; therefore, a simple difference does not make sense. Even after image alignment, it may be realized that the objects in the images moved slightly, and again, image difference becomes problematic. Image alignment and registration is an essential problem of further image analysis.

12.1.3   Ensemble and repeated measurements

In statistical image analysis, we usually deal with a sample of images. This is new to image processing, where one deals with one image at a time. A typical problem of statistical image analysis is that one wants to know if two sets of images, $\{\mathbf{M}_{i1}, i = 1, ..., N_1\}$ and $\{\mathbf{M}_{i2}, i = 1, ..., N_2\}$, belong to the same general population. In this book we use the term *ensemble* to indicate sample images. Typically, ensemble means that the images are independent and identically distributed (iid) up to a transformation. Thus, the notion *iid* for images has a broader sense and just means that images are of the same object and independent. Statistical analysis of images is often complicated by the fact that images may have different resolution, size, viewpoint, position, lighting, and so on. We suggest modeling an ensemble of images using repeated measurements or mixed effects methodology. This methodology was applied to a random sample of shapes in Chapter 11 and is well suited to model within- and between-image variation.

12.1.4 Image and spatial statistics

Statistical image analysis and spatial statistics have much in common. Both work with a planar distribution, and therefore an issue of spatial correlation (local dependence of pixels) is central. Classic reference books for spatial statistics are those of Ripley (1981) and Cressie (1991). Statistical analysis of images is more complicated because it usually deals with an ensemble; in addition, images may be available up to a planar transformation. Image analysis borrows the modeling techniques of spatial correlation from spatial statistics, such as SAR and AR models. To model more general image spatial correlation, the theory of a Markov random field is used (Chellappa and Jain, 1993).

12.1.5 Structured and unstructured images

Images may be divided roughly into two groups: structured and unstructured. Examples of the first group are images of an easily recognized object, such as a human face, building, carrot, rug, and so on. Examples of unstructured images are microscopic images, pieces of painted wall, and aerial images. The human eye is good at differentiating an apple from a TV set, but bad when it comes to comparing hundreds of unstructured images, such as medical histology images. An unstructured image may be well represented by its gray level distribution, and therefore it is image-content independent. An advantage of this approach is that a difficult problem of image alignment is eliminated. On the other hand, it may well happen that images of an apple an a TV set will produce the same gray distribution. Thus, a gray-distribution model assumes that images are of the same type of object.

A structured or content-dependent statistical image analysis is more complex because, in addition to image alignment, it requires specification of the image content and spatial correlation. For example, if cells in a microscopic image are elliptical in shape and one wants to count cells, one has to define the cell shape. The simplest structured image is texture where the pattern repeats in a stochastic manner. Examples of textures are wood and fabric (Cross and Jain, 1983).

Structured images are complex, and unlike unstructured images, a multinomial distribution for gray levels may serve as a uniform probabilistic model. Structured images thus require different statistical techniques.

12.2 Testing for uniform lighting

Digital pictures may be taken at different exposures and lighting. In this section we use the F-test of Section 3.8 to test whether the lighting is uniform . Moreover, we estimate the direction and position of the light.

A 662×621 gray image of a rug is shown in Figure 12.1. The following statistical model is assumed:

$$M(p,q) = \beta_0 + \beta_1 p + \beta_2 q + \varepsilon(p,q), \qquad (12.1)$$

where $p = 1, ..., P = 662$, $q = 1, ..., Q = 621$ are pixel coordinates, and $\varepsilon(p,q)$ is an error term with zero mean and constant variance. In other words, the grayscale level $M(p,q)$ is considered to be a linear function of the pixel coordinates, p and q.

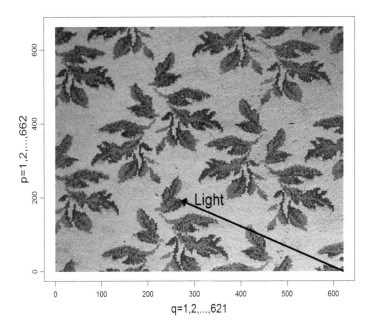

FIGURE 12.1. Rug image and the light direction derived from the linear regression model (the light comes from the bottom-right corner).

The relation may be viewed as a planar regression where β_0 is the intercept, the light intensity at the lower left corner; β_1 is the slope coefficient, the rate at which the light intensity increases or drops vertically; and β_2 is the rate at which the light changes horizontally. If the lighting is uniform, $\beta_1 = 0$ and $\beta_2 = 0$; thus, we can find if the light is uniform by testing the significance of these regression coefficients. In matrix form, (12.1), can be rewritten as

$$\mathbf{M} = \beta_0 \mathbf{1}_P \mathbf{1}'_Q + \beta_1 \mathbf{d}_P \mathbf{1}'_Q + \beta_2 \mathbf{1}_P \mathbf{d}'_Q + \mathbf{E},$$

where $\mathbf{d}_P = (1, 2, ..., P)'$, $\mathbf{d}_Q = (1, 2, ..., Q)'$, and $\mathbf{1}$ is the vector of 1s of the respective dimension. Taking the vec operator of both sides, we rewrite (12.1) as a planar relation in vector form suitable for regression analysis,

$$\mathbf{m} = \beta_0 \mathbf{1}_{PQ} + \beta_1 (\mathbf{d}_P \otimes \mathbf{1}_Q) + \beta_2 (\mathbf{1}_P \otimes \mathbf{d}_Q) + \boldsymbol{\varepsilon},$$

where $\otimes$ indicates the matrix Kronecker product and $\mathbf{m} = \text{vec}(\mathbf{M})$ is the $PQ \times 1$ vector. Applying least squares, we find that $\widehat{M} = 134.4 - 0.0693p + 0.0383q$. As follows from this regression, the average grayscale level is minimum ($\widehat{M} = 88$) when $p = P$ and $q = 1$, corresponding to the upper-left corner of the image (darker). In the lower-right corner the image is lighter ($\widehat{M} = 158$) because maximum $\widehat{M}$ occurs at $p = 1$ and $q = Q$. To test whether the image has uniform lighting we test the null hypothesis: $H_0 : \beta_1 = \beta_2 = 0$ using the F-test (3.57). Since the errors are assumed to be iid, we have $\mathbf{V} = \mathbf{I}$. The residual sum of squares under the null is $RSS_0 = \sum_{p,q} (M(p,q) - \overline{M})^2 = 9.83 \times 10^8$ and the minimal residual sum of squares from regression is $RSS = 8.92 \times 10^8$. For this example, the number of estimated

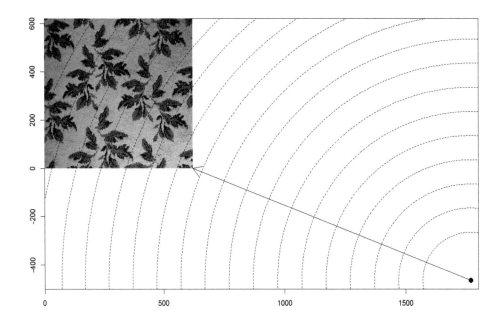

FIGURE 12.2. Source light location with contours via the nonlinear regression model. The linear and nonlinear models yield a close light angle. The location of the light source is estimated at (1770, -465).

parameters is $m = 3$, the total number of observations is $n = P \times Q = 662 \times 621$, and $q = 2$. Formula (3.57) gives $F = 23274$, but the threshold value assuming that the light is uniform is about 3. Thus, the hypothesis that the light is uniformly distributed is rejected overwhelmingly.

12.2.1 Estimating light direction and position

Moreover, having coefficients β_1 and β_2, we may estimate where the light comes from. As noted above, since the first slope coefficient is negative and the second is positive, the light comes from the lower-right corner. Since the tangent of the angle is $0.0693/0.0383$, we estimate that the light comes at the angle $150°$ from the q-axis (indicated by the arrow).The linear model (12.1) assumes that the source light is linear because the levels of the light field are straight lines. Alternatively, one can assume that there is one source of light, say at position (x, y). The levels of the light field are concentric circles. We want to estimate x and y having the rug image in Figure 12.1. As follows from the basic laws of optics, when the light absorption is low, the light intensity is the reciprocal of the distance. To simplify, we take the nonlinear regression model $M(p, q) = 255 - \nu\sqrt{(q - x)^2 + (p - y)^2} + \varepsilon$, where ν is the absorption coefficient and ε is the error term. Estimating parameters of this model by nonlinear least squares gives $\widehat{\nu} = 0.75$, $\widehat{x} = 1770$, and $\widehat{y} = -465$. This means that the estimated location of the light is $(1770, -465)$, see Figure 12.2. Interestingly, the linear and nonlinear models give a similar light angle, indicated by the arrow.

The R function that plots Figure 12.2 and estimates the coordinates of the light source is shown below.

```
carpet=function()
{
    dump("carpet", "c:\\MixedModels\\Chapter12\\carpet.r")
    d <- scan("c:\\MixedModels\\Chapter12\\carpetc.pgm",what="")
    d <- as.numeric(d[2:length(d)])
    K <- d[1] # number of rows
    J <- d[2] # number of columns
    y=d[4:length(d)] # image data
    carp.dat <- matrix(y, nrow = K, ncol = J)
    x1=rep(1:K,times=J);x2=rep(1:J,each=K)
    print("Linear model:")
    o <- lm(y ~x1 + x2)
    print(summary(o))
    print("Nonlinear model:")
    o <- nls(y ~a1 * sqrt(((a2 - x1)^2 + (x2 - a3)^2)),
        start = c(a1 = sqrt(0.006), a2 = 2000, a3 = -500))
    print(summary(o))
    a <- coef(o)
    par(mfrow = c(1, 1), err = -1, mar = c(3, 3, 1, 2))
    image(1:J, 1:K, t(carp.dat), axes = T, xlab = "", ylab = "",
        xlim = c(0, 1800), ylim = c(-500, J),col=gray(0:255/255))
    points(a[2], a[3], pch = 16, cex = 1.5)
    N <- 30
    h <- 3000/N
    theta <- seq(from = 0, to = 8 * atan(1), by = 0.01)
    for(i in 2:(N - 1)) {
        dc <- h * i
        x <- dc * cos(theta)
        y <- dc * sin(theta)
        lines(a[2] + x, a[3] + y, lty = 2)
    }
    arrows(a[2], a[3], J, 0)
}
```

We make a few remarks on this code: (1) the txt file with this code is saved using **dump** command every time the code is issued; and (2) the carpet image is downloaded into an R session using the **scan** command as an array string, the third and fourth elements of the array are the number of rows and columns in the image, and the image itself starts from the fifth element (this is a typical representation of the image in the PGM format).

Problems for Section 12.2

1. Test the hypothesis that the distance from the light source to the bottom-right corner of the rug is more that 2000 pixels. Approximate the squared distance $(\widehat{x} - 621)^2 + \widehat{y}^2$ by a normal distribution and use the delta method to estimate the variance.

2*. Take a picture of an object near the window and measure the location of the window. Save the image in PGM format and repeat the analysis of the light location. Is your estimate close to the actual window location?

12.3   Kolmogorov–Smirnov image comparison

An essential task of image analysis is image comparison. Under the assumption that images are subject to random noise, we want to test if the images are the same. In this and the following section we say that two images are the same if they have the same grayscale distribution. Clearly, if two images are the same, up to a small noise, they should have close grayscale distributions. The reverse is not true. Thus, grayscale distribution analysis is helpful when images of the same content are compared. In this section and the next, nonparametric and parametric approaches are developed.

The image histogram is a frequently used technique of image processing. However, in addition to the histogram, one can compute the distribution, or more specifically, the cumulative distribution function, as the sum of the probabilities that a pixel takes a grayscale level of less than g, where $g = 0, ..., 255$. If $\{h_g\}$ is the image histogram,

$$F_g = \sum_{g'=0}^{g} h_{g'} \tag{12.2}$$

is the empirical cumulative distribution function. As for any distribution function, F_g is nondecreasing within the interval $[0, 1]$.

One advantage of distribution analysis is that it facilitates visual image comparison by plotting grayscale distribution functions on the same scale (it is difficult to plot several histograms on the same scale). Another advantage is that the distribution function allows the application of nonparametric statistical tests, such as Kolmogorov–Smirnov.

12.3.1   Kolmogorov–Smirnov test for image comparison

Let $F^{(1)} = \{F_g^{(1)}, g = 0, ..., 255\}$ and $F^{(2)} = \{F_g^{(2)}, g = 0, ..., 255\}$ be two gray level distributions for the $P_1 \times Q_1$ and $P_2 \times Q_2$ images M_1 and M_2. We compute the maximum, $\widehat{D} = \max_g \left| F_g^{(1)} - F_g^{(2)} \right|$, the distance of one distribution from the other. Kolmogorov and Smirnov proved that if theoretical distributions are the same, then the probability that the observed distance, $\widehat{D}$, is greater than D is

$$Q_{KS}(\lambda) = 2\sum_{j=1}^{\infty}(-1)^{j-1}\exp\left(-2j^2\lambda^2\right),$$

where $\lambda_{KS} = D[\sqrt{J} + 0.11/\sqrt{J} + 0.12]$ and $J = (P_1Q_1P_2Q_2)/(P_1Q_1 + P_2Q_2)$; see Hollander and Wolfe (1999) for more details. Thus, $Q_{KS}(\lambda)$ may be treated as the p-value of the test. The greater the distance between distributions, the less the probability $Q_{KS}(\lambda_{KS})$. For example, if two images yield distance D and the computed probability $Q_{KS}(\lambda_{KS}) < 0.05$, we reject the hypothesis that the two images are the same with a 5% error. We can find λ_{KS} such that $Q_{KS}(\lambda_{KS}) = 0.05$, giving the threshold $\lambda_{KS} = 1.358$.

As a word of caution, all nonparametric tests, including the Kolmogorov–Smirnov, have the alternative $H_A : F_1(x) \neq F_2(x)$ for at least one x. Thus, these tests may be conservative.

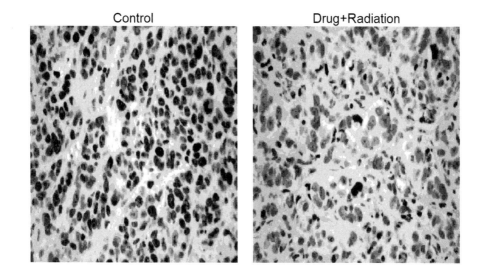

FIGURE 12.3. Histology sections of untreated and treated tumors. The living cancer cells are the dark spots (blobs). To test statistically that the two images have the same grayscale distributions, the Kolmogorov–Smirnov test is used.

12.3.2   Example: histological analysis of cancer treatment

We illustrate the Kolmogorov–Smirnov test with a histological analysis of breast cancer treatment (Sundaram et al., 2003). Two 512×384 images of proliferative-activity tumor tissue sections are shown in Figure 12.3. The dark blobs are cancer cells. In the control tumor (left), no treatment was given. In the treated tumor (right), a combination of drug, EB 1089, and radiation seems to have reduced the number of living cancer cells. We want to confirm this reduction statistically by the Kolmogorov–Smirnov test by computing the p-value.

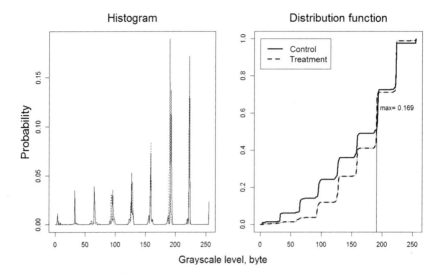

FIGURE 12.4. Histogram and cumulative distribution functions for two histology images. The distribution function of the treated tumor is less (almost everywhere) than that of the control (the maximum difference is 0.169), which means that the control image is darker. The Kolmogorov–Smirnov distribution function distance is used to test the statistical significance.

The grayscale histogram and the distribution functions for these images are shown in Figure 12.4. Clearly, it is difficult to judge the difference in the images by histogram. To the contrary, the distribution functions reveal the difference with the absolute maximum $1/10$. We notice that the treatment distribution function is below control (for most gray levels), which means that the right image is lighter. For these images $P_1 Q_1 = P_2 Q_2 = 512 \times 384 = 1.9661 \times 10^5$, yielding $\lambda_{KS} = 52.882$ and $Q(\lambda_{KS}) < 0.0001$, near zero. Since the p-value is very small, we infer that the null hypothesis that the two images are the same should be rejected.

The R program that plots the two images (Figure 12.3) and computes λ (Figure 12.4) is shown below.

```
KSimage=function(job=1)
{
dump("KSimage","c:\\MixedModels\\Chapter12\\KSimage.r")
if(job==1)
{
par(mfrow = c(1, 2), mar = c(1, 1, 3, 1), omi = c(0, 0, 0, 0))
d <- scan("c:\\MixedModels\\Chapter12\\grp11.pgm",what="")
d <- as.numeric(d[9:length(d)])
nr <- d[1];nc <- d[2]
d <- matrix(d[4:length(d)], nrow = nr, ncol = nc)
```

```
 image(1:nr, 1:nc, d, xlab = "", ylab = "", axes = F,
                col=gray(0:255/255))
 mtext(side = 3, "Control", line = 0.25, cex = 2)
 d <- scan("c:\\MixedModels\\Chapter12\\grp51.pgm",what="")
 d <- as.numeric(d[9:length(d)])
 nr <- d[1];nc <- d[2]
 d <- matrix(d[4:length(d)], nrow = nr, ncol = nc)
 image(1:nr, 1:nc, d, xlab = "", ylab = "", axes = F,
                col=gray(0:255/255))
 mtext(side = 3, "Drug+Radiation", line = 0.25, cex = 2)
}
if(job==2)
{
 par(mfrow = c(1, 2), mar = c(4, 4, 3, 1))
 d <- scan("c:\\kluwer\\image\\sujatha\\grp11.pgm",what="")
 d <- as.numeric(d[9:length(d)])
 nr <- d[1]
 nc <- d[2]
 J1 <- nr * nc
 d1 <- d[4:length(d)]
 d <- scan("c:\\kluwer\\image\\sujatha\\grp51.pgm",what="")
 d <- as.numeric(d[9:length(d)])
 nr <- d[1]
 nc <- d[2]
 print(c(nr, nc))
 J2 <- nr * nc
 d2 <- d[4:length(d)]
 h1 <- f1 <- h2 <- f2 <- rep(0, 256)
 for(i in 0:255) {
 h1[i + 1] <- length(d1[d1 == i])/length(d1)
 h2[i + 1] <- length(d2[d2 == i])/length(d2)
 }
 for(i in 2:256) {
 f1[i] <- f1[i - 1] + h1[i]
 f2[i] <- f2[i - 1] + h2[i]
 }
 f1[256] <- f2[256] <- 1
 matplot(cbind(0:255, 0:255), cbind(h1, h2), type = "l",
                col = 1,xlab="",ylab="")
 mtext(side = 2, "Probability", line = 2.5, cex = 1.75)
 mtext(side = 3, "Histogram", line = 1, cex = 1.75)
```

```
matplot(cbind(0:255, 0:255), cbind(f1, f2), type = "l",
                        col = 1,xlab="",ylab="")
lines(0:255, f1, lwd = 3)
lines(0:255, f2, lwd = 3, lty = 2)
mf <- max(abs(f1 - f2))
jm <- (0:255)[abs(f1 - f2) == mf]
segments(jm, -0.25, jm, 0.6)
text(jm+5, 0.63, paste("max=", round(mf, 3)),adj=0)
mtext(side = 3, "Distribution function", line = 1, cex = 1.75)
legend(0, 1, c("Control", "Treatment"), lty = 1:2, cex = 1.25,
                        lwd = 3)
mtext(side = 1, "Grayscale level, byte", line = -1,
                        outer = T,cex = 1.5)
J <- (J1 * J2)/(J1 + J2)
lambda <- mf * (sqrt(J) + 0.11/sqrt(J) + 0.12)
j <- 1:10000
js <- rep(1, 10000)
js[seq(from = 2, to = 10000, by = 2)] <- -1
Q <- 2 * sum(js * exp(-2 * j^2 * lambda^2))
cat("\nbyte.max =",jm," max.cdf.distance =",round(mf,3),
    " lambda =",round(lambda,3)," QKS =", round(Q,4),"\n")
}
}
```

We make several comments: (1) The two tasks correspond to job=1 (Figure 12.3) and job=2 (Figure 12.4); (2) different software uses different preambules when saving images in PGM format, in this particular case starting from the 9th element; and (3) arrays h1 and h2 contain histograms and f1 and f2 contain cdf values for the two images, alternatively, one can use the cumsum function to compute the cdf.

Problems for Section 12.3

1. Plot $Q_{KS}(\lambda)$ as a function of λ using lambda=seq(from=1,to=2,by=.01). Replace ∞ with 1000 and use matrix operation to avoid the loop: compute the value under the sum as a matrix with 1000 rows and length(lambda) columns. Then use %*% to get $Q_{KS}(\lambda)$. Confirm that $Q_{KS}(1.358) \simeq 0.05$.

2. Use a t-test (Z-score) to test that the treatment image is darker than the control (this is how images are compared using traditional statistics). Does this test confirm the KS test? What test is preferable?

12.4   Multinomial statistical model for images

The aim of this section is to develop a statistical model for gray images based on the grayscale distribution (or simply, gray distribution). As in the previous section, it is assumed that the image is specified by 256 grayscale levels, and therefore our image analysis is content-independent. Based on this model, we shall develop parametric tests for image comparison.

The gray distribution of an image $\{M(p,q), p = 1, ..., P, q = 1, ..., Q\}$ is specified by 256 probabilities $\pi_g = \Pr(M = g)$, where $g = 0, 1, ..., 255$ is the gray level. Assuming that among PQ image pixels there are k_0 black pixels, the k_1 pixels have gray level $g = 1$, k_2 pixels have gray level $g = 2$, etc. the mutual probability can be modeled via the *multinomial* distribution, namely,

$$f(k_0, k_1, ..., k_{255}) = \frac{(PQ)!}{k_0! k_1! ... k_{255}!} \pi_0^{k_0} \pi_1^{k_1} ... \pi_{255}^{k_{255}}, \tag{12.3}$$

Rao (1973), Bickel and Doksum (2001), Agresti (2002). In this formula, the sum of probabilities is 1, $\sum_{g=0}^{255} \pi_g = 1$, and $\sum_{g=0}^{255} k_g = PQ$ is the total number of pixels. Value k_g is called the frequency, so (12.3) specifies the probability that in PQ independent experiments the random variable M takes the value 0 k_0 times, takes the value 1 k_1 times, and so on. An important assumption is that these random experiments are independent. For a binary image, the multinomial distribution reduces to the binomial distribution. Model (12.3) is called a *multinomial* model for gray images.

The log-likelihood function for the multinomial gray level model is

$$l(\pi_0, ..., \pi_{255}) = C + \sum_{g=0}^{255} k_g \ln \pi_g,$$

where $C = \ln(PQ)! - \sum_{g=0}^{255} \ln k_g!$, a constant. To estimate probabilities $\{\pi_g\}$ from a $P \times Q$ image by maximum likelihood, we maximize l with respect to $\{\pi_g\}$ under the restriction that $\sum_{g=0}^{255} \pi_g = 1$. Introducing the Lagrangian

$$\mathcal{L}(\pi_0, ..., \pi_{255}, \lambda) = \sum_{g=0}^{255} k_g \ln \pi_g - \lambda \left(\sum_{g=0}^{255} \pi_g - 1 \right),$$

and taking derivatives with respect to π_g, we obtain $\partial \mathcal{L}/\partial \pi_g = k_g/\pi_g - \lambda = 0$ which implies that $\pi_g = k_q/\lambda$. Hence, the ML estimate of the gth probability is

$$\widehat{\pi}_g = h_g = \frac{k_g}{PQ}. \tag{12.4}$$

This is a familiar estimate of the gray level probability—the ML estimate is just the histogram value, h_g. The variance and covariance of these probability estimates are

$$\text{var}(\widehat{\pi}_g) = \frac{1}{PQ} \pi_g (1 - \pi_g), \quad \text{cov}(\widehat{\pi}_g, \widehat{\pi}_{g'}) = -\frac{1}{PQ} \pi_g \pi_{g'}. \tag{12.5}$$

To estimate the variance and covariance, we use the histogram value h_g instead of π_g in formulas (12.5). As follows from (12.5), $\widehat{\pi}_g$ is consistent because its variance vanishes for large images, $PQ \to \infty$. We shall apply the multinomial model for image comparison and entropy computation.

12.4.1 Multinomial image comparison

Using the notation of Section 12.3, let $M^{(1)}$ and $M^{(2)}$ be $P_1 \times Q_1$ and $P_2 \times Q_2$ gray images. We want to test whether they have the same gray distribution. In other terms, the null hypothesis is $H_0 : \pi_0^{(1)} = \pi_0^{(2)}, ..., \pi_{255}^{(1)} = \pi_{255}^{(2)}$. Two tests can be suggested, assuming that the images are independent: the χ^2 and the likelihood ratio test. Unlike the Kolmogorov–Smirnov test, these tests are parametric because they assume the multinomial distribution specified by the 256 probability parameters.

In the χ^2-test, we estimate $256 \times 2 = 512$ probabilities $\widehat{\pi}_g^{(1)} = h_{1g}$ and $\widehat{\pi}_g^{(2)} = h_{2g}$ as the proportion of pixels with the gray level g. Assuming that images are independent, the variance of the difference is the sum of variances, and as follows from formula (12.5), $\mathrm{var}(h_{1g} - h_{2g}) = h_{1g}(1 - h_{1g})/(P_1 Q_1) + h_{2g}(1 - h_{2g})/(P_2 Q_2)$. Then, under the null hypothesis, the scaled sum of squares approximately has a χ^2-distribution,

$$\sum_{g=0}^{255} \frac{(h_{1g} - h_{2g})^2}{h_{1g}(1 - h_{1g})/(P_1 Q_1) + h_{2g}(1 - h_{2g})/(P_2 Q_2)} \sim \chi^2(255). \qquad (12.6)$$

We take off one degree of freedom because the sum of probabilities is 1. This has little effect because the total degrees of freedom is large. If both h_{1g} and h_{2g}, are zero, the corresponding term is dropped from the summation. One can interpret (12.6) as the squared scaled distance between the two histograms. Following the line of statistical hypothesis testing, if the value on the left-hand side of (12.6) is greater than the $(1 - \alpha)$th quantile of the χ^2-distribution with 255 degrees of freedom, we reject the hypothesis that the two images have the same gray level distribution with error α. Alternatively, one can report the p-value as the χ^2-tail density.

In (12.6) we assumed that $\{h_{1g} - h_{2g}, g = 0, ..., 255\}$ are independent, but as follows from (12.5), they are negatively correlated. To account for correlation, we remove the histogram component with the maximum value $h_{1g} + h_{2g}$ so that $\mathbf{h}_{1*} - \mathbf{h}_{2*}$ is the 255×1 vector of histogram differences with the corresponding 255×255 covariance matrix $\mathbf{V}_{1*} + \mathbf{V}_{2*}$. By construction, the sum of elements is less than 1 and the covariance matrix is nonsingular. Then, in matrix form, similar to (12.6), we have an alternative χ^2-test,

$$(\mathbf{h}_{1*} - \mathbf{h}_{2*})'(\mathbf{V}_{1*} + \mathbf{V}_{2*})^{-1}(\mathbf{h}_{1*} - \mathbf{h}_{2*}) \sim \chi^2(255). \qquad (12.7)$$

In the likelihood ratio test, we need to compute three log-likelihood values, an individual value from each image and a combined value. More precisely, the maximum value of the log-likelihood function from image $i = 1, 2$ can be expressed in terms of frequencies $\{k_{ig}\}$ as follows:

$$
\begin{aligned}
l_i &= \ln n_i! - \sum \ln k_{ig}! + \sum k_{ig} \ln k_{ig} - \ln n_i \sum k_{ig} \\
&= (\ln n_i! - n_i \ln n_i) + \sum (k_{ig} \ln k_{ig} - \ln k_{ig}!),
\end{aligned}
$$

where $n_i = P_i Q_i$ is the number of pixels in the ith image. Next, we combine the two images into one gray level set with $n_3 = P_1 Q_1 + P_2 Q_2$ elements yielding the frequencies $\{k_{3g}, g = 0, ..., 255\}$ and the resulting log-likelihood maximum value

$$l_3 = (\ln n_3! - n_3 \ln n_3) + \sum (k_{3g} \ln k_{3g} - \ln k_{3g}!).$$

According to the likelihood ratio test, under the null hypothesis,

$$2(l_1 + l_2 - l_3) \sim \chi^2(256). \tag{12.8}$$

Again, if the left-hand side of (12.8) is larger than the $(1 - \alpha)$th quantile of the χ^2-distribution, we reject the hypothesis.

Problems for Section 12.4

1. Apply the χ^2 and the likelihood ratio tests to the histologic images in the previous section. Compute the p-values for both tests. Modify the function `KSimage`. Use `lgamma(k+1)` to compute $\ln k!$.

2*. Generate synthetic treatment images from the control image in Figure 12.3 using the formula $M'_\nu(p,q) = \lfloor 255 \times (M(p,q)/255)^\nu \rfloor$, where $M(p,q)$ is the gray intensity of the (p,q)th pixel of the original control image, ν is a positive number ($\nu = 1$ does not change the image), and $\lfloor . \rfloor$ means that the number is rounded to the nearest smallest (R function `floor`); see the function `KSimageR`. Parameter ν is image-specific, e.g. it may take values according to a beta distribution with parameters a and β. Use this method to generate random images for computing the power function of image comparison for three methods: KS, chi-square, and log-likelihood. Make your statement regarding the efficiency of the methods.

12.5   Image entropy

The purpose of an image is to convey information; thus information theory can play an important role in image analysis. Specifically, we use the notion of *entropy* to measure the amount of image information (Resa, 1961; Kulback, 1968). In the image processing literature, image entropy is used in the context of image coding. Here, we apply this concept for optimal image reduction. In this section we show how image entropy can be used for optimal image reduction and enhancement. Although entropy, as the major concept of Shannon communication theory, has some application in image science (see Barrett and Myers, 2004 for a review), we apply it for optimal image reduction. First, we demonstrate the use of entropy for binary images and then for gray and color images.

Recall that if X is a discrete random variable, which takes values $\{x_i, i = 1, 2, ..., n\}$ with probability $\{\Pr(X = x_i) = p_i\}$, the entropy is defined as $\mathcal{E} = -\sum_{i=1}^n p_i \log p_i$. In the special case when X is binary, the entropy is $\mathcal{E} = -[p \log p + (1-p) \log(1-p)]$. Usually, in communication theory, the base of the logarithm is taken to be 2, making interpretation of the entropy a piece of information measured in bits. For example, for a binary random variable with $p = 0$, the entropy is zero. Indeed, by L'Hospital's rule,

$$\begin{aligned} \mathcal{E}(0) &= -\lim_{p \to 0} p \log_2 p - (1 - 0) \log_2(1 - 0) \\ &= -\lim_{p \to 0} \frac{\log_2 p}{p^{-1}} = \frac{1}{\ln 2} \lim_{p \to 0} \frac{1/p}{1/p^2} = 0. \end{aligned}$$

Similarly, one can prove that $\mathcal{E}(1) = 0$. These results have a clear interpretation: when $p = 0$ or $p = 1$, the binary variable takes a constant value, and therefore there is no information in the message. Maximum entropy in a binary message occurs when $p = 1/2$. Indeed, differentiating the entropy, one obtains

$$
\begin{aligned}
\mathcal{E}' &= -1 - \log_2 p + \log_2(1-p) + 1 = \log_2(1-p) - \log_2 p, \\
\mathcal{E}'' &= -p^{-1} - (1-p)^{-1} = -1/[p(1-p)] < 0.
\end{aligned}
$$

The inequality says that $\mathcal{E}$ is a concave function on $(0,1)$. Maximum $\mathcal{E}$ occurs where $\mathcal{E}' = 0$, which yields $p = 1/2$. This means that maximum information contained in a sequence of zeros and ones is attained when they occur with equal probability.

For example, the amount of information in a $P \times Q$ binary image with the proportion of white pixels equal p is

$$
PQ \times \mathcal{E}(p) = -PQ\left[p\log_2 p + (1-p)\log_2(1-p)\right] \text{ bits.} \tag{12.9}
$$

In (12.9) it is assumed that pixel gray levels are uncorrelated. Now we apply the entropy notion to optimal image gray level reduction.

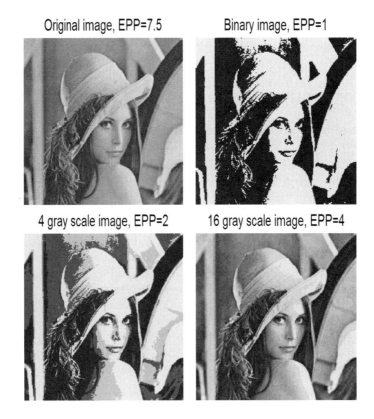

FIGURE 12.5. The original image Lena, the canon of image processing, and three optimal reductions with minimum information loss. The Entropy Per Pixel (EPP) of the original image is close to the absolute maximum, 8 bits. Information in the binary image is almost one-eighth of that in the original image.

12.5.1   Reduction of a gray image to binary

Let M be the original $P \times Q$ gray image with distribution $F = \{F_g, g = 0, ..., 255\}$. We want to reduce this image to a binary image by determining a threshold g_* such that all gray levels less than g_* are set to 0 and all gray levels greater than g_* are set to 255. We want to determine a g_* that reduces the original gray image with minimum information loss. As follows from (12.9), the entropy of a binary image gets maximum when the number of black and white pixels is the same, $p = 1/2$. Thus, g_* is defined by the equation $F_{g_*} = 1/2$, the median. In other words, an optimal threshold is the median of gray distribution. This choice yields minimum information loss.

We illustrate the image reduction in Figure 12.5. This image, *Lena*, is a canon in the image processing community, and many works use this image as an example. The reduction of the original image to binary is such that the number of black and white points in the binary image is the same. The R function that plots Figure 12.5 and computes EPP can be downloaded by issuing

```
source("c:\\MixedModels\\Chapter12\\lena.r")
```

12.5.2   Entropy of a gray image and histogram equalization

Histogram equalization is a well known technique of image processing that helps improve an image. In this section we provide an information basis for this technique and develop a general algorithm to reduce a gray image with minimum information loss.

Assuming that levels of a gray image follow a multinomial distribution (12.3), the entropy of a $P \times Q$ image is defined as

$$\mathcal{E} = -PQ \sum_{g=0}^{255} \pi_g \log_2 \pi_g.$$

Since the theoretical probability, π_g, is estimated by the histogram value, h_g, we come to the following.

Definition 45 *Image Entropy Per Pixel (EPP) is defined as*

$$EPP = -\sum_{g=0}^{255} h_g \log_2 h_g \ bits, \tag{12.10}$$

where h_g is the histogram value.

Theorem 46 *The absolute maximum of EPP is 8 bits. This maximum is attained when each of 256 gray levels occurs with equal probability $1/256$ (i.e., when the histogram is flat).*

Proof. The proof is similar to the maximum likelihood estimation at the beginning of this section. We want to maximize (12.10) over $\{h_g\}$ under the restriction $\sum_{g=0}^{255} h_g = 1$. Introducing the Lagrangian

$$\mathcal{L}(h_0, ..., h_{255}, \lambda) = \sum_{g=0}^{255} h_g \ln h_g - \lambda \left(\sum_{g=0}^{255} h_g - 1 \right)$$

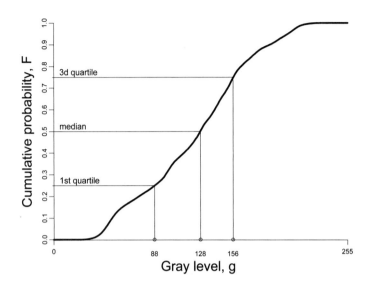

FIGURE 12.6. Optimal reduction of the original image, Lena to a binary and four-level gray image. To reduce Lena to a four-level image with minimum information loss, the thresholds must be 88 (first quartile), 128 (median), and 156 (third quartile).

and taking the derivative with respect to h_g, we obtain h_g =const= $1/256$. This corresponds to the flat histogram. The absolute maximum is

$$EPP = -256\frac{1}{256}\log_2\frac{1}{256} = 8.$$

∎

This theorem creates a theoretical basis for histogram equalization technique: by modifying the gray levels to make the histogram flat, we increase the EPP to a maximum.

For example, as follows from entropy theory, to reduce a gray image to an image with four gray levels with minimum information loss, the thresholds must be the quartiles of the distribution function F, see Figure 12.6. In other words, let q_1 (the first quartile) be the gray level such that $(PQ)/4$ pixels of the original image have gray levels of less than q_1. Let q_2 be the median, i.e., 50% of pixels have gray levels of less than q_2. Finally, let q_3 (the third quartile) be the gray level such that the number of pixels with gray levels greater than q_3 is $(PQ)/4$. This choice of thresholds makes the four-level image the most informative.

For a binary image with an equal number of black and white pixels EPP $= 1$ bit because $-0.5\log_2(1/2) = 1$. For an image with four equal gray levels, EPP $= 2$ bits. Generally, if an image has 2^m equal gray levels, EPP $= m$ bits (see Figure 12.5).

Problems for Section 12.5

1. The frequency of English letters can be downloaded as **read.table("c:\\ MixedModels\\Chapter12\\EnglishLetters.txt")**. Compute the entropy of the statement: *I love statistics* based on the letters frequency.

2. Prove that the maximum enropy of a categorical random variable is attained at $p_i = 1/n$, where $p_i \geq 0$ and $\sum_{i=1}^{n} p_i = 1$.

3. Define a 16-bit image and compute the maximum entropy.

4. The function `histgr` plots the two images depicted in Figure 12.7. Apply histogram equalization to the original image. Compare your result with that produced by commercial software.

Original image

After histogram equalization

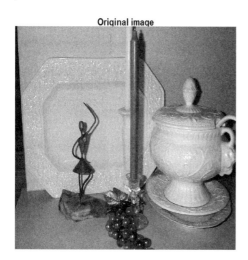 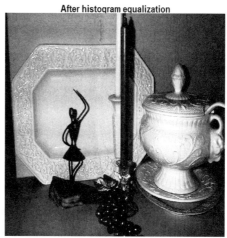

FIGURE 12.7. Two images produced by function `histgr`. Histogram equalization is done by commercial software. Use your own histogram equalization image processing technique to see if the result is the same.

12.6   Ensemble of unstructured images

Usually, one deals with several images of the same object. Then we speak of an *ensemble* of images. Similar to a sample of shapes, we distinguish two features. On one hand, it is assumed that images are *of the same object*, or in statistical terms, they belong to the same general population. On the other hand, they may have image-specific features associated with image variation. For example, if several aerial pictures are taken to assess fire damage, they are all taken over the same area but may differ because the fire damage is not uniform. The same principle was used in the previous chapter, where within- and between-shape variations were recognized. In contrast, in classical statistics, it is assumed that a sample is drawn from one general population and therefore that there would be no room for image-specific variation. In the language of the mixed model methodology, population features are described by population-averaged parameters, and image-specific features are specified by image (or cluster, subject) -specific parameters.

In this section we deal with a sample of independent gray images defined by the $P_i \times Q_i$ integer (gray level) matrices $\mathbf{M}_i, i = 1, 2, ..., N$. Typical questions: (a) Are N images the same? (b) Are two groups of images the same? (c) Does image $(N + 1)$ belong to the same group of images? A statistical test for two gray images was developed in Section 12.3, here we assume that $N > 2$.

There are two extreme approaches to modeling an ensemble of images. First, we can assume that all N images $\mathbf{M}_i$ have *identical* gray level multinomial distributions (12.3). Then one can pool the images and obtain estimates of the probabilities as if we had only one image. Clearly, if all images have the same size, the histogram and the distribution function are the arithmetic means of the individual histograms and the distribution functions. Under this assumption, a comparison of two groups of images reduces to a comparison of two distribution functions, and the Kolmogorov–Smirnov test applies.

Second, we can assume that images have *different* gray level multinomial distributions, and therefore estimation collapses to a separate estimation yielding N vectors $\widehat{\boldsymbol{\pi}}_i$.

Perhaps the most attractive approach would be to assume that, on the one hand, images are from same general population, but on the other hand, they have image-specific variation. Such an approach takes an intermediate position between the two extreme approaches.

In this section we model the image through its gray level distribution, and therefore such analysis is content independent; usually, such images are unstructured. For example, using this approach one may come to the conclusion that images of an apple and an orange are the same because they have the same gray level distribution. However, this approach may be useful when a sample of apples is analyzed. The model for an ensemble of structured (content dependent) images is described in Section 12.8.

The volumetric or mean intensity approach, which can be expressed via histogram values as $\sum_{g=0}^{255} g h_g$, is used traditionally to quantify gray images, especially in the analysis of functional MRI data. One may expect the present approach to be more powerful because it is based on an analysis of all 256 histogram values $\{h_g, g = 0, ..., 255\}$.

Application of the theory of mixed models is crucial to the analysis of an ensemble. Modeling hypotheses reduce image analysis to a linear mixed effects model (Chapters 2 to 4), a generalized linear mixed model (Chapter 7), or a nonlinear mixed effects model (Chapter 8).

12.6.1 Fixed-shift model

The fixed-shift model assumes that the ensemble of N gray images $\{\mathbf{M}_i, i = 1, 2, ... , N\}$, have the same gray level distribution up to an image-specific gray level shift. This model, the fixed-shift intensity model, may be viewed as a generalization of the fixed subject-specific intercept model of Section 7.2.2. This is perhaps the simplest model for an ensemble of images; in the next section we consider a more complex random-shift model. One application of this model is when microscopic images of the same homogeneous tissue are taken at different spots and different exposures. If the images were taken at the same exposure, they would produce the same (up to a random deviation) histogram and distribution function, but a nonconstant exposure implies that some images are darker and some lighter.

We assume that all 256 gray levels are modeled; however, this is not a strict requirement. For example, one can safely omit gray levels with zero frequency for all images.

When modeling a series of dependent images, it is more convenient to parameterize the multinomial distribution (12.3) in a different way, as follows:

$$\pi_0 = \frac{1}{1 + \sum_{j=1}^{255} e^{\rho_j}}, \ \pi_g = \frac{e^{\rho_g}}{1 + \sum_{j=1}^{255} e^{\rho_j}}, \ g = 1, ..., 255, \qquad (12.11)$$

where the $\{\rho_1, ..., \rho_{255}\}$ are new parameters. Obviously, this parameterization implies that all probabilities are positive and the sum is 1. One can easily express the new parameters in terms of the old:

$$\rho_g = \ln \pi_g - \ln \pi_0, \ g = 1, ..., 255, \qquad (12.12)$$

so ρ_g can be interpreted as the relative probability on the log scale. There are some advantages to working with ρ_g rather than π_g: (a) representation (12.11) guarantees that all probabilities are positive for any ρ_g, and (b) there is no restriction on $\{\rho_1, ..., \rho_{255}\}$, unlike $\sum_{g=0}^{255} \pi_g = 1$. The fact that $\{\rho_g\}$ may take any value from $-\infty$ to ∞ makes it possible to assume a normal distribution, substantially simplifying the estimation problem, see the next Section. Transformation (12.12) was used by Besag (1974) but without reference to the multinomial distribution. This transformation is the basis for reduction of a nonlinear multinomial model to a linear mixed effects model, Section 12.6.3. For reasons explained later, this transformation will be called *logit*.

In this section we assume that N images have the same gray level distribution but differ by a constant b_i. Thus, on the log scale the ith image is specified by $\{\rho_g + b_i, g = 1, ..., 255\}$. Then, letting $B_i = \exp(b_i)$, we come to the ith multinomial model, as a straightforward generalization of (12.11),

$$\pi_{i0} = \frac{1}{1 + B_i \sum_{j=1}^{255} e^{\rho_j}}, \ \pi_{ig} = \frac{B_i e^{\rho_g}}{1 + B_i \sum_{j=1}^{255} e^{\rho_j}}, \ g = 1, ..., 255.$$

Assuming that the N images are independent, the joint log-likelihood function, up to a constant, takes the form $l = \sum_{i=1}^{N} \sum_{g=0}^{255} k_{ig} \ln \pi_{ig}$, where k_{ig} is the frequency in the ith image. In terms of ρ_g, we have

$$l = \sum_{i=1}^{N} \left[(n_i - k_{i0}) \ln B_i - n_i \ln \left(1 + B_i \sum_{g=1}^{255} e^{\rho_g} \right) \right] + \sum_{g=1}^{255} d_g \rho_g,$$

where $d_g = \sum_{i=1}^{N} k_{ig}$ is the total frequency of the gth gray level. Our aim is to obtain the maximum likelihood estimators (MLEs) for B_i and ρ_g, as maximizers of l, in closed form. When the $\{\rho_g\}$ are held fixed, we find the maximizer for B_i exactly from the equation $\partial l / \partial B_i = 0$, yielding

$$B_i = \frac{n_i - k_{i0}}{k_{i0} \sum_{g=1}^{255} e^{\rho_g}}, \quad i = 1, ..., N.$$

Plugging this solution back into l, we eliminate nuisance parameters $\{B_i\}$ to obtain a profile log-likelihood function, up to a constant term,

$$l(\rho_1, ..., \rho_{255}) = -(N_T - k_0) \ln \sum_{g=1}^{255} e^{\rho_g} + \sum_{g=1}^{255} d_g \rho_g, \qquad (12.13)$$

where $k_0 = \sum_{i=1}^{N} k_{i0}$ is the frequency of the background and $N_T = \sum n_i$ is the total number of pixels. Taking the derivative with respect to ρ_g we finally come to the MLE,

$$\widehat{\rho}_g = \ln \frac{d_g}{N_T - k_0}, \quad g = 1, ..., 255. \tag{12.14}$$

As the reader can see, this solution follows from $e^{\widehat{\rho}_g} = d_g / \sum_{g=1}^{255} d_g$ as a simple estimator of the probability from the total frequency (note that $\sum_{g=1}^{255} e^{\widehat{\rho}_g} = 1$). Consequently, the MLE for the shift is $\widehat{B}_i = n_i / k_{0i} - 1$.

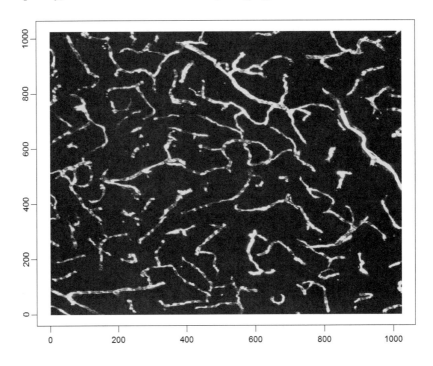

FIGURE 12.8. Typical 1024×1024 gray image of the rat brain. The white bands are vessels filled with oxygenated blood.

12.6.2 Random-shift model

When the number of images (N) is large, a random-shift model may be useful. The similarity to the random intercept model in logistic regression is obvious, see Section 7.2 for a discussion.

Assuming that the random intercepts are iid with normal distribution $b_i \sim \mathcal{N}(0, \sigma^2)$, following the line of Section 7.3, we come to a generalized linear mixed model with a marginal log-likelihood function to maximize

$$l = -\frac{N}{2} \ln \sigma^2 + \sum_{g=1}^{255} d_g \rho_g + \sum_{i=1}^{N} \ln \int_{-\infty}^{\infty} e^{(n_i - k_{i0})b - n_i \ln\left(1 + \sum_{g=1}^{255} e^{b + \rho_g}\right) - \frac{1}{2\sigma^2} b^2} \, db.$$

Several approaches are available. First, one can use numerical integration to evaluate the integral with a given precision. Second, the FSL approach of Section 7.3.2 can be applied. Third, approximation methods such as methods based on Laplace approximation are straightforward to generalize, see the respective sections of Chapter 7.

Hypoxia BOLD MRI data analysis

We illustrate the fixed-shift model with hypoxia BOLD MRI rat brain data, Dunn et al. (2002). The research was concerned with how a shortage of oxygen affects the brain oxygen concentration shortly after hypoxia. First, the MRI images were derived for eight normal rats before treatment (the control group). Next, the rats were shortly put in a hyperbaric chamber with a below-normal oxygen concentration and the MRI images were repeated right after (the hypoxia group). A typical 1024×1024 gray image before treatment is shown in Figure 12.8; the white bands are vessels filled with oxygen. The null hypothesis is that the hypoxia group has the same oxygen concentration as that of the control group. In Figure 12.9 we show all image data for the two groups. Obviously, the animal variation is substantial and overshadows possible differences between groups.

As in image analysis in general, and in this example in particular, quantification is an important step. How should we quantify oxygen in an image: by vessel count, area, length, density? There exists software, such as NIH Image, that facilitates image segmentation and counts the number of vessels (or, more precisely, distinct objects in the image) automatically. However, we should warn the reader that imaging software is far from perfect, and although "automatic" sounds tempting for this example, it is difficult, if not impossible, to count vessels because we are dealing with brain sections. The vessels are cut at an angle, the same vessels are cut twice, and so on. Instead, we prefer to quantify oxygen by the amount of white color, or more precisely, by the density expressed via the gray level distribution. An advantage of this approach versus vessel count is that it reflects the oxygen concentration in the vessel and therefore may be more representative.

For exploratory statistical analysis, we compare the cumulative gray level distribution functions for each rat group in Figure 12.10. As the reader can see, in general, the images from the control group are lighter suggesting that the amount of oxygen in the hypoxia group is higher (note that if X and Y are two random variables such that $X < Y$, then $F_X(t) > F_Y(t)$, where $F(t)$ is the distribution function). To confirm this statistically, we apply the fixed-shift model of Section 12.6.1. This model seems adequate because the distribution functions for each rat are similar up to a shift. Thus, we (a) analyze each group separately, assuming that rat gray distributions are the same up to a shift b_i, $i = 1, ..., 8$, (b) and compare the resulting $\{\widehat{\rho}_g^{control}\}$ and $\{\widehat{\rho}_g^{hypoxia}\}$ using the χ^2-distribution as in Section 12.4.1.

In Figure 12.11 we show the maximum likelihood estimates of ρ_g computed by formula (12.14). Obviously, the control MR images are darker, and therefore right after hypoxia, oxygen flow into the brain exceeds normal. The χ^2-test confirmed this visual finding with a p-value of less than 0.001.

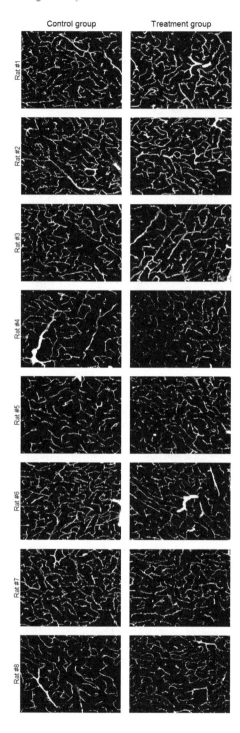

FIGURE 12.9. Rat brain images in two groups of animals (the R function hypoxiaRAT). The variation across animals is substantial and overshadows the difference between groups. A proper statistical model should address animal heterogeneity. The random-shift mixed model seems to be appropriate.

Below we show the R function that reads the data and plots Figure 12.9.

```
hypoxiaRAT=function()
{
dump("hypoxiaRAT", "c:\\MixedModels\\Chapter12\\hypoxiaRAT.r")
n <- 1024
x <- 1:n
# we will save the graph in the file
bmp(file="c:\\MixedModels\\Chapter12\\Hypoxia\\hypoxia.bmp",
                    width=500,height=1500)
par(mfrow=c(8,2),mar=c(1,1,1,1),omi=c(0,0.25,0.25,0))
for(i in 1:8)
for(igr in 1:2)
{
    if(igr==1) cc="c" else cc=""
    fn=paste("c:\\MixedModels\\Chapter12\\Hypoxia\\Group",
                    igr,"\\_",i,cc,"_1a_p.pgm",sep="")
    d <- scan(fn,what="")
    d <- matrix(as.numeric(d[12:length(d)]), n, n)
    image(x, x, d, xlab = "", ylab = "", axes = F,
                    col=gray(0:255/255))
    if(igr==1) mtext(side=2,paste("Rat #",i,sep=""),
                    line=0.25,cex=1.25)
    if(i==1 & igr==1) mtext(side=3,"Control group",
                    line=1,cex=1.5)
    if(i==1 & igr==2) mtext(side=3,"Treatment group",
                    line=1,cex=1.5)
}
dev.off() # saving the graph
}
```

12.6.3   Mixed model for gray images

It is straightforward to generalize the random-shift model to a mixed model with a more complex statistical structure. A statistical model for an ensemble of gray images has a hierarchical structure. In a first-stage model, it is assumed that the gray distribution of each image $i = 1, ..., N$ is specified by the multinomial model (12.11) with random, image-specific probabilities

$$\pi_{i0} = \frac{1}{1 + \sum_{j=1}^{255} e^{\tau_{ij}}}, \ \pi_{ig} = \frac{e^{\tau_{ig}}}{1 + \sum_{j=1}^{255} e^{\tau_{ij}}}, \ g = 1, ..., 255. \quad (12.15)$$

In this model, $\{\tau_{ig}\}$ are random and specified in the linear second-stage model. For example, for the random-shift model of Section 12.6.2, the second-stage model takes the form $\tau_{ig} = \rho_g + b_i$, where b_i is the random effect. More generally, if $\boldsymbol{\tau}_i = (\tau_{i,1}, ..., \tau_{i,255})'$, the second-stage model in vector form can be expressed as

$$\boldsymbol{\tau}_i = \boldsymbol{\rho} + \mathbf{b}_i, \quad i = 1, ..., N, \tag{12.16}$$

where $\boldsymbol{\rho} = (\rho_1, ..., \rho_{255})'$ defines the population-averaged gray distribution. The error term $\mathbf{b}_i$ is the vector of the random effects and has zero mean and a 255×255 covariance matrix $\mathbf{D}_*$, see Section 7.7. For example, for the random-shift model, we have $\mathbf{b}_i = b_i \mathbf{1}$. Obviously, the covariance matrix of the random effects, $\mathbf{D}_*$, should be structured in a parsimonious way because otherwise the number of distinct elements would be too large to estimate, $256 \times (256 + 1)/2 = 32,896$.

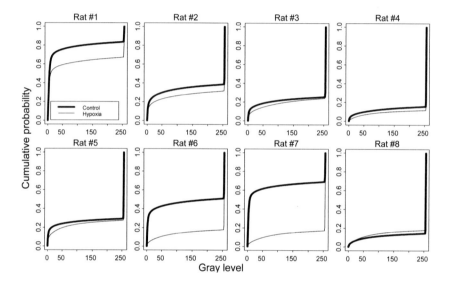

FIGURE 12.10. Cumulative gray-level distributions in two groups for each rat. For most rats the brain images are generally lighter in the control group. We apply the χ^2-distribution to test the overall difference between the groups.

Several covariance structures for $\mathbf{D}_*$ may be suggested:

- Isotropic structure. Matrix $\mathbf{D}_*$ is proportional to the identity matrix, i.e., the off-diagonal elements are zero and all variances are equal.

- Heterogeneous independent structure. The off-diagonal elements are zero, but the diagonal elements are different and unknown. The number of unknown elements in $\mathbf{D}_*$ is 255.

- Toeplitz covariance structure, (11.15). It is assumed that K neighboring gray levels are dependent with $K + 1$ parameters to estimate.

- Band covariance structure such that the covariance between the gth and jth elements of $\mathbf{b}_i$ is zero if $|g - j| > p$. If $p = 0$, we obtain the heterogeneous structure. If $p = 1$, only two neighboring gray levels correlate.

The second-stage model may contain explanatory variables, as did the linear growth curve model of Section 4.1,

$$\boldsymbol{\tau}_i = \mathbf{A}_i\boldsymbol{\rho} + \mathbf{b}_i, \tag{12.17}$$

where $\mathbf{A}_i$ is the design matrix. For example, if two ensembles are compared $\mathbf{A}_i\boldsymbol{\rho} = \boldsymbol{\rho}_1$ if the image is from the first ensemble, and $\mathbf{A}_i\boldsymbol{\rho} = \boldsymbol{\rho}_1 + \boldsymbol{\delta}$ if the image is from the second ensemble. Then, the two ensembles are the same if $H_0 : \boldsymbol{\delta} = \mathbf{0}$. Model (12.17) can incorporate image differences due to gender, age, etc. In functional MRI it may reflect the time when a stimulus occurred.

The statistical model for gray levels specified by (12.15) and (12.17) belongs to the family of generalized linear mixed models studied in Chapter 7. Exact methods of estimation may be computationally intensive, especially when the dimension of the random effect is 255.

12.6.4   Two-stage estimation

It is attractive to apply the two-stage estimation for an ensemble because (a) gray probabilities are random and image-specific, and (b) individual estimates are easy to obtain. The two-stage estimation approach was applied to a nonlinear mixed model in Section 8.5. As follows from (12.4), the individual probability estimate is equal to the histogram value, h_{ig}. Hence, assuming that the image background is black (h_{i0} prevails), we compute logits

$$t_{ig} = \ln h_{ig} - \ln h_{i0}, \quad g = 1, ..., 255 \tag{12.18}$$

as individual estimates of $\{\tau_{ig}\}$ in model (12.15). Having estimates (12.18), we substitute $\boldsymbol{\tau}_i$ with $\mathbf{t}_i = (t_{i,1}, ..., t_{i,255})'$ in model (12.17) and arrive at the second-stage model $\mathbf{t}_i = \mathbf{A}_i\boldsymbol{\rho} + \boldsymbol{\eta}_i$. Notice that the error term $\boldsymbol{\eta}_i$ differs from $\mathbf{b}_i$ because $\mathbf{t}_i$ is an estimate of $\boldsymbol{\tau}_i$, and consequently, the variance of $\boldsymbol{\eta}_i$ is larger than that of $\mathbf{b}_i$. Since the covariance matrix of individual probability estimates has an exact form, (12.5), we can approximate the covariance of $\mathbf{t}_i$ by the delta-method, as is realized below.

Proposition 47 *Let $\widehat{\boldsymbol{\pi}}$ be a 256×1 vector estimate with the variance-covariance matrix specified by (12.5). Let $t_g = \ln\widehat{\pi}_g - \ln\widehat{\pi}_0$, $g = 1, ..., 255$ be components of vector $\mathbf{t}$. Then*

$$\mathrm{cov}(\ln\pi_g - \ln\pi_0, \ln\pi_j - \ln\pi_0) \simeq \frac{1}{PQ} \left\{ \begin{array}{c} 1 + 1/\pi_0 + 1/\pi_g \ \mathit{if} \ g = j \\ 1 + 1/\pi_0 \ \mathit{if} \ g \neq j \end{array} \right.$$

or, in matrix form,

$$\mathrm{cov}(\mathbf{t}) \simeq \frac{1}{PQ} \left[(1 + \pi_0^{-1})\mathbf{1}\mathbf{1}' + \mathbf{D}_1^{-1} \right],$$

where $\mathbf{D}_1 = diag(\pi_1, ..., \pi_{255})$.

Proof. We use the delta-method to approximate the covariance matrix of $\mathbf{t} = (\ln\widehat{\pi}_1 - \ln\widehat{\pi}_0, ..., \ln\widehat{\pi}_{255} - \ln\widehat{\pi}_0)'$. Letting $\boldsymbol{\pi}_1 = (\pi_1, ..., \pi_{255})'$ and $\mathbf{D}_1 = diag(\boldsymbol{\pi}_1)$

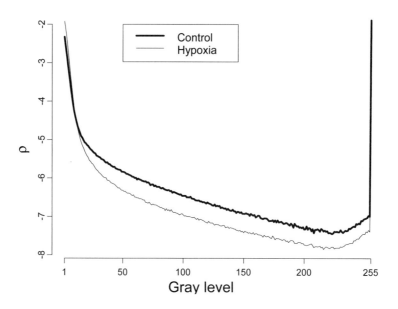

FIGURE 12.11. Maximum likelihood estimates of ρ_g for $g = 1, ..., 255$, for the fixed-shift model, (12.14). Obviously, the MR images of the control group are lighter than those of the hypoxia group. Consequently, the damage to brain vesels by hypoxia is statistically significant.

we express $\partial t/\partial\widehat{\pi} = [-\pi_0^{-1}\mathbf{1}; \mathbf{D}_1^{-1}]$, a 255×256 derivative matrix. The 256×256 covariance matrix of $\widehat{\pi}$ can be partitioned as

$$\mathbf{C} = \begin{bmatrix} \pi_0(1 - \pi_0) & -\pi_0\boldsymbol{\pi}_1' \\ -\pi_0\boldsymbol{\pi}_1 & \mathbf{D}_1 \end{bmatrix}.$$

By the delta-method, the covariance matrix $\mathbf{t}$ can be approximated as

$$(\partial t/\partial\widehat{\pi})\mathbf{C}(\partial t/\partial\widehat{\pi})' = [-\pi_0^{-1}\mathbf{1}; \mathbf{D}_1^{-1}] \begin{bmatrix} \pi_0(1 - \pi_0) & -\pi_0\boldsymbol{\pi}_1' \\ -\pi_0\boldsymbol{\pi}_1 & \mathbf{D}_1 \end{bmatrix} \begin{bmatrix} -\pi_0^{-1}\mathbf{1}' \\ \mathbf{D}_1^{-1} \end{bmatrix}$$

$$= \pi_0^{-2}\pi_0(1 - \pi_0)\mathbf{1}\mathbf{1}' + \pi_0^{-1}\mathbf{1}\pi_0\boldsymbol{\pi}_1'\mathbf{D}_1^{-1} + \mathbf{D}_1^{-1}\pi_0\boldsymbol{\pi}_1\pi_0^{-1}\mathbf{1}' + \mathbf{D}_1^{-1}\mathbf{D}_1\mathbf{D}_1^{-1}$$

$$= \pi_0^{-1}(1 - \pi_0)\mathbf{1}\mathbf{1}' + 2\mathbf{1}\mathbf{1}' + \mathbf{D}_1^{-1} = (1 + \pi_0^{-1})\mathbf{1}\mathbf{1}' + \mathbf{D}_1^{-1}.$$

∎

Applying this result and assuming that the $\{\mathbf{t}_i\}$ have a normal distribution, we arrive at the linear model for logits,

$$\mathbf{t}_i \sim \mathcal{N}(\mathbf{A}_i\boldsymbol{\tau}, \mathbf{D}_* + \mathbf{T}_i), \quad i = 1, ..., N, \tag{12.19}$$

where matrix $\mathbf{T}_i$ is fixed and given by

$$\mathbf{T}_i = \frac{1}{n_i}\left[(1 + h_{i0}^{-1})\mathbf{1}\mathbf{1}' + \mathbf{D}_{i1}^{-1}\right]$$

and $n_i = P_iQ_i$ is the number of pixels and $\mathbf{D}_{i1} = \text{diag}(h_{i1}, ..., h_{i,255})$ is the diagonal matrix of histogram values. In a special case without explanatory variables, (12.16), we have $\mathbf{A}_i = \mathbf{I}$. The unknown parameters are $\boldsymbol{\tau}$ and $\mathbf{D}_*$. If $\mathbf{D}_*$ were known, vector $\boldsymbol{\tau}$ could be estimated by Generalized Least Squares (GLS),

$$\widehat{\boldsymbol{\tau}} = \left(\sum_{i=1}^{N} \mathbf{A}_i'(\mathbf{D}_* + \mathbf{T}_i)^{-1}\mathbf{A}_i \right)^{-1} \left(\sum_{i=1}^{N} \mathbf{A}_i'(\mathbf{D}_* + \mathbf{T}_i)^{-1}\mathbf{t}_i \right)$$

with covariance matrix

$$\mathrm{cov}(\widehat{\boldsymbol{\tau}}) = \left(\sum_{i=1}^{N} \mathbf{A}_i'(\mathbf{D}_* + \mathbf{T}_i)^{-1}\mathbf{A}_i \right)^{-1}.$$

For model (12.16), we have

$$\widehat{\boldsymbol{\tau}} = \left(\sum_{i=1}^{N} (\mathbf{D}_* + \mathbf{T}_i)^{-1} \right)^{-1} \left(\sum_{i=1}^{N} (\mathbf{D}_* + \mathbf{T}_i)^{-1}\mathbf{t}_i \right).$$

Matrix $\mathbf{D}_*$ may be estimated either by maximum likelihood or by the method of moments for the linear growth curve model of Section 4.1. For example, for model (12.16) in the heterogeneous case, compute $s_g^2 = N^{-1}\sum_i (t_{ig} - \bar{t}_g)^2$ and estimate $\mathbf{D}_*$ as $\mathbf{S} - N^{-1}\sum_{i=1}^{N} \mathbf{T}_i$, where $\mathbf{S}$ is the diagonal matrix with the (g, g)th element s_g^2. If matrix $\widehat{\mathbf{D}}_*$ is not positive definite, we apply the projection procedure described in Section 2.15.2.

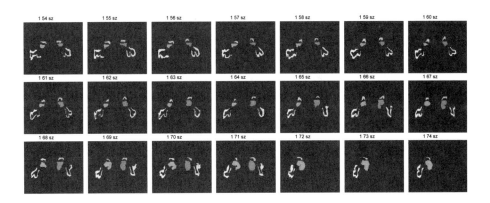

FIGURE 12.12. Typical MR frame images of the amygdala–hippocampal complex of a schizophrenia patient.

12.6.5 Schizophrenia MRI analysis

Schizophrenia is a major mental disorder and is characterized by impaired thinking and hallucinations. It affects about 1% of the general population. Advances in Computerized Tomography (CT) and magnetic resonance imaging (MRI) created a new dimension for brain research, including for schizophrenia (Shenton, 2001). The existing approaches to studying the human brain and its abnormalities using MRI data can be roughly classified into three groups: (1) shape, (2) asymmetry, and (3) volumetric analysis. Here we focus on the latter approach. In the volumetric approach, the organ or region of interest is quantified by one number (Godszal and Pham, 2000). In our approach, we analyze all nonzero gray levels, and therefore the analysis may be more powerful.

In this section we analyze the temporal lobe, or more precisely the amygdala-hippocampal complex, with the MRI data kindly provided by Dr. M. Shenton of Harvard Medical School. The study design description and the appropriate statistical analysis are given in the original article by Shenton et al. (1992). The MRI brain data consist of equidistant frames for 15 schizophrenia patients and 15 matched normal controls. In Figure 12.12 MR frame images of the amygdala–hippocampal complex of the first schizophrenia patient are shown. In Figure 12.13, image frames are shown for the first normal control. All images have the same size, $n_i = P_i Q_i =$const, $i = 1, ..., 30 = N$. We want to determine whether the amygdala-hippocampal complex of the schizophrenia patients and that of controls is different.

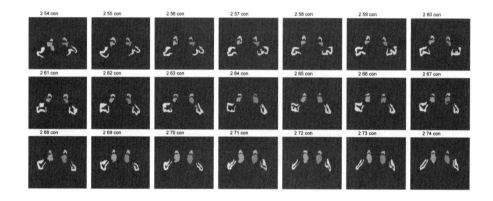

FIGURE 12.13. Typical images of the amygdala-hippocampal complex of a normal control.

The R function below reads 39 cases and plots the MRI frames from 41 to 61 as a 3×7 panel plot (the first 15 cases are controls and the remainder belong to schizophrenia patients).

```
schiz=function ()
{
dump("schiz", "c:\\MixedModels\\Chapter12\\schiz.r")
cc = "c:\\MixedModels\\Chapter12\\schiz\\case"
for (i in 1:30) {
par(mfrow = c(3, 7), mar = c(1, 1, 1, 1),omi=c(0,0,.25,0))
for (j in 1:21) {
d = scan(paste(cc, i, "\\case", i, ".0", j + 50,".pgm",
                sep = ""), what = "", quiet = T)
```

```
dm = matrix(as.numeric(d[12:length(d)]), nrow = 256, ncol = 256)
image(1:256, 1:256, dm, col = gray(0:255/255),xlab="",ylab="",
                  axes=F)
mtext(side=3,paste("Frame",j+50),line=.2,cex=.75)
}
mtext(side=3,paste("Case",i),outer=T,cex=1.25,line=.25)
}
}
```

Each image has only eight different gray levels: 0, 95, 127, 159, 191, 212, 223, and 255 (0 is the black background), so instead of 256 gray levels, we have 8. We start the analysis by computing the logits $t_{ig} = \ln(h_{ig}/h_{i0})$, where h is the histogram value and $i = 1, ..., 30$, $g = 1, ..., 7$. Then we plot the mean logit for each gray level in each group; see Figure 12.14. This plot reveals that for gray levels 95, 127, 159,

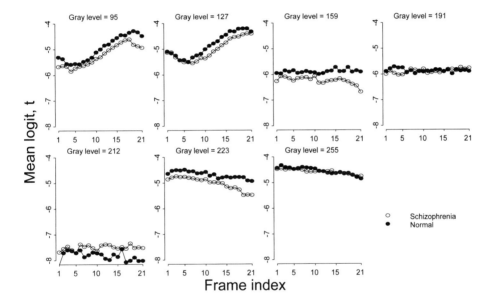

FIGURE 12.14. Mean logit as a function of the frame index for different gray levels in two groups. On average, normals have a higher logit.

and 223 the logits for normals are higher than those for controls. This finding hints of the following linear statistical model for logits

$$t_{ijfg} = \beta_{gf} + \delta(j-1) + b_{ijfg}, \tag{12.20}$$
$$i = 1, 2, ..., 15; \; j = 1, 2; \; f = 1, 2, ..., 21; \; g = 1, 2, 3, 4.$$

where i is the patient index in group j ($j = 1$ codes a schizophrenia patient and $j = 2$ codes a normal control); f is the MRI frame index; and g is the gray level index (gray levels are: 95, 127, 159, and 223). As follows from this model, the logits for each gray level and frame are different, with the mean β_{gf} and the difference between the two groups constant, δ. Assuming that the $\{b_{ijfg}\}$ are iid, we can estimate (12.20) by simple regression analysis, yielding the OLS estimate $\widehat{\delta} = 0.129$ with the t-statistic 9.79 and p-value < 0.00001. The difference in gray levels 95, 127, 159, and 223 for schizophrenia and controls is significant. Model (12.20) can be modified in many ways. For example, one may consider heterogeneous or dependent logits. Also, the logit model may serve as a diagnostic tool to identify schizophrenia using the membership test of Section 3.8.1.

Model (12.20) is easy to apply to compare two samples of images, as a generalization of the standard t-test, where $H_0 : \delta = 0$.

Problems for Section 12.6

1. Develop a for zero-shift test, $H_0 : b_1 = b_2 = ... = b_N = 0$ in the framework of a fixed-shift model.

2*. Develop a maximum likelihood estimation algorithm for maximization l from Section 12.6.2. Write an R function that implements the GH quadrature. Apply Laplace approximation, as discussed in Chapter 7, to approximate the log-likelihood. Write an R function and compare its performance against GH quadrature MLE.

3*. Plot logits and cumulative distribution functions for the rat hypoxia data for the two groups; reproduce Figure 12.10. Compute a two-stage estimate and reproduce the result depicted in Figure 12.11. Use the approximate covariance matrix to test the statistical significance of the treatment effect.

4*. Generalize the two-stage estimation procedure for two groups with different logit parameter δ, the treatment effect. Generalize methods developed in the previous problem to estimate the treatment effect and apply them to the rat hypoxia data. Use the likelihood-ratio test and the Wald test based on the covariance matrix in Proposition 47.

5. The function `bioimage` reads 28 PGM histology image files and plots them as depicted in Figure 12.15. Use the mixed model for grayscale intensities from Section 12.6.3 to compare the treatment effect (the more living cells, the darker the image, see Figure 12.3). Compute the pairwise p-values for image comparison. Is there a synergy between radiation and drug? Use formula (10.17) to estimate the synergy.

6. Modify the function `schiz` to plot 30 cdfs for 15 controls and 15 schizophrenia patients (use the built-in function `cumsum` and use different colors for the two groups). Do the same but for the mean on the logit scale as in Figure 12.14. Apply model (12.20) to discriminate controls from patients. Develop a mixed model with a subject-specific intensity level. Test whether the heterogeneity variance is statistically significant.

12.7   Image alignment and registration

Earlier, we dealt with an image gray level distribution that is content-independent. Starting in this section, we consider content-dependent images. Before doing statistical analysis or image comparison, images must be at the same scale, and consequently, they must be properly aligned and rotated (registered). We use the terms *alignment* and *registration* as synonyms, although sometimes alignment is used when only translation is allowed. For example, if one wants to know the difference between

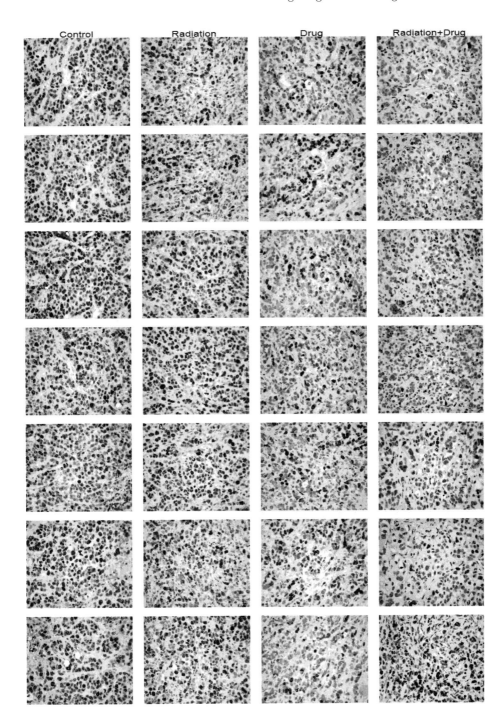

FIGURE 12.15. Twenty eight histology images in four cancer treatment groups ('control' means no treatment). This plot was created by the R function bioimage. Are the differences in the treatments statistically significant?

images (as in the before-and-after analysis), it is tempting to take a pixel-by-pixel difference. The problem is that usually a pixel on one image does not exactly correspond to a pixel on another image. An example of slightly different images is shown in Figure 12.16. Before taking the difference, the images must be aligned (we describe the detail of alignment in Section 12.7.8). Remember that we faced a similar problem with shapes where they must be re-sized and rotated, see Section 11.6.

Image registration is a frequently used technique, especially in medical applications, particularly in the context of brain and medical imaging. See the survey literature by Maintz and Viergever (1998) and a collection of papers in the book by Hajnal et al. (2001). Several commercial software packages for image registration are available, including Automated Image Registration (AIR: http://bishopw.loni.ucla.edu/AIR5) and Statistical Parametric Mapping (SPM: http://www.fil.ion.ucl.ac.uk/spm). The same methodology is also used for image *coregistration*, when images are of the same object or region but derived by different imaging techniques, such as MRI and PET (Kiebel et al., 1997; Ashburner and Friston, 1997).

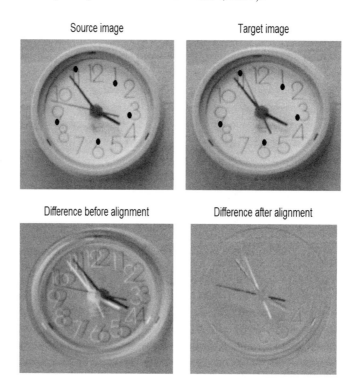

FIGURE 12.16. Two images taken a few seconds apart and their difference before and after alignment. Before computing a pixel-by-pixel difference, the source and target images must be aligned. The first image is 525×504 and the second image is 483×508. Points on the images (black dots) serve as the landmarks for the alignment.

The purpose of this section is to introduce the problem of image registration and discuss several cost functions (registration criteria). To account for coordinate-specific image transformation, random registration is introduced. We show that

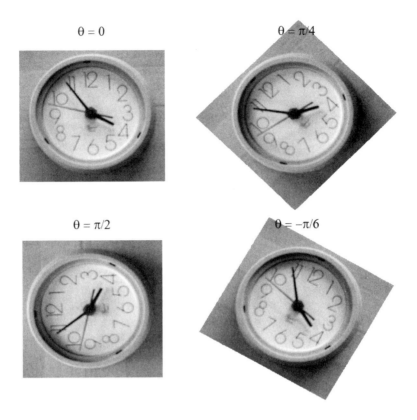

FIGURE 12.17. Rigid transformation of the clock image (rotation by angle θ). This figure was generated by the R function clockROT.

random registration can be studied in the framework of the nonlinear mixed effects model of Chapter 8. To simplify, we consider only planar images.

12.7.1 Affine image registration

Several aspects should be taken into account when two images have to be co-registered: (a) they may have different mean intensity; (b) they may have different scale intensity; (c) the registration may be linear or nonlinear; (d) rotation may be allowed or not allowed; (e) and the transformation may be rigid or general affine (linear). An important step in image registration is the choice of the criterion or cost function (Woods et al., 1998a,b).

Let $\mathbf{M}_i = \{M_i(p,q), p = 1, ..., P_i, q = 1, ..., Q_i\}$ be two images, $i = 1, 2$. Sometimes, $\mathbf{M}_1$ is referred to as the source and $\mathbf{M}_2$ as the target image. We want to find an affine (linear) transformation such that the mean sum of squares,

$$S = \frac{1}{|\mathcal{M}|} \sum_{(p,q) \in \mathcal{M}} [M_1(p,q) - \nu M_2(\beta_1 + \beta_2 p + \beta_3 q, \beta_4 + \beta_5 p + \beta_6 q) - \mu]^2, \quad (12.21)$$

is minimum. Sometimes (12.21) is referred to as the mean-squared error (MSE) criterion or cost function. Eight parameters are to be determined: the intensity shift (μ), the scale intensity (ν), and the vector of affine parameters, $\boldsymbol{\beta} = (\beta_1, ..., \beta_6)'$. Integer indices p and q must satisfy the following restrictions: $1 \le p \le P_1$, $1 \le q \le Q_1$, $1 \le \beta_1 + \beta_2 p + \beta_3 q \le P_2$, $1 \le \beta_4 + \beta_5 p + \beta_6 q \le Q_2$. Apparently, indices for the target image must be rounded to the nearest integer unless the values are interpolated. The set of pairs (p, q) that satisfy these restrictions constitutes the set $\mathcal{M}$, so the summation in (12.21) is over all pairs $(p, q) \in \mathcal{M}$. Since the number of terms in the sum depends on the affine parameters, we normalize it dividing by the number of elements in the set, $|\mathcal{M}|$. Therefore, S is the mean-squared error (MSE) criterion . An implicit assumption of (12.21) is that the variance is constant, otherwise a weighted MSE criterion should be used. Parameters β_2 and β_6 control image zooming or shrinkage; parameters β_3 and β_5 control rotation; parameters β_1 and β_4 control image translation (shift). An advantage of affine transformation is that no restrictions are imposed on $\boldsymbol{\beta}$. If one wants to allow only translation and rigid transformation (rotation and resizing), six parameters are reduced to four by letting $\beta_2 = \beta_6$ and $\beta_3 = -\beta_5$. If the sizes of the source and target images are the same, we come to a nonlinear problem because the coordinates of the target image are $\beta_1 + p\cos\theta + q\sin\theta$ and $\beta_4 - p\sin\theta + q\cos\theta$, where θ is the (clockwise) rotation angle, see Figure 12.17 for an illustration. As with shapes, the choice of transformation should be dictated by the way in which images are sampled. If images have the same or close intensity distribution (histogram), we may assume that $\nu = 1$ and $\mu = 0$, which leads to a simpler MSE.

As is easy to see, criterion S is roughly equivalent to maximization of the correlation coefficient between the two images. Indeed, assuming that the affine parameters are fixed, the minimum of (12.21) in a vector form is attained at the least squares solution for ν and μ, or more precisely,

$$\min_{\nu, \mu} \sum (m_{1i} - \nu m_{2i} - \mu)^2 = (1 - r^2) \sum (m_{1i} - \overline{m}_1)^2$$
$$= \frac{[\sum (m_{1i} - \overline{m}_1)(m_{2i} - \overline{m}_2)]^2}{\sum (m_{2i} - \overline{m}_2)^2}, \tag{12.22}$$

where r^2 is the squared correlation coefficient. This identity implies that instead of S, one can maximize (12.22), with μ and ν eliminated and with m_{1i} substituted for by $M_1(p, q)$ and m_{2i} substituted for by $M_2(\beta_1 + \beta_2 p + \beta_3 q, \beta_4 + \beta_5 p + \beta_6 q)$. However, unlike the MSE, (12.22) is not a quadratic function of parameters even after linearization. To avoid this nonlinearity, one can alternate between the MSE minimization and ν and μ estimation by ordinary least squares. A statistical model-based approach to image registration allows the testing of various hypotheses regarding the type of registration, e.g. whether images are statistically indifferent up to a rigid transformation, see more details in a recent paper by Demidenko (2009).

12.7.2   Weighted sum of squares

From a statistical point of view, registration criterion (12.21) implicitly assumes that the variance of the difference between the two images is the same (gray level independent). Consequently, white will dominate because it has magnitude around

255, and black, 0. We can modify the unweighted criterion, S, by adjusting for the gray level variance, (12.5). Let h_g be the image histogram so that the variance of M is proportional to $h_M(1 - h_M)$. Assuming that the two images are independent, we arrive at the weighted criterion:

$$S_w = \frac{1}{|\mathcal{M}|} \sum_{(p,q) \in \mathcal{M}} \frac{[M_1(p,q) - \nu M_2(\beta_1 + \beta_2 p + \beta_3 q, \beta_4 + \beta_5 p + \beta_6 q) - \mu]^2}{w(p,q)}$$

(12.23)

with the weight $w(p,q) = h_{M_1}(1 - h_{M_1}) + h_{M_2}(1 - h_{M_2})$ as the variance of the difference, $M_1 - M_2$. This weight is parameter independent and can be computed beforehand.

In an alternative approach, we assume that the gray values follow the Poisson distribution, see Section 7.5.1. Since for this distribution the mean equals th evariance, we come to the weight $w(p,q) = M_1(p,q) + M_2(p,q)$.

12.7.3 Nonlinear transformations

Affine transformation may be extended to nonlinear transformation: for example, to account for individual variation. Perhaps the easiest nonlinear transformation is a quadratic transformation of the form $\gamma_1 + \gamma_2 p + \gamma_3 q + \gamma_4 p^2 + \gamma_5 q^2 + \gamma_6 pq$. An advantage of this transformation is that it is still linear in parameters. Polynomials of a higher order can be employed, such as in the package AIR mentioned above.

12.7.4 Random registration

The image registrations discussed so far are rigid because the coordinate system of the target image is expressed as a function of the coordinates of the source image. In real image comparison and registration, the coordinate system may be randomly deformed, as illustrated in Figure 12.18. The aim of this section is to show how random registration can be described in the framework of the nonlinear mixed effects model studied in Chapter 8.

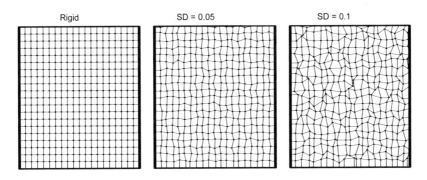

FIGURE 12.18. Regular (rigid) and random registration mapping. The strength of the coordinate system deformation $(p+b_p, q+b_q)$ depends on the standard deviation of random b_p and b_q.

In random registration, we assume that the affine vector $\boldsymbol{\beta}$ is random and location-specific. The statistical model for random registration is written in a hierarchical fashion. To simplify, we shall assume that the identity for the scale intensity, $\nu = 1$, and the intensity shift, $\mu = 0$. In the first-stage model, we express the source through the target image with random coordinates as

$$M_1(p, q) = M_2(\beta_{1pq} + \beta_{2pq}p + \beta_{3pq}q, \beta_{4pq} + \beta_{5pq}p + \beta_{6pq}q) + \varepsilon(p, q), \quad (12.24)$$

where $\boldsymbol{\beta}_{pq} = (\beta_{1pq}, \beta_{2pq}, \beta_{3pq}, \beta_{4pq}, \beta_{5pq}, \beta_{6pq})'$ is a six-dimensional random vector and ε is a random variable with zero mean. It is assumed that the random affine vector $\boldsymbol{\beta}_{pq}$ and the error term $\varepsilon(p, q)$ are independent. In the second-stage model, we specify the affine vector as a random vector with unknown means,

$$\boldsymbol{\beta}_{pq} = \boldsymbol{\beta} + \mathbf{b}_{pq}, \quad p = 1, ..., P, q = 1, ..., Q, \quad (12.25)$$

where $\mathbf{b}_{pq}$ is a vector of random effects with zero mean. Following the line of mixed model terminology, $\boldsymbol{\beta}_{pq}$ is local coordinate-specific and $\boldsymbol{\beta}$ is a global or population-averaged vector of affine parameters. Several assumptions can be made regarding the covariance structure. For example, to address spatial correlation, one may assume that neighboring elements correlate following the planar autoregression or Markov random field scheme

$$b_{h,pq} = \sum_{j=-J}^{J} \sum_{k=-K}^{K} \alpha_{jk} b_{h,p+j,q+k} + \eta_{h,pq}, \quad h = 1, 2, ..., 6. \quad (12.26)$$

This model can be approximated parsimoniously with a Toeplitz covariance matrix as in Section 4.3.4; see more details in Section 12.9.1.

In matrix form, we combine the models (12.24) and (12.25) into one as

$$\mathbf{M}_1 = \mathbf{M}_2(\boldsymbol{\beta} + \mathbf{b}) + \boldsymbol{\varepsilon}. \quad (12.27)$$

This is a nonlinear mixed effects model where $\mathbf{M}_1$ is treated as data and $\mathbf{M}_2$ as a nonlinear function. Although $\mathbf{M}_2$ is a discrete function (matrix), we can assume that the size of this matrix is large enough to treat it as a continuous function of coordinates. To meet this assumption, interpolation methods may be applied. As follows from Sections 8.7 and 8.8.2, assuming normal distribution for the error term and random effects, Laplace approximation leads to minimization of the penalized sum of squares

$$\|\mathbf{M}_1 - \mathbf{M}_2(\boldsymbol{\beta} + \mathbf{b})\|^2 + \mathbf{b}'\mathbf{V}^{-1}\mathbf{b} \Rightarrow \min_{\nu, \mu, \boldsymbol{\beta}, \mathbf{b}}, \quad (12.28)$$

where $\operatorname{cov}(\mathbf{b}) = \sigma^2\mathbf{V}$ and $\operatorname{cov}(\boldsymbol{\varepsilon}) = \sigma^2\mathbf{I}$. Several approximate methods to estimate affine global parameters and covariance matrix $\mathbf{V}$ are suggested in Chapter 8.

12.7.5 Linear image interpolation

So far, we have assumed that the target image is evaluated at the rounded values $\beta_1 + \beta_2 p + \beta_3 q$ and $\beta_4 + \beta_5 p + \beta_6 q$. A more precise evaluation is based on image interpolation. Several methods exist, including B-splines (Gonzalez and Woods, 2002). Here we consider the simplest one—linear interpolation.

Mathematically, the problem is formulated as follows. Let a grayscale image be given by the matrix $\mathbf{M} = \{M(p, q), p = 1, ..., P, q = 1, ..., Q\}$. We want to approximate $M(p + \alpha, q + \beta)$ using the M-values at four neighboring points $\{M(p + s, q + s), s = 0, 1, t = 0, 1\}$, where, without loss of generality, α and β are positive and less than 1. To interpolate, we split the unit square into two triangles and then use the linear interpolation on each of them (sometimes this process is called triangulation). The are two ways to split the square into two triangles—dividing by the diagonal (0,1)–(1,0) or (0,0)–(1,1); to be specific, we take the latter. It is elementary to find that the triangular interpolation formula is given by

$$M(p + \alpha, q + \beta) = M(p, q) \qquad (12.29)$$

$$+ \begin{cases} [M(p+1, q+1) - M(p, q+1)]\alpha + [M(p, q+1) - M(p, q)]\beta \text{ if } \beta > \alpha \\ [M(p+1, q) - M(p, q)]\alpha + [M(p+1, q+1) - M(p+1, q)]\beta \text{ if } \beta \leq \alpha \end{cases}$$

It is elementary to check that this interpolation is continuous and consists of two planes, with the edge at the main diagonal. An example of the triangular interpolation is shown in Figure 12.19 (see the function `imageLI`). Image interpolation is useful when several images of different size are aligned simultaneously, as in Section 12.8.1. To indicate that an image is linearly interpolated, we use a tilde, $\tilde{\ }$.

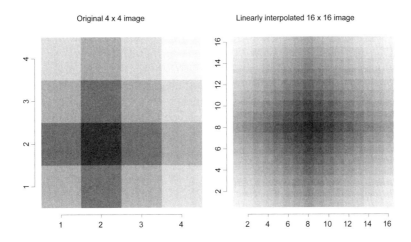

FIGURE 12.19. The original 4×4 image and 16×16 image linearly interpolated by formula (12.29).

12.7.6 Computational aspects

Two issues complicate the minimization of the unweighted or weighted sum of squares of residuals: (a) we deal with discrete minimization (indices are integers), and (b) the function S may have several local minima. If images have different sizes, an interpolation may be applied to reduce the discrete nature (Gonzalez and Woods, 2002). To exclude false minima, several starting points should be used to see whether the minimization converges to the same minimum, see Appendix 13.3 for a general discussion. Below we discuss how to minimize the sum of squares without derivatives.

12.7.7 Derivative-free algorithm for image registration

In the continuous optimization problem $F(\mathbf{x})$, where $\mathbf{x}$ is a vector with continuous elements, the derivative plays the central role. Indeed, many maximization algorithms can be expressed via the update formula $\mathbf{x}_{s+1} = \mathbf{x}_s + \lambda_s \mathbf{H}_s^{-1} \mathbf{g}_s$, where $\mathbf{H}_s$ is a positive definite matrix, $\mathbf{g}_s = \partial F(\mathbf{x} = \mathbf{x}_s)/\partial \mathbf{x}$ is the derivative, λ_s is the step length (typically, $\lambda_s = 1$), and $s = 0, 1, \dots$. Sometimes, computation of the derivative is very complex or even not feasible. Furthermore, in some instances, the derivative does not exist. For those who code in FORTRAN, there is a programming technique that generates a subroutine for derivative computation, *ADIFOR* (Bischof et al., 1992).

Now we discuss a derivative-free optimization technique, or more specifically, a derivative-free approach to the sum of squares minimization in nonlinear regression suggested originally by Ortega and Rheinboldt (1970). Later, Ralston and Jennrich (1978) reinvented the algorithm and called it *DUD*. This algorithm may be useful when the argument is not continuous but takes integer values as in the image registration criteria discussed above. An important by-product result is that this algorithm generates the covariance matrix for the registration parameters so that various statistical hypotheses may be tested; for example, if the transformation is rigid. Parameters ν and μ may be eliminated, but then the criterion function becomes nonsquare, (12.22). Otherwise, one can alternate between S and S_w minimization, when ν and μ are held, finding ν and μ from linear least squares after the transformation parameters are determined.

The derivative-free algorithm DUD is described as follows. We want to minimize the sum of squares (SS) of residuals,

$$S(\boldsymbol{\beta}) = \sum_{i=1}^{n} (y_i - f_i(\boldsymbol{\beta}))^2, \tag{12.30}$$

where $\boldsymbol{\beta}$ is the m-dimensional parameter vector and $f_i = f_i(\boldsymbol{\beta})$ is the regression function; some computational detail was discussed in Section 6.1. For example, for image registration (12.21), y is the gray level, M_1, and f is the gray level, M_2.

The Gauss–Newton algorithm usually works well and has the form

$$\boldsymbol{\beta}_{s+1} = \boldsymbol{\beta}_s + (\mathbf{G}_s' \mathbf{G}_s)^{-1} \mathbf{G}_s' (\mathbf{y} - \mathbf{f}_s), \tag{12.31}$$

where $\mathbf{G}_s = \partial \mathbf{f}/\partial \boldsymbol{\beta}$ is an $n \times m$ matrix evaluated at $\boldsymbol{\beta} = \boldsymbol{\beta}_s$ and $\mathbf{f} = (f_1, ..., f_n)'$, $\mathbf{y} = (y_1, ..., y_n)'$. Can we avoid derivative computation, or, more specifically, can we approximate matrix $\mathbf{G}$ by computing values of function f? Indeed, a finite-difference approach does just that using the approximation $\partial f_i/\partial \boldsymbol{\beta} \approx (f_i(\boldsymbol{\beta} + \Delta\beta \mathbf{1}) - f_i(\boldsymbol{\beta}))/\Delta\beta$, where $\mathbf{1}$ is the $m \times 1$ vector of 1's and $\Delta\beta$ is a scalar. When the components of $\boldsymbol{\beta}$ are integers, the finite-difference approach is, perhaps, the only way to assess the derivative, or, more precisely, the relative change (because the derivative is not defined). The DUD algorithm suggests an economical way to approximate the derivatives based on previous computations of $\mathbf{f}$. Indeed, let the values of the regression vector function be known at $P + 1$ points, $\boldsymbol{\beta}_0, \boldsymbol{\beta}_1, ..., \boldsymbol{\beta}_P$, and we want to approximate matrix $\mathbf{G}$ at $\boldsymbol{\beta}_0$. It is assumed that $P \geq m$ and the $P + 1$ vectors in the m-dimensional space are in *general position*, meaning that vectors $\{\boldsymbol{\beta}_p - \boldsymbol{\beta}_0, p = 1, ..., P\}$ have rank m. From the definition of the derivative, we have

$$\mathbf{f}_p - \mathbf{f}_0 \simeq \mathbf{G}(\boldsymbol{\beta}_p - \boldsymbol{\beta}_0), \qquad (12.32)$$

where $\mathbf{f}_p = \mathbf{f}(\boldsymbol{\beta}_p)$, for $p = 1, ..., P$. The linear system (12.32) for $\mathbf{G}$ has nm unknowns and nP equations. If $P = m$, this system may be solved exactly for $\mathbf{G}$. Otherwise, it is overspecified, so, generally, we find $\mathbf{G}$ using the weighted sum of squares criterion,

$$\operatorname{tr}(\mathbf{G}\mathbf{A} - \mathbf{F})'(\mathbf{G}\mathbf{A} - \mathbf{F})\boldsymbol{\Omega}^{-1} \Rightarrow \min_{\mathbf{G}}, \qquad (12.33)$$

where $\mathbf{A}$ is an $m \times P$ matrix with the pth column $\boldsymbol{\beta}_p - \boldsymbol{\beta}_0$, and $\mathbf{F}$ is an $n \times P$ matrix with the pth column $\mathbf{f}_p - \mathbf{f}_0$. The $P \times P$ weight matrix $\boldsymbol{\Omega}^{-1}$ is positive definite. For example, $\boldsymbol{\Omega}$ may be a diagonal matrix with the pth diagonal element equal to $\|\mathbf{f}_p - \mathbf{f}_0\|^2$. Then points closer to $\mathbf{f}_0$ will have more influence on the derivative approximation. Solving this quadratic optimization problem, we find the LS estimate for the derivative of the regression function based on $P + 1$ function values:

$$\mathbf{G} = \mathbf{F}\boldsymbol{\Omega}^{-1}\mathbf{A}'(\mathbf{A}\boldsymbol{\Omega}^{-1}\mathbf{A}')^{-1}. \qquad (12.34)$$

Matrix $\mathbf{A}$ has full rank, and therefore matrix $\mathbf{A}\mathbf{A}'$ is nonsingular. In fact, formula (12.34) is quite general and may be applied for derivative approximation of any nonlinear function, not necessarily in the nonlinear regression framework. In a special case, when $P = m$, matrix $\mathbf{A}$ is square and then $\mathbf{G} = \mathbf{F}\mathbf{A}^{-1}$. This formula has a clear finite-difference flavor, just expressed in a matrix form. Thus, for $P = m$, weighting is irrelevant.

Now, coming back to the SS minimization, substituting (12.34) into the Gauss–Newton update formula (12.31), we finally obtain the DUD algorithm,

$$\boldsymbol{\beta}_{s+1} = \boldsymbol{\beta}_s + (\mathbf{A}_s\boldsymbol{\Omega}^{-1}\mathbf{A}_s')(\mathbf{A}_s\boldsymbol{\Omega}^{-1}\mathbf{F}_s'\mathbf{F}_s\boldsymbol{\Omega}^{-1}\mathbf{A}_s')^{-1}\mathbf{A}_s\boldsymbol{\Omega}^{-1}\mathbf{F}_s'(\mathbf{y} - \mathbf{f}_{s0}).$$

Several variations of the DUD algorithm exist. First, one can incorporate the step length to provide that the value of the SS drop from iteration to iteration. Second, one may use all previous iteration points or just P, closest to the current beta vector. Third, for a special case, when $P = m$ and $\boldsymbol{\Omega} = \mathbf{I}$, matrix $\mathbf{A}$ becomes an $m \times m$ nonsingular matrix and the derivative matrix (12.34) is approximated as $\mathbf{G} \simeq \mathbf{F}\mathbf{A}^{-1}$. Then formula (12.34) simplifies to

$$\boldsymbol{\beta}_{s+1} = \boldsymbol{\beta}_s + \mathbf{A}_s(\mathbf{F}_s'\mathbf{F}_s)^{-1}\mathbf{F}_s'(\mathbf{y} - \mathbf{f}_{s0}).$$

Clearly, $\mathbf{G}$, approximated by (12.34), may be treated as its continuous counterpart, and therefore, $s^2(\mathbf{G}'\mathbf{G})^{-1}$ serves as a covariance matrix estimate for $\boldsymbol{\beta}$, where s^2 is the minimum SS divided by the degrees of freedom, $n - m$.

12.7.8   Example: clock alignment

In image registration, the choice of the starting point for the affine parameters, $\boldsymbol{\beta}_0$, is very important. It is a good idea to determine this vector from the respective landmarks on both images. We illustrate this technique on clock registration; see Figure 12.16. Aligning two 2D figures requires at least three landmarks, assuming that all six parameters are unknown. If only a rigid transformation is allowed ($\beta_2 = \beta_6$ and $\beta_3 = -\beta_5$), two landmarks would be enough. Generally, more landmarks are better. If there are K landmarks on the first and second images, $\{(x_k, y_k), k = 1, ..., K\}$ and $\{(v_k, u_k), k = 1, ..., K\}$, we approximate $2K$ equations,

$$x_k \simeq \beta_1 + \beta_2 v_k + \beta_3 u_k, \quad y_k \simeq \beta_4 + \beta_5 v_k + \beta_6 u_k,$$

by least squares (if $K = 3$, this system can be solved exactly). When the target and source images are not aligned, the SE $= 32.7$, and after landmark alignment, SE $= 10.7$.

The R function that plots four clock images in Figure 12.16 and uses landmarks for image alignment is shown below. The function matR provides image reflection about the y-axis for correct display. Landmark point coordinates for the original and target images are in arrays cL1 and cL2, respectively. The affine transformation parameters are found from the linear least squares that minimizes the Euclidean norm between the landmarks on the original and target images. The indices should be rounded to avoid image display issues.

```
clockFIG=function()
{
dump("clockFIG", "c:\\MixedModels\\Chapter12\\clockFIG.r")
matR=function(M) #matrix reflection about y-axis
{
nr=nrow(M);nc=ncol(M)
MR=M
for(i in 1:nc) MR[,nc-i+1]=M[,i]
return(MR)
}
c1 <- scan("c:\\MixedModels\\Chapter12\\clock1.pgm",what="")
nr1 <- as.numeric(c1[2]); nc1 <- as.numeric(c1[3])
M1 <- matrix(as.numeric(c1[5:length(c1)]), nrow = nr1, ncol = nc1)
c2 <- scan("c:\\MixedModels\\Chapter12\\clock2.pgm",what="")
nr2 <- as.numeric(c2[2]); nc2 <- as.numeric(c2[3])
M2 <- matrix(as.numeric(c2[5:length(c2)]),nrow=nr2,ncol=nc2)
cL1 <- matrix(c(327, 148, 376, 256, 269, 344, 128,
          280, 191, 101, 252, 111), nrow = 2)
cL2 <- matrix(c(302, 154, 349, 258, 245, 343, 108,
          283, 169, 108, 228, 116), nrow = 2)
cL1 <- cL1[, 1:5]; cL2 <- cL2[, 1:5]
nLc1 <- ncol(cL1)
```

```
 for(i in 1:nLc1) {
i1 <- 1 + 2 * (i - 1)
i2 <- 2 * i
X[i1, 1] <- 1
X[i1, 2:3] <- cL1[1:2, i]
X[i2, 4] <- 1
X[i2, 5:6] <- cL1[1:2, i]
}
xx <- t(X) %*% X
xy <- t(X) %*% as.vector(cL2)
beta <- b <- solve(xx) %*% xy
par(mfrow = c(2, 2), mar = c(1, 1, 3, 1))
image(1:nr1, 1:nc1, matR(M1), xlab = "", ylab = "", axes = F,
                col=gray(0:255/255))
mtext(side = 3, "Source image", line = 0.25, cex = 1.25)
for(i in 1:nLc1)
points(cL1[1+2*(i-1)], nc1-cL1[2*i]+1, pch = 16, cex = 1.25)
image(1:nr2, 1:nc2, matR(M2), xlab = "", ylab = "", axes = F,
                col=gray(0:255/255))
mtext(side = 3, "Target image", line = 0.25, cex = 1.25)
for(i in 1:nLc1)
points(cL2[1+2*(i-1)], nc1-cL2[2*i]+1, pch = 16, cex = 1.25)
del <- matrix(nrow = nr1, ncol = nc1)
r1 <- min(nr1, nr2)
r2 <- min(nc1, nc2)
image(1:r1, 1:nc1, matR(M1[1:r1,1:r2]-M2[1:r1,1:r2]),xlab ="",
                ylab = "", axes = F,col=gray(0:255/255))
mtext(side = 3, "Difference before alignment",line=0.25,cex=1.25)
for(i in 1:nr1)
for(j in 1:nc1) {
p1 <- round(b[1] + b[2] * i + b[3] * j)
q1 <- round(b[4] + b[5] * i + b[6] * j)
if(q1 > 0 & q1 <= nc2 & p1 > 0 & p1 <= nr2)
del[i, j] <- M1[i, j] - M2[p1, q1]
}
image(1:nr1, 1:nc1, matR(del), xlab = "", ylab = "", axes = F,
                col=gray(0:255/255))
mtext(side=3, "Difference after alignment",line=0.25,cex=1.25)
}
```

Problems for Section 12.7

1. Pick the center of the clock as an additional landmark and redo the image alignment (use the `clock` program). Does it improve the image alignment?

2. Apply linear interpolation to the image used in the function `histgr` from Section 12.5 (modify the function `imageLI` for this purpose). Do linear interpolation and histogram equalization commute? (Is the order of operation important?)

3. See the effect of a slight quadratic alignment transformation by modifying the function `clockROT`.

4*. Write an R function which implements the DUD algorithm. Test your function against `nls`.

5. Prove that matrix (12.34) is the solution of minimization problem (12.33).

12.8   Ensemble of structured images

Now we develop a statistical model for an ensemble of structured images following the line of the shape model developed in the previous chapter. Thus, the issue of image registration becomes central. It is assumed that the ensemble consists of N independent images $\{\mathbf{M}_i, i = 1, ..., N\}$ of the same object(s), subject(s), scene, etc. It is allowed to have partial images (showing only part of the scene), but the majority of images should have commonality. Images may have different size, magnification, and viewpoint, so that they are registered up to an affine transformation. Our goal is to reconstruct the true object(s), subject(s), scene, or the *true* image.

Two kinds of assumptions on image-specific transformations may be taken, fixed and random. The first assumption leads to a generalization of the Procrustes model described in Section 11.6, and the second assumption leads to a nonlinear mixed effects model as a generalization of the shape model of Section 11.6.3. To start, we assume that images have the same mean and scale intensity; at the end we relax this assumption.

12.8.1   Fixed affine transformations

Assuming that the images, up to an unknown fixed transformation, differ from the true image by a random error with constant variance, we come to the statistical model,

$$\widetilde{M}_i(\beta_{i1} + \beta_{i2}p + \beta_{i3}q, \beta_{i4} + \beta_{i5}p + \beta_{i6}q) = M(p, q) + \varepsilon(p, q). \tag{12.35}$$

Since images may have different sizes we use the interpolated images indicated by a tilde; see Section 12.7.5. Also, in (12.35), we let

$$p = 1, ..., \overline{P} = \max\{P_i\}, \qquad q = 1, ..., \overline{Q} = \max\{Q_i\}. \tag{12.36}$$

In this model, we treat $\boldsymbol{\beta}_i = (\beta_{i1}, ..., \beta_{i6})'$ as an unknown affine image-specific parameter vector subject to estimation.

The task is to recover the true image M. If errors $\{\varepsilon\}$ are normally distributed, the minimization of the mean-squared error (MSE) is equivalent to maximum likelihood,

$$\frac{1}{|\mathcal{M}|} \sum_{i=1}^{N} \sum_{(p,q)\in\mathcal{M}} \left[\widetilde{M}_i(\beta_{i1} + \beta_{i2}p + \beta_{i3}q, \beta_{i4} + \beta_{i5}p + \beta_{i6}q) - M(p,q) \right]^2, \quad (12.37)$$

where $\mathcal{M}$ is the index set such that the sum of squares is well defined:

$$\mathcal{M} = \{(p,q) : 1 \leq \beta_{i1} + \beta_{i2}p + \beta_{i3}q \leq P_i, 1 \leq \beta_{i4} + \beta_{i5}p + \beta_{i6}q \leq Q_i\}$$

for all $i = 1, ..., N$, where (p,q) are from (12.36) and $|\mathcal{M}|$ denotes the number of elements in the set. Apparently, the images must have a common intersection because otherwise the set $\mathcal{M}$ is null. Obviously, if the affine parameters are fixed, the mean image is simply equal to the ensemble average,

$$\overline{M}(p,q) = \frac{1}{N} \sum_{i=1}^{N} \widetilde{M}_i(\beta_{i1} + \beta_{i2}p + \beta_{i3}q, \beta_{i4} + \beta_{i5}p + \beta_{i6}q). \quad (12.38)$$

There are two ways to minimize (12.37): (1) alternate between N separate MSE minimizations over $\boldsymbol{\beta}_i$ and then substitute M with the mean (12.38), or (2) minimize (12.37) over $6N$ parameters simultaneously with $\overline{M}$ in place of M.

12.8.2 Random affine transformations

If, due to sampling design, images are taken at random angles and have a random size, a model with random affine parameters may be adequate,

$$\boldsymbol{\beta}_i = \boldsymbol{\beta} + \mathbf{b}_i, \quad \mathbf{b}_i \sim \mathcal{N}\left(\boldsymbol{\beta}, \sigma^2 \mathbf{D}\right), \quad i = 1, ...N, \quad (12.39)$$

where $\boldsymbol{\beta}$ is a known vector, say $\boldsymbol{\beta} = (0, 1, 0, 0, 0, 1)'$. Matrix $\mathbf{D}$ is the scaled covariance matrix of the random effects $\mathbf{b}_i$ and determines how "free" $\boldsymbol{\beta}_i$ are. The complete model is written in hierarchical fashion: the first-stage model is the same, (12.35), and the second-stage model is (12.39). Combining these into one model and using matrix notation, we obtain a nonlinear mixed effects (NLME) model,

$$\widetilde{\mathbf{M}}_i(\boldsymbol{\beta} + \mathbf{b}_i) = \mathbf{M} + \boldsymbol{\varepsilon}_i. \quad (12.40)$$

Following the line of argumentation for the random effects shape model of Section 11.6.3, model (12.40) requires a large number of images with a relatively small matrix $\mathbf{D}$. For example, if images are rotated up to 2π, the model with fixed transformations may be more adequate.

Several methods of NLME models are discussed in Chapter 8. Laplace approximation minimizes the penalized MSE,

$$\frac{1}{|\mathcal{M}|} \sum_{i=1}^{N} \left\{ \sum_{(p,q)\in\mathcal{M}} \left[\widetilde{M}_i(b_{i1} + b_{i2}p + b_{i3}q, b_{i4} + b_{i5}p + b_{i6}q) - \overline{M}(p,q) \right]^2 \right.$$
$$\left. + (\mathbf{b}_i - \boldsymbol{\beta})' \mathbf{D}^{-1} (\mathbf{b}_i - \boldsymbol{\beta})' \right\}. \quad (12.41)$$

If $\mathbf{D} \to \mathbf{0}$, the second term dominates in (12.41), resulting in $\mathbf{b}_i = \boldsymbol{\beta}$: All images are the same up to a random error ε. If $\mathbf{D}$ becomes large, the second term vanishes and we arrive at a model with fixed affine parameters, (12.37) and (12.38).

If images have different scale intensity, independent of transformation, we can assume that $\nu_i \sim \mathcal{N}(1, \sigma_\nu^2)$ and incorporate it into (12.40). The mean intensity parameter is unneeded because M is unknown.

Problems for Section 12.8

1. Does the fixed affine image transformation reduce to image alignment from the previous section when $N = 1$?

2*. Develop statistical models for fixed and random rigid transformation of images of different size.

3*. Develop a maximum likelihood estimation of the average true image with images observed up to a random rigid transformation.

12.9   Modeling spatial correlation

So far we have assumed that components of the error term ε in the image models, such as (12.27) or (12.39), are independent. Clearly, this is a very simplifying assumption because in real images neighboring pixels usually correlate. Much research has been done in the area of statistics to address spatial correlation (Ripley, 1981; Cressie, 1991). Two dominant statistical models for spatial correlation are simultaneous and conditional spatial autocorrelation (SAR and CAR). In imaging, the stochastic distribution on the plane is called a random field, and the most popular stochastic model is called a *Markov Random Field (MRF)*. The latter is a variation of spatial autoregression and, similarly to (12.26), can be defined as

$$\varepsilon(p, q) = \sum_{j=-J}^{J} \sum_{k=-K}^{K} \alpha_{jk} \varepsilon(p + j, q + k) + \eta(p, q), \qquad (12.42)$$

where $\{\eta(p, q)\}$ are iid uncorrelated random variables with zero mean, and $\{\alpha_{jk}, j = -J, -J + 1, ..., J, \ k = -K, -K + 1, ..., K\}$ are $(2J + 1)(2K + 1)$ fixed parameters. We refer the reader to a collection of papers edited by Chellappa and Jain (1993) with various applications of the MRF theory to image models.

An important observation is that one can express ε through η from (12.42) via a linear operator. Consequently, if $\{\eta(p, q)\}$ has normal distribution, components of matrix $\boldsymbol{\varepsilon}$ also have joint multivariate normal distributions with the covariance matrix defined by $\{\alpha_{jk}\}$. Hence, instead of modeling (12.42), one can model the covariance matrix of $\boldsymbol{\varepsilon}$. This approach may be more computationally attractive for the estimation of spatial correlation parameters, such as α in (12.42). The desirable correlation structure is simple enough to derive an estimation procedure and complex enough to describe a variety of possible spatial correlations.

A convenient way to generate a normally distributed random (field) matrix with correlated entries is to pre- and postmultiply a matrix with iid elements by fixed matrices. Indeed, let $\boldsymbol{\eta} = \{\eta(p, q), p = 1, ..., P, q = 1, ..., Q\}$ be a $P \times Q$ matrix with iid normally distributed elements with zero mean and variance σ^2. Let $\mathbf{V}_L$ and

$\mathbf{V}_R$ be $P \times P$ and $Q \times Q$ fixed matrices dependent on some parameter vector, $\boldsymbol{\theta}$. Define

$$\boldsymbol{\varepsilon} = \mathbf{V}_L \boldsymbol{\eta} \mathbf{V}_R, \tag{12.43}$$

a $P \times Q$ random matrix. The elements of this matrix have zero mean and correlate. Matrices $\mathbf{V}_L$ and $\mathbf{V}_R$ should fulfill the following requirements: (1) matrices $\mathbf{V}'_R \mathbf{V}_R$ and $\mathbf{V}_L \mathbf{V}'_L$ are invertible, (2) at $\boldsymbol{\theta} = \mathbf{0}$ these matrices turn into identity matrices. The first assumption excludes matrix deficiency and will be justified later. The second assumption means that $\{\boldsymbol{\varepsilon}\}$ become iid as a special case of (12.43). Now we derive the distribution and the covariance matrix implied by (12.43) expressed in terms of the $(PQ) \times 1$ vector, $\mathrm{vec}(\boldsymbol{\varepsilon})$. Using the properties of the Kronecker product, we obtain

$$\mathrm{vec}(\boldsymbol{\varepsilon}) = \mathrm{vec}(\mathbf{V}_L \boldsymbol{\eta} \mathbf{V}_R) = (\mathbf{V}'_R \otimes \mathbf{V}_L)\mathrm{vec}(\boldsymbol{\eta}).$$

But $\mathrm{vec}(\boldsymbol{\eta}) \sim \mathcal{N}\left(\mathbf{0}, \sigma^2 \mathbf{I}_{PQ}\right)$, so we find that

$$\mathrm{vec}(\boldsymbol{\varepsilon}) \sim \mathcal{N}\left(\mathbf{0}, \sigma^2 (\mathbf{V}'_R \mathbf{V}_R \otimes \mathbf{V}_L \mathbf{V}'_L)\right). \tag{12.44}$$

Now it is clear why the first requirement guarantees that matrix $\boldsymbol{\varepsilon}$ has a nondegenerate distribution.

Having found the observation matrix $\boldsymbol{\varepsilon}$ as the difference between the image data and estimated mean, we estimate the parameters of matrices $\mathbf{V}_L$ and $\mathbf{V}_R$ by maximum likelihood. Since the distribution is normal, the log-likelihood, up to a constant, takes the form

$$\begin{aligned} l &= -0.5 \left\{ (PQ)\ln\sigma^2 + \ln|\mathbf{V}'_R \mathbf{V}_R \otimes \mathbf{V}_L \mathbf{V}'_L| \right. \\ &\quad \left. + \sigma^{-2}\mathrm{vec}'(\boldsymbol{\varepsilon})(\mathbf{V}'_R \mathbf{V}_R \otimes \mathbf{V}_L \mathbf{V}'_L)^{-1}\mathrm{vec}(\boldsymbol{\varepsilon}) \right\}. \end{aligned}$$

Using properties of the Kronecker product, we simplify

$$\begin{aligned} \ln|\mathbf{V}'_R \mathbf{V}_R \otimes \mathbf{V}_L \mathbf{V}'_L| &= \ln|\mathbf{V}'_R \mathbf{V}_R| + \ln|\mathbf{V}_L \mathbf{V}'_L|, \\ (\mathbf{V}'_R \mathbf{V}_R \otimes \mathbf{V}_L \mathbf{V}'_L)^{-1} &= (\mathbf{V}'_R \mathbf{V}_R)^{-1} \otimes (\mathbf{V}_L \mathbf{V}'_L)^{-1} \end{aligned}$$

and

$$\begin{aligned} &\mathrm{vec}'(\boldsymbol{\varepsilon})(\mathbf{V}'_R \mathbf{V}_R \otimes \mathbf{V}_L \mathbf{V}'_L)^{-1}\mathrm{vec}(\boldsymbol{\varepsilon}) \\ &= \mathrm{vec}'(\boldsymbol{\varepsilon})[(\mathbf{V}'_R \mathbf{V}_R)^{-1} \otimes (\mathbf{V}_L \mathbf{V}'_L)^{-1}]\mathrm{vec}(\boldsymbol{\varepsilon}) \\ &= \mathrm{tr}((\mathbf{V}'_R \mathbf{V}_R)^{-1}\boldsymbol{\varepsilon}'(\mathbf{V}_L \mathbf{V}'_L)^{-1}\boldsymbol{\varepsilon}). \end{aligned}$$

Thus, function l can be written as

$$l = -0.5\left\{n\ln\sigma^2 + \ln|\mathbf{Q}_R| + \ln|\mathbf{Q}_L| + \sigma^{-2}\mathrm{tr}(\mathbf{Q}_R^{-1}\boldsymbol{\varepsilon}'\mathbf{Q}_L^{-1}\boldsymbol{\varepsilon})\right\}, \tag{12.45}$$

where $n = PQ$ is the number of image pixels, and

$$\mathbf{Q}_R = \mathbf{V}'_R \mathbf{V}_R, \quad \mathbf{Q}_L = \mathbf{V}_L \mathbf{V}'_L.$$

One can easily express σ^2 through $\mathbf{Q}_R$ and $\mathbf{Q}_L$ as

$$\sigma^2 = n^{-1}\mathrm{tr}(\mathbf{Q}_R^{-1}\boldsymbol{\varepsilon}'\mathbf{Q}_L^{-1}\boldsymbol{\varepsilon}). \tag{12.46}$$

As is seen from (12.45), the likelihood is easy to express in terms of the $P \times P$ and $Q \times Q$ matrices $\mathbf{Q}_L$ and $\mathbf{Q}_R$, so we can model those, not the original $\mathbf{V}_L$ and $\mathbf{V}_R$. One can interpret $\mathbf{Q}_L$ and $\mathbf{Q}_R$ as standard deviations and $\mathbf{V}_L$ and $\mathbf{V}_R$ as variances. The log-likelihood function (12.45) is in general form and it requires further specification for matrices $\mathbf{Q}_L$ and $\mathbf{Q}_R$ to estimate parameters of the covariance spatial matrix. Several covariance models can be suggested for $\mathbf{Q}_L$ and $\mathbf{Q}_R$. Below we develop an idea based on the Toeplitz structure used before to model time series in Section 4.3.4 and shape analysis in Section 11.6.3.

12.9.1 Toeplitz correlation structure

A parsimonious way to model matrices $\mathbf{Q}_L$ and $\mathbf{Q}_R$ is to assume that they have a Toeplitz structure, meaning that the elements on the diagonal parallel to the main diagonal are the same. In terms of the elementary Toeplitz matrix, $\mathbf{Q}$ can be expressed as a linear combination with the coefficients subject to estimation:

$$\mathbf{Q} = \mathbf{I} + \sum_{k=1}^{K} \theta_k \mathbf{T}_{k'}. \tag{12.47}$$

To model various correlation lags, we use the index function $k' = k'(k)$. For instance, if the first and the third lags are used, we have $\mathbf{Q} = \mathbf{I} + \theta_1 \mathbf{T}_1 + \theta_2 \mathbf{T}_3$, so that $k'(1) = 1$ and $k'(2) = 3$. In (12.47), $\mathbf{T}_{k'}$ is the k'th elementary $P \times P$ Toeplitz matrix, $\{\theta_k\}$ are unknown parameters, and K is the correlation depth. Examples of the elementary Toeplitz matrix are (4.115). Several isotropic random fields ($\mathbf{Q} = \mathbf{Q}_L = \mathbf{Q}_R$) with Toeplitz spatial correlation (12.47) for different depth, K, and $\theta_k = 0.9^k$, $k' = k$, are shown in Figure 12.20.

Vertically dependent random fields

To illustrate, we consider the vertically dependent random fields, that is when the columns of matrix $\boldsymbol{\varepsilon}$ are independent ($\boldsymbol{\varepsilon} = \mathbf{V}_L \boldsymbol{\eta}$ and $\mathbf{V}_R = \mathbf{I}$), but the rows correlate according to a Toeplitz structure (12.47). If $\boldsymbol{\varepsilon}_i$ denotes the ith column of matrix $\boldsymbol{\varepsilon}$, we have iid $\boldsymbol{\varepsilon}_i \sim \mathcal{N}(\mathbf{0}, \sigma^2 \mathbf{Q})$, where $\mathbf{Q}$ is defined by (12.47), $i = 1, ..., Q$. Two methods of estimation for $\{\theta_k, k = 1, ..., K\}$ are suggested below.

Variance least squares

According to this method, we estimate the variance parameters σ^2 and $\boldsymbol{\theta}$ by minimizing the sum of squares of the difference between the empirical and theoretical covariance matrices, Section 3.12. Since the empirical covariance matrix is $\boldsymbol{\varepsilon}_i \boldsymbol{\varepsilon}_i'$ and the theoretical matrix is $\sigma^2(\mathbf{I} + \sum \theta_k \mathbf{T}_{k'})$, the variance least squares (VLS) estimate minimizes the function

$$S(\sigma^2, \tau_1, ..., \tau_K) = \sum_{i=1}^{Q} \mathrm{tr} \left(\boldsymbol{\varepsilon}_i \boldsymbol{\varepsilon}_i' - \sigma^2 \mathbf{I}_P - \sum_{k=1}^{K} \tau_k \mathbf{T}_{k'} \right)^2,$$

where $\tau_k = \sigma^2 \theta_k$. Differentiating S with respect to σ^2 and noticing that $\mathrm{tr}(\mathbf{T}_{k'}) = 0$, we obtain $\sigma^2 = \mathrm{tr}(\boldsymbol{\varepsilon}\boldsymbol{\varepsilon}')/n$. Differentiating with respect to τ_k, we obtain K linear equations which can be solved for $\tau_1, ..., \tau_K$ as in Section 4.3.

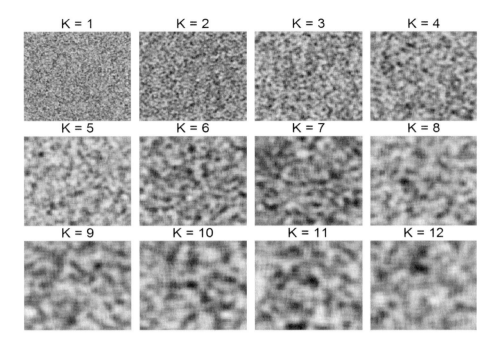

FIGURE 12.20. Random isotropic fields with Toeplitz spatial correlations for different depth, K, and $\theta_k = 0.9^k$.

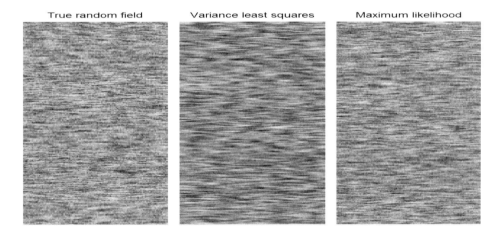

FIGURE 12.21. Three vertically dependent random fields. The first is the true random field with the left Toeplitz correlation structure. The second and third are generated using the variance least squares (VLS) and maximum likelihood (ML) estimates.

Maximum likelihood

Since $\{\varepsilon_i, i = 1, ..., Q\}$ are normally distributed and uncorrelated, the log-likelihood function, up to a constant term, takes the form

$$l = -\frac{1}{2}\left\{n\ln\sigma^2 + Q\ln\left|\mathbf{I} + \sum\theta_k\mathbf{T}_{k'}\right| + \frac{1}{\sigma^2}\sum_{i=1}^{Q}\varepsilon_i'\left(\mathbf{I} + \sum\theta_k\mathbf{T}_{k'}\right)^{-1}\varepsilon_i\right\}.$$

Differentiating with respect to σ^2, we obtain $\sigma^2 = \text{tr}(\varepsilon\mathbf{Q}^{-1}\varepsilon')/n$. The derivatives with respect to θ_k are

$$\frac{\partial l}{\partial\theta_k} = -0.5\left\{Q\text{tr}(\mathbf{Q}^{-1}\mathbf{T}_{k'}) - \sigma^{-2}\text{tr}(\varepsilon'\mathbf{Q}^{-1}\mathbf{T}_{k'}\mathbf{Q}^{-1}\varepsilon_i)\right\}, \quad k = 1, ..., K,$$

and the second derivatives $(j = 1, ..., K)$ are

$$\frac{\partial^2 l}{\partial\theta_k\partial\theta_j} = -0.5\left\{-Q\text{tr}(\mathbf{Q}^{-1}\mathbf{T}_{j'}\mathbf{Q}^{-1}\mathbf{T}_{k'})\right.$$
$$\left. +\sigma^{-2}\text{tr}(\varepsilon'\mathbf{Q}^{-1}\mathbf{T}_{j'}\mathbf{Q}^{-1}\mathbf{T}_{k'}\mathbf{Q}^{-1}\varepsilon) + \sigma^{-2}\text{tr}(\varepsilon'\mathbf{Q}^{-1}\mathbf{T}_{k'}\mathbf{Q}^{-1}\mathbf{T}_{j'}\mathbf{Q}^{-1}\varepsilon)\right\}. \quad (12.48)$$

If $\mathbf{H}$ is the $K \times K$ matrix with the elements $\{-\partial^2 l/\partial\theta_k\partial\theta_j\}$, the Newton's iterations yield

$$\boldsymbol{\theta}_{s+1} = \boldsymbol{\theta}_s + \lambda_s\mathbf{H}^{-1}\left(\frac{\partial l}{\partial\boldsymbol{\theta}}\right), \quad s = 0, 1, ...,$$

where λ_s is the step length to ensure that the l value increases from iteration to iteration. Matrix $\mathbf{H}^{-1}$ is the asymptotic covariance matrix for $\boldsymbol{\theta}$ with the variances on the diagonal. The value $Z_k = \widehat{\theta}_k/SE(\widehat{\theta}_k)$ is a characteristic of statistical significance and serves as guidance for the choice of the right correlation structure.

Example

The two methods of estimation are applied to a vertically dependent random field generated with $K = 5$ and $\theta_k = 0.35 - 0.05k$ and $\sigma^2 = 0.5$, see Figure 12.21. The true values, VLS and ML estimates, are shown in Figure 12.22. As the reader can see, maximum likelihood yields better estimates; also, the random field generated in Figure 12.21 looks closer to the true random field.

12.9.2 Simultaneous estimation of variance and transform parameters

Spatial correlation modifies previous models for image registration and ensemble of images. In particular, the MSE criterion (12.21) or (12.37) will be replaced by the weighted MSE.

To illustrate, we simply assume that we have a uniform image $M(p, q) = \mu + \varepsilon(p, q)$ or in matrix form, $\mathbf{M} = \mu\mathbf{1}_P\mathbf{1}_Q' + \varepsilon$, where ε is the random field defined by (12.43). The parameter of interest is the intensity μ. The log-likelihood function for this image model is given by (12.45) with ε replaced by $\mathbf{M} - \mu\mathbf{1}_P\mathbf{1}_Q'$. Let us assume that the matrices $\mathbf{Q}_L$ and $\mathbf{Q}_R$ are known. Then the MLE for μ minimizes

$$S(\mu) = \text{tr}[\mathbf{Q}_R^{-1}(\mathbf{M} - \mu\mathbf{1}_P\mathbf{1}_Q')'\mathbf{Q}_L^{-1}(\mathbf{M} - \mu\mathbf{1}_P\mathbf{1}_Q')].$$

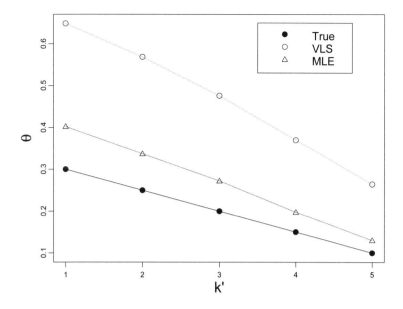

FIGURE 12.22. Estimation by variance least squares (VLS) and maximum likelihood (ML). For this example, the ML estimate is closer to the true θ.

Taking the derivative of S with respect to μ, we find the solution as the generalized least squares estimator,

$$\widehat{\mu}_{ML} = \frac{\mathbf{1}'_P \mathbf{Q}_L^{-1} \mathbf{M} \mathbf{Q}_R^{-1} \mathbf{1}_Q}{(\mathbf{1}'_P \mathbf{Q}_L^{-1} \mathbf{1}_P)(\mathbf{1}'_Q \mathbf{Q}_R^{-1} \mathbf{1}_Q)} = \frac{\sum \left(\mathbf{Q}_L^{-1} \mathbf{M} \mathbf{Q}_R^{-1}\right)_{pq}}{\sum (\mathbf{Q}_L^{-1})_{pq} \sum (\mathbf{Q}_R^{-1})_{pq}}. \tag{12.49}$$

Notice that even a simple model for intensity level leads to a weighted mean. For a proper estimation, matrices $\mathbf{Q}_L$ and $\mathbf{Q}_R$ must be estimated previously and then formula (12.49) applied. In the maximum likelihood approach, μ and these matrices are estimated simultaneously. Consequently, if two images are aligned, the MSE criterion should be replaced by the weighted MSE of the form (12.23), where $w(p, q)$ is the (p, q)th element of the inverse covariance matrix.

Problems for Section 12.9

1. Does the log-likelihood function (12.45) have a maximum; that is, is model (12.43) specified correctly? Does this model turn into a correctly specified model with additional restriction $tr(\mathbf{Q}_R) = tr(\mathbf{Q}_L) = 1$? Maximize l, given by equation (12.45), over $\mathbf{Q}_R$ and $\mathbf{Q}_L$ under these rectrictions.

2. The R function `randmat` plots 36 simulated images with various spatial correlation structure. Identify what correlation structure is used. What correlation model described in this section was used to create those images?

3. Find the information matrix for the log-likelihood by taking the expectation of the Hessian (12.48).

4*. There are three PGM images of the pine bark in the directory `"c:\\MixedModels \\Chapter12\\bark\\`. Write an R function that plots the images. Do they look like vertically dependent random fields in Figure 12.21? Can these images be modeled via the left Toeplitz correlation structure? Compute correlation coefficients between rows and pick those that produce maximum values. These values may be used to construct adequate Toeplitz matrices.

12.10   Summary points

- Mathematically, a gray image is a $P \times Q$ matrix with integer entries that take values from 0 (black) to 255 (white). A color image in the RGB format can be equivalently represented as three grayscale images: Red, Green and Blue.

- *Image processing* is a well-established discipline with a variety of techniques to enhance and restore one image at a time. However, statistical aspects of image estimation and testing are underdeveloped. For example, least squares is used as a criterion of image discrepancy but not as a statistical method of estimation of a statistical model. Consequently, the least squares estimate (LSE) is rarely accompanied by its standard error as a characteristic of how the LSE is sensitive to the data. Statistical hypothesis testing for images is not developed either. For example, there is no analogy of a t-test for images when two sample images are compared.

- Classic statistics deals with numbers; statistical image analysis deals with matrices of numbers. The revolution in digital imaging poses challenging problems to statistical science. A marriage of image processing and statistics creates a new discipline, *Statistical Image Analysis*. This chapter lays out the foundation of this discipline using a model-based approach. In the process, many techniques of image processing receive a theoretical justification, such as histogram equalization and the Karhunen–Loeve transformation.

- We classify images into two groups: structured and unstructured. Structured are images of an object (objects) or easy-to-recognize scene. Unstructured are images without content, such as fabric (textures) or microscopic images. Consequently, for structured images, image registration typically occurs when objects on the first images are aligned with the same objects on the second image. Unstructured images are analyzed using gray level distributions and histograms. Thus, we say that two unstructured images are the same if they have the same gray level distribution.

- The histogram is a standard tool of image processing and is typically used for image enhancement. We apply the cumulative distribution function to compare unstructured images. An advantage of the distribution function is that several distribution functions can be plotted on one graph—a convenient graphical tool for image comparison. A nonparametric Kolmogorov–Smirnov criterion was used to test whether two images are the same.

- We have developed a multinomial distribution for grayscale image. The maximum likelihood estimate for the probability that the gray level of a pixel takes value g is the histogram value $h_g, g = 0, 1, ..., 255$. Two χ^2-tests and one likelihood ratio parametric test were developed to test whether two images have the same gray level distribution.

- Entropy is a milestone of information theory. The entropy of a binary message, as a sequence of 1s and 0s, is zero if the sequence contains only 0 (or 1). The entropy is maximum if the probability of 1 appearing is $\frac{1}{2}$. Based on the multinomial distribution, we have introduced the notion of image entropy. If pixels have the same gray level (blank image), the image entropy is zero.

- We have introduced Entropy Per Pixel (EPP) as a unit for image information, $EPP = -\sum h_g \log_2 h_g$ bits. The absolute maximum of EPP is 8 bits and it is attained when each gray level has the same probability of occurrence, $1/256$. Hence, a popular image enhancement technique known as *histogram equalization* maximizes EPP. Another application of the EPP concept is used to reduce a gray image to a four-gray level image—the thresholds must be quartiles of the distribution function.

- Typically, we deal with an ensemble of unstructured images. Two statistical models based on the multinomial distribution were developed in the framework of mixed model methodology: fixed- and random-shift models. These are analogs of the fixed and random intercept models studied in Sections 2.4 and 7.2, respectively. Logit transformation reduces a nonlinear model to the linear mixed model extensively studied in Chapters 2 through 4. Especially effective is a two-stage estimation method to analyze an ensemble of images. In particular, we have demonstrated how to use this method to compare two samples of images as a generalization of the standard t-test.

- Image alignment and registration is essential for content-dependent image comparison; for example, when a pixel-by-pixel difference is to be taken. Four types of model registration may be suggested: landmark-based, affine, nonlinear, and random (stochastic). In the landmark model, images are aligned such that the landmark points from two images coincide or are as close as can be solved by least squares.

- The affine registration model is the easiest and reduces to the mean squared error minimization over six affine coefficients (parameters) for a 2D image. If the transformation is rigid, it reduces to four parameters. If only rotation is required and the size remains the same, we come to a minimization under a quadratic constraint. Nonlinear registration is typically used a polynomial of a low degree and again reduces to the unconstrained MSE minimization. Random registration is the most complicated and can be accomplished via the nonlinear mixed effects model estimation of Chapter 8.

- A precise image registration requires image interpolation. The easiest is the linear interpolation, although some more elaborate methods, such as B-splines, exist. The derivative-free algorithm for MSE minimization may be preferable because we deal with a discrete function and the derivatives do not exist. The theory of linear statistical hypothesis testing may be applied to affine parameters; for example, to test whether the transformation is rigid.

- If several images of the same object or scene are available, the images must be aligned first to derive the mean image. Two statistical models for the affine parameters can be suggested: fixed and random. The former model assumes that the parameters are fixed and unknown and therefore can be found from individual MSE minimization. The latter model is more complex and assumes that the affine parameters are random with population-averaged values. This model leads to a nonlinear mixed effects model, studied extensively in Chapter 8. In particular, after Laplace approximation, the parameters are found from a penalized MSE.

- A realistic assumption in content-dependent image analysis is to assume spatial correlation that implies treating an image as a random field. Several models for spatial correlation may be suggested. A parsimonious model uses a Toeplitz matrix and can describe complex statistical intra-image dependencies. Methods of estimation developed in the earlier chapters, such as variance least squares or maximum likelihood, apply readily. Spatial correlation complicates image alignment and registration because the variance and transform parameters must be estimated simultaneously. In particular, instead of the mean squared error, one should use the weighted mean-squared error.

- Statistics should play a more important role in image science—from image processing to image reconstruction. For example, little work has been done in applying powerful statistical hypothesis testing to image comparison. Today, image analysis is method-driven. To make further advances, it should be model-driven. A good example of a model-driven image reconstruction is the PET model based on the Poisson distribution. Statistical image modeling not only yields an efficient fitting method but also generates the covariance matrix and/or the likelihood value needed for statistical significance testing, model selection, and verification. We strongly believe that a statistical model-based image analysis will bring image science to the next level.

13
Appendix: Useful Facts and Formulas

13.1 Basic facts of asymptotic theory

13.1.1 Central Limit Theorem

Let $\{a_i, i = 1, 2, ...\}$ be nonzero numbers and $\{\varepsilon_i, i = 1, 2, ...\}$ be independent and identically distributed (iid) random variables with zero mean and variance σ^2. If (a) $\{a_i\}$ are uniformly bounded, i.e., there exists a constant A such that $a_i^2 \le A$ for all $i = 1, 2, ...$ and (b) there exists a limit $\lim_{N \to \infty} N^{-1} \sum_{i=1}^{N} a_i^2 = V > 0$, then the average

$$\bar{\varepsilon}_N = \frac{1}{N} \sum_{i=1}^{N} a_i \varepsilon_i \to 0, \tag{13.1}$$

with probability 1 (almost sure, a.s.), and

$$\frac{1}{\sqrt{N}} \sum_{i=1}^{N} a_i \varepsilon_i \simeq \mathcal{N}(0, \sigma^2 V), \quad N \to \infty. \tag{13.2}$$

Equation (13.1) is referred to as the Law of Large Numbers (LLN) and (13.2) as the Central Limit Theorem (CLT). Convergence with probability 1 (or strong convergence) implies convergence in probability (weak convergence), that is, for any $\delta > 0$, we have $\Pr(|\bar{\varepsilon}_N| > \delta) \to 0$, or symbolically, $p\lim_{N \to \infty} \bar{\varepsilon}_N = 0$. In a special case when $a_i = 1$, we come to a standard formulation. Under formulated conditions, the quadratic convergence also takes place, $\lim_{N \to \infty} \mathrm{var}(\bar{\varepsilon}_N) = 0$. Equation (13.2) means that for any $a < b$, the probability that the random variable at the left belongs to the interval (a, b) converges to $(2\pi V)^{-1/2} \int_a^b e^{-\frac{x^2}{2V}} dx$. Sometimes we say that the left-hand side of (13.2) is asymptotically normally distributed with zero mean and variance V.

   Multivariate formulation: Let $\{\mathbf{A}_i, i = 1, 2, ...\}$ be $m \times k$ matrices and $\{\varepsilon_i, i = 1, 2, ...\}$ iid $k \times 1$ random vectors with zero mean and covariance matrix $\sigma^2 \mathbf{I}_k$. If

(a) matrices $\{\mathbf{A}_i\}$ are uniformly bounded, i.e., there exists a constant A such that $\text{tr}(\mathbf{A}_i'\mathbf{A}_i) \leq A$ for all $i = 1, 2, \ldots$ and (b) there exists a matrix limit $\lim_{N\to\infty} N^{-1} \sum_{i=1}^{N} \mathbf{A}_i\mathbf{A}_i' = \mathbf{V}$, where the $m \times m$ matrix $\mathbf{V}$ is positive definite, then the average vector is asymptotically normally distributed,

$$\overline{\varepsilon}_N = \frac{1}{\sqrt{N}} \sum_{i=1}^{N} \mathbf{A}_i\varepsilon_i \simeq \mathcal{N}(\mathbf{0}, \mathbf{V}) \tag{13.3}$$

as $N \to \infty$, Eicker (1966). We use symbol $\simeq$ to indicate the asymptotic distribution. The multivariate CLT follows from the Lindeberg-Feller conditions (Gnedenko, 1962; Feller, 1966; Rao, 1973). Often, the multivariate CLT is used in combination with the following fact: If $\mathbf{w}_N$ is asymptotically normally distributed with zero mean and covariance matrix $\mathbf{V}$, $\mathbf{w}_N \simeq \mathcal{N}(\mathbf{0}, \mathbf{V})$ and $\mathbf{R}_N$ are fixed matrices with uniformly bounded elements such that $\lim_{N\to\infty} \mathbf{R}_N = \mathbf{R}$, then $\mathbf{R}_N\mathbf{w}_N \simeq \mathcal{N}(\mathbf{0}, \mathbf{R}\mathbf{V}\mathbf{R}')$.

As an example, we prove that if in linear regression $y_i = \boldsymbol{\beta}'\mathbf{x}_i + \varepsilon_i$, the error terms $\{\varepsilon_i\}$ are iid with zero mean and variance σ^2 and the $\mathbf{x}_i$ are $m \times 1$ fixed vectors, then the OLS estimator, $\widehat{\boldsymbol{\beta}}_{OLS} = (\sum_{i=1}^{N} \mathbf{x}_i\mathbf{x}_i')^{-1}(\sum_{i=1}^{N} \mathbf{x}_i y_i)$, is asymptotically normally distributed. To apply (13.3), we assume that there exists a constant A such that $\|\mathbf{x}_i\| \leq A$ and $\lim N^{-1} \sum_{i=1}^{N} \mathbf{x}_i\mathbf{x}_i' = \mathbf{V}$, where $\mathbf{V}$ is a positive definite matrix. Then using the multivariate CLT with $k = 1$, we obtain $\sqrt{N}(\widehat{\boldsymbol{\beta}}_{OLS} - \boldsymbol{\beta}) = (N^{-1} \sum_{i=1}^{N} \mathbf{x}_i\mathbf{x}_i')^{-1}(N^{-1/2} \sum_{i=1}^{N} \mathbf{x}_i\varepsilon_i)$. With certain ambiguity, we usually write $\widehat{\boldsymbol{\beta}}_{OLS} \simeq \mathcal{N}(\boldsymbol{\beta}, \sigma^2(\sum_{i=1}^{N} \mathbf{x}_i\mathbf{x}_i')^{-1})$.

13.1.2 Generalized Slutsky theorem

Let $\mathbf{g}(\boldsymbol{\theta})$ be a continuous vector-valued function of the vector argument $\boldsymbol{\theta}$. The Slutsky (1925) theorem says that $p\lim \mathbf{g}(\widehat{\boldsymbol{\theta}}_n) = \mathbf{g}(p\lim \widehat{\boldsymbol{\theta}}_n)$, or in other words, $p\lim$ and $\mathbf{g}$ are interchangeable. In many applications, the function varies with n, so we deal with $\mathbf{g}_n(\widehat{\boldsymbol{\theta}}_n)$. So the question is: Under what conditions are the functions and limit interchangeable? Usually, the respective result is formulated in terms of uniform convergence. In the theorem below, we show that it suffices for functions $\mathbf{g}_n$ to have uniformly bounded first derivatives, which is easier to check.

Theorem 48 *(Generalized Slutsky Theorem). Let $\{\mathbf{g}_n(\boldsymbol{\theta}), n = 1, 2, \ldots\}$ be a sequence of continuous functions such that $\lim \mathbf{g}_n(\boldsymbol{\theta}) = \mathbf{g}(\boldsymbol{\theta})$ for all $\boldsymbol{\theta}$. Let $\mathbf{g}_n(\boldsymbol{\theta})$ have the first derivative, and for any $\varepsilon > 0$ and $\boldsymbol{\theta}_*$, let there exist a constant $A = A(\varepsilon, \boldsymbol{\theta}_*)$ that $\|\partial\mathbf{g}_n(\boldsymbol{\theta}_*)/\partial\boldsymbol{\theta}\| \leq A$ for all $\|\boldsymbol{\theta} - \boldsymbol{\theta}_*\| \leq \varepsilon$ and uniformly over $n = 1, 2, \ldots$. Let $\widehat{\boldsymbol{\theta}}_n$ be a consistent estimator of $\boldsymbol{\theta}_0$, namely, $p\lim_{n\to\infty} \widehat{\boldsymbol{\theta}}_n = \boldsymbol{\theta}_0$, then $p\lim_{n\to\infty} \mathbf{g}_n(\widehat{\boldsymbol{\theta}}_n) = \mathbf{g}(\boldsymbol{\theta}_0)$.*

Proof. Let ε be any positive number. Using the triangle inequality, it is easy to see that

$$\begin{aligned}
\Pr\left\{\left\|\mathbf{g}_n(\widehat{\boldsymbol{\theta}}_n) - \mathbf{g}(\boldsymbol{\theta}_0)\right\| > \varepsilon\right\} &\leq \Pr\left\{\left\|\mathbf{g}_n(\widehat{\boldsymbol{\theta}}_n) - \mathbf{g}_n(\boldsymbol{\theta}_0)\right\| > \varepsilon/2\right\} \\
&+ \Pr\left\{\left\|\mathbf{g}_n(\boldsymbol{\theta}_0) - \mathbf{g}(\boldsymbol{\theta}_0)\right\| > \varepsilon/2\right\}.
\end{aligned}$$

The second term goes to zero when $n \to \infty$. Thus, it suffices to prove that the first term vanishes. Using the fact that for any events A and B we have $\Pr(A) =$

$\Pr(A \cap B) + \Pr(A \cap B^c) \leq \Pr(A \cap B) + \Pr(B^c)$, we obtain

$$\Pr\left\{\left\|\mathbf{g}_n(\widehat{\boldsymbol{\theta}}_n) - \mathbf{g}_n(\boldsymbol{\theta}_0)\right\| > \varepsilon/2\right\}$$

$$\leq \quad \Pr\left\{\left\|\mathbf{g}_n(\widehat{\boldsymbol{\theta}}_n) - \mathbf{g}_n(\boldsymbol{\theta}_0)\right\| > \varepsilon/2 \cap \left\|\widehat{\boldsymbol{\theta}}_n - \boldsymbol{\theta}_0\right\| \leq \varepsilon\right\} \qquad (13.4)$$

$$+ \Pr\left\{\left\|\widehat{\boldsymbol{\theta}}_n - \boldsymbol{\theta}_0\right\| > \varepsilon\right\}.$$

From multivariate calculus, if $\left\|\widehat{\boldsymbol{\theta}}_n - \boldsymbol{\theta}_0\right\| \leq \varepsilon$, we have

$$\left\|\mathbf{g}_n(\widehat{\boldsymbol{\theta}}_n) - \mathbf{g}(\boldsymbol{\theta}_0)\right\| \leq \max_{\left\|\widehat{\boldsymbol{\theta}}_n - \boldsymbol{\theta}_0\right\| \leq \varepsilon} \left\|\partial \mathbf{g}_n / \partial \boldsymbol{\theta}\right\| \times \left\|\widehat{\boldsymbol{\theta}}_n - \boldsymbol{\theta}_0\right\|, \qquad (13.5)$$

so that probability (13.4) can be bounded from above by $\Pr\{\|\widehat{\boldsymbol{\theta}}_n - \boldsymbol{\theta}_0\| > \varepsilon/(2A)\}$, and therefore

$$\Pr\left\{\left\|\mathbf{g}_n(\widehat{\boldsymbol{\theta}}_n) - \mathbf{g}(\boldsymbol{\theta}_0)\right\| > \varepsilon/2\right\} \quad \leq \quad \Pr\left\{\left\|\widehat{\boldsymbol{\theta}}_n - \boldsymbol{\theta}_0\right\| > \varepsilon/(2A)\right\}$$

$$+ \Pr\left\{\left\|\widehat{\boldsymbol{\theta}}_n - \boldsymbol{\theta}_0\right\| > \varepsilon\right\},$$

vanishes when $n \to \infty$. ∎

This theorem can be generalized to the case when $\{\mathbf{g}_n\}$ are stochastic by applying the Markov and Cauchy inequality to the right-hand side of (13.5). Then we need to have $E(\|\partial \mathbf{g}_n(\boldsymbol{\theta}_*)/\partial \boldsymbol{\theta}\|^2) \leq A$ for all $\|\boldsymbol{\theta} - \boldsymbol{\theta}_*\| \leq \varepsilon$ uniformly over n and $\lim_{n\to\infty} E\left\|\widehat{\boldsymbol{\theta}}_n - \boldsymbol{\theta}_0\right\|^2 = 0$.

We illustrate the generalized Slutsky theorem by proving that an estimated GLS for LME model (2.28), where the true $\mathbf{D}$ is replaced with its consistent estimate $\widehat{\mathbf{D}}$, is consistent. See also Section 3.6.2, where some issues of the asymptotic theory are discussed. In a somewhat tedious but straightforward proof below, we assume the deterministic scheme, that is, matrices $\mathbf{X}_i$ and $\mathbf{Z}_i$ are fixed, and matrix $\sum \mathbf{X}_i' \mathbf{X}_i$ is positive definite.

Let the elements of matrices $\{\mathbf{X}_i, \mathbf{Z}_i\}$ be uniformly bounded when $N \to \infty$, and for every nonnegative definite matrix $\mathbf{D}$, let the positive definite matrix limit, $\lim_{N\to\infty} N^{-1} \sum_{i=1}^{N} \mathbf{X}_i'(\mathbf{I} + \mathbf{Z}_i \mathbf{D} \mathbf{Z}_i')^{-1} \mathbf{X}_i = \mathbf{M}(\mathbf{D})$, exist. Note that we do not require the number of observations per cluster $\{n_i, i = 1, ..., N\}$ to be bounded or go to infinity with N. Since under our assumption

$$\text{cov}(\widehat{\boldsymbol{\beta}}_N) = \sigma^2 \left(\sum \mathbf{X}_i'(\mathbf{I} + \mathbf{Z}_i \mathbf{D} \mathbf{Z}_i')^{-1} \mathbf{X}_i\right)^{-1} \to \mathbf{0}$$

for every $\mathbf{D}$, we have $\lim_{N\to\infty} E\left\|\widehat{\boldsymbol{\beta}}_N - \boldsymbol{\beta}\right\|^2 = 0$. Let ε be positive and $\mathbf{D}_*$ positive definite. Then, according to the generalized Slutsky theorem, we need to prove that the expected value of the norm of the derivative is uniformly bounded in the ε-neighborhood of $\mathbf{D}_*$. Let D_{pq} be an element of $\mathbf{D}$. We want to find A such that $E\left\|d\widehat{\boldsymbol{\beta}}/dD_{pq}\right\|^2 \leq A$ for all $\|\mathbf{D} - \mathbf{D}_*\| \leq \varepsilon$ and N, assuming that $\mathbf{D}$ is a nonnegative definite matrix. Since $\{\mathbf{X}_i, \mathbf{Z}_i\}$ are uniformly bounded, the elements of matrices

$\mathbf{V}_i = \mathbf{I} + \mathbf{Z}_i\mathbf{D}\mathbf{Z}'_i$ and $\mathbf{V}_i^{-1}$ are uniformly bounded as well. Using the chain rule, we find that

$$\frac{d\widehat{\boldsymbol{\beta}}}{dD_{pq}} = \mathbf{T}^{-1}\sum\mathbf{X}'_i\mathbf{V}_i^{-1}\mathbf{z}_{ip}\mathbf{z}'_{iq}\mathbf{V}_i^{-1}\mathbf{X}_i\mathbf{T}^{-1}\sum\mathbf{X}'_i\mathbf{V}_i^{-1}\mathbf{y}_i$$
$$-\mathbf{T}^{-1}\sum\mathbf{X}'_i\mathbf{V}_i^{-1}\mathbf{z}_{ip}\mathbf{z}'_{iq}\mathbf{V}_i^{-1}\mathbf{y}_i,$$

where $\mathbf{T} = \sum\mathbf{X}'_i(\mathbf{I} + \mathbf{Z}_i\mathbf{D}\mathbf{Z}'_i)^{-1}\mathbf{X}_i$, and $\mathbf{z}_{ip}$ and $\mathbf{z}_{iq}$ are the pth and qth columns of matrix $\mathbf{Z}_i$, respectively. It is elementary to show that under our assumptions the elements of matrix $\mathbf{T}^{-1}$ are bounded, and since $\mathrm{cov}(\mathbf{y}_i) = \mathbf{V}_i$, the quantity $E\left\|d\widehat{\boldsymbol{\beta}}/dD_{pq}\right\|^2$ is uniformly bounded as well.

13.1.3 Pseudo-maximum likelihood

Let $\mathbf{y}_1, \mathbf{y}_2, ..., \mathbf{y}_N$ be iid vectors of observations with the common density $f = f(\mathbf{y}; \boldsymbol{\beta}, \boldsymbol{\theta})$ dependent on a pair of vector parameters $(\boldsymbol{\beta}, \boldsymbol{\theta})$. It is assumed that the parameter of interest is $\boldsymbol{\beta}$, and $\boldsymbol{\theta}$ is treated as a nuisance parameter, or the parameter of minor interest. For example, in a mixed model, $\boldsymbol{\beta}$ is the vector of model coefficients and $\boldsymbol{\theta}$ is the variance parameter. The joint information matrix is

$$\mathcal{I} = \begin{bmatrix} \mathcal{I}_{\boldsymbol{\beta}} & \mathcal{I}_{\boldsymbol{\beta\theta}} \\ \mathcal{I}'_{\boldsymbol{\beta\theta}} & \mathcal{I}_{\boldsymbol{\theta}} \end{bmatrix}, \tag{13.6}$$

where

$$\mathcal{I}_{\boldsymbol{\beta}} = -E\left(\frac{\partial^2 l}{\partial^2\boldsymbol{\beta}}\right), \quad \mathcal{I}_{\boldsymbol{\beta\theta}} = -E\left(\frac{\partial^2 l}{\partial\boldsymbol{\beta}\partial\boldsymbol{\theta}}\right), \quad \mathcal{I}_{\boldsymbol{\theta}} = -E\left(\frac{\partial^2 l}{\partial^2\boldsymbol{\theta}}\right),$$

and $l = \sum\ln f$ is the joint log-likelihood function. Under regular conditions, MLE $\widehat{\boldsymbol{\gamma}} = (\widehat{\boldsymbol{\beta}}', \widehat{\boldsymbol{\theta}}')'$, which is the solution to the score equations $\partial l/\partial\boldsymbol{\beta} = \mathbf{0}$ and $\partial l/\partial\boldsymbol{\theta} = \mathbf{0}$, is normally distributed as $N \to \infty$, namely,

$$\widehat{\boldsymbol{\gamma}} - \boldsymbol{\gamma} - \begin{bmatrix} \widehat{\boldsymbol{\beta}} - \boldsymbol{\beta} \\ \widehat{\boldsymbol{\theta}} - \boldsymbol{\theta} \end{bmatrix} \simeq \mathcal{N}(\mathbf{0}, \mathcal{I}^{-1}). \tag{13.7}$$

We admit a certain ambiguity in (13.7) because $\mathcal{I}$ is proportional to N, due to the iid condition, and therefore $\mathcal{I}^{-1} \to \mathbf{0}$. However, we prefer a more general expression (13.7) because the results, under appropriate restrictions, remain true when observations are *not* identically distributed. Since we are interested in $\boldsymbol{\beta}$, we may explicitly find the asymptotic covariance as

$$\mathrm{cov}(\widehat{\boldsymbol{\beta}}) = \left(\mathcal{I}_{\boldsymbol{\beta}} - \mathcal{I}_{\boldsymbol{\beta\theta}}\mathcal{I}_{\boldsymbol{\theta}}^{-1}\mathcal{I}'_{\boldsymbol{\beta\theta}}\right)^{-1} = \mathcal{I}_{\boldsymbol{\beta}}^{-1} + \mathcal{I}_{\boldsymbol{\beta}}^{-1}\mathcal{I}_{\boldsymbol{\beta\theta}}\mathbf{C}_{\widehat{\boldsymbol{\theta}}}\mathcal{I}'_{\boldsymbol{\beta\theta}}\mathcal{I}_{\boldsymbol{\beta}}^{-1}, \tag{13.8}$$

where

$$\mathbf{C}_{\widehat{\boldsymbol{\theta}}} = \mathrm{cov}(\widehat{\boldsymbol{\theta}}) = \left(\mathcal{I}_{\boldsymbol{\theta}} - \mathcal{I}'_{\boldsymbol{\beta\theta}}\mathcal{I}_{\boldsymbol{\beta}}^{-1}\mathcal{I}_{\boldsymbol{\beta\theta}}\right)^{-1}$$

is the asymptotic covariance matrix of the MLE $\widehat{\boldsymbol{\theta}}$. If $\boldsymbol{\theta}$ were known, the asymptotic covariance matrix of $\widehat{\boldsymbol{\beta}}$ would be $\mathcal{I}_{\boldsymbol{\beta}}^{-1}$. This would also be true if $\mathcal{I}_{\boldsymbol{\beta\theta}} = \mathbf{0}$, that is, if the ML estimates $\widehat{\boldsymbol{\beta}}$ and $\widehat{\boldsymbol{\theta}}$ were asymptotically independent. An example of this situation is the LME model, where the estimates of the model coefficients and variance parameters are independent. One can interpret this as saying that the estimated GLS is equivalent to the theoretical GLS (2.28); see more discussion in Section 3.6.2.

Pseudo-maximum likelihood is the name for the situation where, in the score equation, $\partial l / \partial \boldsymbol{\beta} = \mathbf{0}$, a consistent and asymptotically normal estimate, $\widetilde{\boldsymbol{\theta}}$, rather than the MLE, is used (Gong and Samaniego, 1981). The pseudo-MLE, $\widetilde{\boldsymbol{\beta}}$, is also consistent and asymptotically normally distributed but with a variance larger than the MLE variance because the MLE is asymptotically efficient. Parke (1986) derived the formula for the asymptotic covariance matrix of the pseudo-MLE,

$$\operatorname{cov}(\widetilde{\boldsymbol{\beta}}) = \mathcal{I}_{\boldsymbol{\beta}}^{-1} + \mathcal{I}_{\boldsymbol{\beta}}^{-1} \mathcal{I}_{\boldsymbol{\beta\theta}} \mathbf{C}_{\widetilde{\boldsymbol{\theta}}} \mathcal{I}_{\boldsymbol{\beta\theta}}' \mathcal{I}_{\boldsymbol{\beta}}^{-1}, \tag{13.9}$$

where $\mathbf{C}_{\widetilde{\boldsymbol{\theta}}} = \operatorname{cov}(\widetilde{\boldsymbol{\theta}})$ is the asymptotic covariance matrix of $\widetilde{\boldsymbol{\theta}}$. Notice its resemblance to formula (13.8). Since the MLE is efficient, $\mathbf{C}_{\widetilde{\boldsymbol{\theta}}} \geq \mathbf{C}_{\widehat{\boldsymbol{\theta}}}$ and therefore $\operatorname{cov}(\widetilde{\boldsymbol{\beta}}) \geq \operatorname{cov}(\widehat{\boldsymbol{\beta}})$. If the information matrix (13.6) is block diagonal, *any* consistent estimator of $\boldsymbol{\theta}$ will produce a pseudo-MLE asymptotically equivalent to MLE.

13.1.4 Estimating equations approach and the sandwich formula

Maximum likelihood yields asymptotically minimal variances if the distribution is known. The estimating equations approach is very useful for a nonmaximum likelihood estimation, where an estimator is defined as the solution to a system of nonlinear equations. The core of this approach is the estimating function. Historically, the estimating equations approach emerged as a robust technique and is referred to as M-estimation and the corresponding M-estimator (Huber, 1967, 1981). We recommend a recently published paper by Stefanski and Boos (2002) for a transparent introduction to M-estimation and a book by Schervish (1995) or a collection of papers in Matyas (1999) for a rigorous discussion. Maximum likelihood is a special case of the estimating equations approach, with the estimating equation equal to the score equation. It is not our goal to provide complete coverage of the estimating equations approach, particularly in the presence of nuisance parameters; the interested reader is referred to a paper by Yuan and Jennrich (2000). Instead, we would like to draw a big picture and present the key results while putting technical details aside. The sandwich formula plays the central role because it computes the asymptotic variance-covariance matrix of the M-estimator.

Theorem 49 *Let* $\mathbf{y}_1, ..., \mathbf{y}_N$ *be iid* $n \times 1$ *random vectors with a common distribution dependent on an unknown* m-*dimensional parameter* $\boldsymbol{\gamma}$. *Let* $\boldsymbol{\Psi} = \boldsymbol{\Psi}(\mathbf{y}, \boldsymbol{\gamma})$ *be an* $m \times 1$ *vector function defined on* $R^n \times R^m$, *the estimating function. It is assumed that* $\boldsymbol{\Psi}$ *is a continuous function with a piecewise derivative such that*

$$E_{\boldsymbol{\gamma}} \boldsymbol{\Psi}(\mathbf{y}, \boldsymbol{\gamma}) = \mathbf{0}. \tag{13.10}$$

Also, it is assumed that $E_{\boldsymbol{\gamma}} \boldsymbol{\Psi}(\mathbf{y}, \boldsymbol{\gamma}_*) = \mathbf{0}$ *implies that* $\boldsymbol{\gamma}_* = \boldsymbol{\gamma}$. *Let* $\widehat{\boldsymbol{\gamma}}_N$ *be the solution to the estimating equation*

$$\sum_{i=1}^{N} \boldsymbol{\Psi}(\mathbf{y}_i, \boldsymbol{\gamma}) = \mathbf{0}. \tag{13.11}$$

Then, when $N \to \infty$:

1. $\widehat{\boldsymbol{\gamma}}_N$ *is a consistent estimator of* $\boldsymbol{\gamma}$.

2. $\widehat{\boldsymbol{\gamma}}_N$ *has an asymptotic multivariate normal distribution,*

$$\sqrt{N}(\widehat{\boldsymbol{\gamma}}_N - \boldsymbol{\gamma}) \simeq \mathcal{N}\left(\mathbf{0}, \mathbf{A}^{-1}\mathbf{B}\mathbf{A}'^{-1}\right), \tag{13.12}$$

where

$$\mathbf{A} = E_{\boldsymbol{\gamma}}\left(\frac{\partial \boldsymbol{\Psi}}{\partial \boldsymbol{\gamma}}\right), \quad \mathbf{B} = E_{\boldsymbol{\gamma}}\left(\boldsymbol{\Psi}\boldsymbol{\Psi}'\right), \tag{13.13}$$

assuming that the expectations exist and matrix $\mathbf{A}$ *is invertible.*

The major condition for an estimating function to produce a consistent and asymptotically normally distributed estimate is to have zero expectation, $E\boldsymbol{\Psi} = \mathbf{0}$. Thus, sometimes we speak of *unbiased estimating equations.*

Notice that the theorem is formulated under the iid assumption. Often, the estimating function depends on covariates/explanatory variables $\{\mathbf{x}_i\}$. We assume that $\{\mathbf{x}_i\}$ are iid, as in the stochastic scheme of Section 3.6.2 with the common distribution not dependent on parameter $\boldsymbol{\gamma}$. Then we have $\boldsymbol{\Psi}_i = \boldsymbol{\Psi}(\mathbf{y}, \boldsymbol{\gamma}; \mathbf{x}_i)$, and condition (13.10) is rewritten as $E(\boldsymbol{\Psi}_i) = E(\boldsymbol{\Psi}(\mathbf{y}, \boldsymbol{\gamma}; \mathbf{x}_i)|\mathbf{x}_i) = \mathbf{0}$. Thus, although $\mathbf{y}_i|\mathbf{x}_i$ are not iid, $\{\mathbf{y}_i\}$ are iid and Theorem 49 applies. The theorem can be reformulated for the deterministic scheme, but it would require more technical detail, such as the existence of $\lim_{N\to\infty} N^{-1}\sum_{i=1}^{N} \boldsymbol{\Psi}_i$. However, the major condition on the unbiasedness of the estimating functions, $E_{\boldsymbol{\gamma}}\boldsymbol{\Psi}_i = \mathbf{0}$ for all i, remains.

Remarks

- In the expectation $E_{\boldsymbol{\gamma}}\boldsymbol{\Psi}(\mathbf{y}, \boldsymbol{\gamma}_*)$, it is assumed that the true parameter is $\boldsymbol{\gamma}$, and $\boldsymbol{\gamma}_*$ is any other vector from the parameter space. From the implicit function theorem of calculus, it follows that if matrix $\mathbf{A}$ is nonsingular, then in a neighborhood of $\boldsymbol{\gamma}_*$ the solution of $E_{\boldsymbol{\gamma}}\boldsymbol{\Psi}(\mathbf{y}, \boldsymbol{\gamma}_*) = \mathbf{0}$ is $\boldsymbol{\gamma}_* = \boldsymbol{\gamma}$.

- In words, an M-estimator is consistent if the expected value of the estimating function is zero. If the expected value of the estimating function is not zero, the M-estimation produces a biased estimator (sometimes it is called a *biased estimating equations*; Carroll et al., 1995). Specifically, the M-estimator converges to $\boldsymbol{\gamma}_*$ which is the solution to the vector equation, $E_{\boldsymbol{\gamma}}\boldsymbol{\Psi}(\mathbf{y}, \boldsymbol{\gamma}_*) = \mathbf{0}$. A biased estimating equation produces a systematically biased estimate. If $\boldsymbol{\gamma}$ is the true parameter and $E\boldsymbol{\Psi} \neq \mathbf{0}$, the EE estimates from (13.11) converge to $\boldsymbol{\gamma}_*$ as the solution to a nonlinear equation $E_{\boldsymbol{\gamma}}\boldsymbol{\Psi}(\mathbf{y}, \boldsymbol{\gamma}_*) = \mathbf{0}$. We applied this fact to find the bias of the Lindstrom–Bates estimator for a mixed exponential model of Section 8.9.4. Thus, to find an asymptotic bias, one needs to solve a nonlinear equation for $\boldsymbol{\gamma}_*$. Approximately, $\boldsymbol{\gamma}_* = \boldsymbol{\gamma} - \mathbf{A}^{-1}E_{\boldsymbol{\gamma}}\boldsymbol{\Psi}(\mathbf{y}, \boldsymbol{\gamma})$, where matrix $\mathbf{A}$ is defined in (13.13).

- *Sandwich formula* refers to the asymptotic covariance matrix of the M-estimator,

$$\text{cov}(\widehat{\boldsymbol{\gamma}}_N) \simeq \left(\sum_{i=1}^{N} E\frac{\partial \boldsymbol{\Psi}_i}{\partial \boldsymbol{\gamma}}\right)^{-1} \left(\sum_{i=1}^{N} E(\boldsymbol{\Psi}_i \boldsymbol{\Psi}_i')\right) \left(\sum_{i=1}^{N} E\frac{\partial \boldsymbol{\Psi}_i}{\partial \boldsymbol{\gamma}}\right)'^{-1}. \tag{13.14}$$

It is called "sandwich" because matrix $\mathbf{B}$ is between two matrices (Stefanski and Boos, 2002 call matrix $\mathbf{A}$ "bread" and matrix $\mathbf{B}$ "meat"). A *robust* (or empirical) version of the sandwich formula is

$$\text{cov}(\widehat{\boldsymbol{\gamma}}_N) \simeq \left(\sum_{i=1}^{N} \frac{\partial \widehat{\boldsymbol{\Psi}}_i}{\partial \boldsymbol{\gamma}} \right)^{-1} \left(\sum_{i=1}^{N} \widehat{\boldsymbol{\Psi}}_i \widehat{\boldsymbol{\Psi}}'_i \right) \left(\sum_{i=1}^{N} \frac{\partial \widehat{\boldsymbol{\Psi}}_i}{\partial \boldsymbol{\gamma}} \right)^{\prime-1}, \qquad (13.15)$$

where $\widehat{\boldsymbol{\Psi}}_i = \boldsymbol{\Psi}(\mathbf{y}_i, \widehat{\boldsymbol{\gamma}}_N)$. This formula can be justified by the fact that due to the law of large numbers, $N^{-1} \sum_{i=1}^{N} \widehat{\boldsymbol{\Psi}}_i \widehat{\boldsymbol{\Psi}}'_i$ and $N^{-1} \sum_{i=1}^{N} \partial \widehat{\boldsymbol{\Psi}}_i / \partial \boldsymbol{\gamma}$ converge to $E(\boldsymbol{\Psi}\boldsymbol{\Psi}')$ and $E(\partial \boldsymbol{\Psi}/\partial \boldsymbol{\gamma})$. The advantage of the robust formula is that no expectation is taken and therefore no distribution assumption is involved.

13.1.5 Generalized estimating equations approach

Often, we are interested only in parameter $\boldsymbol{\beta}$, which is a part of the total vector parameter $\boldsymbol{\gamma} = (\boldsymbol{\beta}, \boldsymbol{\theta})$. For example, following our notation, $\boldsymbol{\beta}$ is the vector of mixed model coefficients (major interest) and $\boldsymbol{\theta}$ is the random effects variance parameter (minor interest, or nuisance parameter). If there exists a (perhaps simplified) estimator $\widetilde{\boldsymbol{\theta}}$ and $\boldsymbol{\beta}$ is estimated by maximum likelihood, the pseudo-MLE may be employed. In this section we move farther from ML by assuming that parameters are estimated using an estimating function as the solution to an equation.

The generalized estimating equations (GEE) approach is applied to the situation when there are two groups of parameters, $\boldsymbol{\beta}$ and $\boldsymbol{\theta}$. Parameter $\boldsymbol{\beta}$ is viewed as the primary parameter and parameter $\boldsymbol{\theta}$ as minor interest. $\boldsymbol{\beta}$ is estimated from an estimating equation where $\boldsymbol{\theta}$ is replaced by a consistent estimate $\widehat{\boldsymbol{\theta}}$, namely,

$$\sum_{i=1}^{N} \boldsymbol{\Psi}(\mathbf{y}_i, \boldsymbol{\beta}, \widehat{\boldsymbol{\theta}}) = \mathbf{0}. \qquad (13.16)$$

Thus, GEE can be viewed as a generalization of pseudo-MLE, where instead of the score equation, we use a different equation as an estimation device for the primary parameter. Generally, substitution of $\boldsymbol{\theta}$ with $\widehat{\boldsymbol{\theta}}$ should cause estimation of $\boldsymbol{\beta}$ to deteriorate, but in some special cases the asymptotic covariance matrix of GEE is the same as if the true $\boldsymbol{\theta}$ were used. Recall that for pseudo-MLE it was found that pseudo-MLE=MLE when $\mathcal{I}_{\boldsymbol{\beta}\boldsymbol{\theta}} = \mathbf{0}$. A similar condition requires that for the GEE approach,

$$E \frac{\partial \boldsymbol{\Psi}}{\partial \boldsymbol{\theta}} = \mathbf{0}. \qquad (13.17)$$

Namely, under (13.17), the substitution of a consistent estimator $\widehat{\boldsymbol{\theta}}$ in an estimating equation for parameter of interest $\boldsymbol{\beta}$ is equivalent to using the true $\boldsymbol{\theta}$. We illustrate GEE and condition (13.17) with a type II nonlinear marginal model of Section 6.3.

The Iteratively Reweighted Least Squares (IRLS) is a special case of GEE with the estimating equation

$$\sum_{i=1}^{N} \mathbf{K}'_i(\boldsymbol{\beta}, \boldsymbol{\theta})(\mathbf{y}_i - \mathbf{f}_i(\boldsymbol{\beta})) = \mathbf{0}; \qquad (13.18)$$

see Section 6.2.3 for more detail. The estimating equation (13.18) is unbiased because

$$E\frac{\partial \mathbf{K}_i'(\boldsymbol{\beta}, \boldsymbol{\theta})(\mathbf{y}_i - \mathbf{f}_i(\boldsymbol{\beta}))}{\partial \boldsymbol{\theta}} = \frac{\partial \mathbf{K}_i'(\boldsymbol{\beta}, \boldsymbol{\theta})}{\partial \boldsymbol{\theta}} E(\mathbf{y}_i - \mathbf{f}_i(\boldsymbol{\beta})) = \mathbf{0},$$

assuming that (a) the matrix $\mathbf{K}_i$ does not depend on observations $\mathbf{y}_i$, and (b) the model mean, $\mathbf{f}_i(\boldsymbol{\beta})$ does not depend on $\boldsymbol{\theta}$. Liang and Zeger (1986) effectively applied the GEE approach to a generalized linear model with repeated measurements (see Section 7.9).

13.2   Some formulas of matrix algebra

There are many excellent books on matrix algebra with a statistical emphasis: Searle (1982), Graybill (1983), Lancaster and Tismenetsky (1985), Fuller (1987), Magnus (1988), Harville (1997, 2001), Schott (1997), and Turkington (2002).

13.2.1   Some matrix identities

Throughout the book, several matrix identities are used. One of the advantages of those matrix formulas is the dimension-reduction feature, as in Section 2.2.3. The following set of formulas is borrowed from Smith (1973) and scattered through the books on matrix algebra mentioned above:

$$(\mathbf{D} + \mathbf{AB})^{-1} = \mathbf{D}^{-1} - \mathbf{D}^{-1}\mathbf{A}(\mathbf{I} + \mathbf{BD}^{-1}\mathbf{A})^{-1}\mathbf{BD}^{-1},$$

$$(\mathbf{D} + \mathbf{EFE'})^{-1} = \mathbf{D}^{-1} - \mathbf{D}^{-1}\mathbf{E}(\mathbf{E}'\mathbf{D}^{-1}\mathbf{E} + \mathbf{F}^{-1})^{-1}\mathbf{E}'\mathbf{D}^{-1},$$

$$(\mathbf{D} + \mathbf{B})^{-1} = \mathbf{D}^{-1} - \mathbf{D}^{-1}(\mathbf{D}^{-1} + \mathbf{B}^{-1})^{-1}\mathbf{D}^{-1},$$

$$(\mathbf{D} + \mathbf{B})^{-1}\mathbf{B} = \mathbf{I} - (\mathbf{D} + \mathbf{B})^{-1}\mathbf{D}.$$

For example, formula (2.21) follows from the second formula after letting $\mathbf{D} = \mathbf{I}$, $\mathbf{E} = \mathbf{Z}$, and $\mathbf{F} = \mathbf{D}$.

13.2.2   Formulas for generalized matrix inverse

Generalized matrix inverse is a generalization of the standard matrix inverse to singular/deficient and rectangular matrices. Several books cover the topic in depth, Albert (1972) and Rao (1973), amomg others. In this section we present some less known results on the computation of generalized matrix inverse and matrix functions. We have used generalized matrix inverse extensively in Chapters 2 and 3.

Let $\mathbf{Z}$ be any $n \times k$ matrix. We call a $k \times n$ matrix $\mathbf{Z}^-$ the generalized matrix inverse if $\mathbf{ZZ}^-\mathbf{Z} = \mathbf{Z}$. A matrix with this property is not unique. For example, if $\mathbf{Z} = \mathbf{z}$ is a vector column, then $\mathbf{z}^-$ is any vector-row such that $\mathbf{z}^-\mathbf{z} = 1$. Generalized inverse has a direct connection to the solution of an underspecified system of linear equations. If $\mathbf{Zx} = \mathbf{y}$ is a system of linear equations, where $\mathbf{x}$ is an unknown k-vector and $\mathbf{y}$ is a known n-vector, then $\mathbf{x} = \mathbf{Z}^-\mathbf{y}$ is a solution.

The Moore–Penrose inverse defines a *unique* generalized matrix inverse, $\mathbf{Z}^+$, with the following properties: (a) $\mathbf{ZZ}^+\mathbf{Z} = \mathbf{Z}$, (b) $\mathbf{Z}^+\mathbf{ZZ}^+ = \mathbf{Z}^+$, (c) matrix $\mathbf{ZZ}^+$ is symmetric, and (d) matrix $\mathbf{Z}^+\mathbf{Z}$ is symmetric. Since in this book we use only the Moore–Penrose generalized inverse, we call $\mathbf{Z}^+$ the generalized inverse, for brevity. The generalized inverse may be represented as a limit, $\mathbf{Z}^+ = \lim_{\rho \to 0} (\mathbf{Z}'\mathbf{Z}+\rho\mathbf{I})^{-1} \mathbf{Z}'$. In two special cases, the generalized inverse reduces to the standard matrix inverse. First, if $k = n$ and matrix $\mathbf{Z}$ is nonsingular ($|\mathbf{Z}| \neq 0$), then $\mathbf{Z}^+ = \mathbf{Z}^{-1}$. Second, if $k \leq n$ and matrix $\mathbf{Z}$ has full rank k, then $\mathbf{Z}^+ = (\mathbf{Z}'\mathbf{Z})^{-1}\mathbf{Z}'$. In particular, if $\mathbf{Z} = \mathbf{z}$, a vector, then $\mathbf{z}^+ = \mathbf{z}'/ \|\mathbf{z}\|^2$. Another distinctive property of the Moore–Penrose generalized inverse is that $\mathbf{x} = \mathbf{Z}^+\mathbf{y}$ is a solution of $\mathbf{Z}\mathbf{x} = \mathbf{y}$ with minimal length for $\mathbf{x}$.

Now we consider *computation* of the generalized inverse. First, let $\mathbf{Z}$ be a $k \times k$ symmetric matrix and $|\mathbf{Z}| = 0$. To fix the idea, we first assume that $\mathbf{Z}$ is diagonal, $\mathbf{Z} =\text{diag}(z_1, z_2, ..., z_k)$, possibly with some zero elements on the diagonal. Then $\mathbf{Z}^+ =\text{diag}(u_1, u_2, ..., u_k)$, where $u_j = 1/z_j$ if $z_j \neq 0$ and $u_j = 0$ otherwise. Now let $\mathbf{Z}$ be any symmetric matrix. Then from *eigenvalue decomposition,* we can represent $\mathbf{Z} = \mathbf{P}\mathbf{\Lambda}\mathbf{P}'$, where $\mathbf{P}$ is the orthogonal matrix and $\mathbf{\Lambda}$ is the diagonal matrix with eigenvalues of $\mathbf{Z}$ on the diagonal. Then $\mathbf{Z}^+ = \mathbf{P}\mathbf{\Lambda}^+\mathbf{P}'$; the proof is elementary. Second, let $\mathbf{Z}$ be any $n \times k$ matrix with $k \leq n$. Then it is easy to prove that $\mathbf{Z}^+ = (\mathbf{Z}'\mathbf{Z})^+\mathbf{Z}'$.

Eigenvalue decomposition allows us to find a matrix function such as the matrix square root. Indeed, let $\mathbf{M}$ be a (symmetric) nonnegative definite matrix. The square root, $\mathbf{N}$, is a nonnegative definite matrix such that $\mathbf{N}^2 = \mathbf{M}$. Using the notation $\mathbf{N} = \mathbf{M}^{1/2}$, it is easy to see that $\mathbf{M}^{1/2} = \mathbf{P}\mathbf{\Lambda}^{1/2}\mathbf{P}'$, where $\mathbf{\Lambda}^{1/2}$ is the diagonal matrix with square roots on the diagonal. Compare this with the Cholesky decomposition $\mathbf{M} = \mathbf{D}'\mathbf{D}$, where $\mathbf{D}$ is an upper triangular matrix (zero elements under the diagonal). The square root definition can be generalized to find other matrix functions using the rule $f(\mathbf{M}) = \mathbf{P}f(\mathbf{\Lambda})\mathbf{P}'$.

13.2.3 *Vec and vech functions; duplication matrix*

The vec operator/function is used to represent matrix $\mathbf{M}$ as a vector by stacking its vector columns. Thus, if $\mathbf{M}$ is a $k \times m$ matrix, $\text{vec}(\mathbf{M}) = (M_{11}, M_{21}, ..., M_{k1}, M_{12}, ..., M_{km})'$ is a $km \times 1$ vector. The vech operator/function is applied to a symmetric $k \times k$ matrix $\mathbf{M}$ by stacking elements of the matrix starting with the main diagonal, thus vech contains unique matrix elements, $\text{vech}(\mathbf{A}) = (A_{11}, A_{21}, ..., A_{k1}, A_{22}, ..., A_{kk})'$, the $k(k+1)/2 \times 1$ vector. These two functions are related via a linear operator that can be represented through the $k^2 \times k(k+1)/2$ *duplication* matrix $\mathcal{D}_k$: for any symmetric $k \times k$ matrix we have $\text{vec}(\mathbf{M}) =\mathcal{D}_k\text{vech}(\mathbf{M})$, as discussed in Section 3.3. An explicit formula for $\mathcal{D}_k$ is given by Magnus (1988): let $\mathbf{1}_i$ be the $k \times 1$ unit vector with zero components except the ith, which is 1, and let $\mathbf{u}_{ij}$ $(i \geq j)$ be the $k(k+1)/2 \times 1$ unit vector with one at position $(j-1)k + i - j(j-1)/2$. Create matrix $\mathbf{E}_{ij} = \mathbf{1}_i\mathbf{1}_j'$ and define the $k \times k$ matrix $\mathbf{T}_{ij} = \mathbf{E}_{ij} + \mathbf{E}_{ji}$ if $i \neq j$ and $\mathbf{T}_{ii} = \mathbf{E}_{ii}$ if $i = j$. Then $\mathcal{D}_k = \sum_{i \geq j}\text{vec}(\mathbf{T}_{ij})\mathbf{u}_{ij}'$. We have used the duplication matrix throughout the book, starting with Section 3.3, where matrix $\mathcal{D}_k^+$ was introduced: for any symmetric matrix $\mathbf{M}$, we have $\text{vech}(\mathbf{M}) =\mathcal{D}_k^+\text{vec}(\mathbf{M})$. Many matrix operations, such as differentiation, are carried out through the vec function. However, when it comes to computing the covariance matrix, one needs to deal with unique elements of the matrix, and then the vech function is applied. The simplest formula using vec is associated with the trace function:

$$\text{tr}(\mathbf{A}\mathbf{B}) =\text{vec}'(\mathbf{A})\text{vec}(\mathbf{B}). \tag{13.19}$$

The Kronecker product of an $n \times m$ and a $k \times p$ matrix $\mathbf{A}$ and $\mathbf{B}$, is denoted by $\mathbf{A} \otimes \mathbf{B}$. This is an $(nk) \times (mp)$ matrix with the (i,j) block $A_{ij}\mathbf{B}$, where $i = 1, ..., n$ and $j = 1, ..., m$. We can represent the vec of the matrix product via the Kronecker product as

$$\text{vec}(\mathbf{ABC}) = (\mathbf{C}' \otimes \mathbf{A})\text{vec}(\mathbf{B}). \tag{13.20}$$

Sometimes we use a corollary of this formula: $\text{vec}(\mathbf{AB}) = \text{vec}(\mathbf{ABI}) = (\mathbf{I} \otimes \mathbf{A})\text{vec}(\mathbf{B})$ or $\text{vec}(\mathbf{AB}) = \text{vec}(\mathbf{IAB}) = (\mathbf{B}' \otimes \mathbf{I})\text{vec}(\mathbf{A})$. It is easy to show that

$$\mathbf{ab}' = \mathbf{b}' \otimes \mathbf{a} = \mathbf{a} \otimes \mathbf{b}', \quad \text{vec}(\mathbf{ab}') = \mathbf{b} \otimes \mathbf{a} \tag{13.21}$$

for vectors $\mathbf{a}$ and $\mathbf{b}$. The trace of four matrices is linked with the vec operator and Kronecker product through the formula

$$\text{tr}(\mathbf{ABCD}) = \text{vec}'(\mathbf{D})(\mathbf{A} \otimes \mathbf{C}')\text{vec}(\mathbf{B}'). \tag{13.22}$$

We use the following properties of the Kronecker product:

$$
\begin{aligned}
(\mathbf{A} \otimes \mathbf{B})' &= \mathbf{A}' \otimes \mathbf{B}', & (13.23) \\
(\mathbf{A} \otimes \mathbf{B})^{-1} &= \mathbf{A}^{-1} \otimes \mathbf{B}^{-1}, & (13.24) \\
(\mathbf{A} \otimes \mathbf{B})(\mathbf{C} \otimes \mathbf{D}) &= \mathbf{AC} \otimes \mathbf{BD}, & (13.25) \\
\text{tr}(\mathbf{A} \otimes \mathbf{B}) &= \text{tr}(\mathbf{A})\text{tr}(\mathbf{B}), & (13.26) \\
|\mathbf{A} \otimes \mathbf{B}| &= |\mathbf{A}|^k |\mathbf{B}|^p, & (13.27)
\end{aligned}
$$

where matrices are properly defined. In particular, in the last identity it is assumed that matrix $\mathbf{A}$ is $k \times k$ and matrix $\mathbf{B}$ is $p \times p$.

As an illustration of the vec and vech operators, we solve the Lyapunov equation $\mathbf{XA} + \mathbf{AX} = \mathbf{B}$, where all matrices are square and we want to solve for $\mathbf{X}$. Applying the vec operator to an equivalent equation $\mathbf{IXA} + \mathbf{AXI} = \mathbf{B}$ and using identity (13.20), we obtain the linear equation

$$(\mathbf{A}' \otimes \mathbf{I})\text{vec}(\mathbf{X}) + (\mathbf{I} \otimes \mathbf{A})\text{vec}(\mathbf{X}) = \text{vec}(\mathbf{B}).$$

Solving this equation, we obtain $\text{vec}(\mathbf{X}) = (\mathbf{A}' \otimes \mathbf{I} + \mathbf{I} \otimes \mathbf{A})^{-1}\text{vec}(\mathbf{B})$. If matrices $\mathbf{A}$ and $\mathbf{B}$ are symmetric, then matrix $\mathbf{X}$ is symmetric as well. Using the same method, the vec operation transforms an equation $\sum \mathbf{A}_i \mathbf{X} \mathbf{A}_i = \mathbf{B}$ to a linear equation for $\text{vec}(\mathbf{X})$. We solved a similar equation in Section 3.11 when the Method of Moments (MM) estimator was considered.

The commutation matrix $\mathbf{K}_n$ is defined as an $n^2 \times n^2$ matrix such that $\mathbf{K}_n \text{vec}(\mathbf{M}) = \text{vec}(\mathbf{M}')$ for every $n \times n$ matrix $\mathbf{M}$. Magnus (1988) provides an explicit expression $\mathbf{K}_n = \sum_{i,j} \mathbf{H}_{ij} \otimes \mathbf{H}'_{ij}$, where $\mathbf{H}_{ij}$ is the $n \times n$ matrix with 1 in the (i,j)th position and zeros elsewhere. For the commutation matrix, $\mathbf{K}_n(\mathbf{A} \otimes \mathbf{B}) = (\mathbf{B} \otimes \mathbf{A})\mathbf{K}_n$, where $\mathbf{A}$ and $\mathbf{B}$ have the same size, which justifies the name of this matrix. We have used the commutation matrix in Sections 3.3 and 3.10.3.

13.2.4 Matrix differentiation

An easy introduction to matrix differentiation with statistical applications is given in a paper by Wand (2002).

If the matrix $\mathbf{M} = \mathbf{M}(\rho)$ is a function of a scalar, the matrix derivative is simply $d\mathbf{M}/d\rho = \{dM_{ij}/d\rho, i = 1, ..., m, j = 1, ..., n\}$. For example, using the formula $d\mathbf{M}^\alpha/d\rho = \alpha\mathbf{M}^{\alpha-1}(d\mathbf{M}/d\rho)$, we can prove that $f(\rho) = \mathbf{a}'(\mathbf{A}+\rho\mathbf{I})^{-1}\mathbf{a}$ is a decreasing function, where $\mathbf{A}$ is a positive definite matrix. Indeed, $df/d\rho = -\mathbf{a}'(\mathbf{A}+\rho\mathbf{I})^{-2}\mathbf{a} < 0$ for $\mathbf{a} \neq \mathbf{0}$.

To define matrix differentiation with respect to a vector or matrix, we represent the matrix as a vector using the vec function. Let $\mathbf{A}$ and $\mathbf{B}$ be any arbitrary $m \times n$ and $k \times p$ matrices assuming that $\mathbf{A}$ is a function of $\mathbf{B}$; then we define

$$\frac{\partial \mathbf{A}}{\partial \mathbf{B}} = \frac{\partial \text{vec}(\mathbf{A})}{\partial \text{vec}(\mathbf{B})},$$

an $mn \times kp$ matrix. Let $\mathbf{C}$ be an $n \times g$ matrix function; then, using formula (13.20) the chain rule for matrix differentiation takes the form

$$\frac{\partial \mathbf{AC}}{\partial \mathbf{B}} = \frac{\partial \text{vec}(\mathbf{A})}{\partial \text{vec}(\mathbf{B})}(\mathbf{C}' \otimes \mathbf{I}_m) + (\mathbf{I}_g \otimes \mathbf{A})\frac{\partial \text{vec}(\mathbf{C})}{\partial \text{vec}(\mathbf{B})}, \qquad (13.28)$$

where $\mathbf{I}$ is an identity matrix of the appropriate size. As an application of the chain rule formula, we find that

$$\frac{\partial (\mathbf{I} + \mathbf{ZDZ}')}{\partial \mathbf{D}} = \frac{\partial \text{vec}(\mathbf{ZDZ}')}{\partial \text{vec}(\mathbf{D})} = \mathbf{Z} \otimes \mathbf{Z}. \qquad (13.29)$$

Using formula (13.19), we obtain the chain rule for trace,

$$\frac{\partial \text{tr}(\mathbf{AC})}{\partial \mathbf{B}} = \left(\frac{\partial \text{vec}(\mathbf{A})}{\partial \text{vec}(\mathbf{B})}\right)' \text{vec}(\mathbf{C}) + \left(\frac{\partial \text{vec}(\mathbf{C})}{\partial \text{vec}(\mathbf{B})}\right)' \text{vec}(\mathbf{A}).$$

Another application of the chain rule applies to the formula for the derivative of the inverse:

$$\begin{aligned}
\mathbf{0} &= \frac{\partial (\mathbf{MM}^{-1})}{\partial \mathbf{M}} = (\mathbf{M}'^{-1} \otimes \mathbf{I})\frac{\partial \text{vec}(\mathbf{M})}{\partial \text{vec}(\mathbf{M})} + (\mathbf{I} \otimes \mathbf{M})\frac{\partial \text{vec}(\mathbf{M}^{-1})}{\partial \text{vec}(\mathbf{M})} \\
&= (\mathbf{M}'^{-1} \otimes \mathbf{I}) + (\mathbf{I} \otimes \mathbf{M})\frac{\partial \text{vec}(\mathbf{M}^{-1})}{\partial \text{vec}(\mathbf{M})}, \qquad (13.30)
\end{aligned}$$

which finally yields $\partial \text{vec}(\mathbf{M}^{-1})/\partial \text{vec}(\mathbf{M}) = -\mathbf{M}'^{-1} \otimes \mathbf{M}^{-1}$. Analogously, we can derive

$$\frac{\partial \text{vec}(\mathbf{V}^{-1})}{\partial \boldsymbol{\theta}} = -(\mathbf{V}^{-1} \otimes \mathbf{V}^{-1})\frac{\partial \text{vec}(\mathbf{V})}{\partial \boldsymbol{\theta}}, \qquad (13.31)$$

where $\boldsymbol{\theta}$ is a vector. If $\mathbf{M} = \mathbf{M}(\boldsymbol{\theta})$ is a symmetric matrix as a function of vector argument $\boldsymbol{\theta}$, then $\partial \text{tr}\mathbf{M}^{-1}/\partial \boldsymbol{\theta} = (\partial \text{vec}(\mathbf{M})/\partial \boldsymbol{\theta})' \text{vec}(\mathbf{M}^{-2})$. Another application of (13.28) in conjunction with (13.30) gives

$$\begin{aligned}
\frac{\partial (\mathbf{I} + \mathbf{ZDZ}')^{-1}}{\partial \mathbf{D}} &= -\mathbf{V}^{-1}\mathbf{Z} \otimes \mathbf{V}^{-1}\mathbf{Z}, \\
\frac{\partial \mathbf{Z}'(\mathbf{I} + \mathbf{ZDZ}')^{-1}\mathbf{Z}}{\partial \mathbf{D}} &= -\mathbf{Z}'\mathbf{V}^{-1}\mathbf{Z} \otimes \mathbf{Z}'\mathbf{V}^{-1}\mathbf{Z},
\end{aligned}$$

where $\mathbf{V} = \mathbf{I} + \mathbf{ZDZ}'$.

We use several formulas for determinant differentiation. A general formula has the form

$$\frac{\partial \ln |\mathbf{A}|}{\partial \mathbf{B}} = \left(\frac{\partial \text{vec}(\mathbf{A})}{\partial \text{vec}(\mathbf{B})} \right)' \text{vec}(\mathbf{A}^{-1}). \tag{13.32}$$

In a special case when $\mathbf{A} = \mathbf{A}(b)$, where b is a scalar, we have

$$\frac{d \ln |\mathbf{A}|}{db} = \text{vec}' \left(\frac{d\mathbf{A}}{db} \right) \text{vec}(\mathbf{A}^{-1}) = \text{tr} \left(\mathbf{A}^{-1} \frac{d\mathbf{A}}{db} \right).$$

For example, as follows from (13.29),

$$\frac{\partial \ln |\mathbf{I} + \mathbf{ZDZ}'|}{\partial \mathbf{D}} = (\mathbf{Z}' \otimes \mathbf{Z}')\text{vec}(\mathbf{V}^{-1}) = \text{vec}(\mathbf{Z}'\mathbf{V}^{-1}\mathbf{Z}).$$

We use matrix differentiation extensively in Chapter 7, where the Total GEE is introduced.

13.3   Basic facts of optimization theory

Optimization is an important part of statistics. Nonlinear least squares and maximum likelihood estimation are the most common examples of optimization statistical problems. Knowing the basics of optimization theory is a must for a deep understanding of how algorithms work and the reasons for their failure. Typically, optimization theory is overlooked in statistical courses. The aim of this section is to provide basic facts on optimization with a statistical emphasis. More information on optimization theory may be obtained from the books by Ortega and Rheinboldt (1970), Polak (1971), and Dennis and Schnabel (1983).

Optimization problems can be classified by two features: domain of optimization (continuous or integer) and constrained/unconstrained optimization. Paradoxically, integer optimization is usually more difficult than continuous optimization. This is because the solution to an integer optimization problem often requires straightforward enumeration, whereas continuous optimization may be solved iteratively. For example, minimization (or maximization) of a linear function under linear constraints is called linear programming. Here we discuss only continuous optimization problems. First we discuss the unconstrained problem, and then we touch briefly on the unconstrained optimization.

Let $F = F(\mathbf{u})$ be a continuous function of $\mathbf{u} \in R^m$. Maximization and minimization are equivalent optimization problems because maximization of $F(\mathbf{u})$ is equivalent to minimization of $-F(\mathbf{u})$. Thus, without loss of generality, it will be assumed that we want to find a minimum of F on R^m. Classical minimization theory is developed for convex function F. We say that F is strongly *convex* ($\cup$-shaped) if for any $\mathbf{u}_1 \neq \mathbf{u}_2 \in R^m$, we have $F(\lambda \mathbf{u}_1 + (1-\lambda)\mathbf{u}_2) < \lambda F(\mathbf{u}_1) + (1-\lambda)F(\mathbf{u}_2)$ for all $0 < \lambda < 1$. We say that F is strongly *concave* ($\cap$-shaped) if $F(\lambda \mathbf{u}_1 + (1-\lambda)\mathbf{u}_2) > \lambda F(\mathbf{u}_1) + (1-\lambda)F(\mathbf{u}_2)$. To shorten, we omit the word *strongly*. An important feature of a convex function is that it has a unique minimum. Similarly, a concave function has a unique maximum. An example of a concave function is the log-likelihood function of a logistic or Poisson regression if the vectors of covariates have full rank, see Section 7.1. On the other hand, the log-likelihood function of the probit regression is not concave. There is a useful constructive criterion to check if a function is convex:

the Hessian (matrix of second derivatives), $\partial^2 F/\partial \mathbf{u}^2$ should be positive definite at any $\mathbf{u} \in R^m$. Therefore, if the Hessian is positive definite, the minimum is unique; if the negative Hessian is positive definite, the maximum is unique.

Unfortunately, it is quite rare that the optimized function is convex or concave. Even a log-likelihood function for an ordinary linear regression $\mathbf{y} = \mathbf{X}\boldsymbol{\beta} + \boldsymbol{\varepsilon}$, where $\boldsymbol{\varepsilon} \sim \mathcal{N}(\mathbf{0}, \sigma^2 \mathbf{I})$ and matrix $\mathbf{X}$ is of full rank, is not concave. Indeed, the log-likelihood function is $l(\boldsymbol{\theta}) = -0.5n \ln \sigma^2 - \|\mathbf{y} - \mathbf{X}\boldsymbol{\beta}\|^2 / \sigma^2$ with the $(m+1) \times (m+1)$ negative Hessian,

$$\mathbf{H} = \frac{1}{\sigma^6} \left[\begin{array}{cc} \sigma^4 \mathbf{X}'\mathbf{X} & -\sigma^2 \mathbf{X}'(\mathbf{y} - \mathbf{X}\boldsymbol{\beta}) \\ -\sigma^2 \mathbf{X}'(\mathbf{y} - \mathbf{X}\boldsymbol{\beta}) & \|\mathbf{y} - \mathbf{X}\boldsymbol{\beta}\|^2 - 0.5\sigma^2 n \end{array} \right]. \tag{13.33}$$

(Throughout the book, we use the notation $\mathbf{H}$ for the negative Hessian, $\mathbf{H} = -\partial^2 l/\partial \boldsymbol{\theta}^2$.) Obviously, matrix $\mathbf{H}$ is not always positive definite because, for example, the last element may be negative. This means that the log-likelihood function is not concave everywhere, although l has a unique maximum (MLE). However, l is concave on "average" in large samples. By this we mean that the *expected* matrix $\mathbf{H}$ is positive definite. Indeed, since $E \|\mathbf{y} - \mathbf{X}\boldsymbol{\beta}\|^2 = n\sigma^2$ and $E(\mathbf{y} - \mathbf{X}\boldsymbol{\beta}) = \mathbf{0}$, we have

$$E(\mathbf{H}) = \frac{1}{\sigma^6} \left[\begin{array}{cc} \sigma^4 \mathbf{X}'\mathbf{X} & \mathbf{0} \\ \mathbf{0}' & \frac{1}{2}\sigma^2 n \end{array} \right],$$

a positive definite matrix. The reader probably realizes that $E(\mathbf{H})$ is the Fisher information matrix, which is always nonnegative definite.

13.3.1   Criteria for unimodality

Using the standard approach to prove that a function has a unique minimum (is unimodal), one shows that the Hessian matrix is positive definite. As indicated above, the function may have a unique minimum and yet not have a positive definite Hessian. The following result of optimization theory is fundamental yet not well known (Demidenko, 1989, 2000).

Theorem 50 *(Criterion of unimodality). Let $F = F(\mathbf{u})$ be a twice-differentiable function of $\mathbf{u} \in R^m$ such that $\| \mathbf{u} \| \to \infty$ implies that $F(\mathbf{u}) \to \infty$. If at each point where the gradient is zero, the Hessian is positive definite, then F has a unique minimum on R^m (i.e., the function is unimodal).*

Principally, this theorem says that to check whether the function has a unique minimum (maximum), one needs to show that the (negative) Hessian is positive definite *only* on stationary points ($\partial F/\partial \mathbf{u} = \mathbf{0}$), not everywhere, as the standard theory suggests. The condition that F approach infinity when the argument goes to infinity can be facilitated.

To illustrate the criterion of unimodality, we apply it to the log-likelihood function of the ordinary linear regression considered in the previous subsection. We noticed that the negative Hessian (13.33) is not always positive definite, so l is not concave everywhere. However, using the criterion of unimodality, we now prove that l has a a unique maximum. For this we need to show that $\mathbf{H}$ is positive definite where $\partial l/\partial \boldsymbol{\beta} = \mathbf{0}$ and $\partial l/\partial \sigma^2 = 0$. The former equation implies that $\mathbf{X}'(\mathbf{y} - \mathbf{X}\boldsymbol{\beta}) = \mathbf{0}$, so that the off-diagonal block of $\mathbf{H}$ is zero. The latter equation implies that $\|\mathbf{y} - \mathbf{X}\boldsymbol{\beta}\|^2 = \sigma^2 n$, so that the last element is $\sigma^2 n/2 > 0$. Thus, $\mathbf{H}$ is positive definite where the gradient is zero, and therefore l is unimodal.

13.3.2 Criteria for global optimum

The theory of minimization (maximization) is built on an idealistic assumption that the function is convex (concave). This assumption rarely holds in practice, particularly in statistics. Indeed, as was shown at the beginning of this section, even the log-likelihood function of the ordinary linear regression model is not a concave function. On the other hand, the log-likelihood function of the generalized linear model is concave, Section 7.1.4. If the maximized function is not concave, it may have several maxima. Consequently, all algorithms considered in this book can find only a local maximum. Thus, a criterion which verifies that the maximum found is, indeed, the global one is very important. As shown by Demidenko (1989, 2000), there always exists a positive probability that the sum of squares in any nonlinear regression has at least two local minima. The problem of constructing a criterion for the global optimum is a difficult mathematical problem. Some ideas for constructing such criteria for a nonlinear regression, based on the concept of local convexity, have been developed by Demidenko (2000, 2006a, 2008). More curvature of the nonlinear regression increases the chance of encountering several local minima of the sum of squares (linear regression has zero curvature). The unimodality criterion in general form can be formulated as follows: if the value of the sum of squares is less than the minimum squared radius of the regression curvature, the local minimum that is found is the global one. Searle et al. (1992) warn that multiextremality of the log-likelihood function may emerge even in the simple variance components model. The problem of developing relevant criteria for mixed effects models awaits solution.

Since the existence of several minima (maxima) is a reality, good practical advice is to start the iterations from several different parameter values to confirm that they converge to the same point. As a word of caution, do not hurry to assert that the optimization problem has several local minima (maxima) if iterations stop at different locations. Usually, it merely means that the optimization algorithm failed. The gradient and angular criteria (see below) may clarify that the points found are not the local optima but just where the algorithm is stocked.

13.3.3 Criteria for minimum existence

Sometimes, an optimization problem does not have a solution. For example, if in logistic regression there exists $\boldsymbol{\beta}$ such that $\boldsymbol{\beta}'\mathbf{x}_i > 0$ for $y_i - 1$ and $\boldsymbol{\beta}'\mathbf{x}_i < 0$ for $y_i = 0$, the MLE goes to infinity despite the fact that the log-likelihood is concave. In this case, we say that a separation plane exists; constructive criteria to test whether such a plane exists are given in Section 7.10. Criteria for the existence of the optimum are essential and should be checked before launching an optimization process.

To be specific, let us discuss the minimization problem of $F(\mathbf{u})$, where $\mathbf{u} \in D$. Typically, F is a continuous function with continuous derivatives, and the domain of minimization, $D \subset R^m$, is a convex set. Minimization of F seeks a point $\mathbf{u}_*$ on D such that

$$F(\mathbf{u}_*) = \inf_{\mathbf{u} \in D} F(\mathbf{u}). \tag{13.34}$$

If D is a compact set (closed and bounded), then $\mathbf{u}_*$ exists, or more precisely, the infimum is attained. However, in statistics, D is seldom a compact set. For example, the domain of optimization often coincides with the entire space. To develop criteria for existence when $D = R^m$, Demidenko (1981, 1989, 2000) and Nakamura (1984) introduced the notion of the *existence level,*

$$\overline{F}_E = \lim_{r \to \infty} \inf_{\|\mathbf{u}\| \ge r} F(\mathbf{u}). \tag{13.35}$$

Since the function under the limit is a nondecreasing function of r, the limit always exists (it may be $+\infty$; then $\overline{F}_E = \infty$). Having the existence level, it is easy to verify the existence of the minimum: if there exists $\mathbf{u}_0$ such that $\mathbf{u}_0 < \overline{F}_E$, the minimization problem has a solution and $\mathbf{u}_*$ exists. Moreover, if an iteration process starts from $\mathbf{u}_0$, the sequence generated by a descending minimization algorithm, $F(\mathbf{u}_{s+1}) < F(\mathbf{u}_s)$, has at least one limiting point. In particular, if the function F approaches infinity at infinity ($\overline{F}_E = \infty$), any starting point would be successful in this sense. Examples of computation of the existence level for the sum of squares of nonlinear regressions of exponential types are given by Demidenko (1996). The criterion for the existence of the MLE in the linear mixed effects model is developed in Section 2.5. Generalization of the existence level to any convex set D may be found in Demidenko (1989).

13.3.4   Optimization algorithms in statistics

Since minimization of $-F$ is equivalent to maximization of F, without loss of generality, we discuss maximization algorithms. We also refer the reader to Section 2.8, where the algorithms are discussed in the framework of the log-likelihood maximization for the linear mixed effects model. To simplify, we shall assume that the domain of maximization is the entire space R^m, *unconstrained optimization.* At the end of this section we briefly discuss *constrained optimization.*

We classify the optimization algorithms in five categories: (1) Newton–Raphson (NR), (2) Fisher scoring (FS), (3) Empirical Fisher scoring (EFS), (4) Fixed-Point (FP), and (5) Expectation-Maximization (EM). The first three groups iterate as

$$\mathbf{u}_{s+1} = \mathbf{u}_s + \lambda_s \mathbf{H}_s^{-1} \mathbf{g}_s, \tag{13.36}$$

where s is the iteration index, $\mathbf{H}_s$ is a positive definite matrix, $\mathbf{g}_s$ is the gradient of F, namely, $\mathbf{g}_s = \partial F(\mathbf{u} = \mathbf{u}_s)/\partial \mathbf{u}$ evaluated at $\mathbf{u} = \mathbf{u}_s$; and λ_s is a positive scalar, the step length, $0 < \lambda_s \le 1$ used to ensure that at each iteration $F(\mathbf{u}_{s+1}) > F(\mathbf{u}_s)$. Usually, we start from $\lambda_s = 1$ and halve it until the function value becomes greater than at the preceding iteration. As follows from multivariate calculus, for any positive definite matrix $\mathbf{H}_s$ there exists a positive λ_s that increases F if $\mathbf{g}_s \ne \mathbf{0}$. The last two algorithms have the recurrence form

$$\mathbf{u}_{s+1} = \mathbf{R}(\mathbf{u}_s). \tag{13.37}$$

The distinction between (13.36) and (13.37) is somewhat ambiguous because (13.37) can be rewritten in the form (13.36) as $\mathbf{u}_{s+1} = \mathbf{u}_s + \boldsymbol{\delta}_s$, letting $\boldsymbol{\delta}_s = \mathbf{R}(\mathbf{u}_s) - \mathbf{u}_s$. As follows from (13.36), if iterations converge, they converge to a stationary point, i.e., where the gradient vanishes. Indeed, taking the limit of (13.36) as $s \to \infty$, we obtain $\mathbf{u}_* = \mathbf{u}_* + \lambda_* \mathbf{H}_*^{-1} \mathbf{g}_*$, which implies that $\mathbf{g}_* = \mathbf{g}(\mathbf{u}_*)$, where $\lim_{s \to \infty} \mathbf{u}_s = \mathbf{u}_*$. The algorithms mentioned may also be used for an iterative solution of the system of nonlinear equations $\mathbf{g}(\mathbf{u}) = \mathbf{0}$, e.g., estimating equations discussed in Sections 7.9. The algorithms are supposed to increase the function value from iteration to iteration (ascending algorithms), which ensures that iterations do not diverge. In fact, if the starting point $\mathbf{u}_0$ is such that the level set $\{\mathbf{u} : F(\mathbf{u}) \ge F(\mathbf{u}_0)\}$ is compact (bounded), sequence $\{\mathbf{u}_s\}$ generated by (13.36) or (13.37) has at least one limit point. A characteristic feature of the EM algorithm is that it ensures an increase in the likelihood function value so that the step length is redundant.

Below, we consider these algorithms and their modifications in some detail and indicate where we have applied them.

Newton–Raphson (NR). For this algorithm $\mathbf{H} = -\partial \mathbf{g}/\partial \mathbf{u} = -\partial^2 F/\partial \mathbf{u}^2$, assuming that this matrix is positive definite. In fact, it is quite rare that this is true for all $\mathbf{u}$ (then F would be concave). However, one can expect positive definiteness in the neighborhood of a maximum. The condition that $\mathbf{H}$ must be positive definite is a major limitation of this algorithm. Several remedies have been suggested. For example, following Marquardt (1963), one may replace $\mathbf{H}$ with $\mathbf{H}+\mu\mathbf{I}$, where μ is a positive number decreasing to zero as the algorithm progresses (Dennis and Schnabel, 1983). In fact, any approximation of $\mathbf{H}$ may work if the approximate matrix is positive definite. The NR algorithm is especially efficient for concave maximization or in the close neighborhood of the maximum. To illustrate, we apply this algorithm to an iterative solution of the univariate nonlinear equation $g(u) = 0$ on $(-\infty, \infty)$. We assume that the first derivative of the function is positive and the second derivative is negative (the function g is concave, $\cap$-shaped). Also, we assume that $\lim_{u \to \infty} g(u) > 0$ and $\lim_{u \to -\infty} g(u) < 0$, provided that the existence of the solution $u_* : g(u_*) = 0$. Since g is an increasing function, the solution is unique. Let $h(u)$ be another function such that $h(u) \geq g(u)$ and the equation $h(u) = 0$ is easy to solve. Let u_0 be the solution to the latter equation. Then, Newton's iterations $u_{s+1} = u_s + g(u_s)/g'(u_s)$ converge monotonically, $u_s \uparrow u_*$, $s = 0, 1, \ldots$ In fact, one may prove that iterations $u_{s+1} = u_s + g(u_s)/K$ converge monotonically, too, where constant K is an upper bound of $-g'(u)$, namely, $K > -g'(u)$. We have applied this algorithm to VARLINK estimation of the logistic regression with random intercepts in Section 7.3.5. One can generalize this method to multivariate $\mathbf{u}$ by finding an upper bound matrix for $\mathbf{H}$. Thus, if there exists a positive definite matrix $\mathbf{K}$ such that $\mathbf{H} \leq \mathbf{K}$, then (13.36) transforms into $\mathbf{u}_{s+1} = \mathbf{u}_s + \lambda_s \mathbf{K}^{-1} \mathbf{g}_s$. An advantage of this algorithm is that it does not require computation of second derivatives at each iteration; moreover, matrix $\mathbf{K}$ can be inverted just once. We applied this idea to the probit model of Section 7.1.5; the algorithm was called unit step. Although the NR algorithm has a fast convergence in a close neighborhood of the maximum, it requires computation of second derivatives and may fail when the starting point is far from the maximum, so that $\mathbf{H}$ is not positive definite.

Fisher scoring (FS). As mentioned above, the requirement for matrix $\mathbf{H}$ is to be positive definite. If the maximized function is the log-likelihood, one may take matrix $\mathbf{H}$ to be the expected negative Hessian or information matrix. This gives the FS algorithm. Therefore, the FS algorithm may be viewed as the expected NR algorithm, or symbolically, FS $= E(\text{NR})$. There are two major advantages of this algorithm: (a) matrix $\mathbf{H}$ is always positive definite, and (b) $\mathbf{H}^{-1}$ at the final iteration gives the asymptotic covariance matrix of estimated parameters. The FS algorithm for nonlinear regression coincides with the Gauss–Newton algorithm and Iteratively Reweighted Least Squares (IRLS) for the Generalized Linear Model (GLM). See Section 2.11, where this algorithm was applied to the linear mixed effects model; Section 6.2.3, where the nonlinear marginal mixed model was estimated; Section 7.1.4, where the log-likelihood function for GLM was maximized; and Section 7.9, where GEE was applied to clustered GLM. To illustrate the equivalence between IRLS and FS, we consider the problem of estimating parameters of the weighted linear regression using the estimating equation $\sum_{i=1}^{n} \mathbf{x}_i (y_i -$

$\mathbf{x}'_i\boldsymbol{\beta})w_i(\boldsymbol{\beta}) =0$, where w_i is the weight. Since $E(y_i - \mathbf{x}'_i\boldsymbol{\beta}) =0$, the FS algorithm is $\boldsymbol{\beta}_{s+1} = \boldsymbol{\beta}_s + (\mathbf{X}'\mathbf{W}_s\mathbf{X})^{-1}\mathbf{X}'\mathbf{W}_s(\mathbf{y} - \mathbf{X}\boldsymbol{\beta}_s)$, where $\mathbf{W}_s$ is the $n \times n$ diagonal matrix with $W_{ii}(\boldsymbol{\beta}) =w_i(\boldsymbol{\beta})$. After some algebra, we see that these iterations can be rewritten as $\boldsymbol{\beta}_{s+1} = (\mathbf{X}'\mathbf{W}_s\mathbf{X})^{-1}\mathbf{X}'\mathbf{W}_s\mathbf{y}$. But this is IRLS, which at the sth iteration uses the least squares estimate with the weights from the previous iteration. We prefer this algorithm over other algorithms for the log-likelihood maximization or estimating equation solution. It is almost as fast as NR but more reliable because matrix $\mathbf{H}$ is always positive definite.

Empirical Fisher scoring (EFS). From standard asymptotic theory, it follows that $-E(\partial^2 l/\partial\boldsymbol{\theta}^2) = E(\partial l/\partial\boldsymbol{\theta})(\partial l/\partial\boldsymbol{\theta})'$. Thus, instead of taking the expectation, we can estimate the information matrix empirically using only first derivatives. If $\mathbf{d}_i$ denotes the vector of first derivatives of the log-likelihood, iterations (13.36) take the form $\mathbf{u}_{s+1} = \mathbf{u}_s +\lambda_s \left(\sum \mathbf{d}_i\mathbf{d}'_i\right)^{-1}\sum \mathbf{d}_i$, or in matrix notation, $\mathbf{u}_{s+1} = \mathbf{u}_s +\lambda_s(\mathbf{D}'\mathbf{D})^{-1}\mathbf{D}'\mathbf{1}$, where $\mathbf{D}$ is the $n \times m$ matrix with the ith row $\mathbf{d}'_i$. We applied this algorithm for maximum likelihood maximization of logistic regression with random intercepts in Section 7.3.1 and the Fixed Sample Likelihood (FSL) approach of Section 7.8.3. The advantage of the EFS maximization algorithm is that we do not need to compute the second derivatives, and when the sample size is relatively large (say, > 30) this algorithm works as efficiently as the exact version does.

Fixed-Point (FP). This algorithm solves a system of nonlinear equations $\mathbf{g}(\mathbf{u}) = \mathbf{0}$ by recurrence formula (13.37). For a general discussion of this algorithm and, particularly, the contraction-mapping theorem we refer the reader to a classic book by Ortega and Rheinboldt (1970). There are many ways to represent $\mathbf{g}(\mathbf{u}) = \mathbf{0}$ equivalently as $\mathbf{u} = \mathbf{R}(\mathbf{u})$. The solution is the fixed point of the mapping $\mathbf{R} : R^m \to R^m$, which explains the name of the algorithm. The following fact for the univariate case may serve as a guideline for finding a successful fixed-point representation of the original equation. Let $R(u)$ be an increasing function such that $R(0) > 0$ and $\lim_{u\to\infty} R(u) = R_*$ exists. Then the equation $u = R(u)$ has a unique solution u_* in the interval $(0, R_*)$. If the starting point is zero, $u_0 = 0$, the fixed-point iterations $u_{s+1} = R(u_s)$ converge to u_* from below, $u_s \uparrow u_*$. If $u_0 = R_*$, then $u_s \downarrow u_*$ as $s \to \infty$. Note that a necessary condition for R to be an increasing function is $R(0) < R(\infty)$.

To illustrate the FP algorithm, we show how to iteratively find a positive solution, u, to a quadratic equation $u^2 + pu = q$, where p and q are positive constants. Let t be any number such that $t \geq q/p$. Then, letting $R(u) = (q + tu)/(p + t + u)$, we see that the equation $u = R(u)$ is equivalent to the original equation. Also, it is elementary to check that letting $t = q/p$, we obtain $R(0) = q/(p + t) > 0$, $R' > 0$ and $\lim_{u\to\infty} R(u) = t > R(0)$. If we start from $u_0 = 0$, the FP iterations produce an increasing sequence; if we start from $u_0 = t$, the sequence is decreasing. We can obtain function R by rewriting the original quadratic equation as $u_0 u + (p + t)u = q + tu_0$ and solving for u.

In a simpler example, we want to iteratively find the square root of a positive number, $u^2 = q$. Let t be a positive number, then the equation can be rewritten as $u = R(u)$, where

$$R(u) = \frac{q + tu}{t + u}.$$

The function R is increasing if and only if $R(0) = q/t < R(\infty) = t$. Thus, constant t should be chosen such that $t^2 > q$, to ensure convergence of the FP iterations. This method is used below to solve a matrix quadratic equation.

Let $\mathbf{Q}$ be a symmetric positive definite matrix and we want to find a symmetric positive definite matrix $\mathbf{U}$ such that $\mathbf{U}^2 = \mathbf{Q}$, the matrix square root. Higham (1986) developed Newton's iterations to solve the matrix quadratic equation $\mathbf{U}^2 = \mathbf{Q}$ without assuming that $\mathbf{Q}$ is symmetric. A noniterative solution based on the eigenvalue decomposition was mentioned in Section 13.2.2. Here we suggest FP iterations without the eigenvalue solution. Letting $\mathbf{T} = \sqrt{\mathrm{tr}(\mathbf{Q})}\mathbf{I}$, we represent the original equation as $\mathbf{U} = \mathbf{R}(\mathbf{U})$, where

$$\mathbf{R}(\mathbf{U}) = (\mathbf{TU} + \mathbf{Q})(\mathbf{T} + \mathbf{U})^{-1},$$

suitable for FP iterations. This choice of $\mathbf{T}$ guarantees that $\mathbf{R}(\mathbf{0}) = \mathbf{QT}^{-1} < \mathbf{R}(\infty) = \mathbf{T}$ and all $\mathbf{U}$ have the same eigenvectors as matrix $\mathbf{Q}$. This method can be generalized to solve more complicated matrix equations. We used the FP algorithm for the LME model in Section 2.12 and for the Poisson model with random intercepts in Section 7.5.9.

Expectation-Maximization (EM) algorithm is suitable for the likelihood maximization of a hierarchical model. The algorithm was originally introduced by Dempster et al. (1977) on a systematic basis, although particular applications had been known before. See McLachlan and Krishnan (1996) for various extensions and modifications. In particular, we refer the reader to a review paper by Hunter and Lange (2004) where the EM algorithm is viewed in a more general framework of the MM (Minorization–Maximization or Majorization–Minimization) algorithm. The EM algorithm gained much popularity in problems with missing data (Little, 2002). The advantage of the EM algorithm is that it generates parameter values with increasing log-likelihood values. Disadvantages are: (a) that it can be applied only to problems where the expectation is obtained exactly (in closed-form), and (b) that it does not automatically produce an estimate of the asymptotic covariance matrix, so additional computations are required.

13.3.5 *Necessary condition for optimization and criteria for convergence*

If function $F(\mathbf{u})$, $u \in R^m$ has a local minimum or maximum at $\mathbf{u}_0$, the first derivative vanishes at $\mathbf{u}_0$. Sometimes this is called a first-order condition and $\mathbf{u}_0$ is called a *stationary* point. If the derivative, $\mathbf{g} = \partial F/\partial \mathbf{u}$ is zero at $\mathbf{u}_0$ but the function value is neither maximum nor minimum, the point is called a *saddle* point. Since the majority of optimization algorithms have the form (13.36), one may stock at a stationary point; however, the chance is slim (it is possible to show that, excluding pathological cases, the probability of stocking at a saddle point is zero). A good check is to compute the Hessian $\partial^2 F/\partial \mathbf{u}^2 = -\mathbf{H}$: If $\mathbf{u}_0$ is a stationary point and $\mathbf{H}$ is positive definite, a maximum is attained; if $\mathbf{u}_0$ is a point of minimum, $\mathbf{H}$ is negative definite. It is important to remember that the first-order condition holds only for unconstrained optimization. For example, if the function $F(u) = 1 - u^2$ is maximized on $D = \{u : u \geq 1\}$, the point $u = 1$ is maximum but the derivative is not zero. However, if the maximum is attained at an open point of D, the first-order condition works again. If the maximum lies on the boundary, the first-order condition should be replaced by the Kuhn–Tucker condition, see Section 2.15.5.

Next we briefly discuss convergence or stopping criteria. Typically, iterations converge when the change, $|\Delta x|$, is small. What is small? It is better to express the convergence in terms of the *relative* change, $|\Delta x|/(1+|x|)$. Indeed, if $|x|$ close to zero, the change is $|\Delta x|$; if $|x|$ is large, the change is relative to the absolute value of x.

The relative change criterion can be applied to the argument, function value, or gradient. Let $\varepsilon = 10^{-p}$, where, say, $p = 5$. If s and $s + 1$ are two consecutive iterations, then in terms of the function value, convergence holds if $|F_{s+1} - F_s|/(1 + |F_s|) < \varepsilon$. If $|u_{s+1,j} - u_{s,j}|/(1 + |u_{s,j}|) < \varepsilon$ for $j = 1, ..., m$, we say that convergence holds in terms of the argument or parameter. The value p is interpreted as the number of coinciding digits at the two consecutive iterations, so letting $p = 5$ would mean that the first five digits for all parameter values are the same. The same relative criterion can be applied to the gradient,

$$\frac{|\|\mathbf{g}_{s+1}\| - \|\mathbf{g}_s\||}{1 + \|\mathbf{g}_s\|} < \varepsilon.$$

Note that if the log-likelihood function of a mixed model is maximized, the gradient involves all parameters, including the variance parameters of the mixed model.

When the minimization function is the sum of squares, there is an *angular* criterion for convergence with a clear geometrical interpretation (Bates and Watts, 1988; Demidenko, 1989). Geometrically, if the sum of squares, $S(\boldsymbol{\beta}) = \|\mathbf{y} - \mathbf{f}(\boldsymbol{\beta})\|^2$, attains its minimum at $\widehat{\boldsymbol{\beta}}$, the residual vector, $\mathbf{e} = \mathbf{y} - \mathbf{f}(\widehat{\boldsymbol{\beta}})$, is orthogonal to the tangent plane specified by the matrix of first derivatives, $\mathbf{F} = \partial \mathbf{f}/\partial \boldsymbol{\beta}$. Symbolically, we write $\mathbf{e} \perp \mathbf{F}_j$, where $\mathbf{F}_j$ is the jth vector column of matrix $\mathbf{F}$. For a better interpretation we can compute the cosine angle between $\mathbf{e}$ and $\mathbf{F}_j$ as

$$q_j = \frac{\mathbf{e}'\mathbf{F}_j}{\|\mathbf{e}\| \|\mathbf{F}_j\|}, \quad j = 1, 2, ..., m.$$

Due to the fact that $\sin \alpha \simeq \alpha$ for small α, we interpret q_j as the deviation from the right angle.

We can adapt this approach to the marginal model of Chapter 6 with the estimating equation $\mathbf{F}'\mathbf{V}^{-1}(\mathbf{y} - \mathbf{f}(\boldsymbol{\theta})) = \mathbf{0}$. Letting $\mathbf{K} = \mathbf{V}^{-1}\mathbf{F}$, the equation is rewritten as $\mathbf{K}'(\mathbf{y} - \mathbf{f}(\boldsymbol{\theta})) = \mathbf{0}$ with the *total angular* criterion

$$q = \frac{\mathbf{e}'\mathbf{K}(\mathbf{K}'\mathbf{K})^{-1}\mathbf{K}'\mathbf{e}}{\sqrt{m}\|\mathbf{e}\|^2},$$

where m is the dimension of the parameter vector $\boldsymbol{\theta}$ and $\mathbf{e} = \mathbf{y} - \mathbf{f}(\widehat{\boldsymbol{\theta}})$. We prove that $q \leq 1$ using the inequality $\text{tr}(\mathbf{AB}) \leq \sqrt{\text{tr}(\mathbf{A}^2)}\sqrt{\text{tr}(\mathbf{B}^2)}$ and $\text{tr}(\mathbf{AB}) = \text{tr}(\mathbf{BA})$ for any symmetric matrices $\mathbf{A}$ and $\mathbf{B}$ of appropriate size. Indeed,

$$\mathbf{e}'\mathbf{K}(\mathbf{K}'\mathbf{K})^{-1}\mathbf{K}'\mathbf{e} = \text{tr}(\mathbf{e}'\mathbf{K}(\mathbf{K}'\mathbf{K})^{-1}\mathbf{K}'\mathbf{e}) = \text{tr}(\mathbf{K}(\mathbf{K}'\mathbf{K})^{-1}\mathbf{K}'\mathbf{e}\mathbf{e}')$$

$$\leq \sqrt{\text{tr}(\mathbf{K}(\mathbf{K}'\mathbf{K})^{-1}\mathbf{K}'\mathbf{K}(\mathbf{K}'\mathbf{K})^{-1}\mathbf{K}')}\sqrt{\text{tr}(\mathbf{e}\mathbf{e}'\mathbf{e}\mathbf{e}')}$$

$$= \sqrt{\text{tr}(\mathbf{K}(\mathbf{K}'\mathbf{K})^{-1}\mathbf{K}')}\sqrt{\|\mathbf{e}\|^4} = \sqrt{\text{tr}(\mathbf{I}_m)}\|\mathbf{e}\|^2 = \sqrt{m}\|\mathbf{e}\|^2.$$

Thus, if $q < \varepsilon$, we claim that $\widehat{\boldsymbol{\theta}}$ is the solution to the estimating equation. The total angular criterion can be applied to the generalized linear mixed model of Chapter 7 and to some extent to the general nonlinear mixed effects model of Chapter 8.

References

Abramowitz, M. and Stegun, I.A. (Eds.) (1972). *Handbook of Mathematical Functions with Formulas, Graphs and Mathematical Tables.* New York: Wiley.

Acker, H., Carlsson, J., Durand, R., and Sutherland, R.M. (1984). Spheroids in cancer research. *Recent Results in Cancer Research* **95**. Berlin: Springer-Verlag.

Afenya, E. (1996). Acute leukemia and chemotherapy: a modelling approach. *Mathematical Biosciences* **138**, 79–100.

Agresti, A. (2002). *Categorical Data Analysis.* New York: Wiley.

Aherne, W.A., Camplejohn, R.S., and Wright, N.A. (1977). *An Introduction to Cell Population Kinetics.* London: Edward Arnold.

Aitken, M. (1999). Meta-analysis by random effect modelling in generalized linear models. *Statistics in Medicine* **18**, 2343–2351.

Akaike, H. (1974). A new look at the statistical model identification. *IEEE Transactions on Automatic Control* **AC-19**, 716–723.

Albert, A.E. (1972). *Regression and the Moore–Penrose Pseudoinverse.* New York: Academic Press.

Albert, A. and Anderson, J.A. (1984). On the existence of maximum likelihood estimates in logistic regression. *Biometrika* **71**, 1–10.

Albert, M.H., Le, H., and Small, C.G. (2003). Assessing landmark influence of shape variation. *Biometrika* **90**, 669–678.

Amemiya, T. (1977). A note on a heteroscedastic model. *Journal of Econometrics* **6**, 365–370.

682   References

Amemiya, T. (1981). Qualitative response models: a survey. *Journal of Economic Literature* **19**, 1483–1536.

Andersen, E.B. (1970). Asymptotic properties of conditional maximum-likelihood estimators. *Journal of the Royal Statistical Society, ser. B* **2**, 283–301.

Andersen, E.B. (1980). *Discrete Statistical Models with Social Science Application.* Amsterdam: North-Holland.

Anderson, J.A. and Richardson, S.C. (1979). Logistic discrimination and bias correction in maximum likelihood estimation. *Technometrics* **21**, 71–78.

Anderson, T.W. (1969). Statistical inference for covariance matrices with linear structure. In: *Proceedings of the 2nd International Symposium on Multivariate Analysis,* ed. P.R. Krishnaiah. New York: Academic Press, pp. 55–66.

Anderson, T.W. (1971). *The Statistical Analysis of Time-Series.* New York: Wiley.

Anderson, T.W. (1973). Asymptotically efficient estimation of covariance matrices with linear structure. *Annals of Statistics* **1**, 135–141.

Andrews, H.C. and Hunt, B.R. (1977). *Digital Image Restoration.* Englewood Cliffs, NJ: Prentice-Hall.

Ashburner, J. and Friston, K. (1997). Multimodal image coregistration and partitioning: a unified approach. *Neuroimage* **6**, 209–217.

Atkinson, A. and Riani, M. (2000). *Robust Diagnostic Regression Analysis.* New York: Springer-Verlag.

Bajzer, Z. and Vuk-Pavlovic, S. (1997). Mathematical modeling of tumor growth kinetics. In: *A Survey of Models for Tumor-Immune System Dynamics,* ed. J. Adam and N. Bellomo. Boston: Birkhauser.

Banerjee, M. and Frees, E.W. (1997). Influence diagnostics for linear longitudinal models. *Journal of the American Statistical Association* **92**, 999–1005.

Banks, R.B. (1994). *Growth and Diffusion Phenomena.* Berlin: Springer-Verlag.

Bard, Y. (1974). *Nonlinear Parameter Estimation.* New York: IBM.

Baron, J.A., Sandler, R.S., Haile, R.W., Mandel, J.S., Mott, L.A., and Greenberg, E.R. (1998). Folate intake, alcohol consumption, cigarette smoking, and risk of colorectal adenomas. *Journal of the National Cancer Institute* **90**, 57–62.

Barrett, H.H. and Myers, K.J. (2004). *Foundations of Image Science.* New York: Wiley.

Bartlett, M.S. and Hiorus, R.W. (1973). *The Mathematical Theory of the Dynamics of Biological Populations.* New York: Academic Press.

Baserga, R. (1981). The cell cycle. *New England Journal of Medicine* **304**, 453–459.

Bassukas, I.D. (1994). Gompertzian re-evaluation of the growth pattern of transplantable mammary tumor in sialoadenectomized mice. *Cell Proliferation* **27**, 201–211.

Bates, D.M. and Watts, D.G. (1988). *Nonlinear Regression and Its Applications.* New York: Wiley.

Beal, S.L. and Sheiner, L.B. (1982). Estimating population kinetics. *CRC Critical Reviews in Biomedical Engineering* **8**, 195–222.

Beal, S.L. and Sheiner, L.B. (1992). *NONMEM User's Guides.* NONMEM Project Group. San Francisco, CA: University of California.

Beale, E.M.L. (1960). Confidence regions in nonlinear estimation (with discussion). *Journal of the Royal Statistical Society, ser. B* **22**, 41–88.

Beckman, R.J. and Trussel, H.J. (1974). The distribution of an arbitrary studentized residual and the effects of updating in multiple regression. *Journal of the American Statistical Association* **69**, 199–201.

Begg, A.C. (1983). Clinical relevance of experimental end-points. In: *Cancer Treatment: End Point Evaluation*, ed. B.A. Stoll. New York: Wiley, pp. 43–65.

Belsley, D.A., Kuh, E., and Welsh, R.E. (1980). *Regression Diagnostics: Identifying Influential Data and Sources of Collinearity.* New York: Wiley.

Berkey, C.S. and Laird, N.M. (1986). Nonlinear growth curve analyses: estimating population parameters. *Annals of Human Biology* **13**, 111–128.

Berkey, C.S., Hoaglin, D.C., Mosteller, F., and Colditz, G.A. (1995). A random-effects regression model for meta-analysis. *Statistics in Medicine* **14**, 395–411.

Berkson, J. (1950). Are there two regressions? *Journal of the American Statistical Association* **45**, 164–180.

Berlin, J.A., Laird, N.M., Sacks, H.S., and Chalmers, T.C. (1989). A comparison of statistical methods for combining event rates from clinical trials. *Statistics in Medicine* **8**, 154–176.

Besag, J.E. (1974). Spatial interaction and the statistical analysis of lattice systems. *Journal of the Royal Statistical Society, ser. B* **36**, 192–236.

Besag, J.E. (1986). On statistical analysis of dirty pictures. *Journal of the Royal Statistical Society, ser. B* **48**, 259–302.

Besag, J. (1989). Towards Bayesian image analysis. *Journal of Applied Statistics* **16**, 395–407.

Bickel, P.J. and Doksum, K.A. (2001). *Mathematical Statistics*, Vol. 1. 2nd ed. Upper Saddle River, NJ: Prentice Hall.

Biggerstaff, B.J. and Tweedie R.L. (1997). Incorporating variability in estimates of heterogeneity in the random effects model in meta-analysis. *Statistics in Medicine* **16**, 753–768.

Bigun, J. and Smeraldi, F. (Eds.) (2001). *Audio- and Video-Based Biometric Person Authentication.* Berlin: Springer-Verlag.

Birkes, D. and Dodge, Y. (1993). *Alternative Methods of Regression.* New York: Wiley.

Bischof, C., Carle, A., Corliss, G., Griewank, A., and Hovland, P. (1992). ADIFOR: generating derivatives codes from FORTRAN programs. *Scientific Programming* **1**, 11–29.

Bock, R.D. and Aitkin, M. (1981). Marginal maximum likelihood estimation of item parameters: application of an EM algorithm. *Psychometrika* **46**, 443–459.

Bookstein, F.L. (1986). Size and shape spaces for landmark data in two dimensions (with discussion). *Statistical Science* **1**, 181–242.

Bookstein, F.L. (1991). *Morphometric Tools for Landmark Data: Geometry and Biology*. Cambridge, UK: Cambridge University Press.

Bowman, E.T., Soga, K., and Drummond, W. (2001). Particle shape charcterization using Fourier descriptor analysis. *Geotechnique* **51**, 545–554.

Box, M.J. (1971). Bias in nonlinear estimation. *Journal of the Royal Statistical Society, ser. B* **33**, 171–201.

Breslow, N.E. (1984). Extra-Poisson variation in log-linear models. *Applied Statistics* **33**, 38–44.

Breslow, N.E. and Clayton, D.G. (1993). Approximate inference in generalized linear mixed models. *Journal of the American Statistical Association* **88**, 9–25.

Breslow, N.E. and Day, N.E. (1980). *Statistical Methods in Cancer Research*, Vol. 1. Lyon, France: International Agency for Research on Cancer.

Breslow, N.E. and Lee, X. (1995). Bias correction in generalised linear mixed models with single component of dispersion. *Biometrika* **82**, 81–91.

Brockwell, S.E. and Gordon, I.R. (2001). A comparison of statistical methods for meta-analysis. *Statistics in Medicine* **20**, 825–840.

Brown, C.C., Kipnis, V., Freedman, L.S., Hartman, A.M., Schatzkin, A., and Wacholder, S. (1994). Energy adjustment methods for nutritional epidemiology: the effect of categorization. *American Journal of Epidemiology* **139**, 323–336.

Brown, H. and Prescott, R. (1999). *Applied Mixed Models in Medicine*. Chichester, UK: Wiley.

Brown, J.M. (1975). Exploitation of kinetic differences between normal and malignant cells. *Radiology* **114**, 189–197.

Buonaccorsi, J. (1994). Measurement error models for gypsy moth studies. In: *Case Studies in Biometry*, ed. B. Lange et al. New York: Wiley.

Burr, D. (1988). On errors-in-variables in binary regression: Berkson case. *Journal of the American Statistical Association* **83**, 739–743.

Cameron, A.C. and Trivedi, P.K. (1998). *Regression Analysis of Count Data*. Cambridge, UK: Cambridge University Press.

Carlsson, J. and Yuhas, J.M. (1984). Liquid-overlay culture of cellular spheroids. *Recent Results in Cancer Research* **95**, 1–23.

Carroll, R.L. (1982). Adapting for heteroscedasticity in linear models. *Annals of Statistics* **10**, 1224–1233.

Carroll, R.J. and Ruppert, D. (1988). *Transformation and Weighting in Regression.* New York: Chapman & Hall.

Carroll, R.J., Spiegelman, C.H., Lan, K.K., Bailey, K.T., and Abott, R.D. (1984). On errors-in-variables problem for binary regression models. *Biometrika* **71**, 19–25.

Carroll, R.J., Ruppert D., and Stefanski, L.A. (1995). *Nonlinear Measurement Error Models.* New York: Chapman & Hall.

Carter, R.L. and Yang, M.C.K. (1986). Large-sample inference in random coefficient regression models. *Communications in Statistics: Theory and Methods* **8**, 2507–2526.

Casarett, A.P. (1968). *Radiation Biology.* Englewood Cliffs, NJ: Prentice-Hall.

Casella, G. and Berger, R.L. (1990). *Statistical Inference.* 2nd ed. Belmon, CA: Duxbury Press.

Chaganty, R.N. (1997). An alternative approach to the analysis of longitudinal data via generalized estimating equations. *Journal of Statistical Planning and Inference* **63**, 39–54.

Chalmond, B. (2003). *Modeling and Inverse Problems in Image Analysis.* New York: Springer-Verlag.

Chamberlain, G. (1980). Analysis of covariance with quality data. *Review of Economic Studies* **47**, 225–238.

Chambers, E. and Cox, D.R. (1967). Discrimination between alternative binary response models. *Biometrika* **54**, 573–578.

Chatterjee, S. and Hadi, A.S. (1986). Influential observations, high leverage points, and outliers in linear regression. *Statistical Science* **1**, 379–416.

Chatterjee, S. and Hadi, A.S. (1988). *Sensitivity Analysis in Linear Regression.* New York: Wiley.

Chatterjee, S. and Price, B. (1999). *Regression Analysis by Example. 2nd ed.* New York: Wiley.

Chellappa, R. and Jain, A. (Eds.) (1993). *Markov Chain Fields: Theory and Applications.* San Diego, CA: Academic Press.

Chellappa, R., Wilson, C.L., and Sirohey, S. (1995). Human and machine recognition of faces. *Proceedings of the IEEE* **83**, 705–740.

Chen, J. and Shao, J. (1993). Iterative weighted least squares estimators. *Annals of Statistics* **21**, 1071–1092.

Chernoff, H. (1954). On the distribution of the likelihood ratio. *Annals of Mathematical Statistics* **25**, 573–578.

Chi, E.M. and Reinsel, G.C. (1989). Models for longitudinal data with random effects and AR(1) errors. *Journal of the American Statistical Association* **84**, 452–459.

Chignola, R., Schenetti, A., Chiesa, E., Foroni, R., Sartoris, S., Brendolan, A., Tridente, G., Andrighetto, G., and Liberati, D. (1999). Oscillating growth patterns of multicellular tumour spheroids. *Cell Proliferation* **32**, 39–48.

Christensen, R. (1996). *Plane Answers to Complex Questions: The Theory of Linear Models.* New York: Springer-Verlag.

Codington, E.A. and Levinson, A. (1955). *Theory of Ordinary Differential Equations.* New York: McGraw-Hill.

Colton, D., Coyle, J., and Monk, P. (2000). Recent developments in inverse acoustic scattering theory. *SIAM Review* **42**, 369–414.

Conaway, M. (1990). A random effects model for binary data. *Biometrics* **46**, 317–328.

Cook, R.D. (1977). Detection of influential observations in linear regression. *Technometrics* **19,** 15–18.

Cook, R.D. (1986). Assessment of local influence (with discussion). *Journal of the Royal Statistical Society, ser. B* **2**, 139–169.

Cook, R.D. and Weisberg, S. (1982). *Residuals and Influence in Regression.* New York: Chapman & Hall.

Copas, J.B. (1988). Binary regression models for contaminated data (with discussion). *Journal of the Royal Statistical Society, ser. B* **50**, 225–265.

Costa, L.F. and Cesar, R.M. (2001). *Shape Analysis and Classification.* Boca Raton, FL: CRC Press.

Cottle, R.W., Pang, J.-S., and Stone, R.E. (1992). *The Linear Complementarity Problem.* San Diego, CA: Academic Press.

Cox, D.R. (1972). Regression models and life tables. *Journal of the Royal Statistical Society, ser. B* **34**, 178–220.

Cox, D.R. and Hinkley, D.V. (1974). *Theoretical Statistics.* London: Chapman & Hall.

Cox, D.R. and Snell, E.J. (1989). *The Analysis of Binary Data.* 2nd ed. London: Chapman & Hall.

Cressie, N.A. (1991). *Statistics for Spatial Data.* New York: Wiley.

Cressie, N. and Lahiri, S.N. (1993). The asymptotic distribution of REML estimators. *Journal of Multivariate Analysis* **45**, 217–233.

Cross, G.R. and Jain, A.K. (1983). Markov random field texture models. *IEEE Transactions on Pattern Analysis and Machine Intelligence* **PAMI-5**, 25–39.

Crouch, E.A.C. and Spiegelman, D. (1990). The evaluation of integrals of the form $\int f(t) \exp(-t^2) dt$: application to logistic normal models. *Journal of the American Statististical Association* **88**, 464–469.

Crowder, M. (1995). On the use of a working correlation matrix in using generalized linear models for repeated measurements. *Biometrika* **82**, 407–410.

Davey-Smith, G. (2001). *Clinical Meta-analysis.* New York: Wiley.

Davidian, M. and Carroll, R.J. (1987). Variance function estimation. *Journal of the American Statistical Association* **82**, 1079–1091.

Davidian, M. and Giltinan, D.M. (1995). *Nonlinear Models for Repeated Measurement Data.* London: Chapman & Hall.

Davis, C.S. (2002). *Statistical Methods for the Analysis of Repeated Measurements.* New York: Springer-Verlag.

Day, R.S. (1986a). Treatment sequencing, asymmetry, and uncertainty: protocol strategies for combination chemotherapy. *Cancer Research* **46**, 3876–3885.

Day, R.S. (1986b). A branching-process model for heterogeneous cell populations. *Mathematical Biosciences* **78**, 78–90.

Dayton, C.M. (1998). Information criteria for the paired-comparisons problem. *American Statistician* **52**, 144–151.

Demidenko, E. (1981). *Linear and Nonlinear Regression.* Moscow: Finansy and Statistika (in Russian).

Demidenko, E. (1989). *Optimization and Regression.* Moscow: Nauka (in Russian).

Demidenko, E. (1996). On the existence of the least squares estimate in nonlinear growth curve models of exponential type. *Communications in Statistics: Theory and Methods* **25**, 159–182.

Demidenko, E. (1997). Asymptotic properties of nonlinear mixed-effects models. In: *Modelling Longitudinal and Spatially Correlated Data: Methods, Applications, and Future Directions (Springer Lectures in Statistics),* ed. T.G. Gregoire et al. New York: Springer-Verlag.

Demidenko, E. (2000). Is this least squares estimate? *Biometrika* **87**, 437–452.

Demidenko, E. (2001). Computational aspects of probit model. *Mathematical Communications* **6**, 233–247.

Demidenko, E. and Spiegelman D. (1997). A paradox: more measurement error can lead to more efficient estimates. *Communications in Statistics: Theory and Methods* **26**, 1649–1675.

Demidenko, E. and Stukel, T. (2002). Efficient estimation of general mixed effects models. *Journal of Statistical Planning and Inference* **104**, 197–219.

Demidenko, E. and Stukel, T.A. (2005). Influence analysis for linear mixed-effects models. *Statistics in Medicine* **24**, 893–909.

Demidenko, E. and Massam, E. (1999). On the existence of the maximum likelihood estimate in the variance components model and some aspects of the computations. *Sankhya, ser. A* **61**, 431–443.

Demidenko, E. (2006a). The assessment of tumour response to treatment. *Journal of the Royal Statistical Society, ser. C* **55**, 365–377.

Demidenko, E. (2006b). Criteria for global minimum of sum of squares in nonlinear regression. *Computational Statistics and Data Analysis* **51**, 1739-1753.

Demidenko, E. (2007a). Poisson regression for clustered data. *International Statistical Review* **75**, 96–113.

Demidenko, E. (2007b). Sample size determination with logistic regression revisited. *Statistics in Medicine* **26**, 3385–3397.

Demidenko, E. (2008). Criteria for unconstrained global optimization. *Journal of Optimization Theory and Applications* **136**, 375–395.

Demidenko, E. (2009). Statistical hypothesis testing for postreconstructed and postregistered medical images. *SIAM Journal on Imaging Sciences* **2**, 1049–1067.

Demidenko, E. (2010). Three endpoints of in vivo tumour radiobiology and their statistical estimation. *International Journal of Radiation Biology* **86**, 164–173.

Demidenko, E., Sargent, J., and Onega, T. (2012). Random effects coefficient of determination for mixed and meta-analysis models. *Communications in Statistics: Theory and Methods* **41**, 953–969.

Dempster, A.P., Laird, N.M., and Rubin, D.B. (1977). Maximum likelihood from incomplete data via the EM algorithm (with discussion). *Journal of the Royal Statistical Society, ser. B* **39**, 1–38.

Dennis, J.E. and Schnabel, R.B. (1983). *Numerical Methods for Unconstrained Optimization and Nonlinear Equations.* Englewood Cliffs, NJ: Prentice-Hall.

De Pierro, A.R. and Yamagishi, M.E.B. (2001). Fast EM-like methods for maximum "a posteriori" estimates in emission tomography. *IEEE Transactions on Medical Imaging* **20**, 280–288.

DerSimonian, R. and Laird, N.M. (1986). Meta-analysis in clinical trials. *Controlled Clinical Trials* **7**, 177–188.

Dette, H., Pepelyshev, A., and Holland-Letz, T. (2010). Optimal designs for random effect models with correlated errors with applications in population phamacokinetics. *Annals of Applied Statistics* **4**, 1430–1450.

DeVita, V.T., Hellman, S., and Rosenberg, S.A. (1995). *Cancer: Principles and Practice of Oncology,* 5th ed. Philadelphia: J.B. Lippincott.

Diggle, P., Heagerty, P., Liang, K.-Y., and Zeger, S. (2002). *Analysis of Longitudinal Data.* Oxford, UK: Oxford University Press.

Draper, N.R. and Smith, H. (1998). *Applied Regression Analysis,* 3rd ed. New York: Wiley.

Dryden, I.L., Faghihi, M.R. and Taylor, C.C. (1997). Procrustes shape analysis of planar point subsets. *Journal of the Royal Statistical Society, ser B* **59**, 353–374.

Dunn, J.F., O'Hara, J.A., Zaim-Wadghiri, Y., Lei, H., Meyerand, M.E., Grinberg, O.Y., Hou, H., Hoopes, J., Demidenko, E., and Swartz, H.M. (2002). Changes in oxygenation of intracranial tumors with carbogen: a BOLD MRI and EPR oximetry study. *Journal of Magnetic Resonance Imaging* **16**, 511–521.

Durrleman, S. and Simon, R. (1989). Flexible regression models with cubic-splines. *Statistics in Medicine* **8**, 551–561.

Easton, D.M. (1999). X-ray survival as Gompertz growth in number killed. *Journal of Theoretical Biology* **196**, 1–8.

Ehrlich, R. and Weinberg, B. (1970). An exact method for characterization of grain shape. *Journal of Sedimentary Petrology* **40**, 205–212.

Eicker, F. (1966). A multivariate central limit theorem for random linear vector forms. *Annals of Mathematical Statistics* **37**, 1825–1828.

Eisen, M. (1979). *Mathematical Models in Cell Biology and Cancer Chemotherapy.* New York: Springer-Verlag.

Elkind, M.M. (1988). The initial part of the survival curve: Does it predict the outcome of fractionated radiotherapy? *Radiation Research* **114**, 414–425.

Emerson, J.D., Hoaglin, D.C., and Kempthorne, P.J. (1984). Leverage in least squares additive-plus-multiplicative fits for two-way tables. *Journal of the American Statistical Association* **79**, 329–335.

Epstein, C.L. (2003). *Introduction to the Mathematics of Medical Imaging.* Upper Saddle River, NJ: Prentice Hall.

Evans, M. and Swartz, T. (2000). *Approximating Integrals via Monte Carlo and Deterministic Methods.* Oxford, UK: Oxford University Press.

Evans, S.N. and Stark, P.B. (2002). Inverse problems in statistics. *Inverse Problems* **18**, R55–R97.

Ezzet, F. and Whitehead, J. (1991). A random effects model for ordinal responses from a crossover trial. *Statistics in Medicine* **19**, 901–907.

Fahrmeir, L. and Tutz, G. (2001). *Multivariate Statistical Modelling Based on Generalized Linear Models.* New York: Springer-Verlag.

Fay, M.P. (2002). Measuring a binary response's range of influence in logistic regression. *American Statistician* **56**, 5–9.

Feller, W. (1966). *An Introduction to Probability Theory and Its Application.* New York: Wiley.

Ferrante, L., Bompadre, S., Possati, L., and Leone, L. (2000). Parameter estimation in a Gompertzian stochastic model for tumor growth. *Biometrics* **56**, 1076–1081.

Ferrario, V.F., Sforza, C., Tartaglia, G.M., Colombo, A., and Serrao, G. (1999). Size and shape of the human's first permanent molar: a Fourier analysis of the occlusal and equatorial outlines. *American Journal of Physical Anthropology* **108**, 281–294.

Ferson, S., Rohlf, F.J., and Koehn, R.K. (1985). Measuring shape variation of two-dimensional outlines. *Systematic Zoology* **34**, 59–68.

Fessler, J.A. (1994). Penalized weighted least-squares image reconstruction for positron emission tomography. *IEEE Transactions on Medical Imaging* **13**, 290–300.

Finney, D.J. (1971). *Probit Analysis,* 3rd ed. Cambridge, UK: Cambridge University Press.

Fuller, W.A. (1987). *Measurement Error Models.* New York: Wiley.

Fuller, W.A. (1995). *Introduction to Statistical Time-Series.* New York: Wiley.

Fung, W.K. and Kwan, C.W. (1997). A note on local influence on normal curvature. *Journal of the Royal Statistical Society, ser. B* **59**, 839–843.

Fung, W.K. and Tang, M.K. (1997). Assessment of local influence in multivariate regression analysis. *Communications in Statistics: Theory and Methods* **26**, 831–837.

Gallant, A.R. (1975). Testing a subset of the parameters of a nonlinear regression model. *Journal of the American Statistical Association* **70**, 927–932.

Gallant, A.R. (1987). *Nonlinear Statistical Models.* New York: Wiley.

Geman, S. and Geman D. (1984). Stochastic relaxation, Gibbs distributions, and the Bayesian restoration of images. *IEEE Transactions on Pattern Analysis* **6**, 721–741.

Gerald, C.F. and Wheatley, P.O. (1994). *Applied Numerical Analysis,* 5th ed. Reading, MA: Addison-Wesley.

Giampaoli, V. and Singer, J.M. (2009). Likelihood ratio tests for variance components in linear mixed models, *Journal of Statistical Planning and Inference* **139**, 1435–1448.

Gibaldi, M. and Perrier, D. (1982). *Pharmacokinetics,* 2nd ed. New York: Marcel Dekker.

Gill, P.S. (2000). A robust mixed linear model analysis for longitudinal data. *Statistics in Medicine* **19**, 975–987.

Glaholt, S.P., Chen, C.Y., Demidenko, E., Bugge, D.M., Folt, C.L., and Shaw, J.R. (2012). Adaptive iterative design (AID): a novel approach for evaluating the interactive effects of multiple stressors on aquatic organisms. *Science of the Total Environment* **432**, 57–64.

Gnedenko, B.V. (1962). *Theory of Probability.* New York: Chelsea.

Godszal, A.F. and Pham, D.L. (2000). Volumetric segmentation. In: *Handbook of Medical Imaging,* ed. I.N. Bankman. San Diego, CA: Academic Press.

Goldfeld, S.M. and Quandt, R.E. (1972). *Nonlinear Methods in Econometrics*. Amsterdam: North-Holland.

Goldie, J.H. and Coldman, A.J. (1979). A mathematical model for relating the drug sensitivity of tumors to their spontaneous mutation rate. *Cancer Treatment Reports* **66**, 439–449.

Goldstein, H. (1989). Restricted unbiased iterative generalized least-squares. *Biometrika* **76**, 622–623.

Goldstein, H. (1991). Nonlinear multilevel models, with application to discrete response data. *Biometrika* **78**, 45–51.

Goldstein, H. (1995). *Mutilevel Statistical Models*, 2nd ed. London: Edward Arnold.

Golub, G.H. and Pereyra, V. (1973). The differentiation of pseudo-inverses and nonlinear least squares problems whose variables separate. *SIAM Journal on Numerical Analysis* **10**, 413–432.

Golub, G.H. and Pereyra, V. (2003). Separable nonlinear least squares: the variable projection method and its applications. *Inverse Problems* **19**, 1–126.

Gong, G. and Samaniego, F.J. (1981). Pseudo maximum likelihood estimation: theory and applications. *Annals of Statistics* **9**, 861–869.

Gonzalez, R.C. and Woods, R.E. (2002). *Digital Image Processing*, 2nd ed. Upper Saddle River, NJ: Prentice Hall.

Goodall, C.R. (1991). Procrustes methods in statistical analysis of shape. *Journal of the Royal Statistical Society, ser. B* **53**, 285–339.

Goodall, C.R. and Lange, N. (1989). Growth curve models for correlated triangular shapes. In: *Computer Science and Statistics*. Alexandria, VA: American Statistical Association, pp. 445–452.

Gordan, P. (1873). Über die Auflösung linearer Gleichungen mit reelen Coefficienten. *Mathematische Annalen* **6**, 23–28.

Gourieroux, C., Monfort, A., and Trognon, A. (1984). Pseudo maximum likelihood methods: theory. *Econometrica* **52**, 681–700.

Graybill, F.A. (1969). *Matrices with Applications in Statistics*. Belmont, CA: Wadsworth.

Graybill, F.A. (1983). *Matrices with Applications in Statistics*, 2nd ed. Belmont, CA: Wadsworth.

Green, P.J. (1984). Iteratively reweighted least squares for maximum likelihood estimation, and some robust and resistant alternatives. *Journal of the Royal Statistical Society, ser. B* **46**, 149–192.

Green, P.J. (1987). Penalized likelihood for general semi-parametric regression models. *International Statistical Review* **55**, 245–259.

Greenberg, E. (1975). Minimum variance properties of principal components. *Journal of the American Statistical Association* **70**, 194–197.

Grenander, U. and Miller, M.I. (1994). Representations of knowledge in complex systems. *Journal of the Royal Statistical Society, ser. B* **56**, 549–603.

Grizzle, J.E. and Allen, D.M. (1969). Analysis of growth and dose response curves. *Biometrics* **25**, 357–381.

Grömping, U. (1996). A note on fitting of a marginal model to mixed effects log-linear regression data via GEE. *Biometrics* **52**, 280–285.

Gumpertz, M.L. and Pantula, S.G. (1992). Nonlinear regression with variance components. *Journal of the American Statistical Association* **87**, 201–209.

Haberman, S.J. (1974). *The Anaylysis of Frequency Data.* Vol. 1. Chicago: University of Chicago.

Haberman, S.J. (1979). *Analysis of Qualitative Data,* Vol. 2. New York: Academic Press.

Hajnal, J.V., Hill, D.J., and Hawkes, D.L.G. (Eds.) (2001). *Medical Image Registration.* Boca Raton, FL: CRC Press.

Hall, E.J. (2000). *Radiobiology for the Radiobiologist,* 5th ed. Philadelphia: J.B. Lippincott.

Hall, E.L. (1979). *Computer Image Processing and Recognition.* New York: Academic Press.

Hampel, F.R. (1974). The influence curve and its role in robust estimation. *Journal of the American Statistical Association* **69**, 383–393.

Hampel, F. et al. (1986). *Robust Statistics: The Approach Based on Influence Function.* New York: Wiley.

Hanin, L.G., Pavlova, L.V., and Yakovlev, A.Y. (1993). *Biomathematical Problems in Optimization of Cancer Radiotherapy.* Boca Raton, FL: CRC Press.

Hardin, J.W. and Hible, J.M. (2003). *Generalized Estimating Equations.* Boca Raton, FL: Chapman & Hall/CRC Press.

Hardy, R.J. and Thompson, S.G. (1998). A likelihood approach to meta-analysis with random effects. *Statistics in Medicine* **15**, 619–629.

Hartford, A. and Davidian, M. (2000). Consequences of misspecifying assumptions in nonlinear mixed effects models. *Computational Statistics and Data Analysis* **34**, 139–164.

Hartley, H.O. (1961). The modified Gauss–Newton method for the fitting of nonlinear regression function by least squares. *Technometrics* **3**, 269–280.

Hartley, H.O. and Rao, H.N.K. (1967). Maximum likelihood estimation for the mixed analysis of variance components. *Biometrika* **59**, 93–108.

Harville, D.A. (1974). Optimal procedures for some constrained selection problems. *Journal of the American Statistical Association* **69**, 446–452.

Harville, D.A. (1997). *Matrix Algebra from a Statistician's Perspective*. New York: Springer-Verlag.

Harville, D.A. (2001). *Matrix Algebra: Exercises and Solutions*. New York: Springer-Verlag.

Hebert, T. and Leahy, R. (1989). A generalized EM algorithm for a 3-D Bayesian reconstruction from Poisson data using Gibbs priors. *IEEE Transactions on Medical Imaging* **8**, 194–202.

Heckman, I.J. (1981). Statistical models for discrete panel data. In: *Structural Analysis of Discrete Panel Data with Econometric Applications*, ed. C.F. Manski and D. McFadden. Cambridge, MA: MIT Press, pp. 114–178.

Hedeker, D. (2003). A mixed-effects multinomial logistic regression model. *Statistics in Medicine* **22**, 1433–1446.

Heitjan, D.F. (1991). Generalized Norton-Simon models of tumour growth. *Statistics in Medicine* **10**, 1075–1088.

Heitjan, D.F., Manni A., and Simon, A.R. (1993). Statistical analysis of *in vivo* tumor growth experiments. *Cancer Research* **15,** 6042–6050.

Henderson, C.R. (1953). Estimation of variance and covariance components. *Biometrics* **9**, 226–252.

Henderson, C.R. (1963). Selection index and expected genetic advance. In: *Statistical Genetics and Plan Breeding*. Washington, DC: National Acdemy of Science–Natural Research Council, pp. 141–163.

Herman, G.T. (1980). *Image Reconstruction from Projections: The Fundamentals of Computerized Tomography*. New York: Academic Press.

Hestenes, M.R. (1975). *Optimization Theory: The Finite Dimensional Case*. New York: Wiley.

Higashikubo, R., Ragouzis, M., and Roti, J.L. (1996). Flow cytometric BrdUrd-pulse-chase study of x-ray induced alterations in cell cycle progression. *Cell Proliferation* **29**, 43–57.

Higham, N.J. (1986). Newton's method for the matrix square root. *Mathematics of Computation* **46**, 537–549.

Hill, A.A. and Skarsgard, L.D. (1999). Cell-age heterogeneity and deviations from LQ model in the radiation survival responses of human tumour cells. *International Journal of Radiation Biology* **75**, 1409–1420.

Hobolth, A., Pedersen, J., and Jensen, E.B.V. (2003). A continuous parametric shape model. *Annals of the Institute of Statistical Mathematics* **55**, 227–242.

Hodges, S.D. and Moore, P.G. (1972). Data uncertainties and least squares regression. *Applied Statistics* **21**, 185–195.

Hoerl, A.E. and Kennard, R.W. (1970). Ridge regression: biased estimation for non-orthogonal problems. *Technometrics* **12**, 55–67.

Hoffman, K. (1999). *Linear Algebra*, 3d ed. London: Prentice Hall.

Hollander, M. and Wolfe, D.A. (1999). *Nonparametric Statistical Methods*. New York: Wiley.

Hooper, P.M. (1993). Iterative weighted least squares estimation in heteroscedastic linear models. *Journal of the American Statistical Association* **88**, 179–184.

Horgan, G.W. (2001). The statistical analysis of plant part appearence: a review. *Computers and Electronics in Agriculture* **31**, 169–190.

Hsiao, C. (2003). *Analysis of Panel Data*. Cambridge, UK: Cambridge University Press.

Huber, P.J. (1967). The behavior of maximum likelihood estimates under nonstandard conditions. *Proceedings of the 5th Berkley Symposium* **1**, 221–233.

Huber, P.J. (1981). *Robust Statistics*. New York: Wiley.

Huggins, R.M. (1993). A robust approach to the analysis of repeated measures. *Biometrics* **49**, 715–720.

Hunter, D.R. and Lange, K. (2004). A tutorial on MM algorithm. *American Statistician* **58**, 30–37.

Hurvich, C.M. and Tsai, C.L. (1991). Bias of the corrected AIC criterion for underfitted regression and time-series models. *Biometrika* **78**, 499–509.

Hurvich, C.M., Simonoff, J.S., and Tsai, C.L. (1998). Smoothing parameter selection in nonparametric regression using an improved Akaike information criterion. *Journal of the Royal Statistical Society, ser. B* **60**, 271–293.

Ishiguro, M., Sakamoto, Y., and Kitagawa, H. (1997). Bootstrapping log likelihood and EIC, an extension of AIC. *Annals of the Institute of Statistical Mathematics* **49**, 411–434.

Jackson, D. (2006). The power of the standard test for the presence of heterogeneity in meta-analysis. *Statistics in Medicine* **25**, 2688–2699.

Jackson, D., Riley, R., and White, I.R. (2011). Multivariate meta-analysis: Potential and promise. *Statistics in Medicine* **30**, 2481–2498.

Jacqmin-Gadda, H., Joly, P., Commenges, D., Binquet, C., and Chene, G. (2002). Penalized likelihood approach to estimate a smooth mean curve on longitudinal data. *Statistics in Medicine* **21**, 2391–2402.

Jamshidian, M. and Jennrich, R.I. (1993). Conjugate gradient acceleration of the EM algorithm. *Journal of the American Statistical Association* **88**, 221–228.

Jennrich, R.I. (1969). Asymptotic properties of nonlinear least squares estimation. *Annals of Mathematical Statistics* **40**, 633–643.

Jennrich, R.I. and Schluchter, M.D. (1986). Unbalanced repeated-measures models with structured covariance matrices. *Biometrics* **42**, 805–820.

Jobson, J.D. and Fuller, W.A. (1980). Least squares estimation when the covariance matrix and parameter vector are functionally related. *Journal of the American Statistical Association* **75**, 176–181.

Johnson, W. (1985). Influence measures for logistic regression: another point of view. *Biometrika* **72**, 59–65.

Johnson, N.L. and Kotz, S. (1970). *Continuous Univariate Distributions*, Vol. 2. New York: Wiley.

Jones, B. and Dale, R.G. (1995). Cell loss factors and the linear-quadratic model. *Radiotherapy and Oncology* **39**, 136–139.

Kackar, R.N. and Harville D.A. (1984). Approximations for standard errors of estimators of fixed and random effects in mixed linear models. *Journal of the American Statistical Association* **79**, 853–862.

Kagan, A.M., Linnik, Yu.V., and Rao, C.R. (1973). *Characterization Problems in Mathematical Statistics.* New York: Wiley.

Kak, A.C. and Slaney, M. (2001). *Principles of Computerized Tomographic Imaging.* Philadelphia: SIAM.

Kallman, R.F. (Ed.) (1987). *Rodent Tumor Models in Experimental Cancer Therapy.* New York: Pergamon Press.

Kaufman, L. (1993). Maximum likelihood, least squares, and penalyzed least squares for PET. *IEEE Transactions on Medical Imaging* **12**, 200–214.

Kendall, D.G. (1989). A survey of the statistical theory of shape. *Statistical Science* **4**, 87–120.

Kendall, D.G., Barden, D., Carne, T.K., and Le, H. (1999). *Shape and Theory of Shape.* New York: Wiley.

Kendall, M.G. and Stuart, A. (1961). *The Advanced Theory of Statistics*, Vol. 2. New York: Hafner.

Kent, J.T. and Mardia, K.V. (1997). Consistency of Procrustes estimators. *Journal of the Royal Statistical Society, ser. B* **59**, 281–290.

Kenward, M.G. and Roger, J.H. (1997). Small sample inference for fixed effects from restricted maximum likelihood. *Biometrics* **53**, 983–997.

Khatri, C.G. (1966). A note on a MANOVA model applied to problems in growth curve. *Annals of the Institute of Statistical Mathematics* **18**, 75–86.

Khuri, A.I., Mathew, T., and Sinha, B.K. (1998). *Statistical Tests for Mixed Linear Models.* New York: Wiley.

Kiebel, S.J., Ashburner, J., Ploine, J.-B., and Friston, K.J. (1997). MRI and PET coregistration: a cross validation of statistical parametric mapping and automated image registration. *Neuroimage* **5**, 271–279.

Kim, M.G. (1995). Local influence in multivariate regression. *Communications in Statistics: Theory and Methods* **24**, 1271–1278.

Kim, M.G. (1996). Local influence in multivariate normal data. *Journal of Applied Statistics* **23**, 535–541.

Kirsch, A. (1996). *An Introduction to the Mathematical Theory of Inverse Problems.* New York: Springer-Verlag.

Klein, L.R. (1962). *An Introduction to Econometrics.* Englewood Cliffs, NJ: Prentice-Hall.

Knolle, H. (1988). *Cell Kinetic Modelling and Chemotherapy of Cancer.* New York: Springer-Verlag.

Korn, E.L. and Whittemore, A.S. (1979). Methods for analyzing panel studies of acute health effects of air pollution. *Biometrics* **35**, 795–802.

Krailo, M.D. and Pike, M.C. (1984). Conditional multivariate logistic analysis of stratified case–control studies: algorithm AS 196. *Applied Statistics* **33**, 95–103.

Kress, R. (1999). *Linear Integral Equations.* Berlin: Springer-Verlag.

Kullback, S. (1968). *Information Theory and Statistics.* New York: Dover.

Kurz, L. and Benteftifa, M.H. (1997). *Analysis of Variance in Statistical Image Processing.* Cambridge, UK: Cambridge University Press.

Laird, N.M. and Ware, J.H. (1982). Random-effects models for longitudinal data. *Biometrics* **38**, 963–974.

Laird, N., Lange, N., and Stram, D. (1987). Maximum likelihood computations with repeated measures: application of the EM algorithm. *Journal of the American Statistical Association* **82**, 97–105.

Lancaster, P. and Tismenetsky, M. (1985). *The Theory of Matrices,* 2nd ed. New York: Academic Press.

Lange, K.L., Little, R.J.A., and Taylor, J. (1989). Robust statistical modeling using *t*-distribution. *Journal of the American Statistical Association* **84**, 881–896.

Laurent, R.S.S. and Cook, R.D. (1992). Leverage and superleverage in nonlinear regression. *Journal of the American Statistical Association* **87,** 985–990.

Laurent, R.S.S. and Cook, R.D. (1993). Leverage, local influence and curvature in nonlinear regression. *Biometrika* **80**, 99–106.

Lawless, J.F. (1987). Negative binomial and mixed Poisson regression. *Canadian Journal of Statistics* **15**, 209–225.

Lawrence, A.J. (1991). Local and deletion influence. In: *Directions in Robust Statistics and Diagnostics,* ed. W. Stahel and S. Weisberg. New York: Springer-Verlag, pp. 141–157.

Lee, S.Y. and Xu, L. (2004). Influence analysis of nonlinear mixed-effects models. *Computational Statistics and Data Analysis* **45**, 321-341.

Lehmann, E.L. (1986). *Testing Statistical Hypothesis.* New York: Wiley.

Lehmann, E.L. and Casella, G. (1998). *Theory of Point Estimation*. New York: Springer-Verlag.

Lele, S. (1993). Euclidean distance matrix analysis (EDMA): estimation of mean form and mean form difference. *Mathematical Geology* **25**, 573–602.

Lele, S. and Richtsmeier, J.T. (2001). *An Invariant Approach to Statistical Analysis of Shapes*. Boca Raton, FL: Chapman & Hall/CRC Press.

Lessaffre, E. and Kaufmann, H. (1992). Existence and uniqueness of the maximum likelihood estimator for a multivariate probit model. *Journal of the American Statistical Association* **87**, 805–811.

Lestrel, P.E. (1997). An introduction and overview of Fourier descriptors. In: *Fourier Descriptors and Their Application in Biology*, ed. P.E. Lestrel. New York: Cambridge University Press.

Levenberg, K. (1944). A method for the solution of certain non-linear problems in least squares. *Quarterly of Applied Mathematics* **2**, 164–168.

Lewitt, R.M. and Matej, S. (2003). Overview of methods for image reconstruction from projections in emission computed tomography. *Proceedings of the IEEE* **91**, 1588–1611.

Li, Z. and Zhu, L. (2013). A new test for random effects in linear mixed models with longitudinal data. *Journal of Statistical Planning and Inference* **143**, 82–95.

Liang, K.Y. and Liu X.H. (1991). Estimating equations in generalized linear models with measurement error. In: *Estimating Functions*, ed. V.P. Godambe. Oxford: Clarendon Press.

Liang, K.Y. and Zeger, S.L. (1986). Longitudinal data analysis using generalized linear models. *Biometrika* **73**, 13–22.

Lin, X. (1997). Variance component testing in generalised linear models with random effects. *Biometrika* **84**, 309–326.

Lindley, D.V. and Smith, A.F.M. (1972). Bayes estimates for the linear model. *Journal of the Royal Statistical Society, ser. B* **34**, 1–34.

Lindman, H.R. (1992). *Analysis of Variance in Experimental Design*. New York: Springer-Verlag.

Lindstrom, M.J. and Bates, D.M. (1988). Newton–Raphson and EM algorithms for linear mixed-effects models for repeated-measures data. *Journal of the American Statistical Association* **83**, 1014–1022.

Lindstrom, M.J. and Bates, D.M. (1990). Nonlinear mixed-effects models for repeated measures. *Biometrics* **46**, 673–687.

Little, R.J.A. (2002). *Statistical Analysis with Missing Data*. New York: Wiley.

Liu, Q. and Pierce, D.A. (1994). A note on Gauss–Hermite quadrature. *Biometrika* **81**, 624–629.

698   References

Lloyd, T., Andon, M.B., Rollings, N., Martel,. J.K., Landis, J.R., Demers, L.M., Eggli, D.F., Kieslhorst, K., Kulin, H.E. (1993). Calcium supplememtation and bone mineral density in adolescent girls. *Journal of the American Medical Association* **270**, 841–844.

Longford, N.T. (1987). A fast scoring algorithm for maximum likelihood estimation in unbalanced mixed models with nested random effects. *Biometrika* **74**, 817–827.

Longford, N.T. (1994). Logistic regression with random coefficients. *Computational Statistics and Data Analysis* **17**, 1–15.

Looney, W.B., Trefil, J.S., Schaffner, J.C., Kovacs, C.S., and Hopkins, H.A. (1975). Solid tumors models assesement of different treatment modalities: I. Radiation-induced changes in growth rate characteristics of a solid tumor model. *Proceedings of the National Academy of Sciences* **72**, 2662–2666.

Lu, K.H. (1965). Harmonic analysis of the human face. *Biometrics* **21**, 491–505.

Macaskill, G.T. (1993). A note on adjusted profile likelihoods in non-linear regression. *Journal of the Royal Statistical Socierty*, ser. B **55**, 125–131.

Maddala, G.S. (1987). Limited dependent variable models using panel data. *Journal of Human Resources* **22**, 307–338.

Magnus, J.R. (1988). *Linear Structures*. London: Oxford University Press.

Magnus, J.R. and Neudecker, H. (1988). *Matrix Differential Calculus with Applications in Statistics and Econometrics*. New York: Wiley.

Maintz, J.B.A. and Viergever, M.A. (1998). A survey of medical image registration. *Medical Image Analysis* **2**, 1–36.

Malzahn, U. and Böhning, D. (2000). Nonparametric estimation of heterogeneity variance for the standardised difference used in meta-analysis. *Biometrika* **87**, 619–632.

Mao, J.H. and Wheldon, T.E. (1996). A stochastic model for multistage tumorigenesis in developing and adult mice. *Mathematical Biosciences* **129**, 95–110.

Mardia, K.V. (1989). Shape analysis of triangles through directional techniques. *Journal of the Royal Statistical Society, ser. B* **51**, 449–458.

Mardia, K.V. and Dryden I.L. (1989). The statistical analysis of shape data. *Biometrika* **76**, 271–281.

Marquardt, Q.W. (1963). An algorithm for least-squares estimation of nonlinear parameters. *Journal of the Society of Applied Mathematics* **11**, 431–441.

Martin, R. and Teo, K.L. (1994). *Optimal Control of Drug Administration in Cancer Chemotherapy*. Singapore: World Scientific.

Mathew, T. and Sinha, B.K. (1992). Exact and optimum tests in unbalanced split-plot designs under mixed and random models. *Journal of the American Statistical Association* **87**, 192–200.

Matyas, L. (Ed.) (1999). *Generalized Method of Moments Estimation.* Cambridge, UK: Cambridge University Press.

McCulloch, C.E. (1997). Maximum likelihood algorithms for generalized linear mixed models. *Journal of the American Statistical Association* **92**, 330–335.

McCulloch, C.E. and Searle, S.R. (2001). *Generalized, Linear and Mixed Models.* New York: Wiley.

McCullagh, P. and Nelder, J.A. (1989). *Generalized Linear Models,* 2nd ed. New York: Chapman & Hall.

McGilchrist, C.A. (1994). Estimation in generalized mixed models *Journal of the Royal Statistical Society, ser. B* **56**, 61–69.

McLachlan, G.J. and Krishnan, T. (1996). *The EM Algorithm and Extensions.* New York: Wiley.

McLellan, T. and Endler, J.A. (1998). The relative success of some methods for measuring and describing the shape of complex objects. *Systematic Biology* **47**, 264–281.

Meaney, P.M., Demidenko, E., Yagnamurthy, N.K., Li D., Fanning, M.W., and Paulsen, K.D. (2001). A two-stage microwave image reconstruction procedure for improved internal feature extraction. *Medical Physics* **28**, 2358–2369.

Meintz, J.B. and Viergever, M.A. (1998). A survey of medical image registration. *Medical Image Analysis* **2**, 1–36.

Miller, R.G. (1974). An unbalanced jackknife. *Annals of Statistics* **2**, 880–891.

Mittelhammer, R.C., Judge, G.G., and Miller, D.J. (2000). *Econometric Foundations.* Cambridge,UK: Cambridge University Press.

Monahan, J. and Stefanski, L.A. (1991). Normal scale mixture approximations to $F^*(z)$ and computation of the logistic-normal integral. In: *Handbook of Logistic Distribution.* New York: Marcel Dekker, pp. 529–540.

Montgomery, D.C. and Peck, E.A. (1992). *Introduction to Linear Regression Analysis.* New York: Wiley.

Moore, D.F. and Tsiatis, A. (1991). Robust estimation of the variance in moment methods for extra-binomial and extra-Poisson variation. *Biometrics* **47**, 393–401.

Moran, P.A.P. (1971). Maximum likelihood estimators in non-standard conditions. *Proceedings of the Cambridge Philosophical Society* **70**, 441–450.

Morrell, C.H. (1998). Likelihood-ratio testing of variance components in the linear mixed-effects model using restricted maximum likelihood. *Biometrics* **54**, 1560–1568.

Murray, A. and Hunt, T. (1993). *The Cell Cycle.* New York: W.H. Freeman.

Nakamura, T. (1984). Existence theorems of a maximum likelihood estimate from a generalized censored data sample. *Annals of the Institute of Statistical Mathematics* **36**, 375–393.

Nakamura, T. and Lee, C.-S. (1993). On the existence of minimum contrast estimates in a binary response model. *Annals of the Institute of Statistical Mathematics* **45**, 741–758.

Nash, J.C. and Walker-Smith, M. (1987). *Nonlinear Parameter Estimation.* New York: Marcel Dekker.

Neter, J., Kutner, M.H., Nachtsheim, C.J., and Wasserman, W. (1990). *Applied Linear Statistical Models.* Chicago: Irwin.

Neuhaus, J.M. and Lesperance, M.L. (1996). Estimation efficiency in a binary mixed-effects model setting. *Biometrika* **83**, 441–446.

Neyman, J. and Scott, E.L. (1948). Consistent estimates based on partially consistent observations. *Econometrica* **16**, 1–32.

Norton, L. and Day, R. (1991). Potential innovations in scheduling of cancer chemotherapy. In: *Important Advances in Oncology,* ed. V. DeVita, S. Hellman, and S. Rosenberg. Philadelphia: J.B. Lippincott.

Norton, L. and Simon, R. (1977). Growth curve of an experimental solid tumor following radiotherapy. *Journal of the National Cancer Institute* **58**, 1735–1741.

Nuyts, J. and Fessler, J.A. (2003). A penalized-likelihood image reconstruction method for emission tomography, compared to postsmoothed maximum-likelihood with matched spatial resolution. *IEEE Transactions on Medical Imaging* **22**, 1042–1052.

O'Donoghue, J.A. (1997). The response of tumours with Gompertzian growth characteristics to fractionated radiotherapy. *International Journal of Radiation Biology* **72**, 325–339.

O'Hara, J.A., Blumenthal, R.D., Grinberg, O.Y., Demidenko, E., Wilmot, C.M., Taylor, A.M., Goldenberg, D.M., and Swartz, H.M. (2001). Response to radioimmunotherapy correlates with tumor pO_2 measured by EPR oxymetry in human xenografts. *Radiation Research* **155**, 466–473.

Olkin, I. (1996). Meta-analysis: current issues in research synthesis. *Statistics in Medicine* **15**, 1253–1257.

Oman, S.D. and Zucker, D.M. (2001). Modelling and generating correlated binary variables. *Biometrika* **88**, 287–290.

Ortega, J.M. and Rheinboldt, W.C. (1970). *Iterative Solution of Nonlinear Equations in Several Variables.* New York: Academic Press.

Palmer, M.J., Phillips, B.F., and Smith, G.T. (1991). Application of nonlinear models with random coefficients to growth data. *Biometrics* **47**, 623–635.

Pan, J.X. and Fang, K.T. (1996). Influential observation in the growth curve model with unstructured covariance matrix. *Computational Statistics and Data Analysis* **22**, 71–87.

Pan, J.X. and Fang, K.T. (2002). *Growth Curve Models and Statistical Diagnostics.* New York: Springer-Verlag.

Pan, J.X., Fang, K.T., and Rosen, D. (1997). Local influence assessment in the growth curve model with unstructured covariance. *Journal of Statistical Planning and Inference* **62**, 263–278.

Parke, W.R. (1986). Pseudo-maximum likelihood estimation: the asymptotic distribution. *Annals of Statistics* **14**, 355–357.

Parker, J.A. (1990). *Image Reconstruction in Radiology*. Boca Raton, FL: CRC Press.

Patterson, H.D. and Thompson, R. (1971). Recovery of inter-block information when block sizes are unequal. *Biometrika* **58**, 545–554.

Peng, H. and Lu, Y. (2012). Model selection in linear mixed effect models. *Journal of Multivariate Analysis* **109**, 109–129.

Perez, C.A. and Brady, L.W. (1992). *Principles and Practice of Radiation Oncology*. Philadelphia: J.B. Lippincott.

Petrou, M. and Bosdogianni, P. (1999). *Image Processing*. Chichester, UK: Wiley.

Petrou, M. and Petrou, C. (2010). *Image Processing: The Fundamentals*. Chichester, UK: Wiley.

Pinheiro, J.C. and Bates, D.M. (1995). Approximations to the log-likelihood function in the nonlinear mixed-effects model. *Journal of Computational and Graphical Statistics* **4**, 12–35.

Pinheiro, J.C. and Bates, D.M. (2000). *Mixed Effects Models in S-Plus*. New York: Springer-Verlag.

Pinheiro, J.C., Liu, C., and Wu, Y.N. (2001). Efficient algorithms for robust estimation in linear mixed-effects models using multivariate t-distribution. *Journal of Computational and Graphical Statistics* **10**, 249–276.

Pockock, S.J., Cook, D.G., and Beresford, S.A.A. (1981). Regression of area mortality rates on explanatory variables: What weighting is appropriate? *Applied Statistics* **30,** 286–295.

Pogue, B.W., O'Hara, J.A., Demidenko, E., Wilmot, C.M., Goodwin, I.A., Chen, B., Swartz, H.M., and Hasan, T. (2003). Photodynamic therapy with verteporfin in the radiation-induced fibrosarcoma-1 tumor causes enhanced radiation sensitivity. *Cancer Research* **63**, 1025–1033.

Polak, E. (1971). *Computational Methods of Optimization*. New York: Wiley.

Potthoff, R.F. and Roy, S.N. (1964). A generalized multivariate analysis of variance model useful especially for growth curve problems. *Biometrika* **51**, 313–326.

Pregibon, D. (1981). Logistic regression diagnostics. *Annals of Statistics* **4,** 705–724.

Preisler, H.K. (1988). Maximum likelihood estimates for binary data with random effects. *Biometrical Journal* **30**, 339–350.

Preisser, J.S. and Qaqish, B.F. (1996). Deletion diagnostics for generalized estimating equations. *Biometrika* **83,** 551–562.

Prentice, R.L. (1986). Binary regression using an extended beta-binomial distribution, with discussion of correlation induced by covariate measurement errors. *Journal of the American Statistical Association* **81**, 321–327.

Prentice, R.L. (1988). Correlated binary regression with covariates specific to each binary observation. *Biometrics* **44**, 1033–1048.

Press, W.H., Teukolsky, S.A., Vetterling, W.T., and Flannery, B.P. (1992). *Numerical Recipes in C*. New York: Cambridge University Press.

Qi, J. and Huesman, R.H. (2001). Theoretical study of lesion detectability of MAP reconstruction using a computer observer. *IEEE Transactions on Medical Imaging* **20**, 815–822.

R Development Core Team (2011). R: a language and environment for statistical computing. R Foundation for Statistical Computing, Vienna, Austria. http://www.R-project.org/.

Ralston, M.L. and Jennrich, R.I. (1978). DUD: a derivative-free algorithm for nonlinear least-squares. *Technometrics* **20**, 7–14.

Rao, C.R. (1965). The theory of least squares when parameters are stochastic and its application to the analysis of growth curves. *Biometrika* **52**, 447–458.

Rao, C.R. (1971). Estimation of variance and covariance components: MINQUE theory. *Journal of Multivariate Analysis* **1**, 257–275.

Rao, C.R. (1973) *Linear Statistical Inference and Its Application,* 2nd ed. New York: Wiley.

Rao, C.R. and Kleffé, J. (1988). *Estimation of Variance Components and Its Applications*. Amsterdam: North-Holland.

Rao, C.R. and Suryawanshi, S. (1996). Statistical analysis of shape of objects based on landmark data. *Proceedings of the National Academy of Sciences* **93**, 12132–12136.

Rao, C.R. and Toutenburg, H. (1999). *Linear Models: Least Squares and Alternatives*. New York: Springer-Verlag.

Reinsel, G.C. (1985). Mean squared error properties of empirical Bayes estimators in a multivariate random effects general linear model. *Journal of the American Statistical Association* **80**, 642–650.

Reisner, A., Haagensen, J.A.J., Schembri, M.A., Zechner, E.L., and Molin, S. (2003). Development and maturation of *Escherichia coli* K-12 biofilms. *Molecular Microbiology* **48**, 933–946.

Resa, F.M. (1961). *An Introduction to Information Theory*. New York: McGraw-Hill.

Rice, J.A. (1995). *Mathematical Statistics and Data Analysis*, 2nd ed. Belmont, CA: Duxbury Press.

Richardson, A.M. and Welsh, A.H. (1994). Asymptotic properties of restricted maximum likelihood (REML) estimates for a hierarchical mixed linear model. *Australian Journal of Statistics* **36**, 31–43.

Ridout, M.S., Demetrio, C.G.B., and Firth, D. (1999). Estimating intraclass correlation for binary data. *Biometrics* **55**, 137–148.

Ripley, B.D. (1981). *Spatial Statistics.* New York: Wiley.

Ritter, C. and Bates, D.M. (1996). Profile methods. In: *Proceedings in Computational Statistics*, COMPSTAT 1996, ed. A. Prat. Barcelona, Spain: Physica-Verlag, pp. 123–134.

Ritz, J., Demidenko, E., and Spiegelman, D. (2008). Multivariate meta-analysis for data consortia, individual patient meta-analysis, and pooling projects. *Journal of Statistical Planning and Inference* **138**, 1919–1933.

Robert, C.P. and Casella, G. (1999). *Monte Carlo Statistical Methods.* New York: Springer-Verlag.

Roberts, S.A. and Hendry, J.H. (1993). The delay before onset of accelerated tumour cell repopulation during radiotherapy: a direct maximum likelihood analysis of a collection of worldwide tumour control data. *Radiotherapy and Oncology* **29**, 69–74.

Roberts, S.A. and Hendry, J.H. (1998). A realistic closed-form radiobiological model of clinical tumor-control data incorporating intertumor heterogeneity. *International Journal of Radiation Oncology, Biology, and Physics* **41**, 689–699.

Roberts, S.A., Hendry, J.H., Brewsrwe, A.E., and Sleven, N.J. (1994). The influence of radiotherapy treatment time on the control of laryngeal cancer: a direct analysis of data from two British Institute of Radiology trials to calculate the lag period and the time factor. *British Journal of Radiology* **67**, 790–794.

Robinson, G.K. (1991). That BLUP is a good thing: estimation of random effects. *Statistical Science* **6**, 15–51.

Rockwell, S. and Kallman, R.F. (1974). Cyclic radiation-induced variations in cellular radiosensitivity in a mouse mammary tumor. *Radiation Research* **57**, 132–147.

Rodriguez, G. and Goldman, N. (1995). An assessment of estimation procedures for multilevel models with binary responses. *Journal of the Royal Statistical Society, ser. B* **159**, 73-89.

Rofstad, E. (1981). Radiation response of the cells of a human malignant melanoma xenograft: effect of hypoxic cell radiosensitizers. *Radiation Research* **87**, 670–683.

Rohlf, F.J. (1990). Morphometrics. *Annual Review of Ecology and Systematics* **21**, 299–316.

Rohlf, F.J. (2003). Bias and error in estimates of mean shape in geometric morphology. *Journal of Human Evolution* **44**, 665–683.

Rohlf, F.J. and Archie, J.W. (1984). A comparison of Fourier methods for description of wing shape in mosquitoes (diptera: culicadae). *Systematic Zoology* **33**, 302–317.

Ross, S.M. (1993). *Introduction to Probability Models*, 5th ed. San Diego, CA: Academic Press.

Ross, W.H. (1987). The geometry of case deletion and the assessment of influence in nonlinear regression. *Canadian Journal of Statistics* **15**, 91–103.

Ruppert, D., Wand, M.P., and Carroll, R.J. (2003). *Semiparametric Regression.* Cambridge, UK: Cambridge University Press.

Rygaardt, K. and Spang-Thomsen, M. (1997). Quantitation and Gompertzian analysis of tumor growth. *Breast Cancer Research and Treatment* **46**, 303–312.

Sachs, R.K., Heidenreich, W.F., and Brenner, D.J. (1996). Dose timing in tumor radiotherapy: considerations of the cell number stochastically. *Mathematical Biosciences* **138**, 131–146.

Samal, A. and Iyengar, P. (1992). Automatic recognition and analysis of human faces and facial expressions: a survey. *Pattern Recognition* **25**, 65–77.

Sargent, J.D., Tanski, S., and Stoolmiller, M.. (2012). Influence of motion picture rating on adolescent response to movie smoking. *Pediatrics* **130**, 228–236.

Schall, R. (1991). Estimation in generalized linear models with random effects. *Biometrika* **78**, 719–729.

Schall, R.and Dunne, T.T. (1992). A note on the relationship between parameter collinearity and local influence. *Biometrika* **79**, 399–404.

Schervish, M.J. (1995). *Theory of Statistics.* New York: Springer-Verlag.

Schott, J. (1997). *Matrix Analysis for Statistics.* New York: Wiley.

Sclove, S.L. (1987). Application of model-selection criteria to some problems in multivariate analysis. *Psycometrika* **52**, 333–343.

Searle, S.R. (1971a). *Linear Models.* New York: Wiley.

Searle, S.R. (1971b). Topics in variance component estimation. *Biometrics* **27**, 1–76.

Searle, S.R. (1982). *Matrix Algebra Useful for Statistics.* New York: Wiley.

Searle, S.R., Casella G., and McCulloch, C.M. (1992). *Variance Components.* New York: Wiley.

Seber, G.A.F. and Wild, C.J. (1989). *Nonlinear Regression.* New York: Wiley.

Seeram, E. (1994). *Computed Tomography: Physical Principles, Clinical Applications and Quality Control.* Philadelphia: W.B. Saunders.

Self, S.G. and Liang K.-L. (1987). Asymptotic properties of maximum likelihood estimators and likelihood ratio tests under nonstandard conditions. *Journal of the American Statistical Association* **82**, 605–610.

Serfling, R.J. (1980). *Approximation Theorems of Mathematical Statistics.* New York: Wiley.

Seul, M., O'Gorman, L., and Sammon, M.J. (2000). *Practical Algorithms for Image Analysis*. Cambridge, UK: Cambridge University Press.

Shaffer, J.P. (1991). The Gauss–Markov theorem and random regressors. *American Statistician* **45**, 269–273.

Shahine, B.H., Ng, C.E., and Raaphorst, G.P. (1997). Modelling of continuous low dose rate and accelerated fractionated high dose rate irradiation treatments in human glioma cell line. *International Journal of Radiation Biology* **70**, 555–561.

Shao, J. (2010). *Mathematical Statistics,* 2nd ed. New York: Springer-Verlag.

Sheiner, L.B. and Beal, S.L. (1980). Evaluation of methods for estimating population pharmacokinetic parameters. *Journal of Pharmacokinetics and Biopharmaceutics* **8**, 553–571.

Sheiner, L.B. and Beal, S.L. (1985). Pharmacokinetic parameter estimates from several least squares procedures: superiority of extended least squares. *Journal of Pharmacokinetics and Biopharmaceutics* **13**, 185–201.

Shenton, M.E., Kikinis, R., Jolesz, F.A., Pollak, S.D., LeMay, M., Wible, G.C., Hokama, H., Martin, J., Metcalf, D., Coleman, M., and McCarley, R.W. (1992). Abnormalities of left temporal lobe and thought disorder in schizophrenia. *New England Journal of Medicine* **327**, 604–612.

Shenton, M.E., Dickey, C.C., Frumin, M., and McCarley, R.W. (2001). A review of MRI findings in schizophrenia. *Schizophrenia Research* **49**, 1–52.

Shepp, L.A. and Vardi, Y. (1982). Maximum likelihood reconstruction for emission tomography. *IEEE Transactions on Medical Imaging* **MI–1**, 113–122.

Silvapulle, M.J. (1981). On the existence of maximum likelihood estimates for the binomial response models. *Journal of the Royal Statistical Society, ser. B* **43**, 310–313.

Slutsky, E. (1925). Über Stochastische Asymtoten and Grenzwerte. *Metron* **5**, 1–90.

Small, C.G. (1996). *The Statistical Theory of Shapes*. New York: Springer-Verlag.

Smith, A.F.M. (1973). A general Bayesian linear model. *Journal of the Royal Statistical Society, ser. B* **35**, 67–75.

Smith, M. and Kohn, R. (2002). Parsimonious covariance matrix estimation for longitudinal data. *Journal of the American Statistical Association* **97**, 1141–1153.

Solomon, P.J. and Cox, D.R. (1992). Nonlinear component of variance models. *Biometrika* **79**, 1–11.

Spiegelman, D., Rosner, B., and Logan, R. (2000). Estimation and inference for logistic regression with covariate misclassification and measurement error in main study/validation study designs. *Journal of the American Statistical Association* **95**, 51–61.

Starck, J.-L., Murtagh, F., and Bijaoui, A. (1998). *Image Processing and Data Analysis*. Cambridge, UK: Cambridge University Press.

706   References

Steel, G.G. (1977). *Growth Kinetics of Tumors.* Oxford, UK: Clarendon Press.

Stefanski, L.A. and Boos, D.D. (2002). The calculus of M-estimation. *American Statistician* **56**, 29–38.

Stefanski, L.A. and Carroll, R.J. (1985). Covariate measurement error in logistic regression. *Annals of Statistics* **13**, 1335–1351.

Steimer, J.-L., Mallet, A., Golmard, J.L., and Boisvieux, J.F. (1984). Alternative approaches to estimation of population pharmocokinetic parameters: comparison with the nonlinear mixed effect model. *Drug Metabolism Reviews* **15**, 265–292.

Stern, S.E. and Welsh, A.H. (2000). Likelihood inference for small variance components. *Canadian Journal of Statistics* **28**, 517–532.

Stiratelli, R., Laird, N.M., and Ware, J.H. (1984). Random-effects models for serial observations with binary response. *Biometrics* **40**, 961–971.

Stram, D.O. (1996). Meta-analysis of published data using a linear mixed-effects model. *Biometrics* **52**, 536-544.

Stram, D.O. and Lee, J.W. (1994). Variance components testing in the longitudinal mixed effects model. *Biometrics* **50**, 1171–1177.

Stuart, H.C. and Reed, R.B. (1929). Longitudinal studies of child health and development, Harvard School of Public Health, Series II, No. 1, Description of project. *Pediatrics* **24**, 875–885.

Stukel, T. and Demidenko, E. (1997a). Two-stage estimation for general linear growth curve models. *Biometrics* **53**, 340–348.

Stukel, T. and Demidenko, E. (1997b). Comparisons of methods of estimation for nonlinear mixed-effects models. In: *Modelling Longitudinal and Spatially Correlated Data: Methods, Applications, and Future Directions (Springer Lectures in Statistics).* New York: Springer-Verlag, pp. 135–146.

Stukel, T.A., Demidenko, E., Dykes, J., and Karagas, M.R. (2001). Two-stage methods for the analysis of pooled data. *Statistics in Medicine* **20**, 2115–2130.

Sundaram, S., Sea, A., Feldman, S., Strawbridge, R., Hoopes, P.J., Demidenko, E., Binderup, L., and Gewirtz, D.A. (2003). The combination of a potent vitamin D_3 analog, EB 1089, with ionizing radiation reduces tumor growth and induces apoptosis of MCF-7 breast tumor xenografts in nude mice. *Clinical Cancer Research* **9**, 2350–2356.

Sutherland, R.M. (1988). Cell and environment interactions in tumor microregions: the multicellular spheroid model. *Science* **240**, 177–184.

Sutradhar, B.S. and Das, K. (1999). On the efficiency of regression estimators in generalized linear models for longitudinal data. *Biometrika* **86**, 459–465.

Swamy, P.A.V.B. (1971). *Statistical Inference in Random Coefficient Regression Models.* New York: Springer-Verlag.

Takkouche, B., Cadarso-Suarez, C. and Spiegelman, D. (1999). Evaluation of old and new tests of heterogeneity in epidemiologic meta-analysis. *American Journal of Epidemiology* **150**, 206–215.

Thames, H.D., Rozell, M.E., Tucker, S.L., Ang, K., Fisher, D.R., and Travis, E. (1986). Direct analysis of quantal radiation response data. *International Journal of Radiation Biology* **49**, 999–1009.

Thompson, S.G. and Sharp S.J. (1999). Explaining heterogeneity in meta-analysis: a comparison of methods. *Statistics in Medicine* **18**, 2693–2708.

Tikhonov, A.N. and Arsenin, V.Y. (1977). *Solutions of Ill-Posed Problems*. New York: Winston.

Tortora, G., Caputo, R., Damiano, V., Fontanini, G., Melisi, D., Veneziani, B.M., Zunino, F., Bianco, A.R., and Ciardiello, F. (2001). Oral administration of novel taxane, an antisense epidermal growth factor receptor inhibitor iressa causes cooperative antitumor and antiangiogenic activity. *Clinical Cancer Research* **7**, 4156–4163.

Tosteson, T., Stefanski, L.A., and Schaffer, D.W. (1989). A measurement error model for binary and ordinal regression. *Statistics in Medicine* **8**, 1139–1147.

Tubiana, M., Dutreix, J., and Wambersie, A. (1990). *Introduction to Radiology*. London: Taylor & Francis.

Turkan, S. and Toktamis, O. (2012). Influence analysis in the linear mixed model. *Pakistan Journal of Statistics* **28**, 341–349.

Turkington, D.A. (2002). *Matrix Calculus and Zero–One Matrices*. Cambridge, UK: Cambridge University Press.

Venzon, D.J. and Moolgavkar, S.H. (1988). A method for computing profile-likelihood-based confidence intervals. *Applied Statistics* **37**, 87–94.

Verbeke, G. and Molenberghs, G. (2000). *Linear Mixed Models for Longtitudinal Data*. New York: Springer-Verlag.

Verbeke, G. and Molenberghs, G. (2003). The use of score tests for inference on variance components. *Biometrics* **59**, 254–262.

Vogel, C.R. (2002). *Computational Methods for Inverse Problems*. Philadelphia: SIAM.

Vonesh, E.F. (1996). A note on the use of Laplace's approximation for nonlinear mixed-effects models. *Biometrika* **83**, 447–452.

Vonesh, E.F. (2012). *Generalized Linear and Nonlinear Models for Correlated Data: Theory and Applications Using SAS*. Cary, NC: SAS Institute.

Vonesh, E.F. and Carter R.L. (1987). Efficient inference for random-coefficient growth curve models with unbalanced data. *Biometrics* **43**, 617–628.

Vonesh, E.F. and Carter, R.L. (1992). Mixed-effects nonlinear regression for unbalanced repeated measures. *Biometrics* **48,** 1–17.

Vonesh, E.F. and Chinchilli, V.M. (1997). *Linear and Nonlinear Models for the Analysis of Repeated Measurements*. New York: Marcel Dekker.

Vonesh, E.F., Wang, H., Nie, L., and Majumdar, D. (2002). Conditional second-order generalized estimating equations for generalized linear and nonlinear mixed-effects models. *Journal of the American Statistical Association* **97**, 271–283.

Walsh, G.R. (1975). *Methods of Optimization*. New York: Wiley.

Wand, M.P. (2002). Vector differential calculus in statistics. *American Statistician* **56**, 55–62.

Wang, L., Joshi, S.C., Miller, M.I., and Csernansky, J.G. (2001). Statistical analysis of hippocampal asymmetry is schizophrenia. *NeuroImage* **14**, 531–545.

Wang, L., Tan, T., Hu, W., and Ning, H. (2003). Automatic gait recognition based on statistical shape analysis. *IEEE Transactions on Image Processing* **12**, 1120–1131.

Wang, S.G. and Ma, W.Q. (2002). On exact tests of linear hypothesis in linear models with nested error structure. *Journal of Statistical Planning and Inference* **106**, 225–233.

Wang, Y. (1998). Smoothing spline models with correlated random errors. *Journal of the American Statistical Association* **93**, 341–348.

Wang, Y.-G. and Carey, V. (2003). Working correlation structure misspecification, estimation and covariance design: implications for generalized estimating equations performance. *Biometrika* **90**, 29–41.

Watson, G.S. (1986). The shape of a random sequence of triangles. *Advances in Applied Probability* **18**, 159–169.

Weddenburn, R.W.M. (1976). On the existence and uniqueness of the maximum likelihood estimates for certain generalized linear models. *Biometrika* **63**, 27–32.

Wellman, J.M. and Gunst, R.F. (1991). Influence diagnostics for linear measurement error models. *Biometrika* **78**, 373–380.

Wheldon, T.E. (1988). *Mathematical Models in Cancer Research*. Philadelphia: Adam Hilger.

Whitehead, A. and Whitehead, J. (1991). A general parametric approach to the meta-analysis of randomized clinical trials. *Statistics in Medicine* **10**, 1665–1677.

Wiens, D.P. and Zhou, J. (1997). Robust designs based on the infinitesimal approach. *Journal of the American Statistical Association* **92**, 1503–1511.

Willett, W. (1990). *Nutritional Epidemiology*. New York: Oxford University Press.

Wolfinger, R. (1993). Laplace's approximation for nonlinear mixed-effects models. *Biometrika* **80**, 791–795.

Wolfinger, R.D. and Lin, X. (1997). Two Taylor-series approximation methods for nonlinear mixed models. *Computational Statistics and Data Analysis* **25**, 465–490.

Wolfinger, R., Tobias, R., and Sall, J. (1994). Computing Gaussian likelihoods and their derivatives for general linear mixed models. *SIAM Journal of Scientific Computing* **15**, 1294–1310.

Woods, R.P., Grafton, S.T., Holmes, C.J., Cherry, S.R., and Mazziotta, J.C. (1998a). Automated image registration: I. General methods and intrasubject, intramodality validation. *Journal of Computer Assisted Tomography* **22**, 139–152.

Woods, R.P., Grafton, S.T., Watson, J.D.G., Sicotte, N.L., and Mazziotta, J.C. (1998b). Automated image registration: II. Intersubject validation of linear and nonlinear models. *Journal of Computer Assisted Tomography* **22**, 153–165.

Wu, C.-F. (1981). Asymptotic theory of nonlinear least squares estimation. *Annals of Statistics* **9**, 501–503.

Yakovlev, A.Y. and Tsodikov, A.D. (1995). *Stochastic Models of Tumor Latency and Their Applications.* Singapore: World Scientific.

Yakovlev, A.Y. and Zorin, A.V. (1988). *Computer Simulations in Cell Radiobiology.* Berlin: Springer-Verlag.

Yakovlev, A., Muller, W., and Pavlova, L. (1997). Do cells repair precancerous lesions induced by radiation? *Mathematical Biosciences* **142,** 107–117.

Yeap, B.Y. and Davidian, M. (2001). Robust two-stage estimation in hierarchical nonlinear models. *Biometrics* **57**, 266–272.

Yuan, K.-H. and Jennrich, R.I. (2000). Estimating equations with nuisance parameters: theory and applications. *Annals of the Institute of Statistical Mathematics* **52**, 343–350.

Zahn, C.T. and Roskies, R.Z. (1972). Fourier discriptors for plane closed curves. *IEEE Transactions on Computers* **C21**, 269–281.

Zeger, S.L. and Diggle, P.J. (1994). Semiparametric models for longitudinal data with application to CD4 cell numbers in HIV seroconverters. *Biometrics* **50**, 689–699.

Zeger, S.L. and Liang, K.Y. (1986). Longitudinal data analysis for discrete and continuous outcomes. *Biometrics* **42**, 121–130.

Zeger, S.L., Liang, K.Y., and Albert, P.S. (1988). Models for longitudinal data: a generalized estimating equation approach. *Biometrics* **44**, 1049–1060.

Zhang, D., Lin, X., and Sowers, M. (1998). Semiparametric stochastic mixed models for longitudinal data. *Journal of the American Statistical Association* **93**, 710–719.

Zhao, Y.J. and Lee, A.H. (1994). Influence diagnostics for generalized linear measurement error models. *Biometrics* **50**, 1117–1128.

Zhao, Y.J. and Lee, A.H. (1995). Assessment of influence in non-linear measurement error models. *Journal of Applied Statistics* **22**, 215–225.

Index

WILEY SERIES IN PROBABILITY AND STATISTICS

ESTABLISHED BY WALTER A. SHEWHART AND SAMUEL S. WILKS

The *Wiley Series in Probability and Statistics* is well established and authoritative. It covers many topics of current research interest in both pure and applied statistics and probability theory. Written by leading statisticians and institutions, the titles span both state-of-the-art developments in the field and classical methods.

Reflecting the wide range of current research in statistics, the series encompasses applied, methodological and theoretical statistics, ranging from applications and new techniques made possible by advances in computerized practice to rigorous treatment of theoretical approaches.

This series provides essential and invaluable reading for all statisticians, whether in academia, industry, government, or research.

*Now available in a lower priced paperback edition in the Wiley Classics Library.
†Now available in a lower priced paperback edition in the Wiley–Interscience Paperback Series.

BERNARDO and SMITH · Bayesian Theory

BHAT and MILLER · Elements of Applied Stochastic Processes, *Third Edition*

BHATTACHARYA and WAYMIRE · Stochastic Processes with Applications

BIEMER, GROVES, LYBERG, MATHIOWETZ, and SUDMAN · Measurement Errors in Surveys

BILLINGSLEY · Convergence of Probability Measures, *Second Edition*

BILLINGSLEY · Probability and Measure, *Anniversary Edition*

BIRKES and DODGE · Alternative Methods of Regression

BISGAARD and KULAHCI · Time Series Analysis and Forecasting by Example

BISWAS, DATTA, FINE, and SEGAL · Statistical Advances in the Biomedical Sciences: Clinical Trials, Epidemiology, Survival Analysis, and Bioinformatics

BLISCHKE and MURTHY (editors) · Case Studies in Reliability and Maintenance

BLISCHKE and MURTHY · Reliability: Modeling, Prediction, and Optimization

BLOOMFIELD · Fourier Analysis of Time Series: An Introduction, *Second Edition*

BOLLEN · Structural Equations with Latent Variables

BOLLEN and CURRAN · Latent Curve Models: A Structural Equation Perspective

BOROVKOV · Ergodicity and Stability of Stochastic Processes

BOSQ and BLANKE · Inference and Prediction in Large Dimensions

BOULEAU · Numerical Methods for Stochastic Processes

* BOX and TIAO · Bayesian Inference in Statistical Analysis

BOX · Improving Almost Anything, *Revised Edition*

* BOX and DRAPER · Evolutionary Operation: A Statistical Method for Process Improvement

BOX and DRAPER · Response Surfaces, Mixtures, and Ridge Analyses, *Second Edition*

BOX, HUNTER, and HUNTER · Statistics for Experimenters: Design, Innovation, and Discovery, *Second Editon*

BOX, JENKINS, and REINSEL · Time Series Analysis: Forcasting and Control, *Fourth Edition*

BOX, LUCEÑO, and PANIAGUA-QUIÑONES · Statistical Control by Monitoring and Adjustment, *Second Edition*

* BROWN and HOLLANDER · Statistics: A Biomedical Introduction

CAIROLI and DALANG · Sequential Stochastic Optimization

CASTILLO, HADI, BALAKRISHNAN, and SARABIA · Extreme Value and Related Models with Applications in Engineering and Science

CHAN · Time Series: Applications to Finance with R and S-Plus®, *Second Edition*

CHARALAMBIDES · Combinatorial Methods in Discrete Distributions

CHATTERJEE and HADI · Regression Analysis by Example, *Fourth Edition*

CHATTERJEE and HADI · Sensitivity Analysis in Linear Regression

CHERNICK · Bootstrap Methods: A Guide for Practitioners and Researchers, *Second Edition*

CHERNICK and FRIIS · Introductory Biostatistics for the Health Sciences

CHILÈS and DELFINER · Geostatistics: Modeling Spatial Uncertainty, *Second Edition*

CHOW and LIU · Design and Analysis of Clinical Trials: Concepts and Methodologies, *Second Edition*

CLARKE · Linear Models: The Theory and Application of Analysis of Variance

CLARKE and DISNEY · Probability and Random Processes: A First Course with Applications, *Second Edition*

* COCHRAN and COX · Experimental Designs, *Second Edition*

COLLINS and LANZA · Latent Class and Latent Transition Analysis: With Applications in the Social, Behavioral, and Health Sciences

CONGDON · Applied Bayesian Modelling

CONGDON · Bayesian Models for Categorical Data

CONGDON · Bayesian Statistical Modelling, *Second Edition*

CONOVER · Practical Nonparametric Statistics, *Third Edition*

COOK · Regression Graphics

COOK and WEISBERG · An Introduction to Regression Graphics

COOK and WEISBERG · Applied Regression Including Computing and Graphics

CORNELL · A Primer on Experiments with Mixtures

CORNELL · Experiments with Mixtures, Designs, Models, and the Analysis of Mixture Data, *Third Edition*

COX · A Handbook of Introductory Statistical Methods

CRESSIE · Statistics for Spatial Data, *Revised Edition*

---

*Now available in a lower priced paperback edition in the Wiley Classics Library.

†Now available in a lower priced paperback edition in the Wiley–Interscience Paperback Series.

*Now available in a lower priced paperback edition in the Wiley Classics Library.

†Now available in a lower priced paperback edition in the Wiley–Interscience Paperback Series.

MAGNUS and NEUDECKER · Matrix Differential Calculus with Applications in Statistics and Econometrics, *Revised Edition*

MALLER and ZHOU · Survival Analysis with Long Term Survivors

MARCHETTE · Random Graphs for Statistical Pattern Recognition

MARDIA and JUPP · Directional Statistics

MARKOVICH · Nonparametric Analysis of Univariate Heavy-Tailed Data: Research and Practice

MARONNA, MARTIN and YOHAI · Robust Statistics: Theory and Methods

MASON, GUNST, and HESS · Statistical Design and Analysis of Experiments with Applications to Engineering and Science, *Second Edition*

McCULLOCH, SEARLE, and NEUHAUS · Generalized, Linear, and Mixed Models, *Second Edition*

McFADDEN · Management of Data in Clinical Trials, *Second Edition*

* McLACHLAN · Discriminant Analysis and Statistical Pattern Recognition

McLACHLAN, DO, and AMBROISE · Analyzing Microarray Gene Expression Data

McLACHLAN and KRISHNAN · The EM Algorithm and Extensions, *Second Edition*

McLACHLAN and PEEL · Finite Mixture Models

McNEIL · Epidemiological Research Methods

MEEKER and ESCOBAR · Statistical Methods for Reliability Data

MEERSCHAERT and SCHEFFLER · Limit Distributions for Sums of Independent Random Vectors: Heavy Tails in Theory and Practice

MENGERSEN, ROBERT, and TITTERINGTON · Mixtures: Estimation and Applications

MICKEY, DUNN, and CLARK · Applied Statistics: Analysis of Variance and Regression, *Third Edition*

* MILLER · Survival Analysis, *Second Edition*

MONTGOMERY, JENNINGS, and KULAHCI · Introduction to Time Series Analysis and Forecasting

MONTGOMERY, PECK, and VINING · Introduction to Linear Regression Analysis, *Fifth Edition*

MORGENTHALER and TUKEY · Configural Polysampling: A Route to Practical Robustness

MUIRHEAD · Aspects of Multivariate Statistical Theory

MULLER and STOYAN · Comparison Methods for Stochastic Models and Risks

MURTHY, XIE, and JIANG · Weibull Models

MYERS, MONTGOMERY, and ANDERSON-COOK · Response Surface Methodology: Process and Product Optimization Using Designed Experiments, *Third Edition*

MYERS, MONTGOMERY, VINING, and ROBINSON · Generalized Linear Models. With Applications in Engineering and the Sciences, *Second Edition*

NATVIG · Multistate Systems Reliability Theory With Applications

† NELSON · Accelerated Testing, Statistical Models, Test Plans, and Data Analyses

† NELSON · Applied Life Data Analysis

NEWMAN · Biostatistical Methods in Epidemiology

NG, TAIN, and TANG · Dirichlet Theory: Theory, Methods and Applications

OKABE, BOOTS, SUGIHARA, and CHIU · Spatial Tesselations: Concepts and Applications of Voronoi Diagrams, *Second Edition*

OLIVER and SMITH · Influence Diagrams, Belief Nets and Decision Analysis

PALTA · Quantitative Methods in Population Health: Extensions of Ordinary Regressions

PANJER · Operational Risk: Modeling and Analytics

PANKRATZ · Forecasting with Dynamic Regression Models

PANKRATZ · Forecasting with Univariate Box-Jenkins Models: Concepts and Cases

PARDOUX · Markov Processes and Applications: Algorithms, Networks, Genome and Finance

PARMIGIANI and INOUE · Decision Theory: Principles and Approaches

* PARZEN · Modern Probability Theory and Its Applications

PEÑA, TIAO, and TSAY · A Course in Time Series Analysis

PESARIN and SALMASO · Permutation Tests for Complex Data: Applications and Software

PIANTADOSI · Clinical Trials: A Methodologic Perspective, *Second Edition*

POURAHMADI · Foundations of Time Series Analysis and Prediction Theory

POWELL · Approximate Dynamic Programming: Solving the Curses of Dimensionality, *Second Edition*

POWELL and RYZHOV · Optimal Learning

PRESS · Subjective and Objective Bayesian Statistics, *Second Edition*

---

*Now available in a lower priced paperback edition in the Wiley Classics Library.

†Now available in a lower priced paperback edition in the Wiley–Interscience Paperback Series.

PRESS and TANUR · The Subjectivity of Scientists and the Bayesian Approach

PURI, VILAPLANA, and WERTZ · New Perspectives in Theoretical and Applied Statistics

† PUTERMAN · Markov Decision Processes: Discrete Stochastic Dynamic Programming

QIU · Image Processing and Jump Regression Analysis

* RAO · Linear Statistical Inference and Its Applications, *Second Edition*

RAO · Statistical Inference for Fractional Diffusion Processes

RAUSAND and HØYLAND · System Reliability Theory: Models, Statistical Methods, and Applications, *Second Edition*

RAYNER, THAS, and BEST · Smooth Tests of Goodnes of Fit: Using R, *Second Edition*

RENCHER and SCHAALJE · Linear Models in Statistics, *Second Edition*

RENCHER and CHRISTENSEN · Methods of Multivariate Analysis, *Third Edition*

RENCHER · Multivariate Statistical Inference with Applications

RIGDON and BASU · Statistical Methods for the Reliability of Repairable Systems

* RIPLEY · Spatial Statistics

* RIPLEY · Stochastic Simulation

ROHATGI and SALEH · An Introduction to Probability and Statistics, *Second Edition*

ROLSKI, SCHMIDLI, SCHMIDT, and TEUGELS · Stochastic Processes for Insurance and Finance

ROSENBERGER and LACHIN · Randomization in Clinical Trials: Theory and Practice

ROSSI, ALLENBY, and McCULLOCH · Bayesian Statistics and Marketing

† ROUSSEEUW and LEROY · Robust Regression and Outlier Detection

ROYSTON and SAUERBREI · Multivariate Model Building: A Pragmatic Approach to Regression Analysis Based on Fractional Polynomials for Modeling Continuous Variables

* RUBIN · Multiple Imputation for Nonresponse in Surveys

RUBINSTEIN and KROESE · Simulation and the Monte Carlo Method, *Second Edition*

RUBINSTEIN and MELAMED · Modern Simulation and Modeling

RYAN · Modern Engineering Statistics

RYAN · Modern Experimental Design

RYAN · Modern Regression Methods, *Second Edition*

RYAN · Statistical Methods for Quality Improvement, *Third Edition*

SALEH · Theory of Preliminary Test and Stein-Type Estimation with Applications

SALTELLI, CHAN, and SCOTT (editors) · Sensitivity Analysis

SCHERER · Batch Effects and Noise in Microarray Experiments: Sources and Solutions

* SCHEFFE · The Analysis of Variance

SCHIMEK · Smoothing and Regression: Approaches, Computation, and Application

SCHOTT · Matrix Analysis for Statistics, *Second Edition*

SCHOUTENS · Levy Processes in Finance: Pricing Financial Derivatives

SCOTT · Multivariate Density Estimation: Theory, Practice, and Visualization

* SEARLE · Linear Models

† SEARLE · Linear Models for Unbalanced Data

† SEARLE · Matrix Algebra Useful for Statistics

† SEARLE, CASELLA, and McCULLOCH · Variance Components

SEARLE and WILLETT · Matrix Algebra for Applied Economics

SEBER · A Matrix Handbook For Statisticians

† SEBER · Multivariate Observations

SEBER and LEE · Linear Regression Analysis, *Second Edition*

† SEBER and WILD · Nonlinear Regression

SENNOTT · Stochastic Dynamic Programming and the Control of Queueing Systems

* SERFLING · Approximation Theorems of Mathematical Statistics

SHAFER and VOVK · Probability and Finance: It's Only a Game!

SHERMAN · Spatial Statistics and Spatio-Temporal Data: Covariance Functions and Directional Properties

SILVAPULLE and SEN · Constrained Statistical Inference: Inequality, Order, and Shape Restrictions

SINGPURWALLA · Reliability and Risk: A Bayesian Perspective

SMALL and McLEISH · Hilbert Space Methods in Probability and Statistical Inference

SRIVASTAVA · Methods of Multivariate Statistics

STAPLETON · Linear Statistical Models, *Second Edition*

STAPLETON · Models for Probability and Statistical Inference: Theory and Applications

*Now available in a lower priced paperback edition in the Wiley Classics Library.

†Now available in a lower priced paperback edition in the Wiley–Interscience Paperback Series.

STAUDTE and SHEATHER · Robust Estimation and Testing

STOYAN · Counterexamples in Probability, *Second Edition*

STOYAN, KENDALL, and MECKE · Stochastic Geometry and Its Applications, *Second Edition*

STOYAN and STOYAN · Fractals, Random Shapes and Point Fields: Methods of Geometrical Statistics

STREET and BURGESS · The Construction of Optimal Stated Choice Experiments: Theory and Methods

STYAN · The Collected Papers of T. W. Anderson: 1943–1985

SUTTON, ABRAMS, JONES, SHELDON, and SONG · Methods for Meta-Analysis in Medical Research

TAKEZAWA · Introduction to Nonparametric Regression

TAMHANE · Statistical Analysis of Designed Experiments: Theory and Applications

TANAKA · Time Series Analysis: Nonstationary and Noninvertible Distribution Theory

THOMPSON · Empirical Model Building: Data, Models, and Reality, *Second Edition*

THOMPSON · Sampling, *Third Edition*

THOMPSON · Simulation: A Modeler's Approach

THOMPSON and SEBER · Adaptive Sampling

THOMPSON, WILLIAMS, and FINDLAY · Models for Investors in Real World Markets

TIERNEY · LISP-STAT: An Object-Oriented Environment for Statistical Computing and Dynamic Graphics

TSAY · Analysis of Financial Time Series, *Third Edition*

TSAY · An Introduction to Analysis of Financial Data with R

UPTON and FINGLETON · Spatial Data Analysis by Example, Volume II: Categorical and Directional Data

† VAN BELLE · Statistical Rules of Thumb, *Second Edition*

VAN BELLE, FISHER, HEAGERTY, and LUMLEY · Biostatistics: A Methodology for the Health Sciences, *Second Edition*

VESTRUP · The Theory of Measures and Integration

VIDAKOVIC · Statistical Modeling by Wavelets

VIERTL · Statistical Methods for Fuzzy Data

VINOD and REAGLE · Preparing for the Worst: Incorporating Downside Risk in Stock Market Investments

WALLER and GOTWAY · Applied Spatial Statistics for Public Health Data

WEISBERG · Applied Linear Regression, *Third Edition*

WEISBERG · Bias and Causation: Models and Judgment for Valid Comparisons

WELSH · Aspects of Statistical Inference

WESTFALL and YOUNG · Resampling-Based Multiple Testing: Examples and Methods for *p*-Value Adjustment

* WHITTAKER · Graphical Models in Applied Multivariate Statistics

WINKER · Optimization Heuristics in Economics: Applications of Threshold Accepting

WOODWORTH · Biostatistics: A Bayesian Introduction

WOOLSON and CLARKE · Statistical Methods for the Analysis of Biomedical Data, *Second Edition*

WU and HAMADA · Experiments: Planning, Analysis, and Parameter Design Optimization, *Second Edition*

WU and ZHANG · Nonparametric Regression Methods for Longitudinal Data Analysis

YIN · Clinical Trial Design: Bayesian and Frequentist Adaptive Methods

YOUNG, VALERO-MORA, and FRIENDLY · Visual Statistics: Seeing Data with Dynamic Interactive Graphics

ZACKS · Stage-Wise Adaptive Designs

* ZELLNER · An Introduction to Bayesian Inference in Econometrics

ZELTERMAN · Discrete Distributions—Applications in the Health Sciences

ZHOU, OBUCHOWSKI, and McCLISH · Statistical Methods in Diagnostic Medicine, *Second Edition*